SAUNDERS

Q&A

Review for NCLEX-RN

SAUNDERS *Q&A* Review for NCLEX-RN

Linda Anne Silvestri, MSN, RN
Assistant Professor of Nursing
Clinical Coordinator, Nursing Program
Salve Regina University
Newport, Rhode Island

President
Professional Nursing Seminars, Inc.
Charlestown, Rhode Island

W.B. Saunders Company
A Division of Harcourt Brace & Company
Philadelphia London Toronto Montreal Sydney Tokyo

W.B. SAUNDERS COMPANY
A Division of Harcourt Brace & Company

The Curtis Center
Independence Square West
Philadelphia, Pennsylvania 19106

Library of Congress Cataloging-in-Publication Data

Saunders Q&A review for NCLEX-RN / Linda Anne Silvestri.

p. cm.

ISBN 0–7216–7793–2

1. Nursing—Examinations, questions, etc. 2. Nursing—Outlines, syllabi, etc. I. Silvestri, Linda Anne. [DNLM: 1. Nursing, Practical examination questions. WY 18.2 S587s 1999]

RT55. S485 1999 610.73′076—dc21

DNLM/DLC 98-3395

SAUNDERS Q&A REVIEW FOR NCLEX-RN ISBN 0–7216–7793–2

Printed in the United States of America.

Last digit is the print number: 9 8 7 6 5 4 3 2 1

To my father, Arnold Lawrence; my memories of his love, support, and words of encouragement will remain in my heart forever!

To my nursing students, past, present, and future; their inspiration has brought many professional rewards to my life!

NOTICE

Nursing is an ever-changing field. Standard safety precautions must be followed, but as new research and clinical experience broaden our knowledge, changes in treatment and drug therapy become necessary or appropriate. Readers are advised to check the product information currently provided by the manufacturer of each drug to be administered to verify the recommended dose, the method and duration of administration, and the contraindications. It is the responsibility of the treating physician, relying on experience and knowledge of the patient, to determine dosages and the best treatment for the patient. Neither the publisher nor the editor assumes any responsibility for any injury and/or damage to persons or property.

THE PUBLISHER

About the Author

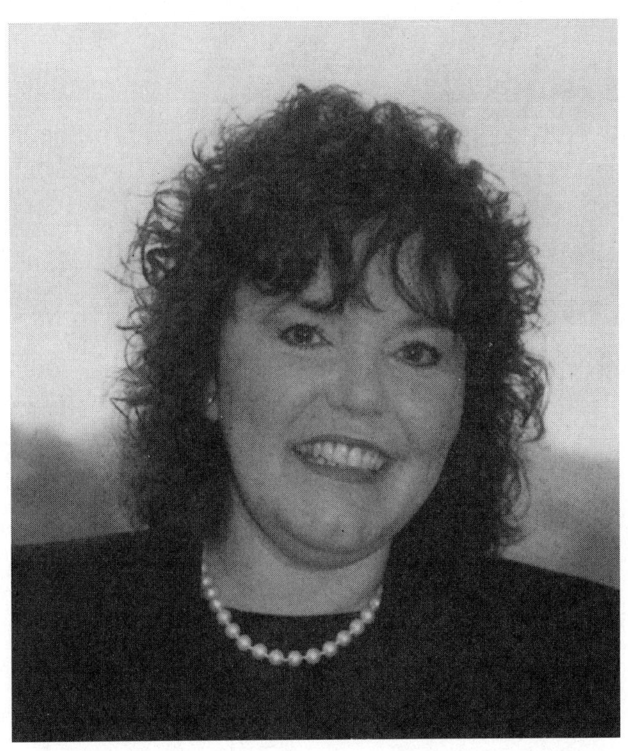

Linda Anne Silvestri received her diploma in nursing at Cooley Dickinson Hospital School of Nursing in Northampton, Massachusetts. Afterwards, she worked at Baystate Medical Center in the trauma center and in the pediatric and acute care units. She later received her BSN from American International College in Springfield, Massachusetts.

A native of Springfield, Massachusetts, Linda began her teaching career as an instructor of medical-surgical nursing and leadership-management nursing at Baystate Medical Center School of Nursing in 1981. In 1985, she earned her MSN from Anna Maria College, Paxton, Massachusetts, with a dual major in Nursing Management and Patient Education.

Linda moved to Rhode Island in 1989 and began teaching advanced medical-surgical nursing and psychiatric nursing to RN and LPN students at the Community College of Rhode Island. While teaching at Community College of Rhode Island, a group of students approached Linda, asking her to help them prepare for the NCLEX. On the basis of her past experience as an NCLEX item writer, she developed a comprehensive review course and hired faculty from the University of Rhode Island, Community College of Rhode Island, and Rhode Island College to teach specific clinical areas for the courses.

In 1991, Linda established Professional Nursing Seminars, Inc., dedicated to conducting NCLEX-RN review courses and assisting nursing graduates to achieve their goals of becoming Registered Nurses. The next year, her company began conducting NCLEX-PN review courses. During 1994, she was courted by Salve Regina University in Newport, Rhode Island, to conduct review courses for their program. Later that same year, Salve Regina University invited her to work as an Assistant Professor and Clinical Coordinator of the Nursing Program, where she teaches in the areas of acute care, community and family health, and NCLEX review. She is currently matriculated at the University of Rhode Island in the PhD in Nursing Program.

Today, Linda Silvestri's company conducts NCLEX review courses throughout New England. She is the successful author of numerous NCLEX-RN and NCLEX-PN review products, including *Saunders Comprehensive Review for NCLEX-RN, Saunders Q&A Review for NCLEX-RN, Saunders Computerized AssessTest for NCLEX-RN,* and *Saunders Instructor's Resource Package for NCLEX-RN.*

Contributors

Marianne P. Barba, MS, RN
Associate Professor of Nursing, Salve Regina University, Newport, Rhode Island

Nancy Blasdell, MSN, RN
Professor/Lecturer and Clinical Laboratory Coordinator, Department of Nursing, Salve Regina University, Newport, Rhode Island

Barbara Bono-Snell, MS, RN, CS
Psychiatric Clinical Nurse Specialist, St. Joseph's Certified Home Health Care Agency, Liverpool, New York

Netta Moncur Bowen, MSN, RN
Nursing Faculty, Seminole Community College, Sanford, Florida

Carolyn Pierce Buckelew, RNCS, NC, CHyp
Nursing Instructor, Charles E. Gregory School of Nursing, Raritan Bay Medical Center, Perth Amboy, New Jersey

Janis M. Byers, MSN, RNC
Nursing Faculty, Sewickley Valley Hospital School of Nursing, Sewickley, Pennsylvania

Penny S. Cass, PhD, RN
Dean, Division of Nursing, Indiana University, Kokomo, Kokomo, Indiana

Deborah H. Chatham, RN, MS, CS
Assistant Professor of Nursing, William Carey College, Gulfport, Mississippi

Tom Christenbery, MSN, RN
Assistant Professor of Nursing, Tennessee State University, Nashville, Tennessee

Anita M. Creamer, RN, MS, CS
Associate Professor of Nursing, Community College of Rhode Island, Warwick, Rhode Island

Barbara A. Dagastine, EdMSN, RN
Associate Professor of Nursing, Hudson Valley Community College, Troy, New York

Jean DeCoffe, MSN, RN
Assistant Professor of Nursing, Salve Regina University, Newport, Rhode Island

DeAnna Jan Emory, MS, RN
Assistant Professor of Nursing, Bacone College, Muskogee, Oklahoma

Mary E. Farrell, MS, RN, CCRN
Associate Professor of Nursing, Salem State College, Salem, Massachusetts

Patsy H. Fasnacht, MSN, RN, CCRN
Nursing Instructor, Lancaster Institute for Health Education, Lancaster, Pennsylvania

Dona Ferguson, MSN, RN, C
Assistant Professor of Nursing and Chair, Nursing and Allied Health, Atlantic Community College, Mays Landing, New Jersey

Thomas E. Folcarelli, MSN, RN
Assistant Professor of Nursing, Community College of Rhode Island, Newport, Rhode Island

Florence Hayes Gibson, MSN, CNS
Associate Professor of Nursing, Northeast Louisiana University, Monroe, Louisiana

Alma V. Harkey, RNC, MSN, ACCE
Instructor of Nursing, Southeast Missouri State University, Cape Girardeau, Missouri

Joyce Ellen Heil, BSN, CCRN
Assistant Instructor of Nursing, St. Margaret School of Nursing, Pittsburgh, Pennsylvania

Barbara Hicks, DSN, RN
Instructor of Nursing, Central Alabama Community College, Coosa Valley School of Nursing, Sylacauga, Alabama

Mary Ann Hogan, MSN, RN
Medical-Surgical Level Coordinator, Baystate Medical Center School of Nursing, Springfield, Massachusetts

Lori Horton, RN
Student, Department of Nursing, Salve Regina University, Newport, Rhode Island

Noreen M. Houck, MS, RN
Assistant Director, Crouse Hospital School of Nursing, Syracuse, New York

Amy Lawyer Hudson, RN, MSN
Nursing Faculty, Phillips Community College, University of Arkansas, Helene, Arkansas

Frances E. Johnson, MS, RNC
Assistant Professor of Nursing, Andrews University, Berrien Springs, Michigan

Deborah Klaas, RN, PhD
Assistant Professor of Nursing, Northern Arizona University, Flagstaff, Arizona

June Peterson Larson, RN, MS
Associate Professor of Nursing, University of South Dakota, Vermillion, South Dakota

Suzanne K. Marnocha, RN, MSN, CCRN
Assistant Professor of Nursing, University of Wisconsin, Oshkosh, Oshkosh, Wisconsin

Ellen Frances McCarty, PhD, RN, CS
Associate Professor of Nursing, Salve Regina University, Newport, Rhode Island

Connie M. Metzler, MSN, RN
Instructor of Nursing, Lancaster Institute for Health Education, Lancaster, Pennsylvania

Patricia A. Miller, MSN, RN
Director, School of Nursing, Baystate Medical Center School of Nursing, Springfield, Massachusetts

Jo Ann Barnes Mullaney, PhD, RN, CS
Professor of Nursing/Returning Registered Nurse Coordinator, Salve Regina University, Newport, Rhode Island

Kathleen Ann Ohman, RN, MS, EdD
Associate Professor of Nursing, College of St. Benedict/St. John's University, St. Joseph, Minnesota

Lynda C. Opdyke, RN, MSN
Facilitator/Academic Affairs, Mercy School of Nursing, Charlotte, North Carolina

MaeDella Perry, RN, MS
Nurse Educator, Medical College of Georgia, Augusta, Georgia

Lisa A. Ruth-Sahd, MSN, RN, CEN, CCRN
Nursing Instructor, Lancaster Institute for Health Education, Lancaster, Pennsylvania, and Adjunct Faculty, York College of Pennsylvania, York, Pennsylvania

Jeanine T. Seguin, MS, RN, CS
Assistant Professor of Nursing, Keuka College, Keuka Park, New York

Alberta Elaine Severs, MSN, MA, RN
Associate Professor of Nursing, Community College of Rhode Island, Lincoln, Rhode Island

Kimberly Sharpe, MS, RN
Instructor of Nursing, Crouse Hospital School of Nursing, Syracuse, New York

Susan Sienkiewicz, MA, RN, CS
Associate Professor of Nursing, Community College of Rhode Island, Lincoln, Rhode Island

Yvonne Marie Smith, MSN, RN, CCRN
Instructor, Aultman Hospital School of Nursing, Canton, Ohio

Judith Stamp, MS, RN
Assistant Professor of Nursing, Hudson Valley Community College, Troy, New York

Yvonne Nazareth Stringfield, EdD, RN
Associate Professor of Nursing, and BSN Program Director, Tennessee State University, Nashville, Tennessee

Mattie Tolley, RN, MS
Instructor of Nursing, Southwestern Oklahoma State University, Weatherford, Oklahoma

Johanna M. Tracy, MSN, RN, CS
Instructor of Nursing, Mercer Medical Center, Trenton, New Jersey

Joyce I. Turnbull, RN, MN
Nursing Lecturer/Clinical Instructor, San Jose State University, San Jose, California

Laurent W. Valliere, BS
Vice President, Professional Nursing Seminars, Inc., Charlestown, Rhode Island

Paula A. Viau, PhD, RN
Assistant Professor of Nursing, University of Rhode Island College of Nursing, Kingston, Rhode Island

Carol Warner, RN, CPN, MSN
Instructor of Nursing, St. Luke's School of Nursing, Bethlehem, Pennsylvania

Deborah Williams, EdD, RN
Associate Professor of Nursing, Western Kentucky University, Bowling Green, Kentucky

Reviewer List

Betty Nash Blevins, MSN, RN, CCRN, CS
Bluefield State College, Bluefield, West Virginia

Clara Willard Boyle, EdD, RN
Salem State College, Salem, Massachusetts

Bonita Eileen Broyles, EdD, BSN, RN
Piedmont Community College, Roxboro, North Carolina

Mary L. Centa, BA, RN, CNOR
Coordinator, Surgical Technology and Perioperative Nursing, Community College of Denver, Denver, Colorado

Marla J. DeJong, MS, RN, CCRN, CEN, Captain
Wilford Hall Medical Center, Lackland Air Force Base, Texas

Lenora D. Follett, MS, RN
Assistant Professor, Department of Nursing, Pacific Union College, Angwin, California

Diane M. Ford, MS, RN, CCRN
Andrews University, Berrien Springs, Michigan

Mary Jo Gay, MSN, RN
Missouri Western State College, St. Joseph, Missouri

Susan V. Gille, PhD, RN, CS, NP-C, FNP
Missouri Western State College, St. Joseph, Missouri

Beth Hammer, MSN, RN, ANP
Zablocki Veterans Affairs Medical Center, Milwaukee, Wisconsin

Ann Putnam Johnson, EdD, RN, CS
Western Carolina University, Cullowhee, North Carolina

Brenda P. Johnson, MSN, RN
Assistant Professor, Southeast Missouri State University, Cape Girardeau, Missouri

Joyce L. Kee, MS, RN
Associate Professor Emerita, College of Nursing, University of Delaware, Newark, Delaware

Denise LeBlanc, BSCN, RN, ENC(c)
Professor, School of Health Sciences, Humber College, Toronto, Ontario

Marquita Lindsey, BSN, RNC
Caddo-Kiowa Vocational Technical School, Ft. Cobb, Oklahoma

Gene Livingston, BS, MEd, RN
Texarkana College, Texarkana, Texas

Mary Jo Melby, BS, RN
Great Plains Area Vo-Tech School, Lawton, Oklahoma

Dorothy M. Obester, PhD, RN
St. Francis College, Loretto, Pennsylvania

Beth Perdue, MSN, RN
Former Instructor, El Centro College, Dallas, Texas

Conchita Quimbo-Rader, MA, RN
Chilton Memorial Hospital, Pompton Plains, New Jersey

Mary E. Sampel, MSN, RN
Saint Louis University, St. Louis, Missouri

Janice G. Sample, MNSc, CNRN, RN
Texarkana College, Texarkana, Texas

Susan T. Sanders, MSN, RN, CNAA
Motlow State Community College, Tullahoma, Tennessee

Karen G. Tarnow, PhD, RN
School of Nursing, University of Kansas, Kansas City, Kansas

David Tilton, BSN, RN
Harrison Hospital, Bremerton, Washington

Linda G. Waite, MN, RN, CCRN
Clinical Nurse Specialist, Kaiser Permanente Medical Center, San Rafael, California

Janice S. Williams, MSN, RN, CS
Department of Nursing, Presentation College, Aberdeen, South Dakota

Marion Yavorka, MSN, RN
School of Nursing, Mercy Hospital, Pittsburgh, Pennsylvania

Student Reviewer List

Melissa D. Ball
Salve Regina University, Newport, Rhode Island

Keri A. Bourassa
Salve Regina University, Newport, Rhode Island

Judith A. Brown
Regis University, Denver, Colorado

Lori Chieka
Salve Regina University, Newport, Rhode Island

Melinda A. Figueiredo
Salve Regina University, Newport, Rhode Island

Michelle Hertz
Salve Regina University, Newport, Rhode Island

MaryAnn Hickey
Salve Regina University, Newport, Rhode Island

Karla Marie Klassen
The College of St. Catherine, St. Paul, Minnesota

Amanda Mandel
Salve Regina University, Newport, Rhode Island

Erica Anne Markey
Salve Regina University, Newport, Rhode Island

Pamela Rosen
University of Rochester, Rochester, New York

Denise J. Servoss
Salve Regina University, Newport, Rhode Island

Tresa K. Vinyard
Southeast Missouri State University, Cape Girardeau, Missouri

Cindy Wilkins
Nebraska Methodist College of Nursing and Allied Health, Omaha, Nebraska

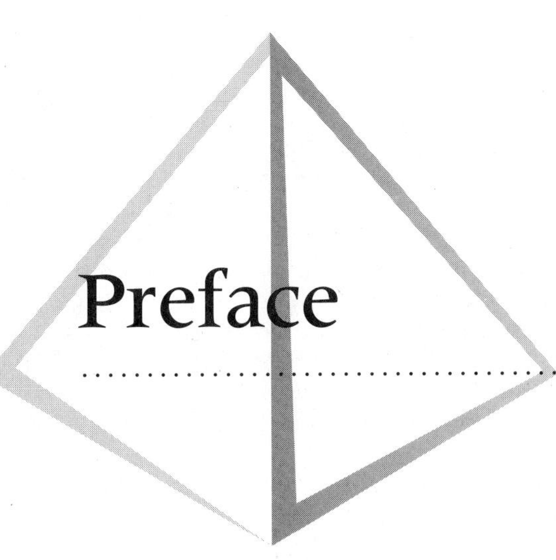

Preface

"Success is climbing a mountain, facing the challenge of obstacles, and reaching the top of the mountain."

—LINDA ANNE SILVESTRI, MSN, RN

Welcome to Saunders Pyramid to Success!

The *Saunders Q&A Review for NCLEX-RN* is one of a series of products designed to assist you in achieving your goal of becoming a registered nurse. The *Saunders Q&A Review for NCLEX-RN* and its accompanying CD-ROM provide you with 3450 practice NCLEX-RN test questions. This book has been uniquely designed and includes 13 chapters containing practice test questions.

CAT NCLEX-RN TEST PREPARATION

This book begins with information regarding NCLEX-RN preparation. Chapter 1 addresses all of the information related to the 1998 CAT NCLEX-RN test plan and the testing procedures related to the examination. This chapter answers all questions that you may have regarding the testing procedures.

Chapter 2 discusses the NCLEX-RN from a nonacademic view and provides an emphasis on a holistic approach to your individual test preparation. This chapter identifies the components of a structured study plan and pattern, anxiety-reducing techniques, and personal focus issues.

Nursing students want to hear what other students have to say about their experiences with CAT NCLEX-RN. Students seek that view with regard to what it is really like to take this examination. Chapter 3 is written by a nursing student who recently took the CAT NCLEX-RN, addresses the issue of what CAT NCLEX-RN is all about, and includes the "story of success." Test-taking strategies are an important component of success in taking the CAT NCLEX-RN examination. Chapter 4, "Test-Taking Strategies," includes all important strategies that will assist in teaching you how to read a question, how not to read into a question, and how to use the process of elimination and various other strategies to select the correct response from the options presented.

The Nursing Process

Chapters 5 to 9 contain practice test questions related to each step of the Nursing Process. Each chapter provides a brief description of the specific step of the Nursing Process. Whether you are currently a nursing student or preparing to take the CAT NCLEX-RN, you may recall that many of the standardized examinations that you have taken in nursing school have reported results that have identified your strengths and areas in need of improvement in the steps of the Nursing Process. Students frequently seek resources and questions related to the particular steps of the Nursing Process to assist them in strengthening these areas. It is difficult for students to find questions addressing a specific step of the Nursing Process. This book is uniquely designed to provide you with just that. Chapter 5 contains questions related to the process of assessment, Chapter 6 contains analysis questions, Chapter 7 contains planning questions, Chapter 8 contains implementation questions, and Chapter 9 contains evaluation questions.

Client Needs

Chapters 10 to 13 contain practice test questions related specifically to each category of Client Needs. In each chapter, the test plan categories and subcategories are specifically identified along with the percentages of test questions in each component of the test plan. Chapter 10 contains questions related to Safe, Effective Care Environment, Chapter 11 contains Physiological Integrity questions, Chapter 12 contains Psychosocial Integrity questions, and Chapter 13 contains Health Promotion and Maintenance questions.

SPECIAL FEATURES OF THE BOOK

Practice Test Questions

While preparing for NCLEX-RN, students have a strong need to review practice test questions. Each chapter contains practice test questions in NCLEX-RN format. This book contains 2700 practice test questions. The accompanying CD-ROM includes all the questions from the book, plus an additional 750 questions, and thus a total of 3450 test questions.

The book is designed with a unique two-column format. The left column presents the practice questions and options, and the right column provides the corresponding answers, rationales, strategies, and references. A special book flap is provided at the back of this book. The book flap is used to cover the answers, rationales, and strategies while the student is answering each question. The two-column format makes review easier so that you do not have to flip through pages in search of answers and rationales.

Each practice question includes the correct answer and the rationale, which provides you with the significant information regarding both correct and incorrect options. The structure of the answer section is unique and provides the following information for every question:

Test-Taking Strategy: The test-taking strategy provides you with the logic for selecting the correct option and assists you in selecting an answer to a question for which you must guess. Specific suggestions for review are identified in the test-taking strategy.

Question Categories: Each question is identified on the basis of the categories used by the CAT NCLEX-RN test plan. Additional content area categories are provided with each question to assist you in identifying areas in need of review. The categories identified with each practice question include Level of Cognitive Ability, Phase of Nursing Process, Client Needs, and the specific nursing Content Area. All categories are identified by their full names so that you do not need to memorize codes or abbreviations.

Reference Source: The reference source and page number are provided for you so that you can easily find the information that you need to review in your undergraduate nursing textbooks.

NCLEX-RN Review CD-ROM

Packaged in the back of this book you will find an NCLEX-RN review CD-ROM. This software contains 3450 questions, 2700 from the book and 750 additional questions. This Windows-compatible program offers three testing modes for review:

Quiz: 10 randomly chosen questions on the Nursing Process, Client Needs, or specific Content Area. Results are given and review is provided after you answer all 10 questions.

Study: 10 randomly chosen questions on the Nursing Process, Client Needs, or specific Content Area. The answer, comprehensive rationale, and test-taking strategy appear after you answer each of the 10 questions. Results are given after you answer all 10 questions.

Examination: 100 randomly chosen questions from the entire pool of 3450 questions chosen by the Nursing Process, Client Needs, or specific Content Area. Results are given and review is provided after you answer all 100 questions.

The CD-ROM allows you to customize your review and determine your areas of strength and weakness. It also provides you with a wealth of practice test questions while at the same time simulating the NCLEX-RN experience on the computer.

HOW TO USE THIS BOOK

Saunders Q&A Review for NCLEX-RN is especially designed to help you with your successful journey to the peak of the Pyramid to Success, becoming a registered nurse. As you begin your journey through this book, you will be introduced to all of the important points regarding the CAT NCLEX-RN, the process of testing, and the unique and special tips regarding how to prepare yourself for this important examination. Read the chapter from the nursing graduate who recently passed the NCLEX-RN, and consider what the graduate had to say about the examination. The test-taking strategy chapter wil provide you with important strategies that will guide you in selecting the correct option or assist you in guessing the answer. Read this chapter and practice these strategies as you proceed through your journey with this book.

Once you have completed reading the introductory components of this book, it is time to remove that special flap found at the back of this book and begin the practice questions. This flap is provided to you with this book to cover the answers, rationales, and strategies while you answer each question. As you read through each question and select an answer, be sure to read the rationale and the test-taking strategy. The rationale provides you with the significant information regarding both the correct and incorrect options, and the test-taking strategy provides you with the logic for selecting the correct option. The strategy also identifies the content area that you need to review if you had difficulty with the question. Use the reference source provided so that you can easily find the information that you need to review.

SAUNDERS PYRAMID TO SUCCESS

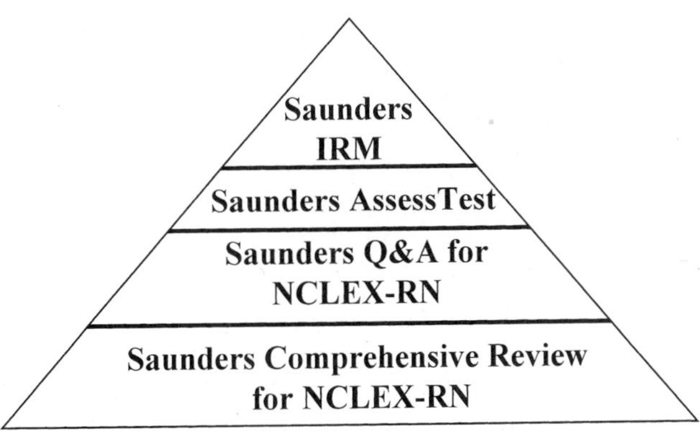

As you work your way through *Saunders Q&A Review for NCLEX-RN* to identify your areas of strength and weakness, you can return to the companion book, *Saunders Comprehensive Review for NCLEX-RN,* to focus your study on these areas. The companion book and its accompanying CD-ROM provide you with a comprehensive review of all areas of the nursing content reflected in the 1998 CAT NCLEX-RN test plan. To determine your readiness for CAT NCLEX-RN, you will use the next step in the Saunders Pyramid to Success, *Saunders Computerized AssessTest for NCLEX-RN,* which is a software program containing 1200 NCLEX-RN–style questions. The software provides detailed analysis similar to that for standardized nursing examinations. The final component of the Saunders Pyramid to Success is the *Saunders Instructor's Resource Package for NCLEX-RN.* This manual and CD-ROM accompany the Saunders program of NCLEX-RN review products. Be sure to ask your nursing program director and nursing faculty about the CD-ROM and its use for a review course or a self-paced review in your school's computer laboratory. Good luck with your journey through the Pyramid to Success!

I wish you continued success throughout your new career as a Registered Nurse!

—Linda Anne Silvestri, MSN, RN

To All Future Registered Nurses,

Congratulations to you!

Whether you are a nursing student in a nursing program completing your studies or a graduate preparing to take the NCLEX-RN, you should be very proud and pleased with yourself for your many accomplishments. I know that you are working very hard to become successful and that you have proved to yourself that you indeed can achieve your goals. I have been teaching nursing students for many years and have been conducting NCLEX-RN Review Courses since 1991. Preparing to take an examination can be an anxiety-producing experience. A component of achieving success in examinations is possessing the knowledge and experience needed to answer a question correctly. An additional component of becoming successful in these examinations is to become comfortable and confident with the ability to face the challenge of a question and to answer the question correctly. In my experience in working with students, it is evident that students strongly need to review practice questions. The more questions, answers, and rationales with which a student can practice, the more proficient the student becomes with test-taking strategies and the ability to answer a question correctly. One of the things that you need to realize is that when you take an examination consisting of multiple-choice questions, the answer is right there in front of you. You need to use your nursing knowledge and skills and become proficient at the strategy involved in reading the question and specifically identifying what the question is asking you. Your knowledge, your experience, and the incorporation of test taking strategies will lead you to success.

On NCLEX-RN, the questions require thought and critical analysis. Consistent practice with the test questions will assist you in becoming comfortable, confident, and proficient with answering the questions correctly.

I am excited and pleased to be able to provide you with Saunders Pyramid To Success products. These products will prepare you for your most important professional goal of becoming a registered nurse. Saunders Pyramid To Success products provide you with everything that you need to prepare for NCLEX-RN. These products include material that is required for examination preparation for all nursing students regardless of educational background, specific strengths, areas in need of improvement, or clinical experience during the nursing program.

Saunders Q&A Review for NCLEX-RN is designed to provide you with questions specifically representative of the components of the 1998 NCLEX-RN test plan. Although the framework for the test plan focuses primarily on Client Needs, the steps of the Nursing Process are an integrated concept and process of the test plan. Therefore, chapters representative of each step of the Nursing Process are included in this book. Each chapter contains questions specifically identifying each component of both the Nursing Process and the categories of Client Needs. So let's get started and begin our journey through the Pyramid To Success!

Welcome to the Profession of Nursing!

Sincerely,

Linda Anne Silvestri MSN, RN

Linda Anne Silvestri, MSN, RN

Acknowledgments

There are many individuals who in their own way have contributed to my success in making my professional dreams become a reality.

First, I wish to acknowledge my mother, Frances Mary; my sister, Dianne Elodia; my brother, Lawrence Peter; and my niece, Gina Marie, who are ever supportive and giving of their love and devotion.

A very special thank you to Sarah Miller for her continuous support and dedication to my work and for her assistance each and every moment as I prepared my work for publication.

I acknowledge Laurent W. Valliere for his continuous love, support, and dedication to my professional endeavors and for his contribution to this publication. I sincerely thank Mary Ann Hogan, MSN, RN, who has always encouraged and supported me through my professional endeavors. Her numerous contributions to this publication are a reflection of her dedication to the profession of nursing and to nursing students. I also acknowledge Patricia Mieg, Senior Educational Representative, who encouraged me to submit my ideas and initial work to the W.B. Saunders Company.

I thank all of the contributors to this publication who provided many of the practice questions contained in this publication and to the many faculty and student reviewers of this publication. A special thank you to Dr. JoAnn Mullaney from Salve Regina University in Newport, Rhode Island, for her numerous and expert contributions to this publication and to Lori Horton, RN, for providing a chapter in this publication regarding her experience with NCLEX-RN.

I want to acknowledge all of the staff at the W.B. Saunders Company for their tremendous assistance throughout the course of this endeavor. A special thank you to all of them.

I want to acknowledge and thank Maura Connor, Senior Acquisitions Editor, for her expert professional guidance and remarkable support throughout this project. Her caring and warm personality, coupled with her energy, enthusiasm, and professional direction, has without a doubt brought this publication to fruition. I thank Victoria Legnini, Editorial Assistant, for her expert organizational skills in maintaining order for all of the work that I submitted for manuscript production. I have also had the fortunate opportunity to work with Anne Ostroff, Copy Editor, whose remarkable editing assisted in finalizing this publication, and with Andrea Stingelin, Director of Marketing, and Cindy Fortunato, Marketing Manager, whose support and creativity assisted with this publication.

I thank Salve Regina University for the opportunity to educate nursing students in the baccalaureate nursing program and for its support during my research and writing of this publication. I especially acknowledge Dr. Eileen Donnelly, Chairperson of the Department of Nursing at Salve Regina University, for her continuous support, academic mentoring, and astute vision regarding the future of the profession of nursing.

I acknowledge the University of Rhode Island, College of Nursing, for providing me with the opportunity for professional growth in my nursing education, particularly Dr. Donna Barcott Swartz and Dr. Suzie Kim, my academic advisors in the doctoral program at the university.

I acknowledge the Community College of Rhode Island, which provided me the opportunity to educate nursing students in the Associate Degree of Nursing Program, and I especially thank Patricia Miller, MSN, RN, and Michelina McClellan, MS, RN, from Baystate Medical Center, School of Nursing, Springfield, Massachusetts, who were my very first mentors in nursing education.

Lastly, a very special thank you to all my nursing students: you light up my life, and your hearts and minds will shape the future of the profession of nursing!

Contents

UNIT I ▽ NCLEX-RN Preparation **1**

1 NCLEX-RN Preparation 3

2 Profiles of Success 14
Laurent W. Valliere, B.S.

3 The NCLEX-RN Examination: From a Student's Perspective 17
Lori Horton, R.N.

4 Test-Taking Strategies 19

UNIT II ▽ The Nursing Process **25**

5 The Process of Assessment 27

6 The Process of Analysis 157

7 The Process of Planning 293

8 The Process of Implementation 425

9 The Process of Evaluation 557

UNIT III ▽ Client Needs **689**

10 Safe, Effective Care Environment 691

11 Physiological Integrity 819

12 Psychosocial Integrity 963

13 Health Promotion and Maintenance 1054

UNIT I

NCLEX-RN Preparation

CHAPTER 1

NCLEX-RN Preparation

THE PYRAMID TO SUCCESS

Welcome to Saunders Q&A for NCLEX-RN, the second component to The Pyramid to Success!

At this time, you have completed your first path toward the peak of the Pyramid with the Saunders Comprehensive Review for NCLEX-RN. Now, it is time to continue that journey to become a Registered Nurse with the Saunders Q&A for NCLEX-RN!

As you begin your journey through this book, you will be introduced to all of the important points regarding the NCLEX-RN examination, the process of testing, and the unique and special tips regarding how to prepare yourself for this very important examination. You will read what a nursing graduate who recently passed NCLEX-RN has to say about the examination. All of those important test-taking strategies are detailed. These details will guide you in selecting the correct option or in selecting an answer to a question you must guess at.

Saunders Q&A for NCLEX-RN contains over 3000 NCLEX-style practice questions. The chapters have been developed to contain questions specific to the categories of Client Needs, as reflected in the NCLEX-RN test plan. In addition, chapters have been prepared to contain questions reflective of each phase of the nursing process to assist you in mastering the process of answering these types of questions.

Each chapter begins with a description of the focus of the chapter, based on the phase of the nursing process or the category of Client Needs. A rationale, test-taking strategy, and reference source containing the page number is provided with each question. Each question is coded on the basis of the level of cognitive ability, the phase of the nursing process, the Client Needs category, and the content area being tested. The rationale provides you with significant information regarding both the correct and incorrect options. The test-taking strategy provides you with the logical path to selecting the correct option. The test-taking strategy also identifies the content area to review, if required. The reference source and page number provide easy access to the information that you need to review.

After the completion of your Saunders Q&A for NCLEX-RN, you are ready for the Saunders AssessTest for NCLEX-RN, a computer disk program containing over 1000 NCLEX-RN style questions that determines your readiness for NCLEX-RN. Let's continue with our journey through The Pyramid to Success!

THE EXAMINATION PROCESS

An important step in the Pyramid to Success is to become as familiar as possible with the examination process. The challenge of this examination can arouse significant anxiety. Knowing what the examination is all about and knowing what you will encounter during the process of testing will assist in alleviating fear and anxiety. The information contained in this chapter addresses the procedures related to the development of the NCLEX-RN Test Plan, the components of the test plan, and the answers to the questions most commonly asked by nursing students and graduates preparing to take the NCLEX-RN. This information was adapted from the *Test Plan for the National Council Licensure Examination for Registered Nurses,* National Council of State Boards of Nursing, Chicago, 1997, and *The NCLEX Process,* National Council of State Boards of Nursing, Chicago, 1995.

DEVELOPMENT OF THE TEST PLAN

As an initial step in the test development process, the National Council of State Boards of Nursing considers the legal scope of nursing practice as governed by state laws and regulations, including the Nurse Practice Act. The National Council uses these laws to define the areas on NCLEX-RN that will assess the competence of candidates for nurse licensure.

The National Council of State Boards of Nursing also conducts a job analysis study to determine the framework for the test plan for NCLEX-RN. Because nursing practice continues to change, this study is conducted every 3 years. The results of the study conducted in 1996 provided the structure for the new test plan implemented in April 1998.

JOB ANALYSIS STUDY

The participants of this study are selected by a stratified random sampling process and include newly licensed registered nurses from all types of basic education programs. The participants are provided a list of nursing activities and are asked how often they performed these activities, called the *frequency rating*. The participants are also asked whether they could sometimes or never omit performing a nursing activity without having a major impact on a client's well-being. This is called the *criticality rating*. The participant is then asked to indicate the setting in which they performed the specific nursing activities. The data obtained from this study are used in developing the framework for NCLEX-RN.

THE TEST PLAN

The content on NCLEX-RN reflects the activities that a minimally competent, newly registered nurse must be able to perform in order to provide clients with safe and effective nursing care. The questions are written to address the levels of cognitive ability, client needs, and integrated concepts and processes as identified in the test plan.

Levels of Cognitive Ability

The NCLEX-RN examination includes questions at the cognitive levels of knowledge, comprehension, application and analysis. Most of the questions are written at the application and analysis levels because the practice of nursing requires the application of knowledge, skills, and abilities. This means that the test taker will be required to analyze and/or apply the facts provided in the test question.

BOX 1-1. Level of Cognitive Ability

A pregnant client is positive for the human immunodeficiency virus (HIV). On the basis of this information, the nurse determines that

1. The client has the herpes simplex virus.
2. HIV antibodies are detected on the enzyme-linked immunosorbent assay (ELISA).
3. The newborn will develop this disease after birth.
4. This client has contacted an airborne disease.

Answer: 2

Level of Cognitive Ability: Analysis

Rationale: This question requires the nurse to analyze knowledge regarding HIV and the data provided in order to answer the question. Option 2 is the correct response. Diagnosis depends on serological studies to detect HIV antibodies. The most commonly used test is the ELISA. Options 1 and 4 are incorrect because HIV stands for human immunodeficiency virus, and it occurs primarily through the exchange of body fluids. Option 3 is incorrect. A neonate born to an HIV-positive mother has a 20%–40% risk of developing this disease.

Reference

Gorrie, T. M., McKinney, E. S., & Murray, S. S. (1994). *Foundations of maternal-newborn nursing*. Philadelphia: W. B. Saunders, p. 728.

Client Needs

In the new test plan implemented in April 1998, the National Council of State Boards of Nursing has identified a test plan framework based on *client needs*. This framework was selected on the basis of the analysis of the findings in the Job Analysis study and because client needs provide a structure for defining nursing actions and competencies across all settings for all clients. The National Council of State Boards of Nursing identifies four major categories of Client Needs. These categories are further divided into subcategories, and the percentage of test questions in each subcategory is identified.

Safe, Effective Care Environment

The Safe, Effective Care Environment category includes two subcategories: (1) Management of Care and (2) Safety and Infection Control. Management of Care (7%–13%) addresses content that tests the knowledge, skills, and ability required to provide integrated cost-effective care to clients by coordinating, supervising care, and/or collaborating with members of the multidisciplinary health care team. Safety and Infection Control (5%–11%) addresses content that tests the knowledge, skills, and ability required to protect clients and health care personnel from environmental hazards.

BOX 1-2. Client Needs and the Percentage of Test Questions

SAFE, EFFECTIVE CARE ENVIRONMENT

Management of care: 7%–13%
Safety and infection control: 5%–11%

HEALTH PROMOTION AND MAINTENANCE

Growth and development through the life span: 7%–13%
Prevention and early detection of disease: 5%–11%

PSYCHOSOCIAL INTEGRITY

Coping and adaptation: 5%–11%
Psychosocial adaptation: 5%–11%

PHYSIOLOGICAL INTEGRITY

Basic care and comfort: 7%–13%
Pharmacological and parenteral therapies: 5%–11%
Reduction of risk potential: 12%–18%
Physiological adaptation: 12%–18%

BOX 1-3. Safe, Effective Care Environment

MANAGEMENT OF CARE

A client with trigeminal neuralgia is undergoing microvascular decompression of the trigeminal nerve. The nurse would plan to have which of the following pieces of equipment at the bedside upon return of the client from the postanesthesia care unit?

1. Padded bed rails, suction equipment
2. Blood pressure cuff, cardiac monitor
3. Flashlight, cardiac monitor, pulse oximeter
4. Cardiac monitor and pulse oximeter

Answer: 3

Rationale: This question addresses the subcategory Management of Care in the Client Needs category Safe, Effective Care Environment. The postoperative care of the client undergoing microvascular decompression of the trigeminal nerve is the same as for the client undergoing craniotomy. This entails hourly neurological assessment, as well as monitoring of cardiovascular and respiratory status. Suctioning is done very cautiously and only when necessary after craniotomy, to avoid increasing the intracranial pressure.

Reference

Black, J., & Matassarin-Jacobs, E. (1997). *Medical-surgical nursing: Clinical management for continuity of care* (5th ed.). Philadelphia: W. B. Saunders, pp. 929–930.

SAFETY AND INFECTION CONTROL

All clients who undergo surgery have the potential to acquire an infection. Which of the following nursing actions is most appropriate to prevent a postoperative wound infection?

1. Adhere to meticulous aseptic techniques
2. Keep the temperature warm to prevent chilling the client
3. Keep the doors to the suite open to improve ventilation
4. Scrub the incision site vigorously to remove all bacteria

Answer: 1

Rationale: This question addresses the subcategory Safety and Infection Control in the Client Needs category Safe, Effective Care Environment. The most important measure in preventing postoperative wound infection is adherence to meticulous aseptic techniques. The temperature in the surgical suite is kept cool to deter bacterial growth. Most pathogenic bacteria metabolize and reproduce at or near normal body temperature. By keeping the room temperature below body temperature, bacterial growth may be inhibited. By keeping air currents and movement to a minimum, airborne contamination can be controlled. Therefore, doors to the surgical suite must remain closed at all times. The skin preparation is performed to free the operative site as much as possible from dirt, skin oils, and transient microbes. This should be accomplished with the least amount of tissue irritation.

Reference

Black, J., & Matassarin-Jacobs, E. (1997). *Medical-surgical nursing: Clinical management for continuity of care* (5th ed.). Philadelphia: W. B. Saunders, p. 490.

Health Promotion and Maintenance

The Health Promotion and Maintenance category includes two subcategories: (1) Growth and Development Through the Life Span and (2) Prevention and Early Detection of Disease. Growth and Development Through the Life Span (7%–13%) addresses content that tests the knowledge, skills, and ability required to assist the client and significant others through the normal expected stages of growth and development from conception through advanced old age. Prevention and Early Detection of Disease (5%–11%) addresses content that tests the knowledge, skills, and ability required to manage and provide care for clients in need of prevention and early detection of health problems.

Psychosocial Integrity

The Psychosocial Integrity category includes two subcategories: (1) Coping and Adaptation and (2) Psychosocial Adaptation. Coping and Adaptation (5%–11%) addresses content that tests the knowledge, skills, and ability required to promote the client's ability to cope with, adapt to, and/or solve problems in situations related to illnesses or stressful events. Psychosocial Adaptation (5%–11%) addresses content that tests the knowledge, skills, and ability required to manage and provide care for clients with acute or chronic mental illnesses.

Physiological Integrity

The Physiological Integrity category includes four subcategories: Basic Care and Comfort; Pharmacological and Parenteral Therapies; Reduction of Risk Potential; and Physiological Adaptation. Basic Care and Comfort (7%–13%) addresses content that tests the knowledge, skills, and ability required to provide comfort and assistance in the performance of activities of daily living. Pharmacological and Parenteral Therapies (5%–11%) addresses content that tests the knowledge, skills, and ability required to manage and provide care related to the administration of medications and parenteral therapies. Reduction of Risk Potential (12%–18%) addresses content that tests the knowledge, skills, and ability required to reduce the likelihood that clients will develop complications or health problems related to existing conditions, treatments, or procedures. Physiological Adaptation

BOX 1–4. Health Promotion and Maintenance

GROWTH AND DEVELOPMENT THROUGH THE LIFE SPAN

The nurse is performing an admission assessment on an elderly client admitted with a diagnosis of cataracts. The nurse assesses for the major symptom associated with cataracts when the nurse

1. Performs an ophthalmoscopic examination.
2. Inserts contact lens.
3. Asks the client to blink.
4. Keeps the lens moist.

Answer: 1

Rationale: This question addresses the subcategory Growth and Development Through the Life Span in the Client Needs category Health Promotion and Maintenance. To assess for cataracts, the nurse would determine whether there is reduced visual acuity. In an ophthalmoscopic examination, the nurse would examine the lens to determine whether it has become more dense. A change in the molecular structure of the cells causes whitish opacities to appear.

Reference

Matteson, M. A., McConnell, E. S., & Linton, A. D. (1997). *Gerontological nursing concepts and practice* (2nd ed.). Philadelphia: W. B. Saunders, p. 360.

PREVENTION AND EARLY DETECTION OF DISEASE

The nurse in a rehabilitation facility is teaching the client with spinal cord injury and the family how to prevent episodes of autonomic dysreflexia. The nurse would evaluate that further clarification is necessary if the client made which of the following statements?

1. "I'm glad I can use my electric fan. I like the cool breeze on me."
2. "I will do the bladder catheterizations on time."
3. "It's important not to let the bedclothes get bunched up underneath me."
4. "I'll make sure to stick to the bowel retraining program."

Answer: 1

Rationale: This question addresses the subcategory Prevention and Early Detection of Disease in the Client Needs category Health Promotion and Maintenance. Causes of autonomic dysreflexia include bladder distention, bowel distention from constipation or fecal impaction, and stimulation of the skin from pain, pressure, or changes in temperature. The client and family should learn the triggering factors, methods of preventing them from occurring, and how to manage an episode.

Reference

Luckmann, J. (1997). *Saunders manual of nursing care*. Philadelphia: W. B. Saunders, pp. 1779–1780.

(12%–18%) addresses content that tests the knowledge, skills, and ability required to manage and provide care to clients with acute, chronic, or life-threatening physical health conditions.

Integrated Concepts and Processes of the Test Plan

The National Council of State Boards of Nursing has identified seven concepts and processes that are fundamental to the practice of nursing. These concepts and processes are a component of the test plan and are incorporated throughout the categories of Client Needs.

ITEM WRITERS

NCLEX-RN item writers are selected by the National Council of State Boards of Nursing, after an extensive application process. The item writers are registered nurses who are clinical experts and experienced in writing test items. Most of the item writers are nursing educators; however, clinical nurse specialists are also selected to participate in this process. These item writers voluntarily submit an application to become an item writer and must meet specific established criteria designated by the National Council in order to be accepted as a participant in the process.

CAT NCLEX-RN

The acronym NCLEX-RN stands for National Council Licensure Examination for Registered Nurses. Computer Adaptive Testing (CAT) NCLEX-RN is a computer-administered multiple-choice examination that the nursing graduate must pass in order to practice in the role as a registered nurse. This examination measures the test candidate's knowledge, skills, and abilities required to perform safely and competently as a newly licensed, entry-level registered nurse.

CAT provides a unique examination for the candidate, because the examination is adapted to each test taker's skill level. The CAT is an examination that is assembled interactively as the candidate answers the questions. All of the test questions are stored in a large test bank and are categorized on the basis of the test plan structure and the level of difficulty of the question. With the CAT method of testing, an examination is created and tailored to test the candidate's knowledge and abilities while fulfilling test plan requirements. In this way, candidates do not waste time answering questions that are far above or below their competency levels.

When a candidate answers a question on CAT NCLEX-RN, the computer will calculate a competency

BOX 1-5. Psychosocial Integrity

COPING AND ADAPTATION

A stillborn was delivered in the Birthing Suite a few hours ago. After the birth, the family has remained together, holding and touching the baby. Which statement by the nurse would further assist them in their initial period of grief?

1. "Don't worry, there is nothing you could do to prevent this from happening."
2. "We need to take the baby from you now so that you can get some sleep."
3. "What have you named your lovely baby?"
4. "We will see to it that you have an early discharge so that you don't have to be reminded of this experience."

Answer: 3

Rationale: This question addresses the subcategory Coping and Adaptation in the Client Needs category Psychosocial Integrity. Nurses should be able to explore measures that help the family create memory of an infant so that the existence of the child is confirmed and the family can complete the grieving process. Option 3 does this and also demonstrates a caring and empathetic response. Options 1, 2, and 4 are blocks to communication and devalue the family's feelings.

Reference

Gorrie, T. M., McKinney, E. S., & Murray, S. S. (1994). *Foundations of maternal-newborn nursing.* Philadelphia: W. B. Saunders, p. 648.

PSYCHOSOCIAL ADAPTATION

The nurse is performing an admission assessment of a family admitted with a diagnosis of violence. Which of the following factors would the nurse initially want to include in the assessment?

1. The family's anger toward the intrusiveness of the nurse
2. The family's denial of the violent nature of their behavior
3. The coping style of each family member
4. The family's current ability to use community resources

Answer: 3

Rationale: This question addresses the subcategory Psychosocial Adaptation in the Client Needs category Psychosocial Integrity. The initial family assessment includes a careful history of each family member. The following factors are part of the nurse's initial assessment of families who are experiencing violence: structure and function of the family, social functioning of each family member, sex role socialization and role strain, each family member's task performance ability, coping style of each family member, daily stresses in the family, resources available to the family in the home and community, expression of frustration and anger, beliefs about aggression and violence, and family's health status.

Reference

Carson, V., & Arnold, E. (1996). *Mental health nursing: The nurse-patient journey.* Philadelphia: W. B. Saunders, pp. 1074–1075.

skill estimate that is based on the answer that the candidate selected. If he or she selected a correct answer to a question, the computer scans the test bank and selects a more difficult question. If he or she selected an incorrect answer, the computer scans the test bank and selects an easier question. This process continues until the test plan requirements are met and a reliable pass or fail decision is made.

THE PROCESS OF REGISTRATION

The initial step in the registration process is that the candidate applies to the State Board of Nursing in the state in which he or she intends to obtain licensure. The candidate needs to obtain information from the board of nursing regarding the specific registration process, because the process may vary from state to state. It is very important that the candidate follow the registration instructions and complete the registration forms precisely and accurately. Registration forms not properly completed or not accompanied by the proper fees in the required method of payment will be returned to the candidate and will delay testing. The initial fee for the application process may vary from state to state. Each board of nursing sets its initial license fee according to its own needs. The registration forms identify the registration and testing service fees. When the board of nursing receives the completed registration form, based on the criteria established by the board, the candidate's eligibility is determined, and the board authorizes his or her admission to the examination. Once eligibility to test has been determined by the board of nursing in the jurisdiction in which licensure is requested, the valid NCLEX registration is processed, and an Authorization to Test form is sent to the candidate. The candidate cannot make an appointment until the board of nursing declares eligibility and he or she receive an Authorization to Test form. The Authorization to Test form provides a candidate identification number and an authorization number, and these numbers are needed in order to make an appointment with the testing center.

SPECIAL TESTING CIRCUMSTANCES

A candidate who requests special accommodations should contact the board of nursing before submitting

BOX 1–6. Physiological Integrity

BASIC CARE AND COMFORT

A client has been taught to use a walker to aid in mobility after internal fixation of a hip fracture. The nurse evaluates that the client is using the walker incorrectly if the client

1. Holds the walker by using the hand grips.
2. Leans forward slightly when advancing the walker.
3. Advances the walker with reciprocal motion.
4. Supports body weight on the hands while advancing the weaker leg.

Answer: 3

Rationale: This question addresses the subcategory Basic Care and Comfort in the Client Needs category Physiological Integrity. The client should use the walker by placing the hands on the hand grips for stability. The client lifts the walker to advance it and leans forward slightly while moving it. The client walks into the walker, supporting the body weight on the hands while moving the weaker leg. A disadvantage of the walker is that it does not allow for reciprocal walking motion. If the client were to try to use reciprocal motion with a walker, the walker would advance forward one side at a time as the client walks; thus the client would not be supporting the weaker leg with the walker during ambulation.

Reference

Lammon, C. B., Foote, A. W., Leli, P. G., et al. (1995). *Clinical nursing skills.* Philadelphia: W. B. Saunders, pp. 245–247.

PHARMACOLOGICAL AND PARENTERAL THERAPIES

A mother is to receive a rubella vaccine on the second postpartum day. Included in the teaching plan are the potential risks of the vaccine. On the basis of these risks, the nurse cautions the client to avoid

1. Sunlight for three days.
2. Scratching the injection site.
3. Pregnancy for 2–3 months after the vaccination.
4. Sexual intercourse for 2–3 months after the vaccination.

Answer: 3

Rationale: This question addresses the subcategory Pharmacological and Parenteral Therapies in the Client Needs category Physiological Integrity. Rubella vaccine is a live attenuated virus that evokes an antibody response that provides immunity for 15 years. Because rubella is a live vaccine, it will act as the virus and is potentially teratogenic in the organogenesis phase of fetal development. The client needs to be informed about the potential effects that this vaccine may have and the need to avoid becoming pregnant for a period of 2–3 months afterwards. Abstinence from sexual intercourse is not necessary, unless another form of effective contraception is not being used. The vaccine may cause local or systemic reactions, but all are mild and shortlived. Sunlight has no effect on the person who is vaccinated.

Reference

Nichols, F. H., & Zwelling, E. (1997). *Maternal-newborn nursing: Theory and practice.* Philadelphia: W. B. Saunders, pp. 1510–1511.

REDUCTION OF RISK POTENTIAL

The nurse is caring for the client who is going to have an arthrogram with a contrast medium. Which of the following assessments by the nurse would be of highest priority?

1. Allergy to iodine or shellfish
2. Ability of the client to remain still during the procedure
3. Whether the client has any remaining questions about the procedure
4. Whether the client wishes to void before the procedure

Answer: 1

Rationale: This question addresses the subcategory Reduction of Risk Potential in the Client Needs category Physiological Integrity. Because of the risk of allergic reaction to contrast dye, the nurse places highest priority on assessing whether the client has an allergy to iodine or shellfish. The nurse also reinforces information about the test, tells the client about the need to remain still during the procedure, and encourages the client to void before the procedure for comfort.

Reference

Black, J., & Matassarin-Jacobs, E. (1997). *Medical-surgical nursing: Clinical management for continuity of care* (5th ed.). Philadelphia: W. B. Saunders, p. 2094.

PHYSIOLOGICAL ADAPTATION

The nurse is positioning the client with increased intracranial pressure (ICP). Which of the following positions would the nurse avoid?

1. Head turned to the side
2. Head midline
3. Neck in neutral position
4. Head of bed elevated 30–45 degrees

Answer: 1

Rationale: This question addresses the subcategory Physiological Adaptation in the Client Needs category Physiological Integrity. The head of the client with increased ICP should be positioned so that the head is in a neutral, midline position. The nurse should avoid flexing or extending the neck or turning the neck side to side. The head of bed should be raised to 30–45 degrees. Use of proper positions promotes venous drainage from the cranium to keep ICP down.

Reference

Ignatavicius, D., Workman, M., & Mishler, M. (1995). *Medical-surgical nursing: A nursing process approach* (2nd ed.). Philadelphia: W. B. Saunders, p. 1273.

BOX 1-7. Integrated Concepts and Processes of the Test Plan

Nursing Process
Caring
Communication
Cultural Awareness
Documentation
Self-Care
Teaching/Learning

a registration form. The board of nursing will provide the candidate with the procedures for the request. Testing accommodations for candidates with disabilities must be authorized by the board of nursing. After board of nursing approval, the National Council of State Boards reviews the requested accommodations to ensure that the proposed modification does not affect the psychometric properties of NCLEX or cause a security risk.

MAKING AN APPOINTMENT TO TEST

The CAT NCLEX-RN examination is administered on a year-round basis. The candidate will be provided with a list of testing centers and the telephone numbers. The expiration date on the Authorization to Test form should be noted; an appointment must be scheduled before this expiration date. The test may be taken at any approved testing center and does not have to be taken in the same jurisdiction in which the candidate is seeking licensure. An eligible candidate taking NCLEX for the first time will be offered an appointment date within 30 days of the telephone call to the testing center. Repeat-testing candidates will be offered an appointment date within 45 days of the telephone call to the testing center. A confirmation notice will not be sent; therefore, it is important to note the date and time of the appointment. When the test center is called, it is also important to verify the address and the directions to the testing center.

CANCELING OR RESCHEDULING AN APPOINTMENT

If for any reason the candidate needs to cancel the appointment to take the test, he or she must remember that 3 business days' (Monday through Saturday) notice is required. The original appointment must be canceled before a new appointment can be scheduled.

LATE ARRIVALS TO THE TEST CENTER

It is important that the candidate arrive at the testing center 30 minutes before the test is scheduled. Candidates arriving late for the scheduled testing appointment may be required to forfeit the NCLEX appointment. If it is necessary for the appointment to be forfeited, the candidate needs to re-register for the examination and pay an additional fee, and the board of nursing will be notified that the candidate will not test.

A few days before the scheduled date of testing, the candidate should take the time to drive to the testing center to determine its exact location, the length of time required to arrive at that destination, and any potential obstacles that might cause a delay, such as road construction, traffic, or parking inaccessibility.

THE TESTING CENTER

The test center is designed to ensure complete security of the testing process. Strict candidate identification requirements have been established. To be admitted to the testing center, the candidate must bring the Authorization to Test form along with two forms of identification. Both forms of identification must be signed by the candidate, and one must contain a photograph of the candidate. The name on the photograph identification must bear the same name as that stated on the Authorization to Test form. Examples of acceptable forms of identification will be included in the information received with the Authorization to Test form. The candidate will be required to sign in and out on the test center log form. Each candidate will be thumbprinted and photographed at the test center, and the photograph will accompany the NCLEX results to confirm the candidate's identity. Personal belongings are not allowed in the testing room. Secure storage will be provided for the candidate; however, storage space is limited, so the candidate must plan accordingly. In addition, the testing center will not assume responsibility for candidates' personal belongings. The testing waiting areas are generally small; therefore, friends or family members who accompany candidates are not permitted to wait in the testing center while candidates are taking the NCLEX-RN.

Once the candidate has completed the admission process and a brief orientation, the proctor will escort the candidate to the assigned computer. The candidate is seated at an individual table with an appropriate work space that includes computer equipment, appropriate lighting, scratch paper, and a pencil. Unauthorized scratch paper may not be brought into or removed from the testing room. Eating, drinking, and smoking are not allowed in the testing room. A video camera is located in the testing room, and full sound and motion videotaping of all test sessions occurs.

Candidates should keep their two forms of identification with them at all times. Candidates cannot leave the testing room without the permission of the proctor. If a candidate leaves the testing room for any reason, he or she will be required to show two forms of identification in order to be readmitted. Candidates must follow the directions given by the test center staff and must remain in their seats during the test, except when authorized to leave. If a candidate believes that there is a problem with the computer, needs more scratch paper, or needs the proctor's attention for any reason, he or she must raise a hand to notify the proctor.

THE COMPUTER

You do not need any computer experience to take a CAT NCLEX-RN examination. Only two computer keys are needed to take the CAT examination: the space bar and the enter key. The space bar key enables you to scroll the options, and the enter key enables you to highlight and select an answer. The enter key must be struck twice in order to record the answer choice and to proceed to the next question. A key board tutorial is provided and administered to all test takers before the start of the examination. In addition, a proctor is present to assist in explaining the use of the computer to ensure your full understanding of how to proceed.

CAT NCLEX-RN TEST QUESTIONS

The examination is composed of individual or "stand alone" test questions. This means that there is no case situation accompanying the question. With this type of question, the candidate can expect the question to appear on the left side of the screen with the four responses on the right side of the screen, or the question appears across the top of the screen and the four responses below.

You must answer the test question presented on the computer screen; otherwise, the test will not move on. This means that you will not be able to skip questions, go back and review questions, or go back and change answers. Students preparing for CAT NCLEX-RN become anxious and frustrated because questions cannot be skipped and returned to at a later time during the examination process. Remember that in a CAT examination, once an answer is recorded, all subsequent answers administered depend to an extent on the response selected for that question. Skipping and returning to earlier questions is not compatible with the logical method of a CAT. In addition, it is important to recall the number of times you may have changed a correct answer to an incorrect one on a pencil and paper nursing examination during your nursing education. The inability to skip questions or go back to change previous answers is not a disadvantage; it actually prevents you from falling into that trap of changing a correct answer to an incorrect one with CAT. There is no penalty for guessing on CAT NCLEX-RN. Remember that the answer to the question will be right there in front of you. If you need to guess, use your nursing knowledge to its fullest extent and all of the test-taking strategies provided to you in Chapter 4 of this book.

BOX 1–8. Appearance of an Individual Test Item on the Computer Screen

The most appropriate method for feeding the infant with cleft lip or palate is

1. With the head in an upright position.
2. With the infant in a lying position.
3. With the infant in a side-lying position.
4. With the infant prone.

The client is admitted with a diagnosis of myasthenia gravis. Pyridostigmine (Mestinon) is prescribed for the client. An adverse effect of this medication is

1. Muscle cramps.
2. Mouth ulcers.
3. Depression.
4. Unexplained weight gain.

TESTING TIME

The maximum testing time will be 5 hours, including the short keyboard tutorial and any rest breaks. There is no minimum amount of examination time. A mandatory 10-minute break will be taken after 2 testing hours, and an optional 10-minute break can be taken after 3 1/2 hours of testing. The computer screen will notify you of the time for these breaks. You must leave the testing room during breaks. You may leave the room for additional, unscheduled breaks, but no additional testing time will be allowed.

THE LENGTH OF THE EXAMINATION

The minimum number of questions that you may need to answer in order to meet adequate testing in each area of the test plan is 75. Sixty of these questions will be real (scored) questions and 15 of these questions will be try-out (unscored) questions. The maximum number of questions you may need to answer will be 265. Again, of these 265 questions, 15 of these questions will be try-out (unscored) questions. The try-out questions are not identified as such. In other words, you do not know which questions are the unscored questions.

COMPLETING THE EXAMINATION

Once the test is completed, you will complete a brief computer-delivered questionnaire about your testing experience. After this questionnaire is completed, the test proctor will collect all scratch paper, sign you out, and permit you to leave.

PROCESSING RESULTS

Upon completion of the examination, results are transmitted electronically to the data center at the

Testing Service. The candidate's results are transmitted to the board of nursing in the U. S. state, district, or territory in which the candidate applied for licensure. A paper copy of the results is mailed to the board of nursing within 48 hours after the examination is completed. The board of nursing will mail the results to the candidate. The candidate should not telephone the Testing Center, the National Council, or the State Board of Nursing for results. The results will not be given to the candidate over the telephone.

INTERSTATE ENDORSEMENT

Because the CAT NCLEX-RN is a national examination, the candidate can apply to take the examination in any state. Once licensure is received, the registered nurse can apply for Interstate Endorsement. The procedures and requirements for Interstate Endorsement may vary from state to state, and these procedures can be obtained from the State Board of Nursing in the state in which endorsement is sought.

STATE BOARDS OF NURSING

Alabama Board of Nursing
P.O. Box 303900
Montgomery, AL 36130-3900
Telephone: (205) 242-4060

Alaska Board of Nursing
3601 C Street, Suite 722
Anchorage, AK 99503
Telephone: (907) 561-2878

American Samoa Health Services Regulatory Board
LBJ Tropical Medical Center
Pago Pago, American Samoa 96799
Telephone: (684) 633-1222

Arizona State Board of Nursing
1651 E. Morton, Suite 150
Phoenix, AZ 85020
Telephone: (602) 255-5092

Arkansas State Board of Nursing
1123 South University, Suite 800
Little Rock, AR 72204
Telephone: (501) 686-2700

California Board of Registered Nursing
P.O. Box 944210
Sacramento, CA 94244-2100
Telephone: (213) 897-3590

Colorado State Board of Nursing
1560 Broadway, Suite 670
Denver, CO 82002
Telephone: (303) 894-2435

Connecticut Department of Public Health
Division of Medical Quality Assurance
P.O. Box 260490
Hartford, CT 06126-0490
Telephone: (860) 509-7603

Delaware Board of Nursing
Cannon Building, P.O. Box 1401
Dover, DE 19901
Telephone: (302) 739-4522

District of Columbia Board of Nursing
614 H Street, N.W.
Washington, DC 20013
Telephone: (202) 727-7856

Florida State Board of Nursing
111 E. Coastline Drive
Jacksonville, FL 32202
Telephone: (904) 798-4858

Georgia Board of Nursing
166 Pryor Street, S.W.
Atlanta, GA 30334
Telephone: (404) 656-3943

Guam Board of Nurse Examiners
P.O. Box 2816
Agana, Guam 96910
Telephone: (671) 734-7295

Hawaii Board of Nursing
Box 3469
Honolulu, HI 99503
Telephone: (808) 586-2695

Idaho State Board of Nursing
P.O. Box 83720
Boise, ID 83720-0061
Telephone: (208) 334-3110

Illinois Department of Professional Regulations
320 W. Washington Street
Springfield, IL 62786
Telephone: (217) 785-9465

Indiana State Board of Nursing
402 W. Washington Street
Indianapolis, IN 46204
Telephone: (317) 233-4405

Iowa Board of Nursing
1223 E. Court Avenue
Des Moines, IA 50319
Telephone: (515) 281-4828

Kansas State Board of Nursing
900 S.W. Jackson Street, Suite 551S
Topeka, KS 66612-1256
Telephone: (913) 296-3782

Kentucky Board of Nursing
312 Whittington Parkway, Suite 300
Louisville, KY 40222-5172
Telephone: (502) 329-7000

Louisiana State Board of Nursing
150 Baronne Street, Suite 912
New Orleans, LA 70112
Telephone: (504) 568-5464

Maine State Board of Nursing
35 Anthony Avenue
State House Station 158

Augusta, ME 04333-0158
Telephone: (207) 264-5275

Maryland Board of Nursing
4140 Patterson Avenue
Baltimore, MD 21215-2254
Telephone: (301) 764-5124

Massachusetts Board of Registration in Nursing
100 Cambridge Street, Room 150
Boston, MA 02202
Telephone: (617) 727-3060

Michigan Board of Nursing
P.O. Box 30018
611 West Ottawa
Lansing, MI 48909
Telephone: (517) 373-1600

Minnesota Board of Nursing
2700 University Avenue, W. 108
St. Paul, MN 55114
Telephone: (612) 643-2565

Mississippi Institution of Higher Learning
3825 Ridgewood Road
Jackson, MS 39211
Telephone: (601) 982-6448

Missouri State Board of Nursing
3605 Missouri Boulevard
Jefferson City, MO 65102
Telephone: (314) 751-0080

Montana State Board of Nursing
Arcade Building—111 Jackson
Helena, MT 59620-0513
Telephone: (406) 444-2071

Nebraska Bureau of Examining Board
P.O. Box 95007
Lincoln, NE 68509
Telephone: (402) 471-2115

Nevada State Board of Nursing
4335 S. Industrial Road, #430
Las Vegas, NV 89103
Telephone: (702) 739-1575

New Hampshire State Board of Nursing
Division of Public Health
6 Hazen Drive
Concord, NH 03301
Telephone: (603) 271-2323

New Jersey Board of Nursing
P.O. Box 45010
Newark, NJ 07101
Telephone: (201) 504-6493

New Mexico Board of Nursing
4206 Louisiana, N.E., Suite A
Albuquerque, NM 87109
Telephone: (505) 841-8340

New York State Board of Nursing
The Cultural Center, Room 3023
Albany, NY 12230
Telephone: (518) 486-2967

North Carolina Board of Nursing
P.O. Box 2129
Raleigh, NC 27602
Telephone: (919) 782-3211

North Dakota Board of Nursing
919 S. 7th Street, Suite 504
Bismarck, ND 58504-5881
Telephone: (701) 224-2974

Ohio Board of Nursing
77 S. High Street, 17th Floor
Columbus, OH 43266-0316
Telephone: (614) 466-9800

Oklahoma Board of Nursing
2915 N. Classen Boulevard, Suite 524
Oklahoma City, OK 73106
Telephone: (405) 525-2076

Oregon State Board of Nursing
800 N.E. Oregon Street, #25
Portland, OR 97232
Telephone: (503) 731-4745

Pennsylvania State Board of Nursing
P.O. Box 2649
Harrisburg, PA 17105
Telephone: (717) 783-7142

Counsel of Higher Education of Puerto Rico
P.O. Box 23305, UPR Station
Rio Piedras, PR 00931-3305
Telephone: (809) 758-3350, extension 2305

Rhode Island Board of Nursing Education and Nurse Registration
3 Capital Hill
Providence, RI 02908-5097
Telephone: (401) 277-2827

State Board of Nursing for South Carolina
220 Executive Center Drive, Suite 220
Columbia, SC 29210
Telephone: (803) 731-1648

South Dakota Board of Nursing
3307 South Lincoln
Sioux Falls, SD 57105
Telephone: (605) 335-4973

Tennessee Board of Nursing
283 Plus Park Boulevard
Nashville, TN 37217
Telephone: (615) 367-6232

Texas Board of Nurse Examiners
9101 Burnett Road, Suite 105
Austin, TX 78752
Telephone: (512) 835-8660

Utah State Board of Nursing
160 E. 300 South, Box 45805
Salt Lake City, UT 84145
Telephone: (801) 530-6736

Vermont Board of Nursing
Licensing and Registration Division
109 State Street
Montpelier, VT 05602
Telephone: (802) 828-2396

Virgin Islands Board of Nursing Licensure
P.O. Box 4247
Charlotte Amalie, VI 00803
Telephone: (809) 776-7397

Virginia State Board of Nursing
6606 W. Broad Street, 4th Floor
Richmond, VA 23230-1717
Telephone: (804) 662-9909

Washington State Nursing Care
Quality Assurance Commission
1300 Quincy, Box 47864
Olympia, WA 98504-7864
Telephone: (206) 753-3726

West Virginia Board of Examiners for Registered Nurses
101 Dee Drive
Charleston, WV 25311-1620
Telephone: (304) 558-3596

Wisconsin Department of Regulation & Licensing
P.O. Box 8935
Madison, WI 53708-8935
Telephone: (608) 267-2357

State of Wyoming Board of Nursing
2301 Central Avenue, Barret Building
Cheyenne, WY 82002
Telephone: (307) 777-7601

REFERENCES

Black, J., & Matassarin-Jacobs, E. (1997). *Medical-surgical nursing: Clinical management for continuity of care* (5th ed.). Philadelphia: W.B. Saunders.

Carson, V., & Arnold, E. (1996). *Mental health nursing: The nurse-patient journey.* Philadelphia: W.B. Saunders.

Gorrie, T. M., McKinney, E. S., & Murray, S. S. (1994). *Foundations of maternal-newborn nursing.* Philadelphia: W.B. Saunders.

Ignatavicius, D., Workman, M., & Mishler, M. (1995). *Medical-surgical nursing: A nursing process approach* (2nd ed.). Philadelphia: W.B. Saunders.

Lammon, C. B., Foote, A. W., Leli, P. G., et al. (1995). *Clinical nursing skills.* Philadelphia: W.B. Saunders.

Luckmann, J. (1997). *Saunders manual of nursing care.* Philadelphia: W.B. Saunders.

Matteson, M. A., McConnell, E. S., & Linton, A. D. (1997). *Gerontological nursing concepts and practice* (2nd ed.). Philadelphia: W.B. Saunders.

National Council of State Boards of Nursing. (1997). *Test plan for the National Council licensure examination for registered nurses.* Chicago: Author.

National Council of State Boards of Nursing. (1995). *The NCLEX process.* Chicago: Author.

National League for Nursing. (1995). *State-Approved Schools of Nursing RN.* New York: Author.

Nichols, F. H., & Zwelling, E. (1997). *Maternal-newborn nursing: Theory and practice.* Philadelphia: W.B. Saunders.

CHAPTER 2

Profiles of Success

Laurent W. Valliere, B.S.

Preparing to take the National Council Licensure Examination for Registered Nurses (NCLEX-RN) can produce a great deal of anxiety in the nursing graduate. You may be thinking that NCLEX-RN is the most important examination that you will ever have to take and that it reflects the culmination of everything that you have worked so hard for. NCLEX-RN is an important examination because receiving that nursing license means that you can begin your career as a Registered Nurse. Your success on NCLEX-RN involves avoiding thoughts that allow this examination to seem overwhelming and intimidating. Such thoughts will take full control over your destiny.

Nursing graduates preparing for NCLEX-RN have difficulty in developing a plan to prepare for this examination. The most important component in developing a plan is to identify your profile that has guided you to your achievements and successes in your nursing education. It is important to begin your venture by reflecting on all the challenges that you experienced during your nursing education. Take time to focus on the thoughts, feelings, and emotions that you experienced before taking an examination while in your nursing program. Scrutinize the very important methods that you used in preparing for that examination both academically and from the standpoint of how you dealt with the anxiety that parallels the experience of facing an examination.

These factors are very important considerations in preparing for NCLEX-RN. These factors are so important because they worked. Think about this for a moment. Your own methods must have worked, or you would not be at the point of preparing for NCLEX-RN.

Every individual requires his or her own methods of preparing for an examination. Graduate nurses who have taken NCLEX-RN will probably share their experiences and methods of preparing for this challenge with you. It is very helpful to listen to what they may tell you. These graduates will provide you with important strategies that they used. Listen to them and hear what they have to say, but remember that this examination is all about you. Your identity and what you require in terms of preparation are most important. Reflect on the methods and strategies that worked for you throughout your nursing program. Do not think that you need to develop new methods and strategies in preparing for NCLEX-RN. Take some time to reflect on these strategies, write them down on a large blank card, sign your name, and write "R.N." after your name. Post this card is a place where you will see it every morning of every day. Commit to your own special strategies. These strategies reflect your profile and identity and will lead you to success!

A frequent concern of graduates preparing for NCLEX-RN relates to deciding whether they should study alone or become a part of a study group. Examining your profile will easily direct you with making this decision. Again, reflect on what has worked for you throughout your nursing program as you prepared for examinations. Remember, your needs are most important. Address your own needs and do not become pressured by peers who are encouraging you to join a study group, if this is not your normal pattern for study. Remember that additional pressure is not what you need at this important time in your life.

Nursing graduates preparing for NCLEX-RN frequently inquire about the best method of preparing for NCLEX-RN. First, remember that you are prepared. In fact, you began preparing for this examination on the first day that you entered your nursing program. The task that you are faced with is to review, in a comprehensive manner, all of the nursing content that you learned in your nursing program. It can become terribly overwhelming to look at your bookshelf, which is overflowing with the nursing books that you used during nursing school, and your challenge becomes monumental when you look at the boxes of nursing lecture notes that you have accumulated. It is unrealistic to even think that you could read all of those nursing books and lecture notes in preparation for NCLEX-RN. These books and lecture notes should be used as a reference source, if needed, during your preparation for NCLEX-RN. *Saunders Comprehensive Review for NCLEX-RN* has identified for you all of the important nursing content areas relevant to the examination. During your review through the comprehensive review, you should have noted the areas that may be unfamiliar or unclear. Be sure that you have taken the time to become familiar with these needed areas. Now progress through the Pyramid to Success and test your knowledge in this book, *Saunders Question & Answer Review for NCLEX-RN.* You may identify nursing content areas that still require further review. Take the time to review, as you are guided to do in this book.

Your profile of success requires that you develop realistic time goals to prepare for NCLEX-RN. It is necessary that you take time to examine your life and all the commitments that you may have. These commitments may include family, work, and friends. As you develop your goals, remember to plan time for fun and exercise. To achieve success, you require a balance of both work time and leisure time. If you do not plan for some leisure time, you will become frustrated and perhaps even angry. These sorts of feelings will block your ability to focus and concentrate. Remember that you need time for yourself.

Goal development may be a relatively easy process because you have probably been juggling your life commitments ever since you entered nursing school. Remember that your goal is to identify a daily time frame and time period for you to use in reviewing and preparing for NCLEX-RN. Open your calendar and identify days on which life commitments will not allow you to spend this time preparing. Block those days off and do not consider them as a part of your review time. Review your normal day. Identify the time that is best for you in terms of your ability to concentrate and focus, so that you can accomplish the most in your identified time frame. Be sure that you consider a time that is quiet and free of distractions. Many people find that the morning hours provide the most productive hours, whereas others may find the afternoon and evening hours most productive. Remember that this examination is all about you, and select the time period that will be most conducive to your success.

The place of study is also very important. Select a place that is quiet and comfortable for study and a place where you normally do your studying and preparing. Some people prefer to study at home in their own environment; if this is your normal pattern, be sure that you are able to free yourself of distractions during your scheduled preparation time. If you are not able to free yourself of distractions, you may consider spending your preparation time at a library. Reflect on what worked best for you during your nursing program in selecting your place of study.

Selecting the amount of daily preparation time has frequently been a dilemma for many graduates preparing for NCLEX-RN. It is very important to set a realistic time period that can be adhered to on a daily basis. Set a time frame that will provide you with quality time and a time frame that can be achieved. If you set a time frame that is not realistic and cannot be achieved every day, you will become frustrated. This frustration will block your journey toward the peak of the Pyramid to Success. The best suggestion to you is to spend at least 2 hours daily for NCLEX-RN preparation. Two hours is a realistic time period both in terms of quality time and a time frame that is achievable. You may find that after 2 hours your ability to focus and concentrate will diminish. You may, however, find that on some days you are able to spend more than the scheduled 2 hours; if you can and feel as though your ability to concentrate and focus is still present, then do so.

Discipline and perseverance will automatically bring control. Control will provide you with the momentum that will sweep you to the peak in the Pyramid to Success. Discipline yourself to spend time preparing for NCLEX-RN every day. Daily preparation is very important because it maintains a consistent pattern and keeps you in synchrony with the mind flow needed the day you are scheduled to take the NCLEX-RN examination. Some days you may think about skipping your scheduled preparation time because you are not in the mood for study or because you just don't feel like studying. On these days, practice discipline and persevere. Stand yourself up, shake off those thoughts of skipping a day of preparation, take a deep breath, and get the oxygen flowing throughout your body. Look in the mirror, smile, and say to yourself "This time is for me and I can do this!" Look at your card that displays your name with "R.N." after it, and get yourself to that special study place. Remember that discipline and perseverance will bring control!

In the profile of success, academic preparation directs the path to the peak of the Pyramid to Success. There are however, additional factors that will influence successful achievement of the peak. These factors include your ability to control anxiety, your physical stamina, the amount of rest and relaxation you have, your self-confidence, and the belief in yourself that you will achieve success on NCLEX-RN. You need to take time to think about these important factors and incorporate these factors into your daily preparation schedule. Anxiety is a common concern among students preparing to take NCLEX-RN. Some anxiety is a normal feeling and will keep your senses sharp and alert. A great deal of anxiety, however, can block your process of thinking and hamper your ability to focus and concentrate. You have already practiced the task of controlling anxiety when you took examinations in nursing school. Now you need to continue with this practice and incorporate this control on a daily basis. Each day, before beginning your scheduled preparation time, sit in your quiet special study place, close your eyes and take a slow deep breath. Fill your body with oxygen, hold your breath to a count of four, then exhale slowly through your mouth. Continue with this exercise and repeat it four to six times. This exercise will relieve your mind of any unnecessary chatter and will deliver oxygen to all of your body tissues and to your brain. On your scheduled day of NCLEX-RN, after the necessary pretesting procedures, you will be escorted to your test computer. Practice this breathing exercise before beginning the examination. Use this exercise during the examination if you feel yourself becoming anxious and distracted and if you are having difficulty focusing and concentrating. Remember that breathing will move that oxygen to your brain!

Physical stamina is a necessary component of readiness for NCLEX-RN. Plan to incorporate a balance of exercise with adequate rest and relaxation time in your preparation schedule. It is important that you maintain healthy eating habits. Begin to practice these healthy habits now, if you haven't already done so. There are a few points to keep in mind each day as you plan your daily meals. Three balanced meals are important, with snacks, such as fruits, included between meals. Remember that food items that contain fat will slow you down and food items that contain caffeine will cause nervousness and sometimes shakiness. These items need to be avoided. Foods high in carbohydrates work best to supply you with your energy needs. Remember that your brain can work like a muscle. It requires those carbohydrates. In addition, don't forget to include your needed fruits and vegetables.

If you are the type of person who is not a breakfast eater, work on changing that habit. Practice the habit of eating breakfast now, as you are preparing for NCLEX-RN. Attempt to provide your brain with energy in the morning with some form of carbohydrate food. It will make a difference. On your scheduled day for NCLEX-RN, feed your brain and eat a healthy breakfast. In addition, on this very important day, bring some form of snack such as fruit or a bagel for break time, and feed your brain again so that you will have the energy to concentrate, focus, and complete your examination.

Adequate rest, relaxation, and exercise are important in your preparation process. Many graduates preparing for NCLEX-RN have difficulty sleeping, particularly the night before the examination. Begin now to develop methods that will assist in relaxing your body and mind and allow you to obtain a restful sleep. You may already have a particular method developed to help you sleep. If not, it may be helpful to try the breathing exercise while you lie in bed to assist in eliminating any mind chatter that is present. It is also helpful to visualize your favorite and most peaceful place while you do these breathing exercises. Graduates have also stated that listening to quiet music and relaxation tapes have helped them relax and sleep. Begin to practice some of these helpful methods now, while you are preparing for NCLEX-RN. Identify those that work best for you. The night before your scheduled examination is an important one. Spend time having some fun, get to bed early, and incorporate the relaxation method that you have been using to help you sleep.

Confidence and belief that you have the ability to achieve success will bring your goals to fruition. Reflect on your profile maintained during your nursing education. Your confidence and belief in yourself, along with your academic achievements, have brought you to the status of graduate nurse. Now you are facing one more important challenge. Can you meet this challenge successfully? Yes, you can! There is no reason to think otherwise, if you have taken all of the necessary steps to ensure that profile of success. Each morning, place your feet on the floor, stand tall, take a deep breath, and smile. Take both hands and imagine yourself brushing off any negative feelings. Look at your card that bears your name with the letters "R.N." after it, and tell yourself, "Yes, I can do this successfully!"

Believe in yourself, and you will reach the peak of the Pyramid to Success!

Congratulations, and I wish you continued success in your career as a Registered Nurse!

CHAPTER 3

The NCLEX-RN Examination: From a Student's Perspective

Lori Horton, R.N.

Taking the NCLEX-RN is the first major step in a nursing graduate's life. I am writing to share with you my experience in preparing for and passing the NCLEX-RN examination. Beginning with my first nursing class, I heard about NCLEX-RN. My nursing professors would consistently remind my classmates and me that in order to transform from graduate nurse to Registered Nurse, we must pass what I called the "dreaded" NCLEX-RN examination. One of the most important factors contributing to my passing the NCLEX-RN was the knowledge that I acquired in nursing school. As simple and routine as that may sound, it is very true.

Other factors that contributed to my success were developing goals and good study habits and maintaining a positive attitude. Always think positive about yourself and about your ability to be successful! Think of this examination as another component to your nursing career and as a positive experience. Your experiences in life can be seen as stepping stones or stumbling blocks, and only you are responsible for how you see them.

Knowing that you have established goals and good study habits helps to build your self-confidence. The more self-confident you are about your goals and about how you have planned your study regimen, the more at ease you will be on the day of the examination.

It is very important to establish a study pattern that will work for you. I found it is best to study for short periods of time each day, never overextending on any given day. If you believe in the goals you have set for yourself, you will achieve them. I believe that a positive attitude is a key to success.

Practice is a major part of taking the NCLEX-RN examination. Practicing questions helped me prepare for the test. The more questions that you practice, the more skilled and confident you will become with regard to the ability to test.

Finally, the day arrives that you have been waiting for. Here are some tips that I found helpful. Be sure that you know how to get to the testing center and what the parking arrangements are. If necessary, take the time to drive to the examination site before your scheduled date so you know exactly where the testing center is located and how long travel time will be. Allow yourself ample time to get to the testing center, because rushing will only add extra stress and disrupt your frame of mind. Get a good night's sleep before the examination. Eat a well-balanced breakfast: avoid fats, and eat complex carbohydrates.

What was the test really like? The day of and the day before the examination, I felt overwhelmed. I thought to myself, "By this point you either know it or you don't." I knew that last-minute cramming was not going to help. I found that the hardest part of this examination was that most of the questions were applying nursing knowledge. The answers were not from memorization, although you must have the nursing knowledge to answer the question accurately. If there are questions that you are not sure of, do not panic. Read the question again, read and think through all of the options given, use test-taking strategies, and select the one that makes the most sense. Remember that the answer is right in front of you. Even though I knew some of the answers immediately, I read through all the options to make sure I was choosing the correct answer. The important thing is not to rush. You owe it to yourself to do your absolute best; after all, becoming a Registered Nurse is your primary goal.

During the test, you may feel frustrated, but try to be patient. I found that taking a deep breath after every few questions helped. The first few questions were the most stressful, not because they were difficult, but because I couldn't believe I was actually to this point of taking my state boards.

I must be honest and tell you that this test is by no means easy. The questions require that you think critically about the information presented in them. When the computer came to question number 75 and shut off, I had a feeling that I had done well. The test had taken me 2 hours to complete, and I thought that no matter what the results were, I knew I had given it my best.

Life after the examination was a waiting game. Every day I would check the mail to see if my results were there. My envelope took 14 days to arrive, and when it finally came, I tore it open, and without reading anything else, I saw the word "PASSED" in big, bold capital letters. It was a great feeling!

Maintain that belief that you will pass the examination and stay positive throughout your review process. Be proud of yourself. The road was long and difficult, but you are now a graduate nurse preparing for NCLEX-RN. This is a great achievement!

Becoming a Registered Nurse is one of the most rewarding accomplishments that I have achieved, thus far, in my life. It is a career that will bring a lifetime of happiness.

Life as a new registered nurse has been very rewarding. I find that I never stop learning. Every day is full of new experiences, and something new is learned. You will surprise yourself with how much you really do know and are able to apply to clinical situations. So, my best advice is to believe in yourself and the rewards will follow!

Best of luck to all future RNs!

CHAPTER 4

Test-Taking Strategies

THE PYRAMID TO SUCCESS

BOX 4–1. The Pyramid to Success

Read the questions and options thoroughly and carefully!
Ask yourself, "What is the question really asking me?"
Be alert to key words and to true and false stems!
Eliminate the incorrect options!
Use all of your nursing knowledge, your clinical experiences, and your test-taking skills to answer the question!

THE COMPONENTS OF THE QUESTION

A. Strategy 1
   1. Identify the components of the question.
   2. Distinguish the "case situation" from the "stem."
   3. Read all of the options carefully and thoroughly.
B. The Case Situation
   1. The case situation gives you the information about a clinical health problem and the information you need to consider in answering the question.
   2. It is extremely important to read all of the information and every word in the case situation.
C. The Stem
   1. The stem usually comes after the case situation and asks you something about it.
   2. The stem asks you to solve a problem and select an answer.
   3. Read the stem very carefully, and specifically identify exactly what the question is asking.
D. The Options
   1. The options are all of the answers, and you must select one.
   2. Read all of the options very carefully, and then reread the stem of the question before selecting the answer.
   3. Use the process of elimination to eliminate the incorrect options.
   4. Once you have eliminated the obviously incorrect options, reread the stem again and identify specifically what the question is asking before making your final choice.

THE CRITICAL ELEMENTS OF THE QUESTION

A. Strategy 2
   1. Identify the critical elements of the case situation and the stem of the question.
   2. The critical elements are the key words or phrases in the case situation and the stem of the question.
B. Key Words or Phrases
   1. The key words or phrases focus your attention on critical ideas in the case, stem, and options.
   2. Key words or phrases that you should look for and focus your attention on include the following:
      a. "Early" or "Late"
      b. "Immediately"
      c. "Most likely" or "Least likely"
      d. "Initial"
      e. "First"
      f. "Best"
      g. "Most appropriate"
      h. "On the day of"
      i. "After several days"
   3. The key words will influence your selection of an answer.

THE CLIENT OF THE QUESTION

A. Strategy 3
   1. Identify the client of the question.
   2. The client is the person who is the focus of the question.

BOX 4–2. Key Words in the Question

- ▲ Which of the following is an *early* sign of shock?
- ▲ Which of the following is a *late sign* of shock?
- ▲ *On the day of* surgery, after a transurethral resection of the prostrate (TURP), the nurse notes that the client's urine is bright red. Which of the following nursing actions is appropriate?
- ▲ *After several days,* after a transurethral resection of the prostrate (TURP), the nurse notes that the client's urine is bright red. Which of the following nursing actions is appropriate?

Noting the key words or phrases in each of these situations will assist in directing you to select the correct option.

- ▲ The *early* signs of shock are quite different from the *late* signs of shock!
- ▲ Bright red urine might be expected *on the day of* surgery after a transurethral resection of the prostrate (TURP) but would not be expected *after several days*!

B. The Client
1. It is important to remember that the client of the question may not necessarily be the person with the health problem.
2. In the test question, the client may be a relative, a friend, a spouse, a significant other, or even another nurse.
3. Identify the client of the question and select an answer that relates to and most directly addresses that client.

THE ISSUE OF THE QUESTION

A. Strategy 4
1. Identify the issue of the question.
2. The issue of the question is the specific subject content that the question is asking about.

B. The Issue
1. Identifying the issue of the question will assist in eliminating the incorrect options and direct you to select the correct response.
2. The issue of the question can include
   a. A drug.
   b. A side effect or toxic effect of a drug.
   c. A procedure.
   d. A complication.
   e. A specific nursing action.

THE TYPE OF STEM IN THE QUESTION

A. Strategy 5
1. Identify the type of stem in the question.
2. The stem can be either a true response stem or a false response stem.

B. True Response Stem
1. True response stems contain key words that prompt you to select an answer that is true with regard to the situation and the question.
2. True response stems may contain the following key words or phrases:
   a. "Most"
   b. "Best"
   c. "Best judgment"
   d. "Initial"
   e. "First"
   f. "Chief"
   g. "Immediate"

C. False Response Stem
1. False response stems contain key words that ask you to select an answer that is *not* true with regard to the situation and question.
2. False response stems may contain the following key words or phrases:
   a. "Except"
   b. "Least likely"
   c. "Need for further education"
   d. "Lowest priority"
   e. "Incorrect"
   f. "Unsafe"

ELIMINATING THE INCORRECT OPTIONS

A. Strategy 6
1. Use the process of elimination and eliminate the incorrect options before selecting an answer.
2. Be alert to the key words or phrases and to the true and the false response stems.

B. Distracters
1. Distracters are options that resemble correct answers but, in fact, are not.
2. They are intended to distract you from the correct answers.
3. Each test item contains three distracters and one correct answer.
4. Use the process of elimination to eliminate the incorrect options.
5. Be alert to the key words and to the true and the false response stems.
6. Once you have eliminated the obviously incorrect options, reread the stem again and identify specifically what the question is asking before making your final choice.

QUESTIONS THAT REQUIRE PRIORITIZING

A. Strategy 7
1. Identify the key words in the question that indicate the need for you to prioritize.
2. Key words include the following:
   a. "Initial"
   b. "Essential"
   c. "Vital"
   d. "Immediate"

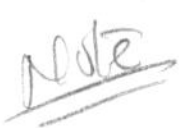

e. "Highest"
f. "Best"
g. "Most"

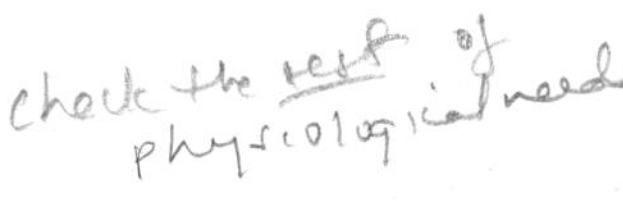

B. Strategy 8
1. Utilize Maslow's "Hierarchy of Needs" theory to prioritize.
2. Physiological needs come *first,* so select an answer that addresses physiological needs.
3. When a physiological need is not addressed in the question, safety needs receive priority, and in this situation, select an answer that addresses safety.

C. Strategy 9
1. Keep in mind the ABCs (airway, breathing, and circulation) when selecting an answer.
2. Remember the order of priority: airway, breathing, and circulation!

D. Strategy 10
1. Use the Nursing Process to prioritize.
2. Remember that assessment is the first step in the Nursing Process.
3. When you are asked to select your first and initial nursing action, use and follow the steps of the Nursing Process to select your response.
4. If an answer contains the concept of assessment or collection of client data, select that answer.

THE NURSING PROCESS (TABLE 4–1)

A. Assessment
1. Assessment questions address the process of gathering subjective and objective data relative to the client, confirming, communicating, and documenting the data.
2. Remember that assessment is the first step in the nursing process.
3. When you are asked a question regarding your initial or first nursing action, select the option that addresses an assessment action.
4. If an assessment action is not one of the options, follow the steps of the nursing process as your guide to select your initial or first action.
5. When answering questions that focus on assessment, look for key words in the options that reflect assessment.

Table 4–1. **Steps of the Nursing Process**

1. Assessment
2. Analysis
3. Planning
4. Implementation
5. Evaluation

Use the nursing process to answer questions!
Follow the steps of the nursing process to select an answer.
The first step of the nursing process is assessment.
When the question asks you what the nurse's initial or most appropriate action is, select the answer that relates to assessment of the client!

6. The following key words or phrases reflect assessment:
   a. "Observe"
   b. "Monitor"
   c. "Check"
   d. "Obtain information"
   e. "Find out"
   f. "Determine"
   g. "Assess"
   h. "Ascertain"

B. Analysis
1. Analysis questions are the most difficult questions because they require an understanding of the principles of physiological responses.
2. Analysis questions require interpretation of the data on the basis of assessment.
3. Analysis questions address formulation of nursing diagnoses and the communication and documentation of the results of the process of analysis.
4. These questions require critical thinking and determining the rationale for therapeutic interventions related to the specific issue addressed in the question.
5. Avoid reading into the question; focus on the data presented in the question.

C. Planning
1. Planning questions require prioritizing nursing diagnoses, determining goals and outcome criteria for goals of care, developing the plan of care, and communicating and documenting the plan of care.
2. Remember that this is a nursing examination and the answer to the question involves something that is included in the nursing care plan rather than in the medical plan.

D. Implementation
1. This examination is about *nursing,* so focus on the nursing action rather than on the medical action, unless the question is asking you what prescribed action is anticipated.
2. Implementation questions address the process of organizing and managing care, counseling and teaching, providing care to achieve established goals, supervising and coordinating care, and communicating and documenting nursing interventions.
3. On NCLEX-RN, the only client that you need to be concerned about is the client in the question that you are answering.
4. When you are answering a question, remember that this client is your only assigned client.
5. Answer the question as if the situation were textbook and ideal and the nurse had all the time and resources needed and readily available at the client's bedside.

E. Evaluation
1. Evaluation questions focus on comparing the actual outcomes of care with the expected outcomes.
2. These questions address evaluation of the client's ability to implement self-care, evaluation of health care team members' ability to imple-

BOX 4–3. Communication Tools and Blocks

Tools	Blocks
Being silent	Giving advice
Offering self to assist client	Showing approval/ disapproval of client's decisions
Showing empathy	Using cliché and false reassurance
Focusing	Requesting an explanation "Why?"
Restatement	
Validation/ clarification	Devaluing the client's feelings
	Being defensive
Giving information	Focusing on inappropriate issues
Dealing with the here and now	Placing the client's issues on hold

Always focus on the client's feelings FIRST!

If an answer reflects the client's feelings, select that answer!

ment care, and the process of communicating and documenting evaluation findings.

3. These questions focus on how the nurse should monitor or make a judgment concerning a client's response to therapy or to a nursing action.
4. In an evaluation question, be alert to false response stems, inasmuch as they are frequently used in evaluation-type questions.
5. The question may ask for the client's statement that indicates *inaccurate* information regarding the issue in the question.

CLIENT NEEDS

A. Safe, Effective Care Environment
   1. These questions address the provision that the nurse meet client needs for a safe and effective care environment by providing and directing nursing care that promotes achievement of coordinated care, environmental safety, and safe and effective treatments and procedures.
   2. Be alert to safety needs addressed in a question!
   3. Remember the importance of handwashing, side rails, and call bells!

B. Physiological Integrity
   1. These questions address the provision that the nurse meet the physiological integrity needs of clients with acute and chronic conditions and of clients at risk for the development of complications from treatments or management modalities.
   2. The nurse provides and directs care to promote physiological adaptation, reduction of risk potential, and provision of basic care.
   3. Be careful not to read into the question; focus on the data presented in the question.
   4. These questions require you to think critically and determine the rationale for the correct response.
   5. Remember that physiological needs are a priority and are addressed first!
   6. Remember to utilize the ABCs—airway, breathing, and circulation—when selecting an answer addressing physiological integrity.
   7. Remember the order of priority: airway, breathing, and circulation!

C. Psychosocial Integrity
   1. These questions address the provision that the nurse meet the psychosocial needs of the client in stress- and crisis-related situations throughout the life span by promoting psychosocial adaptation and coping and promoting adaptation abilities in the client.

BOX 4–4. Pyramid Points

- ▲ If the question asks for an immediate action or response, all answers may be correct; therefore, base your selection on priorities.
- ▲ Reword a difficult question, but if you do so, be careful not to change the intent of the question.
- ▲ Look for the most common or typical response.
- ▲ Relate the situation to something that is familiar to you and try to visualize the client as you go through the case situation and the question.
- ▲ Look for answers that focus on the client as a worthy human being or are directed toward feelings.
- ▲ With medication calculations, talk yourself through each step and be sure the answer makes sense.
- ▲ If there are words in the stem that are unfamiliar, try to figure out the meaning in terms of the context of the sentence, or break down the words by using your medical terminology skills.
- ▲ If one option includes qualifiers such as "generally," "usually," and "tends to" and other options do not, select that option.
- ▲ Absolute terminology such as "always," "never," "all," "every," "none," and "must" tends to render a statement false.
- ▲ Unusual or highly technical language typically indicates that the option is not correct.
- ▲ Remember that lengthy questions are not always the most difficult.
- ▲ Answer all questions as if the situation were ideal and the nurse had all the time and resources needed.
- ▲ Remember, the only client you need to be concerned about is the one in the question you are answering.
- ▲ Pace yourself, and concentrate and focus on one item at a time.
- ▲ Do not become frustrated!
- ▲ Be patient with yourself!

  Optimism!
  Belief!
  Confidence!
  Control!
  Success!

2. Communication Questions
   a. Identify the use of therapeutic communication tools.
   b. When answering communication questions, use of communication tools indicates a *correct* answer.
   c. When answering communication questions, use of communication blocks indicates an *incorrect* answer.

D. Health Promotion and Maintenance
   1. These questions address the provision that the nurse meet client needs for health promotion and maintenance throughout the life span by providing and directing care to clients and significant others.
   2. Nursing care involves promoting growth and development throughout the life span, promoting self-care and providing support systems, and the prevention and early treatment of disease.
   3. Use the teaching/learning theory if the question addresses client education, remembering that client motivation and client readiness to learn are the *first* priority.
   4. Be alert to the true and false response stems with questions that address health promotion and maintenance.

PYRAMID POINTS

A. Unfamiliar Content
   1. Answer questions by using your nursing knowledge, clinical experience, and test-taking skills.
   2. If the content of the question is unfamiliar and you are unable to answer questions by using your nursing knowledge, look for a global response, similar distracters, or similar words in the question and in the options.

B. The Global Response
   1. When more than one option appears to be correct, look for a global response.
   2. A global response is one that is a general statement and may include the ideas of other options within it.

C. Similar Distracters
   1. If you don't know the answer, try looking for similar distracters.
   2. Remember that there is only *one* answer.
   3. If two options say the same thing or include the same idea, then *neither of these options* can be the answer.
   4. The answer has to be an option that is different.

D. Similar Words
   1. If you do not know the answer, look for a similar word or phrase used in the stem or the case situation and in one of the options.
   2. If you find a word, feeling, or behavior that is used in the stem or the case situation and is repeated in one of the options, that option *may* be the correct answer.

REFERENCES

Carson, V., & Arnold, E. (1996). Mental health nursing: The nurse-patient journey. Philadelphia: W. B. Saunders

Leahy, J., & Kizilay, P. (1998). Foundations of nursing practice: A nursing process approach. Philadelphia: W. B. Saunders

National Council of State Boards of Nursing (1997). Plan for the National Council Licensure Examination for Registered Nurses. Chicago: Author.

UNIT II

The Nursing Process

CHAPTER 5

The Process of Assessment

Assessment is the first step of the nursing process. It involves a systematic method of collecting data about a client in order to identify actual and potential client health problems and establish a data base. The data base provides the foundation for the remaining steps of the nursing process; therefore, a thorough and adequate data base is essential.

Data collection begins with the first contact with the client. During all successive contacts, the nurse continues to collect information that is significant and relevant to the needs of the client.

During the assessment process, the nurse collects data about the client from a variety of sources. The client is the primary source of data. Family members and/or significant others are secondary sources of assessment data, and these sources may supplement or verify information provided by the client. Data may also be obtained from the client's record through the medical history, laboratory results, and diagnostic reports. Medical records from previous admissions may provide additional information about the client. The nurse may also obtain data through consultation with other health care team members who have had contact with the client.

A thorough data base is obtained through a health history and a physical assessment. The information collected by the nurse includes both subjective and objective data. Subjective data include the information that the client states. Objective data are the observable, measurable pieces of information about the client. Objective data include measurements, such as vital signs and laboratory findings, and information obtained from observation of the client. Objective data also include clinical manifestations as the signs and symptoms of an illness or disease.

The process of assessment additionally consists of confirming and verifying the client data, communicating information obtained through the assessment process, and documenting assessment findings in a thorough and accurate manner.

PRACTICE TEST

1. During an assessment of a perinatal client with a history of left-sided heart failure, the nurse finds the client experiencing unusual episodes of a nonproductive cough on minimal exertion. The nurse interprets this finding to possibly be the first indicator of which of the following important cardiac problems?

   1 Orthopnea
   2 Decreased blood volume
   3 Right-sided heart failure
   4 Pulmonary edema

Answer: 4

Rationale: Pulmonary edema from heart failure may be first manifested as a cough. The cough occurs in response to fluid filling the alveolar spaces. Pulmonary edema develops as a result of left ventricular failure or acute fluid overload.

Test-Taking Strategy: Look for key phrases in the question, such as "left-sided heart failure" and "nonproductive cough." The stem asks for a cardiac problem. Option 1 is an assessment finding. Option 2 would not result in the data provided in the stem. A nonproductive cough could be a late indicator of left-sided failure, not right-sided failure. For a mnemonic, remember "left" and "lung." Left-sided heart failure produces respiratory symptoms. Option 4 is the best answer.

Level of Cognitive Ability: Analysis
Phase of Nursing Process: Assessment
Client Needs: Physiological Integrity
Content Area: Maternity

References
Lowdermilk, D., Perry, S., & Bobak, I. (1997). *Maternity and women's health care* (6th ed.). St. Louis, MO: Mosby–Year Book, p. 882.
Pillitteri, A. (1995). *Maternal and child health nursing: Care of the childbearing and childrearing family* (2nd ed.). Philadelphia: Lippincott-Raven, p. 353.

---

2. The nurse is caring for a client with a diagnosis of chronic angina pectoris. The client is receiving sotalol (Betapace), 80 mg PO daily. Which of the following would indicate to the nurse that the client is experiencing a side effect related to the medication?

1 Difficulty swallowing
2 Diaphoresis
3 Dry mouth
4 Bradycardia

Answer: 4

Rationale: Sotalol is a beta-adrenergic blocking agent. Side effects include bradycardia, palpitations, difficulty breathing, irregular heart beat, signs of congestive heart failure (CHF), and cold hands and feet. Gastrointestinal disturbances, anxiety and nervousness, and unusual tiredness and weakness can also occur.

Test-Taking Strategy: Note that the question presents a client with chronic angina pectoris, a cardiac disorder. Remember that medications ending with "-lol" are beta-blockers, which are most commonly used for cardiac disorders. Use the process of elimination and note that option 4 is the only option that is directly cardiac related.

Level of Cognitive Ability: Analysis
Phase of Nursing Process: Assessment
Client Needs: Physiological Integrity
Content Area: Pharmacology

Reference
Hodgson, B., & Kizior, R. (1998). *Saunders nursing drug handbook 1998.* Philadelphia: W. B. Saunders, p. 940.

---

3. The nurse is interviewing a client, on admission to the inpatient unit, who was involved in a fire 2 months ago. The client is complaining of insomnia, difficulty concentrating, nervousness, and hypervigilance and is frequently thinking about fires. The nurse correctly assesses these symptoms to be indicative of

1 Obsessive compulsive disorder.
2 Phobia.
3 Post-traumatic stress disorder (PTSD).
4 Dissociative disorder.

Answer: 3

Rationale: PTSD is precipitated by events that are overwhelming, unpredictable, and sometimes life-threatening. Typical symptoms of PTSD include difficulty concentrating, sleep disturbances, intrusive recollections of the traumatic event, hypervigilance, and anxiety.

Test-Taking Strategy: Knowledge about PTSD will assist you in answering this question. If you knew that hypervigilance or hyperalertness and flashbacks of traumatic events were common symptoms of PTSD, you would have chosen the correct response. If you are unfamiliar with this disorder, it is important for you to review it now!

Level of Cognitive Ability: Analysis
Phase of Nursing Process: Assessment
Client Needs: Psychosocial Integrity
Content Area: Mental Health

Reference
Haber, J. (1997). *Comprehensive psychiatric nursing* (5th ed.). St. Louis: Mosby–Year Book, p. 440.

---

4. The home health care nurse is caring for a client with acute pain from cancer. The most appropriate assessment of pain would include which of the following?

1 The client's pain rating
2 The nurse's impression of the client's pain
3 Verbal and nonverbal clues from the client
4 Pain relief after appropriate nursing intervention

Answer: 1

Rationale: The client's perception of pain is the hallmark of pain assessment. Usually noted by the client rating on a scale of 1 to 10, the baseline pain assessment is documented and followed by appropriate medical and nursing intervention. The nurse's impression and the verbal and nonverbal clues are subjective data. Pain relief is an acceptable option but not the best option.

Test-Taking Strategy: Client orientation is required in this question. Nursing impressions are often inaccurate or can be biased, so option 2 can be eliminated. Pain relief after intervention is more appropriately part of the evaluation process. Option 1 is a more inclusive, client-focused answer.

Level of Cognitive Ability: Application
Phase of Nursing Process: Assessment
Client Needs: Physiological Integrity
Content Area: Adult Health/Oncology

Reference
Como, N. (1995). *Home health nursing pocket consultant.* St. Louis: Mosby–Year Book, p. 278.

---

5. Before performing venipuncture to initiate continuous intravenous (IV) therapy, the nurse should

1 Apply a tourniquet below the chosen vein site.
2 Inspect the IV solution for particles or contamination.
3 Secure an armboard to the joint located above the IV site.
4 Place a cool compress over the vein.

Answer: 2

Rationale: All IV solutions should be free of particles or precipitates. A tourniquet is to be applied above the chosen vein site. Cool compresses will cause vasoconstriction, making the veins less visible. Armboards are applied only after the IV is started.

Test-Taking Strategy: The stem contains the key word "before." Each option contains information that pertains to venipuncture. However, by reading each distractor carefully, you can see that each distractor contains incorrect IV initiation information. In addition, option 2 is the only option that reflects assessment, the first step of the nursing process.

Level of Cognitive Ability: Application
Phase of Nursing Process: Assessment
Client Needs: Physiological Integrity
Content Area: Fundamental Skills

Reference
Phillips, L. D. (1997). *Manual of IV therapeutics* (2nd ed.). Philadelphia: F. A. Davis, pp. 239–242.

---

6. A 16-year-old is hospitalized with pneumonia. Which statement by the client would alert the nurse to a potential developmental problem?

1 "Is it okay if I have a couple of friends in to visit me this evening?"
2 "When my friends get here, I would like to play some computer games with them."
3 "Please tell my friends not to visit since I'll see them back at school next week."
4 "I'd like my hair washed before my friends get here."

Answer: 3

Rationale: Adolescents who withdraw from peers into isolation struggle with developing identity, so option 3 should cause the nurse to be concerned. Option 1 shows that the client is eager for companionship. Adolescents often develop special interests within their groups, which may help maximize certain skills, such as with computers. Personal appearance is important to many adolescents.

Test-Taking Strategy: Options 1, 2, and 4 indicate that the client is anticipating the arrival of a peer group, which would be considered appropriate. Option 3 indicates that the client may be withdrawing from appropriate relationships. Review the concepts of growth and development now if you had difficulty answering this question!

Level of Cognitive Ability: Analysis
Phase of Nursing Process: Assessment
Client Needs: Psychosocial Integrity
Content Area: Child Health

Reference
Potter, P. A., & Perry, A. G. (1997). *Fundamentals of nursing: Concepts, process, and practice* (4th ed.). St. Louis: Mosby–Year Book, pp. 530–531.

7. The nurse is caring for a client who received an allogeneic liver transplant. The client is receiving tacrolimus (Prograf) daily. Which of the following would indicate to the nurse that the client is experiencing an adverse reaction to the medication?

1. A decrease in urine output
2. Hypotension
3. Profuse sweating
4. Photophobia

Answer: 1

Rationale: Tacrolimus is an immunosuppressant medication used in the prophylaxis of organ rejection in clients receiving allogeneic liver transplants. Frequent side effects include headache, tremor, insomnia, paresthesia, diarrhea, nausea, constipation, vomiting, abdominal pain, and hypertension. Adverse reactions and toxic effects include nephrotoxicity and pleural effusion, which occur frequently. Nephrotoxicity is characterized by increasing serum creatinine and a decrease in urine output. Neurotoxicity, including tremor, headache, and mental status changes, occurs commonly. It is imperative for the nurse to assess laboratory results, particularly renal function tests, and to monitor input and output closely.

Test-Taking Strategy: Knowledge about tacrolimus is necessary to answer this question. A hint to assist you in selecting the correct option is to use medical terminology in identifying the medication. Look at the medication name Prograf: "Pro" means "for," and "graf" means "graft." This will assist you in identifying the action of the medication as that of preventing transplant rejection. This hint may assist you in identifying the classification as immunosuppressant, which may in turn assist you in remembering side effects and adverse effects of the medication. If you had difficulty with this question, stop now and take the time to review!

Level of Cognitive Ability: Analysis
Phase of Nursing Process: Assessment
Client Needs: Physiological Integrity
Content Area: Pharmacology

Reference

Hodgson, B., & Kizior, R. (1998). *Saunders nursing drug handbook 1998.* Philadelphia: W. B. Saunders, pp. 959–960.

---

8. A client was admitted to the hospital 24 hours ago after pulmonary trauma. Which clinical manifestation would first alert the nurse that the client is experiencing adult respiratory distress syndrome (ARDS)?

1. An increase in respiratory rate
2. Blood-tinged frothy sputum
3. Bronchial breath sounds
4. Diffuse pulmonary infiltrates on the chest x-ray

Answer: 1

Rationale: ARDS usually develops within 24–48 hours after an initiating event. In most cases, tachypnea and dyspnea are the first clinical manifestations. Blood-tinged frothy sputum would manifest later, after the development of pulmonary edema. Breath sounds in the early stages of ARDS are usually clear at the beginning of the syndrome but may change to bronchial breath sounds when pulmonary edema occurs. Chest x-rays may yield normal findings during the early stages but will show infiltrates in the later stages.

Test-Taking Strategy: In this question, you are asked to identify the "initial" clinical manifestation associated with ARDS. It is important to remember that with respiratory conditions, tachypnea and dyspnea are often the initial symptoms along with restlessness as the hypoxia develops. If you had difficulty answering this question, review the signs and symptoms of ARDS now!

Level of Cognitive Ability: Analysis
Phase of Nursing Process: Assessment
Client Needs: Physiological Integrity
Content Area: Adult Health/Respiratory

Reference

Burrell, L. O., Gerlach, M. J., & Pless, B. (1997). *Adult nursing: Acute and community care* (2nd ed.). Stamford, CT: Appleton & Lange, p. 803.

9. Which client behavior should alert the nurse to the need for teaching related to cerebrovascular accident (CVA) prevention?
   1 Eats two bowls of high-fiber grain cereal with skim milk for breakfast
   2 Works as the manager of a busy medical-surgical unit and yet jogs 2 miles daily
   3 Uses oral contraceptives and condoms for pregnancy and disease prevention
   4 Has a blood pressure (BP) of 136/86 and has lost 10 pounds recently

Answer: 3

Rationale: Obesity, hypertension, hypercholesterolemia, smoking, and use of oral contraceptives are all modifiable risk factors for stroke. In option 3, oral contraceptive use is discouraged at times because of a side effect of clot formation. In option 1, the client eats a fairly low-fat meal. In option 2, the client has a stressful job but uses a stress-reduction method. In option 4, the client has borderline BP but has made a change in eating habits.

Test-Taking Strategy: Recognition of stroke risk factors is necessary to answer this question. When taking a health history for a client, the nurse may need to identify risk factors during a general interview. If you had difficulty with this question and are unclear regarding the risk factors related to stroke, review this content now!

Level of Cognitive Ability: Analysis
Phase of Nursing Process: Assessment
Client Needs: Physiological Integrity
Content Area: Adult Health/Neurological

Reference

Black, J. M., & Matassarin-Jacobs, E. (1997). *Medical-surgical nursing: Clinical management for continuity of care* (5th ed.). Philadelphia: W. B. Saunders, p. 986.

10. The nurse reviews the client's electrocardiogram (ECG) rhythm strip. The ECG shows that the rate is 90 beats per minute. What action by the nurse would be most appropriate?
   1 Tell the client the rate is normal
   2 Tell the client not to worry
   3 Tell the client that medication specific to the problem will be prescribed
   4 Tell the client a slower heart rate is preferred

Answer: 1

Rationale: A normal adult resting pulse rate ranges between 60 and 100 beats per minute.

Test-Taking Strategy: This question requires knowing the basic range of pulse rates for an adult. Option 2 tells the client "not to worry," which is not an appropriate action. Options 3 and 4 indicate that there is a problem when clearly there is no problem. Review normal adult vital signs now if you had difficulty with this question!

Level of Cognitive Ability: Application
Phase of the Nursing Process: Assessment
Client Needs: Safe, Effective Care Environment
Content Area: Adult Health/Cardiovascular

Reference

Luckmann, J. (1997). *Saunders manual of nursing care.* Philadelphia: W. B. Saunders, p. 993.

11. The nurse is caring for a client with Buck's traction. Which of the following assessment data would indicate a potential complication associated with Buck's traction?
   1 Weak pedal pulses
   2 Drainage at the pin sites
   3 Warm toes with brisk capillary refill
   4 Redness over the heel area

Answer: 1

Rationale: Weak pedal pulses are a sign of vascular compromise, which can be caused by pressure on the tissues of the leg by the elastic bandage used to secure this type of traction. This type of traction does not involve the use of pins; rather, it is secured by elastic bandages or a prefabricated boot. Warm toes with brisk capillary refill is a normal assessment finding. The heel is usually elevated off the bed; therefore, decubitus over the heel area is not likely.

Test-Taking Strategy: Knowledge about Buck's traction is necessary to assist you in answering this question. You must know that this traction does not require pins and that the heel is kept elevated off the bed, usually by pillows. In addition, if you know the normal assessment findings to assess vascular sufficiency, you would not select option 3. If you had difficulty with this question, take the time now to review Buck's traction!

Level of Cognitive Ability: Analysis
Phase of the Nursing Process: Assessment
Client Needs: Physiological Integrity
Content Area: Adult Health/Musculoskeletal

Reference

Black, J. M., & Matassarin-Jacobs, E. (1997). *Medical-surgical nursing: Clinical management for continuity of care* (5th ed.). Philadelphia: W. B. Saunders, p. 2138.

---

12. The nurse assesses the laboratory results of a client with pheochromocytoma. The magnesium level is 7 mEq/L. On the basis of this laboratory result, the nurse would monitor for

1 Drowsiness.
2 Hypertension.
3 Hyperpnea.
4 Hyperactive reflexes.

Answer: 1

Rationale: The level of hypermagnesemia may be classified as mild (3–5 mEq/L), moderate (6–7 mEq/L), severe (10–11 mEq/L), and emergency (12–15 mEq/L). A client with a mild degree of hypermagnesemia is usually asymptomatic. Neurological manifestations begin to occur at levels of 6–7 mEq/L and are noted as symptoms of neurological depression, such as drowsiness, sedation, lethargy, respiratory depression, muscle weakness, and areflexia. Severe hypotension and nausea and vomiting also occur as early as an increased elevation of 6–7 mEq/L.

Test-Taking Strategy: It is important to be able to identify the signs and symptoms related to a magnesium imbalance. Look at the options and note that options 2, 3, and 4 all relate to a "hyper" related sign. The only option that is different is option 1, which in this situation is the correct option. If you had difficulty with this question, review magnesium imbalances now!

Level of Cognitive Ability: Analysis
Phase of the Nursing Process: Assessment
Client Needs: Physiological Integrity
Content Area: Adult Health/Endocrine

Reference

Lee, C., Barrett, C., & Ignatavicius, D. (1996). *Fluid and electrolytes: A practical approach* (4th ed.). Philadelphia: F. A. Davis, p. 130.

---

13. A perinatal client has received a diagnosis of a vaginal infection with the organism *Candida albicans*. Which of the following assessment findings would be expected by the nurse?

1 Absence of any symptoms
2 Pain, itching, and vaginal discharge
3 Proteinuria, hematuria, edema, and hypertension
4 Costovertebral angle pain

Answer: 2

Rationale: Clinical manifestations of a *Candida* infection include pain, itching, and a thick, white vaginal discharge. Proteinuria, hematuria, edema, hypertension, and costovertebral angle pain are clinical manifestations associated with urinary tract infections.

Test-Taking Strategy: Knowledge of the clinical manifestations of vaginal infections is necessary to answer this question. Avoid option 1 because the word "absence" is absolute terminology. Both options 3 and 4 address urinary tract infections.

Level of Cognitive Ability: Analysis
Phase of Nursing Process: Assessment
Client Needs: Physiological Integrity
Content Area: Maternity

Reference

Lowdermilk, D., Perry, S., & Bobak, I. (1997). *Maternity and women's health care* (6th ed.). St. Louis: Mosby–Year Book, p. 835.

14. A prenatal client was told during a physician office visit that she was positive for human immunodeficiency virus (HIV). The client cried and was significantly distressed about this news. Which of the following nursing diagnoses would these data best support?

1 Pain
2 Noncompliance
3 High Risk for Infection
4 Anticipatory Grieving

Answer: 4

Rationale: A life-threatening diagnosis such as HIV infection will stimulate the anticipatory grief response. Anticipatory grief occurs when the client, family, and loved ones know that the client will die. The prenatal HIV-positive client is forced to make important changes in her life, frequently resulting in grief and diminished self-esteem resulting from inability to achieve life goals.

Test-Taking Strategy: The stem asks the nurse to prioritize according to the data available. Distress and crying are data supporting the nursing diagnosis of anticipatory grieving. The stem does not contain enough information to support options 1 or 2. Option 3 is a possible answer, but the priority nursing diagnosis at this time, according to the information provided, is option 4.

Level of Cognitive Ability: Analysis
Phase of Nursing Process: Assessment
Client Needs: Psychosocial Integrity
Content Area: Maternity

Reference

Pillitteri, A. (1995). *Maternal and child health nursing: Care of the childbearing and childrearing family* (2nd ed.). Philadelphia: Lippincott-Raven, p. 336.

---

15. A prenatal client is suspected of having iron-deficiency anemia. Which of the following would the nurse expect to find with regard to the client's status?

1 A low hemoglobin and hematocrit level
2 A high hemoglobin and hematocrit level
3 Fluid volume excess
4 Fluid volume deficit

Answer: 1

Rationale: When the hemoglobin level is below 11 mg/dL, iron deficiency is suspected. An indirect index of the oxygen-carrying capacity is the packed red blood cell volume or hematocrit level. Pathological anemia of pregnancy is caused primarily by iron deficiency. Without iron therapy, even pregnant women who have excellent nutrition will finish pregnancy with an iron deficit. Iron for the fetus comes from the maternal serum.

Test-Taking Strategy: The stem of the question reflects the assessment phase of the nursing process. Options 3 and 4 are nursing diagnoses and not assessment data. Option 1 reflects the correct answer. The word "deficiency" found in the question and the word "low" found in option 1 are similar, which will assist you in selecting the correct option.

Level of Cognitive Ability: Analysis
Phase of Nursing Process: Assessment
Client Needs: Physiological Integrity
Content Area: Maternity

Reference

Lowdermilk, D., Perry, S., & Bobak, I. (1997). *Maternity and women's health care* (6th ed.). St. Louis: Mosby–Year Book, pp. 845–846.

---

16. The nurse is caring for the postpartum client. Which of the following findings would make the nurse suspect endometritis in this client?

1 Fever over 38°C, beginning on the third postpartum day
2 Lochia rubra on the second postpartum day
3 Elevated white blood cell count
4 Breast engorgement

Answer: 1

Rationale: Fever on the third or fourth postpartum day should raise concerns about possible endometritis until proven otherwise. As a rule, the woman with endometritis demonstrates a rise in temperature well over 38°C. Lochia rubra on the second day postpartum is a normal finding. The white blood cell count of a postpartum woman is normally increased. Thus this conventional method of detecting infection is not of great value in the puerperium. Breast engorgement is also a normal response and is not associated with endometritis.

Test-Taking Strategy: Knowledge about the normal postpartum period is necessary to eliminate options 2, 3, and 4 as possible answers. This leaves option 1 as the only correct option.

Level of Cognitive Ability: Analysis
Phase of Nursing Process: Assessment
Client Needs: Physiological Integrity
Content Area: Maternity

Reference

Pillitteri, A. (1995). *Maternal and child health nursing: Care of the childbearing and childrearing family* (2nd ed.). Philadelphia: Lippincott-Raven, p. 714.

---

17. The nurse is performing an assessment on a post-term neonate. Which physical characteristic would the nurse expect to observe?

1 Vernix that covers the body in a thick layer
2 Desquamation over the body
3 Smooth soles without creases
4 Lanugo covering the entire body

Answer: 2

Rationale: The post-term neonate exhibits dry, peeling, cracked, almost leather-like skin, which is called desquamation, over the body. The preterm neonate exhibits thick vernix covering the body, smooth soles without creases, and lanugo covering the body.

Test-Taking Strategy: In options 1, 3, and 4, the physical characteristics are all of a preterm infant. Option 2 is the only option that describes the post-term infant. By using nursing knowledge, you are able to group the three preterm characteristics together, leaving option 2 as your choice. If you had difficulty with this question, take the time now to review the characteristics of preterm and post-term infants!

Level of Cognitive Ability: Analysis
Phase of Nursing Process: Assessment
Client Needs: Physiological Integrity
Content Area: Maternity

Reference

Pillitteri, A. (1995). *Maternal and child health nursing: Care of the childbearing and childrearing family* (2nd ed.). Philadelphia: Lippincott-Raven, pp. 738–739, 760–761.

---

18. The nurse is performing an admission assessment on a small-for-gestational-age (SGA) full-term infant. The nurse observes tachypnea, grunting, retractions, and nasal flaring. These symptoms are most likely caused by

1 Hypoglycemia.
2 Meconium aspiration syndrome.
3 Respiratory distress syndrome.
4 Transient tachypnea of the newborn.

X

Answer: 2

Rationale: The SGA infant is most prone to meconium aspiration syndrome, evidenced by tachypnea, grunting, retractions, and nasal flaring. In utero, hypoxia can cause the relaxation of the anal sphincter with passage of meconium into the amniotic fluid. The fetus also gasps in response to hypoxia, which can result in aspiration of meconium in utero or with the first breaths after birth. Transient tachypnea of the newborn is primarily found in infants delivered by cesarean section, during which the lung fluid is not squeezed out. Respiratory distress syndrome is a complication of preterm infants.

Test-Taking Strategy: This question requires you to recognize signs of meconium aspiration syndrome and then differentiate between the three listed respiratory conditions (options 2, 3, and 4). Option 1 is easily eliminated because it is not a respiratory condition. Options 3 and 4 can be eliminated because the question states "term" infant, and does not state that a cesarean delivery was performed. If you had difficulty with this question, review this content now.

Level of Cognitive Ability: Analysis
Phase of Nursing Process: Assessment
Client Needs: Physiological Integrity
Content Area: Maternity

Reference

Olds, S., London, M., & Ladewig, P. (1996). *Maternal-newborn nursing: A family-centered approach* (5th ed.). Menlo Park, CA: Addison-Wesley, pp. 923–926.

19. The client had a seizure an hour ago. The family was present during the episode and reported that the client's jaw was moving as though grinding food. In helping to determine the origin of this seizure, the assessment would address the evidence of

1 Prior trauma.
2 Diaphoresis.
3 Rotating eye movements.
4 Loss of consciousness.

Answer: 1

Rationale: Seizures that originate with specific motor phenomena are considered focal/jacksonian and are indicative of a focal structural lesion in the brain often caused by trauma, infection, or drug consumption.

Test-Taking Strategy: The data given by family is the most significant for a diagnosis. The stem asks "to determine the origin of this seizure." Options 2, 3, and 4 address signs and symptoms. Option 1 is the only option that addresses a possible origin.

Level of Cognitive Ability: Application
Phase of Nursing Process: Assessment
Client Needs: Physiological Integrity
Content Area: Adult Health/Neurological

Reference

Luckmann, J. (1997). *Saunders manual of nursing care.* Philadelphia: W. B. Saunders, pp. 697–699.

---

20. The nurse would surmise that a client recovering from a myocardial infarction is exhibiting signs of depression when the client

1 Reports insomnia at night.
2 Consumes 25% of meals and shows little interest in client education.
3 Ignores activity restrictions and does not report the experience of chest pain with activity.
4 Expresses apprehension about leaving the hospital and requests someone to stay with him or her at night.

Answer: 2

Rationale: Signs of depression include withdrawal, crying, anorexia, and apathy. Insomnia may be a sign of anxiety or fear. Ignoring symptoms and activity restrictions is a sign of denial. Apprehension is a sign of anxiety.

Test-Taking Strategy: Use the process of elimination when answering the question. Be careful when you select an answer that contains the word "and." Remember that the entire option needs to be correct. Therefore, carefully read the content before and after the word "and."

Level of Cognitive Ability: Analysis
Phase of the Nursing Process: Assessment
Client Needs: Psychosocial Integrity
Content Area: Adult Health/Cardiovascular

Reference

Lewis, S. M., Collier, I. C., & Heitkemper, M. M. (1996). *Medical-surgical nursing: Assessment and management of clinical problems* (4th ed.). St. Louis: Mosby–Year Book, p. 922.

---

21. The nurse is caring for a client with hypertension receiving torsemide (Demadex), 5 mg PO daily. Which of the following would indicate to the nurse that the client may be experiencing an adverse reaction to the medication?

1 A blood urea nitrogen (BUN) of 15 mg/dL
2 A chloride level of 98 mEq/L
3 A sodium level of 135 mEq/L
4 A potassium level of 3.1 mEq/L

Answer: 4

Rationale: Demadex is a loop diuretic. Overdose of the medication produces acute, profound water loss, volume and electrolyte depletion, dehydration, decreased blood volume, and circulatory collapse. Option 4 is the only option that presents an electrolyte depletion; a normal potassium level is 3.5–5.1 mEq/L. The normal sodium level is 135–145 mEq/L. The normal chloride level is 98–107 mEq/L. The normal BUN is 5–20 mg/dL.

Test-Taking Strategy: Knowledge about Demadex and about normal laboratory values is necessary to answer this question. Knowledge of normal values would assist you in selecting option 4 because this is the only abnormal laboratory value among the four options. If you are unfamiliar with this medication or these laboratory values, take the time now to review this content!

Level of Cognitive Ability: Analysis
Phase of Nursing Process: Assessment
Client Needs: Physiological Integrity
Content Area: Pharmacology

Reference

Hodgson, B., & Kizior, R. (1998). *Saunders nursing drug handbook 1998.* Philadelphia: W. B. Saunders, p. 1008.

---

22. The nurse is performing an admission assessment on a client admitted with a diagnosis of trigeminal neuralgia (tic douloureux). In the assessment, the nurse can expect to discover that the client is experiencing

1 Chronic, intermittent pain in the seventh cranial nerve.
2 Abrupt onset of pain in the fifth cranial nerve.
3 Bilateral pain in the sixth cranial nerve.
4 Unilateral pain in the sixth cranial nerve.

Answer: 2

Rationale: Trigeminal neuralgia is defined as a syndrome of chronic, intermittent pain, involving one or more divisions of the trigeminal nerve, or cranial nerve V. Its etiology can be intrinsic, as in demyelination from multiple sclerosis and herpes virus infection, or extrinsic, as in lesions impinging on the trigeminal nerve (tumors, vascular irregularities, and dental causes).

Test-Taking Strategy: This question assesses your ability to analyze the pathophysiological processes that cause the symptoms of trigeminal neuralgia. Knowing about the cranial nerves and that trigeminal neuralgia affects the fifth cranial nerve would help you to rule out options 1, 3, and 4. If you could not recall which nerve is involved in trigeminal neuralgia, you may remember that Bell's palsy afflicts the seventh cranial nerve. In most cases, the pain is unilateral, so option 3 could be ruled out. You will want to review the cranial nerves and their function and relation to pathophysiology now if you had difficulty with this question!

Level of Cognitive Ability: Analysis
Phase of Nursing Process: Assessment
Client Needs: Physiological Integrity
Content Area: Adult Health/Neurological

Reference

Black, J. M., & Matassarin-Jacobs, E. (1997). *Medical-surgical nursing: Clinical management for continuity of care* (5th ed.). Philadelphia: W. B. Saunders, pp. 915–932.

---

23. A nurse is assessing a client's suicide potential. The most important nursing inquiry would be

1 "Why do you want to hurt yourself ?"
2 "Can you describe how you are feeling right now?"
3 "Has anyone in your family committed suicide?"
4 "Do you have a plan to commit suicide?"

Answer: 4

Rationale: When assessing for suicide risk, the nurse must evaluate whether the client has a suicide plan. Clients who have a definitive plan pose a greater risk for suicide.

Test-Taking Strategy: Knowledge of the importance of assessing for a suicide plan is necessary to assist you in answering this question. If you are unfamiliar with assessment of suicide potential, it would be important to review this information right now!

Level of Cognitive Ability: Analysis
Phase of Nursing Process: Assessment
Client Needs: Psychosocial Integrity
Content Area: Mental Health

Reference

Varcarolis, E. (1998). *Foundations of psychiatric mental health nursing* (3rd ed.). Philadelphia: W. B. Saunders, p. 729.

24. The nurse is performing an admission assessment on a client admitted with newly diagnosed Hodgkin's disease. Which of the following symptoms would the nurse expect the client to report?

1 Night sweats
2 Severe lymph node pain
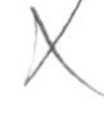
3 Weight gain of 5 pounds
4 Headache with minor visual changes

Answer: 1

Rationale: Assessment of a client with Hodgkin's disease most often reveals enlarged, painless lymph nodes; fever; malaise; and night sweats. Weight loss may be present in metastatic disease.

Test-Taking Strategy: Use the process of elimination in answering the question. In both options 2 and 4, a similarity exists in the sense of pain. If two options are similar, neither one is likely to be the answer. Weight gain is rarely the symptom of any cancer diagnosis, so eliminate option 3. If you had difficulty answering this question, review content related to Hodgkin's disease now!

Level of Cognitive Ability: Analysis
Phase of Nursing Process: Assessment
Client Needs: Physiological Integrity
Content Area: Adult Health/Oncology

Reference

Ignatavicius, D. D., Workman, M. L., & Mishler, M. A. (1995). *Medical-surgical nursing: A nursing process approach* (2nd ed.). Philadelphia: W. B. Saunders, pp. 1069–1070.

---

25. The nurse is assessing a 3-day-old preterm neonate with respiratory distress syndrome (RDS). Which one of the following assessment findings indicates that the neonate's respiratory status is improving?

1 Presence of a systolic murmur
2 Respiratory rate between 60–70 breaths per minute
3 Edema of the hands and feet
4 Urine output of 1–3 mL/kg/hour

Answer: 4

Rationale: Increased urination is an early clue that the neonate's respiratory condition is improving. Lung fluid, which is present in RDS, moves from the lungs into the blood stream as the condition improves and the alveoli open. This extra fluid circulates to the kidneys, which results in increased voiding. Systolic murmurs usually indicate the presence of a patent ductus arteriosus, which is a common complication of RDS. Respiratory rates above 60 breaths per minute are indicative of tachypnea, which is a sign of respiratory distress. Edema of the hands and feet occurs within the first 24 hours as a result of low protein concentrations, a decrease in colloidal osmotic pressure, and transudation of fluid from the vascular system to the tissues.

Test-Taking Strategy: The question asks you to identify an assessment finding that indicates that the neonate's respiratory condition is improving. You might be tempted to choose option 2 because it addresses the respiratory rate, but it is incorrect because the stated rate is too high. Understanding the disease process in RDS with regard to fluid in the lungs should assist you in choosing an option that addresses a normal urine output, which would indicate resolution of excess lung fluid. Review this content now if you had difficulty answering the question!

Level of Cognitive Ability: Analysis
Phase of Nursing Process: Assessment
Client Needs: Physiological Integrity
Content Area: Maternity

Reference

Olds, S., London, M., & Ladewig, P. (1996). *Maternal-newborn nursing: A family-centered approach* (5th ed.). Menlo Park, CA: Addison-Wesley, p. 1169.

26. A nurse practicing in a nurse-managed clinic wants to set up a diabetic teaching seminar. The nurse understands that to meet the needs of the clients, the nurse must first

1 Assess the clients' functional abilities.
2 Ensure that the insurance documentation is up to date.
3 Discuss the focus of the seminar with the multidisciplinary team.
4 Include everyone who comes into the clinic in the teaching sessions.

Answer: 1

Rationale: Nurse-managed clinics focus on individualized disease prevention and on health promotion and maintenance; therefore, the nurse must first assess the clients and their needs in order to effectively plan the seminar.

Test-Taking Strategy: The stem asks for an assessment to fulfill client needs. Options 2 and 3 are important tasks in all agencies but are general options in nature. Option 4 can be eliminated because of the word "everyone." Remember that the first step in the nursing process is assessment. Option 1 reflects assessment!

Level of Cognitive Ability: Application
Phase of Nursing Process: Assessment
Client Needs: Physiological Integrity
Content Area: Adult Health/Endocrine

Reference

Black, J. M., & Matassarin-Jacobs, E. (1997). *Medical-surgical nursing: Clinical management for continuity of care* (5th ed.). Philadelphia: W. B. Saunders, p. 113.

---

27. The nurse is caring for a full-term newborn. Which of the following assessment findings would alert the nurse to suspect the occurrence of jaundice in this newborn?

1 A negative direct Coombs' test result
2 Birth weight of 8 pounds, 6 ounces
3 Presence of a cephalohematoma
4 Infant blood type of O negative

Answer: 3

Rationale: Enclosed hemorrhage, as with cephalohematoma, predisposes the infant to jaundice by producing an increased bilirubin load as the cephalohematoma resolves and is absorbed into the circulatory system. In option 1, the negative direct Coombs' test result indicates that there are no maternal antibodies on fetal erythrocytes. The birth weight in option 2 is within the acceptable ranges for a full-term infant, and therefore does not contribute to an increased bilirubin level. In option 4, the classic Rh incompatibility scenario involves an Rh-negative mother with an Rh-positive fetus/newborn.

Test-Taking Strategy: This question asks you to connect an assessment finding with a risk for the development of jaundice. Knowledge of those risk factors must be applied to this question. If you had difficulty with this question, take time now to review this content!

Level of Cognitive Ability: Analysis
Phase of Nursing Process: Assessment
Client Needs: Physiological Integrity
Content Area: Maternity

Reference

Reeder, S., Martin, L., & Koniak-Griffin, D. (1997). *Maternity nursing: Family, newborn, and women's health care* (18th ed.). Philadelphia: Lippincott-Raven, pp. 1213–1214.

---

28. Which assessment is most important for the nurse to make before advancing a client from liquids to solid food?

1 Food preferences
2 Appetite
3 Presence of bowel sounds
4 Chewing ability

Answer: 4

Rationale: It may be necessary to modify a client's diet to a soft or mechanical chopped diet if the client has difficulty chewing. Food preferences should be ascertained on admission. Appetite will affect the amount of food eaten but not the type of diet ordered. Bowel sounds should be present before introducing any diet.

Test-Taking Strategy: Read the question carefully and identify exactly what the stem is asking. Key words in the question are "liquid" and "solid," focusing on consistency of food. "Chewing" is the only option that addresses a factor affecting food consistency.

Level of Cognitive Ability: Application
Phase of Nursing Process: Assessment
Client Needs: Physiological Integrity
Content Area: Fundamental Skills

Reference

Craven, R. F., & Hirnle, C. J. (1996). *Fundamentals of nursing: Human health and function* (2nd ed.). Philadelphia: J. B. Lippincott, p. 1051.

---

29. The nurse is caring for the client with cystitis. Which of the following assessment findings, if obtained by the nurse, would not be consistent with the typical clinical picture seen with this disorder?

1 Urinary retention
2 Burning on urination
3 Low back pain
4 Hematuria

Answer: 1

Rationale: Clinical manifestations of cystitis usually include urinary frequency, urgency, dysuria, inability to void, or voiding only small amounts. The urine may be cloudy, with hematuria and bacteriuria. The client may complain of pain that is suprapubic or in the lower back. Nonspecific signs include fever, chills, malaise, and nausea and vomiting. Some clients, particularly the elderly, may be asymptomatic.

Test-Taking Strategy: The wording of this question guides you to look for an incorrect response. Begin to answer this question by eliminating options 2 and 4, since they are very commonly associated with cystitis. Knowing that urgency and frequency are typical symptoms (not urinary retention) allows you to choose option 1 over option 3 as the answer.

Level of Cognitive Ability: Analysis
Phase of Nursing Process: Assessment
Client Needs: Physiological Integrity
Content Area: Adult Health/Renal

Reference

Black, J. M., & Matassarin-Jacobs, E. (1997). *Medical-surgical nursing: Clinical management for continuity of care* (5th ed.). Philadelphia: W. B. Saunders, p. 1572.

---

30. What method should the nurse use to most accurately assess the effectiveness of a weight-loss diet for an obese client?

1 Daily weights
2 Serum protein levels
3 Calorie counts every shift
4 Daily intake and output

Answer: 1

Rationale: The most accurate measurement of weight loss is daily weighing of the client at the same time, in the same clothes, and with the same scale. Options 2, 3, and 4 help measure nutrition and hydration status.

Test-Taking Strategy: Look for similar words in question and option: "weight-loss" in question, "weights" in option. Also, two options contain the word "daily." Option 1 measures weight, option 4 measures fluid balance. Assessing weight will most accurately identify weight changes.

Level of Cognitive Ability: Application
Phase of Nursing Process: Assessment
Client Needs: Physiological Integrity
Content Area: Fundamental Skills

Reference

Potter, P. A., & Perry, A. G. (1997). *Fundamentals of nursing: Concepts, process, and practice* (4th ed.). St. Louis: Mosby–Year Book, p. 1105.

31. The client has fallen and sustained a leg injury. Which of the following questions would the nurse ask the client to help determine whether the pain is from fracture?

1 "Does the pain feel like a series of cramps?"
2 "Does the pain feel like pins and needles?"
3 "Is the pain a dull ache?"
4 "Is the pain sharp and piercing?"

Answer: 4

Rationale: Fracture pain is generally described as sharp and piercing. Bone pain is often described as a boring, dull, deep ache. Pain of muscle origin is often described as an aching or cramping pain or soreness. Altered sensations, such as paresthesias (pins and needles), indicate that there is pressure on nerves or impairment of circulation.

Test-Taking Strategy: This question can be analyzed from a viewpoint of common sense. The pain of fracture is likely to be intense and would be least likely to be described as cramps (option 1), pins and needles (option 2), or a dull ache (option 3). A fresh injury such as a fracture is more likely to be described as sharp and piercing. If you had difficulty with this question, take the time now to review the assessment of fractures!

Level of Cognitive Ability: Application
Phase of Nursing Process: Assessment
Client Needs: Physiological Integrity
Content Area: Adult Health/Musculoskeletal

Reference

Smeltzer, S., & Bare, B. (1996). *Brunner and Suddarth's Textbook of medical-surgical nursing* (8th ed.). Philadelphia: Lippincott-Raven, p. 1846.

---

32. A client who has a new feeding gastrostomy tube refuses to participate in the plan of care, will not make eye contact, and does not speak to family or visitors. The nurse assesses that this client is using which type of coping mechanism?

1 Self-control
2 Problem-solving
3 Accepting responsibility
4 Distancing

Answer: 4

Rationale: Self-control is demonstrated by stoicism and hiding feelings. Problem-solving involves making plans and verbalizing what will be done. Accepting responsibility places the responsibility for a situation on oneself. Distancing is an unwillingness or inability to discuss events.

Test-Taking Strategy: The words "refuses," "will not," and "does not" are all indicative of ineffective coping. Option 4, "distancing," is the least effective coping strategy. If you had difficulty with this question, take time now to review coping mechanisms!

Level of Cognitive Ability: Analysis
Phase of Nursing Process: Assessment
Client Needs: Psychosocial Integrity
Content Area: Adult Health/Gastrointestinal

Reference

Ignatavicius, D. D., Workman, M. L., & Mishler, M. A. (1995). *Medical-surgical nursing: A nursing process approach* (2nd ed., Vol. 1). Philadelphia: W. B. Saunders, p. 108.

---

33. The nurse obtains a fingerstick glucose measurement of greater than 400 mg/dL from a client receiving total parenteral nutrition (TPN). What nursing action is most appropriate at this time?

1 Stop the TPN
2 Decrease the flow rate of the TPN
3 Administer insulin
4 Notify the physician

Answer: 4

Rationale: The nurse monitors for complications and reports major changes or abnormalities to the physician. Options 1, 2, and 3 are not done without a physician's being notified for an order.

Test-Taking Strategy: This addresses scope of nursing practice. Options 1, 2, and 3 are not within the scope of nursing practice without first notifying a physician for an order. A blood glucose level greater than 400 mg/dL represents a physiological alteration that necessitates notification of the physician. Do not read into the question. Read only the facts that are stated. The question does not identify orders from a physician; therefore, your best option is to call the physician to report the results.

Level of Cognitive Ability: Application
Phase of Nursing Process: Assessment
Client Needs: Physiological Integrity
Content Area: Fundamental Skills

Reference

Ignatavicius, D. D., Workman, M. L., & Mishler, M. A. (1995). *Medical-surgical nursing: A nursing process approach* (2nd ed., Vol. 2). Philadelphia: W. B. Saunders, p. 1774.

---

34. The nurse is caring for a client who is receiving electroconvulsive therapy (ECT) for a major depressive disorder. Which of the following assessment findings would the nurse identify as an unexpected side effect of ECT necessitating notification of the physician?

1 Memory loss
2 Disorientation
3 Confusion
4 Hypertension

Answer: 4

Rationale: The major side effects of ECT are confusion, disorientation, and memory loss. A change in blood pressure would not be an anticipated side effect and would be a cause for concern. If hypertension occurs after ECT, the physician should be notified.

Test-Taking Strategy: Knowledge about ECT and the side effects of this therapy is necessary to assist you in answering this question. The process of elimination would be used to answer the question. If you are unfamiliar with this treatment modality, it would be important for you to review this information now!

Level of Cognitive Ability: Analysis
Phase of Nursing Process: Assessment
Client Needs: Physiological Integrity
Content Area: Mental Health

Reference

Varcarolis, E. (1998). *Foundations of psychiatric mental health nursing* (3rd ed.). Philadelphia: W. B. Saunders, p. 578.

---

35. The nurse is performing a neurological assessment on a client and is assessing the function of the frontal lobes of the brain. Assessment of which of the following items by the nurse would yield the best information about this area of functioning?

1 Response to verbal stimuli
2 Insight, judgment, and planning
3 Affect or emotions
4 Eye movements

Answer: 2

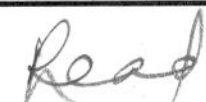

Rationale: Insight, judgment, and planning are part of the function of the frontal lobe, in conjunction with association fibers that connect to other areas of the cerebrum. Level of consciousness is controlled by the reticular activating system as well as by both cerebral hemispheres. Feelings are part of the role of the limbic system and involve both hemispheres. Eye movements are under the control of cranial nerves III, IV, and VI.

Test-Taking Strategy: To answer this question correctly, recall that some of the higher functions of mentation are controlled by or stored in the frontal lobes. This involves not just insight, judgment, and planning but also the bank of information that we call "knowledge." You should be able to eliminate each of the incorrect options if you have this basic knowledge. Review this basic knowledge now if you had difficulty with this question!

Level of Cognitive Ability: Application
Phase of Nursing Process: Assessment
Client Needs: Physiological Integrity
Content Area: Adult Health/Neurological

Reference

Black, J. M., & Matassarin-Jacobs, E. (1997). *Medical-surgical nursing: Clinical management for continuity of care* (5th ed.). Philadelphia: W. B. Saunders, pp. 710–711.

Read

36. Which of the following assessment data items would be most important for a client to modify to lessen the risk for coronary artery disease (CAD)?

1 Elevated high-density lipoprotein (HDL) levels
2 Elevated low-density lipoprotein levels (LDL)
3 Elevated triglyceride levels
4 Elevated serum lipase levels

Good Bad

HDL
LDL

Answer: 2

Rationale: LDL is more directly associated with CAD than are other lipoproteins. LDL levels, along with cholesterol, have a higher associative and predictive value for CAD than do triglyceride levels. In addition, HDL is inversely associated with the risk of CAD. Lipase is a digestive enzyme that breaks down ingested fats in the gastrointestinal tract.

Test-Taking Strategy: Identify and focus on key word "most" in the stem. Identify the key issue as a risk factor. Identify the stem as a true response. Knowledge regarding risk factors related to cardiac disease is necessary to answer this question. It is very important that you are familiar with these risk factors. If you had difficulty answering this question, review this content now!

Level of Cognitive Ability: Analysis
Phase of Nursing Process: Assessment
Client Needs: Physiological Integrity
Content Area: Adult Health/Cardiovascular

Reference

Phipps, W., Cassmeyer, V., Sands J., et al. (1995). *Medical-surgical nursing: Concepts and clinical practice*. St. Louis: Mosby–Year Book, p. 815.

37. The registered nurse finds that a postoperative client has been having difficulty maintaining control of pain with the prescribed narcotics but only while a particular licensed practical nurse (LPN) is assigned to the client. The nurse

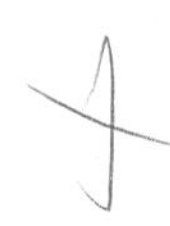

1 Reviews that client's medication administration record and immediately discusses the concern with the nursing supervisor.
2 Notifies the physician that the client needs an increase in narcotic dosage.
3 Decides to avoid assigning that LPN to the care of clients receiving narcotics.
4 Confronts the LPN with the information about the client having pain control problems and asks if the LPN is using the narcotics personally.

Answer: 1

Rationale: The nurse is responsible for the safety of all assigned clients and recognizes the importance of the principle of nonmaleficence (doing or allowing no harm to others). The practice of all peers is monitored by the nurse. The nurse in this situation has noted an unusual occurrence, but before deciding what action to next take, the nurse needs more evidence than suspicion. This can be obtained by reviewing the client record. State and federal labor and narcotic regulations, as well as institutional policies and procedures, must be followed. It is therefore most appropriate that the nurse discuss the situation with the responsible nursing supervisor before taking further action. The client does not need an increase in narcotics but only to receive the full dose ordered; thus option 2 is an incorrect response. Option 3 only ignores the issue and may put the registered nurse in jeopardy as well. A confrontation, as in option 4, is not the most advisable action, as the appropriate administrative authorities need to be consulted first.

Test-Taking Strategy: Two of the options contain the conjunction "and." Be cautious when choosing this type of answer, because both halves of the answer must be correct. The nurse is responsible for protecting clients from the professional misconduct of others, but the charge of misuse of narcotics is a serious one that requires expert input. Option 1 is the only option that includes consultation with an authority figure and thus is the only response that satisfies all conditions. There is nothing in the stem to indicate that the nurse is the sole authority figure, so avoid reading into the question and remember that assessment (gathering data) is the first step!

Level of Cognitive Ability: Application
Phase of Nursing Process: Assessment
Client Needs: Physiological Integrity
Content Area: Fundamental Skills

Reference

Wywialowski, E. F. (1997). *Managing client care* (2nd ed.). St. Louis: Mosby–Year Book, p. 321.

38. The client has received a diagnosis of polycystic kidney disease. The nurse assesses the client for which of the following manifestations, which are the most common for this disorder?

1 Flank pain and hematuria
2 Urinary calculi and renal failure
3 Hypertension and cystic lesions of the bladder
4 Proteinuria and cerebral aneurysm

Answer: 1

Rationale: The most common findings with polycystic disease include hematuria and flank or lumbar pain that is either colicky or dull and aching. Other common findings include proteinuria, calculi, uremia, and palpable kidney masses. Hypertension is another common finding and may be associated with cardiomegaly and heart failure. On occasion, polycystic lesions are found in other organs, such as the liver, thyroid, lungs, pancreas, and bladder. Cerebral aneurysms occur in only 2% of clients with polycystic kidney disease.

Test-Taking Strategy: Note that each of the options contains two items. In order for the option to be correct, both parts of the option must be correct. Knowing that it is not as common for cystic lesions to be present in other parts of the body helps you eliminate option 3. Correspondingly, knowing that coexisting cerebral aneurysms occur infrequently helps you to eliminate option 4. Both options 1 and 2 identify manifestations that occur with polycystic kidney disease. To discriminate between these options, it is necessary to know that flank pain and hematuria are the most common manifestations, which occur with greater frequency than renal failure or urinary calculi. Review assessment findings in polycystic kidney disease now if you had difficulty with this question!

Level of Cognitive Ability: Application
Phase of Nursing Process: Assessment
Client Needs: Physiological Integrity
Content Area: Adult Health/Renal

Reference

Black, J. M., & Matassarin-Jacobs, E. (1997). *Medical-surgical nursing: Clinical management for continuity of care* (5th ed.). Philadelphia: W. B. Saunders, p. 1678.

---

39. The client with urolithiasis is scheduled for extracorporeal shock wave lithotripsy. The nurse ensures that which of the following items are in place or maintained before the client is sent for the procedure?

1 Signed consent, clear liquid restriction, Foley catheter
2 Signed consent, NPO status, intravenous (IV) line
3 IV line, clear liquid restriction, Foley catheter
4 IV line, NPO status, Foley catheter

Answer: 2

Rationale: The client must sign a special consent and status must be NPO for the procedure. The client needs an IV line for the procedure as well.

Test-Taking Strategy: Begin to answer this question by eliminating options 3 and 4, because the client must sign a special consent for this procedure. To discriminate between options 1 and 2, it is necessary to know that the client is premedicated before the procedure. With this in mind, you would realize that the client must be NPO, and you would thus choose option 2 over option 1. If you had difficulty with this question, review the preprocedure preparation for extracorporeal shock wave lithotripsy.

Level of Cognitive Ability: Application
Phase of Nursing Process: Assessment
Client Needs: Safe, Effective Care Environment
Content Area: Adult Health/Renal

Reference

Black, J. M., & Matassarin-Jacobs, E. (1997). *Medical-surgical nursing: Clinical management for continuity of care* (5th ed.). Philadelphia: W. B. Saunders, p. 2070.

40. The client has developed atrial fibrillation with a ventricular rate of 150 per minute. The nurse assesses the client for

1 Hypotension and dizziness.
2 Nausea and vomiting.
3 Hypertension and headache.
4 Flat neck veins.

Answer: 1

Rationale: The client with uncontrolled atrial fibrillation and a ventricular rate of over 100 beats per minute is at risk for low cardiac output from loss of atrial kick. The nurse assesses the client for palpitations, chest pain or discomfort, hypotension, pulse deficit, fatigue, weakness, dizziness, syncope, shortness of breath, and distended neck veins.

Test-Taking Strategy: Flat neck veins are normal or indicate hypovolemia, so option 4 is eliminated. Nausea and vomiting (option 2) would be associated with vagus nerve activity, which does not correlate with a tachycardic state. Of the remaining choices, the correct response can be chosen by thinking of the consequences of falling cardiac output: hypotension and dizziness, not hypertension. Review the symptoms related to atrial fibrillation now if you had difficulty with this question!

Level of Cognitive Ability: Analysis
Phase of Nursing Process: Assessment
Client Needs: Physiological Integrity
Content Area: Adult Health/Cardiovascular

Reference

Ignatavicius, D. D., Workman, M. L., & Mishler, M. A. (1995). *Medical-surgical nursing: A nursing process approach* (2nd ed., Vol. 1). Philadelphia: W. B. Saunders, p. 841.

---

41. A preschooler with a history of cleft palate repair comes to the clinic for a routine well-child checkup. To determine whether this child is experiencing a long-term effect of cleft palate, a nurse should ask which of these questions?

1 "Was the child recently treated for pneumonia?"
2 "Does the child play with an imaginary friend?"

3 "Is the child unresponsive when given directions?"
4 "Has the child had any difficulty swallowing food?"

Answer: 3

Rationale: Unresponsiveness may be an indication that the child is experiencing hearing loss. A child who has a history of cleft palate should be routinely checked for hearing loss. Option 1 is incorrect and unrelated to cleft palate after repair; aspiration might occur before repair. The major concern is to prevent upper respiratory tract infections that lead to middle ear infections. Option 2 is normal behavior for a preschool child. Many preschoolers with vivid imaginations have imaginary friends; this is not indicative of poor socialization skills. Option 4 is incorrect because it is unrelated to cleft palate.

Test-Taking Strategy: This is a difficult question. It requires knowledge of the long-term complications associated with cleft palate as well as knowledge of normal growth and development for a preschooler. Using the process of elimination will assist you in selecting the correct response. If you had difficulty with this question, review content related to cleft palate now!

Level of Cognitive Ability: Application
Phase of Nursing Process: Assessment
Client Needs: Physiological Integrity
Content Area: Child Health

Reference

Pillitteri, A. (1995). *Maternal and child health nursing: Care of the childbearing and childrearing family* (2nd ed.). Philadelphia: Lippincott-Raven, pp. 903, 1128.

42. The nurse is performing a respiratory assessment on an asthmatic client. The nurse is alert to a worsening of the client's respiratory status when which of the following occurs?
   1 Loud wheezing heard throughout the lung field
   2 The absence of wheezing during inhalation
   3 Wheezing heard only during exhalation
   4 Noticeably diminished breath sounds

Answer: 4

Rationale: Wheezing is not a reliable manifestation to determine the severity of an asthma attack. Clients with minor attacks may wheeze loudly, whereas others with severe attacks may not wheeze. The client with severe asthma attacks may have no audible wheezing, because of the decrease of airflow. For wheezing to occur, the client must be able to move sufficient air to produce breath sounds. Wheezing usually occurs first on exhalation. As the asthma attack progresses, the client may wheeze during both inspiration and expiration. Severely decreased breath sounds are an indication of severe obstruction and possible respiratory failure.

Test-Taking Strategy: Remember the ABCs: airway, breathing, and circulation. The stem of the question asks you to identify a "worsening of the client's respiratory status." Remember that diminished breath sounds in a client indicate obstruction and possibly respiratory failure.

Level of Cognitive Ability: Analysis
Phase of Nursing Process: Assessment
Client Needs: Physiological Integrity
Content Area: Adult Health/Respiratory

Reference
Lewis, S. M., Collier, I. C., & Heitkemper, M. M. (1996). *Medical-surgical nursing: Assessment and management of clinical problems* (4th ed.). St. Louis: Mosby–Year Book, p. 686.

---

43. During the admission assessment of a client admitted for esophageal varices, the client says, "I deserve this. I brought it on myself." The nurse's most appropriate response is
   1 "Would you like to talk to the chaplain?"
   2 "Not all esophageal varices are caused by alcohol."
   3 "Is there some reason you feel you deserve this?"
   4 "That is something to think about when you leave the hospital."

Answer: 3

Rationale: Ruptured esophageal varices are often a complication of cirrhosis of the liver, and the most common type of cirrhosis is caused by chronic alcohol abuse. It is important to obtain an accurate history of alcohol intake from the client. If the client is ashamed or embarrassed, he or she may not respond accurately. Option 3 allows the client to discuss feelings about drinking.

Test-Taking Strategy: This question asks for the most appropriate nursing response. Option 1 could block the nurse-client communication process. Options 2 and 4 are somewhat judgmental. The open-ended nature of the question in option 3 allows the nurse and client to communicate. Remember that the client's feelings should be addressed first!

Level of Cognitive ability: Application
Phase of Nursing Process: Assessment
Client Needs: Psychosocial Integrity
Content Area: Adult Health/Gastrointestinal

Reference
Ignatavicius, D. D., Workman, M. L., & Mishler, M. A. (1995). *Medical-surgical nursing: A nursing process approach* (2nd ed., Vol. 2). Philadelphia: W. B. Saunders, p. 1668.

---

44. The nurse is assessing the casted extremity of a client. The nurse would assess for which of the following signs and symptoms indicative of infection?
   1 Coolness and pallor of the extremity
   2 Presence of a "hot spot" on the cast
   3 Diminished distal pulse
   4 Dependent edema

Answer: 2

Rationale: Signs and symptoms of infection under a casted area include odor or purulent drainage from the cast and the presence of "hot spots," which are areas of the cast that are warmer than others. The physician should be notified if any of these occur. Coolness and pallor of the skin, diminished arterial pulse, and edema are signs of impaired circulation in the distal limb.

Test-Taking Strategy: Begin to answer this question by thinking of what you would expect to find with infection: redness, swelling, heat, and purulent drainage. With these in mind, options 1, 3, and 4 can be eliminated easily. The "hot spot" on the cast could signify infection underneath that area and is therefore the correct answer to the question. Review the signs and symptoms of infection now if you had difficulty with this question!

Level of Cognitive Ability: Application
Phase of Nursing Process: Assessment
Client Needs: Physiological Integrity
Content Area: Adult Health/Musculoskeletal

Reference

Black, J. M., & Matassarin-Jacobs, E. (1997). *Medical-surgical nursing: Clinical management for continuity of care* (5th ed.). Philadelphia: W. B. Saunders, p. 2150.

---

45. The nurse assesses the preoperative teaching plan for a client scheduled for radical neck dissection. The nurse's initial assessment should focus on

1 Postoperative communication techniques.
2 Financial status of the client.
3 Client's support systems and coping behaviors.
4 Information given to the client by the surgeon.

Answer: 4

Rationale: The first step in client education is establishing what the client already knows. This allows the nurse not only to correct any misinformation but also to determine the starting point for teaching and to implement the education at the client's level.

Test-Taking Strategy: Look for the key word in the question. In this instance, the key word is "initial." It is likely that all of the options listed may be included in the teaching plan, but you need to determine what the initial assessment action would be. In the teaching-learning process, client motivation and readiness to learn along with what the client knows are initial assessment factors. Review the teaching-learning process now if you had difficulty with this question!

Level of Cognitive Ability: Application
Phase of Nursing Process: Assessment
Client Needs: Psychosocial Integrity
Content Area: Adult Health/Respiratory

Reference

Polaski, A., & Tatro, S. (1996). *Luckmann's Core principles and practice of medical-surgical nursing.* Philadelphia: W. B. Saunders, p. 557.

---

46. The nurse is assessing the client receiving heparin therapy. Which of the following assessments, if made by the nurse, would not indicate a potential complication of the therapy?

1 Dark, tarry stools
2 Hematest-negative nasogastric (NG) drainage
3 Bleeding gums
4 Oozing from the venipuncture site

Answer: 2

Rationale: The nurse monitors the client receiving anticoagulant therapy for adverse effects. These would include internal manifestations such as abdominal pain or swelling; backache; dizziness; headache; hematemesis; hemoptysis; hematuria; black or bloody stools; and Hematest-positive urine, stool, or NG drainage. Overt signs include ecchymoses; petechiae; hematomas; nosebleeds; and bleeding from gums, wounds, and invasive catheter insertion sites.

Test-Taking Strategy: This question is worded to direct you to look for the option that indicates a normal finding. Because the greatest risk associated with anticoagulant therapy is hemorrhage, the correct option is the one that indicates no active bleeding. Review the side effects and adverse effects of heparin therapy now if you had difficulty with this question!

Level of Cognitive Ability: Analysis
Phase of Nursing Process: Assessment
Client Needs: Physiological Integrity
Content Area: Pharmacology

Reference

Hodgson, B. & Kizior, R. (1998). Saunders nursing drug handbook 1998. Philadelphia: W. B. Saunders, pp. 489–491.

47. The medication nurse is supervising a newly hired licensed practical nurse (LPN) during the administration of pyridostigmine (Mestinon) PO to a client with myasthenia gravis. Which assessment, if made by the medication nurse, would demonstrate safe practice by the LPN?

1. Asking the client to lie down on the right side
2. Instructing the client to void before taking the medication
3. Asking the client to take sips of water
4. Asking the client to look up to the ceiling for 30 seconds

Answer: 3

Rationale: Myasthenia gravis can affect the client's ability to swallow. The primary assessment is to determine the client's ability to swallow. Options 1 and 4 are not appropriate. In this situation, there is no reason for the client to lie down to swallow medication or to look up to the ceiling. There is no specific reason for the client to void before this medication.

Test-Taking Strategy: Knowledge about myasthenia gravis and the nursing care involved with the administration of PO medications or other PO substances is necessary to answer this question. Use the process of elimination to answer this question. Note that the case addresses a PO medication. From this, a relationship can be made with option 3, "sips of water." If you had difficulty with this question, review nursing care to the client with myasthenia gravis now!

Level of Cognitive Ability: Analysis
Phase of the Nursing Process: Assessment
Client Needs: Safe, Effective Care Environment
Content Area: Fundamental Skills

Reference

Lehne, R. A. (1998). *Pharmacology for nursing care* (3rd ed.). Philadelphia: W. B. Saunders, p. 132.

---

48. While conducting a prenatal assessment history with a pregnant adolescent, which finding would the nurse assess as not being a risk factor for human immunodeficiency virus (HIV) infection?

1. Development level of client
2. Negative history of IV drug abuse
3. Unprotected sexual contact with multiple partners
4. Residing in an inner city dwelling

Answer: 2

Rationale: Adolescents are particularly susceptible to HIV infection because they often practice high-risk behaviors. In addition, they frequently lack appropriate knowledge regarding disease transmission. According to sociodemographic data, infection rates are more prevalent in urban areas. HIV infection among females is primarily associated with injecting drugs and heterosexual contact with an at-risk partner.

Test-Taking Strategy: This question asks you to apply current concepts of HIV acquisition and sociodemographic characteristics of at-risk populations (adolescent females). This question further relies upon your ability to include questions related to drug abuse and sexual behaviors in all prenatal history-taking interviews. Review risk characteristics for HIV now if you had difficulty with this question!

Level of Cognitive Ability: Analysis
Phase of Nursing Process: Assessment
Client Needs: Physiological Integrity
Content Area: Maternity

Reference

Reeder, S., Martin, L., & Koniak-Griffin, D. (1997). *Maternity nursing: Family, newborn, and women's health care* (18th ed.). Philadelphia: Lippincott-Raven, pp. 284–285.

49. The home care client with chronic obstructive pulmonary disease (COPD) is complaining of increased dyspnea. The client is on home oxygen with a concentrator at 2 liters per minute. The respiratory rate is 22 breaths per minute. The nurse's assessment would focus on

1 Determining the need to increase the oxygen.
2 Conducting further assessment of the client's respiratory status.
3 The need for emergency services to come to the home.
4 The need to reassure the client that there is no need to worry.

Answer: 2

Rationale: Completing an assessment on the client is the first priority, unless of course the client is in respiratory distress, which was not indicated in this question. The client's respiratory rate is 22 breaths per minute. Dyspnea is the client's response to lack of oxygen and is not a quantifiable, objective finding. Reassuring the client is appropriate but not the initial priority, and an assessment must be completed. Calling the emergency services seems premature. The oxygen is not to be increased without the approval of the physician, especially because clients with COPD can retain carbon dioxide.

Test-Taking Strategy: Answers to this question include assessment options with the primary focus on the severity of the situation. There is no immediate need or signs of imminent danger, thus eliminating option 3. Providing reassurance should occur after the assessment has been completed. Remember assessment is the first step of the nursing process. Also remember the ABCs: airway, breathing, and circulation!

Level of Cognitive Ability: Application
Phase of Nursing Process: Assessment
Client Needs: Physiological Integrity
Content Area: Adult Health/Respiratory

Reference

Como, N. (1995). *Home health nursing pocket consultant.* St. Louis: Mosby–Year Book, p. 195.

---

50. The diabetic client has expressed frustration in learning the diabetic regimen and insulin administration. The home health care nurse would

1 Identify the causes of frustration.
2 Continue with diabetic teaching, knowing that the client will overcome any frustrations.
3 Call the physician to discuss termination from home health care services.
4 Offer to administer the insulin on a daily basis until the client is ready to learn.

Answer: 1

Rationale: The home health care nurse must determine what in the teaching is causing the client's frustration. Continuing to teach may only aggravate the learning process, and termination of the client from home care services achieves nothing. Administering insulin may be a short-term solution but not until the assessment has been complete and the reason why the client is frustrated is identified. Terminating services constitutes abandonment unless suitable arrangements have been made for follow-up care.

Test-Taking Strategy: Remember the steps of the nursing process. Assessment is the first step. Of the four options presented, options 2, 3, and 4 represent implementation phases of the nursing process. The only assessment option is option 1.

Level of Cognitive Ability: Application
Phase of Nursing Process: Assessment
Client Needs: Psychosocial Integrity
Content Area: Adult Health/Endocrine

Reference

Zang, S., & Bailey, N. (1997). *Home care manual: Making the transition.* Philadelphia: Lippincott-Raven, p. 514.

Read

51. A client with schizophrenia tells the nurse, "I stopped taking my Thorazine [chlorpromazine] because of the way it made me feel." What side effects is the nurse likely to note during the assessment of the client's complaint?

1 Polyuria, thirst, weight gain, mild nausea
2 Constipation, sedation, hypotension, dizziness
3 Fine hand tremor, hypertension, dry mouth, photophobia
4 Blurred vision, diarrhea, headache, lip smacking

Answer: 2

Rationale: Side effects of chlorpromazine (Thorazine) can include hypotension, dizziness and fainting (especially with parenteral use), drowsiness, blurred vision, dry mouth, lethargy, constipation or diarrhea, nasal congestion, peripheral edema, and urinary retention.

Test-Taking Strategy: Knowledge about chlorpromazine (Thorazine) and side effects is necessary to assist you in answering this question. All of the components of the option must be the side effects of chlorpromazine (Thorazine) for the option to be correct. If you are unfamiliar with the medication addressed and side effects of this medication, it would be important for you to review this information now!

Level of Cognitive Ability: Analysis
Phase of Nursing Process: Assessment
Client Needs: Physiological Integrity
Content Area: Pharmacology

Reference

Hodgson, B., & Kizior, R. (1998). *Saunders nursing drug handbook 1998.* Philadelphia: W. B. Saunders, pp. 212–213.

---

52. The home health nurse is making follow-up visits to the client after renal transplantation. The nurse assesses for signs of acute graft rejection, which include

1 Hypotension, graft tenderness, and anemia.
2 Hypertension, oliguria, thirst, and hypothermia.
3 Fever, vomiting, hypotension, and copious amounts of dilute urine.
4 Fever, hypertension, graft tenderness, and malaise.

Answer: 4

Rationale: Acute rejection usually occurs within the first 3 months after transplantation, although it can occur for up to 2 years after transplantation. The client exhibits fever, hypertension, malaise, and graft tenderness.

Test-Taking Strategy: Use the process of elimination in answering this question. Begin by eliminating options 1 and 3, because hypotension is not part of the clinical picture with graft rejection. You would choose option 4 over option 2 because fever, not hypothermia, accompanies this complication.

Level of Cognitive Ability: Application
Phase of Nursing Process: Assessment
Client Needs: Physiological Integrity
Content Area: Adult Health/Renal

Reference

Black, J. M., & Matassarin-Jacobs, E. (1997). *Medical-surgical nursing: Clinical management for continuity of care* (5th ed.). Philadelphia: W. B. Saunders, p. 1662.

---

53. The nurse is caring for a client with a skin infection. The client is receiving tobramycin sulfate (Nebcin) intravenously every 8 hours. Which of the following would indicate to the nurse that the client is experiencing an adverse reaction to the medication?

1 A blood urea nitrogen (BUN) level of 30 mg/dL
2 A white blood cell count of 6000/μL
3 A sedimentation rate of 15 mm/hour
4 A total bilirubin level of 0.5 mg/dL

Answer: 1

Rationale: Adverse reactions to or toxic effects of tobramycin sulfate (Nebcin) include nephrotoxicity, as evidenced by increases in BUN and serum creatinine; irreversible ototoxicity, as evidenced by tinnitus, dizziness, ringing or roaring in the ears, and reduced hearing; and neurotoxicity, as evidenced by headaches, dizziness, lethargy, tremors, and visual disturbances. A normal white blood cell count is 5,000–10,000/μL; the normal sedimentation rate is 0–30 mm/hour; the normal total bilirubin level is 0.3–1 mg/dL; and the normal BUN is 5–20 mg/dL. Option 1 indicates an elevation in the BUN, which should alert the nurse to the potential of nephrotoxicity related to medication administration.

Test-Taking Strategy: Knowledge about tobramycin sulfate (Nebcin) and of normal laboratory values is necessary to answer this question. Knowledge of normal values would assist you in selecting option 1 because this is the only abnormal laboratory value presented among the four options. If you are unfamiliar with this medication or these laboratory values, take the time now to review this content!

Level of Cognitive Ability: Analysis
Phase of Nursing Process: Assessment
Client Needs: Physiological Integrity
Content Area: Pharmacology

Reference
Hodgson, B., & Kizior, R. (1998). *Saunders nursing drug handbook 1998.* Philadelphia: W. B. Saunders, pp. 998–1000.

---

54. Nursing assessments of the client suspected of carbon monoxide poisoning are directed primarily toward assessment of the

1 Level of consciousness.
2 Cardiac monitor.
3 Respiratory rate.
4 Skin color.

Answer: 1

Rationale: The neurological system is primarily affected by carbon monoxide poisoning. With high levels of carbon monoxide, the neurological status progressively deteriorates.

Test-Taking Strategy: This question requires knowledge that carbon monoxide depresses the nervous system. Note the key words "primarily," and "suspected of." If you are unfamiliar with the assessment findings in carbon monoxide poisoning, review this content now!

Level of Cognitive Ability: Application
Phase of Nursing Process: Assessment
Client Needs: Physiological Integrity
Content Area: Adult Health/Respiratory

Reference
LeMone, P., & Burke, K. (1996). *Medical-surgical nursing: Critical thinking in client care.* Menlo Park, CA: Addison-Wesley, p. 630.

---

55. The nurse is performing cardiovascular assessment of a client. Which of the following items would the nurse assess to gain the best information about the client's left-sided heart function?

1 Breath sounds
2 Peripheral edema
3 Jugular vein distention
4 Hepatojugular reflux

Answer: 1

Rationale: The client with heart failure may exhibit different symptoms, depending on whether the right or the left side of the heart is failing. Peripheral edema, jugular vein distention, and hepatojugular reflux are all indicators of right-sided heart function. Breath sounds are an accurate indicator of left-sided heart function.

Test-Taking Strategy: The client with left-sided heart failure may also have right-sided symptoms if failure is severe. The question asks for the "best" information about left-sided heart function. The correct answer, then, is one that reflects only the left side, which would be breath sounds. Use the mnemonic "left" and "lungs." Options 2, 3, and 4 reflect right-sided heart failure. Take time now to review the signs of right- and left-sided heart failure if you had difficulty with this question!

Level of Cognitive Ability: Application
Phase of Nursing Process: Assessment
Client Needs: Physiological Integrity
Content Area: Adult Health/Cardiovascular

Reference
Smeltzer, S., & Bare, B. (1996). *Brunner and Suddarth's Textbook of medical-surgical nursing* (8th ed.). Philadelphia: Lippincott-Raven, pp. 600, 604.

56. The nurse is obtaining a nursing history from the client admitted with a thrombotic cerebrovascular accident (CVA). The nurse assesses that in the few days before the incident, the client experienced

1. Transient hemiparesis and loss of speech.
2. Throbbing headaches.
3. Unexplained episodes of loss of consciousness.
4. No symptoms at all.

Answer: 1

Rationale: Cerebral thrombosis does not occur suddenly. In the few hours or days preceding a thrombotic CVA, the client may experience a transient loss of speech, hemiplegia, or paresthesias on one side of the body. Signs and symptoms of thrombotic CVA vary but may include dizziness, cognitive changes, and seizures. Headache is rare.

Test-Taking Strategy: This question tests knowledge of premonitory warning signs of CVA. Option 4 should be discarded first because it is not true. Option 3 is irrelevant, and option 2 occurs with sudden-onset CVA. This leaves option 1 as the correct answer. If you had difficulty with this question, take time now to review the signs and symptoms of CVA!

Level of Cognitive Ability: Application
Phase of Nursing Process: Assessment
Client Needs: Physiological Integrity
Content Area: Adult Health/Neurological

Reference
Smeltzer, S., & Bare, B. (1996). *Brunner and Suddarth's Textbook of medical-surgical nursing* (8th ed.). Philadelphia: Lippincott-Raven, p. 1725.

---

57. A client in a long-term care facility has had a series of gastrointestinal (GI) diagnostic tests, including upper GI series and endoscopies. Upon the client's return to the long-term care facility, the priority nursing assessment should focus on

1. Level of consciousness.
2. Activity tolerance.
3. Hydration and nutrition status.
4. Comfort level.

Answer: 3

Rationale: Many of the diagnostic studies to identify GI disorders require that the GI tract be cleaned (usually with laxatives and enemas) before testing. In addition, the client's status is most often NPO before and during the testing period. Because the studies may be done over a period exceeding 24 hours, the client may become dehydrated and/or malnourished.

Test-Taking Strategy: All the options are important and should be part of the assessment process of any client in a long-term care facility. The stem of the question asks for the "priority nursing assessment," which is hydration and nutrition status.

Level of Cognitive Ability: Application
Phase of Nursing Process: Assessment
Client Needs: Physiological Integrity
Content Area: Adult Health/Gastrointestinal

Reference
Lewis, S. M., Collier, I. C., & Heitkemper, M. M. (1996). *Medical-surgical nursing: Assessment and management of clinical problems* (4th ed.). St. Louis: Mosby–Year Book, p. 1097.

---

58. The nurse is assessing a preoperative client. Which of the following questions will help the nurse determine the client's risk for developing malignant hyperthermia postoperatively?

1. "What is your normal body temperature?"
2. "Do you experience frequent infections?"
3. "Do you have a family history of problems with general anesthesia?"
4. "Have you ever suffered from heat exhaustion or heat stroke?"

Answer: 3

Rationale: Malignant hyperthermia is a genetic disorder in which a combination of anesthetic agents (succinylcholine and inhalation agents such as halothane) triggers uncontrolled skeletal muscle contractions. This leads quickly to a potentially fatal hyperthermia. Questioning the client about family history of general anesthesia problems may reveal this as a possibility for the client.

Test-Taking Strategy: To answer this question correctly you must know that malignant hypertension is a complication of anesthesia. Knowing this, you can evaluate each of the options in terms of their connection to general anesthesia. Knowledge of the client's normal body temperature is irrelevant and can be discarded first. Fevers from infection and heat stroke are triggered by environmental factors (organisms and air temperature). The only option that is connected to surgery is option 3. If you had difficulty with this question, take the time now to review postoperative complications!

Level of Cognitive Ability: Application
Phase of Nursing Process: Assessment
Client Needs: Physiological Integrity
Content Area: Fundamental Skills

Reference

Black, J. M., & Matassarin-Jacobs, E. (1997). *Medical-surgical nursing: Clinical management for continuity of care* (5th ed.). Philadelphia: W. B. Saunders, pp. 478–479.

---

59. The nurse is caring for a client who has undergone cystoscopy. The nurse would assess for which of the following abnormal signs in the first few hours after the procedure?

1 Pink-tinged urine
2 Bloody urine with clots
3 Clear yellow urine
4 Urine with a bluish or green tinge

Answer: 2

Rationale: The client may have clear or pink-tinged urine after cystoscopy. If a contrast agent such as methylene blue is used, the urine may have an unusual color such as bluish or green. Grossly bloody urine with clots is always an abnormal finding and should be reported immediately.

Test-Taking Strategy: Begin to answer this question by eliminating option 3, because this is the normal finding. Option 1 is eliminated next, knowing that minor trauma from the procedure could cause pink-tinged urine. To discriminate between the last two options, it is necessary to know that methylene blue might be used for contrast, which could cause the discoloration noted in option 4. If you know that bloody urine with clots indicates active, current bleeding, you would select option 2 as the abnormal sign, which should be reported.

Level of Cognitive Ability: Application
Phase of Nursing Process: Assessment
Client Needs: Physiological Integrity
Content Area: Adult Health/Renal

Reference

Black, J. M., & Matassarin-Jacobs, E. (1997). *Medical-surgical nursing: Clinical management for continuity of care* (5th ed.). Philadelphia: W. B. Saunders, p. 1568.

---

60. A nursing instructor is teaching a student about increased intracranial pressure (ICP). The instructor tells that student that increased ICP is a life-threatening event. The instructor assesses the student's knowledge regarding the three types of noncompressible cranial contents, which would include which of the following?

1 Ventricles, blood volume, and the subarachnoid space
2 Cerebrospinal fluid, the brain, and the foramen ovale
3 Semisolid brain tissue, cerebrospinal fluid, and the intravascular blood
4 Grey matter, white matter, and the extrapyramidal tract

Answer: 3

Rationale: When the volume of any of these three components increases, one or both of the other components must decrease proportionally, or an increase in ICP will occur.

Test-Taking Strategy: This is a difficult question and requires an understanding of the pathophysiological processes associated with ICP. There is only one correct answer. If you had difficulty answering this question, take time now to review the pathophysiological processes associated with increased ICP!

Level of Cognitive Ability: Analysis
Phase of Nursing Process: Assessment
Client Needs: Physiological Integrity
Content Area: Adult Health/Neurological

Reference

Hartshorn, J., Sole, M. L., & Lamborn, M. L. (1997). *Introduction to critical care nursing* (2nd ed.). Philadelphia: W. B. Saunders, p. 271.

61. The client with acute myocardial infarction receives therapy with alteplase recombinant, or tissue plasminogen activator (t-PA). The nurse assesses for complications of this treatment. Which assessment data would the nurse document as indicating a possible complication?

1 Epistaxis
2 Vomiting
3 ST segment elevation on the electrocardiogram (ECG)
4 Absent pedal pulses

Answer: 1

Rationale: Bleeding is a major side effect of t-PA therapy. The bleeding can be superficial or internal and can be spontaneous. The other options are not correlated with the side effects of t-PA therapy. Resolution of ST segment elevation is one of the expected results of t-PA therapy.

Test-Taking Strategy: Identify the key issue of the question as a complication of the medication. Knowledge about the medication and the actions and side effects of t-PA is needed. Knowledge that the medication is a thrombolytic and that bleeding is a common side effect will assist in answering the question. Knowledge that epistaxis is a bloody nose will direct you toward option 1. If you had difficulty with this question, take the time now to review t-PA!

Level of Cognitive Ability: Application
Phase of Nursing Process: Assessment
Client Needs: Physiological Integrity
Content Area: Pharmacology

Reference

Wilson, B., Shannon, M., & Stang, C. (1997). *Nurses drug guide.* Stamford, CT: Appleton & Lange, pp. 30–31.

---

62. The nurse is caring for the client who has returned from the postanesthesia care unit after prostatectomy. The client has a three-way Foley catheter with an infusion of continuous bladder irrigation. The nurse assesses that the flow rate is adequate if the color of the urinary drainage is

1 Dark cherry-colored.
2 Concentrated yellow with small clots.
3 Clear as water.
4 Pale yellow or slightly pink.

Answer: 4

Rationale: The infusion of bladder irrigant is not at a preset rate; rather, it is increased or decreased to maintain urine that is a clear pale yellow color or that has just a slight pink tinge. The infusion rate should be increased if the drainage is cherry-colored or if clots are seen. Correspondingly, the rate can be slowed down slightly if the returns are as clear as water.

Test-Taking Strategy: Use the process of elimination. Begin to answer this question by eliminating option 2 as the least realistic of all the urine characteristics described in the options. You would then systematically eliminate options 1 and 3 as reflecting inadequate and excessive flow, respectively. This leaves option 4 as the correct answer. With proper flow rate of bladder irrigant, the urine should be pale yellow or pale pink.

Level of Cognitive Ability: Application
Phase of Nursing Process: Assessment
Client Needs: Physiological Integrity
Content Area: Adult Health/Renal

Reference

Black, J. M., & Matassarin-Jacobs, E. (1997). *Medical-surgical nursing: Clinical management for continuity of care* (5th ed.). Philadelphia: W. B. Saunders, p. 2361.

---

63. The client has been taking methyldopa (Aldomet) for approximately 2 months. The home care nurse monitoring the effects of therapy would expect to assess tolerance to the medication, if it were to develop, by noting which of the following?

1 Increase in weight
2 Dependent edema
3 Output greater than intake
4 Gradual rise in blood pressure

Answer: 4

Rationale: During the second or third month of therapy, medication tolerance can develop, which is evident by rising blood pressure levels. The physician should be notified.

Test-Taking Strategy: To answer this question correctly, you need to know the definition of medication tolerance: as a client adjusts to a medication, the therapeutic effect diminishes. In addition, knowledge that the medication is an antihypertensive will easily direct you to option 4. If you had difficulty with this question, take time now to review methyldopa.

Level of Cognitive Ability: Application
Phase of Nursing Process: Assessment
Client Needs: Physiological Integrity
Content Area: Pharmacology

Reference

McKenry, L., & Salerno, E. (1995). *Mosby's pharmacology in nursing* (19th ed.). St. Louis: Mosby–Year Book, p. 601.

---

64. The client's vital signs have noticeably deteriorated over the past 4 hours after surgery. The nurse does not recognize the significance of these changes in vital signs and takes no action. The client later requires emergency surgery. The nurse could be prosecuted for that action according to the definition of which of these?

1 Tort
2 Misdemeanor
3 Common law
4 Statutory law

Answer: 1

Rationale: A tort is a wrongful act intentionally or unintentionally committed against a person or his property. The nurse's inaction in the situation described is consistent with the definition of a tort offense. Option 2 is an offense under criminal law; option 3 describes case law that has evolved over time through precedents; option 4 describes laws that are enacted by state, federal, or local governments.

Test-Taking Strategy: This question requires that you understand the differences among the four types of law described. Review the definitions related to these laws now if you had difficulty with this question!

Level of Cognitive Ability: Analysis
Phase of the Nursing Process: Assessment
Client Needs: Physiological Integrity
Content Area: Fundamental Skills

Reference

Catalano, J. T. (1996). *Contemporary professional nursing.* Philadelphia: F. A. Davis, pp. 294–298.

---

65. A client with a history of panic disorder comes to the emergency room and tells the nurse, "Please help me. I think I'm having a heart attack." What nursing assessment is indicated first?

1 Identify the client activity during the pain
2 Assess the signs related to the panic disorder
3 Assess the client's vital signs
4 Determine the client's use of relaxation techniques

Answer: 3

Rationale: Clients with panic disorders experience acute physical symptoms, such as chest pain and palpitations. However, it is critical to assess the physical condition first to rule out a physiological disorder.

Test-Taking Strategy: Assessment of the client's physical status as an initial nursing action is always indicated. Use the ABCs—airway, breathing, and circulation—to answer this question! Be alert to questions that present a psychiatric diagnosis as a distractor that can lead to choosing an incorrect option.

Level of Cognitive Ability: Application
Phase of the Nursing Process: Assessment
Client Needs: Physiological Integrity
Content Area: Mental Health

Reference

Wilson, H., & Kneisl, C. (1996). *Psychiatric nursing* (5th ed.). Menlo Park, CA: Addison-Wesley, p. 373.

66. Which of the following antipsychotic medications can be given in timed-release form and is therefore a good choice for clients in the community who have a history of noncompliance?

1. Fluphenazine decanoate (Prolixin Decanoate)
2. Clozapine (Clozaril)
3. Thioridazine (Mellaril)
4. Haloperidol (Haldol)

Answer: 1

Rationale: The decanoate form of prolixin is an injectable and given every 1–2 weeks. Because it is long-acting and administered by a nurse, it is a good choice for clients who are ambivalent about compliance.

Test-Taking Strategy: Knowledge about medications is necessary to assist you in answering this question. If you know that Prolixin Decanoate is a long-acting antipsychotic, you would select this option. If you are unfamiliar with the medication addressed in this question and the other medications in this classification, it is important to review them now!

Level of Cognitive Ability: Analysis
Phase of Nursing Process: Assessment
Client Needs: Physiological Integrity
Content Area: Pharmacology

Reference
Haber, J. (1997). *Comprehensive psychiatric nursing* (5th ed.). St. Louis: Mosby–Year Book, p. 265.

---

67. Which of the following assessment data would indicate early signs of alcohol withdrawal?

1. Anxiety, tremor, insomnia, tachycardia
2. Disorientation, diaphoresis, insomnia
3. Delusions, fever, vomiting, agitation
4. Clouding of consciousness, tachycardia

Answer: 1

Rationale: Early signs of alcohol withdrawal develop within a few hours after cessation or reduction of alcohol and peak after 24–48 hours. Early signs of withdrawal include anxiety, anorexia, insomnia, tremor, irritability, elevations in pulse and blood pressure, nausea, vomiting, and hallucinations or illusions.

Test-Taking Strategy: Focus your attention to the use of the word "early" in this question. Knowledge of the early signs of withdrawal and alcohol withdrawal delirium will help you choose the correct option. If you are not familiar with the signs and symptoms of alcohol withdrawal and delirium, it is helpful for you to review this content now!

Level of Cognitive Ability: Analysis
Phase of Nursing Process: Assessment
Client Needs: Physiological Integrity
Content Area: Mental Health

Reference
Varcarolis, E. (1998). *Foundations of psychiatric mental health nursing* (3rd ed.). Philadelphia: W. B. Saunders, p. 754.

---

68. Home health care nurses are responsible for the assessment of a client's functional abilities or activities of daily living (ADLs). This assessment requires an evaluation of the client's

1. Self-care needs, such as toileting, feeding, and ambulating.
2. Normal everyday routine in the home.
3. Ability to do light housework, heavy housework, and pay the bills.
4. Abnormal physiological status.

Answer: 1

Rationale: "Activities of daily living" refer to the client's ability to bathe, toilet, ambulate, dress, and feed himself or herself. These functional abilities are always assessed by home health care nurses. The normal routine in the home is not a functional assessment. The ability to do housework relates to instrumental activities of daily living. Abnormal physiological status is related to ADLs but is not the same definitionally.

Test-Taking Strategy: Knowledge of the definitions of ADLs assists in answering this question, thereby eliminating all of the other options. Review the concepts of ADLs now if you had difficulty with this question!

Level of Cognitive Ability: Application
Phase of Nursing Process: Assessment
Client Needs: Physiological Integrity
Content Area: Fundamental Skills

Reference

Como, N. (1995). *Home health nursing pocket consultant.* St. Louis: Mosby–Year Book, p. 98.

---

69. The home health care nurse is admitting a client who has recently received a diagnosis of Alzheimer's disease. The assessment would include which of the following?

1 Problems with concrete thinking
2 Problems with hearing
3 Recent memory loss
4 Difficulty in performing new tasks

Answer: 3

Rationale: Dementia is the hallmark of Alzheimer's disease. Problems with abstract thinking, problems with speech (not hearing), and difficulty in performing familiar tasks are also assessment findings.

Test-Taking Strategy: This question requires basic knowledge of Alzheimer's disease. Review Alzheimer's disease now if you had difficulty with this question.

Level of Cognitive Ability: Application
Phase of Nursing Process: Assessment
Client Needs: Physiological Integrity
Content Area: Adult Health/Neurological

Reference

Rice, R. (1996). *Home health nursing: Practice, concepts and application* (2nd ed.). St. Louis: Mosby–Year Book, p. 317.

---

70. A client is to receive continuous intravenous (IV) fluid replacement for the treatment of dehydration. Which of the following is essential for the nurse to assess before initiating venipuncture?

1 Usual sleep patterns
2 Ability to ambulate
3 Body weight
4 Intake and output

Answer: 3

Rationale: Body weight is a key indicator of fluid status, and a baseline weight should be obtained. Accurate body weight is a better measurement of gains and losses than are intake and output records. An IV line should not greatly alter sleep patterns, and clients will still be able to ambulate with a peripheral IV site.

Test-Taking Strategy: Read the stem carefully for the key terms "essential" and "before." Eliminate the incorrect options that have little pertinence to IV therapy. Remember that body weight is a better measurement of gains and losses.

Level of Cognitive Ability: Application
Phase of Nursing Process: Assessment
Client Needs: Physiological Integrity
Content Area: Fundamental Skills

Reference

Phillips, L. D. (1997). *Manual of IV therapeutics* (2nd ed.). Philadelphia: F. A. Davis, p. 58.

71. The nurse is caring for a client who returns from cardiac surgery with chest tubes in place. The nurse assesses the drainage on an hourly basis and assesses that the client is stable as long as drainage does not exceed how many milliliters over the first 24 hours?

1 100 mL
2 200 mL
3 500 mL
4 1000 mL

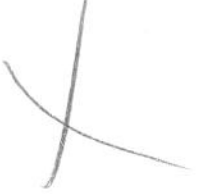

Answer: 3

Rationale: Approximately 500 mL of drainage is expected in the first 24 hours after cardiac surgery. Up to 100 mL may be lost in the first hour postoperatively. The nurse measures and records the drainage on an hourly basis.

Test-Taking Strategy: Options 1 and 2 are least plausible because the values are so small. To discriminate between the remaining options, try converting the drainage to liters (1000 mL = 1 liter; 500 mL = 1/2 liter). Knowing that there are only about 6 liters of blood circulating in the body, this technique may help you choose option 3 over option 4.

Level of Cognitive Ability: Analysis
Phase of Nursing Process: Assessment
Client Needs: Physiological Integrity
Content Area: Adult Health/Cardiovascular

Reference

Black, J. M., & Matassarin-Jacobs, E. (1997). *Medical-surgical nursing: Clinical management for continuity of care* (5th ed.). Philadelphia: W. B. Saunders, p. 1359.

---

72. The nurse is trying to determine the client's adjustment to a new diagnosis of coronary heart disease before discharge. Of the following questions, which one should the nurse ask to elicit the most useful response by the client?

1 "Do you have anyone at home to help with housework and shopping?"
2 "How do you feel about the lifestyle changes you are planning to make?"
3 "Do you understand the use of your new medications?"
4 "Are you going to book your follow-up physician visit?"

Answer: 2

Rationale: All questions relate to aspects of posthospital care, but only option 2 explores the client's feelings about the disease.

Test-Taking Strategy: Open-ended questions are needed to explore client's reactions to or feelings about an identified situation. Closed-ended questions generally elicit a "yes" or "no" response exclusively. All of the incorrect options are closed-ended responses. Avoid closed-ended questions, and always select the option that addresses the client's feelings!

Level of Cognitive Ability: Application
Phase of Nursing Process: Assessment
Client Needs: Health Promotion and Maintenance
Content Area: Adult Health/Cardiovascular

Reference

Potter, P. A., & Perry, A. G. (1997). *Fundamentals of nursing: Concepts, process, and practice* (4th ed.). St. Louis: Mosby–Year Book, pp. 241–242.

---

73. A client is scheduled for an arteriogram with a radiopaque dye. Which of the following assessments is most critical before the procedure?

1 Intake and output before procedure
2 Baseline vital signs
3 Height and weight
4 Allergy to iodine or shellfish

Answer: 4

Rationale: This procedure requires an informed consent, as it involves injection of a radiopaque dye into the blood vessel. The risk of allergic reaction and possible anaphylaxis must be assessed before the procedure.

Test-Taking Strategy: The question asks you for the "most critical" assessment, implying that several options may be plausible. Using the concept of criticality, eliminate options 1 and 3. The remaining options compete for priority, but the risk of anaphylaxis makes option 4 the correct choice. If you had difficulty with this question, review preprocedure care for angiography now!

Level of Cognitive Ability: Application
Phase of Nursing Process: Assessment
Client Needs: Physiological Integrity
Content Area: Adult Health/Neurological

Reference

Ignatavicius, D. D., Workman, M. L., & Mishler, M. A. (1995). *Medical-surgical nursing: A nursing process approach* (2nd ed., Vol. 1). Philadelphia: W. B. Saunders, p. 801.

74. The nurse is caring for a client admitted for subclavian catheter placement. Which of the following psychosocial areas of assessment should the nurse address with the client?

1. Strict restrictions of neck mobility
2. Loss of ability to ambulate as tolerated
3. Possible body image disturbance
4. Continuous pain related to ongoing placement of the subclavian catheter

Answer: 3

Rationale: When a client is going to have a central catheter in the subclavian area, they will be able to move as tolerated. The client may have pain when the catheter is placed, but the pain will not last continuously. The client may, however, be self-conscious with regard to the catheter, experiencing altered body image.

Test-Taking Strategy: The correct answer has to relate to a psychosocial concern. Pain, altered mobility, and restricted neck movements are physical concerns. Remember to key in on client anxieties and concerns and choose the answer that addresses these. Read the question carefully and note that psychosocial is stated in the stem of the question.

Level of Cognitive Ability: Analysis
Phase of Nursing Process: Assessment
Client Needs: Psychosocial Integrity
Content Area: Fundamental Skills

Reference

McFarland, G. & McFarlane, E. (1997). *Nursing diagnosis and intervention* (3rd ed.). St. Louis: Mosby–Year Book, p. 563.

---

75. The nurse continues to assess a client in late first-stage labor for progress and fetal well-being. At the last vaginal examination, there was full effacement, 8 centimeters' dilation, vertex presentation, station 1. Which of the following findings would prompt the nurse to notify the physician that the fetus was in serious fetal distress?

1. Vaginal examination continues to reveal some old meconium staining of the liquid, and the fetal monitor demonstrates a U-shaped pattern of deceleration during contractions, recovering to a baseline of 140
2. Fresh, thick meconium is passed with a small gush of liquid, and the fetal monitor shows late decelerations with a variable descending baseline
3. Fresh meconium is found on the examiner's gloved fingers after a vaginal examination, and the fetal monitor pattern remains essentially unchanged
4. The fetal heart rate slowly drops to 110 during strong contractions, recovering to 138 immediately afterward

Answer: 2

Rationale: Meconium staining alone is not a sign of fetal distress. Old meconium staining may be the result of a prenatal trauma now resolved. It is not unusual for fetal heart rates to drop below the 140–160 range in late labor during contractions, but in a healthy fetus, the heart rate will recover between contractions. Fresh meconium in combination with decelerating nonremediable fetal heart tones is an ominous signal of serious fetal distress from fetal hypoxia.

Test-Taking Strategy: Option 4 can be easily eliminated. Next, eliminate option 1 becasue of the words "old meconium." From the remaining options, noting that option 3 addresses an unchanged fetal pattern will direct you to option 2.

Level of Cognitive Ability: Application
Nursing Process: Assessment
Client Needs: Physiological Integrity
Content Area: Maternity

Reference

Lowdermilk, D., Perry, S., & Bobak, I. (1997). *Maternity and women's health care* (6th ed.). St. Louis: Mosby–Year Book, p. 688.

76. A well-known individual from the community is admitted to the unit with a diagnosis of Parkinson's disease. The nurse gives information regarding the client's condition to a person assumed to be a family member. Later, the nurse realizes that she or he has violated which legal concept of the nurse-client relationship?

1 Invasion of privacy
2 Lack of experience
3 Teaching/learning principles
4 Performing focused physical assessment

Answer: 1

Rationale: Discussing a client's condition without the client's permission violates the client's rights and places the nurse in legal jeopardy. This action by the nurse both is an invasion of privacy and affects the confidentiality issue with client rights.

Test-Taking Strategy: Use the process of elimination in answering this question. Option 2 is a distractor; however, lack of experience could lead to negligence. Teaching-learning principles and physical assessment (options 3 and 4) are considered concepts of standards of practice. Giving false information or performing the assessment incorrectly would constitute negligence. The issue of this question is related to sharing information, which constitutes an invasion of privacy. It is extremely important that you understand client rights. If you had difficulty with this question, take the time now to review client rights!

Level of Cognitive Ability: Application
Phase of Nursing Process: Assessment
Client Need: Safe, Effective Care Environment
Content Area: Adult Health/Neurological

Reference

Potter, P. A., & Perry, A. G. (1997). *Fundamentals of nursing: Concepts, process, and practice* (4th ed.). St. Louis: Mosby–Year Book, p. 66.

---

77. The nurse assesses a client who has a nasogastric tube in place after abdominal surgery. Which of the following observations by the nurse indicates most reliably that the tube is functioning properly?

1 The suction gauge reads low intermittent suction
2 The distal end of the nasogastric tube is pinned to the client's gown
3 The client indicates that pain is a 3 on a 1 to 10 scale
4 The client denies nausea and has 250 mL of fluid in the suction collection container

Answer: 4

Rationale: The nasogastric tube connected to suction is used postoperatively to decompress and rest the bowel. The gastrointestinal tract lacks peristaltic activity as a result of manipulation during surgery. Although the nurse makes pertinent observations of the tube to ensure that it is secure and properly connected to suctioning machinery, the client is assessed for the effect. The client should not experience symptoms of ileus (nausea and vomiting) if the tube is functioning properly.

Test-Taking Strategy: Identify the critical elements in the stem of the question, including the key phrase: "most reliably that the tube is functioning correctly." Option 4 is the only option that relates to the issue: adequate functioning of the tube.

Level of Cognitive Ability: Application
Phase of Nursing Process: Assessment
Client Needs: Physiological Integrity
Content Area: Adult Health/Gastrointestinal

Reference

Black, J. M., & Matassarin-Jacobs, E. (1997). *Medical-surgical nursing: Clinical management for continuity of care* (5th ed.). Philadelphia: W. B. Saunders, pp. 1780–1781.

---

78. The nurse assessing a client with Addison's disease for signs of hyperkalemia would expect to note

1 Polyuria.
2 Dry mucous membranes.
3 Cardiac dysrhythmias.
4 Prolonged bleeding time.

Answer: 3

Rationale: The inadequate production of aldosterone in Addison's disease causes inadequate excretion of potassium and results in hyperkalemia. Potassium ions participate in a number of essential physiological processes, including the maintenance of intracellular tonicity; transmission of nerve impulses; contraction of cardiac, skeletal, and smooth muscles; and maintenance of normal renal function. The clinical manifestations of hyperkalemia are the result of altered nerve transmission. The most harmful consequence of hyperkalemia is its effect on cardiac function.

Test-Taking Strategy: Knowledge of the signs that indicate hyperkalemia is necessary to answer this question. Use of the ABCs—airway, breathing, and circulation—will also assist you in answering this question correctly. If you had difficulty with this question, take time now to review hyperkalemia!

Level of Cognitive Ability: Application
Phase of Nursing Process: Assessment
Client Needs: Physiological Integrity
Content Area: Adult Health/Endocrine

Reference

Polaski, A., & Tatro, S. (1996). *Luckmann's Core principles and practice of medical-surgical nursing.* Philadelphia: W. B. Saunders, p. 58.

---

79. Which of the following should the nurse monitor in a pregnant client with diabetes?

1 Urine for glucose and ketones
2 Blood pressure, pulse, and respirations
3 Urine for specific gravity
4 Evidence of edema

Answer: 1

Rationale: Nurses should assess the pregnant diabetic woman's urine for glucose and ketones at each prenatal visit because the physiological changes of pregnancy can drastically alter insulin requirements. Assessment of blood pressure, pulse and respirations, and urine for specific gravity and evidence of edema are more relevant for the client with pregnancy-induced hypertension.

Test-Taking Strategy: Read the case situation and note that it addresses a client with diabetes. Option 1 is the only option that specifically addresses diabetic assessment. If you had difficulty with this question, take time now to review prenatal care of the client with diabetes!

Level of Cognitive Ability: Application
Phase of Nursing Process: Assessment
Client Needs: Physiological Integrity
Content Area: Maternity

Reference

Olds, S., London, M., & Ladewig, P. (1996). *Clinical handbook for maternal newborn nursing: A family-centered approach* (5th ed.). Menlo Park, CA: Addison-Wesley, pp. 36–37.

---

80. Which of the following assessment data would indicate the onset of an opportunistic protozoan respiratory infection associated with HIV/AIDS?

1 White plaques located on the oral mucosa
2 Fever, exertional dyspnea, and nonproductive cough
3 Ophthalmic nerve involvement causing blindness
4 Ulcerated perirectal lesions

Answer: 2

Rationale: The most common opportunistic infections are protozoan, fungal, viral, and bacterial. The protozoan infection whose symptoms are described in option 2 is *Pneumocystis* pneumonia, the most common, life-threatening opportunistic infection afflicting persons with AIDS/ HIV.

Test-Taking Strategy: This question assess your ability to identify some of the more common infections associated with HIV infection. Option 1 describes a symptom of the fungal infection oral candidiasis (*Candida albicans*), called thrush. Option 3 describes a symptom of the viral infection herpes zoster (shingles), when it has spread to involve the ophthalmic nerve. Option 4 describes symptoms of herpes simplex.

Level of Cognitive Ability: Analysis
Phase of Nursing Process: Assessment
Client Needs: Physiological Integrity
Content Area: Adult Health/Respiratory

Reference

Black, J. M., & Matassarin-Jacobs, E. (1997). *Medical-surgical nursing: Clinical management for continuity of care* (5th ed.). Philadelphia: W. B. Saunders, pp. 614–650.

81. The nurse is caring for a client with trigeminal neuralgia (tic douloureux). The client asks for a snack and something to drink. The nurse assesses that the most appropriate choice for this client to meet nutritional needs is

1 Hot herbal tea with graham crackers.
2 Iced coffee with peanut butter and crackers.
3 Banana and apple juice.
4 Cocoa with honey and toast.

Answer: 3

Rationale: Because mild tactile stimulation of the face of clients with trigeminal neuralgia can trigger pain, the client needs to eat or drink lukewarm, nutritious foods that are soft and easy to chew. Extremes of temperature will also cause trigeminal pain.

Test-Taking Strategy: This question tests your ability to apply knowledge of the appropriate nutrition for clients with trigeminal neuralgia. Use the process of elimination in answering the question. Options 1,2, and 4 contain extremes of temperature and foods that are mechanically difficult to chew and swallow.

Level of Cognitive Ability: Application
Phase of Nursing Process: Assessment
Client Needs: Physiological Integrity
Content Area: Adult Health/Neurological

Reference

Luckmann, J. (1997). *Saunders manual of nursing care.* Philadelphia: W. B. Saunders, pp. 729–733.

---

82. The least important or significant assessment data obtained from the client with peptic ulcer disease is

1 Use of acetaminophen (Tylenol).
2 A history of tarry black stools.
3 Complaints of gastric pain 2–4 hours after meals.
4 History of alcohol abuse.

Answer: 1

Rationale: Unlike aspirin, acetaminophen has little effect on platelet function, doesn't affect bleeding time, and generally produces no gastric bleeding. Therefore, acetaminophen use is not a risk factor for bleeding from peptic ulcers.

Test-Taking Strategy: Use the process of elimination to answer this question. Options 2 and 3 are signs and symptoms of peptic ulcers and bleeding peptic ulcers. Because alcohol may aggravate the stomach mucosa, a history of alcohol abuse is often seen in clients with peptic ulcer disease.

Level of Cognitive Ability: Application
Phase of Nursing Process: Assessment
Client Needs: Physiological Integrity
Content Area: Adult Health/Gastrointestinal

Reference

Lewis, S. M., Collier, I. C., & Heitkemper, M. M. (1996). *Medical-surgical nursing: Assessment and management of clinical problems* (4th ed.). St. Louis: Mosby–Year Book, p. 1192.

83. A child is admitted to the orthopedic unit after a Harrington rod insertion for treatment of scoliosis. Which of the following assessments is the most important in the immediate postoperative period?

1 Capillary refill, sensation, and motion in all extremities
2 Pain level
3 Ability to turn by using the log-roll technique
4 Ability to flex and extend the lower extremities

Answer: 1

Rationale: This question requires you to prioritize. When the spinal column is manipulated during surgery, altered neurovascular status is a possible complication; therefore, neurovascular parameters, including circulation, sensation, and motion, should be checked every 2 hours. Level of pain is an important postoperative assessment, but using the ABCs—airway, breathing, and circulation—will direct you to select option 1 over option 2. Option 4, assessment of flexion and extension of the lower extremities, is incorporated into option 1, which includes checking motion. Log-rolling would be performed by nurses.

Test-Taking Strategy: Use the ABCs to answer this question. The question asks for an appropriate assessment after Harrington rod insertion. Option 1 addresses circulatory status.

Level of Cognitive Ability: Application
Phase of Nursing Process: Assessment
Client Needs: Physiological Integrity
Content Area: Child Health

Reference

Ball, J., & Bindler, R. (1995). *Pediatric nursing: Caring for children.* Stamford, CT: Appleton & Lange, pp. 601–603.

---

84. The nurse has assisted the physician in placing a subclavian catheter. Which of the following is a priority assessment after the procedure?

1 Obtaining an accurate temperature reading to monitor for infection
2 Monitoring blood pressure (BP) to assess for fluid volume overload
3 Labeling the dressing with the date and time of catheter insertion
4 Assessing chest x-ray results

Answer: 4

Rationale: A major risk associated with central catheter placement is the development of a pneumothorax from an accidental puncture of the lung. Assessing the chest x-ray is one of the best methods to determine whether this complication has occurred and to verify tip placement before initiating intravenous (IV) therapy. Although a client may develop an infection at the central catheter site, a temperature elevation would not likely occur immediately after placement. Although BP assessment is always important in evaluating a client's status after an invasive procedure, fluid volume overload is not a concern until IV fluids are started. Labeling the dressing site is important, but it is a nursing intervention, not a top priority assessment that the question asks for.

Test-Taking Strategy: Read the stem carefully to determine which assessment is needed, and immediately eliminate the options that are a nursing intervention. Prioritization and knowledge of postinsertion care are needed to answer this question. Take the time now to review these concepts if you had difficulty with this question!

Level of Cognitive Ability: Application
Phase of the Nursing Process: Assessment
Clinical Needs: Physiological Integrity
Content Area: Fundamental Skills

Reference

Phillips, L. D. (1997). *Manual of IV therapeutics* (2nd ed.). Philadelphia: F. A. Davis, p. 398.

85. The nurse is admitting a client suspected of having tuberculosis (TB). The nurse understands that the most accurate method for diagnosing active TB is

1 The client's long history of hemoptysis.
2 A positive purified protein derivative (PPD) test.
3 A sputum culture positive for mycobacterium.
4 Lung lesions noted on a chest x-ray.

Answer: 3

Rationale: The most accurate means of diagnosing TB is by culture. Establishing the presence of tuberculous bacilli is essential for a definitive diagnosis. Hemoptysis is not a common finding and is usually associated with more advanced cases. A positive PPD test indicates the presence of infection but does not show whether the infection is dormant or active. Other diseases may mimic TB on the chest x-ray.

Test-Taking Strategy: The question asks you to select the most accurate method of diagnosing TB. It is helpful to consider which test or data would be most definitive. The actual presence of live mycobacteria would leave little doubt that the culture is the most accurate method. If you are unfamiliar with the principles and physiology related to TB, review this material now!

Level of Cognitive Ability: Application
Phase of Nursing Process: Assessment
Client Needs: Physiological Integrity
Content Area: Adult Health/Respiratory

Reference

Lewis, S. M., Collier, I. C., & Heitkemper, M. M. (1996). *Medical-surgical nursing: Assessment and management of clinical problems* (4th ed.). St. Louis: Mosby–Year Book, pp. 638–639.

86. A client in late active first-stage labor has just reported a gush of vaginal fluid. The nurse observes a fetal monitor pattern of variable decelerations during contractions, followed by a brief acceleration. There is then a return to baseline until the next contraction, when the pattern is repeated. On the basis of these data, the nurse will continue the client assessment by doing which of the following?

1 Taking the vital signs
2 Performing a manual sterile vaginal examination
3 Performing a Leopold maneuver
4 Testing the vaginal fluid with a nitrazine strip

Answer: 2

Rationale: Moderate variable deceleration with a brief acceleration after a gush of amniotic fluid is a common clinical manifestation of cord compression resulting from occult or frank prolapse of the umbilical cord. A manual vaginal examination can detect the presence of the cord in the vagina, confirming the problem.

Test-Taking Strategy: First identify the client in the case. Analysis of the data in this case points to cord prolapse, and so the at-risk client is the fetus. Thus you would eliminate options that assess maternal risk (option 1), those that do not give you information about the specific risk (option 4), and those that provide you with data not important to the situation (option 3).

Level of Cognitive Ability: Application
Nursing Process: Assessment
Client Needs: Physiological Integrity
Content Area: Maternity

Reference

Lowdermilk, D., Perry, S., & Bobak, I. (1997). *Maternity and women's health care* (6th ed.). St. Louis: Mosby–Year Book, pp. 370, 973.

87. A child has just returned from surgery in a hip spica cast. A nursing priority at this time is to

1 Elevate head of bed.
2 Abduct the hips, using pillows.
3 Check circulation.
4 Turn the child on the right side.

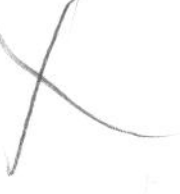

Answer: 3

Rationale: During the first few hours after a cast is applied, the chief concern is swelling that may cause the cast to become a tourniquet and shut off circulation. Therefore, circulatory assessment is a high priority. Elevating the head of bed of a child in a hip spica would cause discomfort. Using pillows to abduct the hips is not necessary because a hip spica immobilizes the hip and knee. Turning the child side to side at least every 2 hours is important because it allows the body cast to dry evenly and prevents complications related to immobility; however, it is not a higher priority than checking circulation.

Test-Taking Strategy: Use the principles associated with prioritizing when answering this question. Use ABCs—airway, breathing, and circulation—to answer this question. Also, use the nursing process to answer this question. The question asks what to do first. Because assessment is the first step in the nursing process, it is likely that the first thing to do with a postoperative client is assess! If you had difficulty with this question, take time now to review nursing care after application of a spica cast.

Level of Cognitive Ability: Application
Phase of Nursing Process: Assessment
Client Needs: Physiological Integrity
Content Area: Child Health

Reference
Wong, D. (1997). Whaley and Wong's *Essentials of pediatric nursing* (5th ed.). St. Louis: Mosby–Year Book, pp. 1130–1131.

---

88. On admission, the nurse assesses the client for the vegetative signs of depression. The nurse does this by determining the client's

1 Ability to think, concentrate, and make decisions.
2 Appetite, weight, sleep patterns, and psychomotor activity.
3 Level of self-esteem.
4 Level of suicidal ideation.

Answer: 2

Rationale: The vegetative signs of depression are changes in physiological functioning during depression. These include those addressed in option 2: appetite, weight, sleep, and psychomotor activity. Options 1, 3, and 4 represent psychological assessment categories.

Test-Taking Strategy: Knowing that the vegetative signs of depression refer to physiological changes directs you to option 2. Use the process of elimination to answer the question. In addition, using the strategy of reading all of the options, you will note that the incorrect options all relate to psychological assessment.

Level of Cognitive Ability: Application
Phase of Nursing Process: Assessment
Client Needs: Physiological Integrity
Content Area: Mental Health

Reference
Wilson, H., & Kneisl, C. (1996). *Psychiatric nursing* (5th ed.). Menlo Park, CA: Addison-Wesley, p. 324.

---

89. The nurse is assessing a client with a brain stem injury. In addition to using the Glasgow Coma Scale, the nurse will

1 Check cranial nerve functioning and respiratory rate and rhythm.
2 Measure arterial blood gases.
3 Assist with a lumbar puncture.
4 Measure pulmonary wedge pressure.

Answer: 1

Rationale: Assessing the respiratory status and cranial nerve function is a critical part of the assessment process in a client with a brain stem injury.

Test-Taking Strategy: Knowledge of the anatomical location of the respiratory center is necessary to answer this question. The respiratory center is located in the brain stem. Option 1 most directly relates to a brain stem injury. If you had difficulty with this question, take time now to review content and nursing care related to brain stem injuries!

Level of Cognitive Ability: Application
Phase of Nursing Process: Assessment
Client Needs: Physiological Integrity
Content Area: Adult Health/Neurological

Reference
Hartshorn, J., Sole, M. L., & Lamborn, M. L. (1997). *Introduction to critical care nursing* (2nd. ed.). Philadelphia: W. B. Saunders, p. 297.

90. The nurse is taking a history from a client suspected of having testicular cancer. Which of the following data will be most helpful in determining risk factors?

1 Number of sexual partners
2 Age and race
3 Geographic location
4 Marital status and number of children

Answer: 2

Rationale: Two basic but important risk factors for testicular cancer are age and race. The disease occurs most frequently in white males between the ages of 18 and 40 years. Other risk factors include a history of undescended testicle and a family history of testicular cancer. Options 1 and 4 are incorrect. Geographic location is rarely a risk factor.

Test-Taking Strategy: Knowledge of the risk factors will assist you in answering the question correctly. Knowing that testicular cancer occurs most often in white males between ages 18 and 40 will help you eliminate other options. If you had difficulty with this question, take time now to review the risk factors related to testicular cancer!

Level of Cognitive Ability: Analysis
Phase of Nursing Process: Assessment
Client Needs: Physiological Integrity
Content Area: Adult Health/Oncology

Reference

Ignatavicius, D. D., Workman, M. L., & Mishler, M. A. (1995). *Medical-surgical nursing: A nursing process approach* (2nd ed.). Philadelphia: W. B. Saunders, pp. 1069–1070.

---

91. The nurse is caring for a client with tuberculosis. The client is receiving rifampin (Rifadin), 600 mg PO daily. Which of the following would indicate to the nurse that the client is experiencing an adverse reaction?

1 A white blood cell count of 6000/μL
2 An alkaline phosphatase level of 25 units/dL
3 A sedimentation rate of 15 mm/hour
4 A total bilirubin level of 0.5 mg/dL

Answer: 2

Rationale: Adverse reactions or toxic effects of rifampin (Rifadin) include hepatotoxicity, hepatitis, blood dyscrasias, Stevens-Johnson syndrome, and antibiotic-related colitis. The nurse should be alert to increased liver function, bilirubin, BUN, and uric acid laboratory results because elevations may indicate an adverse reaction. A normal white blood cell count is 5000–10,000/μL. The normal sedimentation rate is 0–30 mm/hour. The normal total bilirubin level is 0.3–1 mg/dL. The normal alkaline phosphatase level is 4.5–13 King-Armstrong units/dL. Option 2 indicates an elevation in the alkaline phosphatase level, which would alert the nurse to possible hepatotoxicity.

Test-Taking Strategy: Knowledge about rifampin (Rifadin) and about normal laboratory values is necessary to answer this question. Knowing that the medication is metabolized in the liver would assist you in eliminating options 1 and 3 because these laboratory values are not directly related to assessing liver function. This leaves options 2 and 4. Knowledge of normal values would assist you in selecting option 2 because option 4 represents a normal bilirubin value. If you are unfamiliar with this medication or these laboratory values, take the time now to review this content!

Level of Cognitive Ability: Analysis
Phase of Nursing Process: Assessment
Client Needs: Physiological Integrity
Content Area: Pharmacology

Reference

Hodgson, B., & Kizior, R. (1998). *Saunders nursing drug handbook 1998.* Philadelphia: W. B. Saunders, p. 907.

92. A preschool child is placed in traction for treatment of a femur fracture. This child, who reportedly has been toilet-trained for at least 1 year, begins bed-wetting. The nurse recognizes this as

1. Attention-seeking behavior necessitating intervention by the child psychologist.
2. Loss of developmental milestones as a result of prolonged immobilization.
3. Regressing to earlier developmental behavior, which is a normal psychological effect of immobilization.
4. Body image disturbance.

Answer: 3

Rationale: The monotony of immobilization can lead to sluggish intellectual and psychomotor responses. Children may seek the attention of others by reverting to earlier developmental behaviors. Regressive behaviors are not uncommon in immobilized children and usually do not require professional intervention. Although "loss of developmental milestones" may seem like an appropriate response, "regressing to earlier developmental behavior" is a more accurate description of the psychological effects of immobilization. Body image may or may not be affected by long-term immobilization and is not related to the case in question.

Test-Taking Strategy: Option 1 can be eliminated because bed-wetting by an immobilized child is not unusual and a child psychologist is not needed. Option 4 can be eliminated because it does not relate to the question. When reviewing options 2 and 3, note that regression is a normal psychological response to immobilization and is a more accurate description of the psychological effects of immobilization.

Level of Cognitive Ability: Application
Phase of Nursing Process: Assessment
Client Needs: Psychosocial Integrity
Content Area: Child Health

Reference

Ashwill, J. W., & Droske, S. (1997). *Nursing care of children: Principles and practice.* Philadelphia: W. B. Saunders, p. 1112.

93. A client has had a Miller-Abbott tube in place for 24 hours. Which of the following assessment findings is evidence that the tube is located in the intestine?

1. Aspirate from the tube that has a pH of 7
2. The abdominal x-ray report states that the end of the tube is above the pylorus
3. Bowel sounds are absent
4. The client continues to be nauseated

Answer: 1

Rationale: The Miller-Abbott tube is a nasoenteric tube that is used to decompress the intestine, so as to correct a bowel obstruction. The end of the tube should be located in the intestine. The pH of the gastric fluid is acidic, and the pH of the intestinal fluid is 7 or higher. Location of the tube can also be determined by x-ray.

Test-Taking Strategy: The issue of the question is specific content regarding assessment of the client with a Miller-Abbott tube. Read all four options and use the process of elimination. The stem asks for data consistent with placement in the intestine (option 1). The other options do not support that finding. Review the purpose and nursing care of a client with a Miller-Abbott tube now if you had difficulty with this question!

Level of Cognitive Ability: Application
Phase of Nursing Process: Assessment
Client Needs: Physiological Integrity
Content Area: Adult Health/Gastrointestinal

Reference

Black, J. M., & Matassarin-Jacobs, E. (1997). *Medical-surgical nursing: Clinical management for continuity of care* (5th ed.). Philadelphia: W. B. Saunders, pp. 1749–1752.

94. The client with myxedema reports having experienced cold intolerance, puffiness around the eyes and face, and a lack of energy. The nurse knows that these symptoms are caused by a lack of production of which hormone?

1 Luteinizing hormone (LH)
2 Adrenocorticotropic hormone (ACTH)
3 Triiodothyronine (T_3) and thyroxine (T_4)
4 Prolactin (PRL) and growth hormone (GH)

Answer: 3

Rationale: Myxedema results from inadequate peripheral tissue thyroid hormone levels (T_3 and T_4). Low levels of thyroid hormone result in an overall decrease in the basal metabolic rate, affecting virtually every body system and leading to weakness and fatigue. Many metabolic processes are affected, such as a decrease in heat production. There is also an accumulation of hydrophilic proteoglycans in the interstitial space, which causes increased interstitial fluid and subsequent edema. Decrease in LH results in the loss of secondary sex characteristics. A decrease in ACTH is seen in Addison's disease, in which there is a decrease in glucocorticoids and mineralocorticoid hormones, resulting in hypoglycemia and orthostatic hypotension. PRL affects mammary glands to stimulate breast milk production, and GH affects bone and soft tissue by promoting growth through protein anabolism and lipolysis.

Test-Taking Strategy: Read the stem very carefully and specifically identify exactly what the question is asking. Knowing that myxedema is associated with the thyroid gland will assist you in seeing a relationship between what the question is asking and option 3. Review content and laboratory values related to myxedema now if you had difficulty with this question!

Level of Cognitive Ability: Analysis
Phase of Nursing Process: Assessment
Client Needs: Physiological Integrity
Content Area: Adult Health/Endocrine

Reference

Ignatavicius, D. D., Workman, M. L., & Mishler, M. A. (1995). *Medical-surgical nursing: A nursing process approach* (2nd ed., Vol. 2). Philadelphia: W. B. Saunders, pp. 1844–1845.

---

95. A 33-year-old female is admitted with a tentative diagnosis of Graves' disease. Which symptom related to the client's menstrual cycle would she most likely report during the initial assessment?

1 Dysmenorrhea
2 Metrorrhagia
3 Amenorrhea
4 Menorrhagia

Answer: 3

Rationale: Amenorrhea or a decreased menstrual flow is not uncommon with Graves' disease. Dysmenorrhea, metrorrhagia, and menorrhagia are also disorders related to the female reproductive system; however, they are not associated with Graves' disease.

Test-Taking Strategy: Knowledge of the basic clinical manifestations of Graves' disease is necessary to answer this question. Use the process of elimination. A key phrase in the stem to look for and focus your attention on is "most likely to report." The issue of the question is which complication a female with Graves' disease would report. This is a difficult question, and if you had difficulty answering it, take time now to review the clinical manifestations of Graves' disease!

Level of Cognitive Ability: Analysis
Phase of Nursing Process: Assessment
Client Needs: Physiological Integrity
Content Area: Adult Health/Endocrine

Reference

Ignatavicius, D. D., Workman, M. L., & Mishler, M. A. (1995). *Medical-surgical nursing: A nursing process approach* (2nd ed., Vol. 2). Philadelphia: W. B. Saunders, pp. 1834–1836.

96. The nurse is assessing the client for environmental risk factors for neurological disorders. The nurse would not necessarily include which of the following items in the questioning?

1 Exposure to fumes such as paints or bonding agents (glue)
2 Exposure to pesticides
3 Ventilation in the work area
4 Number of windows in the work area

Answer: 4

Rationale: The nurse would assess for risk of exposure to neurotoxic fumes and chemicals. These could include paint, bonding agents, and pesticides. The nurse also inquires about the adequacy of ventilation in the home and work area.

Test-Taking Strategy: Each of the options seems plausible on first reading. The stem clues you to this by asking which may "not necessarily" be included. On closer examination, option 4 is the least reliable option as written. There are many work spaces (such as factories, insurance companies, and operating rooms) which are adequately ventilated without the use of windows. This makes it the correct answer, in view of the wording of this question.

Level of Cognitive Ability: Application
Phase of Nursing Process: Assessment
Client Needs: Health Promotion and Maintenance
Content Area: Adult Health/Neurological

Reference

Black, J. M., & Matassarin-Jacobs, E. (1997). *Medical-surgical nursing: Clinical management for continuity of care* (5th ed.). Philadelphia: W. B. Saunders, p. 714.

---

97. The nurse should expect to observe what major symptom in a pregnant client with pregnancy-induced hypertension (PIH)?

1 Possible decelerations and increased variability of fetal heart rate during labor
2 Possible increase of blood pressure
3 Possible decrease in brachial reflexes
4 Possible increase in urine output during labor and delivery

Answer: 2

Rationale: The major symptom of PIH is increased blood pressure (hypertension). As the disease progresses, it is possible that increased brachial reflexes, decreased fetal heart rate and variability, and decreased urine output will occur, particularly during labor.

Test-Taking Strategy: Knowledge related to PIH is necessary to answer this question. Look at the question and identify the client of the question. The client in this case is the pregnant client; therefore you can eliminate option 1. From here, use the ABCs: airway, breathing, and circulation. This will direct you to selecting option 2. If you had difficulty with this question, it is very important to take time now to review the content related to PIH!

Level of Cognitive Ability: Application
Phase of Nursing Process: Assessment
Client Needs: Physiological Integrity
Content Area: Maternity

Reference

Olds, S., London, M., & Ladewig, P. (1996). *Clinical handbook for maternal-newborn nursing: A family-centered approach* (5th ed.). Menlo Park, CA: Addison-Wesley, pp. 120–121.

---

98. The nurse has just administered a purified protein derivative (PPD) skin test to a client. The nurse will know there is a significant positive reaction when which of the following occurs?

1 An induration of 10 mm or greater
2 A large area of erythema
3 The presence of a wheal
4 Client complaints of constant itching

Answer: 1

Rationale: An induration of 10 mm or greater is usually considered significant. Erythema is not considered significant. The presence of a wheal would indicate that the skin test was administered appropriately. Itching is not an indication of a positive PPD.

Test-Taking Strategy: When answering a question in which you are asked to confirm a diagnosis, it is usually best to select the most objective choice. Option 1 is the most measurable option. If you had difficulty with this question, be sure to review this content. You are likely to see questions similar to this one on NCLEX-RN!

Level of Cognitive Ability: Analysis
Phase of Nursing Process: Assessment
Client Needs: Physiological Integrity
Content Area: Adult Health/Respiratory

Reference

Smeltzer, S., & Bare, B. (1996). *Brunner and Suddarth's Textbook of medical-surgical nursing* (8th ed.). Philadelphia: Lippincott-Raven, pp. 496–497.

---

99. In performing a lethality assessment with a suicidal client, the nurse's best statement is

1 "Do you ever think about ending it all?"
2 "Have you ever thought of killing yourself ?"
3 "Do you wish your life was over?"
4 "Do you have a death wish?"

Answer: 2

Rationale: A lethality assessment requires direct communication between the client and the nurse concerning the client's intent. It is important to provide a question that is directly related to lethality.

Test-Taking Strategy: Note that the stem asks for the "best" statement of the four options. Option 2 is the option that directly addresses the issue of suicide. If you had difficulty with this question, review assessment for suicide risk now!

Level of Cognitive Ability: Application
Phase of Nursing Process: Assessment
Client Needs: Psychosocial Integrity
Content Area: Mental Health

Reference

Wilson, H. S., & Kneisl, C. R. (1996). *Psychiatric nursing* (5th ed.). Menlo Park, CA: Addison-Wesley, pp. 593–595.

---

100. The nurse is caring for a client with cirrhosis of the liver. The client is receiving spironolactone (Aldactone), 50 mg PO daily. Which of the following would indicate to the nurse that the client is experiencing a side effect related to the medication?

1 Hypokalemia
2 Hyperkalemia
3 Constipation
4 Dry skin

Answer: 2

Rationale: Spironolactone (Aldactone) is a potassium-sparing diuretic. Side effects include hyperkalemia, dehydration, hyponatremia, and lethargy. Although the concern with most diuretics is hypokalemia, this medication is potassium-sparing which means that the concern with the administration of this medication is hyperkalemia. Additional side effects include nausea, vomiting, cramping, diarrhea, headache, ataxia, drowsiness, confusion, and fever.

Test-Taking Strategy: Knowledge about spironolactone (Aldactone) is necessary to answer the question. Most of the diuretics produce hypokalemia; however, the potassium-sparing diuretics cause hyperkalemia, particularly in clients taking potassium supplements and in clients with renal insufficiency. If you had difficulty with this question, take the time now to review potassium-sparing diuretics.

Level of Cognitive Ability: Analysis
Phase of Nursing Process: Assessment
Client Needs: Physiological Integrity
Content Area: Pharmacology

Reference

Hodgson, B., & Kizior, R. (1998). *Saunders nursing drug handbook 1998.* Philadelphia: W. B. Saunders, p. 943.

101. The nurse shares with the psychiatrist that he or she believes that a severely depressed client would benefit greatly from electroconvulsive therapy (ECT). This assessment is valid because

1 ECT provides the most rapid relief of any treatment for severe depression.
2 The client has not been started on any medications.
3 The client is well-nourished.
4 The client is not suicidal.

Answer: 1

Rationale: Option 1 is a true statement. Option 2 is incorrect because medications should be attempted before ECT is tried. Most severely ill clients who fail to respond to medications respond to ECT. Option 3 is false; clients at high risk for malnutrition are good candidates for ECT. Option 4 is also false; suicidal clients are equally good candidates for ECT.

Test-Taking Strategy: Read all four options very carefully before selecting an answer. Use the process of elimination. To answer this question correctly, you need to apply characteristics of clients that make them the best candidates for ECT. Option 1 is the only option that addresses the issue in the question. Review ECT now if you had difficulty with this question!

Level of Cognitive Ability: Application
Phase of Nursing Process: Assessment
Client Needs: Psychosocial Integrity
Content Area: Mental Health

Reference

Carson, V., & Arnold, E. (1996). *Mental health nursing: The nurse-patient journey.* Philadelphia: W. B. Saunders, p. 785.

102. Which of the following behaviors is most indicative that the client may be contemplating suicide?

1 The client tells you that he or she plans to use his or her shoelaces to strangle himself or herself
2 The client cries for long periods of time
3 The client spends long periods of time alone
4 The client reports sleep disturbances

Answer: 1

Rationale: If a client displays a suicidal ideation and is able to share a plan, the client should be taken very seriously and suicide precautions should be implemented. Option 1 clearly states such a plan. Options 2, 3, and 4 are indicative of depression but are not as definitive as option 1.

Test-Taking Strategy: In this particular case, it is necessary to assess the client for a cardinal sign of suicidal ideation, and that is the formulation of a specific suicidal plan. A specific suicide plan is addressed in option 1. If you had difficulty with this question, take time now to review assessment of the client for the risk for suicide!

Level of Cognitive Ability: Analysis
Phase of Nursing Process: Assessment
Client Needs: Physiological Integrity
Content Area: Mental Health

Reference

Luckmann, J. (1997). *Saunders manual of nursing care.* Philadelphia: W. B. Saunders Company, p. 1927.

103. The client with myocardial infarction (MI) suddenly becomes tachycardic, shows signs of air hunger, and begins coughing frothy pink-tinged sputum. The nurse expects that the client may be experiencing pulmonary edema, a complication of MI. If pulmonary edema is present, the nurse would, on auscultation of the lungs, hear bilateral

1 Rhonchi.
2 Crackles in bases.
3 Rales to apices.
4 Wheezes.

Answer: 3

Rationale: Pulmonary edema is characterized by extreme breathlessness, dyspnea, air hunger, and the production of frothy pink-tinged sputum. Auscultation of the lungs reveals rales to the apices.

Test-Taking Strategy: Fluid produces sounds that are called rhonchi or crackles, which eliminates options 1 or 4. Option 2 is less plausible than option 3 because bibasilar crackles do not produce such extreme symptoms. Use the process of elimination to answer this question. Review the signs and symptoms of pulmonary edema and the basic adventitious breath sounds if you had difficulty with this question!

Level of Cognitive Ability: Analysis
Phase of Nursing Process: Assessment
Client Needs: Physiological Integrity
Content Area: Adult Health/Cardiovascular

Reference

Luckmann, J. (1997). *Saunders manual of nursing care.* Philadelphia: W. B. Saunders, p. 1072.

---

104. A physical assessment of the suicidal client is performed on admission to the inpatient unit. This is an important part of the admission process because it alerts the nurse to

1 Abnormalities.
2 Evidence of physical self-harm.
3 Existing medical problems.
4 Baseline data.

Answer: 2

Rationale: The physical assessment of a suicidal client should be thorough and should focus on the evidence of self-harm or the formulation of a plan for the suicide attempt. Although all of the options are correct, option 2 is most appropriate in the context of the suicidal client. Clients with a history of self-harm are at greater risk for suicide.

Test-Taking Strategy: This is a difficult question because all the responses are correct. Option 2 is most appropriate in the context of providing care to the suicidal client. Assessing for physical evidence of self-harm is an important component of the assessment process of a suicidal client. Utilize the process of elimination in selecting the correct option. If you had difficulty with this question, take time now to review the characteristics of the client at risk for suicide!

Level of Cognitive Ability: Application
Phase of Nursing Process: Assessment
Client Needs: Physiological Integrity
Content Area: Mental Health

Reference

Wilson, H., & Kneisl, C. (1996). *Psychiatric nursing* (5th ed.). Menlo Park, CA: Addison-Wesley, p. 594.

---

105. A 2-year-old is admitted with juvenile rheumatoid arthritis (JRA). During the focused assessment, the nurse will particularly note

1 Increased irritability and the child's insistence on being carried.
2 Joint tenderness and complaints of joint stiffness.
3 Pallor, coolness, and swelling of joints with a history of daily temperature elevations.
4 The child's description of how difficult it is to move around after periods of inactivity.

Answer: 1

Rationale: Signs and symptoms of JRA include: painful, stiff, swollen, tender, warm involved joints. Joints are especially stiff after sleeping or other periods of inactivity. Children are not always able to clearly identify the problem, and therefore the nurse should be alerted to increased irritability, guarding of the painful joint, or reluctance to walk. The presence of systemic involvement is signaled by daily temperature elevations but not pallor and coolness; thus option 3 is incorrect. Other nonspecific symptoms include anorexia, weight loss, failure to grow, sleep pattern disturbance, lymphadenopathy, and hepatosplenomegaly. The child's age (2 years old) rules out options 2 and 4.

Test-Taking Strategy: Identify the components of the question. The case study presents a 2-year-old with JRA. The stem asks for assessment data. When selecting your answer, be sure to consider the behavior of a 2-year-old, which eliminates options 2 and 4 because children this age typically cannot accurately describe these symptoms. Always note the age of the client when it is stated in a question. If an age is stated, it needs to be considered as you select an option. If you had difficulty with this question, take the time now to review JRA and the normal characteristics associated with growth and development!

Level of Cognitive Ability: Application
Phase of Nursing Process: Assessment
Client Needs: Physiological Integrity
Content Area: Child Health

Reference

Ashwill, J. W., & Droske, S. (1997). *Nursing care of children: Principles and practice.* Philadelphia: W. B. Saunders, p. 1127.

106. In assessing the manic client on admission to the inpatient psychiatric unit, the nurse would expect to find all of the following except

1 Inflated self esteem.
2 Fatigue.
3 Inability to concentrate.
4 Weight gain.

Answer: 4

Rationale: The manic client typically forgets to eat and therefore demonstrates a weight loss rather than a weight gain. The manic client also demonstrates inflated self-esteem, the inability to concentrate, and fatigue.

Test-Taking Strategy: In order to answer this question, you need to know the signs and symptoms of manic behavior. Read the question carefully. Note also that the stem of the question uses the word "except." Review content on bipolar disorders now if you had difficulty with this question!

Level of Cognitive Ability: Analysis
Phase of Nursing Process: Assessment
Client Needs: Physiological Integrity
Content Area: Mental Health

Reference

Wilson, H., & Kneisl, C. (1996). *Psychiatric nursing* (5th ed.). Menlo Park, CA: Addison-Wesley, p. 347.

---

107. The husband of a client who has a Sengstaken-Blakemore tube states to the nurse, " I thought having this tube down her nose the first time would convince my wife to quit drinking." The most appropriate response by the nurse is

1 "Alcoholism is a disease that affects the whole family."
2 "You sound frustrated in dealing with your wife's drinking problem."
3 "Have you discussed this subject at the Al-Anon meetings?"
4 "I think you are a good person to stay with your wife."

Answer: 2

Rationale: The nurse uses therapeutic communication tools in assisting a client (the client's spouse in this question) to express feelings concerning the wife's chronic illness. The nurse listens attentively to the client and uses the tools of clarifying and focusing. Stereotyping (option 1), changing the subject (option 3), and expressing an opinion (option 4) are examples of barriers to communication.

Test-Taking Strategy: Read the stem carefully. Be aware of the key phrase: "most appropriate response." With communication questions, identify the use of therapeutic tools (option 2) and blocks to communication (options 1, 3, 4). Identify the client of the question. The client of the question is the husband. Always focus on client's feelings first!

Level of Cognitive Ability: Application
Phase of Nursing Process: Assessment
Client Needs: Psychosocial Integrity
Content Area: Adult Health/Gastrointestinal

Reference

Black, J. M., & Matassarin-Jacobs, E. (1997). *Medical-surgical nursing: Clinical management for continuity of care* (5th ed.). Philadelphia: W. B. Saunders, pp. 1883–1885.

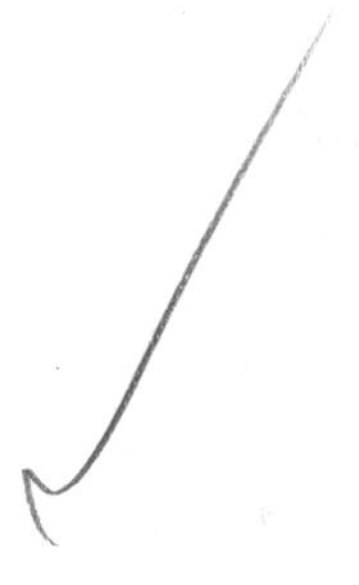

108. The nurse assigned to a postpartum woman in critical condition after an amniotic fluid embolism observes the client's husband sitting slumped by the client's bed holding his head in his hands. Which of the following actions would be the most appropriate for the nurse to take?

1 Administer nursing care to the client silently, allowing the husband to regain his composure
2 Place a hand gently on the husband's shoulder and tell him, "It's going to be all right."
3 Comment to the husband, "You appear to be distressed. While your wife is resting comfortably, how about sitting in the recliner by the window? I'll pull up a chair and we can discuss your concerns."
4 Tell the husband, "I know it's tough, but you need to be strong for your wife. The baby also needs you. Have you been to see the baby today?"

Answer: 3

Rationale: The sudden metamorphosis of an anticipated event of joy into a life-threatening emergency produces anxiety and distress to the client's whole family. The roles of the nurse are to demonstrate empathy and caring while providing opportunities for feelings to be expressed. Therapeutic communication tools that can be used include establishing an environment conducive to trust and open communication, validating or clarifying feelings, showing empathy with touch and voice tone, and giving information about the here and now.

Test-Taking Strategy: In communication questions, options with communication blockers, such as devaluing feelings, implying or showing disapproval, and giving advice or false reassurances, can be eliminated. Silence can be either a therapeutic communication tool that allows the client to verbalize and transmits empathy, or it can be a way of ignoring and placing the client's emotional issues on hold, as it is in this case. Be aware of distractors that mix therapeutic and nontherapeutic techniques. The right option will be ideally therapeutic.

Level of Cognitive Ability: Application
Phase of Nursing Process: Assessment
Client Needs: Psychosocial Integrity
Content Area: Maternity

References

Haber, J. (1997). *Comprehensive psychiatric nursing* (5th ed.). St. Louis: Mosby–Year Book, pp. 128–133.
Lowdermilk, D., Perry, S., & Bobak, I. (1997). *Maternity and women's health care* (6th ed.). St. Louis: Mosby–Year Book, p. 977.

---

109. When a depressed client tells the nurse that he or she would be "far better off dead," the nurse initiates suicide precautions. Which of the following statements is true about suicide?

1 The client who is unsuccessful at suicide will probably not try again
2 Clients who talk about suicide rarely attempt it
3 The more specific the plan, the more likely the client will be successful in the attempt
4 The nurse should not use the word "suicide" in front of the client

Answer: 3

Rationale: The more specific the plan, the greater the likelihood of a successful suicide.

Test-Taking Strategy: Use the process of elimination. You need to understand the dynamics of suicide in order to answer this question. Options 1 and 2 are inaccurate. Option 4 is also inaccurate and not directly related to the issue of the question. Review these concepts now if you had difficulty with this question!

Level of Cognitive Ability: Application
Phase of Nursing Process: Assessment
Client Needs: Safe, Effective Care Environment
Content Area: Mental Health

Reference

Wilson, H., & Kneisl, C. (1996). *Psychiatric nursing* (5th ed.). Menlo Park, CA: Addison-Wesley, p. 593.

110. Which of the following nursing assessments will be included in the plan of care while monitoring for possible complications of total parenteral nutrition (TPN)?

1 Pulse oximetry at 8-hour intervals
2 Hourly vital signs
3 Hemoglobin and hematocrit
4 Blood glucose levels at 6-hour intervals

Answer: 4

Rationale: Major complications of TPN therapy include air embolism, infection, hypoglycemia or hyperglycemia, fluid overload, and electrolyte imbalance. It is standard care to monitor blood glucose levels at 6-hour intervals to prevent complications of hyperglycemia.

Test-Taking Strategy: The issue of this question is specific content: nursing assessment to detect a complication associated with TPN therapy. Read all four options. Consider which problems each assessment would detect. Remember that the base solution for TPN has a higher concentration of dextrose than a normal IV solution would have. Therefore, hyperglycemia is a concern with TPN. Hypoglycemia should be assessed for particularly when TPN is discontinued. Review the complications of TPN now if you had difficulty with this question!

Level of Cognitive Ability: Application
Phase of Nursing Process: Assessment
Client Needs: Physiological Integrity
Content Area: Fundamental Skills

Reference

Black, J. M., & Matassarin-Jacobs, E. (1997). *Medical-surgical nursing: Clinical management for continuity of care* (5th ed.). Philadelphia: W. B. Saunders, pp. 1754–1756.

---

111. A client is admitted to the hospital for a thyroidectomy. While preparing the client for surgery, the nurse assesses for any psychosocial problems that may cause preoperative anxiety. A primary source of anxiety related to a thyroidectomy is fear of

1 Developing gynecomastia and hirsutism postoperatively.
2 Sexual dysfunction and infertility.
3 Imposed dietary restrictions after discharge.
4 Changes in body image secondary to the location of the incision.

Answer: 4

Rationale: Because of the incision being in the neck area, clients are many times afraid of thyroid surgery for fear of having a large scar postoperatively. Having all or part of the thyroid gland removed will not cause the client to experience gynecomastia or hirsutism. Sexual dysfunction and infertility could possibly occur if the entire thyroid were removed and the client were not placed on thyroid replacement medications. The client will not have to abide by dietary restrictions after discharge.

Test-Taking Strategy: The key word in the stem is "primary." Apply your knowledge of thyroid function and anatomical location to answer the question. This should easily direct you to option 4.

Level of Cognitive Ability: Analysis
Phase of Nursing Process: Assessment
Client Needs: Psychosocial Integrity
Content Area: Adult Health/Endocrine

Reference

Ignatavicius, D. D., Workman, M. L., & Mishler, M. A. (1995). *Medical-surgical nursing: A nursing process approach* (2nd ed., Vol. 2). Philadelphia: W. B. Saunders, p. 1840.

112. A client with non–insulin-dependent diabetes mellitus (NIDDM) was recently hospitalized for hyperglycemic hyperosmolar nonketotic (HHNK) syndrome. Upon discharge, the client expresses concerns about the recurrence of HHNK syndrome. Which statement by the nurse is the most appropriate?

1 "Don't worry, your family will help you."
2 "I'm sure this won't happen again."
3 "You have concerns about the treatment for your condition?"
4 "I think you might need to go to the nursing home."

Answer: 3

Rationale: The nursing diagnosis for a client with NIDDM may include a knowledge deficit, potential self-care deficit, and anxiety related to loss of control, inability to manage diabetes, and fear of diabetic complications. The nurse should provide time and attention to hear the client's concerns and questions.

Test-Taking Strategy: The therapeutic response among these options is option 3 because the nurse is attempting to clarify the client's feelings. Options 1, 2, and 4 are inappropriate: options 1 and 2 may give inappropriate false hope, and option 4 disregards the client's concerns and states an opinion that may not be valid. Review the communication tools and blocks now if you had difficulty with this question!

Level of Cognitive Ability: Application
Phase of Nursing Process: Assessment
Client Needs: Psychosocial Integrity
Content Area: Adult Health/Endocrine

Reference

Haber, J. (1997). *Comprehensive psychiatric nursing* (5th ed.). St. Louis: Mosby–Year Book, pp. 128–133.

113. The physician orders intravenous fat emulsion (Intralipid 10%) for a client. Before initiating the solution, the nurse should assess which of the following?

1 The client's blood pressure
2 Hypersensitivity to eggs
3 Fingerstick blood glucose level
4 History of seizures

Answer: 2

Rationale: Before administering any medication, the nurse must assess for allergy or hypersensitivity to substances used in producing the medication. Fat emulsions such as Intralipid 10% contain an emulsifying agent obtained from egg yolks. Clients who are sensitive to eggs are at risk for developing hypersensitivity reactions.

Test-Taking Strategy: The issue of the question is specific content: assessment before administering a medication, intravenous fat emulsion. Read all four options. Eliminate the incorrect options. Option 2 addresses assessment for allergies and hypersensitivity. The other options are not related to fat emulsion. If you had difficulty with this question, review the content related to the administration of intravenous fat emulsions!

Level of Cognitive Ability: Application
Phase of Nursing Process: Assessment
Client Needs: Physiological Integrity
Content Area: Fundamental Skills

Reference

Wilson, B., Shannon, M., & Stang, C. (1997). *Nurses drug guide.* Stamford, CT: Appleton & Lange, pp. 555–557.

114. The nurse is performing an admission assessment on a client admitted with a diagnosis of pheochromocytoma. To assess for the major symptom associated with pheochromocytoma, the nurse

1 Tests the client's urine for glucose.
2 Takes the client's weight.
3 Palpates the skin for its temperature.
4 Takes the client's blood pressure.

Answer: 4

Rationale: Hypertension is the major symptom associated with pheochromocytoma. The blood pressure status would be assessed by measuring the client's blood pressure. Glycosuria, weight loss, and diaphoresis are also clinical manifestations of pheochromocytoma, but hypertension is the major symptom.

Test-Taking Strategy: Use the principles associated with prioritizing when answering this question. Remember your ABCs: airway, breathing, and circulation. A method of assessing circulation is to measure the blood pressure. If you had difficulty with this question, take time now to review the clinical manifestations of pheochromocytoma!

Level of Cognitive Ability: Application
Phase of Nursing Process: Assessment
Client Needs: Physiological Integrity
Content Area: Adult Health/Endocrine

Reference
Luckmann, J. (1997). *Saunders manual of nursing care.* Philadelphia: W. B. Saunders, p. 1411.

---

115. The client is admitted with a myocardial infarction and is experiencing no chest pain at this time. The nurse reviews the ECG rhythm strip and finds that the PR interval is 0.16 seconds. The nurse realizes this is

1 Indicative of first degree atrioventricular (AV) block.
2 An abnormal finding.
3 Indicative of impending reinfarction.
4 A normal finding.

Answer: 4

Rationale: The PR interval represents the time it takes for the cardiac impulse to spread from the atria to the ventricles. The normal PR interval ranges from 0.12 to 0.20 seconds.

Test-Taking Strategy: Use the process of elimination to answer this question. In looking at options 1, 2, and 3, note that there is a similarity: all reflect abnormality. In addition, a rhythm strip is not used to predict occurrences of impending cardiac problems, as option 3 implies. That leaves option 4 as the only correct choice.

Level of Cognitive Ability: Analysis
Phase of Nursing Process: Assessment
Client Needs: Physiological Integrity
Content Area: Adult Health/Cardiovascular

Reference
Black, J. M., & Matassarin-Jacobs, E. (1997). *Medical-surgical nursing: Clinical management for continuity of care* (5th ed.). Philadelphia: W. B. Saunders, pp. 1222–1223.

---

116. The nurse is testing the reflexes of a client. The nurse would assess the pharyngeal reflex by

1 Stimulating the back of the throat with a tongue depressor.
2 Stroking the skin on an abdominal quadrant.
3 Stroking the outer plantar surface of the foot from heel to toe.
4 Stimulating the perianal skin or gently inserting a gloved finger in the rectum.

Answer: 1

Rationale: The pharyngeal (gag) reflex is tested by touching the back of the throat with an object such as a tongue depressor. The abdominal reflex, plantar reflex, and anal reflexes are described in options 2, 3, and 4, respectively. A positive response to each of these reflexes is considered normal.

Test-Taking Strategy: This question is worded in a straightforward manner. Use the process of elimination. Knowing that the word "pharyngeal" refers to the pharynx, or back of the throat, you can readily eliminate each of the incorrect options.

Level of Cognitive Ability: Application
Phase of Nursing Process: Assessment
Client Needs: Physiological Integrity
Content Area: Adult Health/Neurological

Reference
Black, J. M., & Matassarin-Jacobs, E. (1997). *Medical-surgical nursing: Clinical management for continuity of care* (5th ed.). Philadelphia: W. B. Saunders, pp. 726–727.

117. The nurse is caring for a client who is scheduled to have an electroencephalogram (EEG). The nurse would assess that the client is not accurately prepared for the procedure if which of the following items was noted?

1 Client's hair is shampooed
2 Client took morning dose of anticonvulsant
3 Client ate a full breakfast
4 Client verbalizes the test will not give an electric shock

Answer: 2

Rationale: Preprocedure care for EEG involves teaching the client about the procedure, shampooing the client's hair, and giving full meals to prevent hypoglycemia, which could alter brain waves. Antidepressants, tranquilizers, and anticonvulsants are withheld for 24–48 hours before the procedure, as are stimulants such as coffee, tea, cola, alcohol, and cigarettes.

Test-Taking Strategy: Read the stem of the question carefully. The question is worded to direct you to look for an incorrect item. Options 1 and 4 are obviously correct and should be eliminated first. Of the two remaining, you need to know that hypoglycemia and certain medications will interfere with the test results, which should direct you to select option 2 over option 3. If you had difficulty with this question, take time now to review preprocedure care for EEGs!

Level of Cognitive Ability: Analysis
Phase of Nursing Process: Assessment
Client Needs: Physiological Integrity
Content Area: Adult Health/Neurological

Reference

Black, J. M., & Matassarin-Jacobs, E. (1997). *Medical-surgical nursing: Clinical management for continuity of care* (5th ed.). Philadelphia: W. B. Saunders, p. 739.

118. A breastfeeding client, 10 days post partum, telephones the postpartum unit complaining of a reddened, painful breast and elevated temperature. On the basis of the nurse's assessment of the client's complaints, the best direction to give to the client would include which of the following?

1 Stop breastfeeding because you probably have an infection
2 Notify your physician because you may need medication
3 Continue breastfeeding as this is a normal response in breastfeeding mothers
4 Breastfeed only with the unaffected breast

Answer: 2

Rationale: On the basis of the signs and symptoms presented by the client, particularly the elevated temperature, the physician needs to be notified, because an antibiotic that is tolerated by the infant as well as the mother may be prescribed. The mother should continue to nurse on both breasts.

Test-Taking Strategy: Option 1 has been the strategy in the past, but it does not encourage the continuation of breastfeeding or notification of the physician; therefore, another option needs to be considered. Option 3 can be eliminated because it is not a normal response. This leaves options 2 and 4. Option 4 also does not encourage continuation of normal breastfeeding and could possibly lead to engorgement, creating more discomfort and pain for the mother. This leaves option 2 as the correct answer.

Level of Cognitive Ability: Application
Phase of Nursing Process: Assessment
Client Needs: Physiological Integrity
Content Area: Maternity

Reference

Nichols, F., & Zwelling, E. (1997). *Maternal-newborn nursing: Theory and practice.* Philadelphia: W. B. Saunders, p. 1300.

119. The nurse administers 30 units of NPH Insulin to a client with a blood glucose level of 200 mg/dL at 7 A.M. The nurse notes to assess the client at the time when the insulin effects peak, which will be in

1 3–4 hours.
2 4–12 hours.
3 7–15 hours.
4 2 hours.

Answer: 2

Rationale: NPH is an intermediate-acting insulin with an onset in 3–4 hours, a peak in 4–12 hours, and a duration of 18–28 hours.

Test-Taking Strategy: Knowledge of the onset, peak, and duration of this medication is required. If you know NPH is an intermediate-acting insulin, then you can determine which of the options is correct. If you had difficulty with this question, take the time now to review the various types of insulin. You are likely to find a question on NCLEX-RN related to insulin!

Level of Cognitive Ability: Application
Phase of Nursing Process: Assessment
Client Needs: Physiological Integrity
Content Area: Pharmacology

Reference

Hodgson, B., & Kizior, R. (1998). *Saunders nursing drug handbook 1998.* Philadelphia: W. B. Saunders, p. 531.

---

120. The client's ECG telemetry indicated that the client is in ventricular tachycardia. Upon reaching the client's bedside, the nurse assesses for

1 Unresponsiveness.
2 Cyanosis.
3 Lethargy.
4 Unconsciousness.

Answer: 1

Rationale: With ventricular tachycardia, there is a significant decrease in cardiac output. However, assessing for unresponsiveness is a way to determine whether the client is affected by the decreased cardiac output. Recall the steps of basic life support (BLS). Determining unresponsiveness is the first assessment action to take in an unwitnessed situation.

Test-Taking Strategy: Use the steps of BLS when assessing the client in this situation. Determining unresponsiveness is the first action!

Level of Cognitive Ability: Analysis
Phase of Nursing Process: Assessment
Client Needs: Physiological Integrity
Content Area: Adult Health/Cardiovascular

Reference

Luckmann, J. (1997). *Saunders manual of nursing care.* Philadelphia: W. B. Saunders, p. 1048.

---

121. The client is brought to the emergency room after a severe burn caused by a fire at home. The burns are extensive, covering greater than 25% of the total body surface area (TBSA). The nurse reviews the laboratory results and would most likely expect to note which of the following?

1 White blood cell (WBC) count of 6000/μL
2 Hematocrit of 65%
3 Albumin level of 4.0 g/dL
4 Sodium level of 140 mEq/L

Answer: 2

Rationale: Extensive burns over greater than 25% of the TBSA result in generalized body edema in both burned and nonburned tissues and a decrease in circulating intravascular blood volume. Hematocrit levels are elevated in the first 24 hours after injury, demonstrating hemoconcentration from the loss of intravascular fluid. The normal WBC count is 5000–10,000/μL. The normal sodium level is 135–145 mEq/L. The normal albumin level is 3.4–5 g/dL. The normal hematocrit is 40%–54% in the male and 38%–47% in the female.

Test-Taking Strategy: Knowledge regarding physiological alterations and fluid and electrolyte balance during the first 24 hours after injury of a burned client is necessary to answer this question. If you are familiar with normal laboratory values, then by the process of elimination you would be able to identify the correct option. The only abnormal laboratory value is option 2, the hematocrit. If you had difficulty with this question, take time now to review normal laboratory values and the immediate postinjury period for burns!

Level of Cognitive Ability: Analysis
Phase of Nursing Process: Assessment
Client Needs: Physiological Integrity
Content Area: Adult Health/Integumentary

Reference

Black, J. M., & Matassarin-Jacobs, E. (1997). *Medical-surgical nursing: Clinical management for continuity of care* (5th ed.). Philadelphia: W. B. Saunders, p. 2235.

122. A client with angina who responds to the nurse's attempts at teaching about the disease by continually changing the subject is probably exhibiting

1 Denial.
2 Anger.
3 Depression.
4 Anxiety.

Answer: 1

Rationale: Denial is a defense mechanism that allows the client to minimize a threat that may be manifested by refusal to discuss what has happened. Denial is a common early reaction associated with chest discomfort, angina, or myocardial infarction. Anger is often manifested by "acting-out" behaviors. Depression may be manifested by passive behaviors. Anxiety is usually manifested by symptoms of sympathetic nervous system arousal.

Test-Taking Strategy: Knowledge about the mechanism of denial is necessary to answer this question. Read all options. Use the process of elimination and choose the answer on the basis of which behavior best fits the description. The manifestations of anger, depression, and anxiety are different from those of denial. Review these manifestations now if you had difficulty with this question!

Level of Cognitive Ability: Analysis
Phase of Nursing Process: Assessment
Client Needs: Psychosocial Integrity
Content Area: Adult Health/Cardiovascular

Reference

Ignatavicius, D. D., Workman, M. L., & Mishler, M. A. (1995). *Medical-surgical nursing: A nursing process approach* (2nd ed., Vol. 1). Philadelphia: W. B. Saunders, pp. 991, 998.

---

123. The nurse is caring for a client with a diagnosis of rheumatoid arthritis. The client is receiving aspirin (acetylsalicylic acid, or ASA), 5 g PO daily. Which of the following would indicate to the nurse that the client is experiencing an adverse reaction to the medication?

1 Tinnitus
2 Urinary retention
3 Joint pain
4 Constipation

Answer: 1

Rationale: Aspirin is a nonsteroidal anti-inflammatory medication. Adverse reactions include GI bleeding and/or gastric mucosal lesions, ringing in the ears (tinnitus), and generalized pruritus. Headache, dizziness, flushing, tachycardia, hyperventilation, sweating, and thirst are also adverse reactions.

Test-Taking Strategy: Knowledge about aspirin is necessary to answer this question. Remembering that this medication can cause GI disturbances and ototoxicity will assist you in selecting the correct option. If you had difficulty with this question, take the time now to review this medication!

Level of Cognitive Ability: Analysis
Phase of Nursing Process: Assessment
Client Needs: Physiological Integrity
Content Area: Pharmacology

Reference

Hodgson, B., & Kizior, R. (1998). *Saunders nursing drug handbook 1998.* Philadelphia: W. B. Saunders, pp. 75–77.

---

124. A child with hemophilia is brought into the emergency room after being hit on the neck with a baseball. The nurse needs to immediately assess the child for

1 Spontaneous hematuria.
2 Airway obstruction.
3 Headache and slurred speech.
4 Factor VIII deficiency.

Answer: 2

Rationale: Trauma to the neck may cause bleeding into the tissues of the neck, which may compromise the airway. Although hematuria is a symptom of hemophilia, it is not associated with neck injury. Headache and slurred speech are associated with head trauma but is not the priority option in this situation. Factor VIII deficiency is not a symptom of hemophilia but rather a common form of the disease.

Test-Taking Strategy: This question requires prioritization as reflected in the request for the nurse's immediate assessment. Use the ABCs—airway, breathing, and circulation—when selecting this answer. Airway assessment is always a first priority!

Level of Cognitive Ability: Application
Phase of Nursing Process: Assessment
Client Needs: Physiological Integrity
Content Area: Child Health

Reference

Wong, D. (1997). *Whaley and Wong's Essentials of pediatric nursing* (5th ed.). St. Louis: Mosby–Year Book, pp. 918–920.

---

125. The client received a thermal burn caused by the inhalation of steam. The client's mouth is edematous, and the nurse notes blisters in the client's mouth. The priority nursing assessment in the plan of care is focused on which of the following?

1 Difficulty swallowing
2 Pain
3 Fluid and electrolyte imbalances
4 Wheezing heard on auscultation

Answer: 4

Rationale: Thermal burns to the lower airways can occur with the inhalation of steam or explosive gases or with the aspiration of scalding liquids. Thermal burns to the upper airways are more common and generally appear erythematous and edematous with mucosal blisters or ulcerations. The mucosal edema can lead to upper airway obstruction, particularly during the first 24–48 hours after burn injury.

Test-Taking Strategy: Knowledge regarding direct thermal burn injuries would be helpful in answering this question. Use the process of elimination and the ABCs—airway, breathing, and circulation—to assist you in answering this question.

Level of Cognitive Ability: Analysis
Phase of Nursing Process: Assessment
Client Needs: Physiological Integrity
Content Area: Adult Health/Integumentary

Reference

Black, J. M., & Matassarin-Jacobs, E. (1997). *Medical-surgical nursing: Clinical management for continuity of care* (5th ed.). Philadelphia: W. B. Saunders, p. 2237.

---

126. The nurse assesses the client with a diagnosis of thyroid storm. Which of the following classic signs and symptoms associated with thyroid storm would indicate the need for immediate nursing intervention?

1 Fever, tachycardia, and systolic hypertension
2 Polyuria, nausea, and severe headaches
3 Profuse diaphoresis, flushing, and constipation
4 Hypotension, translucent skin, and obesity

Answer: 1

Rationale: The excessive amounts of thyroid hormone cause a rapid increase in the metabolic rate, thereby causing the classic signs and symptoms of thyroid storm such as fever, tachycardia, and hypertension. When these signs are present, the nurse must take quick action to prevent deterioration of the client's health, because death can ensue. Priority interventions include maintaining a patent airway and stabilizing the hemodynamic status. Although some of the other options may contain symptoms associated with thyroid storm, they would not indicate immediate nursing intervention.

Test-Taking Strategy: Use the principles associated with prioritizing when answering this question. Remember the ABCs: airway, breathing, and circulation. Tachycardia, hypertension, and a fever indicate hemodynamic instability and take precedence over other signs and symptoms. Also, by using your knowledge of thyroid storm and knowing that an entire option must be correct, you can eliminate options 2, 3, and 4. Be careful with selections that contain the word "and." Thoroughly read each selection. Option 1 is the only selection in which all the signs and symptoms reflect thyroid storm. If you had difficulty with this question, take time now to review thyroid storm!

Level of Cognitive Ability: Analysis
Phase of Nursing Process: Assessment
Client Needs: Physiological Integrity
Content Area: Adult Health/Endocrine

Reference

Ignatavicius, D. D., Workman, M. L., & Mishler, M. A. (1995). *Medical-surgical nursing: A nursing process approach* (2nd ed., Vol. 2). Philadelphia: W. B. Saunders, pp. 1834–1835.

127. The client was admitted with a diagnosis of frequent symptomatic premature ventricular contractions (PVCs). After sitting up in a chair for a few minutes, the client complains of feeling lightheaded. On cardiac auscultation the nurse would expect to find PVCs

1 A regular apical pulse.
2 An irregular apical pulse.
3 A decrease in cardiac output.
4 An increase in cardiac output.

Answer: 2

Rationale: The most accurate means of assessing pulse rhythm is by auscultation of the apical pulse. When a client has PVCs, the rate is irregular, and if the radial pulse is taken, a true picture of what is happening is not obtained. PVCs also cause a decrease in cardiac output, which cannot be assessed by auscultation. However, the decrease in cardiac output causes the lightheadedness.

Test-Taking Strategy: Read the question carefully. Use the process of elimination. Two options, 2 and 3, are indicative of PVCs. However, look at the stem of the question. The stem indicates the nurse would be auscultating for heart sounds. This action automatically eliminates option 3 (and option 4) as a choice.

Level of Cognitive Ability: Analysis
Phase of Nursing Process: Assessment
Client Needs: Physiological Integrity
Content Area: Adult Health/Cardiovascular

Reference

Black, J. M., & Matassarin-Jacobs, E. (1997). *Medical-surgical nursing: Clinical management for continuity of care* (5th ed.). Philadelphia: W. B. Saunders, p. 1305.

---

128. A major step in bathing a baby is preparing the environment to prevent heat loss and maintain the baby's body temperature. The loss of heat from a wet body surface is known as

1 Convection.
2 Conduction.
3 Radiation.
4 Evaporation.

Answer: 4

Rationale: There are four mechanisms of heat loss. Evaporation of moisture from a wet body surface dissipates heat along with the moisture. In option 1, convection, air moves across the baby's skin and heat is transferred to the air. In option 2, conduction, heat loss occurs when the baby is on a cold surface, such as a table, and the baby's body heat is transferred to the table. Option 3, radiation, occurs when heat from the body radiates to a cooler surface. Preventing heat loss in a baby is an important intervention.

Test-Taking Strategy: Knowledge about the mechanisms of heat loss is important to answer this question. Correlate evaporation with moisture or a wet body surface. This may help you remember the mechanism of evaporation. Review these concepts now if you had difficulty with this question!

Level of Cognitive Ability: Analysis
Phase of Nursing Process: Assessment
Client Needs: Physiological Integrity
Content Area: Child Health

Reference

Nichols, F., & Zwelling, E. (1997). *Maternal-newborn nursing: Theory and practice.* Philadelphia: W. B. Saunders, pp. 1072–1073.

129. The nurse is interviewing a client on her first prenatal visit. She is 6 weeks pregnant, has three living children, and had one spontaneous abortion at 6 weeks. When the nurses assesses family history, the client reports that both her mother and grandmother died of complications from diabetes mellitus. What additional subjective data is important to know at this time in order to plan care for this client?

1 How large her other children were at birth
2 Where she received prenatal care for the previous pregnancies
3 The height of her fundus as compared to her dates of the last menstrual period
4 A 24-hour diet recall

Answer: 1

Rationale: Having previous large newborns of 9 pounds or more is a risk factor for developing gestational diabetes mellitus. Where the client received previous prenatal care will not alter the care given during this pregnancy. The comparison of the fundal height with dates is objective data and is not important data for assessing risk factors for diabetes mellitus at 6 weeks' gestation. A 24-hour diet recall is important information after gestational diabetes has been diagnosed and client teaching has started. However, at this point it is more important to assess for the possibility of gestational diabetes.

Test-Taking Strategy: Eliminate option 4 because this option identifies objective data. Focusing on the issue, the risk for diabetes, will easily direct you to option 1. Review these risks now if you had difficulty with this question!

Level of Cognitive Ability: Application
Phase of Nursing Process: Assessment
Client Needs: Physiological Integrity
Content Area: Maternity

Reference

Reeder, S., Martin, L., & Koniak-Griffin, D. (1997). *Maternity nursing: Family, newborn, and women's health care* (18th ed.). Philadelphia: Lippincott-Raven, pp. 853–860.

---

130. The nurse is caring for a client with chronic obstructive pulmonary disease (COPD) receiving aminophylline (theophylline ethylenediamine) intravenously. The nurse monitors the theophylline blood serum level and assesses that the level is within therapeutic range when it is

1 5 μg/mL.
2 8 μg/mL.
3 15 μg/mL.
4 25 μg/mL.

Answer: 3

Rationale: Aminophylline is a bronchodilator. It is critical that the nurse monitor theophylline blood serum levels daily when a client is receiving this medication to ensure that a therapeutic range is present and to monitor for the potential for toxicity. The therapeutic serum level range is 10–20 μg/mL.

Test-Taking Strategy: Knowledge about aminophylline (theophylline) and the therapeutic serum level range is necessary to answer this question. You are likely to see a question on NCLEX-RN related to this medication. If you are unfamiliar with this medication or the therapeutic serum level, review and learn them now!

Level of Cognitive Ability: Analysis
Phase of Nursing Process: Assessment
Client Needs: Physiological Integrity
Content Area: Pharmacology

Reference

Hodgson, B., & Kizior, R. (1998). *Saunders nursing drug handbook 1998.* Philadelphia: W. B. Saunders, pp. 44–47.

---

131. The client has begun taking divalproex sodium (Depakote) for the management of seizure disorder. The nurse would monitor the results of which of the following serum laboratory tests periodically prescribed for the client?

1 Lactose dehydrogenase (LDH), serum glutamate oxaloacetic transaminase (SGOT), serum glutamate pyruvate transaminase (SGPT)
2 BUN and creatinine
3 Blood glucose
4 Electrolytes

Answer: 1

Rationale: Divalproex sodium (Depakote), an anticonvulsant, can cause hepatotoxicity, which is potentially fatal. The nurse monitors the results of liver function studies, such as LDH, SGOT, SGPT, and ammonia levels. This is especially true in the first 6 months of therapy.

Test-Taking Strategy: To answer this question accurately, recall that this medication can lead to hepatotoxicity. The only laboratory tests that measure liver function are included in option 1, and thus it is the correct answer. Review this medication now if you had difficulty with this question!

Level of Cognitive Ability: Application
Phase of Nursing Process: Assessment
Client Needs: Physiological Integrity
Content Area: Adult Health/Neurological

Reference

Deglin, J., & Vallerand, A. (1997). *Davis's drug guide for nurses* (5th ed.). Philadelphia: F. A. Davis, pp. 1201–1202.

---

132. An anxious client enters the emergency room, seeking treatment for a laceration of the finger while using a power tool. The client's vital signs are as follows: pulse, 96; blood pressure (BP), 148/88; respirations, 24. After the injury is cleansed and the client is reassured, the vital signs are retaken: pulse, 82; BP, 130/80; respirations, 20. The nurse assesses that the change in vital signs is resulting from

1 Reduced stimulation of the sympathetic nervous system.
2 The cooling effects of the cleansing solution.
3 The body's physical adaptation to the air conditioning.
4 Possible impending cardiovascular collapse.

Answer: 1

Rationale: Physical or emotional stress triggers a sympathetic nervous system response. Responses that are reflected in vital signs include increased pulse rate, increased BP, and increased respiratory rate. Stress reduction, then, returns these parameters to baseline.

Test-Taking Strategy: Note the similar ideas in the question and one of the options. The stem tells you that the client is anxious and has an injury. These two elements guide you to think about the body's response to stress. The wording of the stem tells you that the nurse reduced the stress, which guides you to the correct answer.

Level of Cognitive Ability: Analysis
Phase of Nursing Process: Assessment
Client Needs: Physiological Integrity
Content Area: Adult Health/Integumentary

Reference

Black, J. M., & Matassarin-Jacobs, E. (1997). *Medical-surgical nursing: Clinical management for continuity of care* (5th ed.). Philadelphia: W. B. Saunders, p. 1203.

---

133. The nurse is caring for a client with a closed-chest drainage system. The nurse would document that the system is functioning accurately when the nurse notes

1 Tidaling in the water seal compartment.
2 Continuous bubbling in the water seal compartment during both inspiration and expiration.
3 Absence of bubbling in the suction control chamber.
4 The presence of blood clots in the chest tubes.

Answer: 1

Rationale: Fluid in the water seal compartment should rise with inspiration and fall with expiration (tidaling). When tidaling occurs, the drainage tubes are patent and the apparatus is functioning properly. Note that tidaling stops when the lung has reexpanded or if the chest drainage tubes are kinked or obstructed. Continuous bubbling in the water seal compartment during both inspiration and expiration indicates that air is leaking into the drainage system or pleural cavity. This situation must be corrected. Absence of bubbling in a suction control chamber indicates that the system is not functioning properly and that the correct level of suction is not being maintained. Clots noted in a chest tube do require continuous assessment, but this option does not directly relate to what the question is asking.

Test-Taking Strategy: Knowledge about the functioning of chest tube drainage system is necessary to answer this question. You are likely to see questions related to chest tube drainage systems on NCLEX-RN. If you had difficulty with this question, review the functioning of chest tube drainage systems!

Level of Cognitive Ability: Analysis
Phase of Nursing Process: Assessment
Client Needs: Physiological Integrity
Content Area: Adult Health/Respiratory

Reference

Black, J. M., & Matassarin-Jacobs, E. (1997). *Medical-surgical nursing: Clinical management for continuity of care* (5th ed.). Philadelphia: W. B. Saunders, pp. 1163–1166.

134. The nurse is measuring the vital signs of a client with increased intracranial pressure (ICP). The respirations have a variable rate. The cycle of respirations begins shallowly with increasing depth to hyperventilation, followed by decreasing depth to apnea. The cycle then repeats itself. The nurse documents that the client is exhibiting

1 Apneustic respirations.
2 Cheyne-Stokes respirations.
3 Kussmaul respirations.
4 Tachypneic respirations.

Answer: 2

Rationale: The client with increased ICP may exhibit Cheyne-Stokes respirations. Their pattern is as described in the question. Apneustic respirations are rapid and shallow, with prolonged inspiration followed by short, ineffective exhalation. Kussmaul respirations are regular, deep, and rapid. Tachypnea is characterized by respirations that are rapid, regular, and shallow.

Test-Taking Strategy: A baseline knowledge of various types of respirations is needed to answer this question. Begin by eliminating option 4, because by definition that is just a rapid respiratory rate. If you know that Kussmaul breathing occurs with diabetic ketoacidosis, you can eliminate this one quickly, too. Knowledge about the difference between apneustic and Cheyne-Stokes is necessary to discriminate between these two. Review these various types of respirations now if you had difficulty with this question!

Level of Cognitive Ability: Analysis
Phase of Nursing Process: Assessment
Client Needs: Physiological Integrity
Content Area: Adult Health/Neurological

Reference

Black, J. M., & Matassarin-Jacobs, E. (1997). *Medical-surgical nursing: Clinical management for continuity of care* (5th ed.). Philadelphia: W. B. Saunders, p. 238.

---

135. The home health nurse is making a visit to a client with myasthenia gravis. The nurse is inquiring about the client's energy level. The nurse assesses that the client will most likely have fatigue

1 Following exertion and at the end of the day.
2 Following exertion and after meals.
3 After meals and at the end of the day.
4 Early in the morning and late in the day.

Answer: 1

Rationale: The client with myasthenia gravis has weakness after periods of exertion and near the end of the day. The nurse works with the client to space out activities to conserve energy and regain muscle strength by resting between activities.

Test-Taking Strategy: Clients with any form of chronic condition characterized by fatigue experience the greatest amount of fatigue after exertion and at the end of the day. With this global concept in mind, you would eliminate option 4 (early in the morning) and options 2 and 3 (after meals). Remember that in an option with two components, both components must be accurate for the option to be correct.

Level of Cognitive Ability: Analysis
Phase of Nursing Process: Assessment
Client Needs: Physiological Integrity
Content Area: Adult Health/Neurological

Reference

Black, J. M., & Matassarin-Jacobs, E. (1997). *Medical-surgical nursing: Clinical management for continuity of care* (5th ed.). Philadelphia: W. B. Saunders, p. 885.

---

136. The nurse is caring for the client with trigeminal neuralgia (tic douloureux). The nurse would assess the client for

1 Aching pain and ptosis of the eyelid.
2 Burning pain with intermittent facial paralysis.
3 Numbness and tingling accompanied by facial droop.
4 Stabbing pain accompanied by twitching of part of the face.

Answer: 4

Rationale: Trigeminal neuralgia is characterized by spasms of pain that start suddenly and last for seconds to minutes. The pain is often characterized as stabbing or similar to an electric shock. It is accompanied by spasms of facial muscles, which cause twitching of parts of the face or mouth or closure of the eye.

Test-Taking Strategy: This question may be easily interpreted by knowing the common name of the disorder: *tic* douloureux. If you know that a tic is a nervous twitch, then you would automatically select the correct choice. Otherwise, you must recall that trigeminal neuralgia has both sensory and motor aspects: that is, stabbing pain and twitching of part of the face. If you had difficulty with this question, review trigeminal neuralgia now!

Level of Cognitive Ability: Application
Phase of Nursing Process: Assessment
Client Needs: Physiological Integrity
Content Area: Adult Health/Neurological

Reference

Smeltzer, S., & Bare, B. (1996). *Brunner and Suddarth's Textbook of medical-surgical nursing* (8th ed.). Philadelphia: Lippincott-Raven, p. 1815.

---

137. A client arrives at the emergency room with complaints of frequent and excessive urination, excessive thirst, and excessive appetite. The client denies pain. Which of the following laboratory tests would be of greatest significance on the basis of the client's symptoms?

1. Urine culture and sensitivity (C&S)
2. Liver function tests (LFTs)
3. Blood glucose
4. Lipid profile

Answer: 3

Rationale: Polyuria, polydipsia, and polyphagia—the three Ps—are classic signs and symptoms of hyperglycemia. Pain, frequency, and urgency with urination as well as voiding in small amounts may indicate a urinary tract infection, for which a urine C&S would be helpful. LFTs would be indicated if liver disease were suspected. A lipid profile would be helpful to screen this client for cardiac risk factors.

Test-Taking Strategy: Read the question carefully and identify the symptoms that are present in the client. Recalling that the three Ps are associated with diabetes mellitus and hyperglycemia will assist you in selecting the correct option. Review the symptoms of hyperglycemia now if you had difficulty with this question!

Level of Cognitive Ability: Analysis
Phase of Nursing Process: Assessment
Client Needs: Physiological Integrity
Content Area: Adult Health/Endocrine

Reference

Ignatavicius, D. D., Workman, M. L., & Mishler, M. A. (1995). *Medical-surgical nursing: A nursing process approach* (2nd ed., Vol. 2). Philadelphia: W. B. Saunders, p. 1859.

---

138. The nurse is assessing the client with Bell's palsy. The nurse would assess the client for which of the following signs and symptoms related to the disorder?

1. Tingling sensations and ptosis of the eyelid
2. Burning pain with intermittent facial paralysis
3. Speech or chewing difficulties accompanied by facial droop
4. Stabbing pain accompanied by twitching of part of the face

Answer: 3

Rationale: Bell's palsy is a one-sided facial paralysis resulting from compression of the facial nerve (cranial nerve VII). It is accompanied by facial droop from paralysis of the facial muscles; increased lacrimation; painful sensations in the eye, in the face, or behind the ear; and speech or chewing difficulties.

Test-Taking Strategy: Remember that a palsy is a type of paralysis. This would allow you to eliminate option 4. Knowing that the symptoms do not "come and go" (intermittent) helps you eliminate option 2 next. To discriminate between the last two, recall that "facial droop" is much more characteristic of paralysis than just "ptosis," which enables you to choose option 3 as the answer. Review the signs and symptoms of Bell's palsy if you had difficulty with this question!

Level of Cognitive Ability: Application
Phase of Nursing Process: Assessment
Client Needs: Physiological Integrity
Content Area: Adult Health/Neurological

Reference

Smeltzer, S., & Bare, B. (1996). *Brunner and Suddarth's Textbook of medical-surgical nursing* (8th ed.). Philadelphia: Lippincott-Raven, pp. 1818–1819.

139. The nurse is assessing the client's risk for falls. The nurse would assess that which of the following factors does not put the client at added risk?

1 Cataracts
2 Episodes of dizziness
3 Use of nitroglycerin
4 Use of orthopedic shoes

Answer: 4

Rationale: Several factors can increase the client's risk for falls, including impaired vision, medications that cause dizziness or orthostatic hypotension, and problems with balance and coordination. The nurse assesses for these risks and provides preventive teaching. Orthopedic shoes have been specially fitted for the client and are generally sturdy and safe.

Test-Taking Strategy: Use the process of elimination to answer the question. To select the correct option, you should evaluate each of the items in terms of the potential of that item to make the client fall. Cataracts represent a vision impairment, which could increase the client's risk. Dizziness obviously increases the likelihood of a fall. Nitroglycerin could cause orthostatic hypotension, which is also a potential risk. Orthopedic shoes are beneficial to the client, and option 4 is therefore the answer to this question as stated.

Level of Cognitive Ability: Application
Phase of Nursing Process: Assessment
Client Needs: Safe, Effective Care Environments
Content Area: Fundamental Skills

Reference

Black, J. M., & Matassarin-Jacobs, E. (1997). *Medical-surgical nursing: Clinical management for continuity of care* (5th ed.). Philadelphia: W. B. Saunders, p. 2103.

---

140. The client seeks treatment for a fractured radius. There is an open wound on the arm, through which jagged bone edges protrude. The nurse assesses that this client has a

1 Greenstick fracture.
2 Comminuted fracture.
3 Compound fracture.
4 Simple fracture.

Answer: 3

Rationale: A compound fracture, also called an open or complex fracture, is one in which the skin or mucous membrane has been broken and the wound extends to the depth of the fractured bone. A greenstick fracture is an incomplete fracture, which occurs through part of the cross section of a bone; one side of the bone is fractured, and the other side is bent. A comminuted fracture is a complete fracture across the shaft of a bone, with splintering of the bone into fragments. A simple fracture is a fracture of the bone across its entire shaft with some possible displacement but without breaking of the skin.

Test-Taking Strategy: A familiarity with the different types of fractures is necessary to answer this question. Options 1 and 4 should be ruled out first, because they are the least complicated of fractures. To discriminate between the last two, remember that a compound fracture is complex or open. If you remember that a comminuted fracture is broken into minute (small) pieces, it may help to discriminate among options in questions such as these. Review the characteristics of the various types of fractures now if you had difficulty with this question!

Level of Cognitive Ability: Application
Phase of Nursing Process: Assessment
Client Needs: Physiological Integrity
Content Area: Adult Health/Musculoskeletal

Reference

Smeltzer, S., & Bare, B. (1996). *Brunner and Suddarth's Textbook of medical-surgical nursing* (8th ed.). Philadelphia: Lippincott-Raven, p. 1910.

141. The nurse is assessing a client who has expressed suicidal thinking. Which of the following statements would indicate that the client is at highest risk for suicide?

1. "There is nothing left for me in this life. I just wish I could die!"
2. "I tried to kill myself last year at this time by swallowing a bottle of aspirin. This time I'll swallow two bottles!"
3. "God has called on me to come to him. He commands me to jump off the bridge tomorrow."
4. "I'm just useless. I want someone to take me out and shoot me!"

Answer: 3

Rationale: The client with depression or another mental illness has a 3 to 12 times greater risk for suicide than do clients from other populations. The client who commits suicide is usually depressed and has feelings of hopelessness, worthlessness, inadequacy, or guilt. When psychosis is manifested in command auditory hallucinations (or voices telling the client to commit suicide), the likelihood of suicide increases because of increased impulsivity, impaired judgment, and impaired cognitive function. The formulation of a suicide plan indicates the client's intent to commit suicide.

Test-Taking Strategy: This question asks you to apply your knowledge of the risk factors for suicide to the assessment data (presented in the form of a client communication). In all of the client communications, there are risk factors that must not be ignored, but the degree of lethality varies. In option 1, the client expresses hopelessness, a risk factor for suicide. However, the client expresses suicidal ideation as a passive longing rather than an active plan. In option 2, the client reveals a history of a previous suicide attempt and a plan to try again, two risk factors for suicide. However, the suicidal attempt uses a passive method (taking pills rather than jumping off a bridge or shooting a gun) and the suicide plan is vague in that it tells only the method and does not include a date and place in the plan. In option 4, the client expresses hopelessness and despair and a suicidal plan, two risk factors for suicide. However, while the suicidal plan contains a highly lethal method, it is vague as to who will kill the client and the date when the suicide would occur. In option 3, the client identifies an auditory command hallucination and a suicide plan. The nature of the psychosis is highly lethal and the suicide plan includes an active lethal method, the time, and the place.

Level of Cognitive Ability: Analysis
Phase of Nursing Process: Assessment
Client Needs: Psychosocial Integrity
Content Area: Mental Health

Reference

Antai-Otong, D. (1995). *Psychiatric nursing: Biological and behavioral concepts.* Philadelphia: W. B. Saunders, pp. 340–341.

---

142. The client has a diagnosis of atrial fibrillation. During the initial assessment, the nurse assesses for a characteristic of atrial fibrillation by

1. Auscultating the apical pulse for an irregular rate while palpating the radial pulse for pulse deficit.
2. Palpating the radial pulse for quality while auscultating the apical pulse volume.
3. Auscultating the apical pulse for a regular pulse while palpating the radial pulse for quality.
4. Palpating the radial pulse for quality while auscultating the apical pulse for an irregular rate.

Answer: 1

Rationale: In atrial fibrillation, the pulse is irregular. When a pulse rate is irregular, the apical pulse should be auscultated for the irregularity and the radial pulse should be palpated for the pulse deficit.

Test-Taking Strategy: Read the options carefully. Option 1 is the only option that addresses assessment of both the apical and radial rates. Consider the nature of atrial fibrillation. Pulse deficit is a difference between the apical rate and the radial pulse rate, which is a characteristic of this condition. Review the characteristics of atrial fibrillation now if you had difficulty with this question!

Level of Cognitive Ability: Application
Phase of Nursing Process: Assessment
Client Needs: Physiological Integrity
Content Area: Adult Health/Cardiovascular

Reference

Luckmann, J. (1997). *Saunders manual of nursing care.* Philadelphia: W. B. Saunders, p. 135.

143. The newborn is brought to the mother after triple dye has been applied to the baby's umbilical cord. Which explanation of the infant's discolored cord would be best to give the mother?

1. Triple dye is used for initial cord care because it minimizes bacteria and promotes drying
2. Triple dye is used for initial cord care because it makes the cord drop off in 5–7 days
3. Triple dye is used to prevent the cord from hemorrhaging after birth
4. Triple dye is used to prevent *Staphylococcus aureus* colonization

Answer: 1

Rationale: The umbilical cord begins to dry after delivery. The triple dye prevents bacterial colonization and aids in the drying process.

Test-Taking Strategy: Use the process of elimination to answer the question. Option 2 is incorrect: the cord drops off in 7–14 days. Option 3 is incorrect: the dye does not prevent hemorrhaging, but the clamp does. Option 4 is partially correct in that it prevents colonization of *S. aureus;* however, option 1 is more global and therefore correct. Review the principles of cord care if you had difficulty with this question!

Level of Cognitive Ability: Application
Phase of Nursing Process: Assessment
Client Needs: Physiological Integrity
Content Area: Pharmacology

Reference

Nichols, F., & Zwelling, E. (1997). *Maternal-newborn nursing: Theory and practice.* Philadelphia: W. B. Saunders, p. 1147.

---

144. The nurse has been assigned to care for a client with a herniated lumbar disk at the L4–L5 interspace. During the initial client assessment, the nurse would most likely learn that the symptom that first caused the client to seek medical attention was

1. Shoulder pain that radiated from the client's back.
2. Lack of bladder and bowel control.
3. Back pain relieved by resting.
4. Loss of sensation and voluntary muscle control.

Answer: 3

Rationale: A common presenting symptom of herniated lumbar disk is low back pain that is usually aggravated by activity and relieved by rest. Muscle weakness and sensory loss may occur, and there is generally a change in tendon reflexes. Pain in the shoulders is more typical of cervical disk disease or a heart attack. Loss of voluntary muscle movements is not a typical early symptom of lumbar disk disease.

Test-Taking Strategy: Knowledge of the signs and symptoms of lumbar disk disease is pertinent when answering this question. You also must know which symptoms manifest early, as opposed to which symptoms occur later. Noting the area of the herniation (L4–L5 interspace) may assist in directing you to the correct option. By correlating this theoretical material through the process of elimination, you will be able to select the correct answer.

Level of Cognitive Ability: Application
Phase of Nursing Process: Assessment
Client Needs: Physiological Integrity
Content Area: Adult Health/Musculoskeletal

Reference

Black, J. M., & Matassarin-Jacobs, E. (1997). *Medical-surgical nursing: Clinical management for continuity of care* (5th ed.). Philadelphia: W. B. Saunders, p. 917.

---

145. When taking an assessment history from the parents of a 15 month old child suspected of having intussusception, which of these assessment areas would be most important for the nurse to address?

1. Pattern of abdominal pain
2. Known allergies
3. Dietary intake in the past 24 hours
4. Usual pattern of bowel movements

Answer: 1

Rationale: A report of severe colicky abdominal pain in a healthy, thriving child between 3 and 17 months of age is the classic manifestation of intussusception. Typical behavior includes screaming and drawing the knees up to the chest. Options 2, 3, and 4 are important aspects of a health history but are not significant clues to intussusception.

Test-Taking Strategy: Knowledge of the typical pain that occurs in intussusception is necessary to answer this question. This assessment question addresses the gathering of data that will confirm a suspected medical diagnosis of intussusception. The key word in the stem of this question to focus your attention on is "most important." If you had difficulty with this question, take time now to review the characteristics of intussusception!

Level of Cognitive Ability: Application
Phase of Nursing Process: Assessment
Client Needs: Physiological Integrity
Content Area: Child Health

Reference

Wong, D. (1995). *Whaley and Wong's Nursing care of infants and children* (5th ed.). St. Louis: Mosby–Year Book, pp. 1476–1477.

---

146. The client receives a diagnosis of scoliosis. The nurse prepares a nursing care plan for the client who is to undergo Harrington rod fusion. The nurse understands that scoliosis is a condition that is

1 An excessive posterior curvature of the thoracic spine.
2 An abnormal anterior curvature of the lumbar spine.
3 An abnormal lateral curvature of the spine.
4 An abnormal curvature of the spine resulting from inflammation.

Answer: 3

Rationale: Option 1, an excessive posterior curvature of the thoracic spine, is kyphosis. This is also known as "humpback." Option 2, an abnormal anterior curvature of the spine, is lordosis and is usually exaggerated during pregnancy, with obesity, or in persons with tumors of the spine. Scoliosis is defined as abnormal lateral curvature in any area of the spine. The most common place is the right thoracic area, which produces a rib prominence. Scoliosis does not result from inflammation.

Test-Taking Strategy: Knowledge about scoliosis is needed to answer this question. Correlate the term "lateral" with scoliosis, because this may assist you in remembering its description. If you had difficulty with this question, take time now to review its description!

Level of Cognitive Ability: Analysis
Phase of Nursing Process: Assessment
Client Needs: Physiological Integrity
Content Area: Child Health

Reference

Black, J. M., & Matassarin-Jacobs, E. (1997). *Medical-surgical nursing: Clinical management for continuity of care* (5th ed.). Philadelphia: W. B. Saunders, pp. 2120–2121.

---

147. The nurse is sent to the stroke unit to care for a client whose orders include frequent cerebrovascular assessment. The client has a history of cardiac disease. The nurse's assessment would include additional detail regarding

1 Peripheral pulse rate.
2 Apical pulse rhythm.
3 Body temperature.
4 Bowel sounds.

Answer: 2

Rationale: Monitoring the apical heart rhythm is an important component of cerebrovascular assessment. Peripheral pulse rate does not identify significant information for a cardiac disease related to stroke (option 1). Bowel sounds and body temperature (options 3 and 4), although significant to assessments of stroke clients, are not related to information in the stem. Option 2 correctly identifies cerebrovascular assessment.

Test-Taking Strategy: Use the process of elimination and the ABCs—airway, breathing, and circulation—to answer the question. Apical pulse assessment is directly related to the issue of the question, cardiac disease.

Level of Cognitive Ability: Application
Phase of Nursing Process: Assessment
Client Needs: Physiological Integrity
Content Area: Adult Health/Neurological

Reference

Lewis, S. M., Collier, I. C., & Heitkemper, M. M. (1996). *Medical-surgical nursing: Assessment and management of clinical problems* (4th ed.). St. Louis: Mosby–Year Book, pp. 1261, 1742.

148. A black American client with a cerebral hemorrhage is being evaluated for the possibility of a craniotomy. To assess the client's level of anxiety about the possible surgery, the white nurse

1 Interviews the client alone without the presence of the family.
2 Avoids questions concerning the risk of death.
3 Arranges to have a black American colleague assigned to care for the client.
4 Minimizes open-ended questioning concerning finances.

Answer: 3

Rationale: A number of fears are common to all clients anticipating surgery. Assessment of these is critical to a successful outcome. Research literature indicates that black American clients have difficulty communicating their feelings to white doctors and nurses. Family members are rarely excluded (option 1) from discussions. The subjects of death and finances (options 2 and 4) are considered critical to the assessment but may be avoided because of the nurse's lack of comfort in addressing these issues. With interpreting what is important, option 3 addresses most critically the ethnic/cultural side of care, especially when psychosocial needs are threatened.

Test-Taking Strategy: Read the question carefully. Note the similarity in the case of the situation and in the correct answer, option 3. If you had difficulty with this question, take time now to review the cultural considerations related to the care of the black American population!

Level of Cognitive Ability: Application
Phase of Nursing Process: Assessment
Client Needs: Psychosocial Integrity
Content Area: Adult Health/Neurological

Reference

Black, J. M., & Matassarin-Jacobs, E. (1997). *Medical-surgical nursing: Clinical management for continuity of care* (5th ed.). Philadelphia: W. B. Saunders, p. 315.

---

149. An neonate born before the end of 37 weeks of gestation is considered

1 Small for gestational age.
2 Full-term.
3 Preterm.
4 Post-term.

Answer: 3

Rationale: An neonate born before the end of 37 weeks of gestation is considered preterm, regardless of weight. Neonates designated small for gestational age are those whose weights are below the 10th percentile or are 2 standard deviations below normal. A full-term newborn is born between the beginning of week 38 and completion of week 41. A post-term newborn is born at week 42 or after.

Test-Taking Strategy: Option 1 is incorrect, although a preterm baby can be small for gestational age. Options 2 and 4 are incorrect because the gestational age does not match the criteria for preterm. If you can remember that between 38 and 40 weeks is full-term, then anytime before 40 weeks would be preterm and anytime after 41 weeks would be post-term. Review the characteristics of these classifications now if you had difficulty with the question!

Level of Cognitive Ability: Application
Phase of Nursing Process: Assessment
Client Needs: Physiological Integrity
Content Area: Maternity

Reference

Nichols, F., & Zwelling, E. (1997). *Maternal-newborn nursing: Theory and practice.* Philadelphia: W. B. Saunders, p. 1332.

150. The client has a synthetic cast on the right arm for a fractured ulna. The client asks if it would be possible to take a shower. On the basis of the assessment related to the injury and type of cast, the best response to the client would be

1. "The cast padding will not dry."
2. "It is not safe for you to shower alone."
3. "Hot water may soften the synthetic cast."
4. "It may lead to a serious infection."

Answer: 2

Rationale: Water does not damage the synthetic cast; however, the client should know that it may take a while for the cast padding to dry. It may be unsafe for the client to shower alone because the client may slip and fall. Water may soften a plaster cast but has no effect on a synthetic cast. A shower will not cause an infection.

Test-Taking Strategy: Note the key words "best response." Use Maslow's hierarchy of needs theory. Option 2 addresses the issue of safety.

Level of Cognitive Ability: Application
Phase of Nursing Process: Assessment
Client Needs: Safe, Effective Care Environment
Content Area: Adult Health/Musculoskeletal

Reference

Black, J. M., & Matassarin-Jacobs, E. (1997). *Medical-surgical nursing: Clinical management for continuity of care* (5th ed.). Philadelphia: W. B. Saunders, p. 2147.

---

151. The client has sustained a burn injury to the entire right arm, right leg, and anterior thorax. According to the "Rule of Nines," the nurse would assess that this injury constitutes which of the following body percentages?

1. 27%
2. 36%
3. 45%
4. 54%

Answer: 3

Rationale: According to the "Rule of Nines," the right arm is equal to 9% of the body and the left arm is equal to 9%. The right leg is equal to 18%, and the left leg is equal to 18%. The anterior thorax is equal to 18%, and the posterior thorax is equal to 18%. The head is equal to 9%, and the perineum is equal to 1%. The anterior thorax, the right leg, and right arm, according to the "Rule of Nines," constitute 45%.

Test-Taking Strategy: Knowledge of the percentages associated with the "Rule of Nines" is necessary to answer this question. From this point, you would be able to determine the percentage of burn injury and use the process of elimination to select the correct answer. If you had difficulty with this question, take time now to review the "Rule of Nines"!

Level of Cognitive Ability: Analysis
Phase of Nursing Process: Assessment
Client Needs: Physiological Integrity
Content Area: Adult Health/Integumentary

Reference

Black, J. M., & Matassarin-Jacobs, E. (1997). *Medical-surgical nursing: Clinical management for continuity of care* (5th ed.). Philadelphia: W. B. Saunders, p. 2239.

---

152. A newly admitted unconscious client becomes responsive. On assessment, the nurse notes that the client is unable to understand spoken language. A cerebrovascular accident (CVA) is suspected. The nurse understands that the client is likely to have experienced impairment of

1. The voluntary muscle activity of the mouth.
2. Concept formation and abstraction.
3. The auditory association areas.
4. The optic nerve tracts.

Answer: 3

Rationale: Knowledge about the physiology of the cerebral cortex is necessary to answer this question. The frontal lobe controls voluntary muscle activity, including speech. An impairment can result in expressive aphasia. The parietal lobe contains association areas for concept formation, abstraction, spatial orientation, body and object size and shape, and tactile sensation. The occipital lobe contains areas related to vision. The only correct answer is option 3. Auditory association and storage areas are located in the temporal lobe.

Test-Taking Strategy: The question asks you to select specific information related to speech. On that basis, options 2 and 4 can be eliminated. Option 1 relates to expressive, not receptive, aphasia; therefore, option 3 is the only correct answer. If you had difficulty with this question, review the physiology of the cerebral cortex now!

Level of Cognitive Ability: Analysis
Phase of Nursing Process: Assessment
Client Needs: Physiological Integrity
Content Area: Adult Health/Neurological

Reference

Black, J. M., & Matassarin-Jacobs, E. (1997). *Medical-surgical nursing: Clinical management for continuity of care* (5th ed.). Philadelphia: W. B. Saunders, pp. 690–691.

---

153. The assessment and definitive diagnosis of leukemia is based on

1. Suspicion after obtaining the history.
2. Physical manifestations.
3. Results of the white blood cell count.
4. Bone marrow aspiration or biopsy findings.

Answer: 4

Rationale: Bone marrow aspiration or biopsy allows examination of blast cells and other hypercellular activity. Physical manifestations, white blood cell counts, and an accurate history raise suspicion but do not provide a definitive diagnosis. It is important to understand that in leukemia, infiltration of leukemic cells occurs in the bone marrow.

Test-Taking Strategy: The key word is "definitive." Use the process of elimination in selecting the correct option. Eliminate all of the vague answers and look for a specific answer that will address a definitive diagnosis of leukemia. If you had difficulty with this question, take time now to review the assessment findings associated with leukemia!

Level of Cognitive Ability: Application
Phase of Nursing Process: Assessment
Client Needs: Physiological Integrity
Content Area: Adult Health/Oncology

Reference

Wong, D., & Perry, S. (1998). *Maternal-child nursing care.* St. Louis: Mosby–Year Book, p. 1518.

---

154. The recommended ages for the administration of diphtheria-pertussis-tetanus (DPT) vaccine are

1. 2, 4, 6, and 12 months, with a booster at puberty.
2. Birth and 2 and 4 months, with a booster at 4–6 years of age.
3. Birth and 2, 6, and 15 months, with a booster at puberty.
4. 2, 4, 6, and 15 months, with a booster at 4–6 years of age.

Answer: 4

Rationale: Maternal immunoglobulin is transferred primarily during the third trimester, so immunization with DPT is not missing at birth. Newborns have immunity to tetanus, diphtheria, smallpox, measles, and a variety of other viral infections. The period of resistance may vary and last 4–8 months. A booster is needed at 4–6 years of age before the child attends school.

Test-Taking Strategy: Knowledge about the immunization schedule is necessary to answer this question. Read the stem carefully. "Recommended" is the key concept. Use the process of elimination. Eliminate the distracter "birth," used in two of the options. You are likely to see questions on NCLEX-RN related to immunizations. Review this schedule now!

Level of Cognitive Ability: Application
Phase of Nursing Process: Assessment
Client Needs: Psychosocial Integrity
Content Area: Pharmacology

Reference

Ashwill, J., & Droske, S. (1997). *Nursing care of children: Principles and practice.* Philadelphia: W.B. Saunders, pp. 595–596.

155. A client has had arterial bypass surgery. The nurse monitors fluid balance. Of the following, which is the best indicator of fluid balance?

1 Urine output
2 IV fluid infusion
3 Daily weight
4 Nasogastric tube drainage

Answer: 3

Rationale: Daily weight is a reliable indicator of fluid balance. Options 1, 2, and 4 are related to intake or output and are incomplete indicators of fluid balance.

Test-Taking Strategy: Remember that the best indicator of fluid balance is weight. Looking at the similarity between options assists in answering the question. Options 1, 2, and 4 are measurements of intake or output. Option 3, daily weight, is different from the other options.

Level of Cognitive Ability: Application
Phase of Nursing Process: Assessment
Client Needs: Physiological Integrity
Content Area: Adult Health/Cardiovascular

Reference

Black, J. M., & Matassarin-Jacobs, E. (1997). *Medical-surgical nursing: Clinical management for continuity of care* (5th ed.). Philadelphia: W.B. Saunders, p. 1417.

---

156. Which of the following is the best method to use when assessing a client's pupillary reaction to light?

1 Turn the light on directly in front of the eye and watch for a response
2 Check pupil size, then have the client alternate watching the light and the examiner's finger
3 Instruct the client to look straight ahead; then shine the light from the temporal area to the eye
4 Ask the client to follow the light through the six cardinal positions of gaze

Answer: 3

Rationale: Option 2 assesses accommodation of the eye rather than response to light. Option 4 assesses for eye movement related to cranial nerves III, IV, and VI. Options 1 and 3 relate to pupillary response to light; however, shining the light directly into the client's eye without the client's focusing on a distant object is not an appropriate technique.

Test-Taking Strategy: Use the process of elimination to answer the question. Knowledge regarding pupillary assessment is necessary to answer this question. If you are unfamiliar with basic neurological assessments, take time now to review them!

Level of Cognitive Ability: Application
Phase of Nursing Process: Assessment
Client Needs: Physiological Integrity
Content Area: Adult Health/Neurological

Reference

Black, J. M., & Matassarin-Jacobs, E. (1997). *Medical-surgical nursing: Clinical management for continuity of care* (5th ed.). Philadelphia: W. B. Saunders, p. 720.

---

157. An elderly client is admitted to the hospital after falling off a chair at home. During the night the nurse wakes the client up to perform a neurological check. The client states, "I'm so scared. Where am I? What's happening?" On the basis of the assessment, which is the best response by the nurse?

1 "There's no reason to be scared, you're safe here in the hospital."
2 "You fell and hit your head. Your family brought you here."
3 "You're in the hospital after a fall. You feel scared?"
4 "Hold my hand. Try to wake up and tell me your name."

Answer: 3

Rationale: Reflecting is using the client's own words or feelings when responding. In option 3, the nurse gives information to the client as well as reflects feelings. In option 1, the nurse does not demonstrate a value for the client's opinion, thereby blocking communication. In option 2, the nurse gives information but does not deal with the client's emotional need. In option 4, the nurse attempts to calm the client and blocks communication by changing the subject and beginning the neurological assessment.

Test-Taking Strategy: Therapeutic communication aids in facilitating your communication with a client. Remember to respond to the client's emotional needs. Avoid blocks to communication and focus on the client's feelings first!

Level of Cognitive Ability: Application
Phase of Nursing Process: Assessment
Client Needs: Psychosocial Integrity
Content Area: Adult Health/Neurological

Reference

Smeltzer, S., & Bare, B. (1996). *Brunner and Suddarth's Textbook of medical-surgical nursing* (8th ed.). Philadelphia: Lippincott-Raven, p. 29.

---

158. In a post-stroke adult client, which is the best way to elicit the plantar reflex?

1 Firmly stroke the lateral sole of the foot and under the toes with a blunt instrument
2 Tap the Achilles tendon with the reflex hammer
3 Gently prick the client's skin on the dorsum of the foot in two places
4 Hold the sides of the client's great toe and, while moving it, ask what position it is in

Answer: 1

Rationale: The plantar reflex is elicited by option 1. Normally, the toes plantiflex, but when abnormal, the toes dorsiflex and fan out. The other options relate to various neurological assessments: option 2, gastrocnemius muscle contraction; option 3, two-point discrimination; and option 4, proprioception.

Test-Taking Strategies: Knowledge about general neurological assessment is helpful in answering this question. The three distracters in this question are all neurological assessments in the same body area. Review general neurological assessments, especially the plantar reflex and the Babinski reflex. A key in the stem is that the client has had a cerebrovascular accident (CVA). Often, a Babinski reflex is present, indicating upper motor neuron damage. Review general neurological assessment now if you had difficulty with this question!

Level of Cognitive Ability: Application
Phase of Nursing Process: Assessment
Client Needs: Physiological Integrity
Content Area: Adult Health/Neurological

Reference

Black, J. M., & Matassarin-Jacobs, E. (1997). *Medical-surgical nursing: Clinical management for continuity of care* (5th ed.). Philadelphia: W. B. Saunders, pp. 724, 726, 727.

---

159. The nurse is caring for a client with a genitourinary infection who is receiving amoxicillin (Amoxil), 500 mg every 8 hours. Which of the following would indicate to the nurse that the client is experiencing an adverse reaction to the medication?

1 Hypertension
2 Hypotension
3 Constipation
4 Diarrhea

Answer: 4

Rationale: Amoxicillin (Amoxil) is a penicillin. Adverse reactions include superinfections such as potentially fatal antibiotic-associated colitis, which results from altered bacterial balance. Symptoms include abdominal cramps, watery severe diarrhea, and fever. Frequent side effects of amoxicillin include gastrointestinal disturbances, headache, and oral or vaginal candidiasis.

Test-Taking Strategy: Knowledge about amoxicillin (Amoxil) is necessary to answer the question. Antibiotics have a tendency to produce gastrointestinal side effects. If you can remember that this medication is classified as an antibiotic, then by the process of elimination, option 4 would be selected. If you had difficulty with this question, take the time now to review this medication!

Level of Cognitive Ability: Analysis
Phase of Nursing Process: Assessment
Client Needs: Physiological Integrity
Content Area: Pharmacology

Reference

Hodgson, B., & Kizior, R. (1998). *Saunders nursing drug handbook 1998.* Philadelphia: W. B. Saunders, pp. 54–56.

160. The nurse working in a long-term care setting has recently attended a workshop on creating a restraint-free environment for the residents. Several coworkers have been employed in this facility for many years and firmly believe that their current methods are satisfactory. The nurse can be effective in facilitating change by

1. Informing the nursing supervisor that current restraint policies must be changed and requesting that all staff be required to comply.
2. Writing a new restraint policy over the weekend and distributing it to coworkers for immediate implementation on Monday.
3. Asking coworkers to help gather data comparing the facility's restraint procedures and outcomes with those of others using revised procedures.
4. Pointing out to coworkers the various mistakes that they are presently making in adhering to outdated restraint procedures.

Answer: 3

Rationale: To be an effective leader, the nurse must work collaboratively with others to solve common problems. A punitive atmosphere (such as evidenced in option 4) is not effective in promoting change, as it discourages people from taking risks. The nurse who works collaboratively with others to facilitate change has a much greater chance of success than one who unilaterally demands or implements change, such as in options 1 and 2. To focus on errors (perceived or real), as in 4, serves only to alienate others and is not effective in promoting change. Option 3 is an example of collaborative efforts, beginning with assessment of baseline and comparison with outcomes with other facilities. By enlisting the assistance of others, the nurse has a greater chance that they will support proposed changes in procedures.

Test-Taking Strategy: Begin by identifying the critical elements of the stem. In this case, you are being asked to determine the action most likely to lead to change (key words in the stem are "effective" and "facilitating"). Three of the possible answers (1, 2, and 4) focus on unilateral actions by the nurse. Only one answer describes a collaboration between the nurse and coworkers. This response, therefore, is different in content from the remaining three options and is most likely to be the correct response.

Level of Cognitive Ability: Application
Phase of Nursing Process: Assessment
Client Needs: Psychosocial Integrity
Content Area: Fundamental Skills

Reference

Wywialowski, E. F. (1997). *Managing client care* (2nd ed.). St. Louis: Mosby–Year Book, pp. 194–197.

---

161. The physician orders a chemotherapy medication dosage that the nurse believes to be too high. The physician has left the office for the weekend. The nurse

1. Checks with the pharmacist, who agrees the dose is too high and then reduces the dose accordingly.
2. Withholds giving the medication until the physician's partner makes rounds the following day.
3. Reschedules the client's chemotherapy for the following week.
4. Calls the answering service and confers with the on-call physician.

Answer: 4

Rationale: The nurse has a duty to protect the client from harm. If the nurse believes a physician's order to be in error, the nurse is responsible for clarifying before carrying out the order. Checking with the pharmacist (option 1) can assist the nurse in determining whether the dosage ordered is incorrect, but neither the nurse nor pharmacist is licensed to prescribe medications. They therefore cannot alter the dosage without an order from the physician. Withholding the medication (option 2) until the following day is inadvisable, because chemotherapy agents must often be administered in the proper combinations or sequence in order to be effective. Rescheduling the client's chemotherapy (option 3) is similarly inadvisable because chemotherapy must be administered on a specific schedule for maximum positive effect with minimum adverse effects.

Test-Taking Strategy: This question requires you to determine the best response to the situation presented. Some basic understanding of chemotherapy and administration schedules is needed, but you do not have to be an expert in the administration and management of chemotherapy in order to choose the best answer from the four options. With this knowledge, it is easy to recognize that rescheduling or waiting until the next day (options 2 and 3) are poor choices. Conferring with a colleague (option 1) is an appropriate action; however, when the response includes "and," both halves of the response must be acceptable. In this instance, alteration of the dose by the nurse and pharmacist is not appropriate. The remaining answer, option 4, must be correct by process of elimination.

Level of Cognitive Ability: Application
Phase of Nursing Process: Assessment
Client Needs: Physiological Integrity
Content Area: Fundamental Skills

Reference

Potter, P. A., & Perry, A. G. (1997). *Fundamentals of nursing: Theory and practice* (4th ed.). St. Louis: Mosby–Year Book, p. 814.

---

162. The nurse is caring for a client with glaucoma who is receiving acetazolamide (Diamox) daily. Which of the following would indicate to the nurse that the client is experiencing an adverse reaction to the medication?

1 Constipation
2 Difficulty swallowing
3 Dark-colored urine and stools
4 Irritability

Answer: 3

Rationale: Acetazolamide (Diamox) is a carbonic anhydrase inhibitor. Nephrotoxicity and hepatotoxicity may occur and are manifested by dark-colored urine and stools, pain in the lower back, jaundice, dysuria, crystalluria, renal colic, and calculi. Bone marrow depression may also occur.

Test-Taking Strategy: Knowledge about acetazolamide (Diamox) is necessary to answer this question. Remembering that this medication is nephrotoxic and hepatotoxic will assist in directing you to the correct option. If you had difficulty with this question, take time now to review this medication!

Level of Cognitive Ability: Analysis
Phase of Nursing Process: Assessment
Client Needs: Physiological Integrity
Content Area: Pharmacology

Reference

Hodgson, B., & Kizior, R. (1998). *Saunders nursing drug handbook 1998.* Philadelphia: W. B. Saunders, pp. 8–10.

---

163. The nurse auscultates the chest of the client with valvular heart disease every 4 hours. Which breath sound indicates a problem with cardiac output?

1 S3
2 Crackles
3 Bronchial
4 Cardiac gallop

Answer: 2

Rationale: A low cardiac output will cause the backward flow of blood into the heart and pulmonary system, causing crackles to be heard in the lung fields. An S3 heart sound is also termed *ventricular gallop;* therefore, options 1 and 4 are similar. S3 is the third heart sound produced during the rapid filling phase of ventricular diastole when blood flows from the atrium to a noncompliant ventricle. Bronchial breath sounds are normal breath sounds heard over the manubrium in the large tracheal airways. These sounds are loud and high-pitched and have a hollow or harsh quality.

Test-Taking Strategy: Look at the stem of the question. Use the process of elimination. The question asks for identification of a breath sound. Options 1 and 4 are heart sounds and can be eliminated. Option 3 is a normal breath sound and therefore can also be eliminated. This leaves option 2. Crackles, or rales, are an indication of fluid in the lung fields brought on by low cardiac output.

Level of Cognitive Ability: Application.
Phase of Nursing Process: Assessment
Client Needs: Physiological Integrity
Content Area: Adult Health/Cardiovascular

Reference

Black, J. M., & Matassarin-Jacobs, E. (1997). *Medical-surgical nursing: Clinical management for continuity of care* (5th ed.). Philadelphia: W. B. Saunders, p. 1348.

164. The client with cancer of the bladder has a nursing diagnosis of "Fear related to the uncertain outcome of upcoming cystectomy and urinary diversion." The nurse assesses that this diagnosis still applies if the client makes which of the following statements?

1 "I'm so afraid I won't live through all this."
2 "What if I have no help at home after going through this awful surgery?"
3 "I'll never feel like myself once I can't go to the bathroom normally."
4 "I wish I'd never gone to the doctor at all."

Answer: 1

Rationale: In order for Fear to be an actual diagnosis, the client must be able to identify the object of fear. In this question, the client is expressing a fear of death related to cancer. The statement in option 2 reflects Risk for Impaired Home Maintenance Management. Option 3 reflects a Body Image Disturbance. Option 4 is vague and nonspecific. Further exploration would be necessary to associate this statement with a nursing diagnosis.

Test-Taking Strategy: The diagnostic statement includes wording about the uncertain outcome of surgery. Because option 4 is a general statement, it should be eliminated first. Options 2 and 3 focus on the self after surgery but do not contain statements about an uncertain outcome. By elimination, option 1 is correct. The client expresses a fear of dying after enduring the ordeal of surgery.

Level of Cognitive Ability: Application
Phase of Nursing Process: Assessment
Client Needs: Psychosocial Integrity
Content Area: Adult Health/Renal

References

Black, J. M., & Matassarin-Jacobs, E. (1997). *Medical-surgical nursing: Clinical management for continuity of care* (5th ed.). Philadelphia: W. B. Saunders, p. 1552.

Cox, H., Hinz, M., & Lubno, M., et al. (1997). *Clinical applications of nursing diagnosis: Adult, child, women's, psychiatric, gerontic and home health considerations* (3rd ed.). Philadelphia: F. A. Davis, pp. 344, 506, 514.

165. While assessing a client with diabetic ketoacidosis (DKA), the nurse monitors for which of the following gastrointestinal symptoms frequently caused by acidosis?

1 Nausea and vomiting
2 Melena
3 Absolute true borborygmi
4 Constipation

Answer: 1

Rationale: Nausea, vomiting, and diarrhea are secondary to acidosis. There may be increased abdominal bowel sounds secondary to increased peristalsis but true borborygmi primarily suggests a mechanical obstruction of the small intestine. Melena results from bleeding in the upper gastrointestinal tract and is usually a sign of peptic ulcer or small bowel disease.

Test-Taking Strategy: Absolute terminology tends to make a statement false; therefore you can eliminate option 3 as the correct response. Because DKA is an acute situation and melena involves old blood in the stool, you can also eliminate option 2. You are left with options 1 and 4. At this point you need to reread the question and focus on exactly what it is asking about: a symptom caused by acidosis (nausea and vomiting). Constipation could be caused by fluid loss; however, diarrhea is most common during the initial stages of DKA.

Level of Cognitive Ability: Application
Phase of Nursing Process: Assessment
Client Needs: Physiological Integrity
Content Area: Adult Health/Endocrine

Reference

Lewis, S. M., Collier, I. C., & Heitkemper, M. M. (1996). *Medical-surgical nursing: Assessment and management of clinical problems* (4th ed.). St. Louis: Mosby–Year Book, pp. 1076, 1085, 1465.

166. The nurse is caring for a client with a tracheostomy tube. The nurse suspects tracheoesophageal fistula when the nurse notes

1 Abdominal distention.
2 Excess mucus production.
3 Abnormal skin and mucous membrane color.
4 Use of accessory muscles to assist with breathing.

Answer: 1

Rationale: Necrosis of the tracheal wall can lead to an artificial opening between the posterior trachea and esophagus. This problem is called *tracheoesophageal fistula*. The fistula allows air to escape into the stomach, causing abdominal distension. It also promotes aspiration of gastric contents.

Test-Taking Strategy: Use medical terminology to assist you in answering this question. A fistula is an artificial opening. *Tracheoesophageal* means "trachea to esophagus." On the basis of these definitions, review the options and use the process of elimination. This will assist in directing you to the correct option. If you think of air from the trachea moving to the esophagus, you would note that abdominal distention would occur with this condition.

Level of Cognitive Ability: Analysis
Phase of Nursing Process: Assessment
Client Needs: Physiological Integrity
Content Area: Adult Health/Respiratory

Reference

Black, J. M., & Matassarin-Jacobs, E. (1997). *Medical-surgical nursing: Clinical management for continuity of care* (5th ed.). Philadelphia: W. B. Saunders, p. 1069.

167. The mother of a toddler who is hospitalized with mild dehydration must leave her child to go to work. Which behavior would a nurse most likely observe in this child immediately after the mother's departure?

1 Silently curled in bed with a blanket
2 Loudly crying and kicking both legs
3 Playing quietly with a favorite toy
4 Sucking thumb and rocking back and forth

Answer: 2

Rationale: The three stages of separation anxiety are protest, despair, and detachment. Loudly crying and kicking both legs is a protest behavior that is seen in the first stage of separation. Options 1 and 4 are incorrect. Theses are behaviors seen in the stage of despair and at this time the child is withdrawn and employs self-comfort measures. Option 3 is incorrect because the behavior reflects detachment, the third stage of separation.

Test-Taking Strategy: A key phrase in the stem is "immediately after her departure." This directs you to look for the toddler's immediate behavioral response to separation. The reader must be knowledgeable about the three stages of separation anxiety and normal growth and development in a toddler. If you had difficulty with this question, take time now to review normal growth and development and the concepts of separation anxiety!

Level of Cognitive Ability: Analysis
Phase of Nursing Process: Assessment
Client Needs: Psychosocial Integrity
Content Area: Child Health

Reference

Wong, D. (1995). *Whaley and Wong's nursing care of infants and children* (5th ed.). St. Louis: Mosby–Year Book, p. 1065.

168. The nurse is assessing the renal function of the client. After directly noting urine volume and characteristics, the nurse assesses which of the following items as the best indirect indicator of renal status?

1 Bladder distention
2 Level of consciousness
3 Pulse rate
4 Blood pressure

Answer: 4

Rationale: The kidneys normally receive 20%–25% of the cardiac output, even under conditions of rest. In order for kidney function to be optimal, adequate renal perfusion is necessary. Perfusion can best be estimated by the blood pressure, which is an indirect reflection of the adequacy of cardiac output. The pulse rate affects the cardiac output but can be altered by factors unrelated to kidney function. Bladder distention reflects a problem or obstruction that is most often distal to the kidneys. Level of consciousness is an unrelated item.

Test-Taking Strategy: Eliminate level of consciousness first as the item most unrelated to kidney function. Because bladder distention can be affected by a number of factors besides renal function, this is eliminated next. To choose between pulse and blood pressure, remember that the cardiac output = heart rate × stroke volume. The cardiac output overall helps determine the blood pressure and renal perfusion. Thus blood pressure is the more global factor and the one most directly related to kidney perfusion, which makes it the best option.

Level of Cognitive Ability: Application
Phase of Nursing Process: Assessment
Client Needs: Physiological Integrity
Content Area: Adult Health/Renal

Reference

Black, J. M., & Matassarin-Jacobs, E. (1997). *Medical-surgical nursing: Clinical management for continuity of care* (5th ed.). Philadelphia: W. B. Saunders, p. 1537.

---

169. The nurse is caring for a client with a diagnosis of meningitis. The client is receiving amphotericin B (Abelcet or Fungizone) intravenously. Which of the following would indicate to the nurse that the client is experiencing an adverse reaction to the medication?

1 Hypertension
2 Decreased urinary output
3 Muscle weakness
4 Confusion

Answer: 2

Rationale: Amphotericin B is an antifungal. Adverse reactions include nephrotoxicity, which occurs commonly. Cardiovascular toxicity, as evidenced by hypotension and ventricular fibrillation, and anaphylactic reaction occur rarely. Vision and hearing alterations, seizures, hepatic failure, and coagulation defects may also occur. The nurse needs to monitor input and output and renal function tests for potential signs of nephrotoxicity.

Test-Taking Strategy: Knowledge about amphotericin B (Abelcet or Fungizone) is necessary to answer this question. If you can remember that this medication causes nephrotoxicity, cardiovascular toxicity, and vision and hearing alterations, you will be able to select the correct answer. If you had difficulty with this question, take the time now to review this medication!

Level of Cognitive Ability: Analysis
Phase of Nursing Process: Assessment
Client Needs: Physiological Integrity
Content Area: Pharmacology

Reference

Hodgson, B., & Kizior, R. (1998). *Saunders nursing drug handbook 1998.* Philadelphia: W. B. Saunders, pp. 57–59.

---

170. A client is hospitalized for hypoparathyroidism. The nurse assesses the client and notes positive Trousseau's and Chvostek's signs, which are indicative of which electrolyte imbalance?

1 Hypernatremia
2 Hypokalemia
3 Hypocalcemia
4 Hypermagnesemia

Answer: 3

Rationale: Hypoparathyroidism is related to a lack of parathyroid hormone secretion or to a decreased effectiveness of parathyroid hormone on target tissues. The end result of this disorder is hypocalcemia. When serum calcium levels are critically low, the client may exhibit Chvostek's and Trousseau's signs, which indicate potential tetany.

Test-Taking Strategy: Knowledge of which electrolyte imbalance is associated with hypoparathyroidism is necessary to answer this question. Remembering which electrolyte (calcium) is associated with Chvostek's and Trousseau's signs will assist you in answering the question. If you are unfamiliar with these signs, take time to review them now!

Level of Cognitive Ability: Application
Phase of Nursing Process: Assessment
Client Needs: Physiological Integrity
Content Area: Adult Health/Endocrine

Reference

Ignatavicius, D. D., Workman, M. L., & Mishler, M. A. (1995). *Medical-surgical nursing: A nursing process approach* (2nd ed., Vol. 2). Philadelphia: W. B. Saunders, pp. 1853–1854.

171. Which of the following specific assessment findings in a diabetic client would indicate to the nurse that the client is experiencing an episode of hyperglycemia?

1 Mouth sores
2 Diaphoresis
3 Polyuria
4 Anuria

Answer: 3

Rationale: Regular monitoring of the diabetic client may detect signs of hyperglycemia early enough to prevent serious complications. Classic symptoms of hyperglycemia include polydipsia, polyuria, and polyphagia.

Test-Taking Strategy: Knowledge of the signs of hyperglycemia is necessary to answer this question. Remembering the 3 Ps—polyuria, polydipsia, and polyphagia—will assist in directing you to the correct option. If you had difficulty with this question, take time now to review hyperglycemia!

Level of Cognitive Ability: Analysis
Phase of Nursing Process: Assessment
Client Needs: Physiological Integrity
Content Area: Adult Health/Endocrine

Reference

Burrell, L. O., Gerlach, M. J., & Pless, B. (1997). *Adult nursing: Acute and community care* (2nd ed.). Stamford, CT: Appleton & Lange, p. 1166.

---

172. Two weeks after receiving a diagnosis of human immunodeficiency virus (HIV) infection, the client is referred for mental health assessment. In assessing the client, the nurse understands that

1 The shock and disbelief would be followed by anger, self-pity, and malingering.
2 It is uncommon to respond with symptoms similar to those of post-traumatic stress disorder (PTSD) in the first couple of weeks.
3 It is uncommon for the client to experience anxiety and hypervigilance after the first week in which the diagnosis was learned.
4 It is uncommon to become depressed after learning of the diagnosis, inasmuch as anxiety is the prevailing affective response.

Answer: 1

Rationale: The most common response for the client with newly diagnosed HIV infection is shock and disbelief, which is followed by guilt, anger, and depression. A symptom complex resembling PTSD is also common in the first few weeks after notification. The client may experience anxiety, hypervigilance, and malingering.

Test-Taking Strategy: Knowing the stages that clients normally complete with regard to loss and grieving will assist you in discovering the correct and most appropriate option. Note the similarity "uncommon" in each of the incorrect responses. Review the stages of grief and loss now if you had difficulty with this question!

Level of Cognitive Ability: Analysis
Phase of Nursing Process: Assessment
Client Needs: Psychosocial Integrity
Content Area: Fundamental Skills

Reference

Black, J. M., & Matassarin-Jacobs, E. (1997). *Medical-surgical nursing: Clinical management for continuity of care* (5th ed.). Philadelphia: W. B. Saunders, pp. 614–650.

173. The client has an arm cast. The nurse would assess for signs and symptoms of compartment syndrome such as

1 Pain that is relieved by narcotic analgesics.
2 Aggravation of pain with limb elevation.
3 Absence of pain with passive movement.
4 Paralysis of the hand not preceded by paresthesias.

Answer: 2

Rationale: The pain of compartment syndrome is not relieved by narcotic analgesics. The pain is aggravated by limb elevation, which further impairs blood supply. The compartment is painful when moved. Paresthesias occur early in the syndrome, which progresses to paralysis unless pressure in the compartment is not relieved.

Test-Taking Strategy: Familiarity with the signs and symptoms of compartment syndrome is needed to answer this question correctly. By knowing that compartment syndrome occurs with impedance to the arterial circulation, you may be able to deduce that this pain would be aggravated by antigravity measures, such as elevating the limb (option 2). Review the signs of compartment syndrome now if you had difficulty with this question!

Level of Cognitive Ability: Application
Phase of Nursing Process: Assessment
Client Needs: Physiological Integrity
Content Area: Adult Health/Musculoskeletal

Reference

Black, J. M., & Matassarin-Jacobs, E. (1997). *Medical-surgical nursing: Clinical management for continuity of care* (5th ed.). Philadelphia: W. B. Saunders, p. 2139.

174. When assessing risk factors in a client with suspected cervical cancer, the nurse recognizes which risk factor as significant?

1 Late onset of menarche
2 Multiple pregnancies
3 Multiple sexual partners
4 Use of a diaphragm

Answer: 3

Rationale: Risk factors associated with cervical cancer include low economic status, early age of sexual contact or pregnancy, multiple sexual partners, and intrauterine exposure to diethylstilbestrol (DES). Potential risk factors include use of oral contraceptives, cigarette smoking, vitamin A and C deficiencies, and intercourse with men whose previous partners had cervical cancer.

Test-Taking Strategy: Use the process of elimination to answer this question. Multiple pregnancies and onset of menarche have no direct relationship to the cervix, so you can eliminate options 1 and 2. A diaphragm does not increase a client's risk for any type of cancer. If you had difficulty with this question, take time now to review the risk factors associated with cervical cancer!

Level of Cognitive Ability: Analysis
Phase of Nursing Process: Assessment
Client Needs: Physiological Integrity
Content Area: Adult Health/Oncology

Reference

Smeltzer, S. & Bare, B. (1996). *Brunner and Suddarth's Textbook of medical-surgical nursing* (8th ed.). Philadelphia: Lippincott-Raven, pp. 2250–2255.

175. The nurse assesses a client with chronic arterial insufficiency. The client complains of leg pain and cramping after walking three blocks, which is relieved when the client stops and rests. The nurse documents that the client is experiencing

1 Arterial-venous shunting.
2 Deep vein thrombosis.
3 Intermittent claudication.
4 Venous insufficiency.

Answer: 3

Rationale: Intermittent claudication is a classic symptom of peripheral vascular disease, which is also known by other names, including peripheral arterial disease and chronic arterial insufficiency. It is described as a cramp-like pain that occurs with exercise and is relieved by rest. Intermittent claudication is caused by ischemia and is very reproducible; that is, a predictable amount of exercise causes the pain each time.

Test-Taking Strategy: Use the process of elimination to answer the question. The stem tells you that this is an arterial disorder, which rules out options 2 and 4 immediately. The word "intermittent" in option 3 is a clue that it is the correct answer, as it matches the timing in the question. Arterial-venous shunting (option 1) is not an intermittent type of problem.

Level of Cognitive Ability: Analysis
Phase of Nursing Process: Assessment
Client Needs: Physiological Integrity
Content Area: Adult Health/Cardiovascular

Reference

Black, J. M., & Matassarin-Jacobs, E. (1997). *Medical-surgical nursing: Clinical management for continuity of care* (5th ed.). Philadelphia: W. B. Saunders, p. 1406.

---

176. The nurse is assessing the client hospitalized with acute pericarditis. Which of the following assessments, if made by the nurse, would not be indicative of cardiac tamponade?

1 Pulsus paradoxus
2 Distant heart sounds
3 Distended jugular veins
4 Bradycardia

Answer: 4

Rationale: Assessment findings with cardiac tamponade include tachycardia, distant or muffled heart sounds, jugular vein distention, and falling blood pressure, accompanied by pulsus paradoxus (a drop in inspiratory blood pressure by >10 mmHg).

Test-Taking Strategy: If you are unsure of how to answer this question, think of the consequences of the pressure dynamics in the chest when the pericardial sac is rapidly filling with blood or fluid. This will lead you to recognize options 1, 2, and 3 as compatible with the problem. The compensatory response would be tachycardia, not bradycardia, and thus bradycardia is the correct option, given the wording of the question. If you had difficulty with this question, take time now to review the signs of cardiac tamponade!

Level of Cognitive Ability: Analysis
Phase of Nursing Process: Assessment
Client Needs: Physiological Integrity
Content Area: Adult Health/Cardiovascular

Reference

Lewis, S. M., Collier, I. C., & Heitkemper, M. M. (1996). *Medical-surgical nursing: Assessment and management of clinical problems* (4th ed.). St. Louis: Mosby–Year Book, p. 1013.

---

177. The nurse has formulated a nursing diagnosis of Body Image Disturbance for the male client taking spironolactone (Aldactone). The nurse based this diagnosis on assessment of which of the following side effects of the medication?

1 Edema and hirsutism
2 Weight gain and hirsutism
3 Alopecia and muscle atrophy
4 Decreased libido and gynecomastia

Answer: 4

Rationale: The nurse should be alert to the fact that the client taking spironolactone may experience body image changes as a result of threatened sexual identity. These body image changes are related to decreased libido, gynecomastia in males, and hirsutism in females.

Test-Taking Strategy: This question is a good example of why you must read the question carefully. This question specifically states this is a male individual, which cues you to look for an item in the options related to gender. This immediately lets you narrow your choices to options 3 and 4. Spironolactone (Aldactone) may produce the side effects identified in option 4. If you had difficulty with this question, review this medication now!

Level of Cognitive Ability: Application
Phase of Nursing Process: Assessment
Client Needs: Psychosocial Integrity
Content Area: Pharmacology

Reference

Hodgson, B., & Kizior, R. (1998). Saunders nursing drug handbook 1998. Philadelphia: W.B. Saunders, pp. 943–944.

178. The nurse is caring for the client with a history of mild heart failure who is receiving diltiazem (Cardizem) for hypertension. The nurse would assess the client for

1 Tachycardia and rebound hypertension.
2 Wheezing and shortness of breath.
3 Bradycardia, weight gain, and peripheral edema.
4 Chest pain and tachycardia.

Answer: 3

Rationale: Calcium channel–blocking agents, such as diltiazem (Cardizem), are used cautiously in clients with conditions that could be worsened by the medication, such as aortic stenosis, bradycardia, heart failure, acute myocardial infarction, and hypotension. The nurse would assess for signs and symptoms that indicate worsening of these underlying disorders.

Test-Taking Strategy: To answer this question, you must know that diltiazem (Cardizem) is a calcium channel blocker and that these medications decrease the rate and force of cardiac contraction. This helps you to eliminate options 1 and 4, because bradycardia is expected. Option 2 is eliminated because these signs could indicate bronchoconstriction, which occurs not with calcium channel blockers but rather with some beta-adrenergic blockers. If you had difficulty with this question, take time now to review this medication!

Level of Cognitive Ability: Application
Phase of Nursing Process: Assessment
Client Needs: Physiological Integrity
Content Area: Pharmacology

Reference

Hodgson, B., & Kizior, R. (1998). Saunders nursing drug handbook 1998. Philadelphia: W.B. Saunders, p. 329.

179. The nurse has just administered a dose of hydralazine (Apresoline) intravenously to the client. On the basis of the action of this medication, the nurse would initially assess the

1 Cardiac rhythm.
2 Oxygen saturation.
3 Blood pressure.
4 Respiratory rate.

Answer: 3

Rationale: Hydralazine (Apresoline) is a powerful vasodilator that exerts its action on the smooth muscle walls of arterioles. After a parenteral dose, blood pressure is checked every 5 minutes until stable and every 15 minutes thereafter. Although options 1, 2, and 4 may be a component of assessment, they are not directly related to the action of the medication.

Test-Taking Strategy: If you know that hydralazine is an antihypertensive medication, you should be able to select the correct option easily. If you had difficulty with this question, take time now to review it!

Level of Cognitive Ability: Application
Phase of Nursing Process: Assessment
Client Needs: Physiological Integrity
Content Area: Pharmacology

Reference

McKenry, L., & Salerno, E. (1995). *Mosby's pharmacology in nursing* (19th ed.). St. Louis: Mosby–Year Book, p. 612.

180. The nurse is caring for a client 4 days after a pelvic exenteration. The physician has changed the client's diet from NPO to clear liquid. The nurse makes which priority assessment before administering the diet?

1 Gag reflex
2 Urine specific gravity
3 Incision appearance
4 Bowel sounds

Answer: 4

Rationale: Postoperatively, the nurse assesses the client by auscultating lung sounds and assessing bowel sounds before resuming diet and managing pain. Absence of bowel sounds would contraindicate a diet. Options 2 and 3 are unrelated to the issue of the question. The gag reflex, although important immediately postoperatively, would not be the priority because it would have returned by this time.

Test-Taking Strategy: The stem contains key information that indicates that the client underwent surgery 4 days earlier. The gag reflex would have returned by this time, so eliminate option 1. Incision appearance is not related to diet, so eliminate option 3. Any diet will enter the client's bowel so assessment of this area would be key. In addition, note that the type of surgery performed, as identified in the case, was abdominal. This would direct you to selecting option 4.

Level of Cognitive Ability: Application
Phase of Nursing Process: Assessment
Client Needs: Physiological Integrity
Content Area: Adult Health/Oncology

Reference

Smeltzer, S. & Bare, B. (1996). *Brunner and Suddarth's Textbook of medical-surgical nursing* (8th ed.). Philadelphia: Lippincott-Raven, pp. 2250–2255.

---

181. The nurse performs suction on a client with an endotracheal tube. After the procedure, the nurse monitors for side effects related to the suctioning. Which of the following would indicate to the nurse that the client is experiencing a side effect related to this procedure?

1 Hypertension
2 Cardiac irregularities
3 A reddish coloration in the client's face
4 A pulse oximetry level of 95%

Answer: 2

Rationale: The client needs to be assessed closely for side effects related to suctioning. These include hypoxemia, cardiac irregularities caused by vagal stimulation, mucosal trauma, and paroxysmal coughing. If side effects occur during the procedure, especially cardiac irregularities, stop the procedure and reoxygenate the client.

Test-Taking Strategy: Knowledge of the side effects and complications related to suctioning is helpful in answering this question. Use the ABCs—airway, breathing, and circulation—to assist you in answering this question. If you are unfamiliar with the side effects or complications related to suctioning, take the time now to review them!

Level of Cognitive Ability: Analysis
Phase of Nursing Process: Assessment
Client Needs: Physiological Integrity
Content Area: Adult Health/Respiratory

Reference

Black, J. M., & Matassarin-Jacobs, E. (1997). *Medical-surgical nursing: Clinical management for continuity of care* (5th ed.). Philadelphia: W. B. Saunders, p. 1176.

---

182. A nurse is performing a physical assessment on a lethargic client brought to the emergency room by the Emergency Medical Service. The nurse notes a fruity odor to the client's breath. The nurse immediately suspects

1 Hyperglycemic hyperosmolar nonketotic (HHNK) syndrome
2 Diabetic ketoacidosis (DKA)
3 Ethanol oxide intoxication (ETOH)
4 Hypoglycemia

Answer: 2

Rationale: Clients with DKA accumulate large amounts of ketone bodies in extracellular fluids. A fruity odor to the breath develops due to the volatile nature of acetone.

Test-Taking Strategy: Knowledge about DKA and HHNK syndrome is necessary to answer the question. Identify the sign or symptom that is the issue of the question and then eliminate options 3 and 4. If you had difficulty with this question, review the differences between DKA and HHNK syndrome now. Remember to associate a fruity breath odor with DKA!

Level of Cognitive Ability: Application
Phase of Nursing Process: Assessment
Client Needs: Physiological Integrity
Content Area: Adult Health/Endocrine

Reference

Burrell, L. O., Gerlach, M. J., & Pless, B. (1997). *Adult nursing: Acute and community care* (2nd ed.). Stamford, CT: Appleton & Lange, pp. 1168–1169.

183. The nurse assesses the breath sounds of a client with pneumonia. The nurse documents the assessment data as rhonchi located in the left lung. The nurse bases the assessment on the characteristics of rhonchi, which include

1 A musical or hissing noise heard on inspiration.
2 A creaking noise heard on inspiration.
3 A grating noise heard on expiration.
4 A rattling or gurgling noise heard on expiration.

Answer: 4

Rationale: Rhonchi occur as a result of the passing of air through fluid-filled narrow passages. Rhonchi sometimes are referred to as gurgles. Diseases with excess mucus production, such as pneumonia, are associated with rhonchi. Rhonchi are usually heard on expiration and may clear with a cough.

Test-Taking Strategy: Knowledge related to adventitious sounds is necessary to answer this question. Correlate gurgles with rhonchi to assist you in remembering what these sounds would produce. If you had difficulty with this question, take the time now to review adventitious breath sounds!

Level of Cognitive Ability: Analysis
Phase of Nursing Process: Assessment
Client Needs: Physiological Integrity
Content Area: Adult Health/Respiratory

Reference
Black, J. M., & Matassarin-Jacobs, E. (1997). *Medical-surgical nursing: Clinical management for continuity of care* (5th ed.). Philadelphia: W. B. Saunders, p. 1046.

---

184. The nurse is caring for a client with polycystic disease who has just returned to the medical unit after an intravenous pyelography (IVP). Which nursing assessment is of highest priority?

1 Auscultating the lungs
2 Inspecting the groin area
3 Palpating the carotid pulse
4 Measuring intake and output

Answer: 4

Rationale: IVP is used to visualize the kidneys, ureters, and bladder for evaluation of structure and excretory function. As the kidneys clear intravenously injected contrast medium from the blood by glomerular filtration, visualization of the renal parenchyma, collecting system, ureter, and bladder is obtained via multiple x-ray films. This diagnostic test is helpful in the evaluation and diagnosis of renal masses and cysts, ureteral obstruction, retroperitoneal tumors, renal trauma, and other urinary tract abnormalities. In order to recognize a nephrotoxic response to the contrast media after completion of the study, should it occur, closely monitor urinary output and renal function 24–48 hours after the use of radiocontrast material.

Test-Taking Strategy: Knowledge about the IVP procedure is necessary to assist in answering this question. Knowing that the study requires contrast medium to be filtrated from the blood through the kidneys will direct you to option 4. Review postprocedure care after IVP if you had difficulty answering the question!

Level of Cognitive Ability: Application
Phase of Nursing Process: Assessment
Client Needs: Physiological Integrity
Content Area: Adult Health/Renal

Reference
Tilkian, S. M., Conover, M. B., & Tilkian, A. G. (1995). *Clinical and nursing implications of laboratory tests* (5th ed.). St. Louis: Mosby–Year Book, pp. 233–234.

185. The client has received a diagnosis of urolithiasis in the right ureter. The nurse would expect the client to describe the renal colic as

1 Located in the upper right epigastric area, radiating to the right shoulder or back.
2 Occurring 2–3 hours after a meal.
3 Intermittent in the right upper outer abdominal quadrant, radiating to the groin.
4 Worsening with the ingestion of food.

Answer: 3

Rationale: Renal colic is generally associated with acute obstruction of a ureter and resulting ureteral spasm. As the stone moves along the ureter, the pain can be excruciating and is intermittent in character, located in the flank and upper outer quadrant of the affected side. It is caused by the spasm of the ureter and anoxia of the ureter wall from the pressure of the stone. The pain follows the anterior course of the ureter down to the suprapubic area and radiates to the external genitalia.

Test-Taking Strategy: Options 1, 2, and 4 describe pain characteristic of gastrointestinal problems: cholecystitis, duodenal ulcers, and gastric ulcers. Option 3 is the only correct answer according to the pathophysiological characteristics of renal calculi and its excretion through the urinary system. If you had difficulty with this question, review the characteristics of renal colic now!

Level of Cognitive Ability: Analysis
Phase of Nursing Process: Assessment
Client Needs: Physiological Integrity
Content Area: Adult Health/Renal

Reference

LeMone, P., & Burke, K. (1996). *Medical-surgical nursing: Critical thinking in client care.* Menlo Park, CA: Addison-Wesley, p. 897.

---

186. The wound of a client with an extensive burn injury is being treated with the application of 1% silver sulfadiazine (Silvadene). Which of the following signs would indicate to the nurse that the client is experiencing a side effect related to systemic absorption?

1 Pain at the wound site
2 Burning sensation and itching at the wound site
3 A localized rash
4 Photosensitivity

Answer: 4

Rationale: Silver sulfadiazine (Silvadene) is a cream used for burn wounds. Significant systemic absorption may occur if applied to extensive burns. Nonsystemic side effects of the medication include pain, burning sensation, itching, and a localized rash. Systemic side effects include anorexia, nausea, vomiting, headache, diarrhea, dizziness, photosensitivity, and joint pain.

Test-Taking Strategy: Knowledge about silver sulfadiazine (Silvadene) is helpful in answering this question. Note the word "systemic" in the question. This is a key word that will assist you to selecting the correct answer. Pain, burning sensation, itching, and a rash are localized in nature. The only systemic symptom identified in the options is photosensitivity. If you had difficulty with this question, review this medication now!

Level of Cognitive Ability: Analysis
Phase of Nursing Process: Assessment
Client Needs: Physiological Integrity
Content Area: Pharmacology

Reference

Hodgson, B., & Kizior, R. (1998). *Saunders nursing drug handbook 1998.* Philadelphia: W. B. Saunders, pp. 927–928.

---

187. The standardized tool used as a guide in assessing a client with a head injury and increased intracranial pressure (ICP) is

1 Monroe-Kellie hypothesis.
2 Pulse oximetry.
3 Abdominal assessment.
4 Glasgow Coma Scale.

Answer: 4

Rationale: The Glasgow Coma Scale is a fast way to assess consciousness. Its advantages are its simplicity and universality. Each response is given a number (high for normal and low for impaired). The responses are added, and a high number indicates normal functioning. The Monroe-Kellie hypothesis is a theory for understanding the balance of brain tissue, blood, CSF, and ICP. Options 2 and 3 are not related to the assessment of ICP.

Test-Taking Strategy: Knowledge of the purpose of the Glasgow Coma Scale is necessary to answer this question. If you are unfamiliar with this tool, take time now to review its purpose and use!

Level of Cognitive Ability: Application
Phase of Nursing Process: Assessment
Client Needs: Psychosocial Integrity
Content Area: Adult Health/Neurological

Reference

Hartshorn, J., Sole, M. L., & Lamborn, M. L. (1997). *Introduction to critical care nursing* (2nd ed.). Philadelphia: W. B. Saunders, pp. 273–274.

---

188. The client, 26 years old, is being successfully treated for the first episode of major depression. The client says to the nurse, "My mother and grandmother were always getting depressed, so I guess I inherited it. Will I be like them and get sick again?" The most therapeutic response by the nurse is

1. "Although your mother and grandmother got depressed, it doesn't mean you will. You are very different from them. Your early treatment will guarantee a cure. Shall we discuss why you identify so heavily with the female members of your family?"
2. "Today we have learned that if clients are treated early with SSRI's like Prozac for a first episode of depression, they will never experience another depression again. Let's talk of your concerns and make a list of all the worries you are currently experiencing, shall we?"
3. "Although some people with major depression experience only one episode in their lifetime or may not become depressed for 2 years or more, there is a 50%–85% chance of experiencing a second episode within half a year. Knowing when you're becoming depressed and obtaining immediate treatment now eliminates the long illnesses you remember. It seems as if you have some concerns about your illness?"
4. "There is a higher incidence of depression with family history and in women but that does not mean that you are affected. You're doing quite well now. Let's talk about the plans you have, now that you're cured."

Answer: 3

Rationale: The correct answer provides the client with accurate statistical information about depression. It is factual but also provides anticipatory guidance by teaching the client that if there is early recognition of depressive symptoms, treatment will reduce the course of the illness. This information also reduces the client's fears and anxieties arising from the concern that the illness (which does have a high incidence with family history and with female gender) will be as incapacitating as it was for the client's mother and grandmother. The nurse is using the therapeutic communication technique of focusing to assess relevant client needs, to achieve clearer thinking, and to enhance expression of feelings.

Test-Taking Strategy: This question seeks to alert you to answers that contain words that are absolutes, such as "guarantee" and "cured." Remember that the entire option needs to be correct. This knowledge would help you to eliminate options 1 and 4. Option 1 provides inaccurate information. The answer uses a therapeutic communication that is off focus and not pertinent to the concerns vocalized by the client. Although early intervention is key, it does not "guarantee" freedom from illness. Option 2 provides inaccurate information. The therapeutic communication seeks to explore the client's concerns, but the suggestion of making a list is a premature intervention. Option 4 provides inaccurate information. The communication technique makes a judgment of the client's progress and provides false reassurance. As in option 1, the word "cured" is a word that alerts you to the distractor's inaccuracy.

Level of Cognitive Ability: Application
Phase of Nursing Process: Assessment
Client Needs: Physiological Integrity
Content Area: Mental Health

Reference

Johnson, B. (1997). *Adaptation and growth: Psychiatric-mental health nursing* (4th ed.). Philadelphia: Lippincott-Raven, pp. 68–74, 533–562.

189. A client was hospitalized 5 days ago and has developed thrombophlebitis in the right lower extremity. The nurse assigned to this client assesses the client for

1. Bilateral calf tenderness.
2. Unilateral edema.
3. Coolness and pallor of the affected limb.
4. Diminished distal peripheral pulses.

Answer: 2

Rationale: The client with thrombophlebitis, also known as deep vein thrombosis, exhibits redness and/or warmth of the affected leg, tenderness at the site, possible dilated veins (if superficial), low-grade fever, edema distal to the obstruction, and possible positive Homans' sign in the affected extremity. Pedal pulses are unchanged from baseline because this is a venous, not arterial, problem. Often clients silently develop thrombophlebitis; that is, they do not manifest any signs and symptoms unless they experience pulmonary embolism as a complication.

Test-Taking Strategy: This question is worded in the affirmative, and looks for signs and symptoms of thrombophlebitis. Begin by eliminating options 3 and 4, which are symptoms of arterial, not venous, problems. Thrombophlebitis is usually a unilateral problem, which helps you eliminate option 1. In addition, the question states that the client has thrombophlebitis in the right lower extremity. This should direct you to option 2. If you had difficulty with this question, take time now to review the signs of thrombophlebitis!

Level of Cognitive Ability: Application
Phase of Nursing Process: Assessment
Client Needs: Physiological Integrity
Content Area: Adult Health/Cardiovascular

Reference

Black, J. M., & Matassarin-Jacobs, E. (1997). *Medical-surgical nursing: Clinical management for continuity of care* (5th ed.). Philadelphia: W. B. Saunders, p. 1434.

---

190. The nurse assesses that which of the following clients is the least likely to have implantation of an internal automatic cardioverter-defibrillator (AICD)?

1. A client with three episodes of cardiac arrest unrelated to myocardial infarction
2. A client with ventricular dysrhythmias despite medication therapy
3. A client with an episode of cardiac arrest related to myocardial infarction
4. A client with syncopal episodes related to ventricular tachycardia

Answer: 3

Rationale: An AICD detects and delivers an electric shock to terminate life-threatening episodes of ventricular tachycardia and ventricular fibrillation. These devices are implanted in clients who are considered at high risk, including those who have survived sudden cardiac death that is unrelated to myocardial infarction, those whose disease is refractive to medication therapy, and those who have syncopal episodes related to ventricular tachycardia.

Test-Taking Strategy: The question asks you to identify the client least likely to have implantation of the device. Ventricular dysrhythmias that induce syncope or occur while the client is taking medication are likely to be true indications for the AICD, and so you eliminate those first. The last two options are similar, but the main difference is whether the cardiac arrest was related to myocardial infarction (MI). Of these two, the one most likely to be responsive to AICD would be the client without MI, because those dysrhythmias are spontaneous. Thus your answer for the "least" likely client is the one whose dysrhythmias were caused primarily by insult from MI. Review the purpose of AICD now if you had difficulty with this question!

Level of Cognitive Ability: Analysis
Phase of Nursing Process: Assessment
Client Needs: Physiological Integrity
Content Area: Adult Health/Cardiovascular

References

Ignatavicius, D. D., Workman, M. L., & Mishler, M. A. (1995). *Medical-surgical nursing: A nursing process approach* (2nd ed., Vol. 1). Philadelphia: W. B. Saunders, p. 881.

191. The nurse asks the diabetic client to list all the medications that he or she is taking. Which of the following combinations of medications should the nurse report to the physician?

1 Acetohexamide (Dymelor) and trimethoprim-sulfamethoxazole (Bactrim)
2 Chlorpropamide (Diabinese) and amitriptyline (Elavil)
3. Glyburide (DiaBeta) and digoxin (Lanoxin)
4. Tolbutamide (Orinase) and amoxicillin (Amoxil)

Answer: 1

Rationale: Sulfonylureas are hypoglycemic agents that lower blood glucose levels. Dymelor, Diabenese, DiaBeta, and Orinase are sulfonylureas. If administered with a sulfonamide (option 1), increased hypoglycemic effects can occur.

Test-Taking Strategy: Knowledge about these medications and the related medication interactions are necessary to answer this question. If you had difficulty with this question, review these medications now!

Level of Cognitive Ability: Application
Phase of Nursing Process: Assessment
Client Needs: Physiological Integrity
Content Area: Pharmacology

Reference

McKenry, L., & Salerno, E. (1995). *Mosby's pharmacology in nursing* (19th ed.). St. Louis: Mosby–Year Book, pp. 951–953.

---

192. A major symptom associated with Hodgkin's disease is

1 Elevated blood pressure.
2 Unequal respirations.
3 Palpable pedal pulses.
4 Enlarged lymph nodes.

Answer: 4

Rationale: Assessment of Hodgkin's disease most often reveals a greatly enlarged but painless lymph node or nodes, usually the earliest manifestation of Hodgkin's lymphoma. More specific clinical manifestations depend on the site of malignancy and the extent of the disease.

Test-Taking Strategy: Both options 1 and 2 are vital sign measurements and are similar in that manner. Remember if two answers are similar, most often neither one is correct. Knowing that Hodgkin's disease is a lymphoma will help you choose the correct option, enlarged lymph nodes. If you had difficulty with this question, take time now to review the signs of Hodgkin's disease.

Level of Cognitive Ability: Analysis
Phase of Nursing Process: Assessment
Client Needs: Physiological Integrity
Content Area: Adult Health/Oncology

Reference

Ignatavicius D. D., Workman, M. L., & Mishler, M. A. (1995). *Medical-surgical nursing: A nursing process approach* (2nd ed.). Philadelphia: W. B. Saunders, pp. 1069–1070.

---

193. A client is admitted with a diagnosis of left-sided heart failure. What assessment findings would give the nurse the most data about the probability that cardiogenic shock will occur?

1 Tachycardia, hyperventilation, and a pale appearance
2 Peripheral edema, distended neck veins, and hepatic engorgement
3 Tachypnea, confusion, and hypotension
4 Oliguria, bradycardia, and gray skin color

Answer: 3

Rationale: Classical clinical manifestations of cardiogenic shock include altered sensorium; tachycardia; hypotension; tachypnea; oliguria; and cold, clammy, cyanotic skin. Pain and anxiety can cause an increase in respiratory and heart rates as well as a skin color change (option 1). Option 2 presents manifestations of right-sided heart failure. Bradycardia (option 4) occurs in the late stages of shock.

Test-Taking Strategy: Read the question carefully. There are two key phrases: "left-sided heart failure" and "cardiogenic shock." You need to keep both in mind when answering this question. In addition, be careful when the answer stems contain the word "and." Remember that each component of the option needs to be correct. Knowledge of the signs and symptoms of heart failure and cardiogenic shock is needed to assist you in answering this question. Review these now if you had difficulty with the question!

Level of Cognitive Ability: Analysis
Phase of Nursing Process: Assessment
Client Needs: Physiological Integrity
Content Area: Adult Health/Cardiovascular

Reference

Black, J. M., & Matassarin-Jacobs, E. (1997). *Medical-surgical nursing: Clinical management for continuity of care* (5th ed.). Philadelphia: W. B. Saunders, pp. 512, 1266.

---

194. During the admission assessment of a client with ovarian cancer, the nurse recognizes which set of symptoms as typical of the disease?

1 Flatulence and increasing abdominal girth
2 Abdominal fullness and decreased size of one ovary
3 History of birth control pill use and abdominal pain
4 Severe cramping and abnormal discharge

Answer: 1

Rationale: Ovarian cancer is a frustrating disease because of its silent onset and lack of warning symptoms. Some signs and symptoms include irregular menses, abdominal discomfort, flatulence, fullness after a light meal, and increasing abdominal girth.

Test-Taking Strategy: Use the process of elimination to answer the question. Remember that when there are two components to an option, both must be accurate for the option to be correct. Options 3 and 4 are similar in the sense of addressing discomfort; therefore these options can be eliminated. Most tumors of any site increase the organ size, so eliminate option 2. This leaves option 1 as the only correct option. Review the warning signs related to ovarian cancer now if you had difficulty with this question!

Level of Cognitive Ability: Application
Phase of Nursing Process: Assessment
Client Needs: Physiological Integrity
Content Area: Adult Health/Oncology

Reference

Smeltzer, S. & Bare, B. (1996). *Brunner and Suddarth's Textbook of medical-surgical nursing* (8th ed.). Philadelphia: Lippincott-Raven, pp. 1294–1295.

---

195. The nurse administers a fatal dose of digoxin (Lanoxin) to a client. During the subsequent investigation, it is determined that the nurse did not note the client's heart rate of 45 and the high serum digoxin level before administering the medication. This failure to complete an appropriate assessment is addressed under which function of the state's Nurse Practice Act?

1 Defining the specific educational requirements for licensure in this state
2 Describing the scope of practice of licensed and unlicensed care providers
3 Recommending specific terms of incarceration for nurses who violate the law
4 Identifying the process for disciplinary action if standards of care are not met

Answer: 4

Rationale: Options 1, 2, and 4 are all functions of the State Board of Nursing. In the situation described in the stem, acceptable standards of care were not met (the nurse failed to adequately assess the client before administering a medication). Option 4 refers specifically to the situation described in the stem. Option 3 is not a function of a State Board of Nursing.

Test-Taking Strategy: Of the four options, three are functions of the State Board of Nursing, but only one (option 4) is consistent with the error made by the nurse as described in the stem. Option 3 can be discarded immediately, as this power does not reside with a State Board of Nursing. Review information related to the Nurse Practice Act if you had difficulty with this question!

Level of Cognitive Ability: Application
Phase of Nursing Process: Assessment
Client Needs: Physiological Integrity
Content Area: Fundamental Skills

Reference

Zerwekh, J., & Claborn, J. C. (1997). *Nursing today: Transition and trends* (2nd ed.). Philadelphia: W. B. Saunders, pp. 388–390.

196. The assessment data of a client with unstable angina would most likely include

1 Paroxysmal chest discomfort triggered by predictable physical or emotional factors.
2 Chest discomfort that increases when reclining.
3 Chest discomfort associated with rapid eye movement sleep.
4 Chest discomfort that increases in severity over a period of time.

Answer: 4

Rationale: A characteristic of unstable angina is that it tends to increase in number of episodes, duration, and severity over time. Option 1 describes stable angina. Option 2 describes angina decubitus. Option 3 describes nocturnal angina.

Test-Taking Strategy: Knowledge of the characteristics of angina is necessary to answer the question. Identify the key phrase "most likely." Review the characteristics of anginal pain now if you had difficulty with this question!

Level of Cognitive Ability: Analysis
Phase of Nursing Process: Assessment
Client Needs: Physiological Integrity
Content Area: Adult Health/Cardiovascular

Reference

Black, J. M., & Matassarin-Jacobs, E. (1997). *Medical-surgical nursing: Clinical management for continuity of care* (5th ed.). Philadelphia: W. B. Saunders, pp. 1253–1254.

---

197. The mother of a breast-fed newborn calls the nurse to the room and tells the nurse that the baby is having a diarrhea stool. Which of these assessment findings, if present, would validate the mother's concern?

1 Pale, yellow stool
2 Loose, pasty stool
3 Foul stool odor
4 Grimacing with defecation

Answer: 3

Rationale: A sweet- or foul-smelling odor is characteristic of a diarrhea stool, regardless of the feeding method. Options 1 and 2 are incorrect because a breast-fed infant's stool is expected to be loose and to be pale yellow. Option 4 is incorrect because grimacing and grunting during defecation are normal behaviors.

Test-Taking Strategy: The stem cues the reader to discriminate between a normal breast-fed infant's stool and diarrhea stool. The stem also directs the reader to choose an answer that validates the mother's concern regarding diarrhea. If you are unfamiliar with expected stool characteristics in a breast-fed newborn, review this content now!

Level of Cognitive Ability: Analysis
Phase of Nursing Process: Assessment
Client Needs: Physiological Integrity
Content Area: Maternity

Reference

Pillitteri, A. (1995). *Maternal and child health nursing: Care of the childbearing and childrearing family* (2nd ed.). Philadelphia: Lippincott-Raven, pp. 697, 870, 1385.

---

198. The nurse should expect a client with an acute myocardial infarction to first manifest

1 An abnormal Q wave.
2 ST segment elevation on the electrocardiogram.
3 T wave depression.
4 Elevated serum creatine kinase (CK)–MB isoenzyme.

Answer: 2

Rationale: ST segment elevation usually occurs immediately or during the early stages of myocardial infarction. T wave depression and abnormal Q wave changes occur within several hours to several days after the myocardial infarction. The CK-MB isoenzyme begins to rise 3 to 6 hours after myocardial infarction.

Test-Taking Strategy: Identify the key word "first." Use nursing knowledge related to the clinical presentation of myocardial infarction. Whereas all options generally occur with acute myocardial infarction, the first manifestation likely to be seen is the electrocardiographic changes in the ST segment. If you had difficulty with this question, take time now to review the characteristics of myocardial infarction!

Level of Cognitive Ability: Analysis
Phase of Nursing Process: Assessment
Client Needs: Physiological Integrity
Content Area: Adult Health/Cardiovascular

Reference
Ignatavicius, D. D., Workman, M. L., & Mishler, M. A. (1995). *Medical-surgical nursing: A nursing process approach* (2nd ed., Vol. 1). Philadelphia: W. B. Saunders, p. 991.

---

199. The nurse assesses the burn injury and determines that the client sustained a fourth-degree burn. Which of the following assessment data would result in the nurse's conclusion?

1 A wet, shiny, weeping wound surface
2 A dry wound surface
3 Charring at the wound site
4 Decreased wound sensation

Answer: 3

Rationale: In a fourth-degree burn, charring is visible. Extremity movement is limited, and wound sensation is absent.

Test-Taking Strategy: Knowledge of the clinical manifestations associated with the degree of burn injury is necessary to answer this question. Use the process of elimination in selecting the correct option. Knowledge that charring and absence of wound sensation occur in more serious burns would direct you to selecting option number 3. Review burn injury classification according to the depth of injury now if you had difficulty with this question!

Level of Cognitive Ability: Analysis
Phase of Nursing Process: Assessment
Client Needs: Physiological Integrity
Content Area: Adult Health/Integumentary

Reference
Black, J. M., & Matassarin-Jacobs, E. (1997). *Medical-surgical nursing: Clinical management for continuity of care* (5th ed.). Philadelphia: W. B. Saunders, p. 2239.

---

200. The nurse receives a report that a client is depressed about suffering an acute myocardial infarction. The nurse confirms that assessment by noting the client's

1 Hesitancy to be transferred from critical care unit.
2 Ignoring activity restrictions.
3 Talking about rehabilitation measures.
4 Crying off and on during the day.

Answer: 4

Rationale: The emotional and behavioral reactions of clients after myocardial infarction are varied. Depression may be manifested by withdrawal, crying, and apathy. Option 1 is more indicative of dependence and fear. Option 2 is more indicative of denial. Option 3 indicates realistic acceptance.

Test-Taking Strategy: All options are behaviors that may be manifested in the client with myocardial infarction; however, the question is asking about depression. Use the process of elimination. Note that the incorrect options indicate behavioral responses other than depression.

Level of Cognitive Ability: Analysis
Phase of Nursing Process: Assessment
Client Needs: Psychosocial Integrity
Content Area: Adult Health/Cardiovascular

Reference
Lewis, S. M., Collier, I. C., & Heitkemper, M. M. (1996). *Medical-surgical nursing: Assessment and management of clinical problems* (4th ed.). St. Louis: Mosby–Year Book, pp. 921, 922.

---

201. A nurse is assessing a toddler who has a fever of 101°F. Which of these assessment findings, if also present, would be most significant?

1 Malaise
2 Stiff neck
3 Anorexia
4 Weakness

Answer: 2

Rationale: A stiff neck may be indicative of a serious health problem. One such condition is meningitis. Options 1, 3, 4, and an achy feeling are symptoms that frequently accompany fever.

Test-Taking Strategy: The stem asks to identify the "most significant finding." This should give a clue that one of the findings noted in the options is not typically associated with fever. The ability to differentiate an ominous symptom of illness from symptoms that usually occur with a fever will assist you in selecting the correct option!

Level of Cognitive Ability: Application
Phase of Nursing Process: Assessment
Client Needs: Physiological Integrity
Content Area: Child Health

Reference

Smeltzer, S., & Bare, B. (1996). *Brunner and Suddarth's Textbook of medical-surgical nursing* (8th ed.). Philadelphia: Lippincott-Raven, p. 102.

---

202. The nurse is caring for a client with a diagnosis of rheumatoid arthritis. The client is receiving sulindac (Clinoril), 150 mg PO BID. Which of the following would indicate to the nurse that the client is experiencing a side effect related to the medication?

1 Diarrhea
2 Photophobia
3 Fever
4 Tingling in the extremities

Answer: 1

Rationale: Sulindac (Clinoril) is a nonsteroidal anti-inflammatory medication. Frequent side effects include gastrointestinal disturbances, such as constipation or diarrhea, indigestion, and nausea. Dermatitis, rash, dizziness, and headache are also frequent side effects. Occasional side effects include anorexia, gastrointestinal cramps, and flatulence.

Test-Taking Strategy: Knowledge about sulindac (Clinoril) is necessary to answer this question. Nonsteroidal anti-inflammatory medications have a tendency to produce gastrointestinal side effects. If you can remember that this medication is classified as a nonsteroidal anti-inflammatory, then by the process of elimination, option 1 would be selected as the correct answer. If you had difficulty with this question, take the time now to review this medication!

Level of Cognitive Ability: Analysis
Phase of Nursing Process: Assessment
Client Needs: Physiological Integrity
Content Area: Pharmacology

Reference

Hodgson, B., & Kizior, R. (1998). *Saunders nursing drug handbook 1998.* Philadelphia: W. B. Saunders, p. 956.

---

203. The nurse is assessing the client with an abdominal aortic aneurysm (AAA). Which of the following assessment findings by the nurse is probably unrelated to the AAA?

1 Pulsatile abdominal mass
2 Hyperactive bowel sounds in the area
3 Systolic bruit over the area of the mass
4 Subjective sensation of "heart beating" in the abdomen

Answer: 2

Rationale: Only about 40% of clients with AAA exhibit symptoms. Those who do may describe a feeling of the "heart beating" in the abdomen when supine or being able to feel the mass throbbing. A pulsatile mass may be palpated in the middle and upper abdomen. A systolic bruit may be auscultated over the mass. If the mass has thrombi attached, larger vessels could become occluded and smaller vessels blocked by emboli, as in "blue toe syndrome" with digital obstruction.

Test-Taking Strategy: Note the key word "unrelated." Use the process of elimination. Each of the incorrect options contains a circulatory component that suggests a relationship to the AAA. If you had difficulty answering this question, take time now to review the signs and symptoms of AAA!

Level of Cognitive Ability: Application
Phase of Nursing Process: Assessment
Client Needs: Physiological Integrity
Content Area: Adult Health/Cardiovascular

Reference

Smeltzer, S., & Bare, B. (1996). *Brunner and Suddarth's Textbook of medical-surgical nursing* (8th ed.). Philadelphia: Lippincott-Raven, p. 739.

204. The nurse is caring for an elderly client in the home. The client is widowed and competent, but the son, the daughter-in-law, and their three children have unexpectedly moved into the house "to care for him." Which of the following would indicate to the nurse that the client is being exploited?

1. "My son won't let me pay for anything. They're helping me with everything. This is such a help to me as my income's been reduced since the wife died."
2. "Once in a while the children get to be too noisy, but overall it's been the best thing that's happened to me since my wife died."
3. "My son wants me to turn over the deed to the house to him. He says I'll always have a place there, but I'll feel like a tenant in my own home. What do you think?"
4. "It's nice to have my family around me again. Since my wife died, I've been lonely, and they're keeping me young and spoiling me rotten."

Answer: 3

Rationale: Exploitation of the elderly includes charging exorbitant fees for services and goods provided by family members, employees, friends, or caretakers; transferring large sums of money or holdings to family members, caregivers, friends, or employees; adding names of the persons on whom the client is dependent to bank accounts, deeds, stock portfolios, or wills; losses of large sums of money; the elderly person's inability to participate in a decision to move in with adult children; and the elderly person's exclusion from decision making about his or her own health, welfare, and lifestyles although mentally competent.

Test-Taking Strategy: This question assess your knowledge of the issue of exploitation in elder abuse. If you did not know them, they are listed in the rationale, and you will want to review them. In option 1, the client is stating positive reasons that address the reasons that extended families can be helpful today. Option 2 addresses some adjustment to the expansion of the family, but it is expected. Option 4 states the client's complete satisfaction with the expansion of the family. There is no evidence of exploitation in any of the options except option 3.

Level of Cognitive Ability: Analysis
Phase of Nursing Process: Assessment
Client Needs: Safe, Effective Care Environment
Content Area: Fundamental Skills

Reference

Haber, J., (1997). *Comprehensive psychiatric nursing* (5th ed.). St. Louis: Mosby–Year Book, pp. 777–802.

---

205. The nurse is performing an admission assessment of a family admitted with a diagnosis of violence. Which of the following factors would the nurse initially want to include in the assessment?

1. The family's anger toward the intrusiveness of the nurse
2. The family's denial of the violent nature of their behavior
3. The coping style of each family member
4. The family's current ability to use community resources

Answer: 3

Rationale: The initial family assessment includes a careful history of each family member. The following factors are part of the nurse's initial assessment of families who are experiencing violence: structure and function of the family, social functioning of each family member, sex role socialization and role strain, each family member's task performance ability, coping style of each family member, daily stresses in the family, resources available to the family in the home and community, expression of frustration and anger, beliefs about aggression and violence, and family's health status.

Test-Taking Strategy: This question assesses your knowledge of the factors that you would need to consider in an assessment on a family experiencing violence. It is important to recall that family violence results from many interactional factors, so the nurse will need to assess as many issues as possible. Although some family members may regard the nurse's interventions as intrusive (option 1), this is not the focus of an initial assessment of a violent family. Although denial may be one of the coping styles of the family (option 2), it is not specific to every family experiencing violence. Although community resources are important issues (option 4), the current use is not as important as potential resources that may be used to deal with the violent nature of the family.

Level of Cognitive Ability: Analysis
Phase of Nursing Process: Assessment
Client Needs: Safe, Effective Care Environment
Content Area: Mental Health

Reference

Haber, J., (1997). *Comprehensive psychiatric nursing* (5th ed.). St. Louis: Mosby–Year Book, pp. 777–802.

206. When assessing a child with chalasia, which clinical manifestation would a nurse most likely find?

1 Projectile vomiting
2 Visible peristaltic waves
3 Right upper quadrant olive-shaped mass
4 Poor weight gain

Answer: 4

Rationale: A constant reflux of gastric acid into the esophagus results in an irritated esophageal lining. The child experiences esophageal burning. Eating food exacerbates this symptom. Consequently, the child does not eat and loses weight. Options 1, 2, and 3 are incorrect. These are symptoms associated with pyloric stenosis.

Test-Taking Strategy: Focus on the key words in the stem, which are "most likely." Only one option is a true symptom of chalasia. You need to be able to differentiate chalasia from pyloric stenosis. If you had difficulty with this question, review these disorders now!

Level of Cognitive Ability: Application
Phase of Nursing Process: Assessment
Client Needs: Physiological Integrity
Content Area: Child Health

Reference

Wong, D. (1995). *Whaley and Wong's nursing care of infants and children* (5th ed.). St. Louis: Mosby–Year Book, pp. 1460, 1475.

---

207. The diabetic client who has been controlled with daily insulin has been placed on a regimen of atenolol (Tenormin) for control of angina pectoris. Due to the effects of the medication, the nurse assesses that which of the following findings is the most reliable indicator of hypoglycemia?

1 Tachycardia
2 Sweating
3 Low blood glucose level
4 Anxiety

Answer: 3

Rationale: Beta-adrenergic blocking agents, such as atenolol, inhibit the appearance of warning signs and symptoms of acute hypoglycemia, which would include anxiety, increased heart rate, and sweating. Therefore, the client receiving this medication should adhere to the therapeutic regimen and monitor blood glucose levels carefully.

Test-Taking Strategy: Note the use of the word "most reliable" in the stem. This indicates that more than one response could be partially or completely correct. Each of the options is, in fact, a sign or symptom of hypoglycemia. Knowledge of the masking effects of beta-adrenergic blocking agents helps you to choose the blood glucose level as the most reliable indicator. Review the effects of this medication now if you had difficulty with this question!

Level of Cognitive Ability: Application
Phase of Nursing Process: Assessment
Client Needs: Physiological Integrity
Content Area: Adult Health/Endocrine

Reference

Hodgson, B., & Kizior, R. (1998). *Saunders nursing drug handbook 1998.* Philadelphia: W.B. Saunders, p. 80.

---

208. A client is scheduled for elective cardioversion to treat chronic high-rate atrial fibrillation. The nurse assesses that the client is not yet ready for the procedure after determining that

1 The client's digoxin has been withheld for the last 48 hours.
2 The client has received a dose of midazolam (Versed) intravenously.
3 The client is wearing a nasal cannula delivering oxygen at 2 liters per minute.
4 The defibrillator has the synchronizer turned on and is set at 50 joules.

Answer: 3

Rationale: Digoxin may be withheld for up to 48 hours before cardioversion, because it increases ventricular irritability and may cause ventricular dysrhythmias after countershock. The client typically receives a dose of an intravenous sedative or antianxiety agent. The defibrillator is switched to synchronizer mode to time the delivery of the electrical impulse to coincide with the QRS complex and avoid the T wave, which could cause ventricular fibrillation. Energy level is typically set at 50–100 joules. During the procedure, any oxygen is removed temporarily, because oxygen supports combustion, and a fire could result from electrical arcing.

Test-Taking Strategy: The question is worded to look for an incorrect item. A review of the key differences between cardioversion and defibrillation is needed to select the correct answer. The concept of oxygen combustion may prove useful in questions related either to cardioversion or defibrillation. If you had difficulty with this question, review the descriptions and procedures related to defibrillation and cardioversion!

Level of Cognitive Ability: Analysis
Phase of Nursing Process: Assessment
Client Needs: Safe, Effective Care Environment
Content Area: Adult Health/Cardiovascular

Reference

Black, J. M., & Matassarin-Jacobs, E. (1997). *Medical-surgical nursing: Clinical management for continuity of care* (5th ed.). Philadelphia: W. B. Saunders, p. 1313.

---

209. An observation that suggests a physiological problem in a 9-month-old infant is:

1. Head lag when pulled to sitting.
2. Inability to stand without support.
3. Creeping or crawling along the floor.
4. Absence of rooting reflex.

Answer: 1

Rationale: Presence of head lag after the age of 6 months suggests neuromuscular dysfunction and indicates a physiological problem at 9 months. Standing alone is not expected until 10–12 months, and crawling is accomplished by 6–8 months. Basic reflexes such as rooting or startling predominate during the first 3 months and would not be present in late infancy.

Test-Taking Strategy: Knowledge related to normal growth and development is necessary to answer this question. Use the process of elimination to answer the question. Options 2, 3, and 4 are normal assessment findings, whereas option 1 indicates a problem. Review normal growth and development now if you had difficulty with this question!

Level of Cognitive Ability: Analysis
Phase of Nursing Process: Assessment
Client Needs: Physiological Integrity
Content Area: Child Health

Reference

Ball, J., & Bindler, R. (1995). *Pediatric nursing: Caring for children.* Stamford, CT: Appleton & Lange, p. 43.

---

210. The nurse is performing an admission assessment on a client admitted with a diagnosis of Bell's palsy. The nurse assesses for the major symptom associated with Bell's palsy when the nurse observes the affected side for

1. Upward movement of the eyeball when the client closes the eye.
2. Tinel's sign.
3. Phalen's sign.
4. Upper eyelid ptosis and a constricted pupil.

Answer: 1

Rationale: Bell's palsy, the most common type of peripheral facial paralysis, affects the motor aspects of the seventh cranial nerve. The facial nerve is affected by an idiopathic lesion of the peripheral facial nerve (the seventh cranial nerve), causing temporary paralysis of one side of the face, with unilateral paralysis of expression. Clinical manifestations include widened palpebral fissure (distance between upper and lower eyelids), drooping of the mouth, flattened nasolabial fold, a slight lag in closing the eye, and stated difficulty eating. Approximately 85% of clients recover total function.

Test-Taking Strategy: This question tests your knowledge of neurological disorders of the spinal cord. Tinel's sign and Phalen's sign are diagnostic assessment signs for carpal tunnel syndrome. In Tinel's sign, a tingling sensation in the hands and fingers occurs when the wrist is tapped. In Phalan's sign, forceful flexion of the wrists for 20–30 seconds results in numbness and tingling. Option 4 is incorrect because upper eyelid ptosis and a constricted pupil are associated with Horner's syndrome (an early indication of cervical syringomyelia) when coupled with anhidrosis (absence of sweating) and flushing of the face on the affected side. If you are unfamiliar with the signs of Bell's palsy, take time now to review!

Level of Cognitive Ability: Analysis
Phase of Nursing Process: Assessment
Client Needs: Physiological Integrity
Content Area: Adult Health/Neurological

Reference

Black, J. M., & Matassarin-Jacobs, E. (1997). *Medical-surgical nursing: Clinical management for continuity of care* (5th ed.). Philadelphia: W. B. Saunders, pp. 915–932.

---

211. A toddler is scheduled for polio immunization. The inactivated polio vaccine (IPV) should be given instead of the oral polio vaccine (OPV) if the client is

1 Allergic to penicillin.
2 Immunosuppressed by medications or disease.
3 Having loose or frequent stools.
4 Taking oral antibiotics.

Answer: 2

Rationale: OPV is a live vaccine and is contraindicated for clients with decreased immunity (those with congenital decreased immunity, HIV infection, leukemia; those taking immunosuppressing medications) because of the risk of exposure to the virus. IPV is a killed virus. Penicillin allergy, antimicrobial therapy, and diarrhea are not contraindications to childhood immunizations.

Test-Taking Strategy: Knowledge that the OPV is a live virus and is dangerous to administer with immunosuppressed clients is required. If you had difficulty with this question, take time now to review the contraindications associated with immunizations!

Level of Cognitive Ability: Application
Phase of Nursing Process: Assessment
Client Needs: Physiological Integrity
Content Area: Pharmacology

Reference

Ball, J., & Bindler, R. (1995). *Pediatric nursing: Caring for children.* Stamford, CT: Appleton & Lange, p. 43.

---

212. A client is admitted to the hospital with acute myocardial infarction and is given tissue plasminogen activator (t-PA, or alteplase [Activase]) by infusion. Of the following parameters, which one would require the least frequent assessment to detect complications with this therapy?

1 Oxygen saturation
2 Neurological signs
3 Blood pressure and pulse
4 Complaints of abdominal and back pain

Answer: 1

Rationale: Thrombolytic agents dissolve existing clots, and bleeding can occur anywhere in the body. The nurse monitors for any obvious signs of bleeding and also for occult signs of bleeding; this monitoring would include hemoglobin and hematocrit measurement, blood pressure and pulse measurement, assessment of neurological signs, assessment of abdominal and back pain, and evaluation for the presence of blood in the urine or stool.

Test-Taking Strategy: Because bleeding is the prime complication of thrombolytic therapy, the nurse assesses for these signs and symptoms. The question is worded to direct you to look for the least frequent measurement, and therefore you are looking for an option that is not related to bleeding. A change in neurological signs could indicate cerebral bleeding; abdominal and back pain could indicate abdominal bleeding; change in blood pressure and pulse could be general indicators of hemorrhage. Oxygen saturation is not an indicator of bleeding in the respiratory tract; more likely, you would note hemoptysis. Review assessments associated with the administration of this medication if you had difficulty with this question!
Level of Cognitive Ability: Application
Phase of Nursing Process: Assessment
Client Needs: Physiological Integrity
Content Area: Pharmacology

Reference

Ignatavicius, D. D., Workman, M. L., & Mishler, M. A. (1995). *Medical-surgical nursing: A nursing process approach* (2nd ed., Vol. 1). Philadelphia: W. B. Saunders, p. 996.

213. A 4-year-old with cancer is admitted for radiation therapy and surgery. To assess adequacy of support for the child's psychosocial needs, the nurse would ask the parents

1. "What signs and symptoms has your child been having?"
2. "Will a family member be able to stay with the child most of the time?"
3. "How long have you known your child's diagnosis?"
4. "What are your child's favorite books, activities, and toys?"

Answer: 2

Rationale: Separation from family is the most stressful aspect of hospitalization for young children. For children less than 5 years of age, a primary goal is to prevent separation from family. Assessing for the ability and willingness of family members to stay with the child takes priority over determining favorite toys or diversional activities.

Test-Taking Strategy: The key phrases in the stem are "adequacy of support" and "child's psychosocial needs." Option 1 relates to physical problems. Identify the client of the question. Option 3 is focused on the parents, and the client is the child. In choosing between options 2 and 4, use Maslow's hierarchy of needs theory to select the security issue over the diversional activity.

Level of Cognitive Ability: Application
Phase of Nursing Process: Assessment
Client Needs: Psychosocial Integrity
Content Area: Child Health

Reference

Wong, D. (1997). *Whaley and Wong's Essentials of pediatric nursing* (5th ed.). St. Louis: Mosby–Year Book, pp. 629–630.

---

214. In assessing a client who is complaining of angina, the nurse notes a major symptom of a hiatal hernia when the client says, "The pain in my chest . . .

1. Is a tight, burning pain."
2. Is worse after a large meal."
3. Is aggravated by exercise."
4. Is relieved when I lie down."

Answer: 2

Rationale: Hiatal hernia is herniation of a portion of the stomach into the esophagus through an opening in the diaphragm. The cause is unknown, but certain factors have been associated with development. Large meals are associated with clinical manifestations because the full stomach may cause reflux.

Test-Taking Strategy: Knowledge of the signs and symptoms of a hiatal hernia is necessary to answer the question. Use the process of elimination. When reading the four options, note that options 3 and 4 are obviously not true of hiatal hernias. Option 1 may be associated with hiatal hernia, but option 2 is more specific and is the best answer. Review the signs and symptoms of a hiatal hernia now if you had difficulty with this question!

Level of Cognitive Ability: Application
Phase of Nursing Process: Assessment
Client Needs: Physiological Integrity
Content Area: Adult Health/Gastrointestinal

Reference

Lewis, S. M., Collier, I. C., & Heitkemper, M. M. (1996). *Medical-surgical nursing: Assessment and management of clinical problems* (4th ed.). St. Louis: Mosby–Year Book, pp. 1156–1157.

---

215. The school nurse responsible for routine health assessment of 11-year-old children would screen for

1. Meningitis.
2. Congenital hip disorder.
3. Phenylketonuria.
4. Scoliosis.

Answer: 4

Rationale: Scoliosis is a common deformity affecting up to 10% of children who have some degree of spinal curvature. Screening generally begins in the fifth grade. There is no routine screening test for meningitis. Congenital hip disorder and phenylketonuria (PKU) are screened for in newborns.

Test-Taking Strategy: Knowledge of disorders common to school-age children and of routine screenings is needed to select the correct answer. If you are unfamiliar with this information, rely on your clinical experience to eliminate distracters. PKU is screened for in neonates, and the word "congenital" in option 3 suggests that hip disorders would also be screened for in infancy. If you had difficulty with this question, review screening procedures for these disorders now!

Level of Cognitive Ability: Application
Phase of Nursing Process: Assessment
Client Needs: Physiological Integrity
Content Area: Child Health

Reference

Ball, J., & Bindler, R. (1995). *Pediatric nursing: Caring for children.* Stamford, CT: Appleton & Lange, p. 598.

---

216. The female client with a history of chronic infection in the urinary system complains of burning sensation and urinary frequency. To determine whether the current problem is of renal origin, the nurse would assess whether the client has pain or discomfort in the

1 Suprapubic area.
2 Right or left costovertebral angle.
3 Urinary meatus.
4 Labium.

Answer: 2

Rationale: Pain or discomfort from a problem that originates in the kidney is felt at the costovertebral angle on the affected side. Ureteral pain is felt in the ipsilateral labium in the female client and in the ipsilateral scrotum in the male client. Bladder infection is often accompanied by suprapubic pain and by pain or burning sensation at the urinary meatus during voiding.

Test-Taking Strategy: To answer this question accurately, you should know the areas in which pain is felt or referred when it originates in the urinary tract. Knowing that the kidneys sit higher than the level of the bladder and retroperitoneally, you may be able to eliminate each incorrect option by using concepts related to anatomy!

Level of Cognitive Ability: Application
Phase of Nursing Process: Assessment
Client Needs: Physiological Integrity
Content Area: Adult Health/Renal

Reference

Black, J. M., & Matassarin-Jacobs, E. (1997). *Medical-surgical nursing: Clinical management for continuity of care* (5th ed.). Philadelphia: W. B. Saunders, pp. 1548–1549.

---

217. The home care nurse is making home visits to an elderly client with urinary incontinence who is very disturbed by the incontinent episodes. The nurse explores the client's home situation to determine environmental barriers to normal voiding. Which of the following items, as assessed by the nurse, may be contributing to the client's problem?

1 Presence of hand railings in the bathroom
2 Having one bathroom on each floor of the home
3 Nightlight present in the hall between the bedroom and bathroom
4 Bathroom located on the second floor, bedroom on the first floor

Answer: 4

Rationale: Having a bathroom on the second floor and the bedroom on the first floor may pose a problem for the elderly client with incontinence. Both the need to negotiate the stairs and the distance may interfere with reaching the bathroom in a timely manner. It is more helpful to the incontinent client to have a bathroom on the same floor as the bedroom or to have a commode rented for use on the same floor. The presence of night lights and hand railings is helpful to the client in reaching the bathroom quickly and safely.

Test-Taking Strategy: Use the process of elimination. Begin to answer this question by eliminating option 1 as obviously helpful. Option 2 is also helpful and cannot be the answer to the question as stated. Because option 3 is more helpful than option 4, at least for nighttime voiding, option 4 is the correct option!

Level of Cognitive Ability: Analysis
Phase of Nursing Process: Assessment
Client Needs: Psychosocial Integrity
Content Area: Fundamental Skills

Reference

Black, J. M., & Matassarin-Jacobs, E. (1997). *Medical-surgical nursing: Clinical management for continuity of care* (5th ed.). Philadelphia: W. B. Saunders, pp. 1550–1551.

218. The nurse is assessing an electrocardiogram (ECG) rhythm strip of a client. The P waves and QRS complexes are regular. The PR interval is 0.16 seconds, and QRS complexes measure 0.06 seconds. The overall heart rate is 64. The nurse assesses the cardiac rhythm as

1 Normal sinus rhythm.
2 Sinus bradycardia.
3 Sick sinus syndrome.
4 First-degree heart block.

Answer: 1

Rationale: Normal sinus rhythm is defined as a regular rhythm with an overall rate of 60–100 beats/minute. The PR and QRS measurements are normal, measuring 0.12–0.20 seconds and 0.04–0.10 seconds, respectively. Sinus bradycardia is defined as a heart rate below 60 beats per minute.

Test-Taking Strategy: A baseline knowledge of normal ECG measurements can help you answer these questions fairly readily. Be sure to be aware of the characteristics of normal sinus rhythm, atrial fibrillation, premature ventricular contractions (PVCs), ventricular tachycardia, and ventricular fibrillation. Take the time to review these now if needed!

Level of Cognitive Ability: Analysis
Phase of Nursing Process: Assessment
Client Needs: Physiological Integrity
Content Area: Adult Health/Cardiovascular

Reference

Black, J. M., & Matassarin-Jacobs, E. (1997). *Medical-surgical nursing: Clinical management for continuity of care* (5th ed.). Philadelphia: W. B. Saunders, p. 1296.

219. The nurse is caring for a client with a diagnosis of Parkinson's disease. The client is receiving selegiline hydrochloride (Eldepryl), 5 mg PO BID. Which of the following would indicate to the nurse that the client is experiencing an adverse reaction?

1 Tremors
2 Lightheadedness
3 Confusion
4 Abdominal discomfort

Answer: 1

Rationale: Selegiline hydrochloride (Eldepryl) is an antiparkinsonian medication. Side effects of the medication include nausea, dizziness, lightheadedness, faintness, abdominal discomfort, and confusion. Adverse reactions and toxic effects from overdosage may vary from central nervous system depression (sedation, apnea, cardiovascular collapse), to severe paradoxical reaction (hallucinations, tremor, seizures).

Test-Taking Strategy: Knowledge about selegiline hydrochloride (Eldepryl) is necessary to answer this question. The process of elimination is used in answering this question. The stem asks for an adverse reaction to the medication. Side effects are expected symptoms that can occur with some medication. Think of an adverse effect as a toxic effect. Of the four options, option 1 probably represents the adverse reaction. Options 2, 3, and 4 are side effects. If you are unfamiliar with this medication, take the time now to review this content!

Level of Cognitive Ability: Analysis
Phase of Nursing Process: Assessment
Client Needs: Physiological Integrity
Content Area: Pharmacology

Reference

Hodgson, B., & Kizior, R. (1998). *Saunders nursing drug handbook 1998.* Philadelphia: W. B. Saunders, pp. 923–924.

220. The nurse is preparing the client for renal angiography. The nurse would not need to assess for which of the following before the procedure?

1 Baseline circulation to the leg used as the insertion site
2 Allergy to contrast medium, shellfish, or iodine
3 Signed diagnostic procedure consent
4 Signed anesthesia consent

Answer: 4

Rationale: The procedure is performed with local anesthesia, although sedatives may be given before the procedure as well. Therefore, an anesthesia consent is unnecessary. The nurse assesses baseline circulation to the leg if the femoral artery is used and determines whether the client has an allergy to the contrast medium. Because the procedure is invasive, a signed consent is necessary.

Test-Taking Strategy: The key to answer this question is that this procedure is an invasive procedure involving the use of radiopaque dye that is introduced through a large blood vessel. Using these concepts, you would eliminate options 1, 2, and 3 systematically. Using another approach, knowing that the procedure is done in the radiology department also helps you to identify option 4 as the answer to the question as stated. If you are unfamiliar with the preprocedure related to renal angiography, take time now to review!

Level of Cognitive Ability: Application
Phase of Nursing Process: Assessment
Client Needs: Physiological Integrity
Content Area: Adult Health/Renal

Reference

Black, J. M., & Matassarin-Jacobs, E. (1997). *Medical-surgical nursing: Clinical management for continuity of care* (5th ed.). Philadelphia: W. B. Saunders, pp. 1564–1565.

221. The client underwent an upper lobe lobectomy of the right lung 3 hours ago. The closed drainage system has 400 mL of bloody drainage. Vital signs are as follows: blood pressure, 100/50; heart rate, 100; respiratory rate, 26. There is intermittent bubbling in the water seal chamber. One hour after the initial assessment, the nurse notes that the bubbling is now constant and the client appears dyspneic. The nurse should first assess the

1 Lung sounds.
2 Vital signs.
3 Chest tube connections.
4 Amount of drainage.

Answer: 3

Rationale: The change in the client status is most likely related to an air leak caused by a loose connection. Other causes of the change in the client status might be a tear or incision in the pulmonary pleura, which requires physician intervention. Although the other responses are correct, they should be performed after initial attempts to locate and correct the air leak. It takes only a moment to check the connections, and if a leak is found and corrected, the client's symptoms should resolve.

Test-Taking Strategy: This question requires that you have basic knowledge of closed drainage systems and their operation. The key word in the scenario is "first." Knowing that a constant bubbling in the water seal could indicate a leak, you would be directed to select option 3. Review basic knowledge of closed drainage systems now if you had difficulty with this question. You will certainly find similar questions on NCLEX-RN!

Level of Cognitive Ability: Application
Phase of Nursing Process: Assessment
Client Needs: Physiological Integrity
Content Area: Adult Health/Respiratory

Reference

Polaski, A., & Tatro, S. (1996). *Luckmann's Core principles and practice of medical-surgical nursing.* Philadelphia: W. B. Saunders, pp. 609–610.

222. The nurse visits the client at home 2 weeks after a segmental resection of the upper lobe of the left lung. The client is sitting stiffly in a recliner with the right arm held close to the chest. In addition to the reinforcement of postoperative breathing techniques, it is most important that the nurse also assess the

1. Range of motion and compliance with prescribed arm and shoulder exercises.
2. Dietary habits and effectiveness of support services.
3. Physical characteristics of the house and number of steps.
4. Client's ability to drive to the follow-up appointment with the physician.

Answer: 1

Rationale: Failure of the client to perform active range-of-motion exercises as prescribed allows the formation of adhesions of the incised muscle layer and leads to dysfunction syndrome.

Test-Taking Strategy: You are required to read the scenario carefully and analyze the assessment data that is presented in order to identify the client problem. Option 1 is the only option that relates to the scenario in the question. If you had difficulty with this question, review postoperative measures associated with lung surgery!

Level of Cognitive Ability: Application
Phase of Nursing Process: Assessment
Client Needs: Health Promotion and Maintenance
Content Area: Adult Health/Respiratory

Reference
Polaski, A., & Tatro, S. (1996). *Luckmann's Core principles and practice of medical-surgical nursing.* Philadelphia: W. B. Saunders, p. 621.

---

223. The client has received a diagnosis of tumor of the larynx. The nurse determines that the client is in the late stage of the disease process because of the presence of

1. Voice changes.
2. Hoarseness.
3. Hemoptysis.
4. Dyspnea.

Answer: 4

Rationale: Dyspnea is a late sign of a laryngeal tumor that occurs when the tumor growth is beginning to cause airway obstruction. Each of the other signs presented in options 1, 2, and 3 is an early sign.

Test-Taking Strategy: Read the scenario and identify the key elements. In this instance, the key element is the word "late." Consider the anatomy and location of the tumor. This may assist you in identifying the symptom that occurs late. Review these signs now if you had difficulty with this question.

Level of Cognitive Ability: Application
Phase of Nursing Process: Assessment
Client Needs: Physiological Integrity
Content Area: Adult Health/Respiratory

Reference
Polaski, A., & Tatro, S. (1996). *Luckmann's Core principles and practice of medical-surgical nursing.* Philadelphia: W. B. Saunders, p. 549.

---

224. The nurse is caring for the client in traction. The nurse would assess for which of the following potential problems with the traction setup?

1. Ropes are centered in the wheel grooves of the pulleys
2. Ropes are free of frays or shredding
3. Weights are resting against the foot of the bed
4. Knots are secured tightly

Answer: 3

Rationale: The traction setup is checked routinely to ensure that the ropes are in the grooves of the pulleys, ropes are not frayed, knots are tied securely, and weights are hanging freely from the ropes. Weights that rest against another object do not exert the full pulling force that is intended and ordered with the traction.

Test-Taking Strategy: This question exemplifies the basic principles in traction assessment. Use the process of elimination to answer the question. Ropes that are intact and centered in the pulleys and knots that are secure are all needed for proper traction setup and use. Weights that rest against another object do not exert the full pulling force that is intended and ordered with the traction; thus option 3 is the answer to the question as stated. If you had difficulty with this question, take time now to review the principles of traction!

Level of Cognitive Ability: Application
Phase of Nursing Process: Assessment
Client Needs: Physiological Integrity
Content Area: Adult Health/Musculoskeletal

Reference

Smeltzer, S., & Bare, B. (1996). *Brunner and Suddarth's Textbook of medical-surgical nursing* (8th ed.). Philadelphia: Lippincott-Raven, p. 1862.

---

225. The clinic nurse is assessing a client who had a total gastrectomy a few months ago. The nurse is especially careful to assess for

1. Vitamin B_{12} and folic acid deficiencies.
2. Elevated blood urea nitrogen (BUN).
3. Pain.
4. Hypercalcemia.

Answer: 1

Rationale: Common nutritional problems after stomach removal include vitamin B_{12} and folic acid deficiency. This may result from a deficiency of an intrinsic factor and/or inadequate absorption, because food enters the bowel too quickly.

Test-Taking Strategy: Use the process of elimination. Knowledge of the complications associated with gastrectomy will assist in answering the question. If you can recall that vitamin B_{12} deficiency occurs with this type of surgery, then by the process of elimination, you would select option 1. If you had difficulty with this question, take time now to review the complications associated with gastrectomy!

Level of Cognitive Ability: Application
Phase of Nursing Process: Assessment
Client Needs: Physiological Integrity
Content Area: Adult Health/Gastrointestinal

Reference

Black, J. M., & Matassarin-Jacobs, E. (1997). *Medical-surgical nursing: Clinical management for continuity of care* (5th ed.). Philadelphia: W. B. Saunders, p. 1778.

---

226. The nurse is assessing a ventilated client with a diagnosis of acute pulmonary edema. The nurse would determine that the client could be anxious when the client exhibits

1. Tachycardia, clinging to family members, and pupil dilation.
2. Bradycardia, hand clenching, and startling behaviors.
3. Hypotension, confusion, and combative behaviors.
4. Tachypnea, decreased level of consciousness, and palpitations.

Answer: 1

Rationale: Signs of anxiety include behaviors such as clenched hands, heightened awareness, wide eyes, pupil dilation, startle response, furrowed brow, clinging to the family or staff, or physical lashing out. Because anxiety stimulates the sympathetic nervous system, the client may also exhibit palpitations and chest pain, tachycardia, increased respiratory rate, elevated blood glucose levels, and hand tremors. In anxious states, tachycardia, not bradycardia (option 2), is present. The signs noted in option 3 would be seen with hypoxia, not anxiety. Anxiety produces heightened awareness, not a decreased level of consciousness (option 4).

Test-Taking Strategy: Be careful when the answer stems contain the word "and." Remember that each component needs to be correct. If you know that anxiety stimulates the sympathetic nervous system and if you know the effects of sympathetic stimulation, you will easily be directed to option 1. Review the effects of this physiological process now if you had difficulty with this question!

Level of Cognitive Ability: Analysis
Phase of Nursing Process: Assessment
Client Needs: Psychosocial Integrity
Content Area: Adult Health/Cardiovascular

References

Bolander, V. (1994). *Sorensen and Luckmann's Basic nursing: A psychophysiologic approach* (3rd ed.). Philadelphia: W. B. Saunders, p. 287.
Doenges, M. E., Moorhouse, M. F., & Geissler, A. C. (1997). *Nursing care plans: Guidelines for planning and documenting patient care* (4th ed.). Philadelphia: F. A. Davis, pp. 785–786.

227. The client has received a diagnosis of acute pyelonephritis. The nurse assesses the client for which of the following manifestations?

1 Low-grade fever
2 Flank pain on the unaffected side
3 Chills and nausea
4 Pale, dilute urine

Answer: 3

Rationale: Typical manifestations of acute pyelonephritis include high fever, chills, nausea and vomiting, flank pain on the affected side with costovertebral angle tenderness, general weakness, and headache. The client often exhibits the typical signs and symptoms of cystitis, with production of urine that is foul-smelling, cloudy, or bloody and has an increased white blood cell (WBC) count.

Test-Taking Strategy: Use the process of elimination to select the correct answer. The least plausible answer is flank pain on the unaffected side, so option 2 is eliminated first. Pale, dilute urine is the next improbable option, because infection usually causes the urine to become bloody or at least turbid. To discriminate between the last two options, you need to know that pyelonephritis causes high fever, chills, nausea, and vomiting, which would help you discriminate between options 1 and 3. If you had difficulty with this question, take time now to review the clinical manifestations associated with acute pyelonephritis!

Level of Cognitive Ability: Application
Phase of Nursing Process: Assessment
Client Needs: Physiological Integrity
Content Area: Adult Health/Renal

Reference
Black, J. M., & Matassarin-Jacobs, E. (1997). *Medical-surgical nursing: Clinical management for continuity of care* (5th ed.). Philadelphia: W. B. Saunders, p. 1629.

---

228. The nurse is assigned to care for a client with nephrotic syndrome. The nurse assesses which of the following most important parameters on a daily basis?

1 Total protein levels
2 Weight
3 Blood urea nitrogen (BUN)
4 Activity tolerance

Answer: 2

Rationale: The client with nephrotic syndrome typically manifests edema, hypoalbuminemia, and proteinuria. The nurse carefully assesses the fluid balance of the client, which includes daily monitoring of weight, intake and output, edema, and girth measurements. Albumin levels are monitored as they are ordered, as are the BUN and creatinine levels. The client's activity level is adjusted according to the amount of edema and water retention. As edema increases, the client's activity level should be restricted.

Test-Taking Strategy: Begin to answer this question by eliminating options 1 and 3 first. Nephrotic syndrome is a chronic condition, and daily levels of albumin (not total protein or BUN) may be most helpful during acute episodes. Of the two options remaining, knowing that the activity level is adjusted according to the volume of fluid retention helps you choose weight (option 2) as the correct parameter to monitor on a daily basis!

Level of Cognitive Ability: Application
Phase of Nursing Process: Assessment
Client Needs: Physiological Integrity
Content Area: Adult Health/Renal

Reference
Black, J. M., & Matassarin-Jacobs, E. (1997). *Medical-surgical nursing: Clinical management for continuity of care* (5th ed.). Philadelphia: W. B. Saunders, p. 1635.

229. The nurse is assessing the function of cranial nerve XII (hypoglossal nerve). The nurse would assess the function of this nerve by asking the client to

1. Stick out the tongue and move it from side to side.
2. Open the mouth and say "Ah."
3. Swallow a sip of water.
4. Vocalize the sounds "la-la," "mi-mi," and "kuh-kuh."

Answer: 1

Rationale: Cranial nerve XII, the hypoglossal nerve, has motor function only and controls movement of the tongue. To assess its function, the client sticks out the tongue and moves it quickly from side to side. The strength of the tongue can be assessed by having the client push against the inside of the cheek with the tongue while external pressure is applied to that cheek. Options 2, 3, and 4 are assessed as part of glossopharyngeal nerve (cranial nerve IX) and vagus nerve (cranial nerve X) testing, which are done together.

Test-Taking Strategy: Questions related to cranial nerves are difficult unless you know the differences between these nerves. It may help you to associate the word "hypoglossal" with the tongue. Review cranial nerve function and methods of assessment now if you had difficulty with this question!

Level of Cognitive Ability: Application
Phase of Nursing Process: Assessment
Client Needs: Physiological Integrity
Content Area: Adult Health/Neurological

Reference

Black, J. M., & Matassarin-Jacobs, E. (1997). *Medical-surgical nursing: Clinical management for continuity of care* (5th ed.). Philadelphia: W. B. Saunders, p. 721.

---

230. The nurse is assessing the neurological status of a client. The nurse would assess for new memory by asking the client

1. To state the date of birth.
2. What type of transportation was used to get to the hospital.
3. What was on last night's supper meal tray.
4. To repeat three unrelated words spoken to the client immediately and 5 minutes later.

Answer: 4

Rationale: Remote, or long-term, memory is tested by asking the client about something from the past (option 1). The nurse must, however, be able to verify this information. Recent memory is tested by information within days, weeks, or months (options 2 and 3). New memory is tested by asking the client to repeat three unrelated words that the examiner speaks. The client repeats them immediately so the nurse knows that they have been heard correctly, and the nurse asks the client to repeat them again 5 minutes later.

Test-Taking Strategy: This question is fairly straightforward in accordance with the meaning of "new," stated in the question. Each of the incorrect options can be discarded in turn by comparing which of the pieces of information would be "newest" to the client. This should easily direct you to option 4.

Level of Cognitive Ability: Application
Phase of Nursing Process: Assessment
Client Needs: Physiological Integrity
Content Area: Adult Health/Neurological

Reference

Ignatavicius, D. D., Workman, M. L., & Mishler, M. A. (1995). *Medical-surgical nursing: A nursing process approach* (2nd ed., Vol. 2). Philadelphia: W. B. Saunders, p. 1102.

231. The client with renal malignancy is admitted for a diagnostic work-up and probable surgery. During the admission assessment, the nurse inquires about the presence of which of the following common symptoms related to this problem?

1 Flank pain and intermittent hematuria
2 Suprapubic pain and constant slight hematuria
3 Flank pain and foul-smelling urine
4 Abdominal pain and decreased urine output

Answer: 1

Rationale: Renal cancer is commonly manifested by hematuria and flank pain, and a mass may be palpated on physical examination. Because the hematuria is gross but intermittent, the client may delay seeking medical treatment.

Test-Taking Strategy: Begin to answer this question by noting that all of the options contain pain as a component of the option. Knowing that this is a kidney problem, you would eliminate options 2 and 4, expecting that the pain would be felt in the flank area. You could then choose option 1 over option 3, using the knowledge that foul-smelling urine could indicate infection, which is unrelated to this question. You could also choose correctly if you knew that renal cancer causes hematuria that is intermittent in nature, because of tumor growth. If you had difficulty with this question, take time now to review the clinical manifestations associated with renal tumors!

Level of Cognitive Ability: Application
Phase of Nursing Process: Assessment
Client Needs: Physiological Integrity
Content Area: Adult Health/Renal

Reference
Black, J. M., & Matassarin-Jacobs, E. (1997). *Medical-surgical nursing: Clinical management for continuity of care* (5th ed.). Philadelphia: W. B. Saunders, p. 1671.

---

232. The client has undergone urinary diversion after cystectomy for bladder cancer. The nurse assesses the urostomy stoma to ensure that it is

1 Pale and pink.
2 Pink and dry.
3 Red and moist.
4 Dusky to beefy colored.

Answer: 3

Rationale: After urostomy, the stoma should be red and moist. It may be edematous, but this will decrease after the first few days. A dusky or cyanotic color indicates insufficient circulation, with impending necrosis, and warrants immediate notification of the surgeon.

Test-Taking Strategy: Begin to answer this question by eliminating option 2, because a stoma should not be dry. To discriminate among the remaining three items, it is necessary to know the meaning of various color changes in the stoma. Knowing that a dusky stoma indicates insufficient circulation helps you to eliminate option 4 as an answer. Knowing that the color should be red, not pale pink, helps you to choose option 3 correctly.

Level of Cognitive Ability: Application
Phase of Nursing Process: Assessment
Client Needs: Physiological Integrity
Content Area: Adult Health/Renal

Reference
Black, J. M., & Matassarin-Jacobs, E. (1997). *Medical-surgical nursing: Clinical management for continuity of care* (5th ed.). Philadelphia: W. B. Saunders, p. 1590.

---

233. The nurse is assessing the fluid balance of the unconscious client. Which of the following observations indicates the possibility of fluid volume deficit to the nurse?

1 Presence of tongue furrows
2 Moist mucous membranes
3 Intake approximating output
4 Unchanged weight

Answer: 1

Rationale: Signs of fluid balance include equal intake and output for 24, 48, and 72 hours; stable body weight; moist mucous membranes; absence of tongue furrows; good skin turgor; and BUN and electrolytes within normal limits.

Test-Taking Strategy: Some questions related to the care of the unconscious client may be fundamental, inasmuch as so many aspects of care relate to "the basics" of nursing. Each of the three incorrect options illustrates normal fluid balance. Furrows on the tongue indicate dryness and possible dehydration. Review the signs of dehydration now if you had difficulty with this question!

Level of Cognitive Ability: Analysis
Phase of Nursing Process: Assessment
Client Needs: Physiological Integrity
Content Area: Adult Health/Neurological

Reference

Black, J. M., & Matassarin-Jacobs, E. (1997). *Medical-surgical nursing: Clinical management for continuity of care* (5th ed.). Philadelphia: W. B. Saunders, p. 760.

---

234. The nurse is assessing a client with an arm fracture for signs of arterial damage sustained at the time of the fracture. Which of the following signs, if assessed by the nurse, would not be consistent with arterial damage?

1 Pallor or blotchy cyanosis
2 Reddish discoloration of the skin
3 Weakened or absent distal pulse
4 Continued pain despite medication

Answer: 2

Rationale: Signs of arterial damage can result when the artery is contused, thrombosed, or lacerated or when it becomes spastic. These signs include pallor or blotchy cyanosis, variable or absent distal pulse, swelling, pain, poor capillary refill, and distal paralysis or loss of sensation. Reddish discoloration would be more likely to occur with impaired venous return.

Test-Taking Strategy: Read the stem of the question carefully. Impairment of the arterial blood supply results in poor perfusion to the tissues. Options 1 and 3 are definitely arterial signs. Of the two options remaining, knowing that ischemic pain is not relieved with medication helps you to choose the reddened skin as the sign that does not indicate arterial damage. Review the characteristics associated with arterial damage now if you had difficulty with this question!

Level of Cognitive Ability: Analysis
Phase of Nursing Process: Assessment
Client Needs: Physiological Integrity
Content Area: Adult Health/Musculoskeletal

Reference

Black, J. M., & Matassarin-Jacobs, E. (1997). *Medical-surgical nursing: Clinical management for continuity of care* (5th ed.). Philadelphia: W. B. Saunders, p. 2139.

---

235. The nurse is caring for the client in a plaster cast. The cast is white, odorless, and resonant to percussion and feels approximately room temperature to touch. The nurse assesses that the cast is

1 Completely wet.
2 Beginning to dry.
3 About half dry.
4 Fully dry.

Answer: 4

Rationale: A dry plaster cast is white, odorless, close to room temperature, and resonant to percussion. A wet plaster cast, on the other hand, is gray, cool, musty smelling, and dull to percussion.

Test-Taking Strategy: Use the process of elimination to answer this question. Look at the description of the cast in the case and for a relationship in the options. Thinking about the descriptions such as "white" and "resonant" may help you to choose option 4, "fully dry."

Level of Cognitive Ability: Application
Phase of Nursing Process: Assessment
Client Needs: Physiological Integrity
Content Area: Adult Health/Musculoskeletal

Reference

Black, J. M., & Matassarin-Jacobs, E. (1997). *Medical-surgical nursing: Clinical management for continuity of care* (5th ed.). Philadelphia: W. B. Saunders, p. 2148.

236. The nurse inquires about a smoking history while conducting a hospital admission assessment with a client with coronary artery disease. The most important item for the nurse to assess is the

1 Number of pack-years.
2 Brand of cigarettes used.
3 Desire to quit smoking.
4 Number of past attempts to quit smoking.

Answer: 1

Rationale: The number of cigarettes smoked daily and the duration of the habit are used to calculate the number of pack-years, which is the standard method of documenting smoking history. The brand of cigarettes may give a general indication of tar and nicotine levels, but the information has no immediate clinical use. Desire to quit and number of past attempts to quit smoking may be useful when the nurse develops a smoking cessation plan with the client.

Test-Taking Strategy: The question directs you to identify the "most" important item. This indicates that more than one option is correct. The option that would most closely predict the degree of added risk of coronary artery disease is the number of pack-years.

Level of Cognitive Ability: Analysis
Phase of Nursing Process: Assessment
Client Needs: Physiological Integrity
Content Area: Adult Health/Cardiovascular

Reference

Ignatavicius, D. D., Workman, M. L., & Mishler, M. A. (1995). *Medical-surgical nursing: A nursing process approach* (2nd ed., Vol. 1). Philadelphia: W. B. Saunders, p. 787.

---

237. The nurse is screening a 39-year-old white female client. The client has a blood pressure of 152/92 at rest, total cholesterol level of 190 mg/dL, and fasting blood glucose level of 114. The nurse would focus attention on which risk factor for coronary artery disease (CAD)?

1 Age
2 Hyperlipidemia
3 Hypertension
4 Glucose intolerance

Answer: 3

Rationale: Hypertension, cigarette smoking, and hyperlipidemia are major risk factors that have been shown through research to be objective predictors of CAD. Glucose intolerance, obesity, and response to stress are contributing factors. Age greater than 40 is a nonmodifiable risk factor. The nurse places priority on major risk factors that must and can be modified.

Test-Taking Strategy: Risk for CAD is higher with age greater than 40 years, total cholesterol level exceeding 200 mg/dL, and diabetes mellitus (random blood glucose level exceeding 120). The client's age is not a risk factor, and the other values in these areas fall just within the normal ranges. Therefore, hypertension (systolic blood pressure greater than 140 mmHg, diastolic blood pressure greater than 90 mmHg) is the option of choice. Look at the descriptions in the case. Identifying the abnormal finding will assist you in selecting the correct option. If you had difficulty with this question, take time now to review the risk factors associated with CAD!

Level of Cognitive Ability: Analysis
Phase of Nursing Process: Assessment
Client Needs: Health Promotion and Maintenance
Content Area: Adult Health/Cardiovascular

Reference

Black, J. M., & Matassarin-Jacobs, E. (1997). *Medical-surgical nursing: Clinical management for continuity of care* (5th ed.). Philadelphia: W. B. Saunders, pp. 1239, 1962.

238. The client was just told by the primary care physician that the client will have an exercise stress test to evaluate cardiac status after recent episodes of more severe chest pain. As the nurse enters the examining room, the client states, "Maybe I shouldn't bother going. I wonder if I should just take more medication instead." On the basis of the nurse's assessment of the client's comment, the nurse's best response would be

1 "Can you tell me more about how you're feeling?"
2 "Don't worry. Emergency equipment is available if it should be needed."
3 "Most people tolerate the procedure well without any complications."
4 "Don't you really want to control your heart disease?"

Answer: 1

Rationale: Anxiety and fear are often present before stress testing. The nurse uses questioning as a communication method to explore a client's feelings and concerns.

Test-Taking Strategy: Options 2 and 3 are statements, not questions, and therefore limit communication, so eliminate them first. Eliminate option 4 next because it does not focus on the client's feelings. The correct answer is open-ended and is the only one of the options that is phrased to engender trust and sharing of concerns by the client. Focus on clients' feelings first!

Level of Cognitive Ability: Application
Phase of Nursing Process: Assessment
Client Needs: Psychosocial Integrity
Content Area: Adult Health/Cardiovascular

Reference

Potter, P. A., & Perry, A. G. (1997). *Fundamentals of nursing: Concepts, process, and practice* (4th ed.). St. Louis: Mosby–Year Book, pp. 241–242.

239. A neonate receives a diagnosis of Hirschsprung's disease on the basis of failure to pass meconium. The nurse observes that the parents are hesitant to hold their newborn. According to this assessment, an important nursing consideration in working with the parents is to

1 Observe stools for color and character.
2 Help the parents adjust to the congenital disorder.
3 Stabilize the newborn's fluid and electrolyte balance.
4 Teach the parents how to administer a barium enema to their child.

Answer: 2

Rationale: One of the main objectives is to help parents adjust to the congenital disorder in their child and to foster infant-parent bonding. Failure to pass meconium within 24 hours is suggestive of Hirschsprung's disease. A barium enema is a diagnostic tool, which would not be administered by parents. The neonate's fluid and electrolyte status is not likely to be in an imbalanced state at this time.

Test-Taking Strategy: This question specifically asks about a nursing consideration when working with parents. The assessment data reveals the parents are hesitant to hold their newborn. This may indicate a need to help them accept their child even though the child is not perfect. Read all four of the options. Identify the client or clients of the question. Two options refer to interventions appropriate in caring for the child, and the remaining two refer to parental concerns. Of the two referring to parents' concern, option 2 is an appropriate response.

Level of Cognitive Ability: Application
Phase of Nursing Process: Assessment
Client Needs: Psychosocial Integrity
Content Area: Maternity

Reference

Wong, D., & Perry, S. (1998). *Maternal-child nursing care.* St. Louis: Mosby–Year Book, pp. 1399–1401.

240. The nurse is caring for the client with an acute head injury. The nurse carefully assesses which of the following neurological signs as the most sensitive indicator of neurological status?

1 Vital signs
2 Level of consciousness
3 Sensory function
4 Motor function

Answer: 2

Rationale: The level of consciousness is the most sensitive indicator of neurological status. An alteration in the level of consciousness occurs before any other changes in neurological signs or vital signs. Vital signs changes occur late.

Test-Taking Strategy: This question is a classic. If you do not know that the level of consciousness is the most sensitive neurological indicator, memorize it now!

Level of Cognitive Ability: Application
Phase of Nursing Process: Assessment
Client Needs: Physiological Integrity
Content Area: Adult Health/Neurological

Reference
Smeltzer, S., & Bare, B. (1996). *Brunner and Suddarth's Textbook of medical-surgical nursing* (8th ed.). Philadelphia: Lippincott-Raven, p. 1792.

---

241. A pregnant client is admitted to the hospital with a blood pressure of 142/90 and a urine protein measurement of +2. Which one of the following signs would indicate to the nurse that the severity of the client's pre-eclampsia has increased?

1 Deep tendon reflexes
2 Pedal and pretibial edema
3 Fluctuating fetal heart rate
4 Oliguria

Answer: 4

Rationale: Oliguria indicates renal impairment and is a characteristic symptom of severe pre-eclampsia. Renal perfusion is reduced as vasospasm increases, and therefore urine output also decreases. Deep tendon reflexes and fluctuating fetal heart rate are normal assessments. The presence of pedal and pretibial edema does not indicate increasing severity of pre-eclampsia.

Test-Taking Strategy: Knowledge of pre-eclampsia is necessary to answer this question. Knowing that the basic pathophysiology of pre-eclampsia is vasospasm and decreased tissue perfusion will assist you in answering this question. If you are uncertain about the answer, look for similarity in the distracters. There is a similarity in options 1 and 3 in that both options relate to normal assessment findings. If a similarity exists in the answers, then neither one is likely to be the answer. Review the characteristics associated with pre-eclampsia now if you had difficulty with this question!

Level of Cognitive Ability: Analysis
Phase of Nursing Process: Assessment
Client Needs: Physiological Integrity
Content Area: Maternity

Reference
Nichols, F., & Zwelling, E. (1997). *Maternal-newborn nursing: Theory and practice.* Philadelphia: W. B. Saunders, p. 645.

---

242. An infant who has pyloric stenosis is admitted to the hospital. The finding that the nursing assessment is most likely to reveal is

1 Forceful and projectile vomiting.
2 Bile-stained emesis.
3 Peristalsis on auscultation.
4 Hyponatremia.

Answer: 1

Rationale: Pyloric stenosis occurs when the circular muscle of the pylorus becomes grossly enlarged (hypertrophic) and causes constriction of the pylorus and obstruction of the gastric outlet. Infants with hypertrophic pyloric stenosis most commonly manifest forceful and projectile vomiting. The emesis contains milk or formula and is not bile-stained. Bile-stained emesis is a sign of obstruction of the small intestine. Gastric peristalsis visible on examination occurs in some infants. Hypernatremia occurs because of depletion of electrolytes from extensive and prolonged vomiting.

Test-Taking Strategy: Use the process of elimination. The question asks which assessment you are most likely to identify in an infant with pyloric stenosis. Projectile vomiting is present in most infants with pyloric stenosis. Review the clinical manifestations of pyloric stenosis now if you had difficulty with this question!

Level of Cognitive Ability: Application
Phase of Nursing Process: Assessment
Client Needs: Physiological Integrity
Content Area: Child Health

Reference

Wong, D., & Perry, S. (1998). *Maternal-child nursing care.* St. Louis: Mosby–Year Book, pp. 1426–1429.

---

243. The nurse would assess the sensory ability of spinal cord–injured client by asking the client to

1 Spread the fingers.
2 Squeeze the nurse's hand.
3 Discriminate between touch and pinprick stimuli.
4 Move the toes or turn the feet.

Answer: 3

Rationale: Sensation is tested by pinching the skin or pushing on it with a dull object. The nurse starts at the shoulder level and works downward in a systematic manner. The client is asked at which levels sensation is felt and whether it is sharp or dull. Motor function is tested by asking the client to spread the fingers, squeeze the nurse's hands, or move the toes or feet.

Test-Taking Strategy: This question tests the nurse's ability to discriminate between sensory and motor testing of the client with spinal cord injury. The key word in the question is "sensory." Options 1, 2, and 4 are similar in that they all test motor ability. Option 3 is the only option that tests sensory ability. The concept is a basic one. If this item is difficult, a quick review of neurological assessment may be helpful.

Level of Cognitive Ability: Application
Phase of Nursing Process: Assessment
Client Needs: Physiological Integrity
Content Area: Adult Health/Neurological

Reference

Black, J. M., & Matassarin-Jacobs, E. (1997). *Medical-surgical nursing: Clinical management for continuity of care* (5th ed.). Philadelphia: W. B. Saunders, p. 899.

---

244. The client has just had an insertion of skeletal pins and application of leg traction. Initially, the nurse would assess the neurovascular status of the client's affected leg

1 Daily.
2 Every shift.
3 Every 4 hours.
4 Every hour.

Answer: 4

Rationale: Immediately after application of skeletal traction, neurovascular assessment of the affected limb should be completed every hour. The client is told to report any changes in movement or sensation, so that any complications can be detected and treated quickly.

Test-Taking Strategy: Note that the stem asks for the frequency of assessment "initially" after traction setup. This is a clue that the frequency should be greater than usual. Options 1 and 2 are eliminated immediately. To discriminate between every 4 hours and every hour, it is generally correct to choose the more frequent measurement in questions with wording similar to this one.

Level of Cognitive Ability: Application
Phase of Nursing Process: Assessment
Client Needs: Physiological Integrity
Content Area: Adult Health/Musculoskeletal

Reference

Smeltzer, S., & Bare, B. (1996). *Brunner and Suddarth's Textbook of medical-surgical nursing* (8th ed.). Philadelphia: Lippincott-Raven, p. 1863.

245. The nurse is caring for a client with a tracheotomy in whom a respiratory infection has been diagnosed. The client is receiving vancomycin hydrochloride (Vancocin), 500 mg IV every 12 hours. Which of the following would indicate to the nurse that the client is experiencing an adverse reaction to the medication?

1. Decreased hearing acuity
2. Photophobia
3. Hypotension
4. Bradycardia

Answer: 1

Rationale: Vancomycin hydrochloride (Vancocin) is an antibiotic. Adverse reactions and toxic effects include nephrotoxicity, characterized by a change in the amount or frequency of urination and by anorexia, nausea, vomiting, and increased thirst; ototoxicity, characterized by deafness resulting from damage to the auditory branch of the eight cranial nerve; and red-neck syndrome, caused by too-rapid injection of the medication and characterized by chills, fever, fast heartbeat, nausea, vomiting, itching, rash, and redness on the face, neck, arms, and back. When this medication is administered to a client, nursing responsibilities include monitoring renal function laboratory results, input and output, and hearing acuity.

Test-Taking Strategy: Knowledge regarding this medication is necessary to answer this question. Note the key phrase "adverse reactions." This should assist in directing you to option 1. Review this medication now if you had difficulty answering this question!

Level of Cognitive Ability: Analysis
Phase of Nursing Process: Assessment
Client Needs: Physiological Integrity
Content Area: Pharmacology

Reference

Hodgson, B., & Kizior, R. (1998). *Saunders nursing drug handbook 1998.* Philadelphia: W. B. Saunders, pp. 1041–1043.

---

246. The nurse is caring for a recent spinal cord–injured client. The nurse assesses for signs of spinal shock, including

1. Flaccid paralysis of the legs, bowel and bladder incontinence, areflexia.
2. Flaccid paralysis of the legs, bowel and bladder retention, areflexia.
3. Spastic paralysis of the legs, bowel and bladder incontinence, hyperreflexia.
4. Spastic paralysis of the legs, bowel and bladder retention, hyperreflexia.

Answer: 2

Rationale: Signs and symptoms of spinal shock include loss of skeletal muscle movement, loss of bowel and bladder tone, and loss of autonomic reflexes below the level of the injury. Sexual function is also lost. The limbs have a flaccid paralysis, and there is bowel and bladder retention.

Test-Taking Strategy: The simplest way to remember the acute changes in spinal cord injury is to remember that all motor activity is lost below the level of the lesion. This includes loss of skeletal muscle movement (flaccid paralysis), loss of movement of the bowel or bladder wall (bowel and bladder retention), and loss of reflex movements (areflexia). This will help you eliminate each of the incorrect options. If you had difficulty with this question, review the clinical manifestations associated with spinal shock now!

Level of Cognitive Ability: Application
Phase of Nursing Process: Assessment
Client Needs: Physiological Integrity
Content Area: Adult Health/Neurological

Reference

Black, J. M., & Matassarin-Jacobs, E. (1997). *Medical-surgical nursing: Clinical management for continuity of care* (5th ed.). Philadelphia: W. B. Saunders, p. 895.

---

247. The nurse is assessing the client who is practicing crutch walking after a prolonged period of bed rest. The nurse assesses that the client should immediately stop the activity if the client exhibits

1. Slight increase in pulse.
2. Slight increase in respiratory rate.
3. Fatigue of the forearm muscles.
4. Shortness of breath and diaphoresis.

Answer: 4

Rationale: Bed rest decreases the client's strength and endurance. Shortness of breath and diaphoresis are systemic signs of fatigue, indicating that the client needs to rest.

Test-Taking Strategy: Options 1 and 2 are the least plausible and are eliminated first. Option 3 is a viable alternative, but forearm fatigue may or may not be an indication to "immediately" stop the exercise. In addition, forearm fatigue can be minimized with isometric exercise. Option 4 indicates that the client is not tolerating the activity from a cardiopulmonary standpoint and is the better choice of the two. Use the ABCs—airway, breathing, and circulation—to answer the question!

Level of Cognitive Ability: Application
Phase of Nursing Process: Assessment
Client Needs: Physiological Integrity
Content Area: Adult Health/Musculoskeletal

Reference

Smeltzer, S., & Bare, B. (1996). *Brunner and Suddarth's Textbook of medical-surgical nursing* (8th ed.). Philadelphia: Lippincott-Raven, p. 339.

---

248. While counseling a prenatal client about her dietary and drinking habits, the nurse observes that the client has difficulty concentrating and appears agitated. The nurse should proceed with the assessment, using which guideline?

1 Discussion of possible consequences to drinking during pregnancy should be avoided
2 Women respond negatively to a hopeful message of potential benefits of drinking cessation during pregnancy
3 A nonjudgmental approach may help to gain maternal trust
4 Provoking maternal guilt may help a woman recognize her problem and seek support services

Answer: 3

Rationale: The potential effects of alcohol abuse during pregnancy for both mother and fetus have been well documented. The nurse who expresses genuine concern with suspected abuses may motivate positive behavioral changes during the antenatal period. The maternal behaviors of lack of concentration and agitation are frequently seen in childbearing women abusing alcohol.

Test-Taking Strategy: This response reflects your understanding of the behavioral changes that can result from alcohol abuse. By assessing these changes during interactions with clients, the nurse can then employ a nonjudgmental manner in further interactions, which represents a basic tenet of therapeutic nursing care. Remember to display a nonjudgmental attitude!

Level of Cognitive Ability: Application
Phase of Nursing Process: Assessment
Client Needs: Psychosocial Integrity
Content Area: Maternity

Reference

Reeder, S., Martin, L., & Koniak-Griffin, D. (1997). *Maternity nursing: Family, newborn, and women's health care* (18th ed.). Philadelphia: Lippincott-Raven, pp. 913, 917.

---

249. The nurse is assessing the risk of transmission of perinatal infections in a prenatal client. The nurse uses knowledge of which of the following items to guide this assessment?

1 The vaginal pH is decreased during pregnancy, thus reducing the risk of acquiring bacterial infection
2 The mother's immune system is depressed during pregnancy
3 The placenta functions as a filtering system, thus preventing transplacental spread of organisms
4 The vaginal walls become hypertrophied, which reduces the epithelium cell layer to microorganism exposure

Answer: 2

Rationale: The acquisition of neonatal infections can occur during the antenatal, intrapartal, or neonatal period. Infections can occur via two routes: transfer of the infecting agent across the placenta or ascending infection of bacteria from the vagina. Three common alterations during pregnancy may further render the mother or fetus more susceptible to infection: the vaginal wall becomes hypertrophied, exposing more cells to microorganisms; the vaginal epithelium produces more glycogen, which increases the pH of the vagina, resulting in an increased risk for bacterial infection; and the maternal immune system is depressed, as evidenced by suppressed lymphocyte function and decreased counts of $CD4^+$ T lymphocytes.

Test-Taking Strategy: The response to this question is based on applying current knowledge related to the potential acquisition of perinatal infections and your knowledge of the normal maternal physiological changes during pregnancy. Proper understanding of these concepts allows you to eliminate each of the incorrect options systematically. Review these concepts now if you had difficulty with this question!

Level of Cognitive Ability: Application
Phase of Nursing Process: Assessment
Client Needs: Physiological Integrity
Content Area: Maternity

Reference

Nichols, F., & Zwelling, E. (1997). *Maternal-newborn nursing: Theory and practice.* Philadelphia: W. B. Saunders, p. 686.

250. Which of these assessments, identified in a child with celiac disease, would be a critical indicator of the nursing diagnosis Altered Nutrition: Less than Body Requirements?

1 Malodorous stools
2 Muscle wasting in buttocks and extremities
3 Irritability and fretfulness
4 Severe abdominal distention

Answer: 2

Rationale: Option 2 is the only assessment finding that is a critical indicator of altered nutrition. All assessments identified in options 1–4 may be clinical manifestations of celiac disease.

Test-Taking Strategy: Knowledge regarding celiac disease is helpful to answer this question, because you would recognize that the data contained in options 1–4 are all assessment findings in celiac disease. Read the stem of the question carefully. Option 2 is the only option that is a critical indicator of altered nutrition.

Level of Cognitive Ability: Analysis
Phase of Nursing Process: Assessment
Client Needs: Physiological Integrity
Content Area: Child Health

Reference
Wong, D., & Perry, S. (1998). *Maternal-child nursing care.* St. Louis: Mosby–Year Book, pp. 1432–1433.

---

251. A 25-year-old male suffered a fractured femur yesterday. The nurse assesses the client and is particularly alert for the development of which of the following signs and symptoms?

1 Dyspnea, tachycardia, fever
2 Bradycardia, dyspnea, hypertension
3 Fever, malaise, hypotension
4 Hypertension and slow, deep respirations

Answer: 1

Rationale: The young adult male (20–30 years) is especially at risk of development of fat emboli after fractures of the long bones or pelvis, multiple fractures, or crush injuries. Typical signs and symptoms include hypoxia, dyspnea, tachypnea, tachycardia, pyrexia, and signs of cerebral hypoxia. Fat embolus often occurs within 24–72 hours after injury but can occur any time from a few hours after injury to a week later.

Test-Taking Strategy: To answer this question accurately, you need to know that fat embolus is a major complication in an individual of this age and gender, and you need to know what the signs and symptoms are. If you know to look for fat embolism, eliminate at least options 3 and 4, because they do not mention dyspnea. Of the remaining two options, knowing that tachycardia is far more likely to occur than bradycardia may help you choose option 1 as the correct answer. Review the signs and symptoms of fat embolism now if you had difficulty with this question!

Level of Cognitive Ability: Analysis
Phase of Nursing Process: Assessment
Client Needs: Physiological Integrity
Content Area: Adult Health/Musculoskeletal

Reference
Smeltzer, S., & Bare, B. (1996). *Brunner and Suddarth's Textbook of medical-surgical nursing* (8th ed.). Philadelphia: Lippincott-Raven, p. 1917.

---

252. The client has returned to the nursing unit from the postanesthesia care unit after left total knee replacement. Which of the following assessments, if made by the nurse, would be expected?

1 Pallor and coolness of the left foot
2 25 mL/hour drainage from the HemoVac wound suction
3 Inability to flex the left foot
4 Pins-and-needles sensation in the left foot

Answer: 2

Rationale: Following total knee replacement, the neurovascular status of the affected leg is assessed, and findings should be within normal limits. The client should have intact capillary refill and adequate color, temperature, sensation, and motion in the limb. The knee incision has a wound suction drain in place, which is expected to drain up to 200 mL in the first 8 hours after surgery.

Test-Taking Strategy: Each of the incorrect options illustrates an impairment of the neurovascular status of the limb. This leaves the drainage of 25 mL/hr as the only choice, which is reasonable because the wound would be expected to drain after this type of surgery.

Review postoperative expectations after knee replacement now if you had difficulty with this question!

Level of Cognitive Ability: Analysis
Phase of Nursing Process: Assessment
Client Needs: Physiological Integrity
Content Area: Adult Health/Musculoskeletal

Reference

Smeltzer, S., & Bare, B. (1996). *Brunner and Suddarth's Textbook of medical-surgical nursing* (8th ed.). Philadelphia: Lippincott-Raven, pp. 1871, 1877.

---

253. The nurse is assessing the client with chest pain in the emergency room. Which of the following observations by the nurse helps determine that this pain is from myocardial infarction (MI)?

1. The pain, unrelieved by nitroglycerin, was relieved with morphine sulfate
2. The pain was described as substernal and radiating to the left arm
3. The client experienced no nausea or vomiting
4. The client reports the pain began while pushing a lawnmower

Answer: 1

Rationale: The pain of angina may radiate to the left arm, is often precipitated by exertion or stress, has few associated symptoms, and is relieved by rest and nitroglycerin. The pain of MI may radiate to the left arm, left shoulder, jaw, and neck. It typically begins spontaneously, lasts longer than 30 minutes, and is frequently accompanied by associated symptoms (nausea, vomiting, dyspnea, diaphoresis, anxiety). Opioid analgesics are required for relief.

Test-Taking Strategy: The question is seeking an item that differentiates anginal pain from that of MI, which may be similar at the onset. A classic hallmark of the pain from MI is that it is unrelieved by rest and nitroglycerin. If you had difficulty with this question, take time now to review the characteristics of anginal pain and pain related to MI!

Level of Cognitive Ability: Analysis
Phase of Nursing Process: Assessment
Client Needs: Physiological Integrity
Content Area: Adult Health/Cardiovascular

Reference

Ignatavicius, D. D., Workman, M. L., & Mishler, M. A. (1995). *Medical-surgical nursing: A nursing process approach* (2nd ed., Vol. 1). Philadelphia: W. B. Saunders, p. 990.

---

254. A client who has neuroleptic malignant syndrome has been admitted to the hospital. The finding that the nursing assessment is most likely to reveal is

1. Elevation of temperature and parkinsonian symptoms
2. Drop in blood pressure and hot, dry skin
3. Bradycardia and muscle flaccidity
4. Mental acuity and bradypnea

Answer: 1

Rationale: The individual with neuroleptic malignant syndrome experiences an elevation in temperature (sometimes up to 107°F) and parkinsonian symptoms. There can be fluctuations in blood pressure and diaphoresis. The client with neuroleptic malignant syndrome also experiences tachycardia and tachypnea, as well as muscle rigidity. The mental status can deteriorate from stupor to coma.

Test-Taking Strategy: Knowledge regarding the manifestations of neuroleptic malignant syndrome is necessary to assist you in answering the question. The client with neuroleptic malignant syndrome exhibits the parkinsonian symptoms and the elevation in temperature. The other symptoms are the opposite of the actual variations of these entities. If you had difficulty with this question, review neuroleptic malignant syndrome now!

Level of Cognitive Ability: Analysis
Phase of Nursing Process: Assessment
Client Needs: Physiological Integrity
Content Area: Adult Health/Neurological

Reference

Townsend, M. (1996). *Psychiatric mental health nursing: Concepts of care* (2nd ed.). Philadelphia: F. A. Davis, p. 288.

255. The nurse is performing an admission assessment on a client admitted with a diagnosis of fever of unknown origin. The nurse demonstrates competence under a Nurse Practice Act when the nurse

1. Enters the information on the client's record.
2. Writes the information on a worksheet.
3. Informs the supervisor of the client's vital signs.
4. Tells another nurse that the client has a high fever.

Answer: 1

Rationale: Recording the assessment data reflects the requirement of Nurse Practice Acts to maintain adequate records. Verbal information and notes on worksheets are not part of the client's permanent record.

Test-Taking Strategy: Assessment is the first step in the nursing process and includes the collection of data. Recording the data is an essential part of assessment. Review the importance of documentation and the Nurse Practice Act now if you had difficulty with this question!

Level of Cognitive Ability: Application
Phase of Nursing Process: Assessment
Client Needs: Physiological Integrity
Content Area: Fundamental Skills

Reference

Luckmann, J. (1997). *Saunders manual of nursing care.* Philadelphia: W. B. Saunders, pp. 69–71.

256. The charge nurse observes a registered nurse (RN) who is not able to meet client needs in a reasonable time, does not use problem solving in situations, and does not prioritize nursing care. The charge nurse has the responsibility to

1. Supervise the RN more closely so tasks are completed.
2. Provide support and identify the underlying cause.
3. Ask the other staff to help the RN get her work done.
4. Report the RN to the supervisor so that something is done.

Answer: 2

Rationale: Leadership is a social relationship in which one person has a greater ability to influence the behavior of another. Leadership is needed to help everyone reach goals. Option 2 empowers the charge nurse to help the RN while trying to identify and reduce the behaviors that make it difficult for the nurse to function. Options 1, 3, and 4 are punitive, shift the burden to other workers, and do not solve the problem.

Test-Taking Strategy: Remember that assessment is the first step in the nursing process. The charge nurse needs to gather information before making any decisions or deciding on a course of action. "Identifying a cause" is a process of assessment. "Providing support" is a therapeutic nursing action!

Level of Cognitive Ability: Application
Phase of Nursing Process: Assessment
Client Needs: Psychosocial Integrity
Content Area: Fundamental Skills

Reference

Gillies, D. (1994). *Nursing management: A systems approach.* Philadelphia: W. B. Saunders, pp. 333–334.

257. Drug and alcohol use by nurses is the reason for increasing numbers of disciplinary cases. There is a shift in the approach to treating nurses once an assessment is completed: from a punitive approach to treatment for an illness. It is most important to assess the nurse to determine the

1. Physiological impact of the illness on practice.
2. Types of illegal activities related to the abuse.
3. Falsification of client records.
4. Magnitude of drug diversion over time.

Answer: 1

Rationale: Nurses must be able to function at a level that does not affect safe, quality care. The highest priority is to determine how the illness affects the nurse's ability to practice. The other options will be addressed and sorted out as the investigation is carried out.

Test-Taking Strategy: Options 2, 3, and 4 focus on the punitive aspects of the situation. The public must be protected from nurses who cannot function. Assessing the impact of the illness on performance will help determine the treatment plan for each nurse. Option 1 addresses the most immediate concern.

Level of Cognitive Ability: Application
Phase of Nursing Process: Assessment
Client Needs: Physiological Integrity
Content Area: Fundamental Skills

Reference

Brent, N. (1997). *Nurses and the law.* Philadelphia: W. B. Saunders, p. 346.

258. A 55-year-old client with non–insulin-dependent diabetes mellitus (NIDDM) is brought to the immediate care center by the family for evaluation of increasing confusion over the past few weeks and recent onset of weakness. The first diagnostic study to be anticipated would be

1 Computed tomographic (CT) scan of the head.
2 Protime and prothrombin time.
3 Serum sodium and potassium.
4 Serum glucose.

Answer: 4

Rationale: A NIDDM client with gradual development of central nervous system symptoms may be developing hyperglycemic hyperosmolar nonketosis (HHNK). The serum glucose study would yield the most rapid result and would initiate the process of differential diagnosis.

Test-Taking Strategy: Awareness of the time frames for the results of certain diagnostic tests to be obtained, as well as identifying potential causes of the symptoms, will assist you in answering this question. Identifying the relationship between the client diagnosis and option 4 will assist you in selecting the correct answer. If you had difficulty with this question, take time now to review diabetes and its complications!

Level of Cognitive Ability: Analysis
Phase of Nursing Process: Assessment
Client Needs: Psychosocial Integrity
Content Area: Adult Health/Endocrine

Reference

Ignatavicius, D. D., Workman, M. L., & Mishler, M. A. (1995). *Medical-surgical nursing: A nursing process approach* (2nd ed., Vol. 2). Philadelphia: W. B. Saunders, p. 1862.

259. The post–myocardial infarction client is scheduled for a multiple-gated acquisition (MUGA) scan. The nurse would assess to make sure which item is in place before the procedure?

1 Signed consent for cardiac catheterization
2 Notation of allergies to iodine or shellfish
3 An intravenous line
4 A Foley catheter

Answer: 3

Rationale: MUGA is a radionuclide study used to detect myocardial infarction, decreased myocardial blood flow, and left ventricular function. The radioisotope is injected intravenously. The procedure is not the same as cardiac catheterization and does not involve radiopaque dye.

Test-Taking Strategy: Options 1 and 2 can be eliminated, because option 1 necessitates that 2 is also correct. Knowledge that the procedure involves injection of a radioisotope guides you to select option 3. Option 4 is irrelevant. Review preprocedure related to a MUGA scan now if you had difficulty with this question!

Level of Cognitive Ability: Application
Phase of Nursing Process: Assessment
Client Needs: Physiological Integrity
Content Area: Adult Health/Cardiovascular

Reference

Smeltzer, S., & Bare, B. (1996). *Brunner and Suddarth's Textbook of medical-surgical nursing* (8th ed.). Philadelphia: Lippincott-Raven, p. 610.

260. The client with myocardial infarction is going into cardiogenic shock. Because of myocardial ischemia, the nurse would carefully assess the client for

1 Ventricular dysrhythmias.
2 Bradycardia.
3 Rising diastolic blood pressure.
4 Falling central venous pressure (CVP).

Answer: 1

Rationale: Classical signs of cardiogenic shock as they relate to this question include low blood pressure and tachycardia. The CVP would rise as the backward effects of the left ventricular failure became apparent. Dysrhythmias commonly occur as a result of decreased oxygenation to the myocardium.

Test-Taking Strategy: The question is testing the concept of the effect of ischemia on the myocardial cells. Ischemia makes the myocardium irritable, producing dysrhythmias. Knowledge of the classic signs of shock help you systematically eliminate the other responses, which are incorrect.

Level of Cognitive Ability: Application
Phase of Nursing Process: Assessment
Client Needs: Physiological Integrity
Content Area: Adult Health/Cardiovascular

Reference

Smeltzer, S., & Bare, B. (1996). *Brunner and Suddarth's Textbook of medical-surgical nursing* (8th ed.). Philadelphia: Lippincott-Raven, p. 672.

---

261. The nurse is encouraging the client to cough and breathe deeply after cardiac surgery. The nurse would determine that which of the following items is available to maximize the effectiveness of this procedure?

1 Ambu bag
2 Incisional splinting device
3 Suction equipment
4 Nebulizer

Answer: 2

Rationale: The use of an incisional splint such as a "cough pillow" can ease discomfort during coughing and deep breathing, which is indicated every 1–2 hours. The client who is comfortable will do more effective deep breathing and coughing exercises. Use of an incentive spirometer is also indicated.

Test-Taking Strategy: Use the process of elimination to answer the question. This question is part of basic nursing care and may likely be encountered on NCLEX-RN in some form. The question asks for an item that will help the "client," which eliminates options 1 and 3, which are used by the nurse. A nebulizer (option 4) delivers medication, leaving option 2 as the correct answer.

Level of Cognitive Ability: Application
Phase of Nursing Process: Assessment
Client Needs: Physiological Integrity
Content Area: Adult Health/Cardiovascular

Reference

Black, J. M., & Matassarin-Jacobs, E. (1997). *Medical-surgical nursing: Clinical management for continuity of care* (5th ed.). Philadelphia: W. B. Saunders, p. 1361.

---

262. A 24-year-old male seeks medical attention for complaints of claudication in the arch of the foot. Buerger's disease is suspected. The nurse also notes superficial thrombophlebitis of the lower leg. On the basis of this information, which of the following will the nurse include in the psychosocial history?

1 Familial tendency toward peripheral vascular disease
2 Smoking history
3 Recent exposure to allergens
4 History of recent insect bites

Answer: 2

Rationale: The mixture of arterial and venous manifestations (claudication and phlebitis, respectively) in the young male client suggests thromboangiitis obliterans (Buerger's disease). This is a relatively uncommon disorder that is characterized by inflammation and thrombosis of smaller arteries and veins. This disorder is typically found in young adult males who smoke. The cause is unknown but is suspected to have an autoimmune component.

Test-Taking Strategy: A basic knowledge of this disorder is needed to answer this question rapidly and accurately. You can first eliminate options 3 and 4 because they would most likely cause local skin reactions. Note that of the remaining options, option 2 is the modifiable risk factor. It is often better to assess a modifiable factor before a nonmodifiable one so that the appropriate plan of care can be initiated. This may help you prioritize your answer. If you had difficulty with this question, take time now to review Buerger's disease!

Level of Cognitive Ability: Analysis
Phase of Nursing Process: Assessment
Client Needs: Physiological Integrity
Content Area: Adult Health/Cardiovascular

Reference

Smeltzer, S., & Bare, B. (1996). *Brunner and Suddarth's Textbook of medical-surgical nursing* (8th ed.). Philadelphia: Lippincott-Raven, p. 738.

263. The nurse has begun a continuous infusion of dopamine (Intropin) intravenously. The nurse would assess for which adverse effect of this therapy?

1. Falling pulmonary capillary wedge pressure
2. Falling central venous pressure
3. Bradycardia
4. Tachycardia

Answer: 4

Rationale: Dopamine is a positive inotropic agent and vasopressor that is used to improve cardiac output, blood pressure, and urine output. The physician should be notified if the client experiences tachycardia, dysrhythmias, decreasing pulse pressure, and reduced urine output without hypotension. The dose should be reduced or stopped temporarily.

Test-Taking Strategy: The options are divided visually into hemodynamic measurements and effect on heart rate. Usually if there is a cardiac problem, hemodynamic measurements are high (not low), so falling values for central venous pressure and pulmonary capillary wedge pressure would be considered good effects. Because the medication is a beta-adrenergic stimulant, you may reason that the adverse effect you are looking for would be tachycardia. If you had difficulty with this question, review this medication now!

Level of Cognitive Ability: Application
Phase of Nursing Process: Assessment
Client Needs: Physiological Integrity
Content Area: Pharmacology

Reference

Deglin, J., & Vallerand, A. (1997). *Davis's drug guide for nurses* (5th ed.). Philadelphia: F. A. Davis, pp. 408–409.

---

264. The nurse is caring for a client with Alzheimer's disease who is receiving tacrine (Cognex), 20 mg PO QID. Which of the following would indicate to the nurse that the client is experiencing an adverse reaction to the medication?

1. Hypertension
2. Fever
3. Increased salivation
4. Difficulty voiding

Answer: 3

Rationale: Tacrine (Cognex) is a cholinergic agent. Frequent side effects include nausea, vomiting, diarrhea, dizziness, and headache. Overdosage of this medication can cause cholinergic crises, manifested by increased salivation, lacrimation, urination, defecation, bradycardia, hypotension, and increased muscle weakness.

Test-Taking Strategy: Knowledge about tacrine (Cognex) is necessary to answer this question. If you can remember that this medication is a cholinergic agent, it will assist you in identifying that an overdose will cause cholinergic symptoms. Review cholinergic symptoms and this medication now if you had difficulty with this question!

Level of Cognitive Ability: Analysis
Phase of Nursing Process: Assessment
Client Needs: Physiological Integrity
Content Area: Pharmacology

Reference

Hodgson, B., & Kizior, R. (1998). *Saunders nursing drug handbook 1998.* Philadelphia: W. B. Saunders, pp. 958–959.

---

265. The nurse is caring for a client with a diagnosis of metastatic breast carcinoma. The client is receiving tamoxifen citrate (Nolvadex), 10 mg PO BID. Which of the following would indicate to the nurse that the client is experiencing a side effect related to the medication?

1. Hypertension
2. Diarrhea
3. Nose bleeds
4. Vaginal bleeding

Answer: 4

Rationale: Tamoxifen citrate (Nolvadex) is an antineoplastic medication that competes with estradiol for binding to estrogen in tissues containing high concentration of receptors in the breasts, uterus, and vagina. Frequent side effects include hot flashes, nausea, vomiting, vaginal bleeding or discharge, pruritus vulvae, and rash. Adverse or toxic reactions include retinopathy, corneal opacity, and decreased visual acuity.

Test-Taking Strategy: Knowledge about tamoxifen citrate (Nolvadex) is necessary to answer this question. A strategy to answering this question is the relationship of the client's condition, metastatic breast carcinoma, to vaginal bleeding. The breast and vagina are organs of reproduction. If you had difficulty with this question, take the time now to review this medication!

Level of Cognitive Ability: Analysis
Phase of Nursing Process: Assessment
Client Needs: Physiological Integrity
Content Area: Pharmacology

Reference

Hodgson, B., & Kizior, R. (1998). *Saunders nursing drug handbook 1998.* Philadelphia: W. B. Saunders, p. 962.

---

266. The nurse is watching the cardiac monitor and notices that the rhythm suddenly changes. There are no P waves, the QRS complexes are wide, and the ventricular rate is regular but over 100. The nurse assesses that the client is experiencing

1 Premature ventricular contractions (PVCs).
2 Ventricular tachycardia.
3 Ventricular fibrillation.
4 Sinus tachycardia.

Answer: 2

Rationale: Ventricular tachycardia is characterized by absence of P waves, wide QRS complex (usually greater than 0.14 second), and a rate between 100 and 250 impulses per minute. The rhythm usually is fairly regular.

Test-Taking Strategy: Knowing that P waves are absent with ventricular tachycardia will assist you to answer the question. Eliminate option 4 first because the case of the question states that there are no P waves. PVCs are isolated ectopic beats superimposed on an underlying rhythm, so option 1 is eliminated next. There are no true QRS complexes with ventricular fibrillation, which limits your choice to ventricular tachycardia. If you had difficulty with this question, review the characteristics of ventricular tachycardia now!

Level of Cognitive Ability: Analysis
Phase of Nursing Process: Assessment
Client Needs: Physiological Integrity
Content Area: Adult Health/Cardiovascular

Reference

Ignatavicius, D. D., Workman, M. L., & Mishler, M. A. (1995). *Medical-surgical nursing: A nursing process approach* (2nd ed., Vol. 1). Philadelphia: W. B. Saunders, p. 851.

---

267. Which of these organs would be most important to assess for a client who is to start receiving lithium carbonate (Lithobid)?

1 Kidneys
2 Liver
3 Lungs
4 Brain

Answer: 1

Rationale: Before the initiation of lithium treatment, kidney function tests need to be completed, because 95% of the lithium is eliminated through the kidneys. The liver does absorb some of the medication, but the percentage of lithium eliminated through the kidneys is larger. The function of the lungs and brain would not be a priority concern before starting lithium therapy.

Test-Taking Strategy: Knowledge related to the action of the medication is necessary to answer this question. Because the liver and kidneys routinely absorb medications, the test taker would have to know that the elimination of the lithium is mainly through the kidneys. The brain is affected in bipolar disorders but is not a priority in pretreatment for starting lithium. The lungs are an organ but not a priority in this situation. If you had difficulty with this question, be sure to take the time now to review lithium carbonate!

Level of Cognitive Ability: Application
Phase of Nursing Process: Assessment
Client Needs: Physiological Integrity
Content Area: Pharmacology

Reference

Townsend, M. (1996). *Psychiatric mental health nursing: Concepts of Care* (2nd ed.). Philadelphia: F. A. Davis, p. 274.

268. The nurse notes that a client with sinus rhythm has a premature ventricular contraction (PVC) that falls on the T wave of the preceding beat. The client's rhythm suddenly changes to one with no P waves or definable QRS complexes. Instead there are coarse wavy lines of varying amplitude. The nurse assesses this rhythm to be

1 Ventricular tachycardia.
2 Ventricular fibrillation.
3 Atrial fibrillation.
4 Asystole.

Answer: 2

Rationale: Ventricular fibrillation is characterized by irregular, chaotic undulations of varying amplitudes. There is no measurable rate, no visible P waves, and no QRS complexes. It results from electrical chaos in the ventricles.

Test-Taking Strategy: Use the process of elimination to answer the question. The lack of visible QRS complexes eliminates atrial fibrillation and ventricular tachycardia. Asystole is lack of any electrical activity of the heart, which leaves ventricular fibrillation by the process of elimination. If you had difficulty with this question, review the characteristics of ventricular fibrillation now!

Level of Cognitive Ability: Analysis
Phase of Nursing Process: Assessment
Client Needs: Physiological Integrity
Content Area: Adult Health/Cardiovascular

Reference

Ignatavicius, D. D., Workman, M. L., & Mishler, M. A. (1995). *Medical-surgical nursing: A nursing process approach* (2nd ed., Vol. 1). Philadelphia: W. B. Saunders, p. 852.

269. The nurse is caring for a client with a fungal disease of the nails caused by dermatophytes. The client is receiving terbinafine hydrochloride (Lamisil), 250 mg PO daily. Which of the following would indicate to the nurse that the client is experiencing a side effect related to the medication?

1 Constipation
2 Fever
3 Headache
4 Tingling of the extremities

Answer: 3

Rationale: Terbinafine hydrochloride (Lamisil) is an antifungal medication. A frequent side effect of the medication is headache. Occasional side effects include diarrhea, rash, dyspepsia, pruritus, taste disturbances, and nausea. Abdominal pain, flatulence, urticaria, and visual disturbances can occur but are rare.

Test-Taking Strategy: Knowledge about terbinafine hydrochloride (Lamisil) is necessary to answer this question. Other antifungal medications such as terconazole (Terazol), which is administered intravaginally, can also cause a headache. If you had difficulty with this question, stop now and review antifungal medications!

Level of Cognitive Ability: Analysis
Phase of Nursing Process: Assessment
Client Needs: Physiological Integrity
Content Area: Pharmacology

Reference

Hodgson, B., & Kizior, R. (1998). *Saunders nursing drug handbook 1998.* Philadelphia: W. B. Saunders, p. 968.

270. Which of the following assessments indicates the presence of an inguinal hernia in a child?

1 Painless inguinal swelling that appears when the child cries or strains
2 Difficulty in defecating
3 A dribbling stream, indicating an obstruction in the flow of urine
4 Absence of testes within the scrotum

Answer: 1

Rationale: Inguinal hernia is a common defect that appears as a painless inguinal swelling when the infant cries or strains. Option 2 is a symptom indicating obstruction of the herniated loop of intestine that may be partially obstructed. Option 3 describes a sign of phimosis, a narrowing or stenosis of the preputial opening of the foreskin. Option 4 describes cryptorchidism.

Test-Taking Strategy: If you do not know the answer, look for a similar word or phrase used in the stem and in one of the options. Option 1 uses the term "inguinal" (also found in the question) and thus is a good clue that this option is the correct answer. Review the characteristics related to inguinal hernia now if you had difficulty with this question!

Level of Cognitive Ability: Application
Phase of Nursing Process: Assessment
Client Needs: Physiological Integrity
Content Area: Child Health

Reference

Wong, D. (1995). *Whaley and Wong's nursing care of infants and children* (5th ed.). St. Louis: Mosby–Year Book, pp. 492–495.

---

271. A client who has been raped arrives at the emergency room. Which of these observations would be most important for a nurse to consider when planning the immediate care for the client?

1 The victim states she "is numb and feels like it didn't happen."
2 The victim states her last period was 2 weeks ago.
3 The victim states the rapist knows where she lives and has stated, "He will kill me if I tell anyone about the rape."
4 The victim states she knows the rapist well; in fact, they had been dating for several weeks.

Answer: 3

Rationale: The priority statement by the victim is that the rapist will kill her. To provide for her safety is the primary concern for the nurse. The victim who states that she is "numb and feels like it didn't happen" is most likely in the denial stage, and this can be a helpful defense mechanism. The victim who stated that her last period was 2 weeks ago could be concerned about pregnancy, and this is a very real concern for the rape victim. The fact that the rapist and the victim knew each other is a common phenomenon; in most situations of abuse, the victim does know the rapist.

Test-Taking Strategy: All of the distractors could occur after a rape; however, the safety of the client is the priority item. Option 3 presents the issue regarding safety. If you had difficulty with this question, review the data associated with rape victims now!

Level of Cognitive Ability: Analysis
Phase of Nursing Process: Assessment
Client Needs: Physiological Integrity
Content Area: Mental Health

Reference

Varcarolis, E. (1998). *Foundations of psychiatric mental health nursing* (3rd ed.). Philadelphia: W. B. Saunders, p. 424.

---

272. The nurse is caring for a client with a diagnosis of congestive heart failure (CHF). The client is receiving triamterene (Dyrenium), 100 mg PO daily. Which of the following would indicate to the nurse that the client is experiencing an adverse reaction to the medication?

1 Hypokalemia
2 Hyperkalemia
3 Constipation
4 Dry skin

Answer: 2

Rationale: Triamterene (Dyrenium) is a potassium-sparing diuretic. Side effects include frequent urination and polyuria. Occasional side effects include tiredness, nausea, diarrhea, abdominal distress, leg aches, and headache. An adverse reaction or toxic effect is severe hyperkalemia, which may produce irritability, anxiety, heaviness of the legs, paresthesia, hypotension, bradycardia, tented T waves, widening QRS complexes, and ST depression. Although the concern with most diuretics is hypokalemia, this medication is potassium-sparing, which means that the concern with the administration of this medication is hyperkalemia.

Test-Taking Strategy: Knowledge about triamterene (Dyrenium) is necessary to answer the question. This medication is a potassium-sparing diuretic. Most of the diuretics produce hypokalemia; however, the potassium-sparing diuretics cause hyperkalemia. If you had difficulty with this question, take the time now to review the medications in the classification of potassium-sparing diuretics.

Level of Cognitive Ability: Analysis
Phase of Nursing Process: Assessment
Client Needs: Physiological Integrity
Content Area: Pharmacology

Reference

Hodgson, B., & Kizior, R. (1998). *Saunders nursing drug handbook 1998.* Philadelphia: W. B. Saunders, p. 1022.

273. Which psychosocial manifestation should the nurse assess in a new mother whose infant has HIV/AIDS?

1 Reactions of extended family to the AIDS diagnosis
2 Quality of the relationship with other children
3 Degree of parental acceptance of the imperfect child
4 Cause of the mother's fears

Answer: 4

Rationale: The parents of HIV-positive/AIDS infants demonstrate many fears. Assessment of the specific cause of parents' fears (lack of knowledge, loss of ability to breastfeed, financial fears regarding cost of HIV/AIDS treatments, and so forth) can help the nurse plan high-quality care for the family.

Test-Taking Strategy: Use the process of elimination to answer the question. Options 1 and 2 are similar; therefore, eliminate these options. Note the client of the question. The client is the new mother. This will assist in eliminating option 3. In addition, remember that the client's feelings come first!

Level of Cognitive Ability: Application
Phase of Nursing Process: Assessment
Client Needs: Psychosocial Integrity
Content Area: Maternity

Reference

Olds, S., London, M., & Ladewig, P. (1996). *Clinical handbook for maternal-newborn nursing: A family-centered approach* (5th ed.). Menlo Park, CA:, Addison-Wesley, pp. 194–195.

274. The nurse is reviewing the results of the maternal antenatal screening tests ordered for a client. Which of the following tests will provide information regarding the potential for the development of fetal or newborn erythroblastosis fetalis?

1 Hemoglobin and hematocrit levels
2 ABO and Rh blood types with antibody screening
3 Diabetic screening results
4 Alpha-fetoprotein (AFP) levels

Answer: 2

Rationale: Erythroblastosis fetalis is a hemolytic disease of the fetus or newborn that results in excessive destruction of red blood cells (RBCs) and stimulation of immature erythrocytes. It occurs in the majority of cases as a result of blood type (ABO) incompatibilities or the failure to prevent maternal production of Rh antibodies. All pregnant women should be tested for Rh types and ABO groups and should be screened for antibodies to these and other RBC antigens during the antenatal period.

Test-Taking Strategy: By applying knowledge of the purpose of maternal antenatal screening tests, you will find that there is only one correct answer (option 2). Hemoglobin and hematocrit levels measure maternal parameters only. The diabetic screening test assists in the identification of the gestational diabetic mother, and the AFP test screens for the potential of fetal neural tube defects or genetic abnormality (e.g., trisomy 21).

Level of Cognitive Ability: Analysis
Phase of Nursing Process: Assessment
Client Needs: Physiological Integrity
Content Area: Maternity

Reference

Reeder, S., Martin, L., & Koniak-Griffin, D. (1997). *Maternity nursing: Family, newborn, and women's health care* (18th ed.). Philadelphia: Lippincott-Raven, pp. 1081–1082.

275. Which of these actions would be most significant when assessing a client who has depression?

1 Sleeping for 12 hours every day and still complaining about being tired in the day
2 Getting their "old personality back" and being spontaneous and up-lifted after being described as "moody"
3 Requesting to call their significant other who is supportive when they "feel like this"
4 Drinking a glass of wine about twice a week with dinner

Answer: 2

Rationale: The depressed individual who has a sudden mood elevation after a period of being down is identified as at risk to carry out a suicide intent.

Test-Taking Strategy: Use the process of elimination to answer this question. Review the manifestations related to suicide risk now if you had difficulty with this question!

Level of Cognitive Ability: Application
Phase of Nursing Process: Assessment
Client Needs: Psychosocial Integrity
Content Area: Mental Health

Reference

Townsend, M. (1996). *Psychiatric mental health nursing: Concepts of care* (2nd ed.). Philadelphia: F. A. Davis, p. 252.

276. The nurse is caring for an elderly client receiving trimethobenzamide hydrochloride (Tigan) for vomiting. Which of the following would indicate to the nurse that the client is experiencing a side effect related to the medication?

1 Constipation
2 Mental confusion
3 Poor skin turgor
4 Hypertension

Answer: 2

Rationale: Trimethobenzamide hydrochloride (Tigan) is an antiemetic. Elderly clients tend to develop mental confusion, disorientation, agitation, and psychotic-like symptoms. Frequent side effects include drowsiness; dizziness; muscular weakness; dry mouth, nose, throat, and lips; urinary retention; and thickening of bronchial secretions. Sedation, dizziness, and hypotension are more likely to be noted in the elderly.

Test-Taking Strategy: Knowledge regarding trimethobenzamide hydrochloride (Tigan) and the physiological responses of elderly clients to medications is necessary to answer this question. Use the process of elimination to select the correct option. Read all of the responses. Remember that confusion is a concern with elderly clients. Also, note that option 2, mental confusion, is the only option that is directly related to neurological orientation, making this option different from the other options. If you had difficulty with this question, take the time now to review this medication and physiological changes that occur in the elderly.

Level of Cognitive Ability: Analysis
Phase of Nursing Process: Assessment
Client Needs: Physiological Integrity
Content Area: Pharmacology

Reference

Hodgson, B., & Kizior, R. (1998). *Saunders nursing drug handbook 1998.* Philadelphia: W. B. Saunders, p. 1030.

277. The nurse is caring for a client with acute pulmonary emboli who is receiving urokinase (Abbokinase) by intravenous infusion via pump. Which of the following would indicate to the nurse that the client is experiencing an adverse reaction to the medication?

1 Positive peripheral pulses
2 Bradycardia
3 Hypertension
4 Abdominal pain

Answer: 4

Rationale: Urokinase (Abbokinase) is a thrombolytic medication that acts directly on the fibrinolytic system to convert plasminogen to plasmin, an enzyme that degrades fibrin clots, fibrinogen, and other plasma proteins. The nurse needs to monitor the client for bleeding during the administration of this medication. Severe internal hemorrhage can occur as an adverse reaction to the medication. Signs of bleeding or internal hemorrhage would include a drop in blood pressure, a rise in pulse, or client's complaints of abdominal or back pain. Positive peripheral pulses are a normal finding.

Test-Taking Strategy: Knowledge regarding urokinase (Abbokinase) is necessary to answer this question. If you know that this medication is a thrombolytic medication, then you will recall that bleeding is a concern. Use the process of elimination to select the correct option. Option 1 is a normal finding. Options 2 and 3 are not signs of shock.

This leaves option 4 as the only correct response. If a client is bleeding internally, the client will complain of back or abdominal pain. If you had difficulty with this question, take the time now to review this medication and the signs of shock!

Level of Cognitive Ability: Analysis
Phase of Nursing Process: Assessment
Client Needs: Physiological Integrity
Content Area: Pharmacology

Reference

Hodgson, B., & Kizior, R. (1998). *Saunders nursing drug handbook 1998.* Philadelphia: W. B. Saunders, pp. 1035–1036.

---

278. A client with non–insulin-dependent diabetes mellitus (NIDDM) has a glycosylated hemoglobin of 7%. The nurse would deduce that the client's glyburide (Micronase) dosage was

1 Keeping the client in an acceptable range of control.
2 Too low.
3 Too high.
4 Inappropriate; this client needs to be managed with a different medication.

Answer: 1

Rationale: Glycosylated hemoglobin values of less than or equal to 8% are acceptable.

Test-Taking Strategy: Knowledge of the indications for the medication and the normal laboratory value is needed to answer this question correctly. If you had difficulty with this question, take the time now to review this medication and the laboratory test!

Level of Cognitive Ability: Analysis
Phase of Nursing Process: Assessment
Client Needs: Physiological Integrity
Content Area: Adult Health/Endocrine

Reference

Chernecky, C., & Berger, B. (1997). *Laboratory tests and diagnostic procedures* (2nd ed.). Philadelphia; W. B. Saunders, p. 576.

---

279. A client who is being treated for secondary hyperaldosteronism should be asked which of the following questions to assess his or her ability to manage this disease?

1 "How long have you been a cigarette smoker?"
2 "Tell me how you manage your cirrhosis."
3 "Did you ever have gastrointestinal disease in the past?"
4 "Tell me what you do when you are under stress."

Answer: 2

Rationale: Secondary hyperaldosteronism is caused by continuous secretion of aldosterone secondary to high levels of angiotensin II, resulting, in turn, from high plasma renin activity. The risk factors for secondary hyperaldosteronism include chronic heart failure, cirrhosis with ascites, nephrotic syndrome, and hypertension resulting from destructive renal artery disease. The preventive measures, therefore, are successful treatment and control of the causative disease process. The more successfully these factors are controlled, the less secondary hyperaldosteronism will be present.

Test-Taking Strategy: To answer this question, you must apply your knowledge of causes for secondary aldosteronism to the situation. The term "secondary" in the stem should lead you to realize that this disorder is caused by another underlying pathological state. Options 2 and 3 are the only options that identify another disorder. Option 3 asks whether there is a history of gastrointestinal disease, whereas option 2 identifies a current situation. This should direct you to the correct answer, which is option 2. Review secondary hyperaldosteronism now if you had difficulty with this question!

Level of Cognitive Ability: Application
Phase of Nursing Process: Assessment
Client Needs: Psychosocial Integrity
Content Area: Adult Health/Endocrine

Reference

Black, J. M., & Matassarin-Jacobs, E. (1997). *Medical-surgical nursing: Clinical management for continuity of care* (5th ed.). Philadelphia: W. B. Saunders, p. 2055.

280. The nurse is caring for a client with petit mal seizures. The client is receiving valproic acid (Depakene), 250 mg PO daily. Which of the following would indicate to the nurse that the client is experiencing an adverse reaction to the medication?

1 Photophobia
2 Poor skin turgor
3 Lethargy
4 Visual disturbances

Answer: 3

Rationale: Valproic acid (Depakene) is an anticonvulsant. An adverse reaction is hepatotoxicity that may not be preceded by abnormal results of liver function tests but may be noted as loss of seizure control, malaise, weakness, lethargy, anorexia, and vomiting. Blood dyscrasias may also occur. Frequent side effects include nausea, vomiting, and indigestion.

Test-Taking Strategy: Knowledge regarding valproic acid (Depakene) is necessary to answer this question. Read the options carefully and use the process of elimination to select an answer. Note that options 1 and 4 are similar in that both relate to a visual problem. Of options 2 and 3, the best selection is option 3 because it reflects a relationship to the client's diagnosis of a neurological disorder, petit mal seizures. If you had difficulty with this question, take the time now to review this medication!

Level of Cognitive Ability: Analysis
Phase of Nursing Process: Assessment
Client Needs: Physiological Integrity
Content Area: Pharmacology

Reference
Hodgson, B., & Kizior, R. (1998). *Saunders nursing drug handbook 1998.* Philadelphia: W. B. Saunders, pp. 1039–1040.

281. All of the following assessment data were collected from a female client scheduled to undergo an adrenalectomy to treat Cushing's syndrome caused by an adrenal tumor. The nurse assessing the client would expect to note which of the following abnormal data?

1 Hirsutism
2 Hypotension
3 Hypoglycemia
4 Pallor

Answer: 1

Rationale: Increased production of androgens that accompanies a rise in cortisol levels with Cushing's syndrome produces hirsutism and acne in women. Other clinical findings of Cushing's syndrome include hypertension, caused by sodium retention; impaired glucose tolerance or diabetes mellitus, caused by cortisol's anti-insulin effect and ability to enhance gluconeogenesis; and skin changes, including bruising and purplish-red striae, caused by protein catabolism.

Test-Taking Strategy: This question asks you to identify an abnormal assessment data that is indicative of Cushing's syndrome. In both options 2 and 3, a similarity exists in the sense of hypotension and hypoglycemia, which may assist in eliminating these two options. For the remaining options, noting that the question addresses a female client will assist in directing you to option 1. If you had difficulty with this question, take time now to review Cushing's syndrome.

Level of Cognitive Ability: Application
Phase of Nursing Process: Assessment
Client Needs: Physiological Integrity
Content Area: Adult Health/Endocrine

Reference
Burrell, L. O., Gerlach, M. J., & Pless, B. (1997). *Adult nursing: Acute and community care* (2nd ed.). Stamford, CT: Appleton & Lange, p. 1103.

282. The nurse assessing a newborn with congenital hypothyroidism would expect to note

1 Excessive sleepiness.
2 Hypertonic reflexes.
3 Moist skin.
4 Frequent, loose stools.

Answer: 1

Rationale: Signs and symptoms of hypothyroidism may be nonspecific and may include feeding difficulty, prolonged jaundice, respiratory problems, hypotonia, constipation, large posterior fontanel, excess sleep, large tongue, rare crying, umbilical hernia, dry and mottled skin, and slow relaxation of deep tendon reflexes.

Test-Taking Strategy: This question asks you to identify assessment variables that indicate hypothyroidism in a newborn. Knowing that the physiological action of thyroid hormone is the metabolic regulator, you should be able to pick out excessive sleepiness as a consequence of a deficient supply of thyroid hormone. If you had difficulty with this question, review hypothyroidism now!

Level of Cognitive Ability: Analysis
Phase of Nursing Process: Assessment
Client Needs: Physiological Integrity
Content Area: Maternity

Reference

Fox, J. (1997). *Primary health care of children.* Philadelphia: Mosby–Year Book, p. 756.

---

283. The nurse is admitting a client with a medical diagnosis of Addison's disease. Which of these statements if made by the client should be included in the nursing admission notes as a manifestation of this medical condition?

1 "My ankles are swollen most of the time."
2 "I have noted an increase in facial hair."
3 "My blood sugar is lower than normal."
4 "I have episodes of high blood pressure."

Answer: 3

Rationale: Blood glucose levels are low in Addison's disease, as a result of decreased secretion of glucocorticoids (cortisol). Edema is absent and aldosterone secretion is decreased, and so fluid volume deficit develops. Facial hair increases with adrenocortical hyperfunction (Cushing's syndrome). In clients with Addison's disease, hypotension develops as a result of fluid volume deficit.

Test-Taking Strategy: Knowledge of the differences between adrenocortical hyperfunction (Cushing's syndrome) and adrenocortical hypofunction (Addison's disease) is necessary to assist you in answering this question. With C*u*shing's, think "up," or hyperfunction, and with A*d*dison's, think "down," or hypofunction. You must also use your knowledge of the action of cortisol, aldosterone, and sex steroids. Use a blank piece of paper and list the signs and symptoms of hypofunction and hyperfunction of the adrenocortical hormones now to assist in remembering the differences.

Level of Cognitive Ability: Application
Phase of Nursing Process: Assessment
Client Needs: Physiological Integrity
Content Area: Adult Health/Endocrine

Reference

LeMone, P., & Burke, K. (1996). *Medical-surgical nursing: Critical thinking in client care.* Menlo Park, CA: Addison-Wesley, pp. 691, 696.

---

284. The nurse is leading a support group for Alzheimer's disease and related disorders. A participant is worried that his mother may not be taking in sufficient food and water. The nurse correctly assesses the son's understanding of nutritional level when the nurse

1 Asks how much food and fluid the mother is offered during each 24-hour period.
2 Suggests that the son offer his mother small, frequent feedings.
3 Suggests that the son feed his mother and make her clean her plate.
4 Asks the son to weigh his mother tomorrow morning and weekly.

Answer: 4

Rationale: The most reliable information can be obtained by obtaining a baseline weight and weekly weights thereafter. Option 1 is not a reliable assessment because it does not measure how much of the offered food and fluid is ingested. Option 2 may be helpful, but offers of food are no guarantee that she will eat. Option 3 is partially correct; feeding her may be necessary, but forcing her to eat everything makes the situation very stressful and can actually increase the behavior problem.

Test-Taking Strategy: Use the process of elimination and focus on the issue. Option 4 is the only option that is specific, measurable, and directly related to the issue. Remember that the most accurate measure of nutritional status is weight!

Level of Cognitive Ability: Application
Phase of Nursing Process: Assessment
Client Needs: Physiological Integrity
Content Area: Fundamental Skills

Reference

Gorman, L., Sultan, D., & Raines, M. (1996). *Davis's Manual of psychosocial nursing for general patient care.* Philadelphia: F. A. Davis, p. 202.

285. A manic client is placed in seclusion after overturning two tables and throwing a chair against the wall. The most important nursing assessment of the situation would be to

1 Inspect the client for injuries resulting from the incident and initiate appropriate treatment.
2 Document the behavior leading to seclusion.
3 Document the time the client is placed in and released from seclusion.
4 Make sure that there is a written order by the physician allowing for the seclusion.

Answer: 1

Rationale: The primary concern of the nurse should be to ascertain that the client is injury free or to attend to any injuries that may have resulted. Options 2, 3, and 4 are all important tasks for the nurse, but they do not refer to assessment activities.

Test-Taking Strategy: To answer this question, it is necessary to remember Maslow's hierarchy of needs. If a physiological need does not exist, then safety is the most urgent need. In addition, assessment is the first step in the nursing process. Select an assessment option, which is option 1.

Level of Cognitive Ability: Application
Phase of Nursing Process: Assessment
Client Needs: Physiological Integrity
Content Area: Mental Health

Reference

Varcarolis, E. (1998). *Foundations of psychiatric mental health nursing* (3rd ed.). Philadelphia: W. B. Saunders, pp. 611–612.

---

286. A hospitalized adolescent client is angry with the nurse when he or she cannot participate in an activity in the gym because he or she has not successfully achieved level three of the behavior modification program. The client punches the wall and fractures a wrist. The nurse recognizes that the client is using which of the following defense mechanisms?

1 Denial
2 Regression
3 Displacement
4 Reaction formation

Answer: 3

Rationale: In displacement, a client transfers an emotion from its original object to a substitute object. Option 1 would be exemplified when a client denies the existence of some external reality. Option 2 refers to the return to an earlier, more comfortable time in life. Option 4 occurs when a client acts in a way that is the opposite of how he or she feels.

Test-Taking Strategy: The issue of the question is the specific subject content that the question is asking about. In this case, the question is asking about the specific defense mechanism that the client is displaying by the described behavior. If you are unfamiliar with defense mechanisms, review them now!

Level of Cognitive Ability: Analysis
Phase of Nursing Process: Assessment
Client Needs: Physiological Integrity
Content Area: Mental Health

Reference

Townsend, M. (1996). *Psychiatric mental health nursing: Concepts of care.* Philadelphia: F. A. Davis, p. 23.

---

287. In the role of caregiver, the nurse's primary responsibility is to assess the client's ability to

1 Restore emotional and social well-being.
2 Decide the best approach(s) for action.
3 Take steps to prevent injury.
4 Protect human rights.

Answer: 1

Rationale: A primary responsibility of the role as a caregiver is to assess the client's ability to restore social and emotional well-being.

Test-Taking Strategy: Key words in stem are "caregiver" and "assess." Understanding the various roles of a registered nurse is necessary to answer this question. Options 2, 3, and 4 address the nurse's role as a client advocate. Review the roles and responsibilities of the nurse now if you had difficulty with this question!

Level of Cognitive Ability: Application
Phase of Nursing Process: Assessment
Client Needs: Physiological Integrity
Content Area: Fundamental Skills

Reference

Black, J. M., & Matassarin-Jacobs, E. (1997). *Medical-surgical nursing: Clinical management for continuity of care* (5th ed.). Philadelphia: W. B. Saunders, p. 123.

288. A staff nurse has become critical of the unit manager's leadership style. Which assessment by the unit manager would be most appropriate and lead to a democratic resolution?

1 Tell the staff nurse to stop the criticism
2 Propose a tentative solution and discuss it with the staff nurse
3 Invite the staff nurse to discuss the problem and be involved with a solution
4 Persuade the staff nurse to stop being critical and promise better working hours

Answer: 3

Rationale: "Democratic" is the key word of stem. Consulting is the most democratic style, by allowing the staff nurse to be involved from the beginning.

Test-Taking Strategy: Use the process of elimination to select the correct option. Knowledge of the leadership styles is necessary to answer this question. A democratic style allows the individual or group to become involved. Review leadership styles now if you had difficulty with this question!

Level of Cognitive Ability: Application
Phase of Nursing Process: Assessment
Client Needs: Psychosocial Integrity
Content Area: Fundamental Skills

Reference
Potter, P. A., & Perry, A. G. (1997). *Fundamentals of nursing: Concepts, process, and practice* (4th ed.). St. Louis: Mosby–Year Book, p. 301.

---

289. The nurse is assessing a client who has received a diagnosis of Cushing's syndrome. When doing the initial physical assessment, it is essential that the nurse assess for

1 Fluid retention
2 Stretch marks
3 Goiter
4 Melanosis

Answer: 1

Rationale: Excessive secretion of adrenocortical hormones results in water and sodium reabsorption, causing fluid retention. Stretch marks (striae) are a common feature and can result in body image disturbance, but they do not represent a life-threatening situation. Goiter is not a manifestation of Cushing's syndrome. Melanosis is a common sign of Addison's disease.

Test-Taking Strategy: The key word "essential" in the stem indicates the need to prioritize. Options 1 and 2 are manifestations of Cushing's syndrome. However, stretch marks are not life-threatening; therefore, fluid retention should be assessed first. Review the characteristics associated with Cushing's syndrome now if you had difficulty with this question!

Level of Cognitive Ability: Application
Phase of Nursing Process: Assessment
Client Needs: Physiological Integrity
Content Area: Adult Health/Endocrine

Reference
LeMone, P., & Burke, K. (1996). *Medical-surgical nursing: Critical thinking in client care.* Menlo Park, CA: Addison-Wesley, pp. 693, 694.

---

290. When assessing a client who has hypothyroidism, a nurse would expect to identify which of these clinical manifestations?

1 Difficulty sleeping
2 Presence of diarrhea
3 Significant weight loss
4 Intolerance to cold weather

Answer: 4

Rationale: An insufficient level of thyroid hormone causes a decrease in metabolic rate and heat production. Options 1, 2, and 3 are clinical manifestations of hyperthyroidism.

Test-Taking Strategy: Knowledge of the differences between hypothyroidism and hyperthyroidism will assist you in answering this question. You must also use your knowledge of the action of the thyroid hormone. Review the signs and symptoms of hypothyroidism and hyperthyroidism now if you had difficulty with this question!

Level of Cognitive Ability: Analysis
Phase of Nursing Process: Assessment
Client Needs: Physiological Integrity
Content Area: Adult Health/Endocrine

Reference
LeMone, P., & Burke, K. (1996). *Medical-surgical nursing: Critical thinking in client care.* Menlo Park, CA: Addison-Wesley, pp. 673, 682.

291. The client's arterial blood gas measurements are as follows: pH, 7.35; PO_2, 85; PCO_2, 55; HCO_3, 25. The nurse interprets these values as

1 Uncompensated respiratory acidosis.
2 Uncompensated metabolic acidosis.
3 Compensated respiratory acidosis.
4 Compensated metabolic acidosis.

Answer: 3

Rationale: The pH is normal, and therefore compensation has occurred. The O_2 is within normal limits; however, the CO_2 is significantly elevated. The client is hypercapnic. The normal oxygen level is most likely a result of compensatory hyperventilation. The bicarbonate level is normal.

Test-Taking Strategy: Knowledge regarding the interpretation of blood gases is necessary to answer the question. Review the steps of interpreting blood gases now if you had difficulty with this question!

Level of Cognitive Ability: Analysis
Phase of Nursing Process: Assessment
Client Needs: Physiological Integrity
Content Area: Adult Health/Respiratory

Reference

LeMone, P., & Burke, K. (1996). *Medical-surgical nursing: Critical thinking in client care.* Menlo Park, CA: Addison-Wesley, p. 150.

---

292. The nurse is caring for a client with a diagnosis of acute lymphocytic leukemia. The client is receiving asparaginase (Elspar) intravenously. Which of the following would indicate to the nurse that the client is experiencing an adverse reaction related to the medication?

1 White blood cell (WBC) count, 5000/μL
2 Blood urea nitrogen (BUN), 15 mg/dL
3 Platelet count, 200,000 cells/μL
4 Alkaline phosphatase, 25 units/dL

Answer: 4

Rationale: Asparaginase (Elspar) is an antineoplastic medication. Adverse reactions include hepatotoxicity, which usually occurs within 2 weeks of initial treatment. Severe bone marrow depression can also occur, and the risk of allergic reactions can increase after repeated therapy. The normal WBC count is 5000–10,000/μL. The normal platelet count is 150,000–450,000 cells/μL. Normal BUN is 5–20 mg/dL. The normal alkaline phosphatase is 4.5–13 units/dL.

Test-Taking Strategy: Knowledge about asparaginase (Elspar) and normal laboratory values is necessary to answer this question. If you know that this medication is hepatotoxic and that the only abnormal laboratory value presented in the options is the alkaline phosphatase level, by the process of elimination, you would be directed to the correct option. If you had difficulty with this question, take the time now to review this medication!

Level of Cognitive Ability: Analysis
Phase of Nursing Process: Assessment
Client Needs: Physiological Integrity
Content Area: Pharmacology

Reference

Hodgson, B., & Kizior, R. (1998). *Saunders nursing drug handbook 1998.* Philadelphia: W. B. Saunders, pp. 72–74.

---

293. The client is brought to the emergency room after a burn injury. On assessment the nurse notes that the client's eyebrow and nasal hairs are singed. The nurse would identify this type of burn as

1 Thermal.
2 Electrical.
3 Radiation.
4 Chemical.

Answer: 1

Rationale: Exposure to or contact with flames, hot liquids, or hot objects causes thermal burns. Thermal burns are those sustained in residential fires, explosive accidents, scalding, or ignition of clothing or liquids. Chemical burns are caused by tissue contact with strong acids, alkalis, or organic compounds. Electrical burns are caused by heat that is generated by the electrical energy as it passes through the body. Radiation burns are caused by exposure to a radioactive source. If the nurse notes facial burns or singed eyebrow or nasal hairs, the victim likely experienced the burn in an enclosed, smoked-filled space, as in a residential fire.

Test-Taking Strategy: Knowledge about the mechanism of burn injuries is necessary to answer this question. Use the process of elimination in answering the question, considering how each type of burn injury may result in the signs presented in the case of this question. If you had difficulty with this question, review the mechanisms of burn injury now!

Level of Cognitive Ability: Analysis
Phase of Nursing Process: Assessment
Client Needs: Physiological Integrity
Content Area: Adult Health/Integumentary

Reference

Black, J. M., & Matassarin-Jacobs, E. (1997). *Medical-surgical nursing: Clinical management for continuity of care* (5th ed.). Philadelphia: W. B. Saunders, pp. 2233–2237.

---

294. The nurse assesses the carbon monoxide level (COHb) of the client after a burn injury. The nurse notes that the CO_2 level is 8%. Which of the following would the nurse most likely note during the assessment of the client?

1 Tachycardia
2 Tachypnea
3 Coma
4 Impaired visual acuity

Answer: 4

Rationale: Clinical manifestations of carbon monoxide poisoning are related to the levels of COHb saturation. A CO_2 level between 5% and10% would cause impaired visual acuity; between 11% and 20%, flushing and headache; between 21% and 30%, nausea and impaired dexterity; between 31% and 40%, vomiting, dizziness, and syncope; between 41% and 50%, tachypnea and tachycardia; and greater than 50%, coma and death.

Test-Taking Strategy: Knowledge of the clinical manifestations of carbon monoxide poisoning is necessary to answer this question. Use the process of elimination to assist you in answering the question. The nurse would expect, in an uninjured client, that a CO_2 level would be 0%. A CO2 level of 8% is obviously abnormal, but considering the signs presented in the option, select the least serious. If you had difficulty with this question, take time now to review the clinical manifestations associated with carbon monoxide poisoning!

Level of Cognitive Ability: Analysis
Phase of Nursing Process: Assessment
Client Needs: Physiological Integrity
Content Area: Adult Health/Integumentary

Reference

Black, J. M., & Matassarin-Jacobs, E. (1997). *Medical-surgical nursing: Clinical management for continuity of care* (5th ed.). Philadelphia: W. B. Saunders, p. 2237.

---

295. The nurse assesses the burn injury and determines that the client sustained a second-degree burn. Which of the following assessment data would result in the nurse's conclusion?

1 A wet, shiny, weeping wound surface
2 A dry wound surface
3 Charring at the wound site
4 Absence of wound sensation

Answer: 1

Rationale: A second-degree burn appears wet, shiny, and weeping or may contain blisters. The wound blanches with pressure, is painful, and is very sensitive to touch or air currents. Charring would occur in fourth-degree burns. Decreased or absence of wound sensation would occur in third- or fourth-degree burns, respectively.

Test-Taking Strategy: Knowledge of the clinical manifestations associated with the degree of the burn is necessary to answer this question. Use the process of elimination in selecting the correct option. Knowledge that charring, a dry surface, and absence of wound sensation occur in more serious burns would direct you to select option number 1. Review burn injury classification according to the depth of injury now if you had difficulty with this question!

Level of Cognitive Ability: Analysis
Phase of Nursing Process: Assessment
Client Needs: Physiological Integrity
Content Area: Adult Health/Integumentary

Reference

Black, J. M., & Matassarin-Jacobs, E. (1997). *Medical-surgical nursing: Clinical management for continuity of care* (5th ed.). Philadelphia: W. B. Saunders, p. 2239.

296. The nurse assesses the breath sounds of a client with asthma. The nurse documents the assessment data as wheezing located bilaterally. The nurse bases the assessment on the characteristics of wheezing, which include

1 A musical or hissing noise heard on inspiration.
2 A creaking noise heard on inspiration.
3 A grating noise heard on expiration.
4 A rattling or gurgling noise heard on expiration.

Answer: 1

Rationale: A wheeze is a continuous musical or hissing noise that results from the passage of air through a narrowed airway. Wheezes are heard during inspiration or expiration or both. Severe wheezes are audible without a stethoscope. Wheezing is commonly associated with asthma, bronchoconstriction, and edema, but foreign bodies can also cause airway narrowing and wheezing.

Test-Taking Strategy: Knowledge related to adventitious sounds is necessary to answer this question. Correlate wheezing with a musical or hissing noise to assist you in remembering what these sounds would produce. If you had difficulty with this question, take the time now to review adventitious breath sounds!

Level of Cognitive Ability: Analysis
Phase of Nursing Process: Assessment
Client Needs: Physiological Integrity
Content Area: Adult Health/Respiratory

Reference

Black, J. M., & Matassarin-Jacobs, E. (1997). *Medical-surgical nursing: Clinical management for continuity of care* (5th ed.). Philadelphia: W. B. Saunders, p. 1046.

297. The nurse is caring for a client with a tracheostomy tube. The nurse assesses for subcutaneous emphysema, a complication of a tracheotomy. Assessment of this condition is determined by

1 Crackling sounds heard in the upper lobes bilaterally.
2 A puffy and crackling sensation on palpation in the tissues surrounding the tracheotomy site.
3 Signs of respiratory distress.
4 Abnormal skin and mucous membrane color.

Answer: 2

Rationale: Subcutaneous emphysema occurs when air escapes from the tracheotomy incision into the tissues, dissects fascial planes under the skin, and accumulates around the face, neck, and upper chest. These areas appear puffy, and slight finger pressure produces a crackling sound and sensation. In general, this is not a serious condition, because the air will eventually be absorbed.

Test-Taking Strategy: Note the word "subcutaneous" in the case of the question. Correlate this key word with one of the options. The only option that presents a relationship is option 2. Subcutaneous emphysema is also known as *crepitus*. If you had difficulty with this question, take time now to review the signs of subcutaneous emphysema and the complications of a tracheostomy tube.

Level of Cognitive Ability: Analysis
Phase of Nursing Process: Assessment
Client Needs: Physiological Integrity
Content Area: Adult Health/Respiratory

Reference

Black, J. M., & Matassarin-Jacobs, E. (1997). *Medical-surgical nursing: Clinical management for continuity of care* (5th ed.). Philadelphia: W. B. Saunders, p. 1071.

298. The nurse is caring for a client on a ventilator that is set on intermittent mandatory ventilation (IMV). The IMV mode is set at a rate of 8 breaths per minute. The nurse assesses the respiratory rate of the client to be 12 breaths per minute. The nurse documents these assessment findings as

1 The client is "fighting" the ventilator.
2 The client is receiving pressure support ventilation.
3 The client is receiving additional breaths by the ventilator.
4 The client is breathing 4 additional breaths on his or her own.

Answer: 4

Rationale: In the IMV mode, the ventilator delivers a preset number of mechanical breaths. However, it allows the client to breath spontaneously in between with no assistance from the ventilator and at varying tidal volumes. Therefore, if the nurse assesses the respiratory rate to be 12 breaths per minute and the IMV mode is set at 8 breaths per minute, the client is breathing 4 additional breaths on his or her own.

Test-Taking Strategy: Knowledge regarding the modes of ventilation is necessary to answer this question. The term "intermittent mandatory ventilation" may be a clue to assist you in identifying that the mode is preset, allowing the client to breathe spontaneously. If you had difficulty with this question, take time now to review the modes of ventilation!

Level of Cognitive Ability: Analysis
Phase of Nursing Process: Assessment
Client Needs: Physiological Integrity
Content Area: Adult Health/Respiratory

Reference

Black, J. M., & Matassarin-Jacobs, E. (1997). *Medical-surgical nursing: Clinical management for continuity of care* (5th ed.). Philadelphia: W. B. Saunders, p. 1177.

299. The nurse is caring for a client with chronic stable angina receiving amlodipine (Norvasc). Which of the following would indicate to the nurse that the client is experiencing an adverse reaction to the medication?

1 Hypertension
2 Hypotension
3 Constipation
4 Diarrhea

Answer: 2

Rationale: Amlodipine (Norvasc) is a calcium channel blocker. Adverse reactions or toxic effects from overdosage may produce excessive peripheral vasodilation and marked hypotension with reflex tachycardia. Frequent side effects include peripheral edema, headache, and flushing.

Test-Taking Strategy: Knowledge about amlodipine (Norvasc) is necessary to answer this question. If you can remember that this medication is classified as a calcium channel blocker, then by the process of elimination you would be able to select the correct answer. Calcium channel blockers dilate coronary arteries and decrease total peripheral vascular resistance by vasodilation. This will assist you to select option 2, hypotension. If you had difficulty with this question, take the time now to review this medication!

Level of Cognitive Ability: Analysis
Phase of Nursing Process: Assessment
Client Needs: Physiological Integrity
Content Area: Pharmacology

Reference

Hodgson, B., & Kizior, R. (1998). *Saunders nursing drug handbook 1998.* Philadelphia: W. B. Saunders, pp. 51–52.

300. The nurse assesses the breath sounds of a client with pleurisy. The nurse documents the assessment data as a pleural friction rub located in the left lung. The nurse bases the assessment on the characteristics of a pleural friction rub that includes

1 A musical or hissing noise heard on inspiration.
2 A creaking or grating noise heard on inspiration and expiration.
3 Crackles heard during inspiration and expiration.
4 A rattling or gurgling noise heard on expiration.

Answer: 2

Rationale: Pleural friction rubs are the result of pleural inflammation, often associated with pleurisy, pneumonia, or pleural infarct. A rub is described as a creaking, grating noise similar to that made by two pieces of leather rubbing together. A rub is audible on inspiration and expiration over the area of inflammation.

Test-Taking Strategy: Knowledge related to adventitious sounds is necessary to answer this question. Correlate a pleural friction rub with a creaking or grating noise to assist you in remembering what these sounds would produce. If you had difficulty with this question, take the time now to review adventitious breath sounds.

Level of Cognitive Ability: Analysis
Phase of Nursing Process: Assessment
Client Needs: Physiological Integrity
Content Area: Adult Health/Respiratory

Reference
Black, J. M., & Matassarin-Jacobs, E. (1997). *Medical-surgical nursing: Clinical management for continuity of care* (5th ed.). Philadelphia: W. B. Saunders, p. 1046.

REFERENCES

Antai-Otong, D. (1995). *Psychiatric nursing: Biological and behavioral concepts.* Philadelphia: W. B. Saunders.

Ashwill, J. W., & Droske, S. (1997). *Nursing care of children: Principles and practice.* Philadelphia: W. B. Saunders.

Ball, J., & Bindler, R. (1995). *Pediatric nursing: Caring for children.* Stamford, CT: Appleton & Lange.

Bates, B. (1995). *A guide to physical examination and history taking.* Philadelphia: J. B. Lippincott, p. 301.

Black, J. M., & Matassarin-Jacobs, E. (1997). *Medical-surgical nursing: Clinical management for continuity of care* (5th ed.). Philadelphia: W. B. Saunders.

Bolander, V. (1994). *Sorensen and Luckmann's Basic nursing: A psychophysiologic approach* (3rd ed.). Philadelphia: W. B. Saunders.

Brent, N. (1997). *Nurses and the law.* Philadelphia: W. B. Saunders.

Burrell, L. O., Gerlach, M. J., & Pless, B. (1997). *Adult nursing: Acute and community care* (2nd ed.). Stamford, CT: Appleton & Lange.

Carson, V., & Arnold, E. (1996). *Mental health nursing: The nurse-patient journey.* Philadelphia: W. B. Saunders.

Catalano, J. T. (1996). *Contemporary professional nursing.* Philadelphia: F. A. Davis.

Chernecky, C., & Berger, B. (1997). *Laboratory tests and diagnostic procedures* (2nd ed.). Philadelphia; W. B. Saunders.

Como, N. (1995). *Home health nursing pocket consultant.* St. Louis: Mosby–Year Book.

Cox, H., Hinz, M., Lubno, M., et al. (1997). *Clinical applications of nursing diagnosis: Adult, child, women's, psychiatric, gerontic and home health considerations* (3rd ed.). Philadelphia: F. A. Davis.

Craven, R. F., & Hirnle, C. J. (1996). *Fundamentals of nursing: Human health and function* (2nd ed.). Philadelphia: J. B. Lippincott.

Deglin, J., & Vallerand, A. (1997). *Davis's drug guide for nurses* (5th ed.). Philadelphia: F. A. Davis.

Doenges, M. E., Moorhouse, M. F., & Geissler, A. C. (1997). *Nursing care plans: Guidelines for planning and documenting patient care* (4th ed.). Philadelphia: F. A. Davis.

Fortinash, K., & Holoday-Worret, P. (1996). *Psychiatric mental health nursing.* St. Louis: Mosby–Year Book.

Fox, J. (1997). *Primary health care of children.* St. Louis: Mosby–Year Book.

Gillies, D. (1994). *Nursing management: A systems approach.* Philadelphia: W. B. Saunders.

Gorman, L., Sultan, D., & Raines, M. (1996). *Davis's manual of psychosocial nursing for general patient care.* Philadelphia: F. A. Davis.

Haber, J. (1997). *Comprehensive psychiatric nursing* (5th ed.). St. Louis: Mosby–Year Book.

Hartshorn, J., Sole, M. L., & Lamborn, M. L. (1997). *Introduction to critical care nursing* (2nd ed.). Philadelphia: W. B. Saunders.

Hodgson, B., & Kizior, R. (1998). *Saunders nursing drug handbook 1998.* Philadelphia: W. B. Saunders.

Ignatavicius, D. D., Workman, M. L., & Mishler, M. A. (1995). *Medical-surgical nursing: A nursing process approach* (2nd ed., Vols. 1, 2). Philadelphia: W. B. Saunders.

Johnson, B. (1997). *Adaptation and growth: Psychiatric mental health nursing* (4th ed.). Philadelphia: Lippincott-Raven.

Kidd, P., & Wagner, D. (1997). *High acuity nursing* (2nd ed.). Stamford, CT: Appleton & Lange.

Lee, C., Barrett, C., & Ignatavicius, D. (1996). *Fluid and electrolytes: A practical approach* (4th ed.). Philadelphia: F. A. Davis.

Lehne, R. A. (1998). *Pharmacology for nursing care* (3rd ed.). Philadelphia: W. B. Saunders.

LeMone, P., & Burke, K. (1996). *Medical-surgical nursing: Critical thinking in client care.* Menlo Park, CA: Addison-Wesley.

Lewis, S. M., Collier, I. C., & Heitkemper, M. M. (1996). *Medical-surgical nursing: Assessment and management of clinical problems* (4th ed.). St. Louis: Mosby–Year Book.

Lowdermilk, D., Perry, S., & Bobak, I. (1997). *Maternity and women's health care* (6th ed.). St. Louis: Mosby–Year Book.

Luckmann, J. (1997). *Saunders manual of nursing care.* Philadelphia: W. B. Saunders.

May, K. A., & Mahlmeister, L. R. (1994). *Maternal and neonatal family-centered care* (3rd ed.). Philadelphia: J. B. Lippincott.

McFarland, G., & McFarlane, E. (1997). *Nursing diagnosis and intervention* (3rd ed.) St. Louis: Mosby–Year Book.

McKenry, L., & Salerno, E. (1995). *Mosby's pharmacology in nursing* (19th ed.). St. Louis: Mosby–Year Book.

National Council of State Boards of Nursing (Eds.) (1997). *Test plan for the National Council Licensure Examination For Registered Nurses.* Chicago: Author.

Nichols, F., & Zwelling, E. (1997). *Maternal-newborn nursing: Theory and practice.* Philadelphia: W. B. Saunders.

Olds, S., London, M., & Ladewig, P. (1996). *Clinical handbook for maternal-newborn nursing: A family-centered approach* (5th ed.). Menlo Park, CA: Addison-Wesley.

Olds, S., London, M., & Ladewig, P. (1996). *Maternal-newborn nursing: A family-centered approach* (5th ed.). Menlo Park, CA: Addison-Wesley.

Phillips, L. D. (1997). *Manual of IV therapeutics* (2nd ed.). Philadelphia: F. A. Davis.

Phipps, W., Cassmeyer, V., Sands J., et al. (1995). *Medical-surgical nursing: Concepts and clinical practice* (3rd ed.). St. Louis: Mosby–Year Book.

Pillitteri, A. (1995). *Maternal and child health nursing: Care of the*

childbearing and child-rearing family (2nd ed.). Philadelphia: Lippincott-Raven.
Polaski, A., & Tatro, S. (1996). *Luckmann's Core principles and practice of medical-surgical nursing.* Philadelphia: W. B. Saunders.
Potter, P. A., & Perry, A. G. (1997). *Fundamentals of nursing: Concepts, process, and practice* (4th ed.). St. Louis: Mosby–Year Book.
Reeder, S., Martin, L., & Koniak-Griffin, D. (1997). *Maternity nursing: Family, newborn, and women's health care* (18th ed.). Philadelphia: Lippincott-Raven.
Rice, R. (1996). *Home health nursing: Practice, concepts and application* (2nd ed.). St. Louis: Mosby–Year Book.
Ruppert, S., Kernicki, J., & Dolan, J. (1996). *Dolan's critical care nursing: Clinical management through the nursing process* (2nd ed.). Philadelphia: F. A. Davis.
Smeltzer, S., & Bare, B. (1996). *Brunner and Suddarth's Textbook of medical-surgical nursing* (8th ed.). Philadelphia: Lippincott-Raven.
Sullivan, E. J., & Decker, P. J. (1997). *Effective leadership and management in nursing* (4th ed.). Menlo Park, CA: Addison-Wesley.
Tilkian, S. M., Conover, M. B., & Tilkian, A. G. (1995). *Clinical and nursing implications of laboratory tests.* St. Louis: Mosby–Year Book.
Townsend, M. (1996). *Psychiatric mental health nursing: Concepts of care* (2nd ed.). Philadelphia: F. A. Davis.
Varcarolis, E. (1998). *Foundations of psychiatric mental health nursing* (3rd ed.). Philadelphia: W. B. Saunders.
Wilson, B., Shannon, M., & Stang, C. (1997). *Nurses drug guide.* Stamford, CT: Appleton & Lange.
Wilson, H., & Kneisl, C. H. (1996). *Psychiatric nursing* (5th ed.). Menlo Park, CA: Addison-Wesley.
Wong, D. (1995). *Whaley and Wong's Nursing care of infants and children* (5th ed). St. Louis: Mosby–Year Book.
Wong, D. (1997). *Whaley and Wong's Essentials of pediatric nursing* (5th ed.). St. Louis: Mosby–Year Book.
Wong, D., & Perry, S. (1998). *Maternal-child nursing care.* St. Louis: Mosby–Year Book.
Wywialowski, E. F. (1997). *Managing client care* (2nd ed.). St. Louis: Mosby–Year Book.
Zerwekh, J., & Claborn, J. C. (1997). *Nursing today: Transition and trends* (2nd ed.). Philadelphia: W. B. Saunders.
Zang, S., & Bailey, N. (1997). *Home care manual: Making the transition.* Philadelphia: Lippincott-Raven.

CHAPTER 6

The Process of Analysis

Analysis is the second step of the nursing process. In this step, the nurse focuses on the data gathered during the assessment process and identifies actual or potential health care needs, problems, or both.

During this process, the nurse summarizes and interprets the assessment data, organizes and validates the data, and determines the need for additional data. Client assessment data are compared with the normal expected findings and behaviors for the client's age, education, and cultural background. The nurse then draws conclusions regarding the client's unique needs and health care risks or problems.

Client health problems are categorized as potential problems requiring prevention or actual problems being managed or requiring interventions. The nurse reports the results of analysis to relevant members of the health care team and documents the client's unique health care problems, needs, or both.

On the National Council Licensure Examination for Registered Nurses (NCLEX-RN), questions that address the process of analysis are difficult questions because they require an understanding of the principles of physiological responses. These questions require the interpretation of the data based on assessment findings and the formulation of nursing diagnoses. Critical thinking and determining the rationale for therapeutic interventions related to the specific issue addressed in the question are required.

PRACTICE TEST

1. The nurse receives a report that an adult client with delirium has a blood glucose level of 33 mg/dL. The nurse analyzes this report as
   1 Higher than normal, indicating a cause of the delirium.
   2 A normal reading for this client.
   3 A lower than normal reading, indicating a cause for the delirium.
   4 Insignificant and unrelated to the delirium.

Answer: 3

Rationale: Blood glucose levels for an adult normally range between 60 and 120 mg/dL. A blood glucose level of 33 mg/dL indicates hypoglycemia. Metabolic disorders can be an etiological factor of delirium.

Test-Taking Strategy: Knowledge regarding the normal blood level is required to answer the question. Use the process of elimination, and eliminate option 1 (high), option 2 (normal), and option 4 (insignificant). A blood glucose level of 33 mg/dL is certainly significant and indicates a low level or hypoglycemia.

Level of Cognitive Ability: Analysis
Phase of Nursing Process: Analysis
Client Needs: Physiological Integrity
Content Area: Adult Health/Endocrine

Reference

Fishback, F. (1996). *A manual of laboratory and diagnostic tests* (5th ed.). Philadelphia: W. B. Saunders, p. 331.

2. A client who has just been raped is quiet and calm. The nurse would analyze this behavior as indicative of which defense mechanism?

1 Denial
2 Projection
3 Rationalization
4 Intellectualization

Answer: 1

Rationale: Denial is a response by the rape victim. It is described as an adaptive and protective reaction. Projection is blaming or *scapegoating*. Rationalization is justifying the unacceptable attributes about the self. Intellectualization is the excessive use of abstract thinking or generalizations to decrease painful thinking.

Test-Taking Strategy: Knowledge of defense mechanisms is required to answer the question. The key words in the question are "calm" and "quiet." These behaviors are indicative of denial in a rape victim. If you had difficulty with this question, take time now to review content related to the rape victim and defense mechanisms.

Level of Cognitive Ability: Analysis
Phase of Nursing Process: Analysis
Client Needs: Psychosocial Integrity
Content Area: Mental Health

Reference

Varcarolis, E. M. (1998). *Foundations of psychiatric mental health nursing* (3rd ed.). Philadelphia: W. B. Saunders, p. 421.

---

3. After assessment of a child with celiac disease, the nurse analyzes the data and formulates a nursing diagnosis of Altered Nutrition: Less than Body Requirements. Which of the following assessment data would direct the nurse to select this nursing diagnosis?

1 Malodorous stools
2 Muscle wasting in buttocks and extremities
3 Irritability and fretfulness
4 Severe abdominal distention

Answer: 2

Rationale: Option 2 is the only assessment finding that is a specific indicator of altered nutrition. All of the options may be clinical manifestations of celiac disease; however, option 2 is the option that is directly related to altered nutrition.

Test-Taking Strategy: Read the question carefully, noting the nursing diagnosis Altered Nutrition: Less than Body Requirements. Use the process of elimination in selecting the response. This process should assist you in eliminating options 1, 3, and 4. Option 2 is the only option directly related to the nursing diagnosis as stated in the question.

Level of Cognitive Ability: Application
Phase of Nursing Process: Analysis
Client Needs: Physiological Integrity
Content Area: Child Health

Reference

Cox, H., Hinz, M., Lubno, M., et al. (1997). *Clinical applications of nursing diagnosis: Adult, child, women's, psychiatric, gerontic, and home health considerations* (3rd ed.). Philadelphia: F. A. Davis, p. 163.

4. A female client with anorexia nervosa is a member of a predischarge group/support group. The client verbalizes that she would like to buy some new clothes, but her finances are limited. Group members brought some used clothes to the client to replace the client's old clothes. The client believed that the new clothes were much too tight and reduced her calorie intake to 800 calories daily. The nurse analyzes this behavior as

1 Normal behavior.
2 Indicative of the client's ambivalence about hospital discharge.
3 Evidence of the client's altered/distorted body image.
4 Regression as the client is moving toward the community.

Answer: 3

Rationale: Altered/distorted body image is a concern with clients with anorexia nervosa. Although the client may struggle with ambivalence and present with regressed behavior, the client's coping pattern relates to the basic issue of distorted body image. The nurse should address this need in the support group.

Test-Taking Strategy: Read the question carefully. Use the process of elimination to answer the question. The information provided in the question is directly related to an altered body image. This should direct you to the correct option.

Level of Cognitive Ability: Analysis
Phase of Nursing Process: Analysis
Client Needs: Psychosocial Integrity
Content Area: Mental Health

Reference

Stuart, G., & Sundeen, S. (1995). *Principles and practice of psychiatric nursing* (5th ed.). St. Louis: Mosby–Year Book, p. 780.

---

5. The nurse analyzes the assessment data obtained from a client with Parkinson's disease. Which of the following best indicates that the client has a positive Romberg test?

1 Client marches in place
2 Client stands quietly
3 Client sways slightly
4 Client begins to fall

Answer: 4

Rationale: The Romberg test is an assessment for cerebellar functioning related to balance. The client stands with feet together and arms at the side then closes his or her eyes. Slight swaying is normal, but loss of balance indicates a problem and is called a positive Romberg test.

Test-Taking Strategy: A positive Romberg test occurs when the client has a balance problem. A clue in the stem is Parkinson's disease because clients with this disorder often have interferences in balance. In option 1, "marching" can be used to aid a Parkinson's client to start a motion sequence. Additionally, options 2 and 3 do not indicate a concern and do not relate to the Romberg test. Relate the Romberg test to balance. Be sure to monitor and support your client when performing this assessment.

Level of Cognitive Ability: Analysis
Phase of Nursing Process: Analysis
Client Needs: Physiological Integrity
Content Area: Adult Health/Neurological

Reference

Smeltzer, S., & Bare, B. (1996). *Brunner and Suddarth's Textbook of medical-surgical nursing* (8th ed.). Philadelphia: Lippincott-Raven, p. 1691.

6. The nurse is assessing a woman with a diagnosis of amniotic fluid embolus. The woman is 2 hours postpartum. Assessment findings include a blood pressure of 80/50 mmHg, a pulse of 100 beats/minute, bruises at the venipuncture sites, and petechiae in a band around the left mid-deltoid area. The client is saturating an obstetric pad every 10–15 minutes and oozing red serosanguineous fluid from the episiotomy incision. The nurse analyzes that these findings are consistent with

1 Hemorrhage secondary to coagulation failure.
2 Circulatory collapse secondary to right ventricular failure.
3 Pulmonary hypertension secondary to venospasm.
4 Secondary postpartum hemorrhage as a result of uterine atony.

Answer: 1

Rationale: Coagulation failure, particularly disseminated intravascular coagulopathy, is a common result of an amniotic fluid embolus. Manifestations are internal and external hemorrhage clinically determined by bleeding at the site of any trauma (pressure, needle prick, or incision) and petechiae resulting from slight to moderate touch. A postpartum woman who saturates an obstetric sanitary pad in 15 minutes or less is considered to be hemorrhaging, which in this case is caused by lack of coagulation at the placental site.

Test-Taking Strategy: Note the key phrase in the question "amniotic fluid embolism." Read the case situation thoroughly, noting that the case describes hemorrhage. Use the process of elimination to answer the question, and use the key phrases to direct you to the correct option. Eliminate options 2 and 3 because they do not address hemorrhage. Eliminate option 4 because the case situation does not address uterine atony. This leaves option 1 as the correct option. Note that option 1 addresses both hemorrhage and coagulation.

Level of Cognitive Ability: Analysis
Phase of Nursing Process: Analysis
Client Needs: Physiological Integrity
Content Area: Maternity

Reference

Lowdermilk, D., Perry, S., & Bobak, I. (1997). *Maternity and women's health care* (6th ed.). St. Louis: Mosby–Year Book, pp. 445, 792.

---

7. The nurse inserts a nasogastric tube, as prescribed, into the client with a diagnosis of ileus. Which of the following observations is most reliable in determining that the tube is correctly placed?

1 The aspirate is dark green in color
2 The aspirate test is negative for guaiac
3 The tube is inserted the length measured from the client's ear to nose and nose to xiphoid process
4 The pH of the aspirate is 5

Answer: 4

Rationale: After a nurse inserts a nasogastric tube into a client, the correct location of the tube must be verified. The nurse follows the approved procedure for inserting a nasogastric tube, including correct measurement and aspirating fluid with the visible characteristics of gastric fluid. Testing the pH of the gastric fluid and determining its acidity further verify that the tube is in the stomach. The presence of blood (option 2) is unrelated to the location of the tube.

Test-Taking Strategy: Read all four options and reread the stem. Identify the critical elements in the stem of the question, including the key phrase "most reliable." Although options 1 and 3 are true, option 4 is the most exact in determining correct placement of the tube. Option 2 is unrelated to the question. If you had difficulty with this question, take time now to review nasogastric insertion and placement techniques.

Level of Cognitive Ability: Analysis
Phase of Nursing Process: Analysis
Client Needs: Physiological Integrity
Content Area: Adult Health/Gastrointestinal

Reference

Lammon, C. B., Foote, A. W., Leli, P. G., et al. (1995). *Clinical nursing skills.* Philadelphia: W. B. Saunders, pp. 418–422.

8. The client is receiving total parenteral nutrition (TPN). The nurse prepares to call the physician for new TPN orders. Which of the following laboratory results should the nurse analyze and report to the physician when obtaining the new TPN orders?

1 Serum electrolyte levels
2 Arterial blood gas levels
3 Platelet count
4 Differential

Answer: 1

Rationale: TPN solutions contain amino acid and dextrose solutions with electrolytes and trace elements added. The physician uses the electrolyte values to determine if changes are needed in the composition of the TPN solutions that will be administered over the next 24 hours. This prevents the client from developing electrolyte imbalance.

Test-Taking Strategy: Recalling the purpose of TPN assists in answering this question. The issue of this question is specific content, that is, to identify laboratory blood levels that are used to order TPN therapy. Use the process of elimination to answer this question considering the composition of TPN solutions. If you had difficulty with this question, take time now to review the composition of TPN.

Level of Cognitive Ability: Analysis
Phase of Nursing Process: Analysis
Client Needs: Physiological Integrity
Content Area: Fundamental Skills

Reference

Black, J., & Matassarin-Jacobs, E. (1997). *Medical-surgical nursing: Clinical management for continuity of care* (5th ed.). Philadelphia: W. B. Saunders, pp. 1754–1756.

---

9. The home health nurse visits a client who has recently been told that he is positive for human immunodeficiency virus (HIV). The client is having difficulty accepting the diagnosis. The home health care nurse analyzes the client's behavior and

1 Assesses the client's coping skills and knowledge deficit regarding HIV.
2 Acknowledges that psychosocial problems are related to ineffective coping skills.
3 Recognizes that individuals who are HIV positive have less than 1 year to live.
4 Ignores the problem, knowing that over time the client will accept the diagnosis.

Answer: 1

Rationale: The diagnosis of HIV is difficult to hear for the first time. Clients may exhibit a variety of reactions that are not necessarily a direct result of ineffective coping skills. The nurse must also know that persons with HIV are living well beyond 1 year. Ignoring the problem does not eliminate the client's difficulty in understanding the disease process. The nurse must focus on knowledge deficit of a disease process and other psychosocial interventions.

Test-Taking Strategy: Knowledge of HIV, the psychosocial aspects, and longevity of the disease is required to answer the question. Use the process of elimination to answer the question. Options 2 and 3 are factually incorrect. Option 4 is unacceptable nursing practice.

Level of Cognitive Ability: Analysis
Phase of Nursing Process: Analysis
Client Needs: Psychosocial Integrity
Content Area: Adult Health/Respiratory

Reference

Rice, R. (1996). *Home health nursing practice: Concepts and application* (2nd ed.). St. Louis: Mosby–Year Book, p. 336.

---

10. Before the home health care nurse determines the correct position for the client to begin chest physical therapy, which of the following must be ascertained?

1 The client's capability for lung expansion
2 The lung areas involved
3 Deep breathing routines
4 The proximity of oxygen

Answer: 2

Rationale: The goal of chest physical therapy is to mobilize secretions for improved respiratory function. The nurse must be knowledgeable in knowing which areas of the lungs should be targeted for this technique. The client's capability for lung expansion is secondary to the lung assessment. Deep breathing routines and oxygen use do not relate to client positioning.

Test-Taking Strategy: This question requires analytical thinking about the purpose of chest physical therapy and how it relates to the individual client. Eliminate options 3 and 4 first because deep breathing routines and the proximity of oxygen are unrelated to positioning the client. Lung expansion is secondary to the primary purpose (mobilization of secretions) of chest physical therapy. The position for the procedure is based on the area of lung involvement.

Level of Cognitive Ability: Analysis
Phase of Nursing Process: Analysis
Client Needs: Physiological Integrity
Content Area: Adult Health/Respiratory

Reference

Como, N. (1995). *Home health nursing pocket consultant.* St. Louis: Mosby–Year Book, p. 230.

---

11. A client with a C4 spinal cord injury has continuous urinary incontinence. The client's temperature is normal, and the urine is clear. The 24-hour urinary output is 1650 mL. Which additional data must the nurse obtain to confirm a nursing diagnosis?

1 Specific gravity of the urine
2 Hourly urine output
3 Complaints of dysuria
4 Bladder distention

Answer: 4

Rationale: Spinal cord–injured clients may demonstrate urinary atony with retention and overflow dribbling. Another common urinary elimination problem is spastic incontinence. Both problems present with a pattern of continuous incontinence. Bladder palpation for distention permits the nurse to differentiate between the two types of neurogenic bladders. Because the 24-hour output is normal, measurement of hourly output would not provide meaningful information. Urinary tract infection can cause dysuria and incontinence, but spinal cord–injured clients lose bladder sensation. An infection would likely result in pyrexia and cloudy urine.

Test-Taking Strategy: The question requires knowledge of the types of neurogenic bladders, the normal 24-hour urinary output, and the manifestations of urinary tract infection in spinal cord–injured clients. Read the case situation carefully, noting key information to assist in selecting the correct option. Hourly output is initiated only in specific situations when renal failure is impending or when fluid balance must be monitored closely. If you had difficulty with this question, take time now to review the complications associated with a spinal cord injury.

Level of Cognitive Ability: Analysis
Phase of Nursing Process: Analysis
Client Needs: Physiological Integrity
Content Area: Adult Health/Neurological

Reference

Smeltzer, S., & Bare, B. (1996). *Brunner and Suddarth's Textbook of medical-surgical nursing* (8th ed.). Philadelphia: Lippincott-Raven, pp. 1150–1151, 1802.

---

12. The physician aspirates synovial fluid from the client's knee joint. The results are analyzed and would be diagnostic of rheumatoid arthritis if which of the following were observed?

1 Cloudy synovial fluid
2 Microorganisms present in synovial fluid
3 Bloody synovial fluid
4 Urate crystals present in synovial fluid

Answer: 1

Rationale: Cloudy synovial fluid is diagnostic of rheumatoid arthritis. Organisms present in the synovial fluid are characteristic of a septic joint condition. Urate crystals are found in gout. Bloody synovial fluid is seen with trauma.

Test-Taking Strategy: Knowledge that cloudy synovial fluid is indicative of rheumatoid arthritis is necessary to answer the question. Use the process of elimination to answer the question. Remember that organisms indicate infection, blood indicates trauma, and urates indicate gout. Take time now to review the characteristics of rheumatoid arthritis if you had difficulty with this question.

Level of Cognitive Ability: Analysis
Phase of Nursing Process: Analysis
Client Needs: Physiological Integrity
Content Area: Adult Health/Musculoskeletal

Reference

Black, J., & Matassarin-Jacobs, E. (1997). *Medical-surgical nursing: Clinical management for continuity of care* (5th ed.). Philadelphia: W. B. Saunders, p. 661.

13. The nurse is caring for a client with trigeminal neuralgia. Which of the following is a primary nursing diagnosis related to psychosocial dysfunction?

1 Self-Care Deficit: Oral Hygiene related to facial discomfort
2 Anxiety related to sexual dysfunction
3 Cognitive Dysfunction related to memory deficit
4 High risk for Ineffective Coping related to sudden spasms of pain

Answer: 4

Rationale: Trigeminal neuralgia affects cranial nerve V, creating sudden bursts of electric current–like pain in the face. Options 2 and 3 may relate to other neurological disorders but are not characteristic of trigeminal neuralgia. Option 1 is an appropriate diagnosis for trigeminal neuralgia, but it is a physiological not a psychosocial diagnosis.

Test-Taking Strategy: Read the stem of the question carefully, and note that it is asking for psychosocial information. Eliminate option 1 because it relates to a physiological not a psychosocial disorder. A key word is "neuralgia," which relates to nerve pain. Therefore, eliminate options 2 and 3. If you had difficulty with this question, take time now to review trigeminal neuralgia.

Level of Cognitive Ability: Analysis
Phase of Nursing Process: Analysis
Client Needs: Psychosocial Integrity
Content Area: Adult Health/Neurological

Reference

Black, J., & Matassarin-Jacobs, E. (1997). *Medical-surgical nursing: Clinical management for continuity of care* (5th ed.). Philadelphia: W. B. Saunders, pp. 929–930.

14. An adolescent communicates to the nurse at the clinic that using Rollerblades is a new hobby. The client tells the nurse that protective equipment is not being worn. The nurse realizes that this client needs teaching related to the risk factor for

1 A spinal cord injury
2 Multiple sclerosis
3 A cerebrovascular accident
4 Migraine headaches

Answer: 1

Rationale: Trauma, often as a result of falls, is the most common cause of spinal cord injury. Rollerblading, especially without a helmet, is a risk factor. Other risk factors include bicycling, motorcycling, horseback riding, diving into unknown waters, and occupations at heights over 5 feet. Options 2, 3, and 4 are not caused by trauma.

Test-Taking Strategy: Read the question carefully to determine what is being asked. Use the process of elimination to select the correct option. Trauma is the issue of the question. Options 2, 3, and 4 do not occur as a result of trauma.

Level of Cognitive Ability: Analysis
Phase of Nursing Process: Analysis
Client Needs: Health Promotion and Maintenance
Content Area: Child Health

Reference

Black, J., & Matassarin-Jacobs, E. (1997). *Medical-surgical nursing: Clinical management for continuity of care* (5th ed.). Philadelphia: W. B. Saunders, pp. 890, 891.

15. The surgeon is performing an abdominal hysterectomy. The operating room nurse counts the sponges and notes that the sponge count is not correlating with the preoperative count. Which initial action by the nurse will most likely avoid a lawsuit?

1 Recording that the count was correct
2 Informing the surgeon of the situation
3 Looking on the instrument table for the sponge
4 Asking the circulating nurse to look for the sponge

Answer: 2

Rationale: The surgeon has the ultimate responsibility for the safety of the client and can stop the surgery until the sponge is found. Option 1 is illegal and unethical. Options 3 and 4 take time, and if the surgery is nearing completion, the client may have to be opened and explored for the missing sponge.

Test-Taking Strategy: Note the issue of the question and the word "initial" in the stem of the question. The issue of the question is a legal one, and the surgeon is ultimately responsible for the client. Use the process of elimination to answer the question. If you had difficulty with this question, take time now to review legal issues.

Level of Cognitive Ability: Application
Phase of the Nursing Process: Analysis
Client Needs: Physiological Integrity
Content Area: Fundamental Skills

Reference

Brent, N. (1997). *Nurses and the law.* Philadelphia: W. B. Saunders, p. 412.

16. The nurse completes the initial assessment of a client admitted to the psychiatric unit. The nurse analyzes the data and determines that which of the following presents a potential concern?
   1 The presence of bruises on the client's neck
   2 The client's report of not sleeping well
   3 The client's report of suicidal thoughts
   4 The husband stating he does not approve of treatment

Answer: 3

Rationale: The client's thoughts are extremely important when verbalized. Suicidal thoughts direct the nurse to incorporate this information into the plan of care. The nurse has the legal responsibility to protect the client from harm. Options 1, 2, and 4 all affect the treatment of the client but are not of greatest importance at this time.

Test-Taking Strategy: The client is the focus of the question; therefore, eliminate option 4. Use priorities when selecting the correct option. Eliminate option 2 as the least concern of the remaining options. Select option 3 because it is global, and if the client verbalizes suicidal thoughts, it is a priority concern.

Level of Cognitive Ability: Analysis
Phase of the Nursing Process: Analysis
Client Needs: Psychosocial Integrity
Content Area: Mental Health

Reference
Brent, N. (1997). *Nurses and the law.* Philadelphia: W. B. Saunders, p. 415.

---

17. A client in active labor calls the nurse to her bedside to report that when she went to the toilet to urinate she "passed a big gush of clear fluid" and thinks "my water broke." The nurse immediately performs a sterile vaginal examination and discovers a pulsating rope-like object in the vaginal canal. Which of the following would be a priority nursing diagnosis in this situation?
   1 Complication of Labor related to fetal position
   2 Risk for Fetal Injury related to infection secondary to vaginal examination
   3 Potential for Impaired Fetal Gas Exchange related to umbilical cord compression
   4 Fetal Hypoxia related to placental insufficiency

Answer: 3

Rationale: A pulsating rope-like object in the vagina can only be the umbilical cord. Each contraction presses the presenting part downward against the bony pelvis, compressing the prolapsed cord between the presenting part and the bony pelvis. The compression shuts off the fetal circulation at the point of compression leading to decreased fetal tissue perfusion and hypoxia of the fetus.

Test-Taking Strategy: Identify the specific issue addressed in the case and stem. In this instance, cord compression directly cuts off fetal circulation. The placenta is not involved as the cause of the fetal hypoxia, so option 4 is eliminated as a possible choice. Remember the elements in a nursing diagnosis, and rule out any diagnosis that does not speak to an actual or potential client problem or need and identified related factors (etiology) that cause the problem as in option 1. Remember the ABCs (airway, breathing, and circulation) when prioritizing. There is no indication of infection; therefore, eliminate option 2.

Level of Cognitive Ability: Analysis
Nursing Process: Analysis
Client Needs: Physiological Integrity
Content Area: Maternity

Reference
Reeder, S., Martin, L., & Koniak-Griffin, D. (1997). *Maternity nursing: Family, newborn, and women's health care.* (18th ed.). Philadelphia: Lippincott-Raven, p. 1000.

---

18. A client is admitted to a telemetry unit with a potassium level of 6.3 mEq/L. In analyzing the cardiac rhythm, the nurse would anticipate which of the following electrocardiogram (ECG) changes?
   1 A sinus rhythm with a depressed ST segment
   2 A sinus tachycardia with a prolonged QT interval
   3 A sinus tachycardia with an extra U wave
   4 A sinus rhythm with a peaked T wave

Answer: 4

Rationale: Potassium level greater than 5.3 mEq/L constitutes a hyperkalemia that can be detected on ECG by the presence of a tall peaked T wave. A U wave and a depressed ST segment are present with hypokalemia with levels less than 3.5 mEq/L. A prolonged QT interval is indicative of hypocalcemia with calcium levels less than 8.2 mg/dL.

Test-Taking Strategy: Knowledge of basic ECG changes related to electrolyte abnormalities is necessary to answer this question. If you had difficulty with this question, take time now to review ECG changes that occur with hyperkalemia.

Level of Cognitive Ability: Analysis
Phase of Nursing Process: Analysis
Client Needs: Physiological Integrity
Content Area: Adult Health/Cardiovascular

Reference

Hartshorn, J., Sole, M., & Lamborn, M. (1997). *Introduction to critical care nursing* (2nd ed.). Philadelphia: W. B. Saunders, p. 243.

---

19. The client begins to act restless and agitated and complains of shortness of breath and palpitations. The nurse identifies an atrial fibrillation with a rapid ventricular response on the cardiac monitor. Which nursing diagnosis is the most important at this time?

1 Decreased cardiac output
2 Decreased breathing patterns
3 Anxiety
4 Impaired gas exchange

Answer: 1

Rationale: In atrial fibrillation with rapid ventricular response, the atrial chambers quiver, do not contract normally, and fill the ventricles with blood during the last part of diastole. This results in the loss of an important atrial contribution to cardiac output called the *atrial kick*. Loss of the atrial kick and the rapid ventricular rate cause a reduction of cardiac output by as much as 25%.

Test-Taking Strategy: Knowledge of the physiology of atrial fibrillation is required to answer this question. Use the process of elimination to assist in answering this question. Note that the case presents a cardiac problem. Option 1 is the only option that directly addresses a cardiac concern.

Level of Cognitive Ability: Analysis
Phase of Nursing Process: Analysis
Client Needs: Physiological Integrity
Content Area: Adult Health/Cardiovascular

Reference

Huff, J. (1997). *ECG workout: Exercises in arrhythmia interpretation* (3rd ed.). Philadelphia: Lippincott-Raven, pp. 100–101.

---

20. The nurse is caring for a client with Cushing's syndrome who demonstrates withdrawn behavior. The nurse should recognize that this client's behavior is most likely related to which of these nursing diagnoses?

1 Diversional Activity Deficit
2 Powerlessness
3 Hopelessness
4 Body Image Disturbance

Answer: 4

Rationale: Physical changes in the client's appearance can occur with Cushing's syndrome. Such changes include hirsutism, moon face, buffalo hump, acne, and striae and can cause body image disturbance. Options 1, 2, and 3 are not commonly associated with Cushing's syndrome.

Test-Taking Strategy: Note the key phrase "most likely related" in the stem, which indicates an obvious association with the medical condition of the client. Knowledge of the physical changes characteristic of Cushing's syndrome assists you in choosing the correct answer. Options 1, 2, and 3 are not commonly associated with Cushing's syndrome. If you had difficulty with this question, take time now to review the characteristics of Cushing's syndrome.

Level of Cognitive Ability: Analysis
Phase of the Nursing Process: Analysis
Client Needs: Psychosocial Integrity
Content Area: Adult Health/Endocrine

Reference

LeMone, P., & Burke, K. M. (1996). *Medical-surgical nursing: Critical thinking in client care.* Menlo Park, CA: Addison-Wesley, p. 694.

21. Which of the following clinical manifestations would indicate that a client with adult respiratory distress syndrome (ARDS) might need to be mechanically ventilated?

1 The client's PO_2 is 92% on room air
2 The client's pH is 7.38
3 The client requires 50% O_2 to maintain a PaO_2 of 50 mmHg
4 The client's respiratory rate is between 35 and 40 breaths/minute

Answer: 3

Rationale: If blood gas oxygen levels of at least 60 mmHg cannot be maintained, mechanical ventilation must be considered. A required oxygen concentration exceeding 50% would also be a cause for considering mechanical ventilation. A PO_2 of 92% on room air would be desirable for a client with ARDS. A pH of 7.38 is a normal finding, and a respiratory rate of 35–40 breaths/minute would not be a cause by itself for mechanical ventilation.

Test-Taking Strategy: This question requires interpretation of data based on the assessment and identification of abnormal laboratory values. To answer this question, knowledge and understanding of blood gas values are required. If you had difficulty with this question, take time now to review normal blood gas values and the need for mechanical ventilation.

Level of Cognitive Ability: Analysis
Phase of Nursing Process: Analysis
Client Needs: Physiological Integrity
Content Area: Adult Health/Respiratory

Reference

Thompson, J., McFarland, G., Hirsch, J., & Tucker, S. (1997). *Mosby's clinical nursing* (4th ed.). St. Louis: Mosby–Year Book, p. 145.

---

22. A client in the cardiac care unit is receiving tissue plasminogen activator (tPA) for treatment of a myocardial infarction. In analyzing the effects of this treatment, what is the priority nursing diagnosis for this client?

1 Fluid Volume Excess
2 Fluid Volume Deficit
3 High Risk for Infection
4 High Risk for Injury

Answer: 4

Rationale: Clients receiving tPA are at high risk for bleeding and hemorrhage because it is a thrombolytic agent. The nurse needs to assess for overt bleeding and internal bleeding. Vital signs should be closely monitored. The physician should be notified immediately in the event of bleeding.

Test-Taking Strategy: Knowledge of tPA and its actions and side effects is necessary to answer this question. Tissue plasminogen activator should provide you with the clue that directs you to option 4 as the correct option. If you had difficulty with this question, take time now to review this medication.

Level of Cognitive Ability: Analysis
Phase of Nursing Process: Analysis
Client Needs: Safe, Effective Care Environment
Content Area: Adult Health/Cardiovascular

Reference

McKenry, L., & Salerno, E. (1995). *Mosby's pharmacology in nursing* (19th ed.). St. Louis: Mosby–Year Book, p. 661.

23. When performing a nursing assessment on a child, the parents report ribbon-like and foul-smelling stools, constipation since birth, and poor feeding habits. The nurse notes a distended abdomen. Based on these data, the nurse analyzes these signs and symptoms as indicative of

1 Intussusception.
2 Inguinal hernia.
3 Pyloric stenosis.
4 Hirschsprung's disease.

Answer: 4

Rationale: A nurse can help to establish a diagnosis by carefully listening to the client history. In Hirschsprung's disease, frequency of bowel movements, characteristics of stools, onset of constipation, distended abdomen, poor feeding habits, irritability, and signs of undernutrition are significant clues. Constipation and ribbon-like, foul-smelling stools are particularly characteristic of Hirschsprung's disease. Inguinal hernia is indicated by inguinal swelling, pyloric stenosis by projectile vomiting, and intussusception by acute, colicky abdominal pain and currant jelly–like stool.

Test-Taking Strategy: Knowledge of the characteristics of gastrointestinal disturbances in the child is needed to answer this question. If you had difficulty with this question, take time now to review the signs and symptoms of the gastrointestinal disorders presented in the options.

Level of Cognitive Ability: Analysis
Phase of the Nursing Process: Analysis
Client Needs: Physiological Integrity
Content Area: Child Health

Reference

Wong, D., & Perry, S. (1998). *Maternal-child nursing care.* St. Louis: Mosby–Year Book, pp. 1399–1401.

24. The nurse reads the physician's progress notes and notes that the client was diagnosed with cancer. The staging is documented as T3, N2, M1. The nurse analyzes this staging as indicating which of the following?

1 The tumor is in situ.
2 The tumor is 3 cm in size.
3 Nodal involvement cannot be assessed.
4 Distant metastasis was found.

Answer: 4

Rationale: The TNM classification system for staging solid tumors is widely used. M1 indicates distant metastasis present. T refers to the tumor size, with T0 indicating no primary tumor found and T1 to T4 referring to progressively larger tumors. TIS is used to indicate a carcinoma in situ. N refers to regional lymph node involvement. N0 indicates regional nodes were normal, and N1 to N4 indicate increasingly abnormal regional lymph nodes.

Test-Taking Strategy: Knowledge of the TNM classification system for staging solid tumors is required to answer this question. Take time now to review this classification system if you had difficulty with this question.

Level of Cognitive Ability: Analysis
Phase of Nursing Process: Analysis
Client Needs: Physiological Integrity
Content Area: Adult Health/Oncology

Reference

Black, J., & Matassarin-Jacobs, E. (1997). *Medical-surgical nursing: Clinical management for continuity of care* (5th ed.). Philadelphia: W. B. Saunders, pp. 559–560.

25. On entering a new mother's room, the nurse finds the mother crying. The infant is undressed on the bed in front of the mother. The mother looks at the nurse and says, "I can't even dress this baby!" After reassuring the client, the nurse determines that the most appropriate nursing action would be to

1 Diaper the infant while on the bed.
2 Place the infant back in the bassinet.
3 Place the infant in the bassinet and take the infant back to the nursery.
4 Have the mother place the infant in the bassinet and assist the mother in dressing the infant.

Answer: 4

Rationale: The infant needs to be placed in the bassinet for safety. The mother needs to be reassured that she can safely care for her infant. Allow and assist the mother in dressing the infant. Focus on client feelings first.

Test-Taking Strategy: Use the process of elimination in answering this question. A key phrase in the question is "the mother crying." Option 1 is incorrect because the infant needs to be safely placed in the bassinet. Note that options 2 and 3 are similar. Option 2 is incorrect. It places the infant back in the bassinet, but the mother's needs are not met. Option 3 again does not meet the mother's needs. Option 4 is the only option that focuses on the mother's feelings and needs.

Level of Cognitive Ability: Application
Phase of Nursing Process: Analysis
Client Needs: Psychosocial Integrity
Content Area: Maternity

Reference

Nichols, F., & Zwelling, E. (1997). *Maternal-newborn nursing: Theory and practice.* Philadelphia: W. B. Saunders, pp. 1159–1161.

---

26. Which of the following assessment data would the nurse analyze as indicating a potential complication associated with thoracic surgery?

1 Crackles on lung auscultation and frothy sputum
2 Urinary output of 45 mL/hour
3 Chest tube drainage of 100 mL 2 hours after surgery
4 An arterial blood pH of 7.30

Answer: 1

Rationale: The complications associated with thoracic surgery include pulmonary edema, cardiac dysrhythmias, hemorrhage, hemothorax, hypovolemic shock, and thrombophlebitis. Signs of pulmonary edema include dyspnea, crackles, persistent cough, frothy sputum, and cyanosis. A urinary output of 45 mL/hour is an appropriate output. The nurse would become concerned if the output were below 30 mL/hour. Between 100 and 300 mL of drainage may accumulate during the first 2 hours after thoracic surgery. Normal arterial blood pH is 7.35–7.45. An arterial blood pH of 7.30 does not specifically indicate a complication.

Test-Taking Strategy: Knowledge of normal urinary output and laboratory values for arterial blood gases helps to determine the correct answer through the process of elimination. Use the principles associated with prioritizing when answering this question. Use the ABCs. Crackles heard on lung auscultation are associated with edema. If you had difficulty with this question, take time now to review the complications associated with thoracic surgery.

Level of Cognitive Ability: Analysis
Phase of the Nursing Process: Analysis
Client Needs: Physiological Integrity
Content Area: Adult Health/Respiratory

Reference

Black, J., & Matassarin-Jacobs, E. (1997). *Medical-surgical nursing: Clinical management for continuity of care* (5th ed.). Philadelphia: W. B. Saunders, pp. 1159, 1163.

27. The nurse reviews the results of the white blood cell count on a client with Hodgkin's disease after the client received chemotherapy. The results of the test are reported as 2000/mm^3. The nurse analyzes the results as

1 Lower than normal, signifying leukopenia related to chemotherapy.
2 Insignificant and unrelated to Hodgkin's disease.
3 Higher than normal, signifying spread of disease to bone marrow.
4 Normal.

Answer: 1

Rationale: With more extensive Hodgkin's disease, radiation coupled with a multiagent chemotherapy regimen is the most effective treatment. Chemotherapy agents cause drug-induced leukopenia, and treatment focuses on this side effect. Normal white blood cell count is 5000–10,000/mm^3.

Test-Taking Strategy: Knowing that chemotherapy destroys both normal white blood cells and cancer cells is necessary to answer the question. Read the question carefully. The key word is "chemotherapy." The question addresses chemotherapy, and option 1 is the only option that refers to chemotherapy.

Level of Cognitive Ability: Analysis
Phase of Nursing Process: Analysis
Client Needs: Physiological Integrity
Content Area: Adult Health/Oncology

Reference

Ignatavicius, D. D., Workman, M. L., & Mishler, M. A. (1995). *Medical-surgical nursing: A nursing process approach* (2nd ed.). Philadelphia: W. B. Saunders, pp. 1069–1070.

---

28. A preterm newborn is transferred to a tertiary care center because more specialized care is required. The nurse determines that which of the following would be best, in caring for the parents, as the infant is transported?

1 Keep parents out of the way of the transport team
2 Transfer the mother with the infant
3 Allow parents contact with their infant and provide parental support
4 Discuss disposition of the infant in case of death

Answer: 3

Rationale: Option 1 is incorrect. The parents' needs should be respected, and they should be allowed to be within sight of what is going on. They should be kept out of the way, but they can still be present. Option 2 would be the ideal situation, but it is not always necessary or possible and ignores the needs of the father. Option 4 is an incorrect and inappropriate answer. Parents will be grieving the loss of the perfect baby and will be fearful about their infant's condition. Parents should be allowed contact with the infant, and the nurse should provide parental support. Taking a picture of the newborn for the mother to have is one way to provide support. Keeping in constant contact with the receiving unit until the mother can be discharged home also assists in providing support.

Test-Taking Strategy: Identify the client of the question, which is the parents. Use the process of elimination, and eliminate options 2 and 4. From the remaining options, you would be directed to option 3 as the best option. Remember, always focus on the feelings of the client or family first.

Level of Cognitive Ability: Analysis
Phase of Nursing Process: Analysis
Client Needs: Psychosocial Integrity
Content Area: Maternity

Reference

Nichols, F., & Zwelling, E. (1997). *Maternal-newborn nursing: Theory and practice.* Philadelphia: W. B. Saunders, p. 1340.

29. The nurse is caring for a client on a subacute care unit with a diagnosis of heart failure. The client's cardiac monitor shows a regular sinus rhythm with occasional premature atrial contractions. One hour later, the nurse notes on the cardiac monitor screen that the client's QRS complex is now wide and bizarre, the P waves are absent, and the ventricular heart rate is 170 beats/minute. Based on the analysis of these data, what action by the nurse would be unsafe at this time for the client?

1 Checking the client's electrodes
2 Obtaining the defibrillator
3 Assessing the client's pulse
4 Starting cardiopulmonary resuscitation (CPR)

Answer: 4

Rationale: Analysis of the ECG results indicates the client is in ventricular tachycardia. The nurse needs to assess whether or not the client has a pulse. CPR should be initiated only on a pulseless individual. Checking the client's electrodes is not unsafe. If the client were scratching over an electrode site, a pattern similar to ventricular tachycardia can be observed on the monitor. The defibrillator should be available if the client's rhythm is pulseless ventricular tachycardia. The nurse needs to assess the client's pulse to determine whether the client's rhythm is pulseless ventricular tachycardia or ventricular tachycardia with a pulse before intervening.

Test-Taking Strategy: Note that the stem states "unsafe." Eliminate options 1 and 3 because these indicate assessment actions and would be safe interventions. To discriminate between options 2 and 4, review the case situation to determine that the most appropriate action would be as stated in option 2. This leaves option 4 as the correct answer to this question as stated. If you had difficulty with this question, take time now to review ECG patterns and appropriate interventions.

Level of Cognitive Ability: Application
Phase of Nursing Process: Analysis
Client Needs: Safe, Effective Care Environment
Content Area: Adult Health/Cardiovascular

Reference
Black, J., & Matassarin-Jacobs, E. (1997). *Medical-surgical nursing: Clinical management for continuity of care* (5th ed.). Philadelphia: W. B. Saunders, p. 1305.

---

30. The client is brought to the emergency department and is unconscious. From the viewpoint of informed consent, a nurse determines that emergency treatment can be given to the unconscious client because

1 The client's family has given consent.
2 Emergency treatment can be provided under the emergency doctrine.
3 The nurse is covered under liability insurance.
4 The nurse will document the care accurately.

Answer: 2

Rationale: Emergency treatment can be provided under the "emergency doctrine." This doctrine implies that the client would have consented to treatment if able because the alternative would have been death or disability. The emergency doctrine removes the need for obtaining informed consent before emergency treatment and care are initiated.

Test-Taking Strategy: Use the process of elimination to answer the question. Option 1 is an unrealistic answer. The client's family may not be present. Options 3 and 4 are unrelated to the issue of informed consent. Additionally, option 4 is standard nursing procedure regardless of situation. If you had difficulty with this question, take time now to review the emergency doctrine.

Level of Cognitive Ability: Analysis
Phase of Nursing Process: Analysis
Client Needs: Safe, Effective Care Environment
Content Area: Fundamental Skills

Reference
Black, J., & Matassarin-Jacobs, E. (1997). *Medical-surgical nursing: Clinical management for continuity of care* (5th ed.). Philadelphia, W. B. Saunders, p. 2502.

31. The nurse assesses the client with a permanent ventricular pacemaker and observes that the pacing spike is not immediately followed by a QRS complex. The nurse analyzes this occurrence as

1 Normal.
2 Failure to capture.
3 Failure to sense.
4 Microshock.

Answer: 2

Rationale: This question tests knowledge of pacemaker complications. In permanent pacemakers, the pacing wire is usually surgically inserted into the right ventricle transvenously and positioned in the endocardium. The wire is attached to a small, sealed, battery-powered pulse generator, which is either in the abdominal cavity or in the chest wall. Failure to capture is identified if the pacing spike is not immediately followed by a QRS complex (or P wave if it is an atrial pacemaker). Some of the causes of failure to capture include battery or pulse generator failure, increased milliamperage requirements, or poor lead wire position.

Test-Taking Strategy: Knowledge of the complications that can occur with pacemakers is needed to answer the question. Use the process of elimination. Option 1 is incorrect and should be eliminated immediately. Option 4 refers to microshock, a low electric current that passes virtually unnoticed by the client and could permit, in a transvenous pacemaker, stray electric current from surrounding equipment to be conducted in a direct line to the myocardium. Option 3 refers to failure to sense, which occurs when a synchronous pacemaker fails to sense and fires without regard for the client's own rhythm. Causes of failure to sense include sensitivity set too low or failure of the sensing mechanisms located in the pulse generator.

Level of Cognitive Ability: Analysis
Phase of Nursing Process: Analysis
Client Needs: Physiological Integrity
Content Area: Adult Health/Cardiovascular

Reference

Luckmann, J. (1997). *Saunders manual of nursing care.* Philadelphia: W. B. Saunders, pp. 1016–1018.

32. Which of the following client statements indicates an understanding of the measures that can be taken to prevent thrombophlebitis?

1 "I am taking oral contraceptives to avoid pregnancy, which can cause venous stasis."
2 "I avoid sitting or standing in one position for prolonged periods."
3 "I'm glad I don't need to wear those ugly stockings anymore."
4 "I have decreased my fluid consumption to one glass of water a day."

Answer: 2

Rationale: Avoidance of sitting or standing for a prolonged period of time is one measure to prevent venous stasis and thrombophlebitis. Active and passive range of motion exercises, early ambulation, and postoperative deep breathing are additional preventive measures. Taking oral contraceptives causes hypercoagulability. Compression stockings are used to promote venous return, maintain normal coagulability, and prevent injury to the endothelial wall. Adequate hydration is maintained to prevent hypercoagulability.

Test-Taking Strategy: Read the question carefully. This question assesses your ability to recognize measures that can reduce venous stasis. Use the process of elimination to select the correct answer. Remember that avoiding standing or sitting in one position prevents venous stasis. If you had difficulty with this question, take time now to review measures to prevent thrombophlebitis.

Level of Cognitive Ability: Analysis
Phase of Nursing Process: Analysis
Client Needs: Physiological Integrity
Content Area: Adult Health/Cardiovascular

Reference

Black, J., & Matassarin-Jacobs, E. (1997). *Medical-surgical nursing: Clinical management for continuity of care* (5th ed.). Philadelphia: W. B. Saunders, pp. 1321–1322.

33. The client is unwilling to go out of the house for fear of "doing something crazy in public." Because of this, the client remains homebound except when accompanied outside by the spouse. The nurse analyzes these data and determines that the diagnosis would be indicated as

1 Social phobia.
2 Agoraphobia.
3 Claustrophobia.
4 Hypochondria.

Answer: 2

Rationale: Agoraphobia is a fear of open spaces and the fear of being trapped into a situation from which there may not be an escape. Agoraphobia includes the possibility of experiencing a sense of helplessness or embarrassment if an attack occurs. Avoidance of such situations usually results in reduction of social and professional interactions. Social phobia focuses more on a specific situation, such as the fear of speaking, performing, or eating in public. Claustrophobia is a fear of closed-in places. Clients with hypochondriacal symptoms focus their anxiety on physical complaints and are preoccupied with their health.

Test-Taking Strategy: Knowledge of the specific types of phobias and associated client behaviors is required to answer this question. If you had difficulty with this question, take time now to review phobia types and associated client behaviors.

Level of Cognitive Ability: Analysis
Phase of Nursing Process: Analysis
Client Needs: Psychosocial Integrity
Content Area: Mental Health

Reference

O'Toole, M. (1997). *Miller-Keane Encyclopedia & dictionary of medicine, nursing, & allied health* (6th ed.). Philadelphia: W. B. Saunders, p. 1242.

34. Oral polio vaccine (OPV) can be administered to which one of the following infants?

1 Infant with leukemia
2 Infant with lupus on prednisone
3 Infant with acquired immunodeficiency syndrome (AIDS)
4 Infant with cleft palate

Answer: 4

Rationale: OPV is a live attenuated poliovirus and should never be administered to any child who is immunosuppressed. Clients with leukemia or AIDS are immunosuppressed. Prednisone causes immunosuppression. An infant with a cleft palate has a normal functioning immune system.

Test-Taking Strategy: The key to this question is understanding that OPV is a live attenuated poliovirus and that live attenuated vaccines are not to be administered to clients with immunosuppression. From this point, use the process of elimination to select the correct option. If you had difficulty with this question, take time now to review the contraindications to immunizations.

Level of Cognitive Ability: Application
Phase of Nursing Process: Analysis
Client Needs: Physiological Integrity
Content Area: Child Health

Reference

Pillitteri, A. (1995). *Maternal and child health: Nursing care of the childbearing and childrearing family* (2nd ed.). Philadelphia: Lippincott-Raven, p. 1309.

35. Which of the following assessment data, obtained from the client with Raynaud's disease, would indicate to the nurse a need to provide the client with an opportunity to verbalize feelings?

1. "I guess I'll start wearing gloves when I need to."
2. "How does this disease get better?"
3. "I can't stand the way my body looks anymore."
4. "I'm learning to be more careful with my skin."

Answer: 3

Rationale: The client with Raynaud's disease suffers from body image disturbance when the physical changes begin to occur. Therapeutic nursing interventions are implemented to produce verbalized understanding of body image changes, discussion of feelings in the one-to-one relationship, and demonstration of appropriate problem-solving techniques for coping with body changes.

Test-Taking Strategy: This question requires knowledge of the body image disturbances related to the physical changes caused by Raynaud's disease. Read the stem of the question carefully. Option 1 is an example of client verbalization that reflects appropriate coping. Option 2 is an example of the client possibly in denial or without clear understanding of the disease's progression. Option 4 is an example of adequate coping skills being demonstrated related to the physical changes of the disease. Option 3 identifies a client need to verbalize feelings.

Level of Cognitive Ability: Analysis
Phase of Nursing Process: Analysis
Client Needs: Psychosocial Integrity
Content Area: Adult Health/Cardiovascular

Reference

Black, J., & Matassarin-Jacobs, E. (1997). *Medical-surgical nursing: Clinical management for continuity of care* (5th ed.). Philadelphia: W. B. Saunders, pp. 1431–1432.

---

36. The nurse collects a urine specimen for a urinalysis from the client recently diagnosed with polycystic disease of the kidneys. The results of the urinalysis report a urine specific gravity of 1.000. The nurse analyzes this result as

1. Normal.
2. Lower than normal, indicating dilute urine.
3. Higher than normal, indicating concentrated urine.
4. Insignificant and unrelated to polycystic disease.

Answer: 2

Rationale: Specific gravity is a measure of the concentration of particles in the urine. A normal range of urine specific gravity is 1.005–1.030. Early in polycystic disease, the ability of the kidneys to concentrate urine decreases.

Test-Taking Strategy: Knowing that polycystic disease decreases the kidneys' ability to concentrate urine, you would expect the urine to be dilute. In this case, a specific gravity of 1.000, which indicates a low concentration of urine, is the only correct option. If you had difficulty with this question, take time now to review normal specific gravity and the characteristics associated with polycystic disease.

Level of Cognitive Ability: Application
Phase of Nursing Process: Analysis
Client Needs: Physiological Integrity
Content Area: Adult Health/Renal

Reference

Black, J., & Matassarin-Jacobs, E. (1997). *Medical-surgical nursing: Clinical management for continuity of care* (5th ed.). Philadelphia: W. B. Saunders, p. 1678.

37. The nurse must determine how best to assign coworkers (another RN and one LPN) to provide care to a group of clients. Which of the following is the most appropriate assignment?

1 The RN is assigned to care for an unemployed 26-year-old woman, newly diagnosed with AIDS, who has four school-age children.

2 The LPN is assigned to care for a 41-year-old man, post resection of an acoustic neuroma 2 days ago, transferred from intensive care unit this morning.

3 The LPN is assigned to provide discharge teaching on medications and maintenance of a nephrostomy tube to a 35-year-old man.

4 The RN is assigned to care for a 65-year-old woman after assessment of abdominal pain, being discharged today to home with no medications.

Answer: 1

Rationale: To determine what can and cannot be delegated to a coworker, the nurse must carefully consider what level of care each client requires immediately and potentially in the future, what competencies are possessed by coworkers, and what legal limitations there are on the practice of those coworkers. In option 2, the client has undergone a serious neurosurgical procedure that will impair swallowing and gag reflexes, and there is significant risk of increased intracranial pressure in the first few days postoperatively. This situation and the fact that the client has been transferred from the intensive care unit this morning make this an inappropriate assignment for an LPN. The LPN is also not able to provide discharge teaching on medications and treatments to a client. Teaching is a professional responsibility, which the RN cannot delegate to anyone except another RN, making option 3 an incorrect answer. Although under some circumstances the RN might care for the client being discharged after abdominal pain, the stem tells you that there is an LPN available, and the RN would be best used to address the more critical or complicated client needs. Option 4 is therefore incorrect. The newly diagnosed woman with AIDS, unemployed and with small children, is likely to be in need of the skills of an RN in terms of both psychosocial and physiological needs, making option 1 an appropriate assignment.

Test-Taking Strategy: To answer this question, you must understand the differences in practice as defined by law. Knowing that there are professional responsibilities that the RN cannot delegate to anyone other than another RN immediately tells you that delegating teaching to the LPN is inappropriate. Even if you are not familiar with the care of the client after resection of an acoustic neuroma, the fact that the client was just transferred from the intensive care unit this morning is a fairly safe indicator that the client requires a high level of supervision, beyond the scope of the LPN's practice. There is nothing in option 4 to indicate that the client requires the skills of the RN (don't read into the question), and the stem tells you there is an LPN available.

Level of Cognitive Ability: Application
Phase of Nursing Process: Analysis
Client Needs: Safe, Effective Care Environment
Content Area: Fundamental Skills

Reference

Wywialowski, E. F. (1997). *Managing client care* (2nd ed.). St. Louis: Mosby–Year Book, pp. 254–255.

38. A community health nurse has analyzed statistical data and determined that there are several requests for the establishment of a well-baby clinic in various locations. The nurse knows there is funding available for only one clinic. To make a decision about the location of the clinic, what is the first activity the nurse should do?

1 Request more funding to meet the needs of the community
2 Decide to open several clinics offering minimal services and spread the funding around
3 Further analyze the data to document the location with the greatest need
4 Determine whether any locations could offer free services

Answer: 3

Rationale: The question asks about a decision for the one location that can receive funding. The only answer that responds to the question is option 3. All the other options focus on ignoring the funding constraints.

Test-Taking Strategy: Read the stem of the question carefully, and identify the issue of the question. Options 1, 2, and 4 focus the nurse's attention away from the problem at hand. Option 3 is the most global answer, addresses the issue, and provides further assessment, the first step of the nursing process.

Level of Cognitive Ability: Application
Phase of Nursing Process: Analysis
Client Needs: Health Promotion and Maintenance
Content Area: Fundamental Skills

Reference
Clemen-Stone, S., Eigsti, D., & McGuire, S. (1995). *Comprehensive community health nursing: Family, aggregate and community practice* (4th ed.). St. Louis: Mosby–Year Book, pp. 436–437.

39. The nurse is conducting a clinic visit with a prenatal client with heart disease. The nurse carefully evaluates vital signs, weight gain, and fluid and nutritional status to detect complications that can be caused by

1 Hypertrophy and increased contractility.
2 An increase in circulating volume.
3 Fetal cardiomegaly.
4 Rh incompatibility.

Answer: 2

Rationale: Pregnancy taxes the circulating system of every woman because both the blood volume and cardiac output increase approximately 30%. This is especially important to monitor in the client whose heart may not tolerate this normal increase.

Test-Taking Strategy: Knowledge of the pathophysiology associated with the changes that take place during pregnancy is needed to answer this question. Use the process of elimination, and note the client of the question. In option 1, hypertrophy may result in cardiac disease, but the outcome would be a decrease in contractility not an increase. Options 3 and 4 are directed at the fetus, not the prenatal client identified in the stem. If you had difficulty with this question, take time now to review the physiological changes that occur in pregnancy.

Level of Cognitive Ability: Analysis
Phase of Nursing Process: Analysis
Client Needs: Physiological Integrity
Content Area: Maternity

Reference
Pillitteri, A. (1995). *Maternal and child health: Nursing care of the childbearing and childrearing family* (2nd ed.). Philadelphia: Lippincott-Raven, p. 350.

40. The nurse is listening to the lungs of a client who has left lower lobe pneumonia. The nurse interprets that the pneumonia is resolving if which of the following is heard over the affected lung area?

1 Bronchophony
2 Egophony
3 Vesicular breath sounds
4 Whispered pectoriloquy

Answer: 3

Rationale: Vesicular breath sounds are normal sounds that are heard over peripheral lung fields where the air enters the alveoli. A return of breath sounds to normal is consistent with a resolving pneumonia. Bronchophony is an abnormal finding with lung consolidation and is identified if the nurse can clearly hear the client say "ninety-nine" through the stethoscope. (Normally the client's words are unintelligible if heard through a stethoscope.) Egophony occurs when the sound of the letter "e" is heard as an "a" with auscultation and also indicates lung consolidation. Finally, whispered pectoriloquy is present if the nurse hears the client when "one-two-three" is whispered. This is an abnormal finding, again heard over an area of consolidation. Consolidation typically occurs with pneumonia.

Test-Taking Strategy: To answer this question most accurately and quickly, it is necessary to know the differences among these assessment findings. Knowing the areas where normal breath sounds are heard, however, is sufficient to answer this question as stated. If you had difficulty with this question, take time now to review the characteristics of these breath sounds.

Level of Cognitive Ability: Analysis
Phase of Nursing Process: Analysis
Client Needs: Physiological Integrity
Content Area: Adult Health/Respiratory

Reference

Black, J., & Matassarin-Jacobs, E. (1997). *Medical-surgical nursing: Clinical management for continuity of care* (5th ed.). Philadelphia: W. B. Saunders, pp. 1046–1047.

---

41. The nurse collects urine specimens for catecholamine testing from the client with suspected pheochromocytoma. The results of the catecholamine test are reported as 20 μg/100 mL urine. The nurse analyzes these results as

1 Normal.
2 Lower than normal, ruling out pheochromocytoma.
3 Higher than normal, indicating pheochromocytoma.
4 Insignificant and unrelated to pheochromocytoma.

Answer: 3

Rationale: Assays of catecholamines are performed on single-voided urine specimens, 2- to 4-hour specimens, and 24-hour specimens. The normal range of urinary catecholamines is up to 14 μg/100 mL of urine, with higher levels occurring in pheochromocytoma.

Test-Taking Strategy: Knowing that pheochromocytoma is a catecholamine-producing tumor, you would expect that the results of such a test would indicate higher than normal amounts of catecholamine. Additionally the question addresses that the client is suspected of having pheochromocytoma, so if you need to select an answer and you are not sure, select the response that has similarity to a thought in the question. In this case, "suspected pheochromocytoma" is similar to "indicating pheochromocytoma" found in option 3. If you had difficulty with this question, take time now to review this test and its relationship to pheochromocytoma.

Level of Cognitive Ability: Analysis
Phase of Nursing Process: Analysis
Client Needs: Physiological Integrity
Content Area: Adult Health/Endocrine

Reference

Black, J., & Matassarin-Jacobs, E. (1997). *Medical-surgical nursing: Clinical management for continuity of care* (5th ed.). Philadelphia: W. B. Saunders, p. 2058.

---

42. A cooperative, compliant client taking 400 mg of carbamazepine (Tegretol) TID, experienced two seizures at home during the past 2 weeks. The nurse interprets this information as

1 A need to change the dose of the anticonvulsant medication.
2 A possible hysterical response.
3 Not unusual.
4 A need for a second anticonvulsant medication to be added to the treatment plan.

Answer: 4

Rationale: The goal of all therapy for clients with seizures is *no* seizure activity. Because carbamazepine is often the drug of choice and the dose is already high, use of an additional anticonvulsant is not an uncommon practice.

Test-Taking Strategy: Changing an anticonvulsant is not the issue as it would be if the client demonstrated side effects such as a rash (allergic response). The issue is how to control the seizures. Two seizures in 2 weeks requires attention. There are no stem data to support a rash or hysteria, leaving the only choice to be option 4. Adding an additional medication to achieve the goal of absent seizure activity would be attempted. Review content regarding carbamazepine now if you are unfamiliar with this medication. The total dose of 1200 mg/day is a therapeutic dose, and in this client scenario, it is not achieving the goal of preventing seizures.

Level of Cognitive Ability: Analysis
Phase of Nursing Process: Analysis
Client Needs: Physiological Integrity
Content Area: Pharmacology

Reference

Lehne, R. A. (1998). *Pharmacology for nursing care* (3rd ed.). Philadelphia: W. B. Saunders, p. 207.

---

43. The nurse hears a male client who suffered a cerebrovascular accident 2 weeks ago using foul language at his wife. The nurse's interpretation of the situation would be that

1 The client is abusive.
2 The client is frustrated.
3 The wife lacks attention.
4 There is need for family counseling.

Answer: 2

Rationale: Common behavior after stroke is frustration. After a cerebrovascular accident, clients are often emotionally labile, confused, forgetful, and frustrated. Clients may use profanity, which is often termed *automatic language*.

Test-Taking Strategy: Read the question carefully and note that the question specifically addresses a client with a cerebrovascular accident. This along with the client's behavior is the issue of the question. Use the process of elimination, identifying the behavior that commonly occurs after cerebrovascular accident. If you had difficulty with this question, take time now to review client behaviors after cerebrovascular accident.

Level of Cognitive Ability: Analysis
Phase of Nursing Process: Analysis
Client Needs: Psychosocial Integrity
Content Area: Adult Health/Neurological

Reference

Black, J., & Matassarin-Jacobs, E. (1997). *Medical-surgical nursing: Clinical management for continuity of care* (5th ed.). Philadelphia: W. B. Saunders, p. 792.

---

44. Which of the following assessment data would the nurse interpret as an indication of a potential complication associated with severe scoliosis?

1 Fatigue and bradycardia
2 Atelectasis and dyspnea
3 Backache and unlevel shoulders
4 Hypotension and tachycardia

Answer: 2

Rationale: The complications associated with severe scoliosis interfere with respiration. The lungs may not expand fully because of the severe curvature of the spine. The responses in options 1 and 4 are not related to scoliosis. Option 3 includes symptoms of scoliosis. Atelectasis and dyspnea are complications owing to a decreased lung expansion.

Test-Taking Strategy: Use the process of elimination and the ABCs to answer the question. Option 2 addresses airway. Read the question and options carefully. The question asks for complications not symptoms of scoliosis. If you had difficulty with this question, take time now to review the complications associated with scoliosis.

Level of Cognitive Ability: Analysis
Phase of Nursing Process: Analysis
Client Needs: Physiological Integrity
Content Area: Adult Health/Musculoskeletal

Reference

Black, J., & Matassarin-Jacobs, E. (1997). *Medical-surgical nursing: Clinical management for continuity of care* (5th ed.). Philadelphia: W. B. Saunders, p. 2120.

45. The nurse administers a tuberculin test (the Mantoux test) to a person infected with HIV. Seventy-two hours later, the individual has an area of induration measuring 7 mm in diameter. The nurse analyzes these results as

1 Normal.
2 A false-positive result, indicating the test needs to be repeated.
3 A false-negative result, indicating the test needs to be repeated.
4 Positive, indicating the person has been exposed to tuberculosis.

Answer: 4

Rationale: An area of induration 48–72 hours after the Mantoux test is injected measuring 5 mm or greater in people with HIV infection is considered positive. Because the area of induration was 7 mm, the test is positive. Normally an area greater than 10 mm is considered positive. In this case, 7 mm was not a normal, false-positive, or false-negative result. Clients with HIV infection are more likely to have a false-negative result, but 7 mm is not a negative result.

Test-Taking Strategy: Knowledge that the area of induration in a person infected with HIV of 5 mm or greater is considered positive in necessary to answer this question. If you had difficulty with this question, take time now to review the Mantoux test and interpretation of the test results.

Level of Cognitive Ability: Analysis
Phase of Nursing Process: Analysis
Client Needs: Physiological Integrity
Content Area: Adult Health/Respiratory

Reference

Ignatavicius, D. D., Workman, M. L., & Mishler, M. A. (1995). *Medical-surgical nursing: A nursing process approach* (2nd ed.). Philadelphia: W. B. Saunders, p. 720.

---

46. A client is scheduled to have electroconvulsive therapy. Which of the following nursing diagnoses would be most appropriate for this client?

1 Fear
2 Anxiety
3 Risk for Aspiration
4 Body Image Disturbance

Answer: 3

Rationale: Aspiration is safeguarded against by giving the client nothing by mouth for 6–8 hours before the treatment, removing dentures, and administering glycopyrrolate (Robinul) or atropine as prescribed. Although options 1 and 2 could also be contributory diagnoses, they are not the most important ones. There is no reason to imply that option 4 is even a consideration.

Test-Taking Strategy: Use Maslow's hierarchy of needs to answer this question correctly. Physiological needs must come first; therefore, select an answer that addresses these needs. Additionally, use the ABCs. Airway is the concern with the risk of aspiration. If you had difficulty with this question, take time now to review procedures related to electroconvulsive therapy.

Level of Cognitive Ability: Analysis
Phase of Nursing Process: Analysis
Client Needs: Physiological Integrity
Content Area: Mental Health

Reference

Varcarolis, E. M. (1998). *Foundations of psychiatric mental health nursing* (3rd ed.). Philadelphia: W. B. Saunders, p. 579.

---

47. A depressed client is discovered wrapping long shreds of torn sheets around the throat. The most appropriate nursing diagnosis for this client would be

1 Risk for Injury.
2 Ineffective Individual Coping.
3 Hopelessness.
4 Risk for Loneliness.

Answer: 1

Rationale: Option 1 is clearly the correct answer. Knowledge of Maslow's hierarchy of needs dictates that the need for safety is foremost if a physiological need does not exist. Options 2 and 3 could be differential nursing diagnoses but not the most appropriate ones. Option 4 may or may not be a consideration and is not the best choice.

Test-Taking Strategy: This question uses the strategy of key words or phrases. In this case, "most appropriate" is the phrase to pay particular attention to. Also, use Maslow's hierarchy of needs. If a physiological need does not exist, safety is the priority.

Level of Cognitive Ability: Analysis
Phase of Nursing Process: Analysis
Client Needs: Physiological Integrity
Content Area: Mental Health

Reference

Iyer, P., Taptich, B., & Bernocchi-Losey, D. (1995). *Nursing process and nursing diagnosis*. Philadelphia: W. B. Saunders, p. 369.

---

48. An infant crawling on the floor of the playroom suddenly begins to cough and make loud, high-pitched, wheezing sounds when breathing. The nursing diagnosis to consider immediately is

1 Ineffective Airway Clearance related to developmental stage.
2 Risk for Infection related to immature immune function.
3 Risk for Aspiration related to ingestion of a foreign object.
4 Ineffective Breathing Pattern related to inhaled allergen.

Answer: 3

Rationale: The situation describes key signs of airway obstruction caused by aspiration of a foreign object: stridor, wheeze, and cough. The sudden onset and severity of symptoms make infection, allergy, and developmental stage unlikely factors.

Test-Taking Strategy: The key word "immediately" in the stem indicates the need to prioritize. An additional key word is "playroom." Using the ABCs, the most important diagnosis to consider is airway obstruction. Also, options 1, 2, and 4 have related factors that do not result in the sudden signs as described in the situation.

Level of Cognitive Ability: Analysis
Phase of Nursing Process: Analysis
Client Needs: Physiological Integrity
Content Area: Child Health

Reference

Ashwill, J., & Droske, S. (1997). *Nusring care of children: Principles and practice.* Philadelphia: W. B. Saunders, p. 851.

---

49. The nurse is participating in a health screening clinic. The nurse interprets that which of the following clients participating in the screening has the greatest need for instruction to lower the risk of developing respiratory disease?

1 A 50-year-old smoker with cracked asbestos lining on basement pipes in the home
2 A 40-year-old smoker who works in a hospital
3 A 36-year-old who works with pesticides
4 A 25-year-old who does woodworking as a hobby

Answer: 1

Rationale: Smoking greatly enhances the client's risk of developing some form of respiratory disease. Other risk factors include exposure to harmful chemicals, airborne toxins, and dust or fumes. The client at greatest risk, identified in option 1, has two identified risk factors, one of which is smoking.

Test-Taking Strategy: Begin to answer this question by eliminating options 3 and 4 because the most harmful risk factor for the respiratory system is smoking. You would select option 1 over option 2 because asbestos is a substance that is toxic to the lungs if particles are inhaled. In this particular option, there are two risk factors identified, which make this client at greater risk than the others who have one factor identified. If you had difficulty with this question, take time now to review the risk factors associated with respiratory disease.

Level of Cognitive Ability: Analysis
Phase of Nursing Process: Analysis
Client Needs: Health Promotion and Maintenance
Content Area: Adult Health/Respiratory

Reference

Black, J., & Matassarin-Jacobs, E. (1997). *Medical-surgical nursing: Clinical management for continuity of care* (5th ed.). Philadelphia: W. B. Saunders, p. 1039.

50. Which of the following assessment data would the nurse analyze as indicating a potential complication associated with pheochromocytoma?

1. A urinary output of 50 mL/hour
2. Rales heard on auscultation
3. A blood urea nitrogen (BUN) of 20 mg/dL
4. A coagulation time of 5 minutes

Answer: 2

Rationale: The complications associated with pheochromocytoma include hypertensive retinopathy and nephropathy, myocarditis, heart failure, increased platelet aggregation, and cerebrovascular accident. Death can occur from shock, cerebrovascular accident, renal failure, dysrhythmias, and dissecting aortic aneurysm. Rales heard on auscultation are indicative of heart failure. A urinary output of 50 mL/hour is an appropriate output, and the nurse would become concerned if the output was below 30 mL/hour. A BUN of 20 mg/dL is a normal finding. Normal BUN is 11–23 mg/dL. A coagulation time of 5 minutes is normal. Normal coagulation time is 5–15 minutes.

Test-Taking Strategy: Use the principles associated with prioritizing when answering this question. Remember the ABCs. Rales heard on auscultation in the lungs are associated with heart failure. Additionally, if you know normal hourly urine outputs and normal laboratory values for coagulation time and BUN, by the process of elimination, you can determine that option 2 is the correct answer. If you had difficulty with this question, take time now to review the risk factors associated with pheochromocytoma.

Level of Cognitive Ability: Analysis
Phase of Nursing Process: Analysis
Client Needs: Physiological Integrity
Content Area: Adult Health/Endocrine

Reference

Black, J., & Matassarin-Jacobs, E. (1997). *Medical-surgical nursing: Clinical management for continuity of care* (5th ed.). Philadelphia: W. B. Saunders, pp. 2556, 2559.

---

51. A client is hospitalized with a preliminary diagnosis of myxedema. Laboratory studies reveal an elevated thyroid-stimulating hormone (TSH) level and decreased triiodothyronine (T_3) and thyroxine (T_4). The nurse analyzes these results as

1. Supporting the diagnosis of myxedema.
2. Insignificant in regards to the diagnosis of myxedema.
3. Indicating fulminating hyperthyroidism.
4. Revealing hypoparathyroidism, which closely resembles laboratory findings found with myxedema.

Answer: 1

Rationale: Secretion of T_3 and T_4 is regulated by a hypothalamic-pituitary-thyroid gland feedback mechanism. TSH regulates the secretion of thyroid hormone from the thyroid gland. The circulating level of thyroid hormone is the major factor regulating the release of TSH. If the thyroid level is low, TSH release is increased, and if the thyroid level is high, TSH is inhibited. In hyperthyroidism, T_3 and T_4 secretions are elevated because the normal regulatory controls of thyroid hormone are lost. Hypoparathyroidism is associated with a decrease in serum calcium and an increase in serum phosphate.

Test-Taking Strategy: Knowledge of myxedema, hormonal feedback mechanisms, and the associated laboratory values is necessary to answer the question. Remember that in hypothyroidism, T_3 and T_4 are decreased with an elevated TSH. In hyperthyroidism, T_3 and T_4 are elevated with a decreased TSH. If you had difficulty with this question, take time now to review hypothyroidism and hyperthyroidism and the associated laboratory values.

Level of Cognitive Ability: Analysis
Phase of Nursing Process: Analysis
Client Needs: Physiological Integrity
Content Area: Adult Health/Endocrine

Reference

Ignatavicius, D. D., Workman, M. L., & Mishler, M. A. (1995). *Medical-surgical nursing: A nursing process approach* (2nd ed.). Philadelphia: W. B. Saunders, pp. 1793, 1837, 1852.

52. Which of the following would be a priority nursing diagnosis for a client who is experiencing thyroid storm?

1 High Risk for Decreased Cardiac Output
2 Disturbance in Body Image
3 High Risk for Sexual Dysfunction
4 Ineffective Individual Coping

Answer: 1

Rationale: Clients in thyroid storm are experiencing a life-threatening event, which is associated with uncontrolled hyperthyroidism. The signs and symptoms of the disorder develop quickly, and therefore emergency measures must be taken to prevent death. These measures include maintaining hemodynamic status and patency of airway as well as providing adequate ventilation. The criteria for option 1 are appropriate for the client in thyroid storm.

Test-Taking Strategy: The question is asking you to select a priority nursing diagnosis for the client in thyroid storm. Remember the ABCs. Because of the severe nature of this illness and its devastating effects on the cardiopulmonary system, the only likely response is option 1. Options 2, 3, and 4 relate to psychosocial problems, and although they may exist for the client in thyroid storm, they are not a priority.

Level of Cognitive Ability: Analysis
Phase of Nursing Process: Analysis
Client Needs: Physiological Integrity
Content Area: Adult Health/Endocrine

Reference

Ignatavicius, D. D., Workman, M. L., & Mishler, M. A. (1995). *Medical-surgical nursing: A nursing process approach* (2nd ed.). Philadelphia: W. B. Saunders, pp. 1834–1835.

53. Which of the following assessment data would the nurse analyze as an indication of a potential complication associated with varicose veins?

1 Legs are unsightly in appearance and distress the client.
2 The client complains of aching and feelings of heaviness in the legs.
3 The physician finds that the legs become distended when the tourniquet is released during the Trendelenburg test.
4 The client complains of leg edema, and skin breakdown has started.

Answer: 4

Rationale: Complications of varicose veins include leg edema, skin breakdown, ulceration of the legs, trauma leading to rupture of a varicosity, and deep vein thrombosis or chronic insufficiency.

Test-Taking Strategy: Note the key phrase "potential complication." Distinguish between findings that are symptoms of varicose veins and those that represent complications. Options 1 and 2 are common findings in varicosities. Option 3 describes the Trendelenburg test findings that are indicative of varicose veins. In the test, the physician has the client lie down and elevate the legs to empty the veins. A tourniquet is then applied to occlude the superficial veins, after which the client stands and the tourniquet is released. If the veins are incompetent, they quickly become distended owing to backflow. Option 4 identifies a complication and a disruption of skin integrity. If you had difficulty with this question, take time now to review the complications associated with varicose veins.

Level of Cognitive Ability: Analysis
Phase of Nursing Process: Analysis
Client Needs: Physiological Integrity
Content Area: Adult Health/Cardiovascular

Reference

Black, J., & Matassarin-Jacobs, E. (1997). *Medical-surgical nursing: Clinical management for continuity of care* (5th ed.). Philadelphia: W. B. Saunders, pp. 2556, 2559.

54. The nurse inspects the color of the drainage from a nasogastric tube on a postoperative client approximately 24 hours after a laparotomy. The previous shift reported the drainage as "dark red drainage since the surgery." Which of the following current assessment data would the nurse analyze as a potential complication requiring notification of the physician?

1. Light yellowish brown drainage
2. Dark red drainage
3. Coffee-ground granules in the drainage
4. Greenish tinged drainage

Answer: 2

Rationale: For the first 12 hours after a laparotomy, the nasogastric tube drainage may be dark brown to dark red. Later the drainage should change to a light yellowish brown color. The presence of bile may cause a greenish tinge. The physician should be notified at once of the possibility of hemorrhage if the dark red color continues or if bright red blood is observed. Because of the presence of small amounts of blood and the action of gastric secretions, coffee-ground granules may be seen in the nasogastric tube drainage.

Test-Taking Strategy: Use the process of elimination in answering the question. Knowledge of the anticipated postoperative course after a laparotomy, including evolution of the color and character of nasogastric drainage, is helpful in answering this question. Even though option 2 is not a change from the color of the drainage since surgery, after 12 hours, it is an indicator of possible hemorrhage, and the physician should be notified.

Level of Cognitive Ability: Analysis
Phase of Nursing Process: Analysis
Client Needs: Physiological Integrity
Content Area: Adult Health/Gastrointestinal

Reference

Lewis, S., Collier, I., & Heitkemper, M. (1996). *Medical-surgical nursing: Assessment and management of clinical problems* (4th ed.). St. Louis: Mosby–Year Book, p. 1217.

---

55. The client is admitted with acute exacerbation of chronic obstructive pulmonary disease (COPD). Which of the following blood gas results would the nurse most likely expect to note?

1. PO_2 of 68 and PCO_2 of 40
2. PO_2 of 55 and PCO_2 of 40
3. PO_2 of 70 and PCO_2 of 50
4. PO_2 of 60 and PCO_2 of 50

Answer: 4

Rationale: During an acute exacerbation, the arterial blood gases deteriorate with decreasing PO_2 and increasing PCO_2. In early stages of COPD, arterial blood gases demonstrate mild to moderate hypoxemia with the PO_2 in the high 60s to high 70s (mmHg) and normal arterial PCO_2. As the condition advances, hypoxemia increases, and hypercapnia may result.

Test-Taking Strategy: Knowledge regarding the physiological occurrences in COPD and blood gas analysis skills are necessary to answer this question. If you had difficulty with this question, take time now to review the physiological alterations that occur in COPD and the associated blood gas values.

Level of Cognitive Ability: Analysis
Phase of Nursing Process: Analysis
Client Needs: Physiological Integrity
Content Area: Adult Health/Respiratory

Reference

Ignatavicius, D. D., Workman, M. L., & Mishler, M. A. (1995). *Medical-surgical nursing: A nursing process approach* (2nd ed.). Philadelphia: W. B. Saunders, p. 683.

56. The client sustained full-thickness burns to both hands from immersion in scalding water. A sheet graft was surgically applied to the wound. This type of graft is indicated for which of the following primary purposes?

1 Better adherence to wound bed
2 Better cosmetic result
3 Better donor site availability
4 Easier to care for initially

Answer: 2

Rationale: Sheet grafts are often used to graft burns in visible areas. Sheet grafts are done on cosmetically important areas, such as the face and hands, to avoid the meshed pattern that occurs with meshed grafts. A sheet autograft is applied to the excised wound bed without alteration in its integrity.

Test-Taking Strategy: Note the area of the burn as identified in the question. The question addresses burns to both hands, a visible body area. This should direct you to the correct option, option 2, which addresses the cosmetic effect. If you had difficulty with this question, take time now to review the purposes of a sheet graft used in burn clients.

Level of Cognitive Ability: Analysis
Phase of Nursing Process: Analysis
Client Needs: Psychosocial Integrity
Content Area: Adult Health/Integumentary

Reference
Black, J., & Matassarin-Jacobs, E. (1997). *Medical-surgical nursing: Clinical management for continuity of care* (5th ed.). Philadelphia: W. B. Saunders, p. 2255.

---

57. A nurse working in an outpatient clinic receives a call from a 46-year-old African-American client complaining of new-onset, painless vaginal bleeding and watery vaginal discharge. On the basis of this information, the nurse determines that the most appropriate instruction to the client would be to

1 Dial 911 and come to the clinic in an ambulance.
2 Come into the clinic for a Pap smear.
3 Keep her scheduled appointment in 2 months and call the doctor if symptoms worsen.
4 Wait one more menstrual cycle and call if the symptoms persist.

Answer: 2

Rationale: The incidence of invasive cervical cancer in situ peaks around age 45 and occurs twice as often in African-American women. A classical symptom is painless vaginal bleeding and may be accompanied by watery, blood-tinged vaginal discharge that may become dark and foul smelling as the disease progresses. A Pap smear is the initial diagnostic test performed.

Test-Taking Strategy: Use the process of elimination in answering the question. The woman has not reported any immediate life-threatening data, so eliminate option 1. Options 3 and 4 are similar in time frame, and two similar answers are often incorrect. Option 2 is a safe and realistic option. If you had difficulty with this question, take time now to review the risks associated with cervical cancer!

Level of Cognitive Ability: Analysis
Phase of Nursing Process: Analysis
Client Needs: Physiological Integrity
Content Area: Adult Health/Oncology

Reference
Smeltzer, S., & Bare, B. (1996). *Brunner and Suddarth's textbook of medical-surgical nursing* (8th ed.). Philadephia: Lippincott-Raven, p. 798.

58. A client scheduled for a thyroidectomy says to the nurse, "I can't sleep at all because I am so frightened about this surgery, and being cut on my neck." Which of the following nursing diagnoses would be most appropriate?

1 Fear related to inadequate knowledge about the surgical procedure
2 Ineffective Coping related to fear about impending surgery
3 Disturbance in Self-Esteem related to changes in personal appearance
4 Altered Health Maintenance related to hesitancy to complete surgical procedure

Answer: 2

Rationale: The client is having a difficult time coping with the scheduled surgery. The client is able to express her fears but is still anxious. It is most important to address the nursing diagnosis in option 2, to gain the confidence of the client and decrease anxiety. Information regarding a lack of knowledge about the procedure is not available in the question; therefore eliminate option 1. Options 3 and 4 might be correct after obtaining more information. Option 2 is the most correct response based on the information in the question.

Test-Taking Strategy: Use the process of elimination to answer the question. Read the information in the question carefully to select the correct option. Options 3 and 4 can be easily eliminated. Read the question a second time, eliminating option 1 because a knowledge deficit is not addressed in the question.

Level of Cognitive Ability: Analysis
Phase of Nursing Process: Analysis
Client Needs: Psychosocial Integrity
Content Area: Adult Health/Endocrine

Reference

Ignatavicius, D. D., Workman, M. L., & Mishler, M. A. (1995). *Medical-surgical nursing: A nursing process approach* (2nd ed.). Philadelphia: W. B. Saunders, p. 1840.

59. The nurse observes that the client's nasogastric tube (NGT) has suddenly stopped draining. The tube is connected to suction, the machine is on and functioning, and all connections are snug. The tube is secured properly and does not appear to have been dislodged. After checking placement, the nurse gently flushes the tube with 30 mL of normal saline, but the tube still is not draining. The nurse analyzes this problem as

1 Channels of gastric secretions may be bypassing the holes in the tube, and turning the client would promote stomach emptying.
2 Thick gastric secretions may be blocking the tube, and removing this tube and reinserting a new tube will correct the problem.
3 It is normal for an NGT to stop draining, and no action is required.
4 This is a potentially serious complication, and the physician must be notified immediately.

Answer: 1

Rationale: The nurse must check an NGT regularly to maintain tube patency and ensure proper drainage. Nasogastric tubes are used to decompress the stomach. The gastric distention is relieved only if the tube drains properly. One cause of improper tube drainage is due to channels of gastric secretions forming along the walls of the stomach and bypassing the holes in the NGT. Turning the client regularly helps to collapse the channels and promotes gastric emptying. The tube has already been flushed, so it is unlikely that it is still blocked by thick secretions. Although this is a problem that requires attention, it is within the practice of nursing to maintain patency of the NGT.

Test-Taking Strategy: The question addresses that the NGT is not draining properly and asks the nurse to analyze the problem. Option 2 can be ruled out because the tube has just been flushed. Option 4 can be ruled out because there are still some nursing options available to reestablish nasogastric tube patency. Option 3 can be ruled out because it is not acceptable to ignore the tube that has suddenly stopped draining. Steps must be taken to reestablish proper function of the tube. If you had difficulty with this question, take time now to review nursing care of the client with an NGT.

Level of Cognitive Ability: Analysis
Phase of Nursing Process: Analysis
Client Needs: Physiological Integrity
Content Area: Adult Health/Gastrointestinal

Reference

Lewis, S., Collier, I., & Heitkemper, M. (1996). *Medical-surgical nursing: Assessment and management of clinical problems* (4th ed.). St. Louis: Mosby–Year Book, pp. 1237–1238.

60. The nurse is performing nasotracheal suctioning of a client. The nurse interprets that the client is adequately tolerating the procedure if which of the following observations is made?

1 Secretions are becoming bloody.
2 Heart rate decreases from 78 to 54.
3 Coughing occurs with suctioning.
4 Skin color becomes cyanotic.

Answer: 3

Rationale: The nurse monitors for adverse effects of suctioning, which include cyanosis, excessively rapid or slow heart rate, or sudden development of bloody secretions. If they occur, the nurse stops suctioning and reports these signs to the physician immediately. Coughing is a normal response to suctioning for the client with an intact cough reflex and does not indicate that the client cannot tolerate the procedure.

Test-Taking Strategy: The wording of the question asks you to select an option that would be a normal or expected finding while suctioning a client. Cyanosis (option 4) and bradycardia (option 2) are abnormal findings and are eliminated first. Of the two remaining choices, the use of the word "became" in association with bloody secretions tells you that this is a new problem, making this an incorrect option also. Because the cough reflex is normally present, and suction triggers coughing, this is the preferable one of the two remaining options.

Level of Cognitive Ability: Analysis
Phase of Nursing Process: Analysis
Client Needs: Physiological Integrity
Content Area: Adult Health/Respiratory

Reference

Taylor, C., Lillis, C., & LeMone, P. (1997). *Fundamentals of nursing: The art and science of nursing care* (3rd ed.). Philadelphia: Lippincott-Raven, p. 1348.

61. The nurse is reading a client's urinalysis report. The nurse interprets that which of the following items found on the report is considered abnormal?

1 Negative glucose
2 Positive protein
3 pH 6.0
4 Specific gravity 1.018

Answer: 2

Rationale: The urine has a normal pH range of 4.5–8.0 and a specific gravity ranging from 1.010 to 1.025. The urine is typically screened for protein, glucose, ketones, bilirubin, casts, crystals, red blood cells, and white blood cells, all of which should be negative.

Test-Taking Strategy: It is necessary to know the normal urine pH and specific gravity to be able to eliminate options 3 and 4 as possible choices. Knowing that glucose and protein are larger molecules that do not usually spill into the urine helps you to choose option 2 as the abnormal value. If you had difficulty with this question, take time now to review normal urinalysis results.

Level of Cognitive Ability: Analysis
Phase of Nursing Process: Analysis
Client Needs: Physiological Integrity
Content Area: Adult Health/Renal

Reference

Black, J., & Matassarin-Jacobs, E. (1997). *Medical-surgical nursing: Clinical management for continuity of care* (5th ed.). Philadelphia: W. B. Saunders, pp. 1557–1558.

62. The client with AIDS has developed an opportunistic infection of *Pneumocystis carinii* pneumonia. The nurse recognizes that emotional support for the client and caregiver is important. Which of the following statements identifies the least likely purpose or need for emotional support?

1 Providing emotional support will decrease anxiety and improve breathing.
2 As the immune system deteriorates, focus of care is on quality of life issues.
3 The client will be less likely to infect family members with *P. carinii* pneumonia.
4 *P. carinii* pneumonia is associated with a high mortality rate.

Answer: 3

Rationale: Options 1, 2, and 4 are all correct statements. Reduced anxiety reduces oxygen demands. Nursing measures to promote quality of life include emotional support. *P. carinii* pneumonia is associated with a high mortality rate, 40% for the first episode, 75% for the second infection, and 100% if untreated. *P. carinii* pneumonia rarely occurs in a healthy individual.

Test-Taking Strategy: Read the stem of the question carefully. Note that it states the "least likely purpose of emotional support." Use the process of elimination. Option 3 is the only option that does not deal directly with the topic of emotional support. Additionally, options 1, 2, and 4 are all correct statements. If you had difficulty with this question, take time now to review the psychosocial impact associated with AIDS.

Level of Cognitive Ability: Analysis
Phase of Nursing Process: Analysis
Client Needs: Psychosocial Integrity
Content Area: Adult Health/Respiratory

Reference

Lewis, S., Collier, I., & Heitkemper, M. (1996). *Medical-surgical nursing: Assessment and management of clinical problems* (4th ed.). St. Louis: Mosby–Year Book, pp. 250–256, 626.

---

63. An adult client with internal fixation of a fractured femur 1 week ago asks the nurse when he can quit using a cane during ambulation. To respond, the nurse would recognize that

1 Full weight bearing may begin when there is radiographic confirmation of bony fracture fragment union.
2 The client may begin full weight bearing as pain tolerance dictates.
3 After callus formation is complete, the client may begin full weight bearing.
4 When full range of motion and muscle strength are achieved in the affected extremity, the client may begin full weight bearing.

Answer: 1

Rationale: A fractured femur may require up to 20 weeks to heal in an adult. Full weight bearing is permitted as soon as bony union is present. Ambulation with a cane requires at least partial to full weight-bearing status. Full weight bearing is usually restricted until there is radiographic evidence of bony union of the fracture fragments. Callus formation is too weak and the fracture site may refracture with full weight bearing. The stage of fracture healing dictates the amount of weight bearing, not range of motion, muscle strength, or pain.

Test-Taking Strategy: Knowledge of the stages of fracture healing and the various treatments is helpful in answering the question. Use the process of elimination to answer the question. Note that option 1 is the only option that identifies a confirmation of bony union, which would allow the client to bear weight safely. If you had difficulty with this question, take time now to review the stages of fracture healing and the rehabilitation process associated with a fractured femur.

Level of Cognitive Ability: Analysis
Phase of Nursing Process: Analysis
Client Needs: Physiological Integrity
Content Area: Adult Health/Musculoskeletal

Reference

Black, J., & Matassarin-Jacobs, E. (1997). *Medical-surgical nursing: Clinical management for continuity of care* (5th ed.). Philadelphia: W. B. Saunders, p. 2145.

64. Iron dextran (Infed) intramuscularly is prescribed for the client. The nurse prepares the medication and determines that the most appropriate method to administer the medication is via z-track injection. The nurse bases this determination on the fact that this technique is used to

1 Promote drug absorption and inhibit hematoma formation.
2 Prevent skin discoloration by preventing drug seepage.
3 Reduce allergic reactions at the injection site.
4 Administer more than one drug at a single site.

Answer: 2

Rationale: A disadvantage of administering intramuscular iron dextran is that it causes pain and discoloration at the injection site. When intramuscular administration is prescribed, it should be injected deep into the buttock using the z-track technique. Z-track injection keeps the iron dextran deep in the muscle, thereby minimizing leakage and surface discoloration. The z-track technique is used for medications that can stain or irritate the skin.

Test-Taking Strategy: Knowledge regarding the administration of iron dextran is required to answer the question. If you can remember that oral iron preparations stain the teeth, you can, by the process of elimination, select option 2 as the correct answer. If you had difficulty with this question, take time now to review the technique for the administration of intramuscular iron dextran.

Level of Cognitive Ability: Analysis
Phase of Nursing Process: Analysis
Client Needs: Safe, Effective Care Environment
Content Area: Pharmacology

Reference
Lehne, R. A. (1998). *Pharmacology for nursing care* (3rd ed.). Philadelphia: W. B. Saunders, p. 557.

65. The client is to receive medication via patient-controlled analgesia (PCA). The nurse determines that the PCA does not provide for which of the following?

1 PCA enables the client to titrate analgesia.
2 PCA delivers predetermined amounts of analgesia at preset intervals.
3 PCA infusion is initiated by the client, who programs a pump.
4 PCA provides a continuous intravenous solution to keep the vein open between analgesia infusions.

Answer: 3

Rationale: PCA involves the use of a programmed syringe pump that delivers predetermined amounts of analgesia at preset intervals. PCA enables the client to titrate analgesics to maintain a consistent serum level of narcotic rather than experience the peaks and troughs that occur with PRN (as-needed) injections. The pump is programmed by nursing staff as prescribed by the physician. The client has an intravenous infusion running to keep the vein open between analgesia infusions.

Test-Taking Strategy: Knowledge regarding the PCA is required to answer the question. Read the stem of the question carefully, noting the phrase "does not provide." Try to visualize the PCA and its use by the client. Read the wording in the options carefully. Remembering that a client would not program the pump should direct you to the correct option for this question as stated. If you had difficulty answering this question, take time now to review PCA.

Level of Cognitive Ability: Analysis
Phase of Nursing Process: Analysis
Client Needs: Safe, Effective Care Environment
Content Area: Pharmacology

Reference
Lehne, R. A. (1998). *Pharmacology for nursing care* (3rd ed.). Philadelphia: W. B. Saunders, pp. 245–246.

66. The nurse caring for neonates is aware that drug toxicity is more likely to occur in the neonate because

1 The lungs are not developed.
2 The kidneys are smaller than in an adult.
3 Cerebral function is not fully developed.
4 The liver is immature.

Answer: 4

Rationale: The increased medication sensitivity of neonates and infants is due largely to the immature state of five pharmacokinetic processes. These include drug absorption, renal drug excretion, hepatic drug metabolism, protein binding of drugs, and exclusion of drugs from the central nervous system by the blood-brain barrier.

Test-Taking Strategy: Use the process of elimination in answering the question. Knowledge regarding the characteristics of a neonate assists in answering the question. The key word in the correct option is "immature." If you had difficulty with this question, take time now to review the characteristics of a neonate.

Level of Cognitive Ability: Analysis
Phase of Nursing Process: Analysis
Client Needs: Physiological Integrity
Content Area: Pharmacology

Reference

Lehne, R. A. (1998). *Pharmacology for nursing care* (3rd ed.). Philadelphia: W. B. Saunders, pp. 85–86.

---

67. A client with myasthenia gravis is experiencing prolonged periods of weakness. The physician orders a test dose of edrophonium (Tensilon), and the client becomes weaker. The nurse analyzes the results of the test dose as indicative of

1 Normal status.
2 Positive reaction.
3 Myasthenia crisis.
4 Cholinergic crisis.

Answer: 4

Rationale: Tensilon is administered to differentiate overdose of medication (cholinergic crisis) from worsening symptoms of the disease (myasthenic crisis). In cholinergic crisis, muscle tone does not improve after the administration of Tensilon. Instead, weakness may actually increase, and fasciculations (muscle twitching) may be noted around the eyes and face. The Tensilon test poses a danger of ventricular fibrillation and cardiac arrest, although these rarely occur. Atropine sulfate is the antidote for Tensilon and must be available for these complications.

Test-Taking Strategy: Knowledge regarding the Tensilon test is required to answer the question. This is an important test to understand, and you are likely to find questions related to this test on NCLEX-RN. If you had difficulty with this question, take time now to review this important test.

Level of Cognitive Ability: Analysis
Phase of Nursing Process: Analysis
Client Needs: Physiological Integrity
Content Area: Pharmacology

Reference

Ignatavicius, D. D., Workman, M. L., & Mishler, M. A. (1995). *Medical-surgical nursing: A nursing process approach* (2nd ed.). Philadelphia: W. B. Saunders, p. 1223.

---

68. Which of the following assessment data would the nurse analyze as a potential complication associated with Buerger's disease?

1 Discomfort in one digit
2 Cramping in the foot while resting
3 Pain with diaphoresis
4 Numbness and tingling in the legs

Answer: 4

Rationale: Buerger's disease (thromboangiitis obliterans), which affects men between 20 and 40 years of age, has an unknown etiology. It is a recurring inflammation of the small and medium-sized arteries and veins of the upper and lower extremities that results in thrombus formation and occlusion of blood vessels. Option 1 could be an early sign of the disease but probably would not be noticed by the client at this stage, and it is not a complication of the disorder. Option 2 is incorrect because cramping in the legs and feet occurs when exercising and is relieved after rest. Option 3 is neither a complication of the disorder nor a symptom. The most likely assessment data that can be interpreted as a complication of the disorder are numbness and tingling in the legs.

Test-Taking Strategy: This question assesses knowledge of the clinical manifestations associated with Buerger's disease. Read the stem of the question carefully, noting that it is asking for a complication associated with the disorder. Use the ABCs when answering the question. If you had difficulty with this question, take time now to review the complications associated with Buerger's disease.

Level of Cognitive Ability: Analysis
Phase of Nursing Process: Analysis
Client Needs: Physiological Integrity
Content Area: Adult Health/Cardiovascular

Reference

Black, J., & Matassarin-Jacobs, E. (1997). *Medical-surgical nursing: Clinical management for continuity of care* (5th ed.). Philadelphia: W. B. Saunders, pp. 1430–1431.

69. A 9-year-old child with diabetes is attending a band concert in the school gym. The child becomes flushed, hungry, and dizzy. The child goes to the nurse's office, and the nurse performs a blood glucose level that measures 60 mg/dL. The nurse analyzes the assessment data and determines that the most appropriate intervention is

1 Have the child call home to talk to Mom.
2 Contact the health care provider listed on the emergency card.
3 Make sure the child drinks a glass of orange juice.
4 Tell the child to return to the concert.

Answer: 3

Rationale: The child is attending an activity that is different from the normal routine at school. Insulin requirements change with unfamiliar situations. When signs of hypoglycemia occur, the child needs an immediate source of sugar. Options 1 and 2 do not address the hypoglycemic state immediately. Returning to the concert ignores treating the hypoglycemic state.

Test-Taking Strategy: Identify the issue of the question, which is a hypoglycemic state, and the key phrase "most appropriate." The stem of the question is requiring you to interpret the situation as a hypoglycemic state. Options 1 and 2 may be done later but not immediately. Option 4, sending the client back to the concert, may occur after an appropriate intervention is performed. If you had difficulty with this question, take time now to review the assessment data associated with hypoglycemia.

Level of Cognitive Ability: Application
Phase of Nursing Process: Analysis
Client Needs: Physiological Integrity
Content Area: Child Health

Reference

Pillitteri, A. (1995). *Maternal and child health: Nursing care of the childbearing and childrearing family* (2nd ed.). Philadelphia: Lippincott-Raven, p. 1506.

70. The nurse is caring for a client after a colonoscopy. The nurse monitors the client's temperature and notices a sudden temperature elevation. The nurse interprets that this finding may be associated with which potential complication of the procedure?

1 A nosocomial infection
2 Perforation of the intestine
3 Severe dehydration
4 Internal hemorrhage

Answer: 2

Rationale: Perforation of the gastrointestinal wall is a potential complication of any endoscopic procedure. Signs of perforation include abdominal pain, bleeding, and fever. Temperature elevation does not usually accompany internal hemorrhage. The temperature may be elevated with both severe dehydration and a nosocomial infection, but the potential complication that can occur with this procedure is perforation of the intestine.

Test-Taking Strategy: Read the stem of the question carefully, noting that the issue is a potential complication of colonoscopy. Use the process of elimination to answer the question, and note the similarity of "*colon*oscopy" and perforation of the "intestines." If you had difficulty with this question, take time now to review the complications of colonoscopy.

Level of Cognitive Ability: Analysis
Phase of Nursing Process: Analysis
Client Needs: Physiological Integrity
Content Area: Adult Health/Gastrointestinal

Reference

Ignatavicius, D. D., Workman, M. L., & Mishler, M. A. (1995). *Medical-surgical nursing: A nursing process approach* (2nd ed.). Philadelphia: W. B. Saunders, p. 1509.

71. A client has tested positive for HIV antibody. The CD4+ T cell count is 190/μL. Which of the following nursing diagnoses best identifies a potential problem for this client?

1. Risk for Infection related to immunodeficiency
2. Activity Intolerance related to weakness, fatigue
3. Risk for Constipation related to decreased fluid intake
4. Impaired Skin Integrity related to Kaposi's sarcoma

Answer: 1

Rationale: Clients who test positive for HIV antibody are at risk for opportunistic infection. As the CD4+ T cell count falls, the client's risk for infection increases. A CD4+ T cell count of less than 200/μL is an AIDS indicator. AIDS diagnosis is made, in part, on the basis of decreased immune function and signs and symptoms of opportunistic infection. Clients with HIV infection or AIDS commonly are afflicted with diarrhea, not constipation. Options 2 and 4 are incorrect because they describe actual rather than potential problems.

Test-Taking Strategy: When answering questions about actual or potential problems, remember that "risk" problems are potential, not actual. Actual problems generally take higher priority than potential problems. This question asks for a potential problem, however, so options 2 and 4 can be eliminated. An understanding of AIDS would direct you to select option 1 over option 3. If you had difficulty with this question, take time now to review the potential problems associated with AIDS.

Level of Cognitive Ability: Analysis
Phase of Nursing Process: Analysis
Client Needs: Physiological Integrity
Content Area: Adult Health/Respiratory

Reference

Polaski, A., & Tatro, S. (1996). *Luckmann's Core principles and practice of medical-surgical nursing.* Philadelphia: W. B. Saunders, pp. 185–191.

---

72. A 42-year-old client diagnosed with acute viral hepatitis 4 months ago continues to have clinical manifestations of the disease. The client asks, "When will I be able to return to work? I can't stand being tired and not being able to do anything." The spouse confides to the nurse that the client has started drinking a couple of beers every day. The nurse would formulate which of the following nursing diagnoses as most appropriate?

1. Hopelessness related to chronic disease state manifested by despondency
2. Ineffective Individual Coping related to fatigue and inactivity manifested by alcohol use
3. Caregiver Role Strain related to caring for a family member with alcohol addiction
4. Activity Intolerance related to fatigue manifested by the inability to work

Answer: 2

Rationale: Clients with chronic illness often experience feelings of anger and depression. Manifestations of chronic hepatitis include profound fatigue resulting in an inability to pursue normal daily activities. Ineffective coping involves inappropriate use of defense mechanisms (alcohol consumption). It may also include the inability to meet role expectations (working). The destructive use of alcohol contributes to the client's illness and rehabilitation time and further prolongs fatigue and the inability to work. Options 1, 3, and 4 are incorrect. Hopelessness involves the perception that there are no possible solutions to the situation. The client of the question is not the spouse, making option 3 incorrect. Activity Intolerance is relevant; however, this will persist longer if coping styles are not addressed.

Test-Taking Strategy: Determine the client of the question. This would eliminate option 3. Look for the global response. Option 2 includes inactivity, fatigue, alcohol use, and the major problem of ineffective individual coping. Thus, you would choose this option over options 1 and 4, which do not address the concern as described in the question.

Level of Cognitive Ability: Analysis
Phase of Nursing Process: Analysis
Client Needs: Psychosocial Integrity
Content Area: Adult Health/Gastrointestinal

Reference

Ignatavicius, D. D., Workman, M. L., & Mishler, M. A. (1995). *Medical-surgical nursing: A nursing process approach* (2nd ed.). Philadelphia: W. B. Saunders, pp. 1689–1690.

73. A toddler comes into the day care center with "slap marks" on the cheeks and circumoral paleness. Based on these data, the nurse interprets that the initial action would be to

1 Call the supervisor and discuss reporting it to the police for possible child abuse.
2 Complete the assessment and monitor for a fading rash on the trunk.
3 Question the mother about pouring hot water on the toddler's face.
4 Ask the mother to step outside while the examination is completed.

Answer: 2

Rationale: Complete a thorough assessment before deciding on the appropriate nursing intervention. Calling the supervisor before a thorough assessment has been completed and reporting it to police is inappropriate and possibly unfair to the parent. A toddler would become very upset if Mom is asked to step outside (separation anxiety).

Test-Taking Strategy: Use the process of elimination to answer the question. Use the nursing process remembering that assessment is the first step. This should assist in directing you to the correct option.

Level of Cognitive Ability: Application
Phase of Nursing Process: Analysis
Client Needs: Physiological Integrity
Content Area: Child Health

Reference

Wong, D. (1997). *Whaley and Wong's Essentials of pediatric nursing* (5th ed.). St. Louis: Mosby–Year Book, p. 1745.

---

74. A client who has just been diagnosed with a sliding hiatal hernia is being discharged from the outpatient diagnostic area. The client tells the nurse about the concern related to employment. A major responsibility of work involves "wining and dining" customers. The most appropriate response after interpretation of these data is which of the following?

1 "You'd be smart to look for other employment."
2 "Perhaps you could do more lunchtime entertaining."
3 "You should be able to eat all you want as long as you avoid alcohol."
4 "This hiatal hernia doesn't require any lifestyle changes."

Answer: 2

Rationale: Nocturnal attacks of reflux from hiatal hernias are common, especially if the person has eaten near bedtime. Large meals, alcohol, and smoking may also precipitate attacks. Therefore, if the client did more entertaining earlier in the day, attacks might be decreased or eliminated.

Test-Taking Strategy: This question requires you to analyze the characteristics related to hiatal hernia. Use the process of elimination to select the correct response. Option 1 is not an appropriate suggestion for the nurse to make without further assessment of the client's socioeconomic status. Option 3 is incorrect because heavy meals precipitate attacks as does alcohol. Option 4 is incorrect because heavy meals, alcohol, and late meals are all factors that contribute to attacks. If you had difficulty with this question, take time now to review the characteristics associated with hiatal hernia.

Level of Cognitive Ability: Application
Phase of Nursing Process: Analysis
Client Needs: Health Promotion and Maintenance
Content Area: Adult Health/Gastrointestinal

Reference

Lewis, S., Collier, I., & Heitkemper, M. (1996). *Medical-surgical nursing: Assessment and management of clinical problems* (4th ed.). St. Louis: Mosby–Year Book, p. 1157.

75. The client with tuberculosis presents with cough, shortness of breath, and thick purulent secretions. The client stopped taking rifampin (Rifadin) and isoniazid (INH) because he was "feeling better." The client's spouse is crying uncontrollably, stating, "Don't let him die." The client states, "I need to get some sleep. I haven't slept in 3 days. I keep waking up coughing. Whatever is down there is stuck." Which of the following nursing diagnoses is most important for the nurse to address?

1 Ineffective Family Coping
2 Ineffective Airway Clearance
3 Sleep Pattern Disturbance
4 Noncompliance

Answer: 2

Rationale: The most important comment made by the client is "Whatever is down there is stuck." It is most important to maintain a clear airway and breathing. Options 1, 3, and 4 are important but should be addressed after adequate airway clearance is obtained.

Test-Taking Strategy: First determine the client in the question. This should assist in eliminating option 1. Although compliance and sleep may be a problem, the stem of the question is asking for the "most important" nursing diagnosis. Prioritize the client's problems by addressing the ABCs. Additionally, use Maslow's hierarchy of needs as a guide remembering that physiological needs come first.

Level of Cognitive Ability: Analysis
Phase of Nursing Process: Analysis
Client Needs: Physiological Integrity
Content Area: Adult Health/Respiratory

Reference

Polaski, A., & Tatro, S. (1996). *Luckmann's Core principles and practice of medical-surgical nursing.* Philadelphia: W. B. Saunders, pp. 593–595.

---

76. A client with Addison's disease makes all of the following statements. Which one does the nurse analyze as requiring further discussion?

1 "I wear a MedicAlert bracelet at all times."
2 "I need to weigh myself daily and record it."
3 "It's important that I drink enough fluids and increase my salt intake."
4 "I will not need to adjust my medication dose for any reason."

Answer: 4

Rationale: The client with Addison's disease is experiencing deficits of mineralocorticoids, glucocorticoids, and androgens. Aldosterone deficiency affects the ability of the nephrons to conserve sodium, so the client experiences sodium and fluid volume deficit. The client needs to manage this problem with daily hormone replacement and increased fluid and sodium intake. Clients are instructed to weigh themselves daily as a means of monitoring fluid volume balance. Glucocorticoids and mineralocorticoids are essential components of the stress response. Additional doses of hormone replacement therapy are needed with any type of physical or psychological stressor. This information needs to be conveyed to the client and requires that the client wear a MedicAlert bracelet so that health care professionals are aware of this problem if the client were to experience a medical emergency.

Test-Taking Strategy: The question asks you to select the response indicating that the client needs further instruction. Be careful with these types of questions and read them carefully or they can easily confuse you. Look for the option that is an inaccurate statement because this reflects the need for further education. Knowledge of client teaching needs related to the pharmacological management of Addison's disease assists you in answering this question correctly. The pharase "any reason" in option 4 is an absolute and indicates that this may be an incorrect statement. If you had difficulty with this question, take time now to review the treatment associated with Addison's disease.

Level of Cognitive Ability: Analysis
Phase of Nursing Process: Analysis
Client Needs: Physiological Integrity
Content Area: Adult Health/Endocrine

Reference

Black, J., & Matassarin-Jacobs, E. (1997). *Medical-surgical nursing: Clinical management for continuity of care* (5th ed.). Philadelphia: W. B. Saunders, p. 2043.

77. A newly admitted adult client with a fractured femur is placed in skin traction while awaiting surgery. The nurse recognizes that the traction is applied for which of the following purposes?

1. Inhibit bone ossification
2. Prevent hip contracture
3. Decrease muscle spasms
4. Resist peroneal nerve damage

Answer: 3

Rationale: Severe muscle spasms frequently accompany fractures, especially fractures of large bones. The traction helps to decrease these spasms. Ossification is the third stage of fracture healing and is not a purpose of traction. Hip contractures and peroneal nerve damage are complications of traction, not purposes for its application.

Test-Taking Strategy: Knowledge of the purposes of traction, fracture healing stages, and complications of balanced skeletal traction assists you in answering this question correctly. Read the question carefully noting that the question asks for the purpose of the traction. Use the process of elimination, carefully analyzing each option. If you had difficulty with this question, take time now to review the purposes of traction.

Level of Cognitive Ability: Analysis
Phase of Nursing Process: Analysis
Client Needs: Physiological Integrity
Content Area: Adult Health/Musculoskeletal

Reference

Ignatavicius, D. D., Workman, M. L., & Mishler, M. A. (1995). *Medical-surgical nursing: A nursing process approach* (2nd ed.). Philadelphia: W. B. Saunders, p. 1462.

---

78. A hospitalized toddler cries when anyone enters the room and kicks, yells, and clings to the parents if they try to leave. Based on these data, the nurse determines that the priority nursing diagnosis is

1. Anxiety/Fear related to unfamiliar surroundings.
2. Diversional Activity Deficit related to developmental stage.
3. Ineffective Family Coping related to the sick child.
4. Altered Growth and Development related to overprotective parenting.

Answer: 1

Rationale: A toddler derives comfort and security from familiar routines and people. The new sights, sounds, and smells are a source of anxiety during hospitalization. There is no evidence of ineffective coping, altered development, or diversional activity deficit.

Test-Taking Strategy: In test items requiring analysis, be careful not to read into the question. Use the process of elimination to answer the question. Use your knowledge of the nursing process, and look for the assessment data in the question that support the correct nursing diagnosis. Because there is no information supporting the diagnoses in options 2, 3, and 4, these options can be eliminated.

Level of Cognitive Ability: Analysis
Phase of Nursing Process: Analysis
Client Needs: Psychosocial Integrity
Content Area: Child Health

Reference

Wong, D. (1997). *Whaley and Wong's Essentials of pediatric nursing* (5th ed.). St. Louis: Mosby–Year Book, p. 651.

---

79. In analyzing the physiological assessment data of a client presenting with physical injuries and suspected family-related violence, the nurse must first consider

1. The assessment of the type and extent of presenting wounds.
2. The vital signs.
3. The evidence and extent of past injuries.
4. The client's explanations as to how the injuries occurred.

Answer: 2

Rationale: When analyzing data and prioritizing the care of a client suspected of having experienced family violence, the physiological well-being of the client is always considered first. Option 2 is the only option that directly addresses physiological assessment.

Test-Taking Strategy: Note the key words in the question, "physiological" and "first." This question asks for analysis and prioritization of nursing assessment findings. When analyzing data and prioritizing care, the emphasis is always placed on the physical condition. Use the ABCs as a guide in answering the question.

Level of Cognitive Ability: Analysis
Phase of Nursing Process: Analysis
Client Needs: Physiological Integrity
Content Area: Mental Health

Reference

Johnson, B. (1997). *Psychiatric–mental health nursing: Adaptation and growth.* (4th ed.). Philadelphia: Lippincott-Raven, p. 813.

---

80. During an initial assessment of a maternity client, the nurse notes that the laboratory report shows leukopenia, thrombocytopenia, anemia, and an elevated erythrocyte sedimentation rate. The nurse suspects HIV. Which of the following laboratory tests would further support the presence of HIV?

1 T lymphocyte count
2 Angiotensin
3 Glomerular filtration rate
4 Platelet count

Answer: 1

Rationale: HIV has a strong affinity for surface marker proteins on lymphocytes. This affinity of HIV for T lymphocytes leads to significant cell destruction. Angiotensin is produced in the kidney and plays a role in blood pressure control. Glomerular filtration rate indicates kidney function. The platelet count is important and may be used as an indicator of HIV, but the platelet count (thrombocytopenia) has already been addressed in the question.

Test-Taking Strategy: Read the question carefully and use the process of elimination to answer the question. Option 4 has already been identified in the question and can be eliminated. Options 2 and 3 are alike in that they both relate to kidney function. If you had difficulty with this question, review the clinical manifestations and pathology of HIV now.

Level of Cognitive Ability: Analysis
Phase of Nursing Process: Analysis
Client Needs: Physiological Integrity
Content Area: Maternity

Reference

Lowdermilk, D., Perry, S., & Bobak, I. (1997). *Maternity and women's health care* (6th ed.). St. Louis: Mosby–Year Book, p. 735.

---

81. A 9-month-old is admitted to the pediatric unit with a diagnosis of dehydration and malnutrition; rule out failure to thrive. The client weighs 10 pounds, 9 ounces. Child neglect is suspected. Which of the following would be most important for the nurse to observe and analyze during family visiting?

1 The parents' level of concern about the child
2 The parents' patterns of visitation
3 The parents' interactions with one another
4 Clues regarding the nutritional patterns of the other children in the family

Answer: 1

Rationale: Although signs of abusive parents are not always easily identified, there are some behavioral characteristics that emerge. These include a lack of concern for the child's well-being, unreasonable punishments, high demands and unrealistic expectations for the child, and a view of the child as a small adult who can meet his or her personal needs. Assessment of the parents in their role may give the nurse clues as to the family dynamics and assist in determining the educational needs of the parents.

Test-Taking Strategy: The most helpful observations when child abuse is suspected are observations made between the parents and the child. Identify the client of the question. In options 2, 3, and 4, the focus of the assessment does not include the 9-month-old client. If you had difficulty with this question, take time now to review the characteristics of abusing parents.

Level of Cognitive Ability: Analysis
Phase of Nursing Process: Analysis
Client Needs: Psychosocial Integrity
Content Area: Child Health

Reference

Johnson, B. (1997). *Psychiatric–mental health nursing: Adaptation and growth.* (4th ed.). Philadelphia: Lippincott-Raven, pp. 699–700.

82. The client with an endotracheal tube (ETT) gets easily frustrated when trying to communicate personal needs to the nurse. The nurse interprets that which of the following methods for communication may be the easiest for the client?

1 Have the family interpret needs
2 Use a picture or word board
3 Use a pad and paper
4 Devise a system of hand signals

Answer: 2

Rationale: The client with an ETT in place cannot speak. The nurse devises an alternative communication system with the client. Use of a picture or word board is the simplest method of communication because it requires only pointing at the word or object. A pad and pencil is an acceptable alternative, but it requires more client effort and more time. The use of hand signals may not be a reliable method because it may not meet all needs and is subject to misinterpretation. The family should not bear the burden of communicating the client's needs, especially because they may not understand them either.

Test-Taking Strategy: This question is most easily answered by focusing on the words "easily frustrated" and "easiest." Options 3 and 4 are obviously not the "easiest" and are therefore eliminated first. Because the family may not necessarily know what the client is trying to communicate, this option could cause added frustration for the client. By elimination, the picture or word board is the easiest and the least frustrating for the client.

Level of Cognitive Ability: Analysis
Phase of Nursing Process: Analysis
Client Needs: Psychosocial Integrity
Content Area: Adult Health/Respiratory

Reference

Black, J., & Matassarin-Jacobs, E. (1997). *Medical-surgical nursing: Clinical management for continuity of care* (5th ed.). Philadelphia: W. B. Saunders, p. 1175.

---

83. A pregnant woman reports that she has just finished taking prescribed antibiotics for a urinary tract infection (UTI). Which response would the nurse consider to help reduce client fears that her newborn will be born with an infection?

1 "Urinary infections during pregnancy are common. Your baby will be fine."
2 "Your developing baby cannot acquire an infection from you during pregnancy."
3 "Now that you have finished the medication, we will continue to monitor you closely. Repeat the urine culture and review the signs of UTIs before you leave today."
4 "You shouldn't worry about this because you received early prenatal care and are taking your prenatal vitamins."

Answer: 3

Rationale: Symptomatic bacteriuria has been associated with an increased risk of neonatal sepsis after delivery. Appropriate antenatal care of a client with a UTI includes antibiotic treatment and follow-up of repeat cultures and client education.

Test-Taking Strategy: Use the process of communication to answer the question. The correct nursing communication in this situation includes supporting the client's positive behaviors and providing accurate information to help alleviate her concerns. The other options do not realistically address her concerns and hinder further communication between nurse and client.

Level of Cognitive Ability: Application
Phase of Nursing Process: Analysis
Clients Needs: Psychosocial Integrity
Content Area: Maternity

Reference

Reeder, S., Martin, L., & Koniak-Griffin, D. (1997). *Maternity nursing: Family, newborn and women's health care* (18th ed.). Philadelphia: Lippincott-Raven, pp. 1206–1207.

84. The client with Guillain-Barré syndrome asks the nurse what caused the disorder. In formulating a response, the nurse incorporates the understanding that current theories of causation include

1 Mycobacterial infection, nervous system infection, or an unknown cause.
2 Bacterial infection, previous central nervous system injury, or both.
3 Fungal infection, autoimmune disorder, or an unknown cause.
4 Viral infection, autoimmune disorder, some other process, or a combination of these.

Answer: 4

Rationale: Current thinking regarding causation of Guillain-Barré syndrome is that it is caused by a primary viral infection, an immune reaction, some other unidentified cause, or a combination of any of these factors.

Test-Taking Strategy: Options 1 and 3 are the least plausible of all the options and should therefore be eliminated first. Recalling that a popular theory for causation of some nervous system disorders involves the immune system and the role of viruses, you would choose option 4 over option 2. If you had difficulty with this question, take time now to review the causes associated with Guillain-Barré syndrome.

Level of Cognitive Ability: Analysis
Phase of Nursing Process: Analysis
Client Needs: Physiological Integrity
Content Area: Adult Health/Neurological

Reference
Smeltzer, S., & Bare, B. (1996). *Brunner and Suddarth's Textbook of medical-surgical nursing* (8th ed.). Philadelphia: Lippincott-Raven, p. 1820.

85. The nurse is caring for a client after thoracotomy. The client has a chest drainage tube. The nurse would interpret that which of the following findings should be reported to the physician immediately?

1 180 mL of fluid drained in the first hour postoperatively
2 Chest drainage that is grossly bloody directly after surgery
3 Scant bloody drainage on postoperative day 1, followed by increased bloody drainage
4 Rise and fall of fluid in the water seal compartment with inspiration and expiration

Answer: 3

Rationale: Scant or decreasing drainage followed by an increase in bloody drainage may indicate occurrence of a pathological process that may require surgical intervention. Always assess the client further for signs of bleeding or hemorrhagic shock. It is common to see up to 300 mL of drainage from the chest tube in the first postoperative hour. Grossly bloody drainage in the first few hours of surgery is normal. The drainage should become clearer after the initial few hours. Fluid should fluctuate with respiration. This is often called *tidaling*. If no fluctuation occurs, either the lungs have reexpanded or the system has malfunctioned.

Test-Taking Strategy: Read each option carefully, and use the process of elimination. Look for responses that address changes in the client's behavior or physical condition when questioned about the need for the nurse to notify the physician. Option 3 is the only option that describes a change from one condition to another.

Level of Cognitive Ability: Analysis
Phase of Nursing Process: Analysis
Client Needs: Physiological Integrity
Content Area: Adult Health/Respiratory

Reference
Polaski, A., & Tatro, S. (1996). *Luckmann's Core principles and practice of medical-surgical nursing.* Philadelphia: W. B. Saunders, p. 609.

86. A client underwent thoracotomy and right lobectomy 3 days ago. A right anterior chest tube is patent. The client has PCA infusing with morphine. Vital signs are blood pressure, 132/64 mmHg; heart rate, 86 beats/minute; respiratory rate, 22 breaths/minute; temperature, 98.8°F oral. Oxygen saturation is 96% with oxygen at 2 L/minute by nasal cannula. On nursing rounds the nurse assesses the surgical site. The client states, "It looks terrible." The client also states there is mild discomfort when doing range-of-motion exercises on the upper right arm and shoulder. The nurse determines that which of the following is the most relevant current nursing diagnosis?

1. Impaired Gas Exchange related to removal of right lung and ineffective cough
2. Pain related to tissue trauma, chest tube
3. Body Image Disturbance related to actual change in body structure and function
4. Activity Intolerance related to pain in right shoulder

Answer: 3

Rationale: The client is physiologically stable at this point in time with adequate oxygenation on current FIO_2. The client is able to perform range-of-motion exercises with only mild discomfort. Vital signs are within normal limits. Based on Maslow's hierarchy of needs, the client should be able to move from attending to basic needs to higher-level needs. Physiological needs are being met. It is important next to address psychosocial needs. The nurse needs to address Body Image Disturbance. People undergoing thoracotomy have large scars and loss of function related to actual tissue loss.

Test-Taking Strategy: When selecting the appropriate nursing diagnosis, identify the client data as stated in the question. This should guide you to the correct option. Additionally, prioritize client needs using Maslow's hierarchy of needs and the ABCs. When physiological needs are met, as in this situation, it is important to address psychological needs.

Level of Cognitive Ability: Analysis
Phase of Nursing Process: Analysis
Client Needs: Psychosocial Integrity
Content Area: Adult Health/Respiratory

Reference

Ignatavicius, D. D., Workman, M. L., & Mishler, M. A. (1995). *Medical-surgical nursing: A nursing process approach* (2nd ed.). Philadelphia: W. B. Saunders, pp. 746–747.

87. The client with cerebrovascular accident has episodes of coughing while swallowing liquids. The client has developed a temperature of 101°F, oxygen saturation of 92% (down from 97% previously), slight confusion, noticeable dyspnea, and bilateral rhonchi. The nurse interprets that these manifestations are compatible with a diagnosis of

1. Pulmonary edema.
2. Pulmonary embolism.
3. Bacterial pneumonia.
4. Aspiration.

Answer: 4

Rationale: Clinical signs and symptoms of aspiration include fever, dyspnea, crackles or rhonchi, decreased arterial oxygen levels, and confusion. The client may exhibit difficulty in managing saliva or may cough or choke while eating.

Test-Taking Strategy: The signs and symptoms identified in the question are not associated with pulmonary edema or embolism, so these possibilities are eliminated first. The key to answering this question lies in the correct interpretation of the client's coughing. "Coughing while swallowing liquids" points to aspiration as the cause.

Level of Cognitive Ability: Analysis
Phase of Nursing Process: Analysis
Client Needs: Physiological Integrity
Content Area: Adult Health/Neurological

Reference

Black, J., & Matassarin-Jacobs, E. (1997). *Medical-surgical nursing: Clinical management for continuity of care* (5th ed.). Philadelphia: W. B. Saunders, p. 799.

88. The nurse is monitoring the respiratory status of a client after insertion of a tracheostomy. The nurse understands that oxygen saturation measurements obtained by pulse oximetry may be inaccurate if the client has which of the following coexisting problems?

1 Hypotension
2 Fever
3 Respiratory failure
4 Epilepsy

Answer: 1

Rationale: Hypotension, shock, or the use of peripheral vasoconstricting medications may result in inaccurate pulse oximetry readings from impaired peripheral perfusion. Fever and epilepsy would not affect the accuracy of measurement. Respiratory failure would also not affect the accuracy of measurement, although the readings may be abnormally low.

Test-Taking Strategy: Recall that pulse oximetry measures oxygen saturation in blood flowing through the blood vessels in the periphery of the body. Inaccurate measurement may result from any factor that impairs blood flow through the periphery. Evaluating each of the options from this viewpoint helps you to select hypotension as the answer. Epilepsy and fever do not affect the readings adversely. To discriminate between the respiratory failure option and hypotension, look again at the stem. The question asks which item gives an inaccurate reading (not a low reading).

Level of Cognitive Ability: Analysis
Phase of Nursing Process: Analysis
Client Needs: Physiological Integrity
Content Area: Adult Health/Respiratory

Reference

Black, J., & Matassarin-Jacobs, E. (1997). *Medical-surgical nursing: Clinical management for continuity of care* (5th ed.). Philadelphia: W. B. Saunders, p. 1074.

---

89. The nurse in the emergency department is caring for a 28-year-old victim of sexual assault. The client's physical assessment is complete, and physical evidence has been collected. In analyzing the client's psychological reaction to the assault, the nurse notes that the client is withdrawn, fearful, anxious, confused, and at times physically immobile. These behaviors are interpreted by the nurse as

1 Normal reactions to a devastating event.
2 Evidence that the client is a high suicide risk.
3 Indicative of the need for inpatient psychiatric admission.
4 Symptoms of an impending psychotic break.

Answer: 1

Rationale: All of the symptoms noted in the stem of the question indicate a normal reaction to an intensely difficult crisis event. Although the client's initial reactions may be predictive of later problems, they do not indicate an abnormal initial response.

Test-Taking Strategy: The nurse must understand that there is a wide range of *normal* responses to dealing with devastating crisis events. During the acute phase of the rape crisis, the client can display a wide range of emotional and somatic responses. Use knowledge regarding client responses to devastating events and the process of elimination to answer the question. If you had difficulty with this question, take time now to review normal and abnormal client responses to dealing with devastating crisis events.

Level of Cognitive Ability: Analysis
Phase of Nursing Process: Analysis
Client Needs: Psychosocial Integrity
Content Area: Mental Health

Reference

Carson, V., & Arnold, E. (1996). *Mental health nursing: The nurse-patient journey.* Philadelphia: W. B. Saunders, pp. 1090–1092.

90. The nurse is caring for an HIV-positive pregnant woman during the 32nd gestational week clinic visit. The nurse analyzes the assessment data and documents which physical assessment finding as requiring further follow-up?

1 Increased lower extremity edema
2 Increased shortness of breath and bilateral rales
3 Active fetal movement
4 Total weight gain of 22 pounds

Answer: 2

Rationale: HIV infection in pregnant women may cause both maternal and fetal complications. Fetal compromise can occur because of premature rupture of membranes, preterm birth, or low birth weight. Potential maternal side effects during pregnancy include an increased risk of opportunistic infections (i.e., herpes simplex, cytomegalovirus, papillomavirus, toxoplasmosis. and *P. carinii*). Individuals with later stages of HIV are further susceptible to other invasive states, such as tuberculosis and a wide variety of bacterial infections. The information in option 2, increased shortness of breath and bilateral rales, should be followed up by additional questioning (i.e., cough, temperature, mucus production) and testing (i.e., potential sputum analysis, chest x-ray).

Test-Taking Strategy: This question relies on the ability to apply the knowledge of the normal physiological status of the pregnant woman during the third trimester of care. Use the process of elimination, and eliminate options 1, 3, and 4 because these are normal findings. Additionally, using the ABCs directs you to the correct option.

Level of Cognitive Ability: Application
Phase of Nursing Process: Analysis
Clients Needs: Physiological Integrity
Content Area: Maternity

Reference
Nichols, F., & Zwelling, E. (1997). *Maternal-newborn nursing: Theory and practice.* Philadelphia: W. B. Saunders, p. 685.

91. Skin lesions, rashes, and pruritus are frequent symptoms of many systemic communicable diseases experienced by unimmunized children. Which nursing diagnosis statement best identifies the acute potential problem commonly shared by these children?

1 Altered Family Processes related to a child with an acute illness
2 High Risk for Infection related to susceptible host and infectious agents
3 High Risk for Impaired Skin Integrity related to scratching from pruritus
4 Impaired Social Interaction related to isolation from peers

Answer: 3

Rationale: The best option focuses on the acute skin manifestations as stated in the question. There are no data that support options 1 and 4. Option 2 is a diagnosis shared by all of these children because the lack of immunization is a contributing factor. Option 3, the correct option, supports the assessment data identified in the question.

Test-Taking Strategy: The key words here are "acute" and "potential." Use the process of elimination. Options 1 and 4 are actual nursing diagnoses, whereas options 2 and 3 are potential nursing diagnoses. Option 3 supports the assessment data identified in the question. Any option without supporting data in the question should be eliminated.

Level of Cognitive Ability: Analysis
Phase of Nursing Process: Analysis
Client Needs: Physiological Integrity
Content Area: Child Health

Reference
Wong, D. (1997). *Whaley and Wong's Essentials of pediatric nursing* (5th ed.). St. Louis: Mosby–Year Book, p. 412.

92. The nurse is speaking with a group of family members at a local support group regarding the importance of medication compliance. The nurse understands that which of the following may not be feasible to increase medication compliance?

1 Working with the psychiatrist to find the right drug at the right dose that provides the fewest side effects for the client
2 Giving all drugs just once per day
3 Providing clients with the injectable, long-acting form of the drug
4 Including the family in the medication planning process so that compliance can be reinforced at home

Answer: 2

Rationale: Finding the right drug at the right dose that provides the fewest side effects for the client; providing clients with the injectable, long-acting form of the drug; and including the family in the medication planning process are measures that promote compliance. Not all medications can be given on a once-per-day dosing regimen because of the short half-life. Lithium is an example of one such drug that must be dosed throughout the day to maintain steady serum drug levels.

Test-Taking Strategy: Be cautious of words such as "all," "none," "always," and "never." These imply that there are no exceptions, and these words usually indicate an incorrect option. In the case of this question, not "all" drugs may be dosed once a day because of their short half-life. Therefore, it is not appropriate to give all medications once per day.

Level of Cognitive Ability: Analysis
Phase of Nursing Process: Analysis
Client Needs: Psychosocial Integrity
Content Area: Mental Health

Reference

Carson, V., & Arnold, E. (1996). *Mental health nursing: The nurse-patient journey.* Philadelphia: W. B. Saunders, pp. 518, 546, 562–564.

---

93. Which of the following data would indicate a potential complication in a client with AIDS who is receiving intravenous pentamidine isethionate (Pentam)?

1 A hemoglobin of 15 g/dL
2 A blood glucose of 40 mg/dL
3 A coagulation time of 5 minutes
4 A platelet count of 160,000 cells/μL

Answer: 2

Rationale: Pentamidine causes severe hypoglycemia that may be fatal. A blood glucose of 40 mg/dL indicates that the client is hypoglycemic. Normal fasting blood glucose values are 60–120 mg/dL. A hemoglobin of 15 g/dL is a normal value. The normal hemoglobin range in women is 12–16 g/dL and in men is 14–18 g/dL. A coagulation time of 5 minutes is normal. The normal coagulation range is 1–9 minutes. A platelet count of 160,000 cells/μL is normal. The normal platelet range is 150,000–400,000 cells/μL.

Test-Taking Strategy: Knowledge of the normal values for blood glucose, hemoglobin, coagulation time, and platelet count assists in answering the question. By the process of elimination, you would be able to determine that a blood glucose of 40 mg/dL was not normal. Additionally, if you knew that severe hypoglycemia is a side effect of pentamidine, you would be able to select the correct option. If you had difficulty with this question, take time now to review pentamidine isethionate.

Level of Cognitive Ability: Analysis
Phase of Nursing Process: Analysis
Client Needs: Physiological Integrity
Content Area: Pharmacology

Reference

Ignatavicius, D. D., Workman, M. L., & Mishler, M. A. (1995). *Medical-surgical nursing: A nursing process approach* (2nd ed.). Philadelphia: W. B. Saunders, pp. 510–511, 1034–1035, 1869.

94. The nurse is caring for a client with pneumonia who has a history of bleeding esophageal varices. Based on this information, the nurse analyzes the need to prevent

1 Pain and nausea.
2 Nausea and activity.
3 Pain and diarrhea.
4 Constipation and coughing.

Answer: 4

Rationale: Increased intrathoracic pressure contributes to rupturing of varices. Straining at stool, coughing, and vomiting all increase intrathoracic pressure. The nurse needs to implement measures to prevent increased intrathoracic pressure.

Test-Taking Strategy: Use knowledge of esophageal varices to determine the potential complications that can occur. Use the process of elimination to answer the question. Remember, when an option contains two components, both components must be correct. If you had difficulty with this question, take time now to review measures to prevent the rupturing of varices.

Level of Cognitive Ability: Analysis
Phase of Nursing Process: Analysis
Client Needs: Physiological Integrity
Content Area: Adult Health/Gastrointestinal

Reference

Black, J., & Matassarin-Jacobs, E. (1997). *Medical-surgical nursing: Clinical management for continuity of care* (5th ed.). Philadelphia: W. B. Saunders, p. 1884.

95. In reviewing the admission assessment data and physician's orders for the client with peptic ulcer disease, the nurse notes that the client has a history of renal disease. The nurse realizes that the appropriate antacid for the client is

1 Aluminum hydroxide (Amphojel).
2 Magnesium hydroxide (MOM).
3 Aluminum/magnesium combination (Maalox).
4 Calcium carbonate (Tums).

Answer: 1

Rationale: Aluminum hydroxide lowers serum phosphate by binding with dietary phosphorus to form insoluble aluminum phosphate. The phosphate is then excreted in feces. Aluminum hydroxide does not affect the renal system as much as other antacids.

Test-Taking Strategy: Knowledge regarding the absorption and excretion of these medications is required to answer this question. The medications identified in options 2, 3, and 4 are partially excreted by the kidneys and therefore may cause a problem in clients with renal disease. If you had difficulty with this question, take time now to review these medications.

Level of Cognitive Ability: Analysis
Phase of Nursing Process: Analysis
Client Needs: Physiological Integrity
Content Area: Pharmacology

Reference

Black, J., & Matassarin-Jacobs, E. (1997). *Medical-surgical nursing: Clinical management for continuity of care* (5th ed.). Philadelphia: W. B. Saunders, p. 1769.

96. The client with tuberculosis has taken isoniazid (INH) for the past 2 weeks. The client calls to request different medication because of complaints of headache, sweating, and lightheadedness. The client has been trying to take adequate nutrition by eating protein in the form of tuna and aged cheese. The client has been taking the medication on an empty stomach. Based on the interpretation of these findings, the nurse makes which of the following most accurate nursing diagnoses?

1 Noncompliance related to taking medications on an empty stomach
2 Altered Comfort, Pain manifested by headache
3 Altered Health Maintenance related to insufficient knowledge of medication interactions
4 Risk for Infection related to discontinuation of medication

Answer: 3

Rationale: INH interacts with foods containing tyramine and histamine, such as tuna and aged cheese. These foods should be avoided. Common manifestations include headache, diaphoresis, lightheadedness, and hypotension. Medication should be taken on an empty stomach. The client's complaints of headache are real; however, this nursing diagnosis, option 2, focuses on a symptom rather than the cause of the symptom and must be eliminated as a possible answer. The client did not discontinue the medication, making option 4 incorrect.

Test-Taking Strategy: In selecting the correct nursing diagnosis, identify the information in the question that best supports the nursing diagnosis as stated in the option. Eliminate option 1 because the client has been taking the medications on an empty stomach. Eliminate option 2 because this nursing diagnosis focuses on a symptom rather than the cause of the symptom. The client did not discontinue the medication, making option 4 incorrect.

Level of Cognitive Ability: Analysis
Phase of Nursing Process: Analysis
Client Needs: Physiological Integrity
Content Area: Adult Health/Respiratory

Reference

Polaski, A., & Tatro, S. (1996). *Luckmann's Core principles and practice of medical-surgical nursing.* Philadelphia: W. B. Saunders, p. 591.

---

97. The nurse palpates the anterior fontanel of the neonate and notes it as feeling soft. The nurse analyzes assessment data as indicative of

1 Increased intracranial pressure.
2 Dehydration.
3 Decreased intracranial pressure.
4 A normal finding.

Answer: 4

Rationale: The anterior fontanel is normally 2.5–4 cm in width and diamond-like in shape. It can be described as soft, which is normal, or full and bulging, which could be indicative of increased intracranial pressure. Conversely, a depressed fontanel could mean that the neonate is dehydrated.

Test-Taking Strategy: Knowledge regarding normal findings in a neonate is required to answer the question. Use the process of elimination to assist in directing you to the correct option. Remember that the anterior fontanel is soft in the neonate. If you had difficulty answering this question, take time now to review normal neonatal assessment findings.

Level of Cognitive Ability: Analysis
Phase of Nursing Process: Analysis
Client Needs: Physiological Integrity
Content Area: Maternity

Reference

Nichols, F., & Zwelling, E. (1997). *Maternal-newborn nursing: Theory and practice.* Philadelphia: W. B. Saunders, p. 1104.

---

98. The nurse assesses the water seal chamber of a closed chest drainage system and notes fluctuations in the chamber. The nurse analyzes this finding as indicative of which of the following?

1 An air leak is present.
2 The tubing is kinked.
3 The lung has reexpanded.
4 The system is functioning as expected.

Answer: 4

Rationale: Fluctuations (tidaling) in the water seal chamber are normal during inhalation and exhalation. Fluctuations of 5–10 cm (2–4 inches) during normal breathing are common. The absence of fluctuations could mean that the tubing is obstructed by a kink, the client is lying on the tubing, or dependent fluid has filled a loop of tubing. Expanded lung tissue can also block the chest tube eyelets during expiration. The absence of fluctuations could also mean that air is no longer leaking into the pleural space.

Test-Taking Strategy: Knowledge of the functioning of the chest tube drainage system is required to answer the question. If you had difficulty with this question and are unsure of the nursing care related to chest tube drainage systems, stop now, and review this information.

Level of Cognitive Ability: Analysis
Phase of Nursing Process: Analysis
Client Needs: Physiological Integrity
Content Area: Adult Health/Respiratory

Reference

Ignatavicius, D. D., Workman, M. L., & Mishler, M. A. (1995). *Medical-surgical nursing: A nursing process approach* (2nd ed.). Philadelphia: W. B. Saunders, p. 748.

---

99. A mother tells the nurse that her child does not want anything to do with toilet training and yells "no" consistently when she tries to toilet train. The child is 2 years old. According to Erikson, the nurse interprets that the child is experiencing which of the following psychosocial crises?

1 Autonomy versus Shame and Doubt
2 Initiative versus Guilt
3 Industry versus Inferiority
4 Trust versus Mistrust

Answer: 1

Rationale: The crisis of Autonomy versus Shame and Doubt is related to the developmental task of gaining control of self and environment as exemplified by toilet training. Initiative versus Guilt is the crisis of the preschool and early school-age child. Initiative versus Inferiority is the crisis of the 6- to 12-year-old, and Trust versus Mistrust is the crisis of the infant.

Test-Taking Strategy: Knowledge regarding Erikson's stages of psychosocial development is required to answer the question. It is important to be familiar with these stages and the application to nursing assessment and practice. If you had difficulty with this question or are unfamiliar with these stages, take time now to review.

Level of Cognitive Ability: Analysis
Phase of Nursing Process: Analysis
Client Needs: Psychosocial Integrity
Content Area: Child Health

Reference

Ashwill, J., & Droske, S. (1997). *Nursing care of children: Principles and practice.* Philadelphia: W. B. Saunders, pp. 33–35.

---

100. Which of the following assessment data is an indicator of the Somogyi effect in a child with type I diabetes?

1 Glycosylated hemoglobin of 6.5 g/dL
2 Fasting blood glucose of 105 mg/dL
3 A 3:00 A.M. blood glucose of 60 mg/dL followed by a 7:00 A.M. blood glucose of 180 mg/dL
4 Fasting blood glucose of 90 mg/dL and a predinner blood glucose of 210 mg/dL

Answer: 3

Rationale: The Somogyi effect is a rebound hyperglycemia as a result of the secretion of counterregulatory hormones such as epinephrine, growth hormone, and corticosteroids. The 3:00 A.M. blood glucose is low followed by a high level a few hours later, demonstrating the rebound effect. Options 1 and 2 represent normal values. Options 3 and 4 are two-part answers. The fasting blood glucose in option 4 is within normal range but the predinner blood glucose is not.

Test-Taking Strategy: Knowledge of normal laboratory values and the definition of the Somogyi effect assists you in answering this question. If you did not know the definition of the term, the word "effect" should be a clue that the phenomenon is abnormal. Options 1 and 2 are normal levels, and a part of option 4 is within normal range. The process of elimination directs you to option 3, which is the only option that contains two abnormal levels. If you had difficulty with this question, take time now to review normal laboratory values and the description of the Somogyi effect.

Level of Cognitive Ability: Analysis
Phase of Nursing Process: Analysis
Client Needs: Physiological Integrity
Content Area: Child Health

Reference

Wong, D. (1995). *Whaley and Wong's Nursing care of infants and children* (5th ed.). St. Louis: Mosby–Year Book, p. 1772.

101. A client is a 15-year-old gravida I who is 14 weeks pregnant. She comes to the clinic for the first prenatal visit. During the interview, the nurse discovers that the client has been an insulin-dependent diabetic since the age of 9. She tells the nurse, "I'm trying not to eat much so I won't show. I have cut out my insulin so it is okay that I don't eat." The nurse formulates which of the following as the most important nursing diagnosis at this time?

1 Body Image Disturbance related to fear of gaining weight
2 Altered Nutrition: Less Than Body Requirements related to voluntary decrease in food intake
3 Risk for Impaired Skin Integrity related to skin stretching from growing uterus
4 Risk for Injury to fetus related to teenage pregnancy

Answer: 2

Rationale: The decrease in nutritional intake during the first trimester of the pregnancy puts the mother and fetus at jeopardy. The mother is prone to developing ketoacidosis, which can be harmful to the infant. Also, specific nutrients, such as folic acid, may produce fetal anomalies if deficient at this time. Body image disturbance is a problem for this client; however, nutrition is of a higher priority. The client may have a potential risk for skin integrity; however, this will occur later in the pregnancy. The fetus is at risk, but not because the mother is a teenager.

Test-Taking Strategy: The main strategy with this question is to apply Maslow's hierarchy of needs to both the mother and the fetus. Physiological needs are the top priority for both clients. The need for proper nutrition is vital for the fetus at this point as well as for the diabetic mother. Additionally, the stem asks for the most important nursing diagnosis. Option 2 identifies an actual problem, which is physiological in nature and a higher priority than Body Image Disturbance. Options 3 and 4 identify potential problems.

Level of Cognitive Ability: Analysis
Phase of Nursing Process: Analysis
Client Needs: Physiological Integrity
Content Area: Maternity

Reference

Reeder, S., Martin, L., & Koniak-Griffin, D. (1997). *Maternity nursing: Family, newborn, and women's health care* (18th ed.). Philadelphia: Lippincott-Raven, p. 860.

102. Dantrolene (Dantrium) is prescribed for a client with a spinal cord injury for discomfort owing to spasticity. The nurse determines that toxicity is present when which of the following laboratory values is altered?

1 Sedimentation rate
2 White blood cell count
3 Liver function studies
4 Creatinine

Answer: 3

Rationale: The risk of hepatotoxicity can occur with dantrolene, and the liver function studies need to be monitored while the client is taking this medication. The sedimentation rate measures the presence of inflammation and infection. The white blood cell count measures the body's immune defense system. The creatinine measures renal function.

Test-Taking Strategy: Knowledge of the toxic effects of dantrolene is required to answer the question. Correlate this medication with the potential for hepatotoxicity. If you had difficulty with this question, take time now to review the toxic effects of dantrolene.

Level of Cognitive Ability: Analysis
Phase of Nursing Process: Analysis
Client Needs: Physiological Integrity
Content Area: Pharmacology

Reference

Hodgson, B., & Kizior, R. (1998). *Saunders nursing drug handbook 1998.* Philadelphia: W. B. Saunders, pp. 284–286.

103. The client in skeletal traction says to the nurse, "I'm not sure if I want to have skeletal or skin traction to stabilize my fracture." Based on this client statement, the nurse determines that the most appropriate response would be which of the following?

1. "Your fracture is very unstable. You will die if you don't have this surgery performed."
2. "There is no reason to be concerned. I have seen lots of these procedures."
3. "Skeletal traction is much more effective than skin traction in your situation."
4. "You have concerns about skeletal versus skin traction for your type of fracture?"

Answer: 4

Rationale: When answering this type of client question, it is best to use the therapeutic communication technique of paraphrasing. Paraphrasing is restating the client's message in the nurse's own words. Option 1 represents a communication block that reflects a lack of the client's right to an opinion. In option 2, the nurse is offering a false reassurance, and this type of response blocks communication. In option 3, the nurse is expressing disapproval, which does not enhance the therapeutic nurse-client relationship.

Test-Taking Strategy: Therapeutic communication techniques enhance communication. Always select the answer that enhances communication. Avoid responses that block communication. Always address the client's feelings and concerns first.

Level of Cognitive Ability: Application
Phase of Nursing Process: Analysis
Client Needs: Psychosocial Integrity
Content Area: Adult Health/Musculoskeletal

Reference

Elkin, M., Perry, A., & Potter, P. (1996). *Nursing interventions and clinical skills.* St. Louis: Mosby–Year Book, pp. 14–24.

---

104. The client reports that crying spells have been a major problem over the past several weeks and that the physician said depression is probably the reason. The nurse observes that the client is sitting slumped in the chair and the clothes that the client is wearing are not fitting well. The nurse interprets that further assessment should focus next on

1. Sleep patterns.
2. Onset of the crying spells.
3. Weight loss.
4. Medication compliance.

Answer: 3

Rationale: All of the options are possible issues to address. The weight loss, however, is the first item that needs assessment because an obvious ill fit of clothing could signify a substantial problem with physiological integrity. The client has told the nurse that the crying spells have been a problem, and medication has not been mentioned in the information given. Sleep is affected by depression and should be addressed; however, weight loss is the most important with the data given.

Test-Taking Strategy: Use the process of elimination and Maslow's hierarchy of needs to answer the question. Because all of the information is important to assess at some point, the nurse must decide which has priority with the given situation. Significant weight loss is the most serious physiological concern.

Level of Cognitive Ability: Analysis
Phase of Nursing Process: Analysis
Client Needs: Physiological Integrity
Content Area: Mental Health

Reference

Johnson, B. (1997). *Psychiatric–mental health nursing: Adaptation and growth* (4th ed.). Philadelphia: Lippincott-Raven, pp. 545–546.

---

105. Which of the following assessment findings does the nurse interpret as a serious problem associated with Parkinson's disease?

1. Congested cough and coarse rhonchi
2. Last bowel movement 48 hours ago
3. Resting and pill-rolling tremors
4. Shuffling and propulsive gait

Answer: 1

Rationale: Clients with Parkinson's disease are at risk for aspiration. A congested cough and rhonchi may be present after a client aspirates. Although constipation is a problem for clients with Parkinson's disease, concern is greater if the person has not had a bowel movement by the third day. Resting and pill-rolling tremors and shuffling, propulsive gait are expected with Parkinson's disease.

Test-Taking Strategy: The stem of the question asks for a serious problem. Remember the ABCs when prioritizing answers. Aspiration presents a serious risk to the client and may be suspected if the client with Parkinson's develops a congested cough and rhonchi.

Level of Cognitive Ability: Analysis
Phase of Nursing Process: Analysis
Client Needs: Physiological Integrity
Content Area: Adult Health/Neurological

Reference

Ignatavicius, D. D., Workman, M. L., & Mishler, M. A. (1995). *Medical-surgical nursing: A nursing process approach* (2nd ed.). Philadelphia: W. B. Saunders, p. 1152.

---

106. The nurse positions a client for a surgical procedure. For which of the following positions would the nurse be most alert to the potential for decreased lung expansion in the client?

1 Lithotomy
2 Supine
3 Lateral
4 Side lying

Answer: 1

Rationale: The thoracic cage normally expands in all directions except posteriorly. In the lithotomy position, the expansion of the lungs is restricted at the ribs or sternum, and there is a reduction in the ability of the diaphragm to push down against the abdominal muscles. Respiratory function is impaired because of this interference with normal movements. The volume of air that can be inspired is reduced.

Test-Taking Strategy: Knowledge of the positions presented in the options is required to answer this question. Use the process of elimination to answer the question, and try to visualize each position and its effect on lung expansion. The lithotomy position is the one most likely to interfere with the expansion of the lungs. The supine position in option 2 would not interfere with the expansion of the lungs. A similarity exists in the positions noted in options 3 and 4, making it likely that neither is correct. If you had difficulty with this question, take time now to review these positions.

Level of Cognitive Ability: Analysis
Phase of Nursing Process: Analysis
Client Needs: Physiological Integrity
Content Area: Fundamental Skills

Reference

Phipps, W., Cassmeyer, V., Sands, J., et al. (1995). *Medical-surgical nursing: Concepts and clinical practice* (5th ed.). St. Louis: Mosby–Year Book, pp. 619–621.

---

107. The nurse interprets which of the following would indicate normal sinus rhythm in a lead II rhythm strip?

1 An ECG rhythm strip that shows a P-R interval of 0.24
2 An ECG rhythm strip that shows normal PQRST wave forms
3 An ECG rhythm strip with a heart rate of 107 beats/minute
4 An ECG rhythm strip with a heart rate less than 60 beats/minute

Answer: 2

Rationale: A lead II rhythm strip displays a PQRST wave form. P-R interval range is 0.12–0.20 second, which makes option 1 incorrect. The normal rate of firing of the SA node is 60–100 times per minute. Option 3 indicates a sinus tachycardia, whereas option 4 indicates a sinus bradycardia, making these options incorrect.

Test-Taking Strategy: Read all of the information in each of the options. Options 1, 3, and 4 are all abnormal in some way. Option 1 indicates a conduction problem. Both options 3 and 4 are rate related dysrhythmias originating in the sinus node. Additionally, note the word "normal" in the correct option.

Level of Cognitive Ability: Analysis
Phase of Nursing Process: Analysis
Client Needs: Physiological Integrity
Content Area: Adult Health/Cardiovascular

Reference

Luckmann, J. (1997). *Saunders manual of nursing care.* Philadelphia, W. B. Saunders, pp. 993–996

108. The newborn receives naloxone (Narcan) to reverse opiate-induced respiratory depression that occurred after labor and delivery. The nurse continues to monitor the respiratory status of a newborn after the administration of this medication knowing that

1. The infant may demonstrate a gradual reappearance of respiratory depression as the antagonist's short-lived effects diminish.
2. The infant may have an underlying respiratory disorder.
3. The effects of naloxone are long lasting.
4. The use of naloxone in infants produces untoward effects on the respiratory tree.

Answer: 1

Rationale: Naloxone is a short-term opiate antagonist. It reverses the respiratory depression that can be exhibited in newborns whose mothers have been treated with opiates for the pain of labor and delivery. Because it is short-acting, and the newborn's liver is immature, respiratory depression may recur after the duration of effects of naloxone.

Test-Taking Strategy: Knowledge of the medication naloxone is required to answer the question. It is specifically used to reverse respiratory depression. If you had difficulty with this question, take time now to review this medication.

Level of Cognitive Ability: Analysis
Phase of Nursing Process: Analysis
Client Needs: Physiological Integrity
Content Area: Pharmacology

Reference

Hodgson, B., & Kizior, R. (1998). *Saunders nursing drug handbook 1998.* Philadelphia: W. B. Saunders, pp. 719–720.

---

109. An 84-year-old client sustained a major burn injury from flames 3 days ago. Which of the following would be an unanticipated finding at this time?

1. Jugular venous distention and the presence of S3 and S4 heart sounds
2. Polyuria and a decreased urine specific gravity
3. Decreased hematocrit and metabolic acidosis
4. Hyponatremia and hypokalemia

Answer: 1

Rationale: Jugular venous distention and the presence of S3 and S4 heart sounds indicate possible heart failure. Remobilization of fluid from the interstitial to the intravascular space, which may occur beginning 48–72 hours after the injury, can lead to overwhelming strain on cardiac and renal reserve, especially in elderly or otherwise compromised clients. Copious, dilute urine is expected during the diuretic phase of the burn injury. Increased intravascular plasma volume occurs during the diuretic phase causing a relative or dilutional anemia. Metabolic acidosis can occur as the loss of sodium depletes the fixed base, and relative carbon dioxide content increases. Sodium and potassium are lost from fluid shifts. Potassium commonly shifts back into cells as cell membranes stabilize.

Test-Taking Strategy: Knowledge of the pathophysiological occurrences that occur after a burn injury is required to answer the question. Note that the stem of the question asks for the unanticipated finding. Use the ABCs to answer the question. If you had difficulty with this question, take time now to review pathophysiological occurrences after a burn injury.

Level of Cognitive Ability: Analysis
Phase of Nursing Process: Analysis
Client Needs: Physiological Integrity
Content Area: Adult Health/Integumentary

Reference

Smeltzer, S., & Bare, B. (1996). *Brunner and Suddarth's Textbook of medical-surgical nursing* (8th ed.). Philadelphia: Lippincott-Raven, pp. 1558–1563.

110. The nurse notices that a client with trigeminal neuralgia has been withdrawn, is having frequent episodes of crying, and is sleeping excessively. The nurse interprets that the best way to explore issues with the client about this behavior is to

1 Conduct a group discussion with the client's family.
2 Have the client express the feelings in writing.
3 Have the physician speak to the client.
4 Ignore the behavior because it is expected in clients with trigeminal neuralgia.

Answer: 2

Rationale: Speaking can exacerbate the pain with trigeminal neuralgia. Having the client record feelings in writing helps the nurse to gain an understanding of the client's concerns without increasing the pain. Discussing the issue with the family does not provide insight into the client's feelings. It is not in the client's best interest to refer the matter to the physician or to ignore the behavior. The nurse should explore the client's concerns and offer support.

Test-Taking Strategy: Use the process of elimination in answering the question. Identifying the client of the question assists you in eliminating options 1 and 3. Ignoring the behavior blocks any communication and places the client's issues on hold. Remember to address the client's feelings first.

Level of Cognitive Ability: Analysis
Phase of Nursing Process: Analysis
Client Needs: Psychosocial Integrity
Content Area: Adult Health/Neurological

Reference

Lewis, S., Collier, I., & Heitkemper, M. (1996). *Medical-surgical nursing: Assessment and management of clinical problems* (4th ed.). St. Louis: Mosby–Year Book, p. 1794.

---

111. A client is admitted to the cardiac unit. The cardiac monitor indicates normal sinus rhythm. The nurse determines that this finding indicates which of the following?

1 There are several areas responding as the pacemaker of the heart.
2 There is slowed conduction in the bundle of His.
3 The sinoatrial node is responding as the pacemaker of the heart.
4 The atrioventricular node is causing a delay to the bundle of His.

Answer: 3

Rationale: The sinoatrial node is considered the primary pacemaker of the heart because it has the highest rate of automaticity of all potential pacemaker sites. Options 1, 2, and 4 identify rhythms that are abnormal.

Test-Taking Strategy: Knowledge of the conduction system of the heart is required to respond to this question. Use the process of elimination, and eliminate options 2 and 4 first because these options are actually stating the same thing. Remember that the sinoatrial node is the pacemaker of the heart, and eliminate option 1. If you had difficulty with this question, take time now to review information about normal sinus rhythm.

Level of Cognitive Ability: Analysis
Phase of Nursing Process: Analysis
Client Needs: Physiological Integrity
Content Area: Adult Health/Cardiovascular

Reference

Luckmann, J. (1997). *Saunders manual of nursing care.* Philadelphia: W. B. Saunders, pp. 993–996.

112. After an unplanned cesarean section, the nurse finds the client displaying emotional distress. The nurse notes that the woman is tearful, expressing bewilderment, sadness, and feelings of failure and regret because she could not deliver vaginally. The nurse determines that which of the following nursing diagnoses is most appropriate at this time?

1 Situational Low Self-Esteem
2 Knowledge Deficit
3 Ineffective Individual Coping
4 Dysfunctional Grieving

Answer: 1

Rationale: Situational Low Self-Esteem represents temporary negative feelings about the self in response to an event. This is a normal response to cesarean section. Ineffective Individual Coping implies that the person is unable to manage stressors adequately. Dysfunctional Grieving implies prolonged unresolved grief leading to detrimental activities. Knowledge Deficit implies a lack of information or psychomotor skills concerning a condition or treatment. The information provided in the question best supports the nursing diagnosis stated in option 1.

Test-Taking Strategy: When asked to select the most appropriate nursing diagnosis, review the information presented in the question and select the nursing diagnosis that best supports the data presented.

Level of Cognitive Ability: Analysis
Phase of Nursing Process: Analysis
Client Needs: Psychosocial Integrity
Content Area: Maternity

Reference

Lowdermilk, D., Perry, S., & Bobak, I. (1997). *Maternity and women's health care* (6th ed.). St. Louis: Mosby–Year Book, pp. 961–970.

---

113. The nurse is caring for a client experiencing hypotonic labor contractions. The client is discouraged with the progress she is making but adamantly refuses an amniotomy or oxytocin stimulation. The nurse analyzes that the client's behavior may be due to

1 A concern about her own and the baby's well-being.
2 The high level of pain caused by these contractions.
3 The normal "lack of control" clients feel during the transition phase of labor.
4 The client's inability to rest between the frequent contractions.

Answer: 1

Rationale: Clients have concerns when labor does not proceed as expected and often are worried about the effects of treatments and invasive procedures. Hypotonic contractions generally occur during the active phase of labor, after a normal latent phase. These contractions are typically of poor intensity, infrequent, not painful, but causing a slow progression of labor. Therefore, options 2, 3, and 4 are incorrect.

Test-Taking Strategy: Knowledge of the various types of labor dystocias is needed to eliminate the options that are false. Read the case situation carefully. Additionally, always select an option that relates to the client's feelings and concerns.

Level of Cognitive Ability: Analysis
Phase of Nursing Process: Analysis
Client Needs: Psychosocial Integrity
Content Area: Maternity

Reference

Nichols, F., & Zwelling, E. (1997). *Maternal-newborn nursing: Theory and practice.* Philadelphia: W. B. Saunders, pp. 887–891.

114. The community health nurse visits the home of an elderly postoperative cardiovascular client. The caregiver tells the nurse, "The client has fallen out of bed three times." Which of the nurse's observations indicate an increased risk for this client falling out of bed?

1. Client is oriented to person, place, time, and self.
2. Caregiver leaves one side-rail down while the client is in bed.
3. Client's bed is in a low position.
4. Caregiver uses the over-the-bed table for feedings.

Answer: 2

Rationale: Leaving a side-rail down on the bed of an elderly client increases the risk of falling. The aging process also increases this client's potential for falls; therefore, evaluating the safety of the environment is a necessity.

Test-Taking Strategy: Use the process of elimination to answer the question. Option 1 identifies the client is oriented, which would reduce the risk of falling. Option 3 also identifies a safe and appropriate environment. Option 4 does not address the risk of falling.

Level of Cognitive Ability: Analysis
Phase of Nursing Process: Analysis
Client Needs: Safe, Effective, Care Environment
Content Area: Fundamental Skills

Reference

Smith, S., & Duvell, D. (1996). *Clinical nursing skills* (4th ed.). Stamford, CT: Appleton & Lange, p. 120.

---

115. A client with Cushing's syndrome begins to cry and states to the nurse, "I hate the way I look because of this disease." The nurse should identify that the client is at risk for which nursing diagnosis?

1. Body Image Disturbance
2. Anxiety
3. Self-Esteem Disturbance
4. Powerlessness

Answer: 1

Rationale: The nursing diagnosis of Body Image Disturbance refers to a disruption in the way one perceives one's body image. A verbal or nonverbal response to an actual or perceived change in structure or function of the body must be present to justify this nursing diagnosis. The client with Cushing's syndrome experiences many structural and functional changes, including integumentary system changes, mental status changes, and changes in fat distribution, as a result of this disorder.

Test-Taking Strategy: Use the process of elimination to answer the question. The focus is on a client's psychosocial adaptation to a disease that has multiple impacts on body image. The question asks you to interpret the meaning of a client's verbal communication. Use of therapeutic communication skills is helpful in identifying that the client is expressing dissatisfaction with his or her body image.

Level of Cognitive Ability: Analysis
Phase of Nursing Process: Analysis
Client Needs: Psychosocial Integrity
Content Area: Adult Health/Endocrine

Reference

Cox, H., Hinz, M., Lubno, M., et al. (1997). *Clinical applications of nursing diagnosis: Adult, child, women's, psychiatric, gerontic, and home health considerations* (3rd ed.). Philadelphia: F. A. Davis, p. 506.

116. The client had thoracic surgery 2 days ago and has a chest tube in place connected to a Pleur-Evac drainage system. The nurse notes that there is continuous bubbling in the water seal chamber. The nurse interprets that

1 The client has a large amount of fluid that is being evacuated by the system.
2 This is due to the suction applied to the system, which is set at 20 cm of suction pressure.
3 There is a leak in the system, which requires immediate investigation and correction.
4 This is normal on the second postoperative day.

Answer: 3

Rationale: Continuous bubbling in the water seal chamber of a chest tube indicates that there is a leak somewhere in the system, and air is being sucked into the apparatus. The nurse needs to assess the system and initiate corrective action, which may include notifying the physician. Bubbling may occur intermittently with evacuation of pneumothorax, but it should not be continuous, especially with a client who had surgery 2 days earlier. Hemothorax results in accumulation of drainage in the collection chamber but does not cause bubbling in the water seal chamber. Application of suction to the system causes bubbling in the suction control chamber but not the water seal chamber.

Test-Taking Strategy: This question requires knowledge of the function and normal assessment findings for each of the chambers of the Pleur-Evac closed chest drainage system. Continuous bubbling in the water seal chamber indicates leakage of air into the system, whereas intermittent bubbling indicates drainage of pneumothorax. This knowledge requires you to select option 3 as the only possible correct choice. If you had difficulty with this question or are unfamiliar with the chest tube drainage system, stop now and review.

Level of Cognitive Ability: Analysis
Phase of Nursing Process: Analysis
Client Needs: Physiological Integrity
Content Area: Adult Health/Respiratory

Reference

Black, J., & Matassarin-Jacobs, E. (1997). *Medical-surgical nursing: Clinical management for continuity of care* (5th ed.). Philadelphia: W. B. Saunders, pp. 1163–1164.

---

117. A client comes into the clinic stating, "I spend hours each evening reviewing the events of the day to see if I behaved appropriately or if I should have done something differently. I am amazed when I check my watch after one of these reviews and find that 2–3 hours have gone by. I tell myself to 'snap out of it' but I continue to do it. I also take 2–3 hours each morning to get dressed because I want my clothes to be 'just right.' " The nurse analyzes the client's statements and determines that the client's behavior is indicative of which of the following?

1 A personality disorder
2 Agoraphobia
3 An obsessive-compulsive disorder
4 Attention deficit disorder

Answer: 3

Rationale: Obsessions are defined as persistent thoughts that are intrusive that the person tries to ignore or suppress. This client wants to "snap out of" this daily review, but the thoughts continue for hours. Compulsions are defined as repetitive behaviors that the client feels driven to perform, such as changing clothes frequently until the client gets it "just right."

Test-Taking Strategy: Read the client's statements carefully, noting the client behaviors. Noting the repetitiveness of behaviors that the client describes should provide you with the clue that directs you to the correct option. If you had difficulty answering this question, take time now to review the characteristics of obsessive-compulsive disorders.

Level of Cognitive Ability: Analysis
Phase of Nursing Process: Analysis
Client Needs: Psychosocial Integrity
Content Area: Mental Health

Reference

Carson, V., & Arnold, E. (1996). *Mental health nursing: The nurse-patient journey.* Philadelphia: W. B. Saunders, p. 701.

---

118. The nurse determines that which of the following assessment data indicates a negative effect on the fetus?

1 Increased baseline variability
2 Late decelerations
3 Accelerations
4 Fetal heart rate between 120–160 beats/minute

Answer: 2

Rationale: Signs of impaired fetal oxygenation, which would occur when uterine integrity is disturbed, include late decelerations, decreased baseline variability, and tachycardia or bradycardia. A normal fetal heart rate is 120–160 beats per minute. Accelerations occur in a fetus with a mature central nervous system and who is well oxygenated.

Test-Taking Strategy: Use the process of elimination to answer the question. Options 1, 3, and 4 are indications of fetal well-being and can be eliminated as an effect of a complication causing hypoxia. Knowing that late decelerations are accompanied by decreased fetal blood flow and oxygenation leads you to choose option 2. If you had difficulty with this question, take time now to review late decelerations.

Level of Cognitive Ability: Analysis
Phase of Nursing Process: Analysis
Client Needs: Physiological Integrity
Content Area: Maternity

Reference

Nichols, F., & Zwelling, E. (1997). *Maternal-newborn nursing: Theory and practice.* Philadelphia: W. B. Saunders, p. 953.

---

119. A child is admitted to the hospital with a diagnosis of acute rheumatic fever. The nurse analyzes the laboratory results. Which of the following blood laboratory findings would confirm the likelihood of rheumatic fever?

1 Increased leukocyte count
2 Decreased hemoglobin count
3 Increased antibody level
4 Decreased erythrocyte sedimentation rate

Answer: 3

Rationale: Children suspected of having rheumatic fever are tested for the evidence of a recent streptococcal infection. An increased antibody level evidenced by an elevated or rising antistreptolysin O titer assists in confirming the diagnosis. An increased erythrocyte sedimentation rate occurs in rheumatic fever. The leukocyte count and hemoglobin count do not confirm the diagnosis of rheumatic fever.

Test-Taking Strategy: Knowledge of the clinical manifestations related to rheumatic fever is required to answer the question. Take the time now to review the clinical manifestations and diagnostic tests that confirm the presence of rheumatic fever.

Level of Cognitive Ability: Analysis
Phase of Nursing Process: Analysis
Client Needs: Physiological Integrity
Content Area: Child Health

Reference

Ashwill, J., & Droske, S. (1997). *Nursing care of children: Principles and practice.* Philadelphia: W. B. Saunders, p. 658.

---

120. The client scheduled for pulmonary angiography is fearful about the procedure and asks the nurse if the procedure involves significant pain and radiation exposure. The nurse gives a reassuring response to the client, based on the understanding that

1 The procedure is somewhat painful, but there is minimal exposure to radiation.
2 Discomfort may occur with needle insertion, and there is minimal exposure to radiation.
3 There is absolutely no pain, although a moderate amount of radiation must be used to get accurate results.
4 There is mild pain throughout the procedure, and the exposure to radiation is negligible.

Answer: 2

Rationale: Pulmonary angiography involves minimal exposure to radiation. The procedure is painless, although the client may feel discomfort with insertion of the needle for the catheter that is used for dye injection.

Test-Taking Strategy: Knowledge regarding the procedure assists in answering the question. Knowing that radiation exposure is minimal helps you to eliminate option 3 first. It is necessary to know that the only discomfort occurs with needle insertion to discriminate among the other three options. If you had difficulty with this question, take time now to review the description of pulmonary angiography.

Level of Cognitive Ability: Application
Phase of Nursing Process: Analysis
Client Needs: Psychosocial Integrity
Content Area: Adult Health/Respiratory

Reference

Black, J., & Matassarin-Jacobs, E. (1997). *Medical-surgical nursing: Clinical management for continuity of care* (5th ed.). Philadelphia: W. B. Saunders, p. 1062.

121. The nurse is caring for a client experiencing a partial placental abruption. The client is uncooperative and refusing any interventions until her husband arrives at the hospital. The nurse analyzes the client's behavior as most likely the result of

1. Acute anxiety and the need for support.
2. An undiagnosed psychiatric disorder.
3. Emotional immaturity.
4. A stubborn personality.

Answer: 1

Rationale: Any of the situations identified in the options may contribute to the reason for the client's behavior, but the most likely is stress. Option 1, however, is the only option that supports the information identified in the question. Clients can be anxious about the unknown effects of complications, and the presence of a support person while dealing with a crisis is crucial.

Test-Taking Strategy: The key phrase in the stem of the question is "most likely." When answering questions dealing with client behavior, choose the option dealing with the client's anxiety and the need for support. Remember the client's feelings and concerns are the priority.

Level of Cognitive Ability: Analysis
Phase of Nursing Process: Analysis
Client Needs: Psychosocial Integrity
Content Area: Maternity

Reference

Gorrie, T. M., McKinney, E. S., & Murray, S. S. (1994). *Foundations of maternal newborn nursing.* Philadelphia: W. B. Saunders, pp. 674–675.

---

122. The client with the diagnosis of major depression becomes more anxious on the unit, reports sleeping poorly, and seems be more irritable with staff and family. The nurse interprets the client's behavior as

1. Being at increased risk for suicide.
2. A normal response to hospitalization.
3. An attempt to deal with pertinent issues.
4. Indicating a need for time off the unit.

Answer: 1

Rationale: The behaviors mentioned may be manifested by the client who is contemplating suicide. Many of these symptoms are symptoms of the depressed client; however, with this client these behaviors have increased. Hospitalization should lessen these symptoms in the depressed client because a feeling of hope or relief may occur once treatment begins. Facing issues may be traumatic, but this is not the best answer for the question. Time off the unit for this client could put the client at risk for injury. Only when anxiety and irritability can be controlled could the client safely leave the unit.

Test-Taking Strategy: Identify the client behaviors addressed in the question. Use the process of elimination in answering the question. Additionally, use Maslow's hierarchy of needs to assist in answering the question. Of the options presented, option 1 is the priority. If you had difficulty with this question, take time now to review the characteristics and client behaviors related to suicide.

Level of Cognitive Ability: Analysis
Phase of Nursing Process: Analysis
Client Needs: Physiological Integrity
Content Area: Mental Health

Reference

Carson, V., & Arnold, E. (1996). *Mental health nursing: The nurse-patient journey.* Philadelphia: W. B. Saunders, pp. 932–936.

---

123. The nurse enters the client's room and finds the client slumped down in the chair. Breathing is shallow, and a pulse is present. Based on these data, the nurse analyzes that the priority would be to

1. Call the physician immediately.
2. Check the vital signs and level of consciousness.
3. Have the nursing assistant call a Code Blue.
4. Ask the unit clerk to call the family immediately.

Answer: 2

Rationale: The client is breathing and has a pulse; therefore, the nurse must determine that further assessment is needed before any other action. The vital signs and level of consciousness should be assessed. Once that assessment is made, the physician does need to be notified as well as the family. Code Blue is not indicated at the present time. Further assessment might warrant that later.

Test-Taking Strategy: This question asks the nurse to prioritize based on the analysis of the data. Use the steps of the nursing process and the ABCs to answer the question.

Level of Cognitive Ability: Analysis
Phase of Nursing Process: Analysis
Client Needs: Physiological Integrity
Content Area: Adult Health/Cardiovascular

Reference

Ignatavicius, D. D., Workman, M. L., & Mishler, M. A. (1995). *Medical-surgical nursing: A nursing process approach* (2nd ed.). Philadelphia: W. B. Saunders, pp. 874–875.

---

124. A client experiencing delusions is taken to the laboratory for routine blood work and begins shouting, "You're all vampires. Take me home." Based on the client's behavior, the nurse determines that the most therapeutic response would be

1 "No one wants to hurt you. This is a hospital where we help people."
2 "What makes you think we're vampires?"
3 "I'll leave until you calm down."
4 "It must be scary to think others want to hurt you."

Answer: 4

Rationale: This response helps the client to focus on the emotion underlying the delusion but does not argue with it. A danger in directly attempting to change the client's mind is that the delusion may, in fact, be even more strongly held.

Test-Taking Strategy: Knowledge of the dynamics of delusions and how delusions meet the client's underlying needs is helpful to answer the question. Option 4 recognizes the need and realizes that arguing with the client reinforces the need, thereby allowing the client to cling to further abnormal or illogical thinking. Additionally, option 4 focuses on the client's feelings.

Level of Cognitive Ability: Application
Phase of Nursing Process: Analysis
Client Needs: Psychosocial Integrity
Content Area: Mental Health

Reference

Haber, J. (1997). *Comprehensive psychiatric nursing* (5th ed.). St. Louis: Mosby–Year Book, p. 592.

---

125. A client received a dose of regular insulin (Humulin R) today at 7 A.M. At what time could the nurse most likely anticipate the potential for a hypoglycemic reaction to occur?

1 8 A.M.
2 10 A.M.
3 12 noon
4 2 P.M.

Answer: 2

Rationale: Humulin R is a rapid-acting insulin with a peak action at 2–4 hours after injection. Hypoglycemic reactions are most likely to occur during the peak action of insulin.

Test-Taking Strategy: Knowledge regarding the general action (onset, peak, and duration) of rapid-acting insulin is required to answer the question. Remember Humulin R (*R* meaning *rapid*). If you had difficulty with this question, take time now to review regular insulin.

Level of Cognitive Ability: Analysis
Phase of Nursing Process: Analysis
Client Needs: Physiological Integrity
Content Area: Adult Health/Endocrine

Reference

Ignatavicius, D. D., Workman, M. L., & Mishler, M. A. (1995). *Medical-surgical nursing: A nursing process approach* (2nd ed.). Philadelphia: W. B. Saunders, p. 1897.

---

126. A home health nurse observes a mother providing care to an infant who has diarrhea. Which of these observations would require the nurse's immediate intervention?

1. The mother checks the diaper for evidence of elimination every hour.
2. The mother allows the buttocks to dry before applying a clean diaper.
3. The mother applies petroleum jelly to the perineal area after cleansing.
4. The mother uses a damp wash cloth to clean the buttocks after a stool.

Answer: 4

Rationale: A diarrhea stool has an alkaline pH that can cause skin breakdown. A damp wash cloth is an ineffective way to clean the skin. The mother should be taught to clean the skin thoroughly under running water using a mild soap. Options 1, 2, and 3 are correct measures to promote skin integrity.

Test-Taking Strategy: This question asks for the observations that would require the nurse's immediate intervention. Read each option carefully, and eliminate the incorrect options. Options 1, 2, and 3 are actions that maintain skin integrity, and option 4 is an action that causes skin breakdown. If you had difficulty with this question, take time now to review skin care for an infant who has diarrhea.

Level of Cognitive Ability: Analysis
Phase of Nursing Process: Analysis
Client Needs: Physiological Integrity
Content Area: Child Health

Reference

Wong, D. (1995). *Whaley and Wong's Nursing care of infants and children* (5th ed.). St. Louis: Mosby–Year Book, p. 1241.

---

127. A primigravida is receiving magnesium sulfate for pregnancy-induced hypertension. The nurse performs client assessments every 30 minutes. Which of the following assessments would the nurse analyze as the greatest concern?

1. Urinary output of 20 mL
2. Deep tendon reflexes of 2+
3. Respirations of 10 breaths/minute
4. Fetal heart tones of 116 beats/minute

Answer: 3

Rationale: Option 1 identifies an adequate output because the criterion is at least 30 mL/hour, and this client's output is 20 mL in 30 minutes. Deep tendon reflexes of 2+ are normal. Magnesium sulfate depresses the respiratory rate. If the respiratory rate is less than 12 breaths/minute, the continuation of the medication needs to be reassessed. The fetal heart tone is within normal limits for a resting fetus.

Test-Taking Strategy: Note the key phrase "greatest concern" in the stem of the question. Use the process of elimination to answer the question. Identify the assessment finding that is abnormal. If you had difficulty with this question, take time now to review client assessments during the administration of magnesium sulfate.

Level of Cognitive Ability: Analysis
Phase of Nursing Process: Analysis
Client Needs: Physiological Integrity
Content Area: Maternity

Reference

Lowdermilk, D., Perry, S., & Bobak, I. (1997). *Maternity and women's health care* (6th ed.). St. Louis: Mosby–Year Book, p. 714.

128. The nurse monitors the laboratory data on a client with coronary artery disease. A fasting blood glucose reading of 200 mg/dL is recorded on the chart. The nurse would properly analyze these results as

1 Elevated, signaling the presence of diabetes, a risk factor for coronary artery disease.
2 Decreased, indicating decreased risk of coronary artery disease.
3 Normal, indicating adequate blood glucose control with no risk for coronary artery disease.
4 Elevated but no apparent association with coronary disease.

Answer: 1

Rationale: A fasting blood glucose of 200 mg/dL signals the presence of diabetes. Diabetes predisposes a client to coronary artery disease.

Test-Taking Strategy: Knowledge of the normal blood glucose level and that an elevated fasting blood glucose may indicate diabetes mellitus is required to answer the question. Use the process of elimination to answer the question. If you had difficulty with this question, take time now to review the normal blood glucose level and the risk factors associated with coronary artery disease.

Level of Cognitive Ability: Analysis
Phase of Nursing Process: Analysis
Client Needs: Physiological Integrity
Content Area: Adult Health/Cardiovascular

Reference

Black, J., & Matassarin-Jacobs, E. (1997). *Medical-surgical nursing: Clinical management for continuity of care* (5th ed.). Philadelphia: W. B. Saunders, p. 1241.

---

129. The client with a rib fracture resists directions by the nurse to cough and deep breathe because of the pain. The nurse interprets that the most appropriate nursing action would be to

1 Continue to give the client gentle encouragement to do so.
2 Request that the physician perform a nerve block to deaden the pain.
3 Explain in detail the potential complications from lack of coughing and deep breathing.
4 Premedicate the client and assist the client to splint the area during these exercises.

Answer: 4

Rationale: Shallow respirations and splinting that occur with rib fracture predispose the client to developing atelectasis and pneumonia. It is essential that the client perform coughing and deep breathing to prevent these complications. The nurse accomplishes this most effectively by premedicating the client with pain medication and assisting the client with splinting during the exercises.

Test-Taking Strategy: Use the process of elimination to answer the question. Options 2 and 3 are likely to be the most extreme or unrealistic options and should be eliminated first. Of the remaining two, premedication and assistance are more likely to be effective than continued gentle encouragement.

Level of Cognitive Ability: Application
Phase of Nursing Process: Analysis
Client Needs: Health Promotion and Maintenance
Content Area: Adult Health/Cardiovascular

Reference

Black, J., & Matassarin-Jacobs, E. (1997). *Medical-surgical nursing: Clinical management for continuity of care* (5th ed.). Philadelphia: W. B. Saunders, p. 2526.

---

130. A client with a diagnosis of angina pectoris who has been pain-free for 2 days complains of recurrent chest pain. The nurse notes a sinus tachycardia on the cardiac monitor. Based on these data, analysis of the standing physician orders would most likely direct the nurse to do which of the following initially?

1 Obtain an ECG
2 Administer oxygen by nasal cannula
3 Notify the physician
4 Establish an intravenous access

Answer: 2

Rationale: Myocardial ischemia is expressed symptomatically as angina (chest pain). The pain is related to an imbalance of myocardial oxygen supply and demand. Oxygen administration would help to correct this imbalance. Oxygen administration can be accomplished quickly and can be working to provide relief while the other nursing actions are being implemented.

Test-Taking Strategy: This item involves prioritizing nursing activities identified in the options. The key word is "initially." Although all of the options may be performed, the first activity would be to administer oxygen to the client to facilitate pain relief. Use nursing knowledge and knowledge of the situation to answer the question. The actions identified in the remaining options would also be performed, but oxygen is the first priority. Remember the ABCs.

Level of Cognitive Ability: Application
Phase of Nursing Process: Analysis
Client Needs: Physiological Integrity
Content Area: Adult Health/Cardiovascular

Reference

Lewis, S., Collier, I., & Heitkemper, M. (1996). *Medical-surgical nursing: Assessment and management of clinical problems* (4th ed.). St. Louis: Mosby–Year Book, pp. 894, 896, 903.

---

131. On admission to the nursery, the nurse observes jitteriness in a 42-week gestation infant. The infant's vital signs are temperature, 98.0°F; pulse, 148 beats/minute; respirations, 62 breaths/minute. The nurse interprets these data as being supportive of which nursing diagnosis?

1 High Risk for Injury related to hypoglycemia
2 High Risk for Hypothermia related to diminished subcutaneous fat
3 High Risk for Infection related to immaturity of the immune system
4 High Risk for Impaired Gas Exchange related to lack of surfactant

Answer: 1

Rationale: The symptoms of jitteriness and tachypnea (respiratory rate of 62 breaths/minute) in a 42-week gestation infant are indicative of hypoglycemia. Hypoglycemia may develop in this infant because of the insufficient stores of glycogen, which may have been depleted during the postterm time period. Insufficient amounts of glucose to the infant's brain could possibly cause central nervous system damage. Options 2 and 3 are applicable to the postterm infant, although the data presented are not supportive of those diagnoses. Option 4 is inappropriate because postterm infants have adequate surfactant.

Test-Taking Strategy: Knowledge of the complications of the postterm infant is required to answer the question. When answering a question related to a nursing diagnosis, determine that the symptoms presented are defining criteria for the listed nursing diagnoses. Options 1, 2, and 3 are applicable to the postterm infant; however, the symptoms of jitteriness and tachypnea are classic for hypoglycemia, not hypothermia or infection.

Level of Cognitive Ability: Analysis
Phase of Nursing Process: Analysis
Client Needs: Physiological Integrity
Content Area: Maternity

Reference

Pillitteri, A. (1995). *Maternal and child health: Nursing care of the childbearing and childrearing family* (2nd ed.). Philadelphia: Lippincott-Raven, pp. 760–761.

---

132. The nurse analyzes that the wife of an alcoholic client is benefiting from attending an Al-Anon group when the nurse hears the wife say

1 "My attendance at the meetings has helped me to see that I provoke my husband's violence."
2 "I no longer feel that I deserve the beatings my husband inflicts on me."
3 "I can tolerate my husband's destructive behaviors now that I know they are common with alcoholics."
4 "I enjoy attending the meetings because they get me out of the house and away from my husband."

Answer: 2

Rationale: Al-Anon support groups are a protected, supportive opportunity for spouses and significant others to learn what to expect and to obtain excellent pointers about successful behavioral changes. Option 2 is the most healthy response because it exemplifies an understanding that the alcoholic partner is responsible for his behavior and cannot be allowed to blame family members for loss of control. In option 1, the nonalcoholic partner should not feel responsible when the spouse loses control. Option 3 indicates that the wife remains codependent. Option 4 indicates that the group is being seen as an escape, not a place to work on issues.

Test-Taking Strategy: Use the process of elimination to answer the question. Identify the client of the question, and identify the option that most directly addresses the issue of the question, that is, benefiting from attending an Al-Anon group.

Level of Cognitive Ability: Analysis
Phase of Nursing Process: Analysis
Client Needs: Psychosocial Integrity
Content Area: Mental Health

Reference

Carson, V., & Arnold, E. (1996). *Mental health nursing: The nurse-patient journey.* Philadelphia: W. B. Saunders, p. 1013.

133. Early assessment of the infant of a diabetic mother includes a blood glucose screening. The nurse performs a blood glucose screening and obtains a result of 40 mg/dL. The nurse analyzes that this result indicates

1 Hypoglycemia.
2 A borderline normal level.
3 Hyperglycemia.
4 Hypotonia.

Answer: 2

Rationale: Infants of diabetic mothers are at risk for hypoglycemia. An acceptable level for newborns is 40 mg/dL and greater. That places the finding noted in the question at the normal level. The finding is neither hypoglycemia nor hyperglycemia. Hypotonia refers to muscle tone and is not relevant to this blood glucose screening.

Test-Taking Strategy: Knowledge regarding the normal blood glucose level is required to answer the question. Take time to review this normal laboratory value now, if you had difficulty with this question.

Level of Cognitive Ability: Analysis
Phase of Nursing Process: Analysis
Client Needs: Physiological Integrity
Content Area: Maternity

Reference

Nichols, F., & Zwelling, E. (1997). *Maternal-newborn nursing: Theory and practice.* Philadelphia: W. B. Saunders, pp. 1357–1358.

134. An 8-day-old male infant is irritable, has a high-pitched persistent cry, and has a temperature of 99.4°F. He is also tachypneic, is diaphoretic, continues to lose weight, and is hyperreactive to environmental stimuli. The nurse analyzes these behaviors as consistent with

1 Hypercalcemia.
2 Drug withdrawal.
3 Sepsis.
4 Intraventricular hemorrhage.

Answer: 2

Rationale: Drug withdrawal causes a hyperresponse in the infant because of the increased central nervous system stimulation (tachypnea, elevated temperature, increased use of calories). These signs seem to be most apparent at around 1 week of age. Hypercalcemia, sepsis, and intraventricular hemorrhage are characterized by symptoms of central nervous system depression.

Test-Taking Strategy: Use the process of elimination to answer the question. The majority of these symptoms are *hyper* (high-pitched cry, increased temperature, increased respirations, activity levels) and are reflective of central nervous system stimulation. Selection of drug withdrawal matches these symptoms. Sepsis, intraventricular hemorrhage, and hypercalcemia produce central nervous system depression symptoms (bradycardia, apnea, lethargy). Select the problem that would exhibit the central nervous system irritability. If you had difficulty with this question, take time now to review the symptoms of drug withdrawal in the newborn.

Level of Cognitive Ability: Analysis
Phase of Nursing Process: Analysis
Client Needs: Physiological Integrity
Content Area: Child Health

Reference

Ashwill, J., & Droske, S. (1997). *Nursing care of children: Principles and practice.* Philadelphia: W. B. Saunders, pp. 575–576.

135. A 12-month-old infant has just returned to the hospital room from surgery after a palatoplasty. The nurse performs an assessment and determines that which of these findings require the need for further intervention?

1 The child is in a prone position.
2 The respiratory rate is 30 breaths/minute.
3 Oral palate packing is in place.
4 Clove-hitch restraints are secured to the arms.

Answer: 4

Rationale: Elbow restraints are generally used to prevent the child from putting anything into the mouth. Clove-hitch restraints unnecessarily restrict movement of the child's extremities. The prone position prevents aspiration. A respiratory rate of 30 breaths/minute is within normal parameters for a 12-month-old infant. Oral packing may remain in place for 48–72 hours after surgery.

Test-Taking Strategy: Knowledge of postoperative care of a child with palatoplasty and ways to meet basic human need is essential. Focus on the phrase "most significant" when reading the stem of the question. Use the process of elimination, identifying the data not requiring further intervention. If you had difficulty with this question, take time now to review the postoperative care after palatoplasty.

Level of Cognitive Ability: Analysis
Phase of Nursing Process: Analysis
Client Needs: Physiological Integrity
Content Area: Child Health

Reference

Wong, D. (1995). *Whaley and Wong's Nursing care of infants and children* (5th ed.). St. Louis: Mosby–Year Book, pp. 476, 1171.

---

136. An inebriated client in the emergency department becomes loud and offensive when told there will be a short delay before treatment. The nurse analyzes the situation and determines that which approach is most helpful?

1 Attempt to talk with the client to deescalate behavior
2 Watch the behavior escalate before intervening
3 Inform the client that he will be asked to leave if the behavior continues
4 Offer to take the client to an examination room until the client can be treated

Answer: 4

Rationale: Safety of the client, other clients, and staff is of prime concern. When dealing with an impaired individual, trying to talk may be out of the question. Medication may be needed, and it may be necessary to restrain or seclude a client temporarily until he or she is no longer a danger to others. Eliminate option 1, because the client is inebriated and may not be able to be reasoned with. Option 2 is incorrect because waiting to intervene could cause the client to become even more agitated and a threat to others. Option 3 would only further aggravate an already agitated individual. Option 4 is in effect an isolation technique that allows for separation from others and provides a less stimulating environment where the client can maintain dignity.

Test-Taking Strategy: Identifying that the client is inebriated makes a tremendous difference in the option that is selected. Use these data and the process of elimination in selecting the correct option. Option 4 most directly addresses the situation and the behavior and feelings of the client.

Level of Cognitive Ability: Analysis
Phase of Nursing Process: Analysis
Client Needs: Psychosocial Integrity
Content Area: Mental Health

Reference

Carson, V., & Arnold, E. (1996). *Mental health nursing: The nurse-patient journey.* Philadelphia: W. B. Saunders, p. 348.

---

137. The school nurse conducts a health teaching session with 5- and 6-year-old children. The nurse determines that which of the following will best prevent spread of infection in a 5- or 6-year-old attending school and should be taught to the children?

1 Children should obtain optimal sleep and rest.
2 Children should wash hands thoroughly and frequently.
3 Children should avoid playing with coughing or sneezing children.
4 Children should eat a diet high in fruits and vegetables.

Answer: 2

Rationale: Effective handwashing is the most effective way to prevent the transmission of infection. Although rest and diet are important, these measures do not prevent the spread of infection. Option 3 is unrealistic in a school setting and reduces transmission of airborne infections only, making option 2 the best answer.

Test-Taking Strategy: The key word "best" indicates that all options may be correct, so read all four options carefully and select the most important one. Relying on the knowledge that handwashing is most important in reducing transmission of pathogens helps in selecting the correct option.

Level of Cognitive Ability: Analysis
Phase of Nursing Process: Analysis
Client Needs: Physiological Integrity
Content Area: Child Health

Reference

Wong, D. (1997). *Whaley and Wong's Essentials of pediatric nursing* (5th ed.). St. Louis: Mosby–Year Book, p. 393.

138. A nurse, who feels guilty about strong negative feelings toward a fellow employee, tends to use the defense mechanism of projection. This nurse is most likely to react to a disagreement with a fellow employee by

1 Slamming cupboards in the office.
2 Telling a friend that this employee hates him.
3 Getting angry at the supervisor.
4 Apologizing and offering to go out to lunch together.

Answer: 2

Rationale: The defense mechanism of projection is an unconscious process that rejects emotionally unacceptable feelings to other people, objects, or situations and casts the blame onto another. Options 1 and 3 describe displacement, in which the feeling is transferred to another person or object. Option 4 describes reaction formation in which a behavior is used that is directly opposite to a person's unacceptable trait.

Test-Taking Strategy: Knowledge of defense mechanisms is needed to select the correct option. Use the process of elimination to answer the question. Be careful to read the question carefully and identify the defense mechanism that corresponds to the case situation. If you had difficulty with this question, take time now to review defense mechanisms.

Level of Cognitive Ability: Analysis
Phase of Nursing Process: Analysis
Client Needs: Psychosocial Integrity
Content Area: Fundamental Skills

Reference

Haber, J. (1997). *Comprehensive psychiatric nursing* (5th ed.). St. Louis: Mosby–Year Book, pp. 389–391.

---

139. A 47-year-old client is being treated with atenolol (Tenormin) for hypertension. The client tells the nurse, "I am very tired since I began taking the medication." This is reflective of which nursing diagnosis?

1 Activity Intolerance
2 Cardiac Output, Decreased
3 Health Maintenance, Altered
4 Self-Care Deficit

Answer: 2

Rationale: Atenolol is a beta-blocker that causes a decreased heart rate and blood pressure and a decrease in cardiac output. Fatigue is the most common side effect. If this fatigue interferes with the client's activity level, dosage can be adjusted to eliminate this side effect. Activity intolerance is the state in which an individual has insufficient energy to complete activities of daily living. This is not described in this question.

Test-Taking Strategy: When the question asks to select the appropriate nursing diagnosis, identify the data presented in the question, and use these data to select the nursing diagnosis. Defining characteristics of decreased cardiac output include complaints of fatigue or weakness. Use the process of elimination to select the correct option.

Level of Cognitive Ability: Analysis
Phase of Nursing Process: Analysis
Client Needs: Physiological Integrity
Content Area: Pharmacology

Reference

Hodgson, B., & Kizior, R. (1998). *Saunders nursing drug handbook 1998.* Philadelphia: W. B. Saunders, pp. 78–81.

---

140. The nurse performs an assessment on a client taking an antipsychotic medication. Which of the following assessment data would the nurse identify as indicating neuroleptic malignant syndrome?

1 Hypothermia, polyuria, dizziness
2 Hypotension, confusion, nausea
3 Vomiting, headache, diarrhea
4 Hyperthermia, muscular rigidity, hypertension

Answer: 4

Rationale: Neuroleptic malignant syndrome is a serious, potentially fatal reaction to antipsychotics. The classic symptoms include hyperthermia; severe extrapyramidal symptoms, such as muscular rigidity; and autonomic dysfunction, such as hypertension and tachycardia.

Test-Taking Strategy: Knowledge of this serious reaction to antipsychotics is required to assist you in answering this question. If you are unfamiliar with this serious and potentially fatal reaction, review this information now.

Level of Cognitive Ability: Analysis
Phase of Nursing Process: Analysis
Client Needs: Physiological Integrity
Content Area: Pharmacology

Reference

Varcarolis, E. M. (1998). *Foundations of psychiatric mental health nursing* (3rd ed.). Philadelphia: W. B. Saunders, p. 651.

---

141. The home care nurse has been visiting a client with lung cancer weekly for 1 month. Over time, the nurse assesses increasing dyspnea as well as increasing edema of the face and arms of the client. The nurse analyzes these symptoms and finds them consistent with

1. Superior vena cava syndrome.
2. Spinal cord compression.
3. Distant metastasis.
4. Renal failure.

Answer: 1

Rationale: The superior vena cava is the large vessel that accepts blood from the head, neck, and arms, returning it to the heart. Therefore, compression of this vessel by a tumor or enlarged lymph nodes can cause decreased blood return from these areas resulting in swelling. Although spinal cord compression is another oncologic emergency, it does not cause these symptoms. Distant metastasis would, by definition, not be near the lungs in this case. The edema of renal failure would not be confined to these specific areas of the body.

Test-Taking Strategy: Read the case situation and consider every word when answering the question. In this case, no other option would be manifested by the exact findings described in the case situation except option 1, superior vena cava syndrome. Note the location of the cancer, and consider the anatomical structures nearby to assist in selecting the correct option.

Level of Cognitive Ability: Analysis
Phase of Nursing Process: Analysis
Client Needs: Physiological Integrity
Content Area: Adult Health/Oncology

Reference

Smeltzer, S., & Bare, B. (1996). *Brunner and Suddarth's Textbook of medical-surgical nursing* (8th ed.). Philadelphia: Lippincott-Raven, pp. 309–310.

---

142. The nurse is caring for a client with Addison's disease. The nurse assesses the vital signs and determines that the client has orthostatic hypotension. The nurse analyzes this finding as related to which of the following?

1. A decrease in cortisol release
2. A decreased secretion of aldosterone
3. An increase in epinephrine secretion
4. Increased levels of androgens

Answer: 2

Rationale: A decreased secretion of aldosterone results in a limited reabsorption of sodium and water; therefore, the client experiences fluid volume deficit. A decrease in cortisol, an increase in epinephrine, and an increase in androgen secretion do not result in postural hypotension.

Test-Taking Strategy: Knowledge of the action of aldosterone in the regulation of intravascular volume and blood pressure assists in answering this question. Try to sense the relationship between blood pressure control and aldosterone when selecting the correct option. If you had difficulty with this question, take time now to review the action of aldosterone.

Level of Cognitive Ability: Analysis
Phase of Nursing Process: Analysis
Client Needs: Physiological Integrity
Content Area: Adult Health/Endocrine

Reference

LeMone, P., & Burke, K. M. (1996). *Medical-surgical nursing: Critical thinking in client care.* Menlo Park, CA: Addison-Wesley, p. 697.

143. The nurse is taking pulmonary artery catheter measurements on the client with adult respiratory distress syndrome (ARDS). The pulmonary capillary wedge pressure (PCWP) reading is 12 mmHg. The nurse interprets that this reading is:

1 High and expected.
2 Low and unexpected.
3 Normal and expected.
4 Uncertain and unexpected.

Answer: 3

Rationale: The normal PCWP is 8–13 mmHg, and the client is considered to have high readings if they exceed 18–20 mmHg. The client with ARDS has a normal PCWP, which is an expected finding because the edema is in the interstitium of the lung and is noncardiac in origin.

Test-Taking Strategy: To answer this question correctly, it is necessary to know the normal PCWP and that in this situation it is normal. This makes sense, knowing that fluid accumulates in the interstitium of the lung in ARDS and not in the vascular bed. Thus, the answer could only be option 3, that the reading is normal and expected. If you had difficulty with this question, take time now to review the normal PCWP.

Level of Cognitive Ability: Analysis
Phase of Nursing Process: Analysis
Client Needs: Physiological Integrity
Content Area: Adult Health/Respiratory

Reference

Black, J., & Matassarin-Jacobs, E. (1997). *Medical-surgical nursing: Clinical management for continuity of care* (5th ed.). Philadelphia: W. B. Saunders, p. 1233.

---

144. An elderly client with advanced Alzheimer's disease is placed in balanced suspension traction. The physician expects to internally fixate the client's femur in 7–10 days. Based on this information, the nurse determines that the first priority relates to which of the following nursing diagnoses?

1 Constipation, Risk for
2 Activity Intolerance, Risk for
3 Diversional Activity Deficit, Risk for
4 Thought Process, Altered

Answer: 1

Rationale: Although all of these diagnoses may apply to this client, 7–10 days of lying supine, being elderly, and having cognitive impairment put the client at extreme risk for constipation and possibly impaction. Although the client likely does have altered thought processes because of the Alzheimer's disease, the nurse is least likely to reverse this process. The client is immobilized, making Risk for Activity Intolerance an irrelevant point. Diversional Activity Deficit represents psychosocial needs, which become important once physiological needs are met.

Test-Taking Strategy: This question requires the analysis of several factors, including cognitive impairment; skeletal traction; and the effects of analgesics, immobility, and aging on the gastrointestinal tract. The clues in the stem are the number of days before surgery is performed, combined with the fact that the client is elderly and is probably unable to communicate basic physiological needs.

Level of Cognitive Ability: Analysis
Phase of Nursing Process: Analysis
Client Needs: Physiological Integrity
Content Area: Adult Health/Musculoskeletal

Reference

Lewis, S., Collier, I., & Heitkemper, M. (1996). *Medical-surgical nursing: Assessment and management of clinical problems* (4th ed.). St. Louis: Mosby–Year Book, p. 1858.

---

145. The nurse is reading the purified protein derivative (PPD) skin test (Mantoux's test) for a client with no documented health problems. The site has no induration and a 1-mm area of ecchymosis. The nurse interprets that the result is

1 Positive.
2 Negative.
3 Uncertain.
4 Borderline.

Answer: 2

Rationale: A positive PPD reading has induration measuring 10 mm or more and is considered abnormal. A small area of ecchymosis is insignificant and is probably related to the injection technique.

Test-Taking Strategy: Use the process of elimination to answer the question. To answer this question accurately, you need to know that induration is necessary for a positive response. Because the client in this question has no induration, the result can only be negative.

Level of Cognitive Ability: Analysis
Phase of Nursing Process:Analysis
Client Needs: Physiological Integrity
Content Area: Adult Health/Respiratory

Reference

Black, J., & Matassarin-Jacobs, E. (1997). *Medical-surgical nursing: Clinical management for continuity of care* (5th ed.). Philadelphia: W. B. Saunders, p. 720.

---

146. Which of these behaviors, if present in a client's history, would the nurse determine as being most likely related to manifestations of hypothyroidism?

1 Depression
2 Nervousness
3 Irritability
4 Anxiety

Answer: 1

Rationale: Hypothyroid clients experience a slow metabolic rate, and its manifestation includes apathy, fatigue, sleepiness, and depression. Options 2, 3, and 4 represent clinical manifestations of hyperthyroidism.

Test-Taking Strategy: Knowledge of the differences between hypothyroidism and hyperthyroidism assists in answering this question. Remember *hypo* meaning *down* and *hyper* meaning *up*. This may assist you in remembering the symptoms that occur in each condition. If you had difficulty with this question, take time now to review the differences between these disorders.

Level of Cognitive Ability: Analysis
Phase of the Nursing Process: Analysis
Client Needs: Psychosocial Integrity
Content Area: Adult Health/Endocrine

Reference

Black, J., & Matassarin-Jacobs, E. (1997). *Medical-surgical nursing: Clinical management for continuity of care* (5th ed.). Philadelphia: W. B. Saunders, pp. 2008, 2014, 2015.

---

147. An elderly client is transferred to the nursing unit after a graft to a stage IV decubitus ulcer. Which dietary items would the nurse encourage the client to eat to promote wound healing?

1 Chicken breast, broccoli, strawberries, milk
2 Peanut butter and jelly, cantaloupe, tea
3 Pork, potatoes, Jell-O, orange juice
4 Spaghetti with clam sauce, garlic bread, cola

Answer: 1

Rationale: Protein and vitamin C are necessary for wound healing. Poultry and milk are good sources of protein. Broccoli and strawberries are good sources of vitamin C. Peanut butter is a source of niacin. Jell-O and jelly have no nutrient value. Spaghetti is a complex carbohydrate.

Test-Taking Strategy: Knowledge of nutrition related to wound healing is needed to answer the question. Recall that protein and vitamin C are necessary for wound healing. When an option contains more than one item, be sure that all items in the option relate to what the question is asking. Use the process of elimination with the items in each option.

Level of Cognitive Ability: Application
Phase of Nursing Process: Analysis
Client Needs: Physiological Integrity
Content Area: Integumentary

Reference

Craven, R. F., & Hirnle, C. J. (1996). *Fundamentals of nursing: Human health and function* (2nd ed.). Philadelphia: Lippincott-Raven, p. 1028.

148. A client receiving enteral feedings develops diarrhea shortly after initiation of the feedings. When reviewing the nursing history for this client, which of these notations would the nurse interpret as a need to call the physician?

1 Prior history of enteral feedings
2 Difficulty swallowing
3 History of hemorrhoids
4 Lactose intolerance since childhood

Answer: 4

Rationale: Research has shown that causes for the onset of diarrhea with the use of enteral feedings include drug therapy, lactose intolerance, decreased serum albumin levels, osmotic overload, and too-rapid infusion rate. Prior history of enteral feedings, difficulty swallowing, and a history of hemorrhoids are not significant in this situation, warranting a need to contact the physician.

Test-Taking Strategy: Use priority setting to answer this question, seeking the response that addresses physiological integrity. This question is looking for the physiological cause of an adverse reaction to enteral feedings. Option 1 is not physiological and indicates that the client has tolerated this treatment before. Option 2 is an indication for enteral feeding. Option 3 is most commonly associated with constipation, not diarrhea. Option 4 warrants notifying the physician to change to a lactose-free formula.

Level of Cognitive Ability: Analysis
Phase of Nursing Process: Analysis
Client Needs: Physiological Integrity
Content Area: Fundamental Skills

Reference

Burrell, L. O., Gerlach, M. J., & Pless, B. (1997). *Adult nursing: Acute and community care* (2nd ed.). Stamford, CT: Appleton & Lange, p. 1347.

149. A client is admitted to the hospital with acute pancreatitis. Based on the nursing knowledge associated with this condition, a nursing diagnosis most appropriate for this client would be

1 Fluid Volume Excess related to sodium retention.
2 Alteration in Fluid and Electrolyte Balance related to hyperkalemia.
3 Alteration in Comfort related to abdominal pain.
4 Potential for Hypoglycemia related to low blood glucose secondary to too much insulin.

Answer: 3

Rationale: Abdominal pain is the predominant symptom of pancreatitis. Shock and hypovolemia may occur from hemorrhage, toxemia, or loss of fluid into peritoneal space. Potassium and sodium may be lost because of gastric suction and frequent vomiting. Hyperglycemia may result from impaired carbohydrate metabolism.

Test-Taking Strategy: Knowledge of the common signs and symptoms associated with pancreatitis as well as actual and potential health care needs is needed to answer this question. If you had difficulty with this question, take time now to review the signs and symptoms associated with acute pancreatitis.

Level of Cognitive Ability: Analysis
Phase of Nursing Process: Analysis
Client Needs: Physiological Integrity
Content Area: Adult Health/Gastrointestinal

Reference

Black, J., & Matassarin-Jacobs, E. (1997). *Medical-surgical nursing: Clinical management for continuity of care* (5th ed.). Philadelphia: W. B. Saunders, p. 1923.

150. The nurse is caring for a client with hyperaldosteronism. Based on the physiological responses that occur in this condition, the nurse determines that the priority nursing diagnosis is

1 Risk for Injury related to impaired immune response.
2 Fluid Volume Excess related to hypernatremia.
3 Impaired Tissue Integrity related to protein catabolism.
4 Pain related to demineralization of bones.

Answer: 2

Rationale: Hyperaldosteronism produces sodium and water reabsorption resulting in hypertension from blood volume expansion. These clinical manifestations place the client at risk for the nursing diagnosis of fluid volume excess. Excess cortisol production produces an altered immune response, protein catabolism, and bone demineralization, thus placing the client at risk for injury.

Test-Taking Strategy: Knowledge regarding the physiological responses that occur in hyperaldosteronism is required to answer this question. If you had difficulty with this question, take time now to review the physiological responses that occur in this condition.

Level of Cognitive Ability: Analysis
Phase of Nursing Process: Analysis
Client Needs: Physiological Integrity
Content Area: Adult Health/Endocrine

Reference

Luckmann, J. (1997). *Saunders manual of nursing care.* Philadelphia: W. B. Saunders, pp. 1405–1407.

151. While performing a preoperative physical assessment of a client being prepared for an adrenalectomy, the nurse obtains a temperature reading of 99.4°F. The nurse analyzes this temperature reading as

1 Within normal limits.
2 A finding that needs to be reported to the physician immediately.
3 An expected finding caused by the operative stress response.
4 Slightly abnormal but an insignificant finding.

Answer: 2

Rationale: An adrenalectomy is performed because of excess adrenal gland function. Excess cortisol production impairs the immune response, making the client at risk for infection. Because of this, clients need to be protected from infection, and minor variations in normal vital sign values need to be reported so that infections are detected before they become overwhelming.

Test-Taking Strategy: This question asks you to interpret the meaning or severity of a slightly elevated temperature finding in a client being prepared to undergo an adrenalectomy. Knowing that a low-grade temperature is an indication of infection and keeping in mind that the adrenal glands are needed to fight infection should direct you to select option 2 as the correct answer. If you had difficulty with this question, take time now to review preoperative nursing care and the preoperative care of the client undergoing adrenalectomy.

Level of Cognitive Ability: Analysis
Phase of Nursing Process: Analysis
Client Needs: Physiological Integrity
Content Area: Adult Health/Endocrine

Reference

Burrell, L. O., Gerlach, M. J., & Pless, B. (1997). *Adult nursing: Acute and community care* (2nd ed.). Stamford, CT: Appleton & Lange, p. 1106.

152. A client admitted to a psychiatric unit for a psychotic episode is observed running around, banging on doors, yelling, "Let me out. There's nothing wrong with me. I don't belong here." The nurse analyzes these behaviors as

1 Projection.
2 Denial.
3 Regression.
4 Rationalization.

Answer: 2

Rationale: Denial is refusal to admit to a painful reality, which is treated as if it does not exist. In projection, a person unconsciously rejects emotionally unacceptable features and attributes them to other people, objects, or situations. In regression, the client returns to an earlier, more comforting, although less mature way of behaving. Rationalization is justifying illogical or unreasonable ideas, actions, or feelings by developing acceptable explanations that satisfy the teller as well as the listener.

Test-Taking Strategy: Remember that defense mechanisms are misused by clients who are dealing with threats to their esteem. The key phrase in the question that should direct you to the correct option is "There's nothing wrong with me." Select the response that recognizes an attempt to avoid looking at the reality of the situation. If you had difficulty with this question, take time now to review defense mechanisms.

Level of Cognitive Ability: Analysis
Phase of Nursing Process: Analysis
Client Needs: Psychosocial Integrity
Content Area: Mental Health

Reference

Carson, V., & Arnold, E. (1996). *Mental health nursing: The nurse-patient journey.* Philadelphia: W. B. Saunders, pp. 695–698.

---

153. A nurse is working in a tuberculosis screening clinic. The nurse understands that which of the following populations are the high-priority candidates for tuberculosis?

1 Persons admitted to the hospital for day surgery
2 Children over 6 years of age in a summer school program
3 Residents of a nursing home
4 A family who has recently emigrated from Australia

Answer: 3

Rationale: Residents of long-term care facilities are considered high-risk candidates for tuberculosis. Children under 4 would also be considered a high-priority group. Persons admitted for day surgery are not high-risk candidates. Persons from Asia, Africa, Latin America, and the Caribbean are considered high risk but not persons from Australia.

Test-Taking Strategy: Use the process of elimination to answer the question. A general understanding of susceptibility for infection is needed to answer this question. The very young and very old are often susceptible to infection, as are persons with chronic or debilitating diseases. Persons residing in nursing homes may fall into the category of being elderly, having chronic health problems, and living in group settings. If you had difficulty with this question, take time now to review high-risk candidates for tuberculosis.

Level of Cognitive Ability: Analysis
Phase of Nursing Process: Analysis
Client Needs: Physiological Integrity
Content Area: Adult Health/Respiratory

Reference

Thompson, J., McFarland, G., Hirsch, J., & Tucker, S. (1997). *Mosby's clinical nursing* (4th ed.). St. Louis: Mosby–Year Book, p. 1130.

---

154. Rh_o (D) immune globulin (RhoGAM) is prescribed for the client after delivery. The nurse reviews the client's history and determines that this medication is contraindicated

1 In persons who have experienced a severe reaction to human globulin.
2 When it is known or suspected that Rh-positive fetal blood cells have entered the circulation of an Rh-negative woman.
3 When exposure to Rh sensitization occurs during amniocentesis.
4 When exposure to Rh sensitization occurs because of abortion.

Answer: 1

Rationale: RhoGAM is not given when a client has experienced a severe reaction to its component human globulin. Administration predisposes the client to fever, myalgia, and irritation at the injection site. RhoGAM is indicated when Rh-negative clients are exposed to Rh-positive fetal blood cells in any way, including amniocentesis and abortion.

Test-Taking Strategy: Knowledge regarding RhoGAM is required to answer the question. You are likely to see questions related to this medication on NCLEX-RN. Take time now to review this medication if you had difficulty with this question.

Level of Cognitive Ability: Analysis
Phase of Nursing Process: Analysis
Client Needs: Physiological Integrity
Content Area: Maternity

Reference

Nichols, F., & Zwelling, E. (1997). *Maternal-newborn nursing: Theory and practice.* Philadelphia: W. B. Saunders, pp. 652–658.

155. A client with suspected Guillain-Barré syndrome has a lumbar puncture performed. The cerebrospinal fluid (CSF) protein is 750 mg/dL. The nurse analyzes these results as

1 Normal.
2 Lower than normal, ruling out Guillain-Barré syndrome.
3 Higher than normal, supporting the diagnosis of Guillain-Barré syndrome.
4 Not significant and unrelated to Guillain-Barré syndrome.

Answer: 3

Rationale: Seven to 10 days after the onset of symptoms of Guillain-Barré syndrome, the CSF protein levels become extremely high. Normal CSF protein is 15–45 mg/dL.

Test-Taking Strategy: Knowledge regarding the diagnostic results associated with Guillain-Barré syndrome and the normal level of CSF protein is required to answer the question. If you are unsure about the normal level of CSF protein, select the response that is similar to the focus of the question. A CSF protein of 750 mg/dL is certainly an elevated level. If you had difficulty with this question, take time now to review the diagnostic results associated with Guillain-Barré syndrome and the normal level of CSF protein.

Level of Cognitive Ability: Analysis
Phase of Nursing Process: Analysis
Client Needs: Physiological Integrity
Content Area: Adult Health/Neurological

Reference

Black, J., & Matassarin-Jacobs, E. (1997). *Medical-surgical nursing: Clinical management for continuity of care* (5th ed.). Philadelphia: W. B. Saunders, p. 877.

156. A female client with myasthenia gravis expresses concern over her inability to smile, her drooping eyelids, and how the disease has made her weak and changed the way she looks. The most appropriate nursing diagnosis for this client would be which of the following?

1 High Risk for Injury related to muscle weakness and visual disturbances
2 Activity Intolerance related to muscle weakness and fatigue
3 Impaired Verbal Communication related to muscle weakness
4 Body Image Disturbance related to muscle weakness

Answer: 4

Rationale: Although each of the options may apply to clients with myasthenia gravis, the data in the stem best support option 4, the diagnosis related to body image.

Test-Taking Strategy: When answering questions related to selecting a nursing diagnosis, identify the data presented in the question to determine the appropriate nursing diagnosis. Remember the answer is often in the case of the question. The client expressed concern over how the disease changed her looks. This statement supports the altered body image.

Level of Cognitive Ability: Analysis
Phase of Nursing Process: Analysis
Client Needs: Psychosocial Integrity
Content Area: Adult Health/Neurological

Reference

Ignatavicius, D. D., Workman, M. L., & Mishler, M. A. (1995). *Medical-surgical nursing: A nursing process approach* (2nd ed.). Philadelphia: W. B. Saunders, p. 1224.

157. The nurse is caring for a client with Paget's disease. The nurse understands that the client is to receive calcitonin (Calcimar) for which of the following purposes?

1 To decrease bone reabsorption
2 To promote the urine excretion of calcium
3 To decrease gastrointestinal absorption of calcium
4 To increase bone metabolism

Answer: 1

Rationale: Calcitonin works in conjunction with parathyroid hormone to regulate calcium by decreasing the rate of bone turnover and regulating bone metabolism.

Test-Taking Strategy: This question requires knowledge related to the purpose and action of medications used to treat Paget's disease. Option 4 is the opposite action to the correct action. Options 2 and 3 describe the actions related to other medications, furosemide (Lasix) and glucocorticoids. If you had difficulty with this question, take time now to review the action and purpose of calcitonin and the treatment for Paget's disease.

Level of Cognitive Ability: Analysis
Phase of Nursing Process: Analysis
Client Needs: Physiological Integrity
Content Area: Pharmacology

Reference

Hodgson, B., & Kizior, R. (1998). *Saunders nursing drug handbook 1998.* Philadelphia: W. B. Saunders, pp. 137–138.

---

158. A client has just had a cesarean section to deliver a nonviable fetus owing to abruptio placentae. She has just been told that she is developing disseminated intravascular coagulopathy. She begins to cry and screams, "God, just let me die now." Which of the following nursing diagnoses would the nurse determine as most appropriate for this client?

1 Hopelessness related to the loss of the baby and personal health
2 Knowledge Deficit related to the disease process
3 Self-Esteem Disturbance related to being ill
4 Grief related to the loss of the baby

Answer: 1

Rationale: By seeing no way out of the situation except for death, the client meets the criteria for hopelessness. A person who lacks hope feels that life is too much to handle. Option 2 is a possible nursing diagnosis later, but there are not enough data to support it at this point. The data provided in the question do not support the nursing diagnosis in option 3, Self-Esteem Disturbance. Option 4 may be a possible nursing diagnosis at a later time; at this time, however, the diagnosis of hopelessness should take precedence.

Test-Taking Strategy: This question addresses formulating and prioritizing nursing diagnoses. Identify the data addressed in the question to select the correct response. The key phrase that should direct you to the correct option is "God, just let me die now."

Level of Cognitive Ability: Analysis
Phase of Nursing Process: Analysis
Client Needs: Psychosocial Integrity
Content Area: Maternity

Reference

McFarland, G., & McFarlane, E. (1997). *Nursing diagnosis and intervention: Planning for patient care.* St. Louis: Mosby–Year Book, pp. 577–578.

---

159. The clinic nurse is caring for a pregnant client with AIDS. The nurse determines that which one of the following is the most appropriate nursing diagnosis for this client?

1 Altered Health Maintenance
2 High Risk for Infection
3 Sensory/Perceptual Alterations
4 Fluid Volume Deficit

Answer: 2

Rationale: HIV infection decreases the body's immune response, making the infected person susceptible to infections. HIV affects helper T lymphocytes, which are vital to the body's defense system. Opportunistic infections are a primary cause of death in persons affected with AIDS. Therefore, preventing infection is a priority of nursing care.

Test-Taking Strategy: A knowledge of the pathophysiology of AIDS is needed to answer this question. Knowing that AIDS affects the body's immune system assists in selecting the correct answer. The key phrase is "most appropriate." If you had difficulty with this question, take time now to review the potential concerns related to the client with AIDS.

Level of Cognitive Ability: Analysis
Phase of Nursing Process: Analysis
Client Needs: Physiological Integrity
Content Area: Maternity

Reference

Nichols, F., & Zwelling, E. (1997). *Maternal-newborn nursing: Theory and practice.* Philadelphia: W. B. Saunders, p. 685.

160. A woman with pre-eclampsia delivered a healthy son and continued to receive magnesium sulfate therapy postpartum. Twenty-four hours after delivery, the client began to diurese with more than 100 mL of urine every hour. Based on the knowledge of pre-eclampsia, the nurse analyzes that this volume of urine output indicates that

1 Edema and vasoconstriction in the brain and kidneys have decreased.
2 Convulsions are imminent.
3 High-output renal failure has occurred.
4 Hyperkalemia is present.

Answer: 1

Rationale: Diuresis is a positive prognostic sign that indicates that edema and vasoconstriction in the brain and kidneys have decreased. As vasospasm is decreased, edema also lessens, and tissue perfusion increases. Diuresis reflects this increasing tissue perfusion to the kidneys. Clients who have severe pre-eclampsia are not considered to be out of danger until birth and diuresis occurs. Diuresis is not an indication of impending seizure. Although renal failure is a complication of severe pre-eclampsia, it is not of the high-output type of kidney failure. Potassium is lost through the urine; therefore, hyperkalemia is not associated with diuresis.

Test-Taking Strategy: A knowledge about the pathophysiology of pre-eclampsia is necessary to answer this question correctly. Knowing that oliguria is associated with severe pre-eclampsia can help you determine that diuresis would be associated with improvement of the condition. If you had difficulty with this question, take time now to review the expected responses to treatment of pre-eclampsia.

Level of Cognitive Ability: Analysis
Phase of Nursing Process: Analysis
Client's Needs: Physiological Integrity
Content Area: Maternity

Reference

Nichols, F., & Zwelling, E. (1997). *Maternal-newborn nursing: Theory and practice.* Philadelphia: W. B. Saunders, pp. 650–652.

---

161. The client has requested and undergone testing for HIV. The client now asks what will be done next, since the results of two enzyme-linked immunosorbent assay (ELISA) tests have been positive. The nurse's response is based on the understanding that

1 The client will probably have a bone marrow biopsy done.
2 A Western blot will be done to confirm these findings.
3 A CD4 cell count will be done to measure T helper lymphocytes.
4 The client will be definitively diagnosed as HIV positive at this point.

Answer: 2

Rationale: If the results of two ELISA tests are positive, the Western blot is done to confirm the findings. If the result of the Western blot is positive, the client is considered to be positive for HIV and infected with the HIV virus.

Test-Taking Strategy: Knowledge of the procedural steps in diagnosing HIV is needed to answer this question. Review these now if they are unfamiliar to you. This is a subject of great concern to clients, and you would want to have the appropriate information to share. The increasing incidence of HIV as a major health problem also makes it a reasonably frequent area for testing on NCLEX-RN.

Level of Cognitive Ability: Analysis
Phase of Nursing Process: Analysis
Client Needs: Physiological Integrity
Content Area: Adult Health/Respiratory

Reference

Black, J., & Matassarin-Jacobs, E. (1997). *Medical-surgical nursing: Clinical management for continuity of care* (5th ed.). Philadelphia: W. B. Saunders, p. 611.

162. The nurse is caring for the following group of clients on the clinical nursing unit. The nurse interprets that which of them is most at risk for development of pulmonary embolism?

1 A 65-year-old man out of bed 1 day after prostate resection
2 A 73-year-old woman who has just had pinning of a hip fracture
3 A 25-year-old woman with diabetic ketoacidosis
4 A 38-year-old man with pulmonary contusion after an auto accident

Answer: 2

Rationale: Clients frequently at risk for pulmonary embolism include clients who are immobilized. This is especially true in the immobilized postoperative client. Other at-risk clients include those with conditions that are characterized by hypercoagulability, endothelial disease, and advancing age.

Test-Taking Strategy: These options can best be compared by evaluating the degree of immobility that each client has and also the age of the client, which is given in each option. The clients in options 1 and 3 have the least long-term anticipated immobility, and therefore they should be eliminated first. Of the two remaining, the younger client with the lung contusion would be expected to be less immobile than the elderly woman with hip fracture, leaving option 2 as the answer. If you had difficulty with this question, take time now to review the risks for the development of pulmonary embolism.

Level of Cognitive Ability: Analysis
Phase of Nursing Process: Analysis
Client Needs: Physiological Integrity
Content Area: Adult Health/Respiratory

Reference
Smeltzer, S., & Bare, B. (1996). *Brunner and Suddarth's Textbook of medical-surgical nursing* (8th ed.). Philadelphia: Lippincott-Raven, p. 526.

---

163. The client who had a lung resection for cancer has been told that bone metastasis has occurred. The client is considering megavitamin and diet therapy because the original surgery did not provide a cure. The client asks the nurse for an opinion of these therapies. In formulating a response, the nurse incorporates which of the following concepts?

1 The client's right to justice, and the nurse's obligation to project parentalism
2 The client's right to privacy, and the nurse's obligation to uphold the law
3 The client's right to freedom of speech, and the nurse's obligation to support the client
4 The client's right to autonomy, and the nurse's obligation to behave ethically

Answer: 4

Rationale: The client has the right to autonomy, or the exercise of personal choice. At the same time, the nurse has the obligation to behave ethically. Unconventional cancer treatments have not been proven to be effective, may be toxic to the client, and may be extremely expensive. The nurse balances the client's right to self-determination with the obligation to share with the client knowledge about the ineffectiveness of these methods. Privacy is the right of a client to be free from intrusion by someone into their own personal affairs. Justice is the ethical principle of treating people fairly.

Test-Taking Strategy: Use the process of elimination to answer the question. Begin to answer this question by eliminating options 1 and 2, which are the two options that have the smallest degree of "fit" with the wording of the question. Of the remaining two, you would select option 4 by knowing that the nurse must behave ethically and that the client ultimately has freedom of choice.

Level of Cognitive Ability: Analysis
Phase of Nursing Process: Analysis
Client Needs: Psychosocial Integrity
Content Area: Adult Health/Oncology

Reference
Bolander, V. (1994). *Sorenson and Luckmann's Basic nursing: A psychophysiologic approach* (3rd ed.). Philadelphia: W. B. Saunders, p. 47.

164. The client has had a radical neck dissection for cancer of the throat, and the physician is about to remove the dressing. The client indicates to the nurse and physician an unwillingness to look at the incision with the mirror in the bedside stand. The nurse formulates which of the following nursing diagnoses for this client?

1. Anxiety
2. Fear
3. Body Image Disturbance
4. Ineffective Family Coping

Answer: 3

Rationale: The client who has experienced extensive surgery of the head or neck is often sensitive to personal appearance in the early postoperative period. The nurse identifies that the client is experiencing Body Image Disturbance. This diagnosis is used when the client has either a verbal or a nonverbal response to a change in body image that is either actual or perceived. Ineffective Family Coping is not appropriate because the stem gives no information about the family. The diagnoses Anxiety and Fear are used when the client has a vague (Anxiety) or an identified (Fear) sense of unease or dread.

Test-Taking Strategy: When asked to select a nursing diagnosis, use the information presented in the question as a guide to the correct response. The stem of the question gives no information about any fear or anxiety that the client may have, so options 1 and 2 are eliminated first. Option 3 is chosen over option 4 because the stem also gives no information about the family.

Level of Cognitive Ability: Analysis
Phase of Nursing Process: Analysis
Client Needs: Psychosocial Integrity
Content Area: Adult Health/Oncology

Reference

Cox, H., Hinz, M., Lubno, M., et al. (1997). *Clinical applications of nursing diagnosis: Adult, child, women's, psychiatric, gerontic, and home health considerations* (3rd ed.). Philadelphia: F. A. Davis, pp. 496, 506, 514.

---

165. A young pregnant woman with diabetes has lost 10 pounds during the first 15 weeks of gestation. The client tells the nurse, "I do not eat regular meals." Based on the client's statement, the nurse determines that the best response would be

1. "If you do not eat regular meals you will hurt your baby."
2. "Can you tell me more about what you are eating?"
3. "I'll have the doctor review your diet history?"
4. "It does not matter anymore how much weight you gain."

Answer: 2

Rationale: It is important for the nurse to get more information from the client. In option 2, the nurse is using the therapeutic communication tool of validation and clarification to obtain more information. The other options block communication. Option 1 devalues the client and shows disapproval, option 3 is avoiding the issue, and option 4 provides false reassurance.

Test-Taking Strategy: When answering communication questions, identify the use of therapeutic communication techniques and communication blocks. Therapeutic communication tools are those that enhance communication and indicate a correct response. Avoid selecting responses that block communication. Additionally, option 2 identifies the process of gathering assessment data, the first step in the nursing process.

Level of Cognitive Ability: Analysis
Phase of Nursing Process: Analysis
Client Needs: Psychosocial Integrity
Content Area: Maternity

Reference

Nichols, F., & Zwelling, E. (1997). *Maternal-newborn nursing: Theory and practice.* Philadelphia: W. B. Saunders, p. 671.

166. The nurse answers a call light to the room of a woman just admitted in early latent labor. The client is lying flat on her back on the bed. The husband states excitedly, "I think my wife is going into shock or something. She was just lying there and she turned so pale and her hands are so clammy. She's dizzy and sick to her stomach." The nurse notes on the noninvasive blood pressure machine that the client's pulse is 58 beats/minute and her blood pressure is 90/50 mmHg. The nurse interprets that the client is experiencing

1. Altered tissue perfusion related to hypotensive syndrome (vena cava syndrome).
2. Progression from latent to active first-stage labor.
3. Hyperventilation related to excitement secondary to first labor experience.
4. Anxiety related to situational crisis: onset of labor.

Answer: 1

Rationale: The supine position of the woman is adding gravity pressure onto the inferior vena cava, which is already displaced and partially compressed by the full-term gravid uterus. The increased compression has decreased the cardiac output, leading to beginning tissue hypoxia bringing on the symptoms as described in the question.

Test-Taking Strategy: Read the case situation carefully, identifying key assessment information. Be cautious about a client or family member's conclusions, in this case the husband's, because it may be false information. Use the process of elimination in selecting the correct option. Read all of the information in the options, and eliminate options that are not supported by data stated in the case situation.

Level of Cognitive Ability: Analysis
Phase of Nursing Process: Analysis
Client Needs: Physiological Integrity
Content Area: Maternity

Reference

Reeder, S., Martin, L., & Koniak-Griffin, D. (1997). *Maternity nursing: Family, newborn, and women's health care* (18th ed.). Philadelphia: Lippincott-Raven, p. 374.

---

167. Which of the following is an appropriate nursing diagnosis for an adolescent being admitted to the nursing unit for treatment of slipped capital femoral epiphysis (SCFE)?

1. Anticipatory Grieving related to life-threatening diagnosis
2. Chronic Impaired Self-Image related to immobilization
3. Diversional Activity Deficit related to impaired mobility/confinement to bed
4. High Risk for Fluid Volume Deficit related to negative nitrogen balance

Answer: 3

Rationale: SCFE refers to spontaneous displacement of the proximal femoral epiphysis and is treated by skeletal traction followed by surgical repair and casting. The monotony of immobilization can lead to sluggish intellectual and psychomotor responses, which can be overcome or prevented by engaging the adolescent in diversional activities. The stem of the question does not indicate that this adolescent has Chronic Low Self-Esteem, Body Image Disturbance, or Situational Low Self-Esteem, even though these are possible diagnoses. Option 1 is inappropriate because SCFE is not a life-threatening disorder. There is not enough information in the stem to suggest Fluid Volume Deficit (option 4) as an appropriate nursing diagnosis, and although negative nitrogen balance is a complication of immobility, it is not directly related to fluid balance.

Test-Taking Strategy: Read all four options carefully, and use the process of elimination to rule out the incorrect options. Identify the information in the question, and use this information as a guide in selecting the appropriate nursing diagnosis.

Level of Cognitive Ability: Analysis
Phase of Nursing Process: Analysis
Client Needs: Psychosocial Integrity
Content Area: Child Health

Reference

Wong, D. (1997). *Whaley and Wong's Essentials of pediatric nursing* (5th ed.). St. Louis: Mosby–Year Book, pp. 1122–1123, 1125, 1145.

168. The nurse measures the head circumference of an infant after the surgical placement of a ventricular peritoneal shunt for the correction of hydrocephalus. The result of the head circumference measurement is reported as having increased by 1 cm in the last 24 hours on the fifth postoperative day. The nurse analyzes this result as

1 Normal for this postoperative period.
2 A complication of the proper functioning of the shunt.
3 Insignificant and unrelated to the patency of the ventricular peritoneal shunt.
4 Subcutaneous tissue swelling owing to the surgical procedure.

Answer: 2

Rationale: The head circumference should be decreasing slightly every day as the superficial tissue fluid is reabsorbed after surgical trauma. An increase in the head circumference indicates a lack of proper shunting of CSF owing to either a blockage or defect in the ventricular peritoneal shunt apparatus. Medical or surgical intervention is required.

Test-Taking Strategy: Knowledge that a ventricular peritoneal shunt is surgically placed to divert the collection of CSF from the ventricular part of the brain to the peritoneal cavity is required to answer the question. From this point, use the process of elimination, selecting option 2, as one would then expect the head circumference to decrease in size by the fifth postoperative day.

Level of Cognitive Ability: Analysis
Phase of Nursing Process: Analysis
Client Needs: Physiological Integrity
Content Area: Child Health

Reference

Ashwill, J., & Droske, S. (1997). *Nursing care of children: Principles and practice.* Philadelphia: W. B. Saunders, pp. 1238–1241.

---

169. This morning a client sustained a fractured right proximal fibula and tibia that was casted in a long leg plaster cast. During evening rounds, the nurse notes right lower extremity capillary refill greater than 3 seconds and toes that are edematous and dusky. The client states that the pain medication is not working anymore and that the right foot feels like it is asleep. The nurse analyzes the information and determines that the client's symptoms are most clearly an example of

1 Fat embolism.
2 Volkmann's thrombosis.
3 Venous thrombosis.
4 Compartment syndrome.

Answer: 4

Rationale: In this situation, structures within the leg are being compressed by edema and the cast. As pressure within the fascia compartment increases, nerves and blood vessels are occluded resulting in ischemia and unrelieved pain, which is called *compartment syndrome.* Fat embolism may result from a fracture, but the client is not experiencing any signs or symptoms of this. Venous thrombosis may occur after fractures but would not affect sensation. Volkmann's contracture is a result of compartment syndrome in an upper extremity after a fractured humerus.

Test-Taking Strategy: Knowledge of the complications associated with lower extremity trauma and with casting is helpful in answering this question. Also, knowledge of fat embolism, contractures, and venous thrombosis is helpful. If you had difficulty with this question, take time now to review the complications associated with a fracture.

Level of Cognitive Ability: Analysis
Phase of Nursing Process: Analysis
Client Needs: Physiological Integrity
Content Area: Adult Health/Musculoskeletal

Reference

Black, J., & Matassarin-Jacobs, E. (1997). *Medical-surgical nursing: Clinical management for continuity of care* (5th ed.). Philadelphia: W. B. Saunders, pp. 2139–2141.

170. A client has a newly fractured fibula that is plaster casted in the emergency department. Which of the following crutch walking gaits should the nurse anticipate teaching the client before discharge?

1 Four-point alternate gait
2 Three-point gait
3 Two-point gait
4 Swing-through gait

Answer: 2

Rationale: The client with a new fracture that is casted with a plaster cast needs to avoid weight bearing. Option 2 is the only option that identifies a gait that allows non–weight bearing on the affected extremity. The client should not bear weight on the affected extremity until the physician evaluates the client on the follow-up examination.

Test-Taking Strategy: Knowledge of the different crutch walking gaits and the amount of weight bearing necessary for each gait is helpful in answering this question. Remember that plaster casts are weak until they dry in about 48–72 hours, so non–weight bearing is essential until follow-up by the physician. If you had difficulty with this question and are unfamiliar with the different types of crutch walking gaits, take time now to review them.

Level of Cognitive Ability: Application
Phase of Nursing Process: Analysis
Client Needs: Physiological Integrity
Content Area: Adult Health/Musculoskeletal

Reference

Lammon, C. B., Foote, A. W., Leli, P. G., et al. (1995). *Clinical nursing skills.* Philadelphia: W. B. Saunders, pp. 240–245.

---

171. The nurse is interviewing the parents of a newborn with spina bifida (meningomyelocele). Which of the following statements, by the parents, would the nurse analyze as a need to prepare for coping issues?

1 "Will our baby ever be normal?"
2 "What is the best position to feed our baby?"
3 "Will our baby be incontinent all the time?"
4 "Should we tell our friends about the baby?"

Answer: 4

Rationale: Spina bifida occurs during fetal growth and development and has genetic predispositions. Parents who have children with congenital defects blame themselves for their children's defects. Parents, at times, have difficulties bonding with their newborn because they are grieving the loss of their perfect baby. It is a stressful adjustment. Integrating the new baby with special needs into the parents' life causes many different stressors. Option 4 best describes coping issues. The parents have not stated "their baby" but "the baby," which could indicate some difficulties with acceptance at this time. It is also difficult to anticipate others' reactions to children with special needs. Options 1, 2, and 3 are all appropriate questions to seek additional knowledge regarding the care for the newborn safely and to establish a reference of growth and development potential.

Test-Taking Strategy: Identify the option that addresses the coping needs of the parents. This information makes option 4 the correct response. Use the process of elimination, reading each option carefully. The parents have not stated "their baby" but "the baby" in option 4, which could indicate some difficulties with acceptance at this time.

Level of Cognitive Ability: Analysis
Phase of Nursing Process: Analysis
Client Needs: Psychosocial Integrity
Content Area: Child Health

Reference

Ashwill, J., & Droske, S. (1997). *Nursing care of children: Principles and practice.* Philadelphia: W. B. Saunders, pp. 1233–1237.

172. The nurse performs an assessment on a child with pertussis (whooping cough). Which of the following assessment data would the nurse analyze as indicative of a potential complication?

1 A weight gain
2 A urinary output of 30 mL/hour
3 Decreased breath sounds of the lung bases
4 A white blood cell count of 10.0 × 1000 cells/mm^3

Answer: 3

Rationale: Complications from pertussis include pneumonia, atelectasis, otitis media, convulsions, and subarachnoid bleeding. Decreased breath sounds are indicative of both pneumonia and atelectasis. A weight gain is normal, as is a urine output of 30 mL/hour and a white blood cell count of 10.0 × 1000 cells/mm^3.

Test-Taking Strategy: Use the principles associated with prioritizing when answering this question. Remember the ABCs. Decreased breath sounds are associated with the airway. Option 3 addresses airway.

Level of Cognitive Ability: Analysis
Phase of Nursing Process: Analysis
Client Needs: Physiological Integrity
Content Area: Child Health

Reference

Ashwill, J., & Droske, S. (1997). *Nursing care of children: Principles and practice.* Philadelphia: W. B. Saunders, pp. 612–613.

173. A client with quadriplegia complains bitterly about the nurse's slow response to the call bell and the rigidity of the therapy schedule. Which analysis of this behavior should serve as a basis for planning care?

1 The client is reacting to loss of control.
2 The client's complaints indicate depression.
3 The client must adjust to institutional schedules.
4 Limits must be set on staff response time to call bells.

Answer: 1

Rationale: Clients who feel a sense of control over their situation adapt to their limitations more readily that those who think that they have lost control. Both of the client's complaints indicate a need for greater control. Clients should be offered an opportunity for input into scheduling and planning for staff response to their needs.

Test-Taking Strategy: Read the question carefully, identifying adequate data to support each option. There are not sufficient data to indicate depression. Because self-care is usually a desired outcome, interventions that limit client control, such as option 3, should be avoided. Option 4 addresses only one of the client's complaints without focus on the real problem. It would not serve as the basis for a plan of care.

Level of Cognitive Ability: Analysis
Phase of Nursing Process: Analysis
Client Needs: Psychosocial Integrity
Content Area: Adult Health/Neurological

Reference

Smeltzer, S., & Bare, B. (1996). *Brunner and Suddarth's Textbook of medical-surgical nursing* (8th ed.). Philadelphia: Lippincott-Raven, p. 1808.

174. A client with a T-4 spinal cord injury is to be monitored for autonomic dysreflexia (hyperreflexia). Which of the following assessment findings indicates to the nurse that the problem is occurring?

1 Knee jerk reaction is absent bilaterally.
2 The client complains of a headache, and the blood pressure is elevated.
3 100 mL of residual urine remains after the client voids.
4 Pupil responses are brisk bilaterally.

Answer: 2

Rationale: Exaggerated autonomic nervous system reactions to stimuli that occur in autonomic dysreflexia result in sudden hypertensive episodes with severe headache. The client may sweat profusely above the level of the cord lesion and complain of a stuffy nose. Pupil and knee jerk response are not affected. Although a distended bladder is often the precipitating event, not all clients with bladder distention exhibit dysreflexia.

Test-Taking Strategy: The key word in the stem is "autonomic," which indicates that involuntary organ function is involved. Because knee jerk reactions involve skeletal muscles, option 1 can be ruled out. Option 3 is a tempting option, but read carefully; catheterization is a treatment of dysreflexia, not an assessment technique. Pupils are above the level of the lesion and so are unlikely to be affected. Because blood pressure is an autonomic function and headache can result from hypertension, option 2 is correct. If you had difficulty with this question, take time now to review autonomic dysreflexia (hyperreflexia).

Level of Cognitive Ability: Analysis
Phase of Nursing Process: Analysis
Client Needs: Physiological Integrity
Content Area: Adult Health/Neurological

Reference

Smeltzer, S., & Bare, B. (1996). *Brunner and Suddarth's Textbook of medical-surgical nursing* (8th ed.). Philadelphia: Lippincott-Raven, p. 1804.

---

175. The nurse is assessing a client with spinal shock. Which of the following assessment findings is inconsistent with spinal shock in a client with a C-5 cord injury?

1 The blood pressure rises when the client sits up.
2 There is bladder distention with overflow dribbling.
3 The client's lung sounds and PO_2 are diminished.
4 The client's abdomen is distended with absent bowel sounds.

Answer: 1

Rationale: During the period of areflexia that characterizes spinal shock, the blood pressure may fall when the client sits up. The bowel and bladder often become flaccid and fail to empty spontaneously. Accessory muscles of respiration may become areflexic as well, diminishing respiratory excursion and oxygenation.

Test-Taking Strategy: Knowledge regarding the assessment findings in spinal shock is needed to answer the question. Be careful when selecting the response, noting the key word "inconsistent" in the question. If you had difficulty with this question, take time now to review the signs and symptoms of spinal shock.

Level of Cognitive Ability: Analysis
Phase of Nursing Process: Analysis
Client Needs: Physiological Integrity
Content Area: Adult Health/Neurological

Reference

Smeltzer, S., & Bare, B. (1996). *Brunner and Suddarth's Textbook of medical-surgical nursing* (8th ed.). Philadelphia: Lippincott-Raven, p. 1800.

---

176. The nurse who is caring for a client with a ruptured cerebral aneurysm keeps the room darkened, restricts visitors, and turns the television off. Which nursing diagnosis should the nurse explore first, when the client exhibits a mild tachycardia, reports difficulty sleeping, and seems withdrawn?

1 Sleep Pattern Disturbance related to recurrent nightmares
2 Risk for Altered Health Maintenance related to depression
3 Anxiety related to illness and isolation
4 Impaired Social Interaction related to inability to maintain personal attachments

Answer: 3

Rationale: The environmental restrictions used to prevent bleeding as well as the serious nature of the illness are likely to create anxiety in most clients, and this client is showing several manifestations of anxiety. There is insufficient evidence to suggest that clinical depression or nightmares are present. The social isolation is imposed by the nurse and is not a client response to the situation.

Test-Taking Strategy: When asked to select a nursing diagnosis, use the data presented in the question to guide you in selecting the correct option. In this situation, the client presents signs of anxiety.

Level of Cognitive Ability: Analysis
Phase of Nursing Process: Analysis
Client Needs: Psychosocial Integrity
Content Area: Adult Health/Neurological

Reference

McFarland, G., & McFarlane, E. (1997). *Nursing diagnosis and intervention: Planning for patient care.* St. Louis: Mosby–Year Book, p. 552.

177. A client with a diagnosis of symptomatic premature ventricular contractions (PVCs) complains of dizziness. The nurse obtains a rhythm strip. A review of the rhythm strip shows the client is in ventricular bigeminy. The nurse recognizes that these subjective and objective findings are also associated with

1 An increase in cardiac output.
2 A decrease in cardiac output.
3 Normal sinus rhythm.
4 Normal pacemaker activity.

Answer: 2

Rationale: When PVCs occur, there is also a decrease in cardiac output. This occurs because there is a premature depolarization of the cardiac cells. The prematurity does not allow for optimal filling of the ventricular chambers, causing reduced stroke volume and hence decreased cardiac output.

Test-Taking Strategy: This question requires knowing what physiological changes take place when PVCs occur. Eliminate options 3 and 4 because these options indicate a normal rhythm. If you are unfamiliar with PVCs and the physiological changes that occur, review this content now.

Level of Cognitive Ability: Analysis
Phase of Nursing Process: Analysis
Client Needs: Physiological Integrity
Content Area: Adult Health/Cardiovascular

Reference
Black, J., & Matassarin-Jacobs, E. (1997). *Medical-surgical nursing: Clinical management for continuity of care* (5th ed.). Philadelphia: W. B. Saunders, p. 1304.

178. The nurse reviews an ECG rhythm strip and finds there is an irregular baseline with no identifiable P waves. Additionally the QRS complexes are irregular. The nurse analyzes this as

1 A normal finding on an ECG.
2 A major ventricular dysrhythmia.
3 A characteristic of atrial fibrillation.
4 A cause of increased cardiac output.

Answer: 3

Rationale: Atrial fibrillation is a disorganized twitching of the atria at a rate greater than 350 beats/minute. The ventricular response is irregular because of the low percentage of atrial impulses that are actually conducted. Characteristic of atrial fibrillation is an absent P wave.

Test-Taking Strategy: Look for the option that directly addresses the situation. Use the process of elimination. First, eliminate the option that has no relationship to the ECG rhythm interpretation, option 4. Because the QRS rate is irregular, it cannot be a normal pattern, eliminating option 1. Because the question does identify the P wave, which represents depolarization of the atria, as being problematic, eliminate option 2. Therefore, the only correct response is option 3.

Level of Cognitive Ability: Analysis
Phase of Nursing Process: Analysis
Client Needs: Physiological Integrity
Content Area: Adult Health/Cardiovascular

Reference
Luckmann, J. (1997). *Saunders manual of nursing care.* Philadelphia: W. B. Saunders, p. 1008.

179. The nurse is caring for a newly admitted client who has severe dyspnea, tachypnea, and diffuse crackles on lung auscultation. The client is extremely agitated. Arterial blood gas measurements indicate a pH, 7.48; PCO_2, 25; HCO_3, 24; and PO_2, 84. After analysis of the arterial blood gases, the most appropriate first action for the nurse is to

1. Initiate a dopamine hydrochloride drip
2. Notify the physician of the arterial blood gas results
3. Initiate continuous pulse oximetry
4. Place the client in high Fowler's position

Answer: 4

Rationale: Improving the client's gas exchange is the priority nursing action. Placing the client in high Fowler's position promotes diaphragmatic expansion and ventilation. Dopamine would be used for low-output failure. Because no information is available on the client's vital signs, this would not be an appropriate first action. Although notifying the physician is important, promoting diaphragmatic expansion and ventilation is the priority. The arterial blood gas analysis already reveals hypoxemia. Once immediate measures are taken to improve gas exchange, continuous monitoring of the client's oxygen saturation with pulse oximetry should be initiated.

Test-Taking Strategy: Use the principles associated with prioritizing when answering this question. Remember the ABCs. Placing the client in high Fowler's position facilitates the client's breathing.

Level of Cognitive Ability: Analysis
Phase of Nursing Process: Analysis
Client Needs: Physiological Integrity
Content Area: Adult Health/Cardiovascular

Reference

Black, J., & Matassarin-Jacobs, E. (1997). *Medical-surgical nursing: Clinical management for continuity of care* (5th ed.). Philadelphia: W. B. Saunders, pp. 334, 1288.

---

180. Fluoxetine (Prozac) is prescribed for a client being treated for depression. Two weeks after starting the treatment, the client tells the nurse that the medication is not working. Based on the information provided by the client, the nurse determines that the most appropriate response would be which of the following?

1. "You may need a stronger dose than the one prescribed."
2. "The oral route of administration delays the therapeutic effects."
3. "Prozac is not effective for all clients."
4. "It takes approximately 2–4 weeks before clinical improvement is noted."

Answer: 4

Rationale: Comprehensive client teaching regarding medications includes, among other topics, the time frame in which expected results are realized. The time frame in which the therapeutic effects of Prozac are seen is usually 2–4 weeks after initiation of therapy. It is important to advise clients to comply with the prescribed regimen so that therapeutic levels are maintained.

Test-Taking Strategy: Identify the issue of the question, which in this situation is the effect of a medication. The nurse's reply would be based on the knowledge of the drug's action, eliminating options 1 and 3. Option 2 can also be eliminated as a viable response because Prozac is always administered orally. Option 4 is the correct option.

Level of Cognitive Ability: Application
Phase of Nursing Process: Analysis
Client Needs: Psychosocial Integrity
Content Area: Pharmacology

Reference

Hodgson, B., & Kizior, R. (1998). *Saunders nursing drug handbook 1998.* Philadelphia: W. B. Saunders, p. 431.

---

181. A client with dissecting abdominal aortic aneurysm is being prepared for surgery. The client asks the nurse, "Will I be okay?" Based on the client's question, the nurse determines that the best response would be

1. "You have to have this surgery."
2. "Would you like to talk about the surgery?"
3. "Don't worry. You'll be fine."
4. "I hope you will be fine."

Answer: 2

Rationale: Option 2 is an open-ended question and allows the nurse to explore the client's feelings and fears. Option 1 blocks communication as does option 4. Option 3 offers false reassurance. The client wants to and needs to talk about the impending surgery.

Test-Taking Strategy: Therapeutic communication techniques help provide the answer to this question. The client is expressing a desire to discuss the surgery and possible outcomes. Recognizing open-ended questions enhances the ability to answer this question correctly. Additionally, option 2 addresses the client's feelings.

Level of Cognitive Ability: Application
Phase of Nursing Process: Analysis
Client Needs: Psychosocial Integrity
Content Area: Fundamental Skills

Reference

Potter, P., & Perry, A. (1997). *Fundamentals of nursing: Concepts, process and practice* (4th ed.). St. Louis: Mosby–Year Book, pp. 234–238.

---

182. The nurse caring for a client with pericarditis monitors for cardiac tamponade. Which symptom does the nurse determine is most indicative of cardiac tamponade?

1 Chest pain
2 Paradoxical pulse
3 Hypertension
4 Bradycardia

Answer: 2

Rationale: Cardiac tamponade is a life-threatening complication caused by accumulation of fluid in the pericardium. In cardiac tamponade, assessment reveals hypotension, tachycardia, jugular venous distention, cyanosis of the lips and nails, dyspnea, muffled heart sounds, diaphoresis, and paradoxical pulse. Cardiac tamponade requires immediate intervention.

Test-Taking Strategy: Knowledge of the signs associated with cardiac tamponade is required to answer the question. Cardiac tamponade is a life-threatening condition. If you had difficulty with this question, take time now to review the signs associated with this complication.

Level of Cognitive Ability: Analysis
Phase of Nursing Process: Analysis
Client Needs: Physiological Integrity
Content Area: Adult Health/Cardiovascular

Reference

Black, J., & Matassarin-Jacobs, E. (1997). *Medical-surgical nursing: Clinical management for continuity of care* (5th ed.). Philadelphia: W. B. Saunders, p. 1337.

---

183. Which of the following assessment data would indicate a potential complication associated with Bell's palsy?

1 Partial facial paralysis
2 Crocodile tears while eating
3 Negative outcomes on electromyography 2 weeks after symptom onset
4 The ability to taste food 1 week after symptom onset

Answer: 2

Rationale: Complications of Bell's palsy include abnormal regeneration of nerves; *crocodile tears* (autonomic fibers reconnect to lacrimal duct instead of salivary glands so the client develops excessive tearing while eating); abnormal facial movements owing to reinnervation of inappropriate muscles; and incomplete motor fiber reinnervation leading to spasms, atrophy, and contractures.

Test-Taking Strategy: This question tests your knowledge about the complications that can occur in Bell's palsy. In option 1, partial facial paralysis is a factor indicating good recovery, whereas total facial paralysis indicates a poor prognosis. In option 3, the electromyography performed 2 weeks after symptom onset indicates that nerve regeneration is present (negative test outcome indicating a positive prognostic outcome). In option 4, tasting food 1 week after symptom onset indicates a good prognosis for recovery.

Level of Cognitive Ability: Analysis
Phase of Nursing Process: Analysis
Client Needs: Physiological Integrity
Content Area: Adult Health/Neurological

Reference

Black, J., & Matassarin-Jacobs, E. (1997). *Medical-surgical nursing: Clinical management for continuity of care* (5th ed.). Philadelphia: W. B. Saunders, pp. 915–932.

184. The nurse caring for a client with HIV notes that the physician has documented middle-stage HIV in the client's record. In the middle stage of HIV disease, the nurse would expect the client's clinical status to consist of

1. Swollen lymph nodes of the neck, armpit, and groin with no other signs of a related infectious disease.
2. A combination of protozoan, fungal, bacterial, and viral infections along with Kaposi's sarcoma.
3. Constipation and weight loss.
4. Anhedonia in both lungs.

Answer: 1

Rationale: In the middle stage of HIV disease, after an asymptomatic period, HIV-infected clients develop a generalized lymphadenopathy causing the lymph nodes of the neck, armpit, and groin areas to swell and to remain swollen for months, with no other signs of a related infectious disease. This syndrome usually occurs within a few months of seroconversion for HIV antibody. Other symptoms of middle-stage HIV disease include fever, night sweats, chronic diarrhea, fatigue, minor oral infections (*Candida albicans*), and headache. Opportunistic infections, which may be protozoan, viral, fungal, and bacterial, are common in the late stage, as is AIDS-related malignancies such as Kaposi's sarcoma and AIDS dementia complex. Anhedonia refers to an absence of pleasure in activities, sports, and interpersonal relationships.

Test-Taking Strategy: This question tests your knowledge of HIV and the symptoms that accompany its stages. The key phrase in the stem is "middle stage." This implies that the client has symptoms, but it will not be the most severe of all the options listed. Take a few moments to review the content area if this question was difficult.

Level of Cognitive Ability: Analysis
Phase of Nursing Process: Analysis
Client Needs: Physiological Integrity
Content Area: Adult Health/Respiratory

Reference

Black, J., & Matassarin-Jacobs, E. (1997). *Medical-surgical nursing: Clinical management for continuity of care* (5th ed.). Philadelphia: W. B. Saunders, pp. 621–623.

---

185. The client states, "I have decided to stop blaming myself and to mobilize my depression like my doctor said. I intend to take my son's rifle and shoot my husband and his new girlfriend tonight while they're working late at the office." Which of the following reflects the most appropriate nursing action?

1. "I will need to report your intentions to the law and to your husband. Let's call your husband and son and talk about your feelings and intentions."
2. "I disagree with your conclusion that this is the way to 'mobilize your depression.' Nevertheless, I will respect your confidentiality."
3. "How can you come to the conclusion that this is how to 'mobilize your depression'? This is not an appropriate decision."
4. "I will respect your confidentiality, but I am going to commit you immediately."

Answer: 1

Rationale: The ethical dilemma is to decide whether to respect the client's confidentiality or to follow the "duty to warn" in serious intention to inflict harm. The Tarasoff decision (*Tarasoff versus Regents of University of California,* 1974) states that "protective privilege ends where public peril begins." Consequently, any clear threats by psychiatric clients to specific people must be reported to the authorities (law enforcement) and the intended victims by mental health care providers and psychotherapists. Generally, caregivers are less liable if they opt for preventing violence. Although the Tarasoff decision is being used, it is preferable to include the client in the decision to warn. This action strengthens the therapeutic alliance and improves the client's relationship with the person being threatened. Although involuntary commitment is usually allowed for those diagnosed mentally ill or if there is anticipation of harm to self or others, the clinician must use the client's statements to justify the commitment, so the confidentiality statement contradicts the actions that need to be taken for commitment.

Test-Taking Strategy: This question tests your knowledge of legal issues in psychiatric nursing and your ability to reflect on the steps involved in ethical decision making. Use the process of elimination to answer the question. Option 2 is incorrect. The client has a specific plan for homicide, which includes the potential victims, the method, the time, and the place. With such high lethality, the nurse is responsible to take appropriate action. Option 3 uses a judgmental attitude and is overly controlling. Option 4 contains a contradictory message and inaccurate information.

Level of Cognitive Ability: Application
Phase of Nursing Process: Analysis
Client Needs: Physiological Integrity
Content Area: Mental Health

Reference

Antai-Otong, D., & Kongale, G. (1995). *Psychiatric nursing: Biological and behavioral concepts.* Philadelphia: W. B. Saunders, pp. 86–87.

---

186. Which of the following assessment data would the nurse determine as indicating that the client is experiencing a major depressive episode?

1 The client is a man
2 The client states, "Since my wife died last week, I've been waking up hours before I should and I'm tired all day"
3 The client uses marijuana
4 The client states, "The last 3 weeks, I'm doing all the things I used to do but I'm not enjoying them"

Answer: 4

Rationale: Major depression occurs twice as frequently in women as in men. Reacting to loss by experiencing altered sleep for 1 week is a normal grief response, whereas early morning awakening that extends over 2 weeks along with other symptoms would constitute major depression. Although depression is often associated with substance abuse, it would, in and of itself, not constitute a major depression. Option 4 is the correct answer because it describes anhedonia (loss of pleasure in activities previously or usually enjoyed) that has extended over 3 weeks, a cardinal criterion for major depression according to *Diagnostic and Statistical Manual of Mental Disorders*, 4th edition (DSM-IV).

Test-Taking Strategy: Knowledge of the epidemiology of and criteria for major depression assists you to analyze the options accurately. Use the process of elimination in selecting the correct option. If you were unfamiliar with the content, you might be able to determine the correct option by considering the time frame noted in the option, which is one of the factors to be considered in the criterion for major depression according to DSM-IV. Take time now to review the assessment data related to depression if you had difficulty with this question.

Level of Cognitive Ability: Analysis
Phase of Nursing Process: Analysis
Client Needs: Psychosocial Integrity
Content Area: Mental Health

Reference

Antai-Otong, D., & Kongale, G. (1995). *Psychiatric nursing: Biological and behavioral concepts.* Philadelphia: W. B. Saunders, p. 171.

---

187. The nurse calls the laboratory for the dexamethasone suppression test (DST) results performed on the client to determine the presence of depression. The pathologist says, "Tell the doctor that the DST shows nonsuppression, the urinary MHPG levels are high, and the TRH stimulation test is blunted." The nurse analyzes these results as

1 Consistent with those found in healthy clients.
2 Insufficient without a serotonin test.
3 Unrelated to those found in depression.
4 Consistent with those found in major depression.

Answer: 4

Rationale: The DST, used to diagnose adrenal function, involves the oral administration of 1 mg of dexamethasone (a synthetic glucocorticoid) at 11:00 P.M. to challenge the hypothalamic-pituitary-adrenal axis. Blood levels of the hormone cortisol are drawn at 4:00 P.M. on the day before administering dexamethasone and at 8:00 A.M. (highest level for normal rhythm), 4:00 P.M. (lowest level of rhythm), and 11:00 P.M. the day after taking the dexamethasone. Fifty percent of depressed clients do not suppress dexamethasone. The results of urinary methoxyhydroxyphenylglycol (MHPG) levels, used to measure a norepinephrine metabolite, may be high or low in depression. If the results are high, the depression responds best to antidepressants that affect the serotonin system, and if the results are low, the depression responds best to antidepressants that stimulate the norepinephrine system. Thyrotropin-releasing hormone (TRH) is used to measure thyroid function. In healthy clients, TSH increases two times the baseline in 30 minutes after the administration of an intravenous bolus of TRH. In the majority of clients with primary depression, TSH is blunted.

Test-Taking Strategy: This question asks you to select the response that makes the correct interpretation of the laboratory findings. Knowledge and understanding of the blood and urine studies that are used to diagnose the presence of depression assist you to answer this question correctly. Options 1, 2, and 3 are incorrect analyses for the findings reported by the pathologist. If you had difficulty with this question, take time now to review these diagnostic tests.

Level of Cognitive Ability: Analysis
Phase of Nursing Process: Analysis
Client Needs: Physiological Integrity
Content Area: Mental Health

Reference
Haber, J. (1997). *Comprehensive psychiatric nursing* (5th ed.). St. Louis: Mosby–Year Book, p. 234.

---

188. The nurse is caring for a 5-year-old child with tetralogy of Fallot. The nurse notes that the child has clubbed fingers and understands that the clubbing is most likely due to

1 Peripheral hypoxia.
2 Delayed physical growth.
3 Chronic hypertension.
4 Destruction of bone marrow.

Answer: 1

Rationale: Clubbing, a thickening and flattening of the tips of the fingers and toes, is thought to occur because of a chronic tissue hypoxemia and polycythemia. There is no relationship between clubbing and delayed physical growth, chronic hypertension, or destruction of bone marrow.

Test-Taking Strategy: Note the relationship between clubbed "fingers" in the case situation and "peripheral" hypoxia in the correct option. Additionally, use the ABCs in selecting the correct option. Hypoxia certainly relates to oxygenation. If you had difficulty with this question, take time now to review the physiology associated with clubbed digits.

Level of Cognitive Ability: Analysis
Phase of Nursing Process: Analysis
Client Needs: Physiological Integrity
Content Area: Child Health

Reference
Ashwill, J., & Droske, S. (1997). *Nursing care of children: Principles and practice.* Philadelphia: W. B. Saunders, pp. 887, 924.

---

189. The nurse is preparing the client for skin grafting. The nurse notes that the physician has documented that the client is scheduled for heterograft. The nurse understands that heterograft used for the burned client is

1 Skin from another species.
2 Skin from a cadaver.
3 Skin from the burned client.
4 Skin from a skin bank.

Answer: 1

Rationale: Biologic dressings are obtained from living or deceased humans (homograft or allograft) or animals (heterograft or xenograft). Heterograft is skin from another species. The most commonly used type of heterograft is pigskin because of its relative compatibility with human skin. Homograft is skin from another human, which is usually obtained from a cadaver and is provided through a skin bank.

Test-Taking Strategy: Knowledge regarding the types of biologic dressings is helpful to answer the question. Note that options 2, 3, and 4 all refer to donor skin from the human species. Option 1, the correct option, identifies skin from a different species. If you had difficulty with this question, take time now to review the types of skin grafting.

Level of Cognitive Ability: Analysis
Phase of Nursing Process: Analysis
Client Needs: Physiological Integrity
Content Area: Adult Health/Integumentary

Reference
Ignatavicius, D. D., Workman, M. L., & Mishler, M. A. (1995). *Medical-surgical nursing: A nursing process approach* (2nd ed.). Philadelphia: W. B. Saunders, p. 1998.

190. The nurse is caring for a client that is comatose. The nurse notes in the client's chart that the client is exhibiting decerebrate posturing. The nurse understands that decerebrate posturing can best be observed as

1 The extension of the extremities and pronation of the arms.
2 The flexion of the extremities and pronation of the arms.
3 Upper extremity flexion with lower extremity extension.
4 Upper extremity extension with lower extremity flexion.

Answer: 1

Rationale: Decerebrate posturing (abnormal extension), which is associated with dysfunction in the brain stem area, is the extension of the extremities and the pronation of the arms.

Test-Taking Strategy: Knowledge regarding the identification of posturing is required to answer the question. Posturing is a late sign of deterioration in the client's neurological status and warrants immediate physician notification. If you had difficulty with this question, take time now to review assessment related to posturing.

Level of Cognitive Ability: Analysis
Phase of Nursing Process: Analysis
Client Needs: Physiological Integrity
Content Area: Adult Health/Neurological

Reference
Black, J., & Matassarin-Jacobs, E. (1997). *Medical-surgical nursing: Clinical management for continuity of care* (5th ed.). Philadelphia: W. B. Saunders, p. 723.

---

191. A postgastrectomy client who is being discharged from the hospital tells the nurse, "I hope my stomach problems are over. I need to get back to work right away. I've missed a lot of work and I'm really behind. If I don't get my act together, I may lose my job." Based on the client's statement, the nurse determines that at this time, it is most appropriate to discuss

1 Reducing stressors in life.
2 The postgastrectomy diet.
3 An exercise program.
4 Wound care.

Answer: 1

Rationale: Some clients need help reducing stressors in their lives. This may be extremely important for recovery. Clients may expect a rapid recovery and are disappointed with complications. The client introduces concerns in the statement made. This provides an opportunity for the nurse to discuss stress and its relationship to gastrointestinal disorders.

Test-Taking Strategy: The key phrase in the question is "most appropriate." Use the process of elimination in answering the question. All options should be discussed with the client before discharge, but because the client has introduced concerns, Option 1 is the best answer.

Level of Cognitive Ability: Analysis
Phase of Nursing Process: Analysis
Client Needs: Psychosocial Integrity
Content Area: Adult Health/Gastrointestinal

Reference
Black, J., & Matassarin-Jacobs, E. (1997). *Medical-surgical nursing: Clinical management for continuity of care* (5th ed.). Philadelphia: W. B. Saunders, p. 1780.

---

192. The client recovering from a craniotomy complains of a "runny nose." Based on the analysis of the client's complaint, the best nursing action is to

1 Provide the client with tissues.
2 Tell the client not to blow the nose.
3 Monitor the client for signs of a cold.
4 Notify the physician immediately.

Answer: 4

Rationale: If the client has sustained a craniocerebral injury or is recovering from a craniotomy, careful observation of any drainage from the eyes, ears, nose, or traumatic area is critical. CSF is colorless and generally nonpurulent, and its presence is indicative of a serious breach of cranial integrity. Any suspicious drainage should be reported immediately.

Test-Taking Strategy: Use the process of elimination in answering the question. In a client with cranial trauma and injury, the nurse should suspect CSF leakage if drainage is noted from the eyes, ears, nose, or traumatic area. Eliminate options 1 and 3 as the least plausible choices. Note the phrase "best nursing action" in the stem of the question. Although the nurse would discourage the client from blowing the nose, in this serious situation, the best nursing action is to notify the physician immediately.

Level of Cognitive Ability: Application
Phase of Nursing Process: Analysis
Client Needs: Physiological Integrity
Content Area: Adult Health/Neurological

Reference

Ignatavicius, D. D., Workman, M. L., & Mishler, M. A. (1995). *Medical-surgical nursing: A nursing process approach* (2nd ed.). Philadelphia: W. B. Saunders, p. 1287.

---

193. The client with bipolar disorder is receiving lithium carbonate. The nurse knows that medication is used primarily to treat

1. The depressive phase of bipolar disorder.
2. The manic phase of bipolar disorder.
3. Both depressive and manic episodes.
4. Hypertensive emergencies.

Answer: 2

Rationale: Lithium is an antimanic medication and is used to treat the manic phase of a manic-depressive disorder.

Test-Taking Strategy: Knowledge regarding lithium is required to answer the question. If you know that lithium is an antimanic medication, by the process of elimination, you can easily select the correct option, option 2. If you had difficulty with this question, take time now to review this important medication. You are likely to see questions related to this medication on NCLEX-RN.

Level of Cognitive Ability: Analysis
Phase of Nursing Process: Analysis
Client Needs: Physiological Integrity
Content Area: Pharmacology

Reference

Hodgson, B., & Kizior, R. (1998). *Saunders nursing drug handbook 1998.* Philadelphia: W. B. Saunders, pp. 598–600.

---

194. Chlorpromazine (Thorazine) is prescribed for the client with psychotic disorder. The nurse understands that this medication produces its desired effect by

1. Initiating peripheral muscle relaxation.
2. Blocking dopamine neurotransmission.
3. Stimulating cholinergic synapses in the cerebrum.
4. Inactivating basal ganglia cells.

Answer: 2

Rationale: Chlorpromazine blocks dopamine neurotransmission at postsynaptic dopamine receptor sites, thus reversing psychotic symptoms.

Test-Taking Strategy: Knowledge regarding the action and use of chlorpromazine is required to answer this question. If you can remember that this medication is an antipsychotic, you may be able to recall the action of the medication. If you had difficulty with this question, take time now to review its use and action.

Level of Cognitive Ability: Analysis
Phase of Nursing Process: Analysis
Client Needs: Physiological Integrity
Content Area: Pharmacology

Reference

Hodgson, B., & Kizior, R. (1998). *Saunders nursing drug handbook 1998.* Philadelphia: W. B. Saunders, pp. 210–213.

195. A visiting nurse says, "Now that the client is responding to the antidepressant, the suicidal risk is over and I can stop my visits." After analyzing this nurse's statement, which of the following is the most appropriate response by the psychiatric nurse?

1. "I agree, clients who want to kill themselves are only suicidal for a limited time. No one can feel self-destructive forever."
2. "I disagree, your comment reflects a lack of knowledge that this disease runs in families."
3. "I agree, the suicidal threats were really attention-seeking. Continuing to visit would reinforce the client's use of manipulation."
4. "I disagree, most suicides occur within about 3 months after improvement begins because the client now has the energy to carry out the suicidal intentions."

Answer: 4

Rationale: The statement made by the visiting nurse is a classic example of one of the myths or fables about suicide. The facts presented by the psychiatric nurse in the correct option are accurate. Most suicides do occur within 3 months after the beginning of the improvement when the client has the energy to carry out the suicidal intentions. At all visits, the nurse would want to assess for the continuation of suicidal ideation.

Test-Taking Strategy: Knowledge regarding the facts of suicide is required to answer the question. In option 1, although it is true that suicidal ideation is usually time-limited, this depends on whether the feelings of self-destruction are eradicated. A small segment of the population with mental illness learns to live successfully despite of the persistence of self-destructive ideas throughout their lives. In option 2, the information is incorrect because suicide is not inherited. In addition, the communication is hypercritical and puts down the visiting nurse. Option 3 presents a myth about suicide. All threats and gestures must be approached with the gravity of the potential act in mind.

Level of Cognitive Ability: Application
Phase of Nursing Process: Analysis
Client Needs: Physiological Integrity
Content Area: Mental Health

Reference

Carson, V., & Arnold, E. (1996). *Mental health nursing: The nurse-patient journey.* Philadelphia: W. B. Saunders, pp. 932–936.

---

196. The client recovering from cardiogenic shock is experiencing alteration in level of consciousness. The nurse suspects the client's decreased level of consciousness is due to a decrease in cardiac output. What other finding would support this nurse's analysis?

1. Urinary output of 60 mL/hour
2. Blood pressure of 108/60 mmHg
3. Pedal pulses faintly palpable
4. Lung fields clear with respirations of 22 breaths/minute

Answer: 3

Rationale: In cardiogenic shock, the client's heart is unable to generate cardiac output to meet the body's demand. If the client is experiencing a decrease in cardiac output, the nurse would expect to see a decrease in urinary output (<30 mL/hour for an adult); a decrease in blood pressure; adventitious breath sounds; a decrease in the strength and quality of peripheral pulses; and cool, pale skin.

Test-Taking Strategy: Use the process of elimination to answer this question. Analyze each option carefully. Option 3 is the only option that presents an abnormal finding, the faint, barely palpable pedal pulses. If you had difficulty with this question, take time now to review the signs and symptoms of decreased cardiac output.

Level of Cognitive Ability: Analysis
Phase of Nursing Process: Analysis
Client Needs: Physiological Integrity
Content Area: Adult Health/Cardiovascular

Reference

Smeltzer, S., & Bare, B. (1996). *Brunner and Suddarth's Textbook of medical-surgical nursing* (8th ed.). Philadelphia: Lippincott-Raven, p. 251.

197. The nurse is assessing the client admitted with suspected carbon monoxide poisoning. The client behaves as if intoxicated. The nurse interprets that

1 The client must also have a high blood alcohol level.
2 The client probably suffers from alcoholism.
3 The carbon monoxide has caused the blood glucose to fall.
4 The behavior is most likely the result of hypoxia.

Answer: 4

Rationale: The client with carbon monoxide poisoning may appear intoxicated. This is the end result of hypoxia on the central nervous system. With carbon monoxide poisoning, oxygen cannot easily bind onto the hemoglobin, which is carrying strongly bound carbon monoxide. Because cerebral tissue has a critical need for oxygen, sustained hypoxia may yield this typical finding.

Test-Taking Strategy: Use the process of elimination in answering the question. Options 1 and 2 should be eliminated first. There are several conditions in which the client may appear intoxicated from the central nervous system effects of a neurological disorder, with no involvement of alcohol. In comparing the remaining options, you would choose option 4 over option 3 if you know that carbon monoxide displaces oxygen on the hemoglobin molecule. Additionally, option 4 addresses oxygen, the first priority.

Level of Cognitive Ability: Analysis
Phase of Nursing Process: Analysis
Client Needs: Physiological Integrity
Content Area: Adult Health/Respiratory

Reference

Smeltzer, S., & Bare, B. (1996). *Brunner and Suddarth's Textbook of medical-surgical nursing* (8th ed.). Philadelphia: Lippincott-Raven, p. 2024.

198. The client with carbon dioxide narcosis has a potassium level of 6.2 mEq/L. The nurse interprets that this result is

1 Unexpected, and indicates a concurrent history of renal insufficiency.
2 Unexpected, and indicates a deficit of hydrogen ions in the bloodstream.
3 Expected, and indicates the result of massive hemolysis.
4 Expected, and indicates that acidosis has driven hydrogen ions into the cell, forcing potassium out.

Answer: 4

Rationale: With severe respiratory acidosis, compensatory mechanisms fail. As hydrogen ion concentrations continue to rise, they are driven into the cell, forcing intracellular potassium out. This is an expected finding in this situation.

Test-Taking Strategy: With a buildup of carbon dioxide, the body attempts to eliminate hydrogen ions from the circulation because they are another source of body acid. The blood buffer system tries to buffer them as the first line of defense. With a rapid buildup of carbon dioxide, this is insufficient, and the body needs to find another way to lose hydrogen ions. Because the renal system doesn't begin to function for almost 24 hours, the hydrogen ions are driven into the cells, and potassium comes out. With these concepts in mind, hyperkalemia is an expected finding, which eliminates options 1 and 2. Because this disorder has nothing to do with hemolysis, the only correct choice is option 4.

Level of Cognitive Ability: Analysis
Phase of Nursing Process: Analysis
Client Needs: Physiological Integrity
Content Area: Adult Health/Respiratory

Reference

Smeltzer, S., & Bare, B. (1996). *Brunner and Suddarth's Textbook of medical-surgical nursing* (8th ed.). Philadelphia: Lippincott-Raven, p. 234.

199. The nurse analyzes the results of laboratory tests of a child with hemophilia A. The laboratory test most likely to be abnormal in a client diagnosed with hemophilia A would be

1 White blood cell count.
2 Sedimentation rate.
3 Clot retraction time.
4 Partial thromboplastin time.

Answer: 4

Rationale: In hemophilia A, factor VIII assay is 0%–30% of normal; activated partial thromboplastin time is prolonged; and the platelet count, bleeding time, and prothrombin time are normal. The white blood cell count, sedimentation rate, and clot retraction time are unrelated to the diagnosis of hemophilia A.

Test-Taking Strategy: Knowledge of the diagnostics related to hemophilia is required to answer this question. If you had difficulty with this question, take the time now to review abnormal diagnostic findings in hemophilia A.

Level of Cognitive Ability: Analysis
Phase of Nursing Process: Analysis
Client Needs: Physiological Integrity
Content Area: Child Health

Reference

Luckmann, J. (1997). *Saunders manual of nursing care.* Philadelphia: W. B. Saunders, p. 1162.

---

200. A 2-year-old child is admitted to the pediatric unit with a diagnosis of celiac disease. Based on the diagnosis, the nurse expects that the child's stools will be

1 Dark in color.
2 Abnormally small in amount.
3 Unusually hard.
4 Foul smelling.

Answer: 4

Rationale: The stools of a child with celiac disease are characteristically malodorous, pale, fatty, large (bulky), and soft (loose). Excessive flatus is common, and bouts of diarrhea may occur.

Test-Taking Strategy: Knowledge of the clinical manifestations associated with celiac disease is required to answer the question. Take time now to review the clinical manifestations of the disease if you had difficulty with this question.

Level of Cognitive Ability: Analysis
Phase of Nursing Process: Analysis
Client Needs: Physiological Integrity
Content Area: Child Health

Reference

Ashwill, J., & Droske, S. (1997). *Nursing care of children: Principles and practice.* Philadelphia: W. B. Saunders, p. 734.

---

201. The nurse gathers assessment data from the client admitted with gastroesophageal reflux disease (GERD). The client is scheduled for a Nissen repair. Based on an understanding of this disease, the nurse determines that the client may be at risk for which of the following?

1 Diarrhea
2 Belching
3 Aspiration
4 Abdominal pain

Answer: 3

Rationale: The primary symptom of GERD is heartburn, also called *pyrosis.* Another symptom is regurgitation. If the fluid reaches the level of the pharynx, the client notes a sour or bitter taste in the mouth. This effortless regurgitation frequently occurs when the client is in the upright position. If regurgitation occurs when the client is recumbent, the client is at risk for aspiration. Belching may be a symptom of the disease. Diarrhea and abdominal pain are not specifically associated with the disease.

Test-Taking Strategy: Use the process of elimination and the ABCs in answering the question. Note that option 3 identifies the priority concern and relates to airway.

Level of Cognitive Ability: Analysis
Phase of Nursing Process: Analysis
Client Needs: Physiological Integrity
Content Area: Adult Health/Gastrointestinal

Reference

Ignatavicius, D. D., Workman, M. L., & Mishler, M. A. (1995). *Medical-surgical nursing: A nursing process approach* (2nd ed.). Philadelphia: W. B. Saunders, p. 1540.

202. A client has a blood glucose level drawn for suspected hyperglycemia. The nurse, on interviewing the client, determines that the client ate lunch approximately 2 hours ago. The laboratory reports the blood glucose to be 180 mg/dL. The nurse analyzes these results to be

1 Normal.
2 Lower than the normal value.
3 Elevated from the normal value.
4 A value that indicates immediate physician notification.

Answer: 3

Rationale: Normal fasting blood glucose values range from 70 to 120 mg/dL. Two-hour postprandial blood glucose level should be less than 140 mg/dL. In this situation, the blood glucose value was 180 mg/dL 2 hours after the client ate, which is an elevated value. This value does not require physician notification.

Test-Taking Strategy: Knowledge of normal blood glucose values assists in answering this question. It is also important to read the question carefully, noting that the client ate 2 hours before the blood test. If you had difficulty with this question, take time now to review normal fasting blood glucose and 2-hour postprandial blood glucose values.

Level of Cognitive Ability: Analysis
Phase of Nursing Process: Analysis
Client Needs: Physiological Integrity
Content Area: Adult Health/Endocrine

Reference
Ignatavicius, D. D., Workman, M. L., & Mishler, M. A. (1995). *Medical-surgical nursing: A nursing process approach* (2nd ed.). Philadelphia: W. B. Saunders, p. 1869.

---

203. The home care nurse visits a client diagnosed with cancer of the esophagus. The nurse focuses the assessment of the client based on which of the following most appropriate nursing diagnoses?

1 Pain related to the presence of the tumor mass
2 Spiritual Distress related to impending death
3 Ineffective Individual Coping related to the disease effects
4 Altered Nutrition Less Than Body Requirements related to impaired swallowing

Answer: 4

Rationale: The most common nursing diagnosis associated with cancer of the esophagus is Altered Nutrition Less Than Body Requirements related to impaired swallowing. Pain, Spiritual Distress, and Ineffective Individual Coping may also be additional nursing diagnoses if appropriate for the client.

Test-Taking Strategy: Identify the key phrase "most appropriate" in the stem of the question. Use Maslow's hierarchy of needs to select the correct option. Eliminate options 2 and 3 because they are not physiological in nature. Knowledge regarding the most common nursing diagnosis is helpful in choosing between options 1 and 4. The best option is option 4. Pain may or may not be present or may occur with varying degrees. Altered Nutrition is the most common problem.

Level of Cognitive Ability: Analysis
Phase of Nursing Process: Analysis
Client Needs: Physiological Integrity
Content Area: Adult Health/Oncology

Reference
Ignatavicius, D. D., Workman, M. L., & Mishler, M. A. (1995). *Medical-surgical nursing: A nursing process approach* (2nd ed.). Philadelphia: W. B. Saunders, p. 1555.

---

204. The client has facial asymmetry, drooling, loss of tearing on one side, and inability to close the eye. The nurse interprets that the client has impaired function of which cranial nerve (CN)?

1 CN III
2 CN V
3 CN VI
4 CN VII

Answer: 4

Rationale: The facial nerve (CN VII) has both motor and sensory divisions. Common abnormalities of this nerve include loss of the nasolabial fold, an inability to close the eye and to blink automatically, facial asymmetry, drooling and inability to swallow secretions, loss of the ability to form tears, and possible loss of taste on the anterior two thirds of the tongue. Bell's palsy, fracture of the temporal bone, and parotid lacerations or contusions are often responsible for this dysfunction.

Test-Taking Strategy: Questions related to cranial nerves are difficult unless you know the differences between them. If you remember that CN VII is the facial nerve, you can eliminate each of the other incorrect responses. Review cranial nerves now if you had difficulty with this question.

Level of Cognitive Ability: Analysis
Phase of Nursing Process: Analysis
Client Needs: Physiological Integrity
Content Area: Adult Health/Neurological

Reference

Black, J., & Matassarin-Jacobs, E. (1997). *Medical-surgical nursing: Clinical management for continuity of care* (5th ed.). Philadelphia: W. B. Saunders, pp. 720–721.

---

205. The nurse is preparing to administer TPN via a central line. The nurse realizes that use of a central line is better than a peripheral site for TPN therapy because

1 The high glucose content of TPN increases the client's risk of infection.
2 Major electrolyte imbalances are associated with TPN.
3 TPN contains trace elements and vitamins.
4 TPN is a hyperosmotic solution.

Answer: 4

Rationale: TPN solution is a hyperosmotic solution and thus needs to be diluted as much as possible to prevent vein irritation. Large central veins are used because they are less likely to be affected by the high solute concentration. The other options are correct regarding TPN but are not the logical rationale for choosing a central line over a peripheral site.

Test-Taking Strategy: Read the question and options carefully to be certain that the option is answering the question asked. The question is asking why a central line is used with TPN. Although the other options provide correct information regarding TPN, only option 4 identifies the rationale for preference of a central line.

Level of Cognitive Ability: Analysis
Phase of Nursing Process: Analysis
Clinical Needs: Physiological Integrity
Content Area: Fundamental Skills

Reference

Phillips, L. D. (1997). *Manual of IV therapeutics* (2nd ed.). Philadelphia: F. A. Davis, pp. 563–564.

---

206. The nurse should anticipate that the client may develop shock postoperatively owing to the preoperative medications, anesthetic agents, or fluid or blood loss. Which of the following would indicate the development of shock?

1 Cold skin, drowsiness, and hypertension
2 Fever, irritability, and rapid respirations
3 Tachycardia, cold skin, and hypotension
4 Slow pulse, warm skin, and restlessness

Answer: 3

Rationale: Postoperative hypotension or shock can have numerous causes, such as inadequate ventilation, side effects of anesthetic agents or preoperative medications, and fluid or blood loss. A significant drop in blood pressure, accompanied by an increase or decrease in heart rate, may indicate hemorrhage, circulatory failure, or fluid shifts. The manifestations of shock include hypotension; tachycardia; cold, moist, pale, or cyanotic skin; and increased restlessness and apprehension.

Test-Taking Strategy: Knowledge of the physiology of shock is helpful in determining the correct signs of shock. Remember when an option has more than one part, all, of the parts must be correct. Remembering that a drop in blood pressure and a rise in pulse are indicative of shock assists in eliminating options 1 and 4. Restlessness is one of the first indications of shock, and it is important to remember this; however, option 4, which contains the sign of restlessness, does not identify additional signs of shock. Option 2 does not identify indicators of shock; therefore, this option should be eliminated. If you had difficulty with this question, take time now to review the signs of shock.

Level of Cognitive Ability: Analysis
Phase of Nursing Process: Analysis
Client Needs: Physiological Integrity
Content Area: Adult Health/Cardiovascular

Reference

Black, J., & Matassarin-Jacobs, E. (1997). *Medical-surgical nursing: Clinical management for continuity of care* (5th ed.). Philadelphia: W. B. Saunders, p. 483.

207. The nurse analyzes the results of laboratory studies performed on a client with peptic ulcer disease. Which of the following laboratory values would indicate a complication associated with the disease?

1 White blood cell count of 5000/μL
2 Hemoglobin 10.2 g/dL
3 Platelet count of 400,000 cells/μL
4 Creatinine 1 mg/dL

Answer: 2

Rationale: The most common complications of peptic ulcer disease are hemorrhage, perforation, pyloric obstruction, and intractable disease. Low hemoglobin and hematocrit levels indicate bleeding. The normal hemoglobin range in women is 12–16 g/dL and in men is 14–18 g/dL. A white blood cell count is performed to indicate the presence of infection or inflammation. The normal white blood cell count is 5000–10,000/μL. A platelet count of 160,000 cells/μL is normal. The normal platelet range is 150,000–400,000 cells/μL. The creatinine measures renal function. The normal value is 0.6–1.3 mg/dL.

Test-Taking Strategy: Knowledge regarding the complications associated with peptic ulcer disease is required to answer the question. Knowledge of normal laboratory values would also assist in directing you to the correct option. The only abnormal laboratory value in the options is the hemoglobin, which is low, indicating bleeding. If you had difficulty with this question, take time now to review both the complications of peptic ulcer disease and the normal laboratory values presented in the options.

Level of Cognitive Ability: Analysis
Phase of Nursing Process: Analysis
Client Needs: Physiological Integrity
Content Area: Adult Health/Gastrointestinal

Reference

Ignatavicius, D. D., Workman, M. L., & Mishler, M. A. (1995). *Medical-surgical nursing: A nursing process approach* (2nd ed.). Philadelphia: W. B. Saunders, p. 1570.

---

208. The nurse collects blood glucose samples every shift for the child with Reye's syndrome. The result of the 10 A.M. blood glucose is 40 mg/dL by glucometer reading. The nurse analyzes this result as

1 Normal.
2 Lower than normal, indicating Reye's syndrome.
3 Higher than normal, ruling out Reye's syndrome.
4 Insignificant and unrelated to Reye's syndrome.

Answer: 2

Rationale: Blood glucose values are obtained by either drawn blood or finger stick with the use of a glucometer apparatus. Normal blood glucose values range from 50 to 60 mg/dL for an infant, 60 to 100 mg/dL for a child, and 70 to 105 mg/dL for an adolescent. A blood glucose level of 40 mg/dL is lower than normal. Hypoglycemia is a major symptom of Reye's syndrome.

Test-Taking Strategy: Knowledge of the clinical manifestations associated with Reye's syndrome and normal blood glucose levels assists in answering the question. Because the question addresses a child with Reye's syndrome, the best option is option 2, which states "indicating Reye's syndrome." If you had difficulty with this question, take time now to review the clinical manifestations associated with Reye's syndrome.

Level of Cognitive Ability: Analysis
Phase of Nursing Process: Analysis
Client Needs: Physiological Integrity
Content Area: Child Health

Reference

Ashwill, J., & Droske, S. (1997). *Nursing care of children: Principles and practice.* Philadelphia: W. B. Saunders, pp. 1250–1251.

209. The nurse reviews the health history of a preschooler with conjunctivitis. Which of the following symptoms prompts the nurse to investigate allergy as the probable cause?

1 Photophobia
2 Purulent discharge
3 Itching
4 Ptosis

Answer: 3

Rationale: Itching is most often associated with allergy. Photophobia or purulent discharge could be the result of bacterial or viral infection. Ptosis refers to drooping eyelids and is unrelated to allergy. The nurse needs to understand the causative agent to determine if infection control measures versus allergen precautions need to be taken.

Test-Taking Strategy: Look for key words as clues to eliminate options. Purulent suggests infection. Sensitivity to light (photophobia) is a broad response that could signal tiredness, infection, or even trauma. Ptosis is unrelated to allergy. Itching is a classic allergic reaction.

Level of Cognitive Ability: Analysis
Phase of Nursing Process: Analysis
Client Needs: Physiological Integrity
Content Area: Child Health

Reference
Ashwill, J., & Droske, S. (1997). *Nursing care of children: Principles and practice.* Philadelphia: W. B. Saunders, pp. 1336–1337.

---

210. A client is admitted with diabetic ketoacidosis (DKA). The daughter says to the nurse, "My mother died last month, and now this. I've been taking care of my father and trying to follow all of the instructions from his doctor. What have I done wrong?" Based on this statement, the nurse analyzes that the best response would be:

1 "Maybe we can keep your father in the hospital for a while longer to give you a rest."
2 "An emotional stress, such as your mother's death, can trigger diabetic ketoacidosis even though you are following the prescribed regimen."
3 "You should talk to the social worker about getting someone at home who is more capable in managing a diabetic's care."
4 "Tell me what you think you did wrong."

Answer: 2

Rationale: Environment, infection, or an emotional stressor can initiate the pathophysiologic mechanism of DKA. Option 1 is not cost-effective. Options 3 and 4 substantiate the daughter's feelings of guilt and incompetence. Option 2 assists in relieving the daughter's guilt and provides an accurate statement regarding diabetic ketoacidosis.

Test-Taking Strategy: Use the process of elimination to answer the question. Identify and eliminate statements that would demean the daughter and block therapeutic communication. Additionally, identify accuracy in the statement, which option 2 provides.

Level of Cognitive Ability: Application
Phase of Nursing Process: Analysis
Client Needs: Psychosocial Integrity
Content Area: Adult Health/Endocrine

Reference
Ignatavicius, D. D., Workman, M. L., & Mishler, M. A. (1995). *Medical-surgical nursing: A nursing process approach* (2nd ed.). Philadelphia: W. B. Saunders, p. 1860.

---

211. The client sustained a high-voltage electrical injury. The nurse analyzes the laboratory results. Which of the following laboratory values would the nurse interpret as increasing the client's risk of developing acute tubular necrosis?

1 Myoglobin in the urine
2 Carbonaceous sputum
3 Hyperkalemia
4 Cloudy CSF

Answer: 1

Rationale: Myoglobin can be released from damaged muscles and precipitate out in the renal tubules causing acute tubular necrosis. Carbonaceous sputum occurs as a result of inhalation of smoke, as during a fire. This finding would indicate an inhalation injury. Hyperkalemia commonly occurs after any cellular trauma or as a result of deteriorating renal function, and cardiac dysrhythmias, not renal damage, would occur as a result of hyperkalemia. Cloudy CSF indicates meningitis. Additionally, assessing CSF is not routinely performed in a burn injury.

Test-Taking Strategy: Look for a similarity in the question and in the options. Note that the question asks about acute tubular necrosis. This is a *renal* disorder. The only option that relates to this complication is option 1, myoglobin in the *urine*.

Level of Cognitive Ability: Analysis
Phase of Nursing Process: Analysis
Client Needs: Physiological Integrity
Content Area: Adult Health/Integumentary

Reference

Black, J., & Matassarin-Jacobs, E. (1997). *Medical-surgical nursing: Clinical management for continuity of care* (5th ed.). Philadelphia: W. B. Saunders, p. 2241.

---

212. Three days after the client undergoes pelvic exenteration, the nurse assesses the client, and breath sounds are decreased in the lung bases bilaterally. Arterial blood gases indicate a pH of 7.39, PO_2 of 93, and PCO_2 of 40. On the basis of the analysis of these findings, the nurse's first action would be to

1 Ask the client to cough and deep breathe.
2 Notify the physician.
3 Order that the blood gases be remeasured.
4 Do nothing because these results are expected.

Answer: 1

Rationale: Postoperative pneumonia is a complication caused by atelectasis in the lungs. The blood gas results presented in the question are in the normal ranges except for a slightly decreased O_2 level. Decreased breath sounds indicate possible atelectasis that may be cleared by coughing and deep breathing.

Test Taking Strategy: The ability to interpret blood gas results is helpful in identifying the correct answer. Eliminate option 4 because the situation presents a client with decreased breath sounds in the lung bases bilaterally. Eliminate option 2 because notifying a physician is rarely the nurse's first action, unless the situation is a life-threatening one, without first gathering more data or using a nursing intervention. There is no reason to order the blood gases to be remeasured; in fact, this option is not within the realm of the nurse's role. Option 1 is a safe, noninvasive intervention and addresses the priority issue of airway!

Level of Cognitive Ability: Application
Phase of Nursing Process: Analysis
Client Needs: Physiological Integrity
Content Area: Adult Health/Respiratory

Reference

Smeltzer, S., & Bare, B. (1996). *Brunner and Suddarth's textbook of medical-surgical nursing* (8th ed.). Philadelphia: Lippincott-Raven, pp. 2250–2255.

---

213. The nurse is caring for a client with type I diabetes. The client is hyperglycemic. Which of the following nursing diagnoses is most important to consider first, when planning care for this client?

1 Altered Health Maintenance
2 Altered Urinary Patterns
3 Alteration in Nutrition
4 Fluid Volume Deficit

Answer: 4

Rationale: Type I diabetics with hyperglycemia can develop ketoacidosis and lose large amounts of fluid. Polyuria develops as the body attempts to get rid of the excess glucose. Because glucose is hyperosmotic, fluid is pulled from the tissue. Nausea and vomiting, a result of hyperglycemia, can lead to a loss of sodium and water. Water is also lost from the lungs in an attempt to get rid of excess carbon dioxide. Severe dehydration can lead to hypovolemic shock. Of all the nursing diagnoses listed, Fluid Volume Deficit is the most serious.

Test-Taking Strategy: This question requires prioritization of basic needs. Using the ABCs, fluid balance becomes an important client need. A good way of selecting the correct option is to rank the nursing diagnoses in order of importance: (1) Fluid Volume Deficit, (2) Altered Nutrition, (3) Altered Urinary Elimination, and (4) of least importance considering the case situation, Altered Health Maintenance.

Level of Cognitive Ability: Analysis
Phase of Nursing Process: Analysis
Client Needs: Physiological Integrity
Content Area: Adult Health/Endocrine

Reference

Ignatavicius, D. D., Workman, M. L., & Mishler, M. A. (1995). *Medical-surgical nursing: A nursing process approach* (2nd ed.). Philadelphia: W. B. Saunders, p. 1885.

214. A client who is currently taking levothyroxine (Synthroid) complains of cold intolerance, constipation, dry skin, weight gain, and puffy eyes. The nurse analyzes these findings and anticipates that the physician will order which of the following?

1. Increased levothyroxine dosage after checking T_4 level
2. Decreased levothyroxine dosage after checking T_4 level
3. Discontinuing levothyroxine because the client is having an adverse reaction
4. No changes in medication because these are common side effects that diminish with time

Answer: 1

Rationale: Manifestations of hypothyroid syndrome include cold intolerance; constipation; loss of initiative; thick, dry skin; notably puffy appearance of the skin around the eyes; slowed intellectual function, including retarded speech and apathy; and low metabolic rate. Levothyroxine is used to correct hypothyroid syndrome. This dosage would appear to be subtherapeutic.

Test-Taking Strategy: Knowledge regarding levothyroxine is required to answer the question. Use the process of elimination to select the correct option. Knowing that this medication is used for hypothyroidism, analyzing the client symptoms in this case can assist you in determining that the client requires additional medication. If you had difficulty with this question, take time now to review the signs and symptoms of hypothyroidism and the use of the medication levothyroxine.

Level of Cognitive Ability: Analysis
Phase of Nursing Process: Analysis
Client Needs: Physiological Integrity
Content Area: Pharmacology

Reference

Hodgson, B., & Kizior, R. (1998). *Saunders nursing drug handbook 1998.* Philadelphia: W. B. Saunders, pp. 589–590.

---

215. A client with newly diagnosed diabetes mellitus has had several hypoglycemic reactions in the last few days. The client now refuses to take insulin stating, "Every time I take insulin it makes me sick." Which of the following nursing diagnoses must be addressed first?

1. Altered Health Maintenance related to the inability to take insulin
2. Fear (Insulin) related to a history of blood glucose levels identifying hypoglycemic reactions
3. Altered Health Maintenance, Insulin Administration, related to the lack of information about insulin and its complications
4. Noncompliance related to taking insulin

Answer: 2

Rationale: The nurse must remember that clients with newly diagnosed diabetes go through stages of grieving, with fear being the first stage. A client must be helped to understand his or her feelings for the client to become compliant and accept teaching.

Test-Taking Strategy: There are several key words in this question that should direct you to the correct option. That the client is newly diagnosed and has had several hypoglycemic reactions are key phrases in the question. Option 2 addresses the key phrases. Fear is the most common reason for the refusal to take insulin, and this must be addressed first.

Level of Cognitive Ability: Analysis
Phase of Nursing Process: Analysis
Client Needs: Psychosocial Integrity
Content Area: Adult Health/Endocrine

Reference

Ignatavicius, D. D., Workman, M. L., & Mishler, M. A. (1995). *Medical-surgical nursing: A nursing process approach* (2nd ed.). Philadelphia: W. B. Saunders, p. 1874.

216. The client was evacuated from under a burning car and transported to the emergency department (ED). En route to the ED, the client received oxygen via nasal cannula at 2 L/minute. An 18-gauge intravenous line was initiated in the antecubital area, and lactated Ringer's solution was infused at 125 mL/hour. The initial assessment on arrival at the ED revealed pulse, 130 beats/minute; respirations, 32 breaths/minute and labored; and blood pressure, 100/70 mmHg. The oxygen saturation was 84%, and lung sounds were diminished on the left side. An obvious deformity of the left femur was present with an absent dorsalis pedis pulse. The total burn surface area was 50%. The nurse analyzes this information and determines that the priority intervention is to

1 Cover the burn wounds to decrease the risk of contamination and prevent hypothermia.
2 Increase the intravenous infusion rate to help perfusion to vital organs.
3 Increase oxygen delivery by placing a 100% oxygen mask on the client.
4 Place a splint on the left leg to stabilize the fracture.

Answer: 3

Rationale: The client is exhibiting numerous symptoms, but the inadequate oxygenation, low oxygen saturation, tachypnea, labored respirations, and decreased breath sounds are the priority. Ensuring adequate oxygenation is always a priority intervention. Although burn wound contamination and hypothermia are concerns, they are not the first priority at this time. Although adequate fluid resuscitation is also an important intervention, it is a secondary concern to oxygenation. Stabilization of the fracture is not the first priority but would be the second intervention considering the absent dorsalis pedis pulse.

Test-Taking Strategy: Read the client information in the question carefully, noting the oxygen saturation is 84%. Use the ABCs and the process of elimination in answering the question. This strategy can direct you to the correct option.

Level of Cognitive Ability: Analysis
Phase of Nursing Process: Analysis
Client Needs: Physiological Integrity
Content Area: Adult Health/Integumentary

Reference

Ignatavicius, D. D., Workman, M. L., & Mishler, M. A. (1995). *Medical-surgical nursing: A nursing process approach* (2nd ed.). Philadelphia: W. B. Saunders, p. 1981.

---

217. The student nurse examines an Asian-American infant's eyes and notes apparent strabismus. Which of the following is the most appropriate statement for interpreting findings to the registered nurse?

1 "It probably isn't strabismus but appears that way because of the baby's ethnic background."
2 "You will want to call the pediatrician immediately because this could lead to a detached retina."
3 "It probably is strabismus because the baby's mother has abused tranquilizers."
4 "Strabismus isn't life-threatening, but it requires surgery in the first 2 months to prevent the crossed eyes from being a lifelong condition."

Answer: 1

Rationale: This question assesses knowledge of ethnic physical variations and ability to provide an accurate and appropriate report of assessment findings. Asian-American, Native American, and Alaskan Native infants often have a pseudostrabismus because of a flattened nasal bridge. It needs to be distinguished from a true strabismus in the assessment. Additionally, the correct option contains accurate information and avoids devaluing statements.

Test-Taking Strategy: Knowledge of ethnic physical variations in the eyes of infants and the use of therapeutic communication techniques are required to answer this question. Use the process of elimination in answering the question. Options 2, 3, and 4 provide incorrect information. If you selected any of these responses, review the appropriate topic now.

Level of Cognitive Ability: Analysis
Phase of Nursing Process: Analysis
Client Needs: Physiological Integrity
Content Area: Child Health

Reference

Jarvis, C. (1996). *Physical examination and health assessment* (2nd ed.). Philadelphia: W. B. Saunders, pp. 300–349.

218. The nurse is performing an initial physical examination on a young female client who complains of fatigue, weakness, malaise, muscle and joint pain, anorexia with slight weight loss, and photosensitivity. The physician suspects systematic lupus erythematosus (SLE). Which of the following symptoms would the nurse determine as supporting data related to this diagnosis?

1 Presence of two hemoglobin S genes
2 Ascites
3 Emboli
4 Butterfly rash on cheeks and bridge of nose.

Answer: 4

Rationale: SLE, chiefly occurring in females 10–35 years of age, is a chronic inflammatory disease that affects multiple body systems. A butterfly rash on the cheeks and the bridge of nose is a key symptom of SLE. Other symptoms observed in SLE include alopecia, Raynaud's phenomenon, pericarditis, pleural effusion, myocarditis, nephritis, hepatomegaly, splenomegaly, mental status alterations, and convulsive disorders. Option 1 is found in sickle cell anemia. Options 2 and 3 are found in many conditions but not usually in SLE.

Test-Taking Strategy: Knowledge of the symptoms associated with SLE is required to answer the question. If you are unfamiliar with this disease and had difficulty with this question, take time now to review the signs and symptoms of SLE.

Level of Cognitive Ability: Analysis
Phase of Nursing Process: Analysis
Client Needs: Physiological Integrity
Content Area: Adult Health/Musculoskeletal

Reference

Ignatavicius, D. D., Workman, M. L., & Mishler, M. A. (1995). *Medical-surgical nursing: A nursing process approach* (2nd ed.). Philadelphia: W. B. Saunders, p. 488.

219. Which of the following assessment data would the nurse analyze as indicating a potential complication associated with secondary skin lesions?

1 Fluid-filled lesion greater than 2 cm (3/4 inch) in diameter
2 Circumscribed lesion consisting of loss of superficial epidermis
3 Semisolid or fluid-filled encapsulated mass extending deep into the dermis
4 Raised, circumscribed lesion less than 1 cm (3/8 inch) in diameter that contains yellow-white purulent material

Answer: 2

Rationale: Primary skin lesions appear on healthy skin in response to disease or external irritation. Secondary skin lesions are due to changes in the primary lesion that are usually related to the disease process. Erosions are secondary skin lesions involving the circumscribed loss of superficial epidermis, such as a rug burn or an abrasion. Other secondary skin lesions include atrophy, crusts, excoriation, fissure, keloid, lichenification, scales, scars, and ulcers. Option 1 describes a bulla, which is also called a blister. Bullae appear in cases of severe poison oak or ivy dermatitis and second-degree burns. Option 3 describes a cyst that can occur with acne. Option 4 describes a pustule that appears with acne, impetigo, and furuncles. Other primary skin lesions include comedos, macules, nodules, papules, patches, plaques, tumors, vesicles, and wheals.

Test-Taking Strategy: Read the question carefully, noting that the question asks for the potential complication associated with secondary skin lesions. Use the process of elimination to answer the question. Fluid-filled lesions or lesions containing yellow-white purulent material are not associated with secondary skin lesions. If you had difficulty with this question, take time now to review secondary skin lesions.

Level of Cognitive Ability: Analysis
Phase of Nursing Process: Analysis
Client Needs: Physiological Integrity
Content Area: Adult Health/Integumentary

Reference

Jarvis, C. (1996). *Physical examination and health assessment* (2nd ed.). Philadelphia: W. B. Saunders, p. 230.

220. The nurse notes that a client's urinalysis report contains a notation of positive red blood cells. The nurse interprets that this finding is unrelated to which of the following items that is part of the client's clinical picture?

1 Diabetes mellitus
2 Concurrent anticoagulant therapy
3 History of kidney stones
4 History of recent blow to the right flank

Answer: 1

Rationale: Hematuria can be caused by trauma to the kidney, such as with blunt trauma to the lower posterior trunk or flank. Kidney stones can cause hematuria as they scrape the endothelial lining of the urinary system. Anticoagulant therapy can cause hematuria as a side effect. Diabetes mellitus does not cause hematuria, although it can lead to renal failure from prerenal causes.

Test-Taking Strategy: Read the stem of the question carefully, noting the key word "unrelated." Begin to answer this question by eliminating options 2 and 4, which are most likely to cause red blood cells in the urine. To discriminate between the last two options, knowing that the scraping of the stones against mucosa could cause minor trauma and bleeding helps you to eliminate this option as well. Thus, diabetes mellitus is the item unrelated to positive red blood cells in the urine.

Level of Cognitive Ability: Analysis
Phase of Nursing Process: Analysis
Client Needs: Physiological Integrity
Content Area: Adult Health/Renal

Reference

Black, J., & Matassarin-Jacobs, E. (1997). *Medical-surgical nursing: Clinical management for continuity of care* (5th ed.). Philadelphia: W. B. Saunders, pp. 1548–1550.

---

221. A client was admitted to a medical unit with acute blindness. Many tests are performed, and there seems to be no organic reason why this client cannot see. The nurse later learns that the client became blind after witnessing a hit-and-run car accident, when a family of three were killed. The nurse suspects that the client may be experiencing a

1 Psychosis.
2 Conversion disorder.
3 Dissociative disorder.
4 Repression.

Answer: 2

Rationale: A conversion disorder is the alteration or loss of a physical function that cannot be explained by any known pathophysiological mechanism. It is thought to be an expression of a psychological need or conflict. In this scenario, the client witnessed an accident that was so psychologically painful the client became blind. A dissociative disorder is a disturbance or alteration in the normally integrative functions of identity, memory, or consciousness. Psychosis is a state in which a person's mental capacity to recognize reality, communicate, and relate to others is impaired, thus interfering with the person's capacity to deal with life demands. Repression is a coping mechanism in which unacceptable feelings are kept out of awareness.

Test-Taking Strategy: The key to the answer lies in the fact that the client evidences no organic reason to account for the blindness, hence a conversion disorder. If you had difficulty with this question, take time now to review defense mechanisms.

Level of Cognitive Ability: Analysis
Phase of Nursing Process: Analysis
Client Needs: Psychosocial Integrity
Content Area: Mental Health

Reference

Carson, V., & Arnold, E. (1996). *Mental health nursing: The nurse-patient journey.* Philadelphia: W. B. Saunders, pp. 697, 963–964.

222. The nurse reprimands the unit secretary for the overuse of clerical supplies. Later that afternoon, the unit secretary is overheard reprimanding the temporary secretary and the student nurses for "wasting supplies." This behavior is an example of

1 Denial.
2 Repression.
3 Suppression.
4 Displacement.

Answer: 4

Rationale: Ego defense mechanisms are operations outside of a person's awareness that the ego calls into play to protect against anxiety. Displacement is the discharging of pent-up feelings on persons less dangerous than those who initially aroused the emotion. In this scenario, the nurse reprimands the unit secretary for overuse of clerical supplies. The secretary lashes out at the temporary secretary and student nurses for wasting supplies. These are much "safer targets" to become angry with than the nurse. Denial is the blocking out of painful or anxiety-inducing events or feelings. Suppression is consciously keeping unacceptable feelings and thoughts out of awareness. Repression is unconsciously keeping unacceptable feelings out of awareness.

Test-Taking Strategy: Knowledge of ego defense mechanisms is necessary to answer the question. Read the behavior identified in the question to assist you in determining the type of ego defense mechanism. If you had difficulty with this question, take time now to review defense mechanisms.

Level of Cognitive Ability: Analysis
Phase of Nursing Process: Analysis
Client Needs: Psychosocial Integrity
Content Area: Mental Health

Reference

Carson, V., & Arnold, E. (1996). *Mental health nursing: The nurse-patient journey.* Philadelphia: W. B. Saunders, p. 697.

---

223. The nurse is monitoring the fetal heart rate (FHR). The nurse documents and reports that a reassuring FHR pattern is present. Which of the following is indicative of a reassuring FHR pattern?

1 Late decelerations are present.
2 Short-term variability averages 6 to 10 beats/minute, and long-term variability averages two to six cycles per minute.
3 FHR does not change as a result of fetal activity.
4 Average baseline rate ranges between 80 and 100 beats/minute.

Answer: 2

Rationale: Short-term variability averages 6–10 beats/minute, and long-term variability averages two to six cycles per minute. The FHR should accelerate with fetal movement. The baseline range for the FHR is 120–160 beats/minute. Late decelerations are a result of decreased uteroplacental perfusion, which causes a decrease in the fetal PO_2.

Test-Taking Strategy: Use the process of elimination in answering the question. Eliminate option 3 because any movement increases FHR. Eliminate option 4 because 80–100 beats/minute is too low for a FHR. Eliminate option 1 because late decelerations indicate a perfusion problem. This leaves option 2 as the correct option. If you had difficulty with this question, take time now to review the characteristics of a normal and abnormal FHR.

Level of Cognitive Ability: Analysis
Phase of Nursing Process: Analysis
Client Needs: Physiological Integrity
Content Area: Maternity

Reference

Nichols, F., & Zwelling, E. (1997). *Maternal-newborn nursing: Theory and practice.* Philadelphia: W. B. Saunders, pp. 947–953.

224. The client with acute glomerulonephritis has had a urinalysis sent to the laboratory. The report reveals that there is hematuria and proteinuria. The nurse interprets that these results are

1. Consistent with glomerulonephritis.
2. Inconsistent with glomerulonephritis.
3. Unclear, and no conclusion can be drawn.
4. Indicative of impending renal failure.

Answer: 1

Rationale: Gross hematuria and proteinuria are the cardinal signs of glomerulonephritis. The urine may be small in volume, dark or smoky in color from the hematuria, and foamy from the proteinuria. Concurrent serum studies reveal elevated blood urea nitrogen, creatinine, C-reactive protein levels, and antistreptolysin O titer.

Test-Taking Strategy: Use the process of elimination to answer the question. Option 4 should be eliminated first because the results identified in the question do not indicate impending renal failure. Option 3 is not a likely answer. To choose correctly between options 1 and 2, it is necessary to know that these findings are consistent with glomerulonephritis. If you had difficulty with this question, take time now to review assessment findings in glomerulonephritis.

Level of Cognitive Ability: Analysis
Phase of Nursing Process: Analysis
Client Needs: Physiological Integrity
Content Area: Adult Health/Renal

Reference

Black, J., & Matassarin-Jacobs, E. (1997). *Medical-surgical nursing: Clinical management for continuity of care* (5th ed.). Philadelphia: W. B. Saunders, p. 1631.

---

225. The nurse is caring for a toddler who sustained second-degree burns. Which of the following would the nurse assess in determining the adequacy of fluid resuscitation in the child?

1. Blood pressure
2. Urinary output
3. Apical rate
4. Respiratory pattern

Answer: 2

Rationale: Urinary output is the best indicator of perfusion and adequate fluid resuscitation. If a child does not have adequate urine output, the reason is insufficient administration of resuscitative fluids. Sensorium is also an important guide to the adequacy of fluid resuscitation. Neither the blood pressure nor respiratory pattern is a sufficient guide regarding the adequacy of fluid resuscitation.

Test-Taking Strategy: Note the similarity with the key phrase "fluid resuscitation" in the question and "urinary output" in the correct option. If you had difficulty with this question, take time now to review burn shock and fluid resuscitation.

Level of Cognitive Ability: Analysis
Phase of Nursing Process: Analysis
Client Needs: Physiological Integrity
Content Area: Child Health

Reference

Ashwill, J., & Droske, S. (1997). *Nursing care of children: Principles and practice.* Philadelphia: W. B. Saunders, p. 1071.

226. The client with acute pyelonephritis is scheduled for a voiding cystourethrogram. The client is timid and modest by nature. The nurse interprets that this client would most likely benefit from increased support and teaching about the procedure because

1 Radiopaque contrast material is injected into the bloodstream.
2 Radioactive material is inserted into the bladder.
3 The client must lie on an x-ray table in a cold, barren room.
4 The client must void while the micturition process is filmed.

Answer: 4

Rationale: Having to void in the presence of others can be embarrassing for clients and may actually interfere with the client's ability to void. The nurse teaches the client about the procedure to try to minimize stress from lack of preparation and gives the client encouragement and emotional support. Screens may be used in the radiology department to try to provide an element of privacy during this procedure.

Test-Taking Strategy: Begin to answer this question by eliminating options 1 and 2 because the contrast material is inserted into the bladder by means of a catheter. To discriminate between options 3 and 4, you must know that the client has to void to allow filming of the movement of urine through the lower urinary tract. Note the key phrase "timid and modest" in the question. This assists in directing you to the correct option.

Level of Cognitive Ability: Analysis
Phase of Nursing Process: Analysis
Client Needs: Psychosocial Integrity
Content Area: Adult Health/Renal

Reference
Black, J., & Matassarin-Jacobs, E. (1997). *Medical-surgical nursing: Clinical management for continuity of care* (5th ed.). Philadelphia: W. B. Saunders, pp. 1564, 1629.

227. The nurse is caring for a child with a suspected diagnosis of aplastic anemia. Which of the following tests would the nurse anticipate to be performed to confirm the diagnosis?

1 Bone marrow aspiration
2 Complete blood count
3 Sickle cell screen
4 Schilling test

Answer: 1

Rationale: Bone marrow aspirations identify aplastic anemia and show pancytopenia, a deficiency in erythrocytes, leukocytes, and thrombocytes. A Schilling test is diagnostic for pernicious anemia. A sickle cell screen is diagnostic for sickle cell anemia. A complete blood count identifies anemia but may not identify the specific type.

Test-Taking Strategy: If you have no idea of the correct option, use your logical thinking processes and remember that anemias originate in the bone marrow. Select option 1, which mentions bone marrow.

Level of Cognitive Ability: Analysis
Phase of Nursing Process: Analysis
Client Needs: Physiological Integrity
Content Area: Child Health

Reference
Ashwill, J., & Droske, S. (1997). *Nursing care of children: Principles and practice.* Philadelphia: W. B. Saunders, p. 987.

228. A pregnant woman at 38 weeks' gestation arrives at the emergency department. She reports fresh, bright red vaginal bleeding and denies any pain. Based on this information, the nurse would determine that the client may be experiencing

1 Passage of the mucus plug.
2 Abruptio placentae.
3 Rupture of the amniotic sac.
4 Placenta previa.

Answer: 4

Rationale: The key symptom in placenta previa is painless vaginal bleeding in the second or third trimester of pregnancy. Passage of the mucus plug appears as pink or blood-tinged mucus. Findings of abruptio placentae include dark red blood and abdominal pain. A ruptured amniotic sac includes findings of a watery vaginal drainage.

Test-Taking Strategy: Knowledge regarding the symptoms associated with placenta previa and abruptio placentae assists in answering the question. Eliminate options 1 and 3 because these conditions would not produce bloody discharge. Remember the phrases "placenta previa and painless" and "abruptio and acute." If you had difficulty with this question, take time now to review the assessment signs associated with both disorders.

Level of Cognitive Ability: Analysis
Phase of Nursing Process: Analysis
Client Needs: Physiological Integrity
Content Area: Maternity

Reference

Nichols, F., & Zwelling, E. (1997). *Maternal-newborn nursing: Theory and practice.* Philadelphia: W. B. Saunders, pp. 872–873.

---

229. During inspection of a client's skin, the nurse notes redness and an abrasion-type wound on the sacrum area. The nurse determines that this assessment finding is indicative of a

1 Stage I pressure ulcer.
2 Stage II pressure ulcer.
3 Stage III pressure ulcer.
4 Stage IV pressure ulcer.

Answer: 2

Rationale: In a stage I pressure ulcer, the skin is intact, and the area is red and does not blanch with external pressure. In a stage II pressure ulcer, the skin is not intact, and the ulcer is superficial and may be characterized as an abrasion, blister, or shallow crater. In a stage III pressure ulcer, skin loss is full thickness, and there is a deep crater-like appearance. In a stage IV pressure ulcer, skin loss is full thickness with extensive destruction; tissue necrosis; or damage to muscle, bone, or supporting structures.

Test-Taking Strategy: Remembering that in stage I the skin is intact and that the skin disruption worsens as the stage increases may assist in directing you to the correct option. If you had difficulty with this question, take time now to review the characteristics of pressure ulcers.

Level of Cognitive Ability: Analysis
Phase of Nursing Process: Analysis
Client Needs: Physiological Integrity
Content Area: Adult Health/Integumentary

Reference

Ignatavicius, D. D., Workman, M. L., & Mishler, M. A. (1995). *Medical-surgical nursing: A nursing process approach* (2nd ed.). Philadelphia: W. B. Saunders, p. 1936.

---

230. A client has undergone left heart catheterization using the right femoral approach and is returned to the nursing unit. Thirty minutes later, the client complains of numbness and tingling of the right foot. The pedal pulse is weak, and the foot is pale. The nurse notifies the physician immediately because these symptoms are consistent with

1 Femoral artery thrombus or hematoma.
2 Local allergic reaction to the contrast dye.
3 Right sciatic nerve damage.
4 Early massive infection at the catheter insertion site.

Answer: 1

Rationale: Adverse changes, such as numbness and tingling, coolness, pallor, cyanosis, or sudden loss of peripheral pulses, indicate serious circulatory impairment and are reported to the physician at once. Allergic reaction to the dye is a systemic problem, not local. The timing of the symptoms is not consistent with sciatic pain. Infection does not become apparent this quickly.

Test-Taking Strategy: Use the ABCs to answer the question. The symptoms and timing all point to a circulatory problem. Evaluation of the possible options guides you to the correct answer. The correct option is the only one that involves circulatory compromise.

Level of Cognitive Ability: Analysis
Phase of Nursing Process: Analysis
Client Needs: Physiological Integrity
Content Area: Adult Health/Cardiovascular

Reference

Black, J., & Matassarin-Jacobs, E. (1997). *Medical-surgical nursing: Clinical management for continuity of care* (5th ed.). Philadelphia: W. B. Saunders, p. 1232.

231. The client admitted with coronary artery disease complains of dyspnea at rest. The nurse determines that which of the following items would be of most help to the client?

1. Placing an oxygen cannula at the bedside for use if needed
2. Performing continuous monitoring of oxygen saturation
3. Elevating the head of the bed to at least 45 degrees
4. Providing a walker to aid in ambulation

Answer: 3

Rationale: The management of dyspnea is generally directed toward alleviating the cause. Symptom relief may be achieved or at least aided by placing the client at rest with the head of bed elevated. In severe cases, supplemental oxygen is used.

Test-Taking Strategy: The phrase "of most help to the client" directs you to look for the item that is going to have the best immediate effect from the client's perspective. Therefore, eliminate options 1 and 4 first. Of the remaining two, option 3 is of most help to the client, whereas option 2 is of most help to the nurse.

Level of Cognitive Ability: Analysis
Phase of Nursing Process: Analysis
Client Needs: Physiological Integrity
Content Area: Adult Health/Cardiovascular

Reference

Ignatavicius, D. D., Workman, M. L., & Mishler, M. A. (1995). *Medical-surgical nursing: A nursing process approach* (2nd ed.). Philadelphia: W. B. Saunders, p. 789.

---

232. A client with ARDS had been recently placed on a ventilator. The most current arterial blood gas results are PO_2, 75 mmHg; PCO_2, 30 mmHg; pH, 7.45; SaO_2, 90%; HCO_3, 20. The nurse analyzes these results and determines that which of the following acid-base conditions exist?

1. Compensated respiratory alkalosis
2. Compensated metabolic acidosis
3. Respiratory alkalosis
4. Metabolic acidosis

Answer: 1

Rationale: Remember that when a respiratory condition exists, an opposite effect is found between the pH and the PCO_2. In respiratory alkalosis, the pH is elevated with a decrease in the PCO_2 level. In this case, the pH is at the high end of normal range (7.35–7.45). When the pH is within normal range, the condition is compensated.

Test-Taking Strategy: Use the process of elimination to answer the question. Remember that when the pH is within normal range, the condition is compensated. This assists in eliminating options 3 and 4. Normal pH is 7.35–7.45. In acidosis, the pH is down, and in alkalosis, the pH is elevated. Therefore, eliminate option 2.

Level of Cognitive Ability: Analysis
Phase of Nursing Process: Analysis
Client Needs: Physiological Integrity
Content Area: Adult Health/Respiratory

Reference

Ignatavicius, D. D., Workman, M. L., & Mishler, M. A. (1995). *Medical-surgical nursing: A nursing process approach* (2nd ed.). Philadelphia: W. B. Saunders, p. 337.

---

233. The nurse is caring for a client with a suspected diagnosis of Cushing's syndrome. Which of the following would the nurse interpret as being indicative of this condition?

1. Butterfly rash and peripheral edema
2. Weight loss and polydipsia
3. Dysphasia and polyuria
4. Truncal obesity and translucent-like skin

Answer: 4

Rationale: Clients with Cushing's syndrome experience weight gain with truncal obesity. The extremities appear thin with the presence of muscle wasting and weakness. The skin is often described as being thin and translucent. A butterfly rash across the cheeks of the face is seen in SLE. Polydipsia and polyphagia are seen in diabetes mellitus. Weight loss and peripheral edema may be seen in a number of conditions.

Test-Taking Strategy: When a question contains two components, be sure that each component is correct before selecting the option. Additionally, if you can associate a part of the option with the disorder presented in the question and can eliminate other options, select that option. If you can associate the first part of option 4, truncal obesity with Cushing's syndrome, and you cannot recall any of the other findings, select option 4. If you had difficulty with this question, take time now to review the clinical manifestations associated with Cushing's syndrome.

Level of Cognitive Ability: Analysis
Phase of Nursing Process: Analysis
Client Needs: Physiological Integrity
Content Area: Adult Health/Endocrine

Reference

Ignatavicius, D. D., Workman, M. L., & Mishler, M. A. (1995). *Medical-surgical nursing: A nursing process approach* (2nd ed.). Philadelphia: W. B. Saunders, p. 1824.

---

234. The nurse is caring for a child in sickle cell crisis. After gathering the assessment data, which of the following would the nurse analyze as being the most likely cause of the crisis?

1 A change in fluid intake
2 Increased intake of vitamin C
3 Minimal rest periods over the last several days
4 Dehydration occurring during strenuous exercise

Answer: 4

Rationale: Situations that precipitate sickling include hypoxia, vascular stasis, low environmental or body temperature, acidosis, strenuous exercise, anesthesia, dehydration, and infections.

Test-Taking Strategy: Use the process of elimination, using knowledge related to the physiology associated with sickle cell crisis. Eliminate options 2 and 3 because these are unrelated to sickle cell crisis. Option 1 is vague and does not describe if the change in fluid intake includes an increase or decrease; therefore, eliminate that option. If you had difficulty with this question, take time now to review the causes of sickle cell crisis.

Level of Cognitive Ability: Analysis
Phase of Nursing Process: Analysis
Client Needs: Physiological Integrity
Content Area: Child Health

Reference

Ashwill, J., & Droske, S. (1997). *Nursing care of children: Principles and practice.* Philadelphia: W. B. Saunders, pp 972–974.

---

235. The client with a leaking intracranial aneurysm has been placed on subarachnoid precautions. The client says, "I feel so isolated in here. Why can't I walk in the hall and have the telephone connected?" In formulating a response, the nurse incorporates the understanding that

1 The aneurysm will heal more quickly in a quiet environment.
2 Ischemic brain tissue cannot process large amounts of information at one time.
3 Clients with aneurysms need isolation to cope with labile emotions.
4 Environmental stimuli are minimized to prevent aneurysm rupture or bleed.

Answer: 4

Rationale: Subarachnoid precautions (or aneurysm precautions) are intended to minimize environmental stimuli that could increase intracranial pressure and trigger bleeding or rupture of the aneurysm.

Test-Taking Strategy: It is important to understand the nature and use of aneurysm precautions in a client with intracranial aneurysm or with subarachnoid hemorrhage. If you are unfamiliar with aneurysm precautions, take a few moments now to review them.

Level of Cognitive Ability: Analysis
Phase of Nursing Process: Analysis
Client Needs: Psychosocial Integrity
Content Area: Adult Health/Neurological

Reference

Smeltzer, S., & Bare, B. (1996). *Brunner and Suddarth's Textbook of medical-surgical nursing* (8th ed.). Philadelphia: Lippincott-Raven, p. 1766.

236. The client with a hip fracture asks the nurse why Buck's extension traction is being applied before surgery. The nurse's response is based on the understanding that Buck's extension traction primarily

1 Provides rigid immobilization of the fracture site.
2 Provides comfort by reducing muscle spasms and provides fracture immobilization.
3 Lengthens the fractured leg to prevent severing of blood vessels.
4 Allows bony healing to begin before surgery.

Answer: 2

Rationale: Buck's extension traction is a type of skin traction often applied after hip fracture before the fracture is reduced in surgery. It reduces muscle spasms and helps to immobilize the fracture. It does not lengthen the leg for the purpose of preventing blood vessel severance. It also does not allow for bony healing to begin.

Test-Taking Strategy: Options 3 and 4 are the least plausible of all the choices and should be eliminated first. To discriminate between the last two, look at the words "rigid immobilization" in option 1. Because skin traction uses lighter weights than skeletal traction, this type of traction cannot be said to provide rigid immobilization. At the same time, skin traction is useful in reducing muscle spasms while immobilizing an area, which makes option 2 the correct answer. If you had difficulty with this question, take time now to review the purpose of Buck's traction.

Level of Cognitive Ability: Analysis
Phase of Nursing Process: Analysis
Client Needs: Physiological Integrity
Content Area: Adult Health/Musculoskeletal

Reference
Black, J., & Matassarin-Jacobs, E. (1997). *Medical-surgical nursing: Clinical management for continuity of care* (5th ed.). Philadelphia: W. B. Saunders, p. 2138.

237. The nurse tests the urine of a client with acute renal failure with a multitest reagent strip. The strip tests highly positive for proteinuria. The nurse analyzes that this result is consistent with which of the following types of renal failure?

1 Atypical renal failure
2 Prerenal failure
3 Intrinsic renal failure
4 Postrenal failure

Answer: 3

Rationale: With intrinsic renal failure, there is a fixed specific gravity, and the urine tests definitely positive for proteinuria. In prerenal failure, the specific gravity is high, and there is little or no proteinuria. In postrenal failure, there is a fixed specific gravity and little or no proteinuria.

Test-Taking Strategy: Begin to answer this question by eliminating option 1 as a nonexistent entity. Knowing that proteinuria occurs because of leakage at the basement membrane of the glomerulus helps you to choose option 3 over options 2 and 4 as the correct answer. If you had difficulty with this question, take time now to review the types and characteristics of renal failure.

Level of Cognitive Ability: Analysis
Phase of Nursing Process: Analysis
Client Needs: Physiological Integrity
Content Area: Adult Health/Renal

Reference
Black, J., & Matassarin-Jacobs, E. (1997). *Medical-surgical nursing: Clinical management for continuity of care* (5th ed.). Philadelphia: W. B. Saunders, p. 1638.

238. During a prenatal visit, a pregnant woman in the second trimester complains of constipation. Which of the following would the nurse determine as a harmful measure in preventing constipation?

1 Daily activity such as walking or swimming
2 Drinking six to eight glasses of water daily
3 Increasing whole grains and fresh vegetables in the diet
4 Adding 1 tablespoon of mineral oil to a bowl of cereal daily

Answer: 4

Rationale: Mineral oil should never be used as a stool softener because it inhibits the absorption of fat-soluble vitamins from the body. Constipation should be treated with increased fluids (six to eight glasses per day) and a diet high in roughage and fiber. Increasing exercise is also an excellent way to improve gastric motility.

Test-Taking Strategy: Note that options 1, 2, and 3 are natural methods for increasing gastric motility. Option 4 is an unnatural measure and needs to be avoided. If you had difficulty with this question, take time now to review measures to prevent constipation.

Level of Cognitive Ability: Analysis
Phase of Nursing Process: Analysis
Client Needs: Health Promotion and Maintenance
Content Area: Maternity

Reference

Nichols, F., & Zwelling, E. (1997). *Maternal-newborn nursing: Theory and practice.* Philadelphia: W. B. Saunders, pp. 504–505.

239. A nurse is conducting an assessment on a child suspected of having Reye's syndrome. Which of the following data, as reported by the mother, would the nurse interpret as being most associated with Reye's syndrome?

1 The child had food poisoning 6 months ago.
2 The child had influenza 2 weeks ago.
3 The child has food allergies.
4 The child has a history of meningitis.

Answer: 2

Rationale: The exact cause of Reye's syndrome is not clear. Many theories of susceptibility exist. Some theories point to the exposure of viral agents or toxins, whereas others suggest that such exposure merely precipitates the disease in infants and children already at risk. The role of salicylates is also unknown. It may be a synergistic cofactor, with an unknown host factor in combination with a viral illness, such as varicella or influenza.

Test-Taking Strategy: Use the process of elimination, remembering that the cause is not clear but is most closely associated with the exposure of a viral illness. If you had difficulty with this question, take time now to review Reye's syndrome.

Level of Cognitive Ability: Analysis
Phase of Nursing Process: Analysis
Client Needs: Physiological Integrity
Content Area: Child Health

Reference

Ashwill, J., & Droske, S. (1997). *Nursing care of children: Principles and practice.* Philadelphia: W. B. Saunders, p. 1250.

240. The nurse is changing the diaper of a 1-day-old full-term newborn girl. The nurse notes that the genitalia are red and swollen and that a thick white mucoid vaginal discharge is present. Based on these findings, the nurse determines that the best action would be to

1 Obtain a specimen of the discharge for culture.
2 Document the findings.
3 Notify the physician.
4 Review the mother's record to determine a history of gonorrhea.

Answer: 2

Rationale: The genitalia of a newborn girl are frequently red and swollen. This edema disappears in a few days. A vaginal discharge of thick white mucus is seen in the first week of life. The mucus is occasionally blood tinged about the third or fourth day, staining the diaper. The cause of the pseudomenstruation, similar to that of breast engorgement, is the withdrawal of maternal hormones.

Test-Taking Strategy: Knowledge of the normal findings in a newborn is required to answer the question. Knowing that this is a normal expected finding directs you to option 2, the correct option. If you had difficulty with this question, take time now to review normal newborn findings.

Level of Cognitive Ability: Application
Phase of Nursing Process: Analysis
Client Needs: Physiological Integrity
Content Area: Maternity

Reference

Nichols, F., & Zwelling, E. (1997). *Maternal-newborn nursing: Theory and practice.* Philadelphia: W. B. Saunders, p. 1107.

---

241. The nurse develops a nutritional plan for the client with ulcerative colitis. Based on the physiological processes associated with this disorder, the nurse determines that which of the following diets is best for this client?

1 High-fat diet
2 Low-fat diet
3 High-residue diet
4 Low-residue diet

Answer: 4

Rationale: Clients with significant but less severe symptoms of ulcerative colitis are restricted to a low-fiber or low-residue diet. The low-fiber diet provides all four food groups and essential nutrients and is limited in high roughage content, which causes further bowel irritation. Clients following a low-fiber diet should avoid foods such as whole wheat grains, nuts, and raw fruits and vegetables.

Test-Taking Strategy: Use the process of elimination in selecting the correct option, keeping in mind the pathophysiology associated with ulcerative colitis. Think about the disorder, remembering that for clients with an ulcerated and inflamed bowel, avoidance of stimulation and further irritation is an aim of therapy. If you had difficulty with this question, take time now to review the dietary measures used in treating ulcerative colitis.

Level of Cognitive Ability: Analysis
Phase of Nursing Process: Analysis
Client Needs: Physiological Integrity
Content Area: Adult Health/Gastrointestinal

Reference

Ignatavicius, D. D., Workman, M. L., & Mishler, M. A. (1995). *Medical-surgical nursing: A nursing process approach* (2nd ed.). Philadelphia: W. B. Saunders, p. 1642.

---

242. The nurse is assessing the client admitted with suspected carbon monoxide poisoning. The nurse anticipates that which of the following will be prescribed for the client?

1 Acetylcysteine (Mucomyst)
2 Vitamin K
3 Naloxone (Narcan)
4 Oxygen

Answer: 4

Rationale: With carbon monoxide poisoning, oxygen cannot easily bind onto the hemoglobin, which is carrying strongly bound carbon monoxide. Option 1 is the antidote for acetaminophen (Tylenol) overdose. Option 2 is the antidote for warfarin (Coumadin) overdose. Option 3 is the antidote for narcotic overdose.

Test-Taking Strategy: Recalling that carbon monoxide displaces oxygen on the hemoglobin molecule will easily direct you to option 4. Review treatment measures for this disorder now if you had difficulty with this question!

Level of Cognitive Ability: Analysis
Phase of Nursing Process: Analysis
Client Needs: Physiological Integrity
Content Area: Adult Health/Respiratory

Reference

Black, J., & Matassarin-Jacobs, E. (1997). *Medical-surgical nursing: Clinical management for continuity of care* (5th ed.). Philadelphia: W. B. Saunders, p. 2538.

243. The client has had a bowel resection, and a colostomy is created. The client indicates to the nurse an unwillingness to look at the colostomy. The nurse formulates which of the following nursing diagnoses for this client?

1 Anxiety
2 Fear
3 Body Image Disturbance
4 Ineffective Family Coping

Answer: 3

Rationale: The nurse identifies that the client is experiencing a Body Image Disturbance. This diagnosis is used when the client has either a verbal or a nonverbal response to a change in body image that is either actual or perceived. Ineffective Family Coping is not appropriate because the stem gives no information about the family. Anxiety or Fear is used when the client has a vague (Anxiety) or an identified (Fear) sense of unease or dread.

Test-Taking Strategy: When a question asks you to select the appropriate nursing diagnosis, use the information provided in the question to assist in directing you to the correct option. The question gives no information about any fear or anxiety that the client may have, so options 1 and 2 are eliminated first. Option 3 is chosen over option 4 because the stem also gives no information about the family.

Level of Cognitive Ability: Analysis
Phase of Nursing Process: Analysis
Client Needs: Psychosocial Integrity
Content Area: Adult Health/Gastrointestinal

References

Cox, H., Hinz, M., Lubno, M., et al. (1997). *Clinical applications of nursing diagnosis: Adult, child, women's, psychiatric, gerontic, and home health considerations* (3rd ed.). Philadelphia: F. A. Davis, pp. 496, 506, 514.

244. The client receiving therapy with carbidopa/levodopa (Sinemet) is upset and tells the home health nurse that his urine has turned a darker color since beginning to take this medication. The client wants to discontinue its use. In formulating a response to the client's concerns, the nurse interprets that this change is

1 Indicative of developing toxicity.
2 A sign of interaction with another drug.
3 A harmless side effect of the medication.
4 A result of taking the medication with milk.

Answer: 3

Rationale: With carbidopa/levodopa therapy, a darkening of the urine or sweat may occur. The client should be reassured that this is a harmless effect of the medication, and its use should be continued.

Test-Taking Strategy: Knowledge of the side effects of this medication is needed to answer this question. If you are unfamiliar with carbidopa/levodopa, you may want to take a few moments now to review this medication. It is always helpful to alert the client to side effects that could possibly be considered distasteful to the client.

Level of Cognitive Ability: Analysis
Phase of Nursing Process: Analysis
Client Needs: Psychosocial Integrity
Content Area: Pharmacology

Reference

Deglin, J., & Vallerand, A. (1997). *Davis's drug guide for nurses* (5th ed.). Philadelphia: F. A. Davis, p. 692.

245. A client with a history of simple partial seizures is taking clorazepate (Tranxene). The client asks the nurse if there is a risk of addiction. The nurse's response is based on the understanding that clorazepate

1 Is not habit forming either physically or psychologically.
2 Leads to physical and psychological dependence with prolonged high-dose therapy.
3 Leads to physical tolerance, but only after 10 or more years of therapy.
4 Can result in psychological dependence only, owing to the nature of the medication.

Answer: 2

Rationale: Clorazepate is classified as an anticonvulsant, antianxiety agent, and sedative/hypnotic (benzodiazepine). One of the nursing implications of clorazepate therapy is that the medication can lead to physical or psychological dependence when there is prolonged therapy at high doses. For this reason, the amount of medication that is readily available to the client at any one time is restricted.

Test-Taking Strategy: Knowing that the medication is a benzodiazepine leads you to conclude that this medication can lead to physical as well as psychological dependence. This helps you eliminate each of the incorrect options in turn.

Level of Cognitive Ability: Analysis
Phase of Nursing Process: Analysis
Client Needs: Physiological Integrity
Content Area: Pharmacology

Reference

Deglin, J., & Vallerand, A. (1997). *Davis's drug guide for nurses* (5th ed.). Philadelphia: F. A. Davis, pp. 286–287.

---

246. The client with Raynaud's phenomenon asks the nurse what causes the disorder. In formulating a response, the nurse incorporates the knowledge that this disorder is often seen in clients with

1 Collagen disorders, such as rheumatoid arthritis and systemic lupus erythematosus.
2 Early stage of lung disorders, such as chronic airflow limitation.
3 Microemboli from atrial fibrillation.
4 Peripheral arterial insufficiency.

Answer: 1

Rationale: Raynaud's phenomenon is frequently seen associated with collagen disorders, such as rheumatoid arthritis, scleroderma, and SLE. Other factors that may contribute to the disorder include occupationally related trauma or pressure to the fingertips (typists, pianists, use of handheld vibrating tools) and exposure to heavy metal.

Test-Taking Strategy: Familiarity with this disorder is necessary to answer this question. Briefly review Raynaud's phenomenon if needed. Eliminate option 2 immediately. Option 4 is incorrect because pulses are normal in a majority of these clients. Atrial fibrillation (option 3) is not a predisposing disorder.

Level of Cognitive Ability: Analysis
Phase of Nursing Process: Analysis
Client Needs: Physiological Integrity
Content Area: Adult Health/Cardiovascular

Reference

Lewis, S., Collier, I., & Heitkemper, M. (1996). *Medical-surgical nursing: Assessment and management of clinical problems* (4th ed.). St. Louis: Mosby–Year Book, p. 1053.

---

247. The nurse has done a neurovascular assessment on the client with peripheral arterial disease. Which of the following signs or symptoms would be of greatest concern to the nurse?

1 Pallor and coolness of the toes of the affected limb
2 Weakly palpable pedal pulses
3 Blanching of the feet when elevated above heart level
4 Complaints of rest pain by the client

Answer: 4

Rationale: Classic manifestations of peripheral arterial disease include color changes (pallor, rubor, cyanosis), temperature changes, and trophic changes in the affected extremity. Pedal pulse diminishes and becomes absent as the disease progresses. Progression of pain from intermittent claudication to rest pain indicates a severe degree of occlusion and a critical state of ischemia.

Test-Taking Strategy: This is a difficult question and requires the discrimination of mild symptoms and more severe symptoms associated with this disorder. The phrase "of greatest concern" indicates that there is more than one partially or completely correct option. Options 1, 2, and 3 indicate milder symptoms of the disease, whereas rest pain indicates a severe degree of ischemia.

Level of Cognitive Ability: Analysis
Phase of Nursing Process: Analysis
Client Needs: Physiological Integrity
Content Area: Adult Health/Cardiovascular

Reference

Smeltzer, S., & Bare, B. (1996). *Brunner and Suddarth's Textbook of medical-surgical nursing* (8th ed.). Philadelphia: Lippincott-Raven, pp. 726–727.

---

248. The client who takes chlorothiazide (Diuril) every evening expresses frustration with the drug and wants to stop therapy. When the home care nurse explores the reasoning, the client says, "It keeps me up all night. I feel as though I should bring my pillow into the bathroom." The nurse interprets that the client can best be assisted to adapt to this therapy successfully by

1 Switching to a morning administration of the medication.
2 Taking a sleep aid with the medication.
3 Limiting oral fluids before bedtime.
4 Asking the physician for a new brand of medication.

Answer: 1

Rationale: Diuretic therapy should be administered in the morning to cause the least disruption as is possible in the client's sleep cycle.

Test-Taking Strategy: Note the key phrase in the question "every evening." Begin to answer this question by eliminating options 2 and 4 as the least likely solutions. Option 3 may be of limited use, but the nighttime scheduling of the diuretic is what is causing the nocturia. Thus, option 1 is the best choice. This question addresses a fundamental point in diuretic therapy, regardless of the specific type of agent used.

Level of Cognitive Ability: Analysis
Phase of Nursing Process: Analysis
Client Needs: Psychosocial Integrity
Content Area: Pharmacology

Reference

Deglin, J., & Vallerand, A. (1997). *Davis's drug guide for nurses* (5th ed.). Philadelphia: F. A. Davis, p. 403.

---

249. The nurse is scheduled to administer a dose of digoxin (Lanoxin) to a client with atrial fibrillation. The client has a potassium level of 4.6 mEq/L. The nurse interprets that the

1 Dose should be omitted for that day.
2 Client needs a dose of potassium before receiving the digoxin.
3 Dose should be withheld and the physician notified.
4 Dose should be administered as ordered.

Answer: 4

Rationale: Hypokalemia can make the client more susceptible to digitalis toxicity. The nurse monitors the results of potassium levels drawn on the client. The normal reference range of potassium for an adult is 3.5–5.1 mEq/L. If the potassium level is low, the dose is withheld, and the physician is notified.

Test-Taking Strategy: To answer this question correctly, you must know that hypokalemia potentiates digitalis and what the normal values for potassium are. Options 1 and 2 are eliminated first because these options are the least prudent actions based on the way they are worded. Knowing the normal potassium level helps you choose option 4 over option 3. The potassium level is within normal limits; therefore, administer the medication as prescribed.

Level of Cognitive Ability: Analysis
Phase of Nursing Process: Analysis
Client Needs: Physiological Integrity
Content Area: Pharmacology

Reference

Deglin, J., & Vallerand, A. (1997). *Davis's drug guide for nurses* (5th ed.). Philadelphia: F. A. Davis, p. 370.

250. The client newly diagnosed with Parkinson's disease exhibits bradykinesia, rigidity, and tremors. The client asks the nurse what causes the symptoms. The nurse's response is based on an understanding that

1. Antibodies against acetylcholine receptors impair neuromuscular transmission.
2. There is loss of dopamine in the substantia nigra and basal ganglia.
3. Viral infection triggers an autoimmune reaction in the nervous system.
4. It is caused by compression of peripheral nerves.

Answer: 2

Rationale: Parkinson's disease is characterized by depletion of dopamine levels in the substantia nigra, whose nerve fibers carry dopamine to the corpus striatum. When the dopamine levels in the basal ganglia drop, the symptoms of Parkinson's disease occur. Option 1 describes myasthenia gravis. Option 3 describes Guillain-Barré syndrome. Option 4 is nonspecific.

Test-Taking Strategy: To answer this question easily, you need to know what causes Parkinson's disease. It may be helpful to remember that one of the medications used to treat the disorder is levo*dopa*. This may help you to recall that an insufficient amount of *dopa*mine is responsible for the signs and symptoms.

Level of Cognitive Ability: Analysis
Phase of Nursing Process: Analysis
Client Needs: Physiological Integrity
Content Area: Adult Health/Neurological

Reference

Smeltzer, S., & Bare, B. (1996). *Brunner and Suddarth's Textbook of medical-surgical nursing* (8th ed.). Philadelphia: Lippincott-Raven, pp. 1771, 1776, 1820.

251. The nurse observes the client as seizure activity begins. The client's entire body becomes rigid, and jerky alternations between muscle relaxation and contraction occur in all four extremities bilaterally. The nurse interprets the client is experiencing

1. Simple partial seizures.
2. Complex partial seizures.
3. Partial seizures secondarily generalized.
4. Generalized tonic-clonic seizures.

Answer: 4

Rationale: Generalized seizures are seizures that are bilaterally symmetrical and have no focal point of onset. There are seven subtypes, including tonic-clonic, tonic, clonic, absence, atonic, myoclonic, and infantile spasms. The tonic-clonic pattern is as described in the stem. Partial seizures are seizures that begin locally. They are divided into three subtypes: simple partial seizures (without impaired level of consciousness), complex partial seizures (with impaired level of consciousness), and partial seizures secondarily generalized.

Test-Taking Strategy: Knowledge of different types of seizure activity is needed to differentiate quickly among the various options. If you look at the description in the stem, however, you can see that the seizure affects all four extremities and therefore cannot be *partial*. This effectively eliminates each of the incorrect options.

Level of Cognitive Ability: Analysis
Phase of Nursing Process: Analysis
Client Needs: Physiological Integrity
Content Area: Adult Health/Neurological

Reference

Smeltzer, S., & Bare, B. (1996). *Brunner and Suddarth's Textbook of medical-surgical nursing* (8th ed.). Philadelphia: Lippincott-Raven, pp. 1784–1785.

252. The nurse admits a newborn with a diagnosis of myelomeningocele to the nursery. The nurse determines that which of these nursing diagnoses would be the initial priority in this newborn's plan of care?

1. Altered Parenting
2. Altered Skin Integrity
3. Risk for Infection
4. Risk for Injury

Answer: 2

Rationale: A myelomeningocele is a neural tube defect caused by failure of the posterior neural tube to close. The meninges are exposed through the surface of the skin in a herniated sac that may be either healed or leaking. Skin integrity is altered because a thin membrane covers the protruding sac. Therefore, option 2 is the best answer. Options 3 and 4 are the next best answers. The sac houses the meninges, CSF, and part of the spinal cord. If injury to the sac occurs, an infection is a risk. Although parenting may be affected, it is not the initial priority.

Test-Taking Strategy: Read the stem of the question carefully, noting the phrase "initial priority." Remember that physiological needs and actual needs take priority over any risk of potential problems. Eliminate option 1 because the question does not address information about the parents. Options 3 and 4 are possible complications. If you had difficulty with this question, take time now to review the initial care of a newborn with myelomeningocele.

Level of Cognitive Ability: Analysis
Phase of Nursing Process: Analysis
Client Needs: Physiological Integrity
Content Area: Maternity

Reference

Nichols, F., & Zwelling, E. (1997). *Maternal-newborn nursing: Theory and practice.* Philadelphia: W. B. Saunders, p. 1371.

---

253. The nurse analyzes the laboratory results of a client taking lithium. Which of the following does the nurse identify as a precipitating factor of lithium toxicity?

1 Hyponatremia
2 Hypernatremia
3 Hypocalcemia
4 Hypercalcemia

Answer: 1

Rationale: Sodium depletion decreases renal excretion of lithium, thereby causing the medication to accumulate and potentiating toxicity. Clients need to be instructed to maintain a normal sodium intake. Diuretics promote sodium loss, and these medications need to be used with caution in the client taking lithium. Sodium loss secondary to diarrhea can cause lithium accumulation, and the client should be forewarned of this possibility.

Test-Taking Strategy: If you can remember that a client taking lithium concurrently with a diuretic is at risk for toxicity, this may assist you in selecting the correct option. Additionally, remembering that lithium has properties in common with potassium and sodium assists in directing you to the correct option.

Level of Cognitive Ability: Analysis
Phase of Nursing Process: Analysis
Client Needs: Physiological Integrity
Content Area: Pharmacology

Reference

Lehne, R. A. (1998). *Pharmacology for nursing care* (3rd ed.). Philadelphia: W. B. Saunders, p. 609.

---

254. The nurse is caring for a client with acute pancreatitis. Which of the following nursing diagnoses would the nurse determine as the priority?

1 Pain related to the effects of pancreatic inflammation and enzyme leakage
2 Fluid Volume Deficit related to blood and gastrointestinal losses
3 High Risk for Altered Skin Integrity related to pruritus
4 High Risk for Activity Intolerance related to debilitation

Answer: 1

Rationale: Abdominal pain is the most prominent symptom of acute pancreatitis. The main focus of nursing care is aimed at reducing discomfort and pain by the use of measures that decrease gastrointestinal tract activity, thus decreasing pancreatic stimulation. Although options 2, 3, and 4 are also appropriate nursing diagnoses related to a client with acute pancreatitis, they are not the priority.

Test-Taking Strategy: Note the key word "priority" in the question. Eliminate options 3 and 4 because these describe potential rather than actual problems. Note that option 1 directly addresses the issue of pancreatic inflammation. If you had difficulty with this question, take time now to review the clinical manifestations associated with acute pancreatitis.

Level of Cognitive Ability: Analysis
Phase of Nursing Process: Analysis
Client Needs: Physiological Integrity
Content Area: Adult Health/Gastrointestinal

Reference

Ignatavicius, D. D., Workman, M. L., & Mishler, M. A. (1995). *Medical-surgical nursing: A nursing process approach* (2nd ed.). Philadelphia: W. B. Saunders, p. 327.

255. A client with cancer is being sent home with TPN. As part of the discharge teaching, the client and family members are taught how to start, stop, and control the infusion system. The nurse determines that this teaching best meets what need of the client and family?

1 Self-esteem
2 Independence
3 Compliance
4 Acceptance

Answer: 2

Rationale: Allowing the client to control the treatment promotes self-care and independence. Teaching the client and family how to start, stop, and control the infusion system does not address self-esteem, acceptance, or compliance needs.

Test-Taking Strategy: Client-focused care promotes self-care. The key word in the question is "control." Additionally the stem of the question addresses the "need" of the client and family. Giving the client control promotes independence. Always read the question carefully to eliminate those options that do not address content identified in the question.

Level of Cognitive Ability: Analysis
Phase of Nursing Process: Analysis
Client Needs: Psychosocial Integrity
Content Area: Fundamental Skills

Reference

Burrell, L. O., Gerlach, M. J., & Pless, B. (1997). *Adult nursing: Acute and community care* (2nd ed.). Stamford, CT: Appleton & Lange, pp. 1353–1354.

---

256. A client just had a subclavian central line inserted. Which of the following would the nurse analyze as the best determinant of correct placement of the catheter tip?

1 Chest x-ray
2 Blood flow return
3 Patent flush with normal saline
4 Auscultation of lung sounds

Answer: 1

Rationale: After placement of a subclavian line, a chest x-ray is the only method listed that verifies tip placement of the catheter. Flushing and blood return help to determine that the line is in a vein but do not identify any information concerning where exactly the tip is located. Auscultation of lung sounds may be helpful in identifying a pneumothorax, but it does not provide information regarding actual catheter tip location.

Test-Taking Strategy: Read the stem carefully to determine what the question is asking for. It is clearly asking for a way to determine tip placement, and there is only one correct answer. Note the key phrase "best determinant." This assists you in the process of elimination. If you had difficulty with this question, take time now to review nursing care after insertion of a subclavian catheter.

Level of Cognitive Ability: Analysis
Phase of Nursing Process: Analysis
Client Needs: Physiological Integrity
Content Area: Fundamental Skills

Reference

Phillips, L. D. (1997). *Manual of IV therapeutics* (2nd ed.). Philadelphia: F. A. Davis, p. 398.

257. The nurse is assigned to care for a client that had a thoracentesis 2 hours ago. The nursing assessment notes state that the client has bilateral chest expansion, bilateral breath sounds, no nasal flaring, and the presence of crepitus in the area of the thoracentesis. The nurse interprets these findings to mean

1 The client is exhibiting normal findings.
2 The client is exhibiting signs of subcutaneous emphysema.
3 The client is beginning to develop a respiratory infection.
4 The client is exhibiting signs of respiratory distress.

Answer: 2

Rationale: Subcutaneous emphysema may follow a thoracentesis because air in the pleural cavity leaks into subcutaneous tissues. The tissues feel like lumpy paper and crackle when palpated (crepitus). Usually, subcutaneous emphysema causes no problem unless it is increasing and constricting vital organs such as the trachea.

Test-Taking Strategy: Knowledge that crepitus relates to subcutaneous emphysema is helpful in answering the question. Use the process of elimination in answering the question. Additionally, note the similarity of the term "crepitus" in the question and "subcutaneous emphysema" in the correct option, option 2. Analyze the data presented in the question, and note the abnormal data. This assists in directing you to the correct option. If you had difficulty with this question, take time now to review normal respiratory assessment findings after thoracentesis.

Level of Cognitive Ability: Analysis
Phase of Nursing Process: Analysis
Client Needs: Physiological Integrity
Content Area: Adult Health/Respiratory

Reference
Black, J., & Matassarin-Jacobs, E. (1997). *Medical-surgical nursing: Clinical management for continuity of care* (5th ed.). Philadelphia: W. B. Saunders, pp. 1063–1064.

---

258. A client has returned from the radiology department after a pulmonary angiography. For the procedure, a catheter was inserted into the femoral vein and was removed at the end of the procedure. The nurse inspects the client's catheter insertion site and notes a dark bulge that is tender to touch. The nurse is unable to locate the pedal pulse and the foot is cool. Based on these findings, what interpretation would the nurse make?

1 The pressure dressing was applied too tight.
2 The client needs additional blankets.
3 An occlusion of the femoral artery could have possibly occurred from a hematoma in the area of the femoral vein stick.
4 The room is too cool for the client.

Answer: 3

Rationale: The signs identified in the question indicate an occlusion of the femoral artery. Before the procedure, mark the peripheral pulses distal to the cannulation sites with a felt-tipped pen, and record the quality of the pulses in the chart. This aids in locating the pulses after the procedure. Pulses are checked preprocedure for postprocedure comparisons and to detect possible occlusion of the vessel undergoing cannulation. Postcatheterization care is similar for all catheterizations. Notify the physician at once if the client experiences numbness or tingling. Also note if the extremity becomes cool, pale, or cyanotic or if sudden loss of peripheral pulses occurs. These manifestations represent serious impairment of circulation.

Test-Taking Strategy: Use knowledge regarding pulmonary angiography and what the procedure entails to answer this question. Options 2 and 4 are similar; therefore, eliminate both of these options. A cool room would cause vasoconstriction but not to the point of obliteration of arterial pulses. A tight dressing may cause a problem with obliteration, but the best interpretation of the signs presented in the question is found in option 3.

Level of Cognitive Ability: Analysis
Phase of Nursing Process: Analysis
Client Needs: Physiological Integrity
Content Area: Adult Health/Respiratory

Reference
Black, J., & Matassarin-Jacobs, E. (1997). *Medical-surgical nursing: Clinical management for continuity of care* (5th ed.). Philadelphia: W. B. Saunders, pp. 1062, 1231–1232.

259. The physician is about to cardiovert a client who has a cardiac rhythm of unstable ventricular tachycardia. The physician tells the nurse to turn the synchronizer switch to the "on" position. The nurse understands that this is necessary so that

1 The correct amount of energy will be delivered to the client.
2 The machine will switch to battery operation during the procedure.
3 The paddles will become charged.
4 The electric shock will be delivered on the client's R wave.

Answer: 4

Rationale: The synchronizer switch ensures that the electric shock is released on the client's R wave. This is done to prevent the shock from being delivered on the vulnerable T wave, which could result in ventricular fibrillation.

Test Taking Strategy: If you are relatively unfamiliar with the particulars of this procedure, look at the word "synchronizer." In everyday language, if something is synchronized, it is timed with something else. Using that perspective, you can eliminate the incorrect options fairly easily. Review cardioversion now if you had difficulty with this question!

Level of Cognitive Ability: Analysis
Phase of Nursing Process: Analysis
Client Needs: Physiological Integrity
Content Area: Adult Health/Cardiovascular

Reference

Ignatavicius, D. D., Workman, M. L., & Mishler, M. A. (1995). *Medical-surgical nursing: A nursing process approach* (2nd ed.). Philadelphia: W. B. Saunders, p 874.

260. A recently admitted trauma client has an immediate portable chest x-ray ordered. Surgery or a chest tube insertion may be required depending on the findings. The client is aware of the implications and states, "I'm afraid of what they will find." In analyzing the current data, the nurse arrives at the nursing diagnosis of

1 Anxiety related to impending surgery
2 Anxiety related to perceived threat of health status
3 Anxiety related to lack of knowledge of medical management
4 Anxiety related to lack of knowledge of chest x-ray procedure

Answer: 2

Rationale: Anxiety may be related to any threat to the individual's physical or psychological integrity. Analysis of the situation and client statement reveals that the anxiety is most closely related to the perceived threat of health status. The "unknown" in this situation is what is the concern of the client. Anxiety is defined as a vague uneasy feeling whose source is often nonspecific or unknown to the individual.

Test-Taking Strategy: Note the key phrase in the question, "I'm afraid of what they will find." When selecting the appropriate nursing diagnosis, look at the information presented in the question carefully. The client's statement supports option 2.

Level of Cognitive Ability: Analysis
Phase of Nursing Process: Analysis
Client Needs: Psychosocial Integrity
Content Area: Adult Health/Respiratory

Reference

Bolander, V. (1994). *Sorensen and Luckmann's Basic nursing: A psychophysiologic approach* (3rd ed.). Philadelphia: W. B. Saunders, p. 287.

261. A postoperative client is using an incentive spirometer. The nurse observes the client to inhale slowly with the mouthpiece placed between the teeth and the lips closed. The client inhales to the preset inspiratory goal and holds the breath for about 3 seconds, then exhales slowly. The client takes one breath and returns the incentive spirometer to the bedside. Based on this observation, what interpretation should the nurse make?

1 The client is using the incentive spirometer correctly.
2 The client should be repeating the sequence 10–20 times in each session.
3 The client should be inhaling and exhaling quickly.
4 The client should not be holding the breath after inhalation.

Answer: 2

Rationale: Incentive devices use a concept of sustained maximal inspiration. Each device has a means of setting an inspiratory goal. Correct use requires a spontaneous, slow, voluntary, deep breath. When full inhalation is reached, the breath is held for at least 3 seconds. This sequence is repeated 10–20 times an hour. Incentive exercises are most effective when used every hour while the client is awake.

Test-Taking Strategy: Options 3 and 4 describe incorrect technique. The client should be inhaling and exhaling slowly and should hold the breath about 3 seconds at the end of inhalation. For the technique to be effective, it must be repeated 10–20 times in a session and performed every hour. Thus, option 1 is incorrect because the client performed the technique only once. If you had difficulty with this question, take time now to review the correct procedure for the use of an incentive spirometer.

Level of Cognitive Ability: Analysis
Phase of Nursing Process: Analysis
Client Needs: Physiological Integrity
Content Area: Fundamental Skills

Reference
Bolander, V. R. (1994). *Sorensen and Luckmann's Basic nursing: A psychophysiologic approach* (3rd ed.). Philadelphia: W. B. Saunders, p. 1237.

---

262. During the postoperative assessment of a client, the nurse notices that the client is crying softly. Based on this observation, which of the following would the nurse determine as being the most appropriate response?

1 "Oh, honey, you don't need to worry. Everything will be okay."
2 "You are crying. Tell me about your feelings."
3 "Don't be upset. You have the best surgeon in town."
4 "You seem upset. I'll leave you alone for a while."

Answer: 2

Rationale: Taking time to discuss the client's concerns is as important a nursing action in many instances as any intervention for physical care. Therapeutic communication should focus on the client's nonverbal cues and encourage the client to express feelings or concerns about surgery. False reassurance blocks therapeutic communication with the client. Changing the subject is a communication technique that also blocks therapeutic communication with the client.

Test-Taking Strategy: Therapeutic communication techniques are required to answer this question. Use the process of elimination, and select an answer that enhances communication, as in option 2. Remember the client's feelings are the priority.

Level of Cognitive Ability: Analysis
Phase of Nursing Process: Analysis
Client Needs: Psychosocial Integrity
Content Area: Fundamental Skills

Reference
Potter, P., & Perry, A. (1997). *Fundamentals of nursing: Concepts, process and practice* (4th ed.). St. Louis: Mosby–Year Book, pp. 242, 245, 1424.

263. A client's preoperative vital signs are temperature, 37.0°C (98.6°F) orally; apical pulse, 80 beats/minute with regular rhythm; respiration rate, 22 breaths/minute; and blood pressure, 168/94 mmHg in the right arm. Based on the interpretation of these findings, which of the following actions should the nurse take first?

1. Report the vital signs immediately to the surgeon
2. Compare these values to those recorded previously
3. Recheck the blood pressure in 5 minutes
4. Report only the apical pulse because it is above the normal range

Answer: 2

Rationale: Preoperative assessment of vital signs provides important baseline data with which to compare after surgery. Anxiety and fear commonly cause elevations in heart rate and blood pressure. Anesthetic agents typically depress all vital functions. The vital signs as stated in the question do not need to be reported to the physician immediately. The apical pulse is not above the normal range. Rechecking the blood pressure in 5 minutes is likely to show an unchanged blood pressure measurement.

Test-Taking Strategy: Knowledge of the normal ranges for vital signs is important in answering this question. Also, knowledge of the effects of anxiety and fear on the vital signs is necessary. The principles of prioritizing should be used to answer this question. Note that the stem states to select the first action. The first action should be to compare the values with those recorded previously.

Level of Cognitive Ability: Application
Phase of Nursing Process: Analysis
Client Needs: Physiological Integrity
Content Area: Fundamental Skills

Reference

Potter, P., & Perry, A. (1997). *Fundamentals of nursing: Concepts, process and practice* (4th ed.). St. Louis: Mosby–Year Book, p. 1386.

264. A diabetic client is on a mixed-dose insulin protocol of 8 units regular insulin and 12 units of NPH insulin at 7 A.M. At 10:30 A.M., the client reports feeling uneasy and shaky. Which of the following is the probable explanation for this?

1. The NPH insulin's action is peaking, and there is an insufficient blood glucose level.
2. The regular insulin's action is peaking, and there is an insufficient blood glucose level.
3. The client consumed too many calories at breakfast and now has an elevated blood glucose level.
4. The symptoms are unrelated to the insulin or diet, and the client is at risk of a cardiovascular emergency.

Answer: 2

Rationale: Feeling uneasy and shaky indicates signs of hypoglycemia. NPH insulin peaks in 6–12 hours; therefore, option 1 is incorrect. Regular insulin peaks in 2–4 hours, which indicates the probable cause of the hypoglycemic reaction. Consuming too many calories does not cause a hypoglycemic reaction. Option 4 has no relationship to the information in the question.

Test-Taking Strategy: The client is manifesting signs and symptoms of hypoglycemia. At this point, knowledge of the peak action of both NPH and regular insulin is necessary to select between options 1 and 2. Eliminate option 3 based on the knowledge of the signs of hypoglycemia and the actions of insulin. Eliminate option 4 because this option does not present a relationship to the information in the question. If you had difficulty with this question, take time now to review the signs of hypoglycemia and the peak times of NPH and regular insulin.

Level of Cognitive Ability: Analysis
Phase of Nursing Process: Analysis
Client Needs: Physiological Integrity
Content Area: Adult Health/Endocrine

Reference

Lehne, R. A. (1998). *Pharmacology for nursing care* (3rd ed.). Philadelphia: W. B. Saunders, p. 580.

265. The client is awake but disoriented to place and time, responds slowly to questions, and is restless. Arterial blood gas results show a pH of 7.33, PCO_2 of 48, PO_2 of 93, and HCO_3 of 24. Based on the analysis of the client's symptoms and the blood gas results, the most appropriate nursing diagnosis is

1 Anxiety related to hypercapnea and respiratory acidosis.
2 Sensory/Perceptual Alteration related to physiological changes of respiratory acidosis.
3 Risk for Injury related to metabolic alkalosis and confusion.
4 Impaired Gas Exchange related to hypoventilation secondary to respiratory arrest.

Answer: 2

Rationale: The client's blood gas results indicate respiratory acidosis. Symptoms of respiratory acidosis include headache, irritability, muscle twitching, behavioral changes, confusion, lethargy, and coma. Anxiety, hypoventilation, and respiratory arrest are not addressed in the question.

Test-Taking Strategy: This question requires the ability to interpret arterial blood gas results and relate that interpretation to the client's clinical presentation. Read the question and all the options carefully. When selecting an appropriate nursing diagnosis, use the data presented in the question to do so. The client data reflect a sensory/perceptual problem, which should direct you to option 2.

Level of Cognitive Ability: Analysis
Phase of Nursing Process: Analysis
Client Needs: Physiological Integrity
Content Area: Adult Health/Respiratory

Reference

LeMone, P., & Burke, K. M. (1996). *Medical-surgical nursing: Critical thinking in client care.* Menlo Park, CA: Addison-Wesley, p. 156.

---

266. The nurse is caring for a client who recently had a jugular line placed. After changing the tubing at the insertion site, the client states, "I feel light-headed, weak, and somewhat short of breath." Which of the following does the nurse suspect may be occurring?

1 Fluid overload
2 Pneumothorax
3 Air embolism
4 Septicemia

Answer: 3

Rationale: The most likely occurrence based on the given situation is an air embolism. An air embolism can occur when an inaccurate technique is used to change intravenous tubing. Options 1, 2, and 4 are potential complications of intravenous therapy; however, there are not enough data presented in the question to assume that these complications are likely to be occurring.

Test-Taking Strategy: Read the case situation carefully. It reveals that the problem is occurring after an intravenous tubing was recently changed. Knowledge that a major complication that occurs with central line tubing changes is air embolism is needed to answer this question. Eliminate options 1 and 4, which do not correlate with the signs and symptoms presented in the case situation. Review the complications and causes of intravenous therapy now if you had difficulty with this question.

Level of Cognitive Ability: Analysis
Phase of Nursing Process: Analysis
Client Needs: Physiological Integrity
Content Area: Fundamental Skills

Reference

Phillips, L. D. (1997). *Manual of IV therapeutics* (2nd ed.). Philadelphia: F. A. Davis, pp. 294–295.

267. A client has an intravenous infusion started before surgery for a right below-the-knee amputation. Which of the following nursing diagnoses is most appropriate for the nurse to consider in providing preoperative care?

1 Fluid Volume Deficit related to intravenous therapy
2 Fluid Volume Excess related to intravenous therapy
3 High Risk for Pain related to surgery
4 Possible Anxiety related to coping with preoperative therapies

Answer: 4

Rationale: Client anxiety is a top priority concern before treatments and surgery. Before procedures (intravenous therapy) and surgery, most clients experience anxiety. There are no data given in the situation to indicate signs of actual fluid volume deficit or overload. High-risk postoperative concerns, such as pain, should be addressed in the preoperative period but are not the issue of the question.

Test-Taking Strategy: Read the stem carefully and determine that preoperative care is the concern. With nursing diagnosis questions, be certain that there are enough data in the situation to support the use of an actual diagnosis. The key phrase is "most appropriate for the nurse to consider." Eliminate options 1 and 2 because they relate to actual nursing diagnoses. Remember also to focus on client concerns as a priority in the preoperative period.

Level of Cognitive Ability: Analysis
Phase of Nursing Process: Analysis
Client Needs: Psychosocial Integrity
Content Area: Fundamental Skills

Reference

McFarland, G., & McFarlane, E. (1997). *Nursing diagnosis and intervention: Planning for patient care.* St. Louis: Mosby–Year Book, pp. 552–553.

---

268. The nurse is caring for a client who had a small bowel resection yesterday. The client has continuous gastric suction. Which of the following intravenous solutions would the nurse anticipate as most likely being prescribed for the client?

1 25% albumin
2 5% dextrose in water (D5W)
3 Lactated Ringer's solution
4 Normal saline (0.9% NaCl)

Answer: 3

Rationale: Multiple electrolyte solutions such as lactated Ringer's are used to replace fluid from alimentary tract losses. Albumin is used for shock and protein replacement. D5W contains only glucose and no electrolytes to replace gastrointestinal losses. Normal saline contains no glucose, and glucose is essential for calories when a client is unable to take anything by mouth.

Test-Taking Strategy: The case situation of this question contains key information related to the client's condition and the type of fluid losses the client is experiencing (gastric). Knowledge of the various types of intravenous fluids is required to answer this question. You need to know that multiple electrolytes need to be replaced, which are contained in lactated Ringer's solution alone. Lactated Ringer's solution is also a more global response because lactated Ringer's solution contains sodium, potassium, and glucose, which are identified in options 2 and 4. If you had difficulty with this question, take time now to review the components of these intravenous solutions.

Level of Cognitive Ability: Analysis
Phase of Nursing Process: Analysis
Client Needs: Physiological Integrity
Content Area: Fundamental Skills

Reference

Phillips, L. D. (1997). *Manual of IV therapeutics* (2nd ed.). Philadelphia: F. A. Davis, pp. 137–139.

269. The client has carboxyhemoglobin levels greater than 50%. Physical assessment reveals the client is unresponsive and has an irregular breathing pattern with periods of apnea. The nurse analyzes these data and determines that the priority nursing diagnosis is

1 High Risk for Ineffective Airway Clearance related to excessive secretions.
2 Ineffective Breathing Pattern secondary to neural hypoxia.
3 Potential for Altered Tissue Perfusion secondary to insufficient oxygen transport.
4 Potential for Impaired Gas Exchange secondary to insufficient oxygen transport.

Answer: 2

Rationale: When the carboxyhemoglobin levels are greater than 50%, the respiratory center becomes depressed because of inadequate oxygenation, and hypoxia occurs. Option 2 is the only option that identifies an actual problem, and the question does identify clinical manifestations.

Test-Taking Strategy: The only option that identifies an actual problem is option 2. Note the relationship between the phrase "irregular breathing pattern" in the question and "ineffective breathing pattern" in the option.

Level of Cognitive Ability: Analysis
Phase of Nursing Process: Analysis
Client Needs: Physiological Integrity
Content Area: Adult Health/Respiratory

Reference

Thompson, J., McFarland, G., Hirsch, J., & Tucker, S. (1997). *Mosby's clinical nursing* (4th ed.). St. Louis: Mosby–Year Book, p. 149.

---

270. The nurse notices that a client who had a Mantoux tuberculin skin test yesterday is frequently inspecting and touching the injection site. Even though the client was instructed that the test would not be read until 48 hours later, the client has asked numerous questions about a positive reaction and even asks the nurse if the test results look like it might be positive. Initially the nurse analyzes these data to mean

1 The client has an inquisitive nature.
2 The client wants to increase personal knowledge in the area of tuberculin skin testing.
3 The client is demonstrating obsessive-compulsive tendencies.
4 The client is anxious that the test results may be significant.

Answer: 4

Rationale: People experience anxiety in certain situations and not in others. Anxiety varies with an individual's perception, which, in turn, depends on a person's psychosocial makeup, education, degree of maturity, and life experiences. The nurse should know that anxiety is exhibited in many forms. People may communicate their anxiety both verbally and nonverbally. The nurse needs to pick up on cues, interpret them, and seek to validate those first impressions. A person's voice may shake or break, pitch may change, and speed may fluctuate. There is no indication in the question that the client is exhibiting obsessive-compulsive tendencies.

Test-Taking Strategy: Use the process of elimination to answer the question. Initially the nurse would analyze the client's behavior as possibly indicating that the client is anxious related to the skin test and results. It is important that the nurse seek to understand the situation from the client's perspective, rather than her own. Option 4 considers the client's behavior from the client's perspective.

Level of Cognitive Ability: Analysis
Phase of Nursing Process: Analysis
Client Needs: Psychosocial Integrity
Content Area: Adult Health/Respiratory

Reference

Black, J., & Matassarin-Jacobs, E. (1997). *Medical-surgical nursing: Clinical management for continuity of care* (5th ed.). Philadelphia: W. B. Saunders, pp. 1141–1142.

271. The client with thromboangiitis obliterans (Buerger's disease) asks the nurse what can be done to alleviate the symptoms. In formulating a response, the nurse incorporates the understanding that

1 There is no current treatment.
2 Surgery is the most successful therapy.
3 Intervention is predominantly aimed at pain control with analgesics.
4 Treatment is essentially the same as for peripheral vascular disease.

Answer: 4

Rationale: The main goals of treatment are to improve circulation to the affected areas, prevent disease progression, and protect the extremities from infection and trauma. In essence, treatment is the same as for peripheral arterial insufficiency.

Test-Taking Strategy: Option 1 is an unrealistic statement and is eliminated first. With arterial and venous involvement, surgery is not a likely choice; therefore, eliminate option 2. Pain is caused by ischemia, so option 3 would be of limited use. The correct option is option 4. All measures used to treat peripheral vascular disease are useful in treating thromboangiitis obliterans (Buerger's disease).

Level of Cognitive Ability: Analysis
Phase of Nursing Process: Analysis
Client Needs: Physiological Integrity
Content Area: Adult Health/Cardiovascular

Reference

Smeltzer, S., & Bare, B. (1996). *Brunner and Suddarth's Textbook of medical-surgical nursing* (8th ed.). Philadelphia: Lippincott-Raven, p. 738.

---

272. The nurse is caring for an adolescent with sickle cell anemia hospitalized for the treatment of vaso-occlusive crisis. The nurse determines that which of these nursing diagnoses should receive priority in the client's plan of care?

1 Ineffective Family Coping
2 Altered Tissue Perfusion
3 Pain
4 Social Interaction, Impaired

Answer: 2

Rationale: In vaso-occlusive crisis, impaired tissue perfusion to the brain, the kidneys, and the peripheral areas occurs. The priority is to correct or minimize the occlusions to prevent necrosis. Treatment includes hydration, oxygenation, and measures to decrease metabolism. A second priority is to address the pain caused by the vaso-occlusion. Options 1 and 4, although appropriate to include in the plan of care, are not considered to be a priority.

Test-Taking Strategy: Use Maslow's hierarchy of needs and the process of elimination to answer the question. The question asks for the priority nursing diagnosis. Additionally, use the ABCs to answer the question. Altered tissue perfusion, which relates to oxygenation, is the priority. If you had difficulty with this question, take time now to review the physiology associated with sickle cell crisis.

Level of Cognitive Ability: Analysis
Phase of Nursing Process: Analysis
Client Needs: Physiological Integrity
Content Area: Child Health

Reference

Ashwill, J., & Droske, S. (1997). *Nursing care of children: Principles and practice.* Philadelphia: W. B. Saunders, p. 971.

---

273. Which of the following nursing diagnoses would the nurse identify as the priority in caring for a child hospitalized with HIV?

1 Altered Family Processes related to a terminal disease.
2 Risk for Altered Nutrition: Less Than Body Requirements
3 Risk for Infection related to impaired body defenses
4 Impaired Social Interaction related to social stigma

Answer: 3

Rationale: Options 1 and 4 relate to psychosocial needs, which are secondary after addressing physical needs. Prevention of the occurrence of opportunistic infections and treatment of opportunistic infections are the priority for clients with HIV. Nutritional support is also a priority concern; however, infection would be most life-threatening.

Test-Taking Strategy: Use the process of elimination and Maslow's hierarchy of needs to answer the question. This assists in eliminating options 1 and 4 because these options relate to psychosocial needs. Options 2 and 3 relate to physiological needs. Both options 2 and 3 are potential nursing diagnoses, but infection would present the most immediate life-threatening concern. If you had difficulty with this question, take time now to review HIV.

Level of Cognitive Ability: Analysis
Phase of Nursing Process: Analysis
Client Needs: Physiological Integrity
Content Area: Child Health

Reference

Ashwill, J., & Droske, S. (1997). *Nursing care of children: Principles and practice.* Philadelphia: W. B. Saunders, p. 648.

---

274. The client who was started on anticonvulsant therapy with clonazepam (Klonopin) tells the nurse of increasing clumsiness and unsteadiness since starting the medication. The client is visibly upset by these manifestations and asks the nurse what to do. The nurse's response is based on the understanding that these symptoms

1 Are most severe during initial therapy and decrease or disappear with long-term use.
2 Indicate that the client is experiencing a severe untoward reaction to the drug.
3 Are probably the result of interaction with another medication.
4 Usually occur when the client takes the medication with food.

Answer: 1

Rationale: Drowsiness, unsteadiness, and clumsiness are expected effects of the drug during early therapy. They are dose related and usually diminish or disappear altogether with continued use of the drug. These effects do not indicate a severe side effect is occurring. They are also unrelated to interaction with another medication. The client is encouraged to take this medication with food to minimize gastrointestinal upset.

Test-Taking Strategy: To answer this question successfully, knowledge of this medication is needed. You need to know that the effects described in the question occur early in the course of therapy and decrease or disappear with long-term use. If you had difficulty with this question, review this medication now.

Level of Cognitive Ability: Analysis
Phase of Nursing Process: Analysis
Client Needs: Psychosocial Integrity
Content Area: Pharmacology

Reference

Deglin, J., & Vallerand, A. (1997). *Davis's drug guide for nurses* (5th ed.). Philadelphia: F. A. Davis, pp. 282–283.

---

275. The client has been prescribed cyclobenzaprine (Flexeril) in the treatment of painful muscle spasms accompanying a herniated intervertebral disk. The nurse would withhold the medication and question the order if the client had concurrent orders to take

1 Furosemide (Lasix).
2 Valproic acid (Depakene).
3 Ibuprofen (Motrin).
4 Tranylcypromine (Parnate).

Answer: 4

Rationale: The client should not receive cyclobenzaprine if the client has taken monoamine oxidase inhibitors, such as tranylcypromine or phenelzine (Nardil), within the last 14 days. Otherwise the client could experience hypertensive crisis, convulsions, or death.

Test-Taking Strategy: Knowledge regarding cyclobenzaprine and the contraindications in its use is required to answer the question. It is necessary to know that cyclobenzaprine may not be taken with monoamine oxidase inhibitors within the last 14 days. If you had difficulty with this question, review this medication and the contraindications associated with it.

Level of Cognitive Ability: Application
Phase of Nursing Process: Analysis
Client Needs: Physiological Integrity
Content Area: Pharmacology

Reference

Hodgson, B., & Kizior, R. (1998). *Saunders nursing drug handbook 1998.* Philadelphia: W. B. Saunders, pp. 269–270.

276. The nurse is urging the client to cough and deep breathe after nephrectomy. The client tells the nurse, "That's easy for you to say. You don't have to do this." The nurse interprets that the client's statement is most likely a result of

1 A stress response to the ordeal of surgery.
2 A latent fear of needing dialysis if the surgery is unsuccessful.
3 Effects of circulating metabolites that have not been excreted by the remaining kidney.
4 Pain that is intensified because the location of the incision is near the diaphragm.

Answer: 4

Rationale: The client after nephrectomy may be in considerable pain. This is due to the size of the incision and its location near the diaphragm, which makes coughing and deep breathing so uncomfortable. For this reason, narcotics are used liberally and may be most effective when provided as PCA or through epidural analgesia.

Test-Taking Strategy: The question asks for the "most likely" reason for the client's statement, which implies that more than one option may be partially correct. Begin to answer the question by eliminating options 2 and 3 as the least plausible options. Knowing that coughing and deep breathing intensify pain after many surgical procedures helps you to choose option 4 over option 1.

Level of Cognitive Ability: Analysis
Phase of Nursing Process: Analysis
Client Needs: Physiological Integrity
Content Area: Fundamental Skills

Reference

Black, J., & Matassarin-Jacobs, E. (1997). *Medical-surgical nursing: Clinical management for continuity of care* (5th ed.). Philadelphia: W. B. Saunders, pp. 1672–1673.

---

277. The client is being evaluated as a potential kidney donor for a family member. The potential donor asks the nurse why different teams are evaluating the donor and recipient. In formulating a response, the nurse understands that this is being done to

1 Save the client and recipient valuable preoperative time.
2 Avoid a conflict of interest by the team evaluating the recipient and team evaluating the donor.
3 Help reduce the cost of the preoperative workup.
4 Have a sufficient number of people reviewing the case, so no information is overlooked.

Answer: 2

Rationale: Both the kidney donor and recipient need thorough medical and psychological evaluation before transplant surgery. To avoid conflict of interest, evaluation of the donor is done by a team different from that caring for the donor. The psychosocial issues in living-related organ donation may be complex, and conversations with the donor are held in strict confidence to preserve family relations.

Test-Taking Strategy: Begin to answer this question by eliminating options 3 and 4, which are the least plausible. You would choose option 2 over option 1 using knowledge of concepts regarding client advocacy. One group cannot advocate for both parties simultaneously. If you had difficulty with this question, take time now to review the concepts related to donor selection.

Level of Cognitive Ability: Analysis
Phase of Nursing Process: Analysis
Client Needs: Psychosocial Integrity
Content Area: Adult Health/Renal

Reference

Black, J., & Matassarin-Jacobs, E. (1997). *Medical-surgical nursing: Clinical management for continuity of care* (5th ed.). Philadelphia: W. B. Saunders, p. 1661.

278. The nurse is caring for a client who has been diagnosed as having a kidney mass. The client asks the nurse the reason for renal biopsy, when other tests such as computed tomography scan and ultrasound are available. In formulating a response, the nurse incorporates the knowledge that renal biopsy

1. Helps differentiate between a solid mass and a fluid-filled cyst.
2. Provides an outline of the renal vascular system.
3. Gives specific cytological information about the lesion.
4. Determines if the mass is growing rapidly or slowly.

Answer: 3

Rationale: Renal biopsy is a definitive test that gives specific information about whether the lesion is benign or malignant. An ultrasound scan discriminates between a fluid-filled cyst and a solid mass. Renal arteriography outlines the renal vascular system.

Test-Taking Strategy: Begin to answer this question by eliminating options 1 and 2 first. Basic knowledge of the purposes of biopsy helps you discard these quickly. To discriminate between options 3 and 4, remember that with biopsy the cells are examined under a microscope. This examination then yields specific information about the type of neoplastic cell. Although some types of cancer grow more quickly than others, it is not possible to determine this by biopsy. Thus, you would choose option 3 as the better answer.

Level of Cognitive Ability: Analysis
Phase of Nursing Process: Analysis
Client Needs: Physiological Integrity
Content Area: Adult Health/Renal

Reference

Black, J., & Matassarin-Jacobs, E. (1997). *Medical-surgical nursing: Clinical management for continuity of care* (5th ed.). Philadelphia: W. B. Saunders, p. 1671.

---

279. The client with diabetes mellitus verbalizes that it is difficult to adhere to the diabetic treatment plan. The nurse interprets the client's concern and determines that the most appropriate response is

1. "If you don't take your insulin you will develop diabetic ketoacidosis."
2. "Let's go over your diet again to be sure it contains foods you like."
3. "Do you understand what noncompliance can mean to your future health?"
4. "Let's check your blood glucose now."

Answer: 2

Rationale: It is important to determine and deal with a client's concerns and to identify measures that can assist the client to comply with the diabetic regimen. The nurse should determine if a knowledge deficit exists and if the client's treatment plan maintains normalcy as much as is possible with the client's lifestyle. Scare tactics as described in options 1 and 3 should not be used. Positive reinforcement is necessary instead of focusing on negative behaviors. Option 4 does not address the issue of the question.

Test-Taking Strategy: Identify the issue of the question. The key phrase is "difficult to adhere to the diabetic treatment plan." This leads the nurse to assist the client in identifying measures that promote compliance. When answering communication questions, you should choose the option that gives information or clarifies. Options 1 and 3 are incorrect because they show disapproval and could scare the client. Option 4 places the client's issues on "hold."

Level of Cognitive Ability: Application
Phase of Nursing Process: Analysis
Client Needs: Psychosocial Integrity
Content Area: Adult Health/Endocrine

Reference

Black, J., & Matassarin-Jacobs, E. (1997). *Medical-surgical nursing: Clinical management for continuity of care* (5th ed.). Philadelphia: W. B. Saunders, p. 1965.

---

280. A newly diagnosed diabetic is admitted to the hospital for evaluation and control of the disease. When analyzing the assessment data, which of the following would the nurse most likely expect to find?

1. Hyperglycemia
2. Hypoglycemia
3. Weight gain
4. Hematuria

Answer: 1

Rationale: Hyperglycemia identifies the disease of diabetes. Clients with this finding are a new diabetic, have been previously diagnosed as a diabetic and have not been following their diet, have become too sedentary, or have failed to take medication. Newly diagnosed diabetics present with a variety of symptoms, which may include polydipsia, polyuria, polyphagia, weakness, weight loss, and dehydration. Definitive diagnosis is verified by hyperglycemia.

Test-Taking Strategy: Use the process of elimination in answering the question. Knowing that diabetes is a lack of insulin and therefore results in hyperglycemia is important in determining the answer. If you had difficulty with this question, take time now to review the characteristics associated with diabetes.

Level of Cognitive Ability: Analysis
Phase of Nursing Process: Analysis
Client Needs: Physiological Integrity
Content Area: Adult Health/Endocrine

Reference

Black, J., & Matassarin-Jacobs, E. (1997). *Medical-surgical nursing: Clinical management for continuity of care* (5th ed.). Philadelphia: W. B. Saunders, pp. 1960–1961.

---

281. The family of a spinal cord–injured client asks if spinal shock will go away quickly. The nurse's response is based on the understanding that spinal shock

1 Is gone within 1 week.
2 Can last from 7 days to 3 months.
3 Typically resolves in 6 months.
4 May come and go for almost a year.

Answer: 2

Rationale: The client who suffers a spinal cord injury experiences spinal shock at the time of the injury. The client loses all motor, bowel, bladder, and sexual function and loses all reflexes below the level of the injury. Spinal shock resolves in 7 days to 3 months. Indications of resolving spinal shock include hyperreflexia and positive Babinski's reflex.

Test-Taking Strategy: When spinal shock develops, it remains until it starts to resolve. Knowing that it cannot "come and go" helps to eliminate option 4. The time frame for option 1 is absurdly short and should also be eliminated. To differentiate between the last two options, you must know that it usually resolves within 3 months.

Level of Cognitive Ability: Analysis
Phase of Nursing Process: Analysis
Client Needs: Physiological Integrity
Content Area: Adult Health/Neurological

Reference

Black, J., & Matassarin-Jacobs, E. (1997). *Medical-surgical nursing: Clinical management for continuity of care* (5th ed.). Philadelphia: W. B. Saunders, p. 895.

---

282. The client with thrombotic cerebrovascular accident experiences periods of emotional lability. The family asks the nurse why the client alternately laughs and cries and is irritable and demanding. The nurse formulates a response based on the understanding that

1 The client is not adapting well to the disability.
2 The client is experiencing side effects of prescribed anticoagulants.
3 The problem is likely to get worse before it gets better.
4 This is an expected, although troublesome, finding after cerebrovascular accident.

Answer: 4

Rationale: The emotional aspects of care for the client with cerebrovascular accident can be difficult for the family. The client often experiences periods of emotional lability, which are characterized by sudden bouts of laughing or crying or by irritability, depression, confusion, or being demanding.

Test-Taking Strategy: Eliminate option 3 first as being the most unlikely. Anticoagulants do not cause emotional lability, so this option can be eliminated as well. Option 1 is plausible, but you would pick option 4 as the correct answer by knowing the emotional changes that accompany cerebrovascular accident.

Level of Cognitive Ability: Analysis
Phase of Nursing Process: Analysis
Client Needs: Psychosocial Integrity
Content Area: Adult Health/Neurological

Reference

Smeltzer, S., & Bare, B. (1996). *Brunner and Suddarth's Textbook of medical-surgical nursing* (8th ed.). Philadelphia: Lippincott-Raven, p. 1734.

283. The client with myasthenia gravis begins to experience abdominal cramps, diarrhea, and excessive pulmonary secretions. The client also has sweating, blurred vision, and excessive production of saliva and tears. The nurse interprets that the client is experiencing

1 Cholinergic crisis.
2 Myasthenic crisis.
3 Concurrent infection.
4 Reaction to plasmapheresis.

Answer: 1

Rationale: Signs and symptoms of cholinergic crisis include general weakness and difficulty chewing, swallowing, speaking, and breathing. Nausea and vomiting, abdominal cramping, diarrhea, and increased production of body secretions also occurs. It is due to overmedication and is treated by withholding all medications and supporting the client's respiratory function until symptoms improve.

Test-Taking Strategy: If you can remember that anticholinergic medications slow the gastrointestinal tract and decrease production of body secretions, you may be able to deduce that the client in this question is experiencing cholinergic crisis. The client's symptoms are the opposite of the effects that anticholinergic medications would have. This may be the most helpful way to remember this information.

Level of Cognitive Ability: Analysis
Phase of Nursing Process: Analysis
Client Needs: Physiological Integrity
Content Area: Adult Health/Neurological

Reference

Black, J., & Matassarin-Jacobs, E. (1997). *Medical-surgical nursing: Clinical management for continuity of care* (5th ed.). Philadelphia: W. B. Saunders, p. 886.

---

284. The nurse notes ventricular fibrillation on the client's cardiac monitor. The nurse hurries to the client's room, expecting the client to be

1 Dizzy and nauseated.
2 Complaining of severe palpitations.
3 Hypotensive and pale.
4 Pulseless and unresponsive.

Answer: 4

Rationale: With onset of ventricular fibrillation, the client loses consciousness and becomes pulseless and apneic. There are no heart sounds or blood pressure. Death occurs if not treated.

Test-Taking Strategy: To answer this question correctly, you need to know that with ventricular fibrillation there is no organized contraction of the ventricles and thus no cardiac output. This knowledge helps you select the correct response. If you had difficulty with this question, take time now to review the clinical manifestations and the interventions for ventricular fibrillation.

Level of Cognitive Ability: Analysis
Phase of Nursing Process: Analysis
Client Needs: Physiological Integrity
Content Area: Adult Health/Cardiovascular

Reference

Ignatavicius, D. D., Workman, M. L., & Mishler, M. A. (1995). *Medical-surgical nursing: A nursing process approach* (2nd ed.). Philadelphia: W. B. Saunders, p. 852.

---

285. The nurse is reviewing a rhythm strip obtained from the cardiac monitor. The strip shows ectopic beats that are premature, have no P wave, and have QRS complexes that are wide and bizarre. There is a compensatory pause. The nurse interprets these ectopic beats to be

1 Premature atrial contractions.
2 Premature ventricular contractions.
3 Atrial fibrillation.
4 Ventricular fibrillation.

Answer: 2

Rationale: Premature ventricular contractions are generally easily recognizable on the ECG. They occur early in relation to the timing of previous normal beats, have no visible P wave, and have a characteristically wide and bizarre QRS complex. There is a compensatory pause.

Test-Taking Strategy: Because there is no P wave, the activity cannot be atrial in origin, so eliminate options 1 and 3 first. The terms "contraction" and "fibrillation" may help you to choose option 2 over 4 because there is a QRS complex. Know the baseline descriptions of key ventricular dysrhythmias to answer questions such as these.

Level of Cognitive Ability: Analysis
Phase of Nursing Process: Analysis
Client Needs: Physiological Integrity
Content Area: Adult Health/Cardiovascular

Reference

Black, J., & Matassarin-Jacobs, E. (1997). *Medical-surgical nursing: Clinical management for continuity of care* (5th ed.). Philadelphia: W. B. Saunders, p. 1305.

---

286. The nurse is caring for an infant diagnosed with hydrocephalus. Which manifestation would the nurse interpret as the earliest finding of increased intracranial pressure?

1 Irritability
2 Sunset sign
3 Separated cranial sutures
4 Tachycardia

Answer: 1

Rationale: The earliest finding associated with increased intracranial pressure would be irritability. Options 2, 3, and 4 are findings of increased intracranial pressure and are likely to progress slowly over a longer time period. Additional findings include poor feeding or vomiting, lethargy, a bulging fontanel, a high-pitched cry, increased head circumference, distended scalp veins, and an increased or decreased response to pain.

Test-Taking Strategy: Note that the question asks for the "earliest" clinical manifestation. Early manifestations include changes in mentation. This should assist in directing you to option 1, the correct option. If you had difficulty with this question, take time now to review the clinical manifestations associated with intracranial pressure.

Level of Cognitive Ability: Analysis
Phase of Nursing Process: Analysis
Client Needs: Physiological Integrity
Content Area: Child Health

Reference

Ashwill, J., & Droske, S. (1997). *Nursing care of children: Principles and practice.* Philadelphia: W. B. Saunders, p. 1231.

---

287. The nurse is caring for a child hospitalized with laryngotracheal bronchitis. Which of the following, if assessed, most clearly indicates respiratory distress?

1 Brassy respirations
2 Agitation
3 Nasal flaring
4 Dehydration

Answer: 3

Rationale: Signs of respiratory distress include the use of accessory muscles; substernal, intercostal, and suprasternal retractions; nasal flaring; and restlessness. Option 1 describes an early and classic manifestation of laryngotracheal bronchitis. Option 2 may be an indication of increasing respiratory distress but can also indicate several other clinical problems. Option 4 is not a sign of respiratory distress.

Test-Taking Strategy: Use the process of elimination in answering the question. Note the key phrase "most clearly" in the question. This should assist in directing you to the correct option. If you had difficulty with this question, take time now to review the signs of respiratory distress in a child.

Level of Cognitive Ability: Analysis
Phase of Nursing Process: Analysis
Client Needs: Physiological Integrity
Content Area: Child Health

Reference

Ashwill, J., & Droske, S. (1997). *Nursing care of children: Principles and practice.* Philadelphia: W. B. Saunders, p. 834.

288. The nurse is assessing a pregnant woman to determine whether labor has begun. Which of the following would indicate signs of true labor?

1 Contractions are irregular in rhythm and duration.
2 Uterus is soft with indentable contractions.
3 Cervical changes are not apparent.
4 Contractions are most intense in the upper uterine segment or fundus.

Answer: 4

Rationale: Discomfort and pain associated with true labor contractions typically begins in the lower abdomen and back then radiates over the entire abdomen. Options 1, 2, and 3 all describe findings associated with uterine contractions of false labor.

Test-Taking Strategy: Note that the question asks for the signs associated with true labor. Eliminate option 3 first because cervical changes are expected in true labor. Option 1 is incorrect because in true labor, contractions are regular. Eliminate option 4 because a firm uterus is present when contractions occur. If you had difficulty with this question, take time now to review the characteristics of true and false labor.

Level of Cognitive Ability: Analysis
Phase of Nursing Process: Analysis
Client Needs: Physiological Integrity
Content Area: Maternity

Reference

Nichols, F., & Zwelling, E. (1997). *Maternal-newborn nursing: Theory and practice.* Philadelphia: W. B. Saunders, p. 737.

289. An athlete comes to the ambulatory care center for treatment of a sports injury. Vital signs are pulse, 53 beats/minute; respiratory rate, 20 breaths/minute; and blood pressure, 110/64 mmHg. The nurse interprets these vital signs as

1 Normal, as a result of the abstinence from caffeine by the athlete.
2 Normal, as a result of the cardiovascular response to physical conditioning.
3 Abnormal, as a result of stimulation of the vagus nerve with injury.
4 Abnormal, as a result of the body's response to physical injury.

Answer: 2

Rationale: Athletes often have sinus bradycardia because exercise increases the stroke volume of the heart. Because the cardiac output is a product of stroke volume and heart rate, fewer beats are needed per minute at rest to maintain the normal cardiac output.

Test-Taking Strategy: Injury to the body triggers a sympathetic nervous system response, which includes tachycardia, so eliminate options 3 and 4 first. The question mentions nothing about caffeine intake, so eliminate that option, leaving option 2 as the remaining viable alternative.

Level of Cognitive Ability: Analysis
Phase of Nursing Process: Analysis
Client Needs: Physiological Integrity
Content Area: Adult Health/Cardiovascular

Reference

Black, J., & Matassarin-Jacobs, E. (1997). *Medical-surgical nursing: Clinical management for continuity of care* (5th ed.). Philadelphia: W. B. Saunders, p. 1299.

290. The female client who has been receiving radiation therapy for bladder cancer tells the nurse that it feels as if she is voiding through the vagina. The nurse interprets that the client may be experiencing

1 Extreme stress as a result of the diagnosis of cancer.
2 Altered perineal sensation as a side effect of radiation therapy.
3 The development of a vesicovaginal fistula.
4 Rupture of the bladder.

Answer: 3

Rationale: A complication of radiation therapy for bladder cancer is fistula formation. In women, this is frequently manifested as a vesicovaginal fistula, which is an opening between the bladder and the vagina. With this complication, the client senses that urine is flowing out of the vagina. In men, a colovesical fistula may develop, which is an opening between the bladder and the colon. This is manifested as voiding urine that contains fecal material.

Test-Taking Strategy: Eliminate options 1 and 4 first as the least plausible of all the options. Specific knowledge of the usual effects of radiation therapy directs you to choose option 3 over option 2 as the correct answer. Additionally, note the similarity of the phrase "voiding through the vagina" in the question and "vesicovaginal fistula" in the correct option. If you had difficulty with this question, take time now to review the complications associated with radiation and bladder cancer.

Level of Cognitive Ability: Analysis
Phase of Nursing Process: Analysis
Client Needs: Physiological Integrity
Content Area: Adult Health/Oncology

Reference

Black, J., & Matassarin-Jacobs, E. (1997). *Medical-surgical nursing: Clinical management for continuity of care* (5th ed.). Philadelphia: W. B. Saunders, p. 1584.

---

291. A client who has been diagnosed with chronic renal failure has been told that hemodialysis is required. The client becomes angry and withdrawn and states, "I'll never be the same now." The nurse formulates which of the following nursing diagnoses for this client?

1 Altered Thought Processes
2 Body Image Disturbance
3 Anxiety
4 Noncompliance

Answer: 2

Rationale: The client with any renal disorder, such as renal failure, may become angry and depressed because of the permanence of the alteration. Because of the physical change and the change in lifestyle that may be required to manage a severe renal condition, the client may experience Body Image Disturbance.

Test-Taking Strategy: Use the process of elimination in answering the question. Options 1 and 4 are eliminated first because the client is not cognitively impaired (option 1) or stating refusal to undergo therapy (option 4). To discriminate between the last two, note that the client's statement focuses on self, which is consistent with Body Image Disturbance. Therefore, select option 2 rather than option 3 (Anxiety) because the client is able to identify the cause of concern.

Level of Cognitive Ability: Analysis
Phase of Nursing Process: Analysis
Client Needs: Psychosocial Integrity
Content Area: Adult Health/Renal

Reference

Black, J., & Matassarin-Jacobs, E. (1997). *Medical-surgical nursing: Clinical management for continuity of care* (5th ed.). Philadelphia: W. B. Saunders, p. 1552.

---

292. A client with angina pectoris tells the nurse that chest pain usually occurs after going up two flights of stairs. Recently the client had three more severe episodes of chest pain while watching television, while going down stairs, and after falling asleep. The nurse interprets that the client is now experiencing

1 Nocturnal angina.
2 Unstable angina.
3 Variant angina.
4 Intractable angina.

Answer: 2

Rationale: Unstable angina is triggered by an unpredictable amount of exertion or emotion and may occur at night. The attacks increase in number, duration, and severity over time. Variant angina is triggered by coronary artery spasm, and the attacks are of longer duration than classic angina, tend to occur early in the day, and tend to occur at rest. Intractable angina is chronic and incapacitating and is refractory to medical therapy. Nocturnal angina may be associated with dreaming that occurs with rapid-eye-movement sleep.

Test-Taking Strategy: Knowledge regarding the definitions of these forms of angina is needed to answer the question. If necessary, you can look at the adjectives before the word "angina" in each option to help guide you to the correct answer. If you had difficulty with this question, take time now to review the characteristics of the various types of angina.

Level of Cognitive Ability: Analysis
Phase of Nursing Process: Analysis
Client Needs: Physiological Integrity
Content Area: Adult Health/Cardiovascular

Reference

Black, J., & Matassarin-Jacobs, E. (1997). *Medical-surgical nursing: Clinical management for continuity of care* (5th ed.). Philadelphia: W. B. Saunders, p. 1254.

293. A client is brought to the emergency department with suspected spinal cord damage. The client has flaccid paralysis, the blood pressure is 70/50 mmHg, and the pulse is 62 beats/minute. What do these findings indicate?

1. Autonomic dysreflexia
2. Spinal shock
3. Infection
4. Stable vital signs

Answer: 2

Rationale: Spinal shock occurs immediately after injury as a result of disruption of the communication pathways. These assessment findings indicate spinal shock. Hypertension is evidenced in autonomic dysreflexia. Infection could cause the above-mentioned findings; however, the question states that the client has a spinal cord trauma, which should immediately alert the nurse to consider spinal shock. These are not stable vital signs.

Test-Taking Strategy: Knowledge of spinal shock assists you to answer this question correctly. Options 3 and 4 can easily be eliminated. Spinal cord injury should prompt you to think of spinal shock and autonomic dysreflexia. From this point, your best selection is option 2, spinal shock, considering the blood pressure as noted in the question. If you had difficulty with this question, take time now to review the signs and symptoms of spinal shock and autonomic dysreflexia.

Level of Cognitive Ability: Analysis
Phase of Nursing Process: Analysis
Client Needs: Physiological Integrity
Content Area: Adult Health/Neurological

Reference

Hartshorn, J., Sole, M., & Lamborn, M. (1997). *Introduction to critical care nursing* (2nd ed.). Philadelphia: W. B. Saunders, p. 299.

---

294. The manic client announces to everyone in the dayroom that a stripper is coming to perform this evening. When the psychiatric orderly firmly states that this will not happen, the manic client becomes verbally abusive and threatens physical violence to the orderly. Based on the analysis of this situation, the nurse determines that the most appropriate action would be to

1. With assistance, escort the manic client to his room and administer as-needed haloperidol (Haldol).
2. Tell the client that smoking privileges are revoked for 24 hours.
3. Orient the client to time, person, and place.
4. Tell the client that the behavior is not appropriate.

Answer: 1

Rationale: The client is at risk for injury to self and others and therefore should be escorted out of the dayroom. Hyperactive and agitated behavior usually responds to haloperidol (Haldol). Antipsychotic medications are useful to manage the manic client as lithium takes 1–3 weeks to become effective. Option 2 may increase the agitation that already exists in this client. Orientation would not halt the behavior. Telling the client that the behavior is not appropriate has already been attempted by the orderly.

Test-Taking Strategy: Use Maslow's hierarchy of needs and the process of elimination to answer the question. Look for the response that promotes safety of the client, other clients, and staff. Knowledge of psychopharmacology is also helpful to answer this question correctly. If you had difficulty with this question, take time now to review the appropriate interventions in dealing with a manic client.

Level of Cognitive Ability: Application
Phase of Nursing Process: Analysis
Client Needs: Psychosocial Integrity
Content Area: Mental Health

Reference

Wilson, H. S., & Kneisl, C. R. (1996). *Psychiatric nursing* (5th ed.). Menlo Park, CA: Addison-Wesley, pp. 347, 349.

295. The client has a nursing diagnosis of Risk for Violence: Self-Directed. The physician has placed the client on basic suicide precautions. The nurse finds the client in the dayroom burning his arm with a lighted cigarette. After removing the cigarette and attending to the burn, the nurse determines that the next most appropriate action would be to

1. Call the psychiatrist and report the incident.
2. Put the client in a locked seclusion room.
3. Institute one-on-one nursing supervision.
4. Restrain the client.

Answer: 3

Rationale: When a client harms himself, immediate one-on-one nursing supervision is instituted. This meets the safety needs of the client. After doing this, the psychiatrist is notified of the incident. The client should not be restrained or placed in seclusion.

Test-Taking Strategy: Use Maslow's hierarchy of needs in thinking about how to answer this question. Note that the stem of the question asks for the nurse's "next" action. The nurse's action is based on meeting the physiological and safety needs of the client first. Option 3 is the option that would meet the safety need for this client.

Level of Cognitive Ability: Application
Phase of Nursing Process: Analysis
Client Needs: Physiological Integrity
Content Area: Mental Health

Reference

Wilson, H. S., & Kneisl, C. R. (1996). *Psychiatric nursing* (5th ed.). Menlo Park, CA: Addison-Wesley, p. 599.

---

296. The client diagnosed with pneumonia has a poor appetite because of dyspnea and becomes fatigued with minimal amounts of exertion. The nurse formulates which of the following nursing diagnoses for this client?

1. Impaired Physical Mobility
2. Ineffective Breathing Pattern
3. Activity Intolerance
4. Ineffective Airway Clearance

Answer: 3

Rationale: The client with pneumonia may have an Activity Intolerance related to insufficient available oxygen to meet metabolic needs. The client may also have insufficient energy reserves from omitting food intake during dyspneic periods. This diagnosis is often used in the client with pneumonia.

Test-Taking Strategy: Use the process of elimination to answer the question. The stem mentions nothing about clearance of respiratory secretions or the client's pattern of breathing, so options 2 and 4 may be eliminated first. Read the information provided in the question to select between the remaining options. Of the two remaining, you would choose Activity Intolerance over Impaired Physical Mobility because the effort of movement and eating is causing the client's respiratory symptoms.

Level of Cognitive Ability: Analysis
Phase of Nursing Process: Analysis
Client Needs: Physiological Integrity
Content Area: Adult Health/Respiratory

Reference

Black, J., & Matassarin-Jacobs, E. (1997). *Medical-surgical nursing: Clinical management for continuity of care* (5th ed.). Philadelphia: W. B. Saunders, p. 1137.

---

297. The nurse is preparing to institute intravenous heparin therapy for a client. The nurse questions the physician's order because of which of the following active problems listed on the client's medical record?

1. Deep vein thrombosis
2. Degenerative arthritis
3. Cerebral aneurysm
4. Chronic obstructive lung disease

Answer: 3

Rationale: Heparin therapy is contraindicated with preexisting health conditions such as threatened abortion, active hemorrhage, cerebrovascular hemorrhage, cerebral or aortic aneurysm, severe hypertension, hemophilia, thrombocytopenia, pericarditis, and recent or upcoming ophthalmic surgery or neurosurgery. Caution should be used if risk of hemorrhage is present, such as recent childbirth; severe diabetes; vasculitis; trauma; significant renal impairment; and active lesions of the respiratory, gastrointestinal, or genitourinary tracts.

Test-Taking Strategy: When answering questions of this nature, look for options in which a risk of bleeding is present. This helps you narrow the choices fairly quickly. In this instance, eliminate option 1 first (because it is a reason to institute heparin therapy). There is no associated risk of bleeding with options 2 and 4, which leads you to the correct choice, which is cerebral aneurysm.

Level of Cognitive Ability: Application
Phase of Nursing Process: Analysis
Client Needs: Physiological Integrity
Content Area: Pharmacology

Reference

Hodgson, B., & Kizior, R. (1998). *Saunders nursing drug handbook 1998.* Philadelphia: W. B. Saunders, pp. 489–491.

---

298. The client with an abdominal aortic aneurysm complains of lightheadedness, nausea, and abdominal and flank pain. The client's pulse rate has climbed from 78 to 116 beats/minute. Blood pressure has dropped from 136/88 to 98/68 mmHg. The nurse interprets these signs and symptoms as consistent with

1 Acute glomerulonephritis.
2 Vasovagal reaction.
3 Rupture of the abdominal aortic aneurysm.
4 Lower gastrointestinal bleed.

Answer: 3

Rationale: The client with ruptured abdominal aortic aneurysm typically presents with a pulsating abdominal mass; intense abdominal pain accompanied by flank, back, or scrotal pain; and signs and symptoms of shock.

Test-Taking Strategy: The client is exhibiting signs of shock, which eliminates options 1 and 2 immediately. Of the two remaining options, the client's history and pattern of pain point to rupture of the aneurysm. There is no other information in the stem that would guide you to suspect a gastrointestinal bleed. If you had difficulty with this question, take time now to review signs and symptoms of a ruptured abdominal aortic aneurysm.

Level of Cognitive Ability: Analysis
Phase of Nursing Process: Analysis
Client Needs: Physiological Integrity
Content Area: Adult Health/Cardiovascular

Reference

Black, J., & Matassarin-Jacobs, E. (1997). *Medical-surgical nursing: Clinical management for continuity of care* (5th ed.). Philadelphia: W. B. Saunders, p. 1426.

---

299. The male client being treated for urethritis from chlamydial infection asks the nurse how long it will be necessary to refrain from sexual relations. The nurse's response is based on the knowledge that the client

1 May immediately resume sexual relations as long as there is no discomfort.
2 Should refrain from sexual activity until fully cured.
3 Can resume sexual relations immediately as long as a condom is used.
4 Should refrain from sexual activity for 24 hours after initiation of antibiotic therapy.

Answer: 2

Rationale: The client with urethritis from chlamydial infection should not engage in any form of sexual activity (intercourse as well as oral-genital or oral-anal contact) until the client is fully cured. At that point, the client should also use condoms to prevent reinfection.

Test-Taking Strategy: Use the process of elimination in answering the question. Using the basic principles of infection control, eliminate options 1 and 4. To discriminate between the last two options, recall that condoms can break or tear. This would guide you to choose option 2 over option 3. If you had difficulty with this question, take time now to review client teaching related to chlamydial infection.

Level of Cognitive Ability: Analysis
Phase of Nursing Process: Analysis
Client Needs: Physiological Integrity
Content Area: Adult Health/Renal

Reference

Black, J., & Matassarin-Jacobs, E. (1997). *Medical-surgical nursing: Clinical management for continuity of care* (5th ed.). Philadelphia: W. B. Saunders, p. 2470.

300. The client has a chest tube that is attached to a Pleur-Evac closed-chest drainage system. The client asks the nurse "Can the tube come out faster if you turn the wall suction up higher?" The nurse's response is based on the understanding that turning up the wall suction

1. Would not increase the actual suction in the system but would cause more air to be pulled through the air vent and suction chamber to the suction source.
2. Would not increase the actual suction in the system but could cause the client to suffer injury.
3. Would increase the actual suction in the system but could damage lung tissue.
4. Would increase the actual suction in the system and is a good idea.

Answer: 1

Rationale: The amount of suction in the Pleur-Evac drainage system is controlled by the amount of sterile water that is poured into the suction control chamber. Increasing the wall suction will only cause vigorous bubbling in the suction chamber, as more air is pulled through the air vent and suction control chamber to the suction source. The only effect this would have is to increase the rate of water evaporation from the suction control chamber, so sterile water would have to be added to the system more frequently.

Test-Taking Strategy: Basic knowledge of the functioning of the chambers of a closed-chest drainage system is needed to answer this question. Knowing that it is the water level in the chamber that regulates the amount of suction (not the level of the wall suction control) helps you to eliminate options 3 and 4. To discriminate between options 1 and 2, recall that the only effect of added wall suction is the evaporation of the water at a faster rate, which would cause you to choose option 1 over option 2. If you had difficulty with this question, take time now to review chest tube drainage systems.

Level of Cognitive Ability: Analysis
Phase of Nursing Process: Analysis
Client Needs: Physiological Integrity
Content Area: Adult Health/Respiratory

Reference

Black, J., & Matassarin-Jacobs, E. (1997). *Medical-surgical nursing: Clinical management for continuity of care* (5th ed.). Philadelphia: W. B. Saunders, p. 1164.

REFERENCES

Ashwill, J., & Droske, S. (1997). *Nursing care of children: Principles and practice.* Philadelphia: W. B. Saunders.

Antai-Otong, D., & Kongale, G. (1995). *Psychiatric nursing: Biological and behavioral concepts.* Philadelphia: W. B. Saunders.

Black, J., & Matassarin-Jacobs, E. (1997). *Medical-surgical nursing: Clinical management for continuity of care* (5th ed.). Philadelphia: W. B. Saunders.

Bolander, V. (1994). *Sorenson and Luckmann's Basic nursing: A psychophysiologic approach* (3rd ed.). Philadelphia: W. B. Saunders.

Brent, N. (1997). *Nurses and the law.* Philadelphia: W. B. Saunders.

Burrell, L. O., Gerlach, M. J., & Pless, B. (1997). *Adult nursing: Acute and community care* (2nd ed.). Stamford, CT: Appleton & Lange.

Carson, V., & Arnold, E. (1996). *Mental health nursing: The nurse-patient journey.* Philadelphia: W. B. Saunders.

Clemen-Stone, S., Eigsti, D. G., & McGuire, S. (1995). *Comprehensive community health nursing: Family, aggregate and community practice* (4th ed.). St. Louis: Mosby–Year Book.

Como, N. (1995). *Home health nursing pocket consultant.* St. Louis: Mosby–Year Book.

Cox, H., Hinz, M., Lubno, M., et al. (1997). *Clinical applications of nursing diagnosis* (3rd ed.). Philadelphia: F. A. Davis.

Craven, R. F., & Hirnle, C. J. (1996). *Fundamentals of nursing: Human health and function* (2nd ed.). Philadelphia: Lippincott-Raven.

Deglin, J., & Vallerand, A. (1997). *Davis's drug guide for nurses* (5th ed.). Philadelphia: F. A. Davis.

Elkin, M., Perry, A., & Potter, P. (1996). *Nursing interventions and clinical skills.* St. Louis: Mosby–Year Book.

Fishback, F. (1996). *A manual of laboratory and diagnostic tests* (5th ed.). Philadelphia: W. B. Saunders.

Gorrie, T. M., McKinney, E. S., & Murray, S. S. (1994). *Foundations of maternal newborn nursing.* Philadelphia: W. B. Saunders.

Haber, J. (1997). *Comprehensive psychiatric nursing* (5th ed.). St. Louis: Mosby–Year Book.

Hartshorn, J., Sole, M., & Lamborn, M. (1997). *Introduction to critical care nursing* (2nd ed.). Philadelphia: W. B. Saunders.

Hodgson, B., & Kizior, R. (1998). *Saunders nursing drug handbook 1998.* Philadelphia: W. B. Saunders.

Huff, J. (1997). *ECG workout: Exercises in arrhythmia interpretation* (3rd ed.). Philadelphia: Lippincott-Raven.

Ignatavicius, D. D., Workman, M. L., & Mishler, M. A. (1995). *Medical-surgical nursing: A nursing process approach* (2nd ed.). Philadelphia: W. B. Saunders.

Iyer, P., Taptich, B., & Bernocchi-Losey, D. (1995). *Nursing process and nursing diagnosis.* Philadelphia: W. B. Saunders.

Jarvis, C. (1996). *Physical examination and health assessment* (2nd ed.). Philadelphia: W. B. Saunders.

Johnson, B. (1997). *Psychiatric–mental health nursing: Adaptation and growth* (4th ed.). Philadelphia: Lippincott-Raven.

Lammon, C. B., Foote, A. W., Leli, P. G., et al. (1995). *Clinical nursing skills.* Philadelphia: W. B. Saunders.

Lehne, R. A. (1998). *Pharmacology for nursing care* (3rd ed.). Philadelphia: W. B. Saunders.

LeMone, P., & Burke, K. M. (1996). *Medical-surgical nursing: Critical thinking in client care.* Menlo Park, CA: Addison-Wesley.

Lewis, S., Collier, I., & Heitkemper, M. (1996). *Medical-surgical nursing: Assessment and management of clinical problems* (4th ed.). St. Louis: Mosby–Year Book.

Lowdermilk, D., Perry, S., & Bobak, I. (1997). *Maternity and women's health care* (6th ed.). St. Louis: Mosby–Year Book.

Luckmann, J. (1997). *Saunders manual of nursing care.* Philadelphia: W. B. Saunders.

McFarland, G., & McFarlane, E. (1997). *Nursing diagnosis and intervention: Planning for patient care.* St. Louis: Mosby–Year Book.

McKenry, L., & Salerno, E. (1995). *Mosby's pharmacology in nursing* (19th ed.). St. Louis: Mosby–Year Book.

National Council of State Boards of Nursing (1997). *Test plan for the National Council Licensure Examination for Registered Nurses.* Chicago: Author.

Nichols, F., & Zwelling, E. (1997). *Maternal-newborn nursing: Theory and practice.* Philadelphia: W. B. Saunders.

O'Toole, M. (1997). *Miller-Keane Encyclopedia & dictionary of medicine, nursing, & allied health* (6th ed.). Philadelphia: W. B. Saunders.

Phillips, L. D. (1997). *Manual of IV therapeutics* (2nd ed.). Philadelphia: F. A. Davis.

Phipps, W., Cassmeyer, V., Sands, J., et al. (1995). *Medical-surgical nursing: Concepts and clinical practice* (5th ed.). St. Louis: Mosby–Year Book.

Pillitteri, A. (1995). *Maternal and child health: Nursing care of the childbearing and childrearing family* (2nd ed.). Philadelphia: Lippincott-Raven.

Polaski, A., & Tatro, S. (1996). *Luckmann's Core principles and practice of medical-surgical nursing.* Philadelphia: W. B. Saunders.

Potter, P., & Perry, A. (1997). *Fundamentals of nursing: Concepts, process and practice* (4th ed.). St. Louis: Mosby–Year Book.

Reeder, S., Martin, L., & Koniak-Griffin, D. (1997). *Maternity nursing: Family, newborn, and women's health care* (18th ed.). Philadelphia: Lippincott-Raven.

Rice, R. (1996). *Home health nursing practice: Concepts and application* (2nd ed.). St. Louis: Mosby–Year Book.

Smeltzer, S., & Bare, B. (1996). *Brunner and Suddarth's Textbook of medical-surgical nursing* (8th ed.). Philadelphia: Lippincott-Raven.

Smith, S., & Duvell, D. (1996). *Clinical nursing skills* (4th ed.). Stamford, CT: Appleton & Lange.

Stuart, G., & Sundeen, S. (1995). *Principles and practice of psychiatric nursing* (5th ed.). St. Louis: Mosby–Year Book.

Taylor, C., Lillis, C., & LeMone, P. (1997). *Fundamentals of nursing: The art and science of nursing care* (3rd ed.). Philadelphia: Lippincott-Raven.

Thompson, J., McFarland, G., Hirsch, J., & Tucker, S. (1997). *Mosby's clinical nursing* (4th ed.). St. Louis: Mosby–Year Book.

Varcarolis, E. M. (1998). *Foundations of psychiatric mental health nursing* (3rd ed.). Philadelphia: W. B. Saunders.

Wilson, H. S., & Kneisl, C. R. (1996). *Psychiatric nursing* (5th ed.). Menlo Park, CA: Addison-Wesley.

Wong, D. (1995). *Whaley and Wong's Nursing care of infants and children* (5th ed.). St. Louis: Mosby–Year Book.

Wong, D. (1997). *Whaley and Wong's Essentials of pediatric nursing* (5th ed.). St. Louis: Mosby–Year Book.

Wong, D., & Perry, S. (1998). *Maternal-child nursing care.* St. Louis: Mosby–Year Book.

Wywialowski, E. F. (1997). *Managing client care* (2nd ed.). St. Louis: Mosby–Year Book.

CHAPTER 7

The Process of Planning

Planning is the third step of the nursing process. This step involves the functions of setting priorities, determining goals of care, planning actions, collaborating with other health team members, establishing evaluative criteria, and communicating the plan of care.

Setting priorities assists the nurse in organizing and planning care that solves the most urgent problems. Priorities may change as the client's level of wellness changes. Both actual and potential problems should be considered when priorities are established. Actual problems are usually more important than potential problems. However, potential problems may at times take precedence over actual problems.

Once priorities are established, the client and nurse mutually decide on the expected goals. The selected goals serve as a guide in the selection of nursing interventions and in determining the criteria for evaluation. Before nursing actions are implemented, mechanisms to determine goal achievement and the effectiveness of nursing interventions are established. Unless criteria have been predetermined, it is difficult to know whether the goal has been achieved and the problem is resolved.

It is important for the nurse both to identify health or social resources available to the client and to collaborate with other health care team members when planning the delivery of care. The nurse needs to communicate the plan of care, review the plan of care with the client, and document the plan of care thoroughly and accurately.

PRACTICE TEST

1. The nurse is caring for a 4-week-old infant who is scheduled for a pyloromyotomy. The nurse should include which of the following in the plan of care?

1 Position infant prone with the head of the bed elevated
2 Restrain infant in a high chair
3 Feed infant in a lying-down position
4 Feed infant one mashed banana

Answer: 1

Rationale: Preoperatively, the infant's status is NPO (nothing by mouth), and the infant is stabilized with intravenous fluids and electrolytes. The head of the bed is elevated and the infant is placed prone to reduce the risk of aspiration. Options 3 and 4 are not accurate during the preoperative period, because the infant is kept NPO. An infant would not be restrained in a high chair.

Test-Taking Strategy: Use the process of elimination to answer the question. Eliminate options 3 and 4 first. The infant would not be fed lying down and would not be fed mashed bananas at this age. Next, eliminate option 2 because you would not restrain an infant in a high chair. If you had difficulty with this question, take time now to review preoperative positioning for an infant scheduled for pyloromyotomy.

Level of Cognitive Ability: Application
Phase of Nursing Process: Planning
Client Needs: Safe, Effective Care Environment
Content Area: Child Health

Reference
Ashwill, J., & Droske, S. (1997). *Nursing care of children: Principles and practice.* Philadelphia: W. B. Saunders, p. 719.

2. When a client is at high risk for suicide, the nurse should include which of these measures in the client care plan?
   1 Day hall supervision
   2 Constant observation
   3 Checks every 15 minutes
   4 One-to-one supervision at night

Answer: 2

Rationale: Providing constant observation will provide the client a sense of security until he or she can regain control of the desire to commit suicide. The client who receives only day hall and one-to-one supervision at night will be alone during some time periods. With checks only every 15 minutes, the client also has time to attempt suicide when no staff is present.

Test-Taking Strategy: Use knowledge regarding care of a suicidal client and the process of elimination to answer the question. Options 1, 3, and 4 are similar in that there are time periods in which the client will be alone. Option 4 is different, and the only accurate choice for a high-risk client is to maintain constant supervision. If you had difficulty with this question, take time now to review nursing care for a client at risk for suicide!

Level of Cognitive Ability: Application
Phase of Nursing Process: Planning
Client Needs: Safe, Effective Care Environment
Content Area: Mental Health

Reference

Townsend, M. (1996). *Psychiatric–mental health nursing: Concepts of care* (2nd ed.). Philadelphia: F. A. Davis, p. 255.

3. A child with Hirschsprung's disease has surgery that results in the creation of a temporary colostomy. The nurse plans to monitor the nasogastric (NG) tube, which is attached to suction, because the primary purpose of the NG tube postoperatively is to
   1 Maintain adequate hydration and electrolyte balance.
   2 Initiate enteral feedings.
   3 Decompress the abdomen until intestinal motility returns.
   4 Minimize electrolyte losses through vomiting.

Answer: 3

Rationale: Early in the postoperative period, the client has a high risk for injury related to the absence of bowel motility. Nasogastric suctioning is initiated to decompress the abdomen in order to prevent abdominal distention and vomiting until bowel motility returns.

Test-Taking Strategy: Options 1 and 2 are incorrect because the nasogastric tube in this situation is for suctioning rather than enteral feedings. Option 4 is incorrect because electrolytes are lost as easily from suctioned stomach contents as from vomiting.

Level of Cognitive Ability: Application
Phase of Nursing Process: Planning
Client Needs: Physiological Integrity
Content Area: Child Health

Reference

Wong, D., & Perry, S. (1998). *Maternal-child nursing care.* St. Louis: Mosby–Year Book, pp. 1399–1401.

4. The nurse is meeting a client who will receive electroconvulsive therapy (ECT) on an out-patient basis in about 1 hour. The client's father has brought the client into the hospital for the first treatment. As the client is being prepared for the treatment, the nurse notices that the client is chewing something. The nurse explores what the client is eating. The client responds that another client has given out breath mints in the waiting room, saying "It was only a few small mints... can't hurt me. " The nurse would immediately plan to

   1 Notify the professional staff in the department to prevent anyone who had eaten mints from receiving a treatment.
   2 Return to the waiting area and request that the client relinquish the package of breath mints, reinforcing to the client that no one can eat anything before ECT.
   3 Place another staff member in the waiting room to monitor clients' activity, safety, and behavior within the environment.
   4 Inform the client that the client will not be receiving electroconvulsive therapy (ECT) and call the client's father to take the client home.

Answer: 1

Rationale: The nurse's priority action would be to inform the professional staff in the department to prevent anyone who had eaten mints from receiving a treatment. Next, the nurse would request that the mints be given to the nurse. It would be determined which other clients had already ingested mints. Then the nurse would place an attendant in the waiting room to monitor client safety and behavior in the environment. Last, the nurse would call the client's father, explain the situation, and have the father take the client home. All nursing actions would involve addressing safety and promoting safety in the environment.

Test-Taking Strategy: Use Maslow's hierarchy of needs theory to prioritize. Note the key word "immediately." This implies that more than one option may be partially or totally correct. You must prioritize which of the options must be completed first. The nurse is addressing safety needs to promote safe and effective treatments and procedures.

Level of Cognitive Ability: Application
Phase of Nursing Process: Planning
Client Needs: Safe, Effective Care Environment
Content Area: Mental Health

Reference

Johnson, B. (1997). *Psychiatric–mental health nursing: Adaptation and growth* (4th ed.). Philadelphia: Lippincott-Raven, p. 660.

5. The client is scheduled to have a lumbar puncture. The nurse plans to teach the client that the reason for the knee-chest positioning is that it

   1 Provides for greater client comfort.
   2 Prevents leakage of cerebrospinal fluid.
   3 Allows for a smaller puncture site to be made.
   4 Increases the spacing between the vertebrae.

Answer: 4

Rationale: The anatomy of the vertebral column is such that curving the structure provides for more open spacing in the area of L3 to L5. The choice of the size of the needle for puncture is not dependent on position. Also, client position is not related to leakage of cerebrospinal fluid. The size of the dural tear depends on the position of the needle in relation to the dural fibers. Pillows and support of the nursing staff aid in client comfort.

Test-Taking Strategy: Knowledge of the anatomy of the vertebral column is essential to answer this question. Try to visualize this client's position and the procedure to assist in selecting the correct option. If you had difficulty with this question, take time now to review the rationale for the position required for this procedure!

Level of Cognitive Ability: Application
Phase of Nursing Process: Planning
Client Needs: Safe, Effective Care Environment
Content Area: Adult Health/Neurological

Reference

Black, J., & Matassarin-Jacobs, E. (1997). *Medical-surgical nursing: Clinical management for continuity of care* (5th ed.). Philadelphia: W. B. Saunders, p. 734.

6. A client with a cerebral vascular accident (CVA) is admitted to the hospital. Which measure should the nurse include in the plan of care to prevent an increase in intracranial pressure (ICP)?

 1 Keep the head of bed in a slightly elevated, neutral position
 2 Maintain ventilation to keep the arterial carbon dioxide tension ($PaCO_2$) 35–40 mmHg
 3 Institute vigorous suction at least every 30 minutes
 4 Control temperature with a hypothermia blanket to the point that shivering begins

Answer: 1

Rationale: A number of factors can affect intracranial pressure. In option 2, the $PaCO_2$ leads to vasodilation of the cerebral blood vessels, raising the pressure. In option 3, the client should be suctioned to prevent hypoxia, which can lead to vasodilation; however, the suctioning should not be vigorous. The frequency of suctioning should be as needed (PRN), not on a fixed time schedule. In option 4, the body temperature should be controlled but not to the point of shivering, which raises metabolism and ICP. Keeping the head positioned as in option 1 promotes venous drainage from the head, which in turn helps control ICP.

Test-Taking Strategy: Read the stem carefully and note that the question asks for the plan to prevent increased ICP. Note the critical words in the options. In option 1, note the number of descriptors for the head position. Often a very specific answer may be the correct one. The frequency of suctioning (every 30 minutes) for a client in this condition is excessive. The word "vigorous" in this option is another clue that this option is incorrect. In option 4, "shivering" is a key word. If you had difficulty with this question, take time now to review the measures that will prevent ICP!

Level of Cognitive Ability: Application
Phase of Nursing Process: Planning
Client Needs: Safe, Effective Care Environment
Content Area: Adult Health/Neurological

References

Black, J., & Matassarin-Jacobs, E. (1997). *Medical-surgical nursing: Clinical management for continuity of care* (5th ed.). Philadelphia: W. B. Saunders, pp. 775, 782, 783.

Smeltzer, S., & Bare, B. (1996). *Brunner and Suddarth's Textbook of medical-surgical nursing* (8th ed.). Philadelphia: Lippincott-Raven, pp. 1710, 1712.

---

7. The client comes to the emergency room with complaints of severe abdominal pain. The client does not have any insurance. The nurse develops a plan of care for the client because legally the hospital must

 1 Refer the client to the nearest public hospital.
 2 Have a physician see the client before admission.
 3 Provide uncompensated care in emergency situations.
 4 Respect family's request to admit the family member.

Answer: 3

Rationale: Federal law and many state laws require that hospitals must provide emergency care. Only after the client has been medically screened and stabilized can the client be transferred. The client must give consent for the transfer, and there must be a facility that will accept the client. Options 1, 2, and 4 do not fully address the legal requirements for emergency care and are therefore incorrect.

Test-Taking Strategy: Note the key phrase "does not have insurance" and the word "legally" found in the stem. This should provide you with the clue regarding the issue of the question. Option 3 is the option that addresses the legal scope of providing emergency care.

Level of Cognitive Ability: Application
Phase of Nursing Process: Planning
Client Needs: Safe, Effective Care Environment
Content Area: Fundamental Skills

Reference

Brent, N. (1997). *Nurses and the law.* Philadelphia: W. B. Saunders, pp. 406–407.

8. The nurse is collaborating with other health professionals to plan a community program that addresses end-of-life issues. An important document to include and discuss in the program is a "living will," which

1 Delegates the legal authority to act on the client's behalf in the event the client is incapacitated.
2 Is a "do not resuscitate" order in the event the client is on a respirator and there is no hope of recovery.
3 Sets out which life-sustaining treatments will be accepted if there is no hope of recovery.
4 Describes the types of organ donation that the client and family will accept in case of accidental death.

Answer: 3

Rationale: The nurse needs to be familiar with the current laws and processes regarding end-of-life decisions. A "living will" is designed to identify the life-sustaining treatments that are acceptable and under what conditions. There are several specific documents and processes that the nurse must be familiar with in order to meet legal requirements as well as individualized client needs and decisions.

Test-Taking Strategy: It is important to know the current laws and processes to work effectively with clients who need to address end-of-life issues. Option 3 is the broadest and the most global answer. Options 1, 2, and 4 are more specific. If you had difficulty with this question, take time now to review the components of a "living will"!

Level of Cognitive Ability: Application
Phase of Nursing Process: Planning
Client Needs: Health Promotion and Maintenance
Content Area: Fundamental Skills

Reference

Bandman, E., & Bandman, B. (1995). *Nursing ethics through the life span.* Stamford, CT: Appleton & Lange, pp. 284–285.

---

9. After identifying an umbilical cord prolapse during a vaginal examination of a client in active late first-stage labor, the nurse initiates an emergency plan of care by applying upward pressure with a gloved hand on the presenting part and calling for assistance. The nurse would plan to do which of the following as the next step of the emergency nursing care plan?

1 Adjusting the labor bed to the Trendelenburg position
2 Encouraging the woman to push with each contraction
3 Setting up for an emergency cesarean section
4 Calmly reassuring the woman and her partner that all possible measures are being taken

Answer: 1

Rationale: Adjusting the labor bed into Trendelenburg (mattress flat, foot of bed elevated) position uses gravity to reverse the direction of the pressure, keeping the presenting part off the umbilical cord. In addition to pushing the fetal head away from the cervix and bony pelvis, positioning of the woman into the Trendelenburg, knee-chest, or modified Sims' position is the most urgent action the nurse can take. Pushing with the contractions is contraindicated because it will push the presenting part against the cord. Not all prolapsed cords lead to a cesarean section.

Test-Taking Strategy: Read the case situation carefully, noting key words that identify priority actions. In this case the key word is "next." Remember that this is a nursing examination and focus on nursing rather than medical actions. Use Maslow's hierarchy of needs theory to guide you in determining levels of priority. On the basis of the pathophysiology of this situation, option 2 would worsen the situation by causing greater pressure on the cord. Option 4 does not address a physiological need. Select the option that addresses the physiological safety of the primary client (the fetus).

Level of Cognitive Ability: Application
Phase of Nursing Process: Planning
Client Needs: Safe, Effective Care Environment
Content Area: Maternity

Reference

Lowdermilk, D., Perry, M., & Bobak, I. (1997). *Maternity & women's health care* (6th ed.). St. Louis: Mosby–Year Book, p. 975.

10. The nursing educator of a series of birthing classes is preparing a request for the equipment and space needs of the classroom. Which of the following, if listed on the request, will enable clients to avoid supine hypotension (vena cava syndrome)?

1. An 8 × 4 foot floor space for each client
2. A mat, three or four pillows, and a covered foam wedge
3. A series of posters demonstrating common minor disorders of pregnancy
4. A tape player and several compact disks with soft, relaxing music

Answer: 2

Rationale: Supine hypotension (vena cava, or hypotensive, syndrome) is brought about by pressure of the gravid uterus on the blood vessels of the abdomen. Birthing clients usually recline on a mat to practice exercises that will be used in labor. The covered foam wedge and pillows can be used to support the pregnant woman in a nonsupine position, such as a modified Sims' or semi-Fowler's, which will put less pressure on the inferior vena cava and iliac vessels and reduce the potential for supine hypotension.

Test-Taking Strategy: Remember the physiological process underlying the problem identified in the case situation. In a client safety question, consider which adaptation of the environment will prevent the pathophysiological response that initiated the problem. Reread the stem to confirm what is being asked. Do not be misled by mention of other events or items that might be used for other purposes in the same situation. Focus on the issue of the question. If you had difficulty with this question, take time now to review the precipitators of vena cava syndrome!

Level of Cognitive Ability: Application
Phase of Nursing Process: Planning
Client Needs: Safe, Effective Care Environment
Content Area: Maternity

Reference

Reeder, S., Martin, L., & Koniak-Griffin, D. (1997). *Maternity nursing: Family, newborn and women's health care* (18th ed.). Philadelphia: Lippincott-Raven, p. 374.

---

11. The physician orders a nasogastric tube to low suction for a client admitted with uncontrolled vomiting. In preparing for the procedure, the nurse plans to

1. Wear sterile gloves and follow aseptic technique during the procedure.
2. Determine the length to insert the tube by measuring from ear to nose and then nose to navel.
3. Explain to the client that he or she will be asked to swallow water during the insertion procedure.
4. Position the client with the head of the bed elevated to 30 degrees.

Answer: 3

Rationale: When the nurse inserts a nasogastric tube in a client, the approved procedure must be followed. Determining the correct length to insert the tube, placing the client in a high Fowler's position, and gaining client cooperation in passing the tube are essential to the insertion process. Using sterile and aseptic technique is not indicated because the gastrointestinal tract is not sterile. The correct length of the tube is determined by measuring from the tip of the client's nose to the earlobe and then from the nose to the xiphoid process, not the navel. The client is asked to swallow water so that the tube will enter the esophagus and not the trachea.

Test-Taking Strategy: Identify the critical elements in the stem of the question, including the key phrase: most reliable. Read all four options, and reread the stem. Option 1 is unnecessary; 2 and 4 are incorrect and could result in harm to the client. Option 3 is the only correct choice.

Level of Cognitive Ability: Application
Phase of Nursing Process: Planning
Client Needs: Safe, Effective Care Environment
Content Area: Adult Health/Gastrointestinal

Reference

Lammon, C. B., Foote, A. W., Leli, P. G., et al. (1995). *Clinical nursing skills.* Philadelphia: W. B. Saunders, pp. 418–422.

12. A nurse caring for a client with a Sengstaken-Blakemore tube in place should have which of the following items in close proximity in case of an emergency?

   1 Intravenous dose of magnesium sulfate
   2 The obturator
   3 Scissors
   4 A 60-mL syringe

Answer: 3

Rationale: A Sengstaken-Blakemore tube is inserted in cirrhosis clients with ruptured esophageal varices. It has esophageal and gastric balloons. It is important to ensure that the gastric balloon is inflated to prevent migration of the tube. If the gastric balloon deflates with the esophageal balloon inflated, complete or partial airway obstruction could develop. A pair of scissors should be available to deflate the balloons and allow for tube removal in such an emergency situation.

Test-Taking Strategy: The issue of this question is specific content: equipment for emergency use at the bedside of a client with a Sengstaken-Blakemore tube in place. Read all four options. Option 3 identifies the equipment. All other options are incorrect. Take the time now to review the nursing care related to this type of tube if you are unfamiliar with it!

Level of Cognitive Ability: Application
Phase of Nursing Process: Planning
Client Needs: Safe, Effective Care Environment
Content Area: Adult Health/Gastrointestinal

Reference

Black, J., & Matassarin-Jacobs, E. (1997). *Medical-surgical nursing: Clinical management for continuity of care* (5th ed.). Philadelphia: W. B. Saunders, p. 1885.

---

13. The client is recovering at home from a cerebrovascular accident (CVA) that has left the client with severe right-sided hemiplegia. In conducting a home environmental assessment and developing the plan of care, the home health care nurse would

   1 Evaluate the use of assistive devices for ambulation and transferring activities.
   2 Assess the client's performance of the activities of daily living.
   3 Evaluate the home for electrical and mechanical safety.
   4 Assess environmental needs for safe functioning in the home.

Answer: 4

Rationale: Environmental assessment is analogous to assessment of the home. This is necessary to ensure safety for clients in the home. This assessment is especially important for clients who have compromised health, as does this client with a CVA. The use of assistive devices in the home is related to home assessment in an indirect way and not related to planning for care. Electrical and mechanical safety are part of the home assessment inventory. The client's activities of daily living, although important for assessment, are not part of the environmental assessment of the home.

Test-Taking Strategy: The focus here is on environmental or home assessment. In developing the plan of care for home assessment, the nurse concentrates on the home and how the client functions in the home. Remember that assessment is the first step of the nursing process. Therefore, eliminate options 1 and 3. Of the remaining two options, option 4 is the most global response and is most directly related to the issue of the question.

Level of Cognitive Ability: Application
Phase of Nursing Process: Planning
Client Needs: Safe, Effective Care Environment
Content Area: Adult Health/Neurological

Reference

Como, N. (1995). *Home health nursing pocket consultant.* St. Louis: Mosby–Year Book, p. 107.

14. The physician has just ordered oxygen via concentrator for the client who has chronic obstructive pulmonary disease (COPD). What information about safety precautions should the nurse provide to the client and family?

1 Smoking is permissible 10 feet from the client
2 Oxygen tubing should not be kinked
3 The client may adjust the oxygen settings as desired
4 The oxygen needs to be shut off when the client is eating

Answer: 2

Rationale: Open flame is not permissible around oxygen. Clients are generally instructed not to adjust their oxygen settings but to call the home health care nurse or physician if there is difficulty breathing. Unless otherwise indicated, oxygen can be used while eating and is often encouraged if the client is short of breath as a result of increased oxygen demand. If the tubing is kinked, the client will not receive the desired oxygen.

Test-Taking Strategy: This question focuses on safety issues and oxygen therapy principles in the home. It requires that the home health care nurse understand safety and oxygen efficacy. You should eliminate option 1 on the basis of misinformation and oxygen safety. Client teaching for oxygen and physician orders would dictate compliance with oxygen settings, which eliminates option 3. Basic oxygenation principles allow clients to perform activities of daily living when using oxygen, and it is generally encouraged because more oxygen is required when the client is performing activities. Finally, for oxygen to be effective, the tubing cannot be kinked, which would obstruct the flow of oxygen.

Level of Cognitive Ability: Application
Phase of Nursing Process: Planning
Client Needs: Safe, Effective Care Environment
Content Area: Fundamental Skills

Reference
Potter, P., & Perry, A. (1997). *Fundamentals of nursing: Concepts, process, and practice* (4th ed.). St. Louis: Mosby–Year Book, pp. 1236, 1243.

---

15. The cardiac monitor alarm sounds for an asystole rhythm, and a straight line is noted on the screen. The nurse's first plan of action is to

1 Call a code.
2 Turn the amplitude up to pick up the QRS complexes.
3 Assess the client.
4 Confirm the rhythm by using a second lead.

Answer: 3

Rationale: Regardless of the system used for monitor observation, certain practices should always be followed. If the monitor alarm sounds, the nurse should evaluate the clinical status of the client before anything else, to see whether the problem is an actual dysrhythmia or a malfunction of the monitoring system. Asystole should not be mistaken for an unattached electrocardiographic wire. Assess the client first!

Test-Taking Strategy: The key word in the stem is "first." The question requires that the nurse prioritize nursing actions. Each of the options are possible responses to observing a straight line on the monitor. Although the monitor interprets the rhythm as an asystole, the first thing the nurse must do is determine whether the analysis is correct. The only way this can be done is by using the first step of the nursing process and assessing the client. All the other options follow as a result of this assessment.

Level of Cognitive Ability: Application
Phase of Nursing Process: Planning
Client Needs: Safe, Effective Care Environment
Content Area: Adult Health/Cardiovascular

Reference
Ignatavicius, D. D., Workman, M. L., & Mishler, M. A. (1995). *Medical-surgical nursing: A nursing process approach* (2nd ed.). Philadelphia: W. B. Saunders, p. 853.

16. The nurse is planning care for a client with congestive heart failure being treated with digoxin (Lanoxin) and furosemide (Lasix). Which of the following dinners would be the best choice from the daily menu?

1 Beef vegetable soup, macaroni and cheese, and a dinner roll
2 Beef ravioli, spinach soufflé, and Italian bread
3 Baked pollack, mashed potatoes, and carrot-raisin salad
4 Roasted chicken breast, brown rice, and stewed tomatoes

Answer: 3

Rationale: Lasix depletes potassium stores, and a client taking digoxin and furosemide needs to maintain normal potassium levels and moderate salt intake. Hypokalemia may make the client more susceptible to digitalis toxicity. The recommended daily intake for potassium is 2000 mg. Potassium toxicity only occurs with supplements, not from consuming an excess from foods. As long as a person has normally functioning kidneys, potassium toxicity is not a concern. Option 1 is not the best choice because beef vegetable soup contains 1002 mg of sodium and only 76 mg of potassium. Macaroni with cheese has 1029 mg of sodium and no potassium. Option 2 is not the best choice because beef ravioli has 1150 mg of sodium and no potassium. Spinach soufflé is a good source of potassium (345 mg) but also contains 820 mg of sodium. Option 4 is not the best choice because although roasted chicken contains very little sodium (63 mg), it also contains very low levels of potassium (218 mg). Stewed tomatoes contain 125 mg of potassium and 230 mg of sodium. Brown rice contains only 42 mg of potassium. Option 3 is the best choice because all three foods are high in potassium: potato (314 mg), pollack (388 mg), and raisins (600 mg). All are low in sodium. Other good sources include tomatoes, oranges, apricots, avocadoes, and all-bran cereal.

Test-Taking Strategy: Use the process of elimination, focusing on the client's condition when answering nutrition questions. In nutrition questions that ask you to select foods or food groups, the items in the correct response have to contain the sources of the desired electrolyte. Look at each food item in the option, eliminating the options that do not contain the desired food source. If you had difficulty with this question, take time now to review the foods that are high in potassium and low in sodium!

Level of Cognitive Ability: Application
Phase of Nursing Process: Planning
Client Needs: Physiological Integrity
Content Area: Adult Health/Cardiovascular

Reference

Ignatavicius, D. D., Workman, M. L., & Mishler, M. A. (1995). *Medical-surgical nursing: A nursing process approach* (2nd ed.). Philadelphia: W. B. Saunders, pp. 256, 902.

17. The physician prescribes an intravenous infusion of isoproterenol hydrochloride (Isuprel) for a client. In planning care, the nurse will include which of the following nursing interventions?

1 Administer Isuprel via an infusion pump
2 Dilute Isuprel only in normal saline
3 Maintain a separate IV line for Isuprel infusion
4 Use only Isuprel with epinephrine for intravenous use

Answer: 1

Rationale: For continuous infusion, Isuprel solution may be diluted in 5% dextrose in water (D5W), 10% dextrose in water (D10W), normal saline, 5% dextrose in lactated Ringer's (D5LR), or lactated Ringer's solution. The medication should be administered through a Y-site to ensure accurate dosage. Always administer with an infusion pump to ensure delivery of precise amount of medication. A separate IV line is not necessary. Isuprel with epinephrine is a different type of medication.

Test-Taking Strategy: The key to the correct option is to remember that in order to safely administer a cardiac medication intravenously, an infusion pump should always be used!

Level of Cognitive Ability: Application
Phase of Nursing Process: Planning
Client Needs: Safe, Effective Care Environment
Content Area: Adult Health/Cardiovascular

Reference

Hodgson, B., & Kizior, R. (1998). *Saunders nursing drug handbook 1998*. Philadelphia: W. B. Saunders, p. 553.

18. The nurse plans to change the dressing of the client who has had arterial bypass surgery. Which technique is most important for the nurse to follow?

1 Universal precautions
2 Aseptic technique
3 Clean technique
4 Reverse isolation

Answer: 2

Rationale: Aseptic technique is important to reduce risk of infection. Universal precautions are important but not specifically to this procedure. Reverse isolation is not necessary, and clean technique would be poor practice and put the client at risk for infection.

Test-Taking Strategy: The key to the question is identifying the most important technique to follow for the client who has had surgery. Although universal precautions are important, they do not protect the client from infection. Preventing infection is the issue of the question and the key concept to understand in selecting the correct option.

Level of Cognitive Ability: Application
Phase of Nursing Process: Planning
Client Needs: Safe, Effective Care Environment
Content Area: Fundamental Skills

Reference

Black, J., & Matassarin-Jacobs, E. (1997). *Medical-surgical nursing: Clinical management for continuity of care* (5th ed.). Philadelphia: W. B. Saunders, pp. 1415–1417.

---

19. A client has an inoperable abdominal aortic aneurysm (AAA). The nurse should plan to teach the client about the need for

1 Antihypertensives.
2 Bed rest.
3 Restricting fluids.
4 Maintaining a low-fiber diet.

Answer: 1

Rationale: The medical treatment for AAA is controlling blood pressure. Hypertension creates added stress on the blood vessel wall, increasing the likelihood of rupture. There is no need for the client to cut back on fluids or to be on bed rest. A low-fiber diet is not helpful.

Test-Taking Strategy: The relationship between AAA and hypertension is the key to choosing the correct answer to this question. If this question was difficult, take a few moments to review AAA and its treatment now!

Level of Cognitive Ability: Application
Phase of Nursing Process: Planning
Client Needs: Health Promotion and Maintenance
Content Area: Adult Health/Cardiovascular

Reference

Ignatavicius, D. D., Workman, M. L., & Mishler, M. A. (1995). *Medical-surgical nursing: A nursing process approach* (2nd ed.). Philadelphia: W. B. Saunders, p. 951.

---

20. The nurse is developing a teaching plan for a pregnant diabetic. Which of the following instructions has highest priority for inclusion in the plan?

1 How to test for proteinuria
2 How to assess and manage preterm bleeding
3 How to manage the discomfort of early labor
4 How to assess signs of hypoglycemia and required treatment

Answer: 4

Rationale: In diabetes, the pancreas does not produce enough insulin for necessary carbohydrate metabolism. The physiological changes of pregnancy drastically alter insulin requirements. Pregnant diabetics should be taught to monitor themselves for hypoglycemia to control the disease and minimize potential maternal and fetal side effects. Testing for proteinuria is important to the mother with pregnancy-induced hypertension. Management of preterm bleeding is taught to the mother with placenta previa. Managing the discomforts of early labor is important for all pregnant women.

Test-Taking Strategy: Use the process of elimination identifying the key phrases. In this question, the key word "diabetic" and key phrase "highest priority" guide you to select option 4 as the best choice. Note the relationship between "diabetic" in the question and "hypoglycemia" in the correct response!

Level of Cognitive Ability: Application
Phase of Nursing Process: Planning
Client Needs: Health Promotion and Maintenance
Content Area: Maternity

Reference

Olds, S., London, M., & Ladewig, P. (1996). *Clinical handbook for maternal-newborn nursing: A family-centered approach* (5th ed.). Menlo Park, CA: Addison-Wesley, pp. 35–39.

---

21. The hospital experience strongly influences the process of breast-feeding. Which one of the following factors does the nurse recognize as most favorable when planning to teach a client to breast-feed?

1 Brief separation of infant and mother after birth to allow the mother to rest
2 A client with previous breast-feeding experience
3 A physician who encourages clients to breast-feed
4 A positive nurse-client relationship

Answer: 4

Rationale: Because hospital stays are short, all contacts with the mother become teachable moments. The nurse-client relationship becomes a growth-fostering experience so that the mother feels confident in her ability to breast-feed. Brief separation decreases the chance of correct latch and suck in the immediate postpartum period. Infants should be placed at the breast immediately after delivery. Physician encouragement is helpful but is not critical for successful breast-feeding. Although previous breast-feeding experience is helpful, the most significant factor is the nurse-client relationship!

Test-Taking Strategy: Use the process of elimination when answering the question, noting the key phrase "most significant." Option 1 is totally incorrect. Option 3 is eliminated next as being least plausible. Of the remaining two options, the more significant factor is a positive nurse-client relationship.

Level of Cognitive Ability: Application
Phase of Nursing Process: Planning
Client Needs: Health Promotion and Maintenance
Content Area: Maternity

Reference

Nichols, F., & Zwelling, E. (1997). *Maternal newborn nursing: Theory and practice.* Philadelphia: W. B. Saunders, pp. 1238–1239.

---

22. After a newborn undergoes circumcision, which of the following would the nurse include in the postprocedure plan of care?

1 Preventing the infant from eating for several hours
2 Ensuring consent is obtained
3 Restraining the infant on a Circumstraint board
4 Observing for bleeding and assessing for pain

Answer: 4

Rationale: To care for the newborn's circumcision, the nurse should observe for bleeding, which is the most common complication. A common protocol is to assess the site every hour for 8 to 12 hours. Wearing gloves is consistent with standard precautions. Assessing the infant's facial expression, body movements, and character of crying will indicate the need to minimize or lessen pain. Nutrition is important. The consent is to be obtained before the procedure. Restraints are not necessary after the procedure.

Test-Taking Strategy: Read the options carefully. Use the process of elimination when selecting the correct option. Options 1, 2, and 3 are nursing actions required before the procedure. In addition, use the ABCs—airway, breathing, and circulation—to answer the question!

Level of Cognitive Ability: Application
Phase of Nursing Process: Planning
Client Needs: Physiological Integrity
Content Area: Maternity

Reference

Nichols, F., & Zwelling, E. (1997). *Maternal-newborn nursing: Theory and practice.* Philadelphia: W. B. Saunders, pp. 1164–1168.

23. The nurse from a previous shift reports to an oncoming nurse that a client with congestive heart failure appears anxious and is reluctant to ask questions. Which action should the nurse plan to do first when caring for this client?

1. Minimize the time spent talking to the client, thus respecting the client's wishes
2. Request a family member to be present when caring for the client
3. Discuss with the client common fears and questions expressed by other clients
4. Ask the client about the reluctance to ask questions

Answer: 3

Rationale: Imparting the common fears and questions expressed by other clients often encourages the client to ask questions that were thought of but not spoken. The nurse should plan to spend additional time with the client. Requesting a family member to be present may reduce the client's anxiety and may be tried after the nurse has talked to the client. However, communication with the client is needed to determine the source of the anxiety. Requesting an explanation is a nontherapeutic technique of communication. The client may not know the reason.

Test-Taking Strategy: Therapeutic communication techniques enhance communication. When answering questions related to communication, always select the answer that will enhance communication. Use the process of elimination with this question. Avoid selecting responses that will block communication. Always address the client's concerns and feelings.

Level of Cognitive Ability: Application
Phase of Nursing Process: Planning
Client Needs: Psychosocial Integrity
Content Area: Adult Health/Cardiovascular

Reference

Black, J., & Matassarin-Jacobs, E. (1997). *Medical-surgical nursing: Clinical management for continuity of care* (5th ed.). Philadelphia: W. B. Saunders, p. 1289.

---

24. The nurse is assigned to a client with acute pulmonary edema who is receiving digoxin (Lanoxin) and heparin therapy. In planning care for this client, which of the following nursing actions would be unsafe?

1. Withholding digoxin if heart rate is less than 60
2. Administering heparin with a 25-gauge needle
3. Restricting the client's potassium intake
4. Encouraging the client to rest after meals

Answer: 3

Rationale: Clients with acute pulmonary edema are on a sodium-restricted, not potassium-restricted, diet. Restricting potassium makes the client more prone to digitalis toxicity. Digitalis should be withheld and the physician notified when the client's heart rate is less than 60 unless orders indicate otherwise. Heparin should be administered with a 25- or 27-gauge needle to reduce tissue trauma. Resting after meals decreases the demands placed on the heart and should be encouraged.

Test-Taking Strategy: Knowledge regarding the care of clients with acute pulmonary edema is needed to answer this question. Note the word "unsafe" in the stem of the question. If you had difficulty with this question, take time now to review the administration and effects of digoxin and heparin!

Level of Cognitive Ability: Application
Phase of Nursing Process: Planning
Client Needs: Safe, Effective Care Environment
Content Area: Adult Health/Cardiovascular

Reference

Black, J., & Matassarin-Jacobs, E. (1997). *Medical-surgical nursing: Clinical management for continuity of care* (5th ed.). Philadelphia: W. B. Saunders, pp. 1288–1289.

25. The nurse is planning care for a client with Hodgkin's disease who is neutropenic as a result of radiation and chemotherapy. Which of the following plans would be most effective in decreasing the risk of infection?

1 Limiting visitors to immediate family only
2 Providing a diet high in protein
3 Meticulous handwashing
4 Monitoring electrolyte levels daily

Answer: 3

Rationale: Specific nursing management of the client undergoing treatment for Hodgkin's disease focuses on minimizing the risks or side effects of therapy. Risk for infection is significant, and handwashing is the most effective means of decreasing risk of infection.

Test-Taking Strategy: Use the process of elimination. Eliminate options 2 and 4 because diet and electrolytes do not directly relate to infection. Limiting visitors to immediate family will not help because an immediate family member may transmit an infection. Handwashing is often the answer to a safe, effective care environment question.

Level of Cognitive Ability: Application
Phase of Nursing Process: Planning
Client Needs: Safe, Effective Care Environment
Content Area: Adult Health/Oncology

Reference

Ignatavicius, D. D., Workman, M. L., & Mishler, M. A. (1995). *Medical-surgical nursing: A nursing process approach* (2nd ed.). Philadelphia: W. B. Saunders, pp. 1069–1070.

---

26. In planning care for a client who has undergone pelvic exenteration, which statement by the nurse would be most therapeutic?

1 "Would you like to talk?"
2 "How do you feel about your body?"
3 "You are looking good today."
4 "Will your family help you deal with this?"

Answer: 2

Rationale: Postoperatively, a client begins to deal with the trauma of the surgery by expressing grief about the mutilated body. Later, the client may become depressed or withdrawn, even angry or hostile. The client needs intense emotional support to adapt to the altered body image and functions.

Test-Taking Strategy: Open-ended questions are most therapeutic, so eliminate options 1 and 4. Responses should be client-based and avoid false reassurance, so option 3 is incorrect. Option 2 is open-ended and focuses on client feelings. Remember, focus on client's feelings first!

Level of Cognitive Ability: Application
Phase of Nursing Process: Planning
Client Needs: Psychosocial Integrity
Content Area: Adult Health/Oncology

Reference

Smeltzer, S., & Bare, B. (1996). *Brunner and Suddarth's Textbook of medical-surgical nursing* (8th ed.). Philadelphia: J. B. Lippincott, pp. 2254–2255.

---

27. In planning safe, effective care for a client admitted to the cardiac unit with a medical diagnosis of cardiovascular insufficiency, the nurse would include as a priority

1 Maintenance of good body alignment while the client is on bed rest.
2 Maintenance of as large a fluid intake as allowed.
3 Family instruction on how to obtain medical assistance.
4 Evaluation of tolerance for new activities.

Answer: 1

Rationale: Good body alignment promotes rest and relaxation and decreases the workload of the cardiovascular system. Adequate fluid intake is important, but a large fluid intake could stress the heart. Option 3 addresses the family, not the client. Eliminate option 4 because although it is important, it is not timely immediately after admission to a cardiac unit.

Test-Taking Strategy: Read the question carefully, noting the client of the question. This will help you eliminate option 3. Eliminate option 2 because it addresses large amounts of fluids. The question asks for a priority plan on admission to a cardiac unit. This implies that the client's activity would be limited, allowing you to choose option 1 over option 4.

Level of Cognitive Ability: Application
Phase of Nursing Process: Planning
Client Needs: Safe, Effective Care Environment
Content Area: Adult Health/Cardiovascular

Reference

Luckmann, J. (1997). *Saunders manual of nursing care.* Philadelphia: W. B. Saunders, pp. 1052–1055.

---

28. The nurse formulates a nursing diagnosis of Dysfunctional Grieving for the client. The nurse plans to assist the client in achieving the goal of gaining self-esteem by encouraging

1. Preventative measures against tooth decay.
2. Maintaining a daily diary of negative feelings.
3. Maintaining a well-groomed appearance.
4. Verbalizing feelings of being unloved.

Answer: 3

Rationale: The client may demonstrate increased feeling of self-worth through outward appearance. Options 2 and 4 focus on negative issues and should be avoided. Option 1 is indirectly related to self-esteem.

Test-Taking Strategy: To answer this question correctly, it is necessary to understand the concept of self-esteem. Eliminate options 2 and 4 as they focus on negative issues. Option 3 is directly related to self-esteem and is the most global response!

Level of Cognitive Ability: Analysis
Phase of Nursing Process: Analysis
Client Needs: Psychosocial Integrity
Content Area: Mental Health

Reference

Potter, P., & Perry, A. (1997) *Fundamentals of nursing: Concepts, process, and practice* (4th ed.). St. Louis: Mosby–Year Book, p. 470.

---

29. The nurse is planning stress management strategies for the client with irritable bowel syndrome. Which of the following suggestions would the nurse plan to give the client?

1. Try to avoid every possible stressful situation
2. Learn measures such as biofeedback or progressive relaxation
3. Limit exercise to reduce bowel stimulation
4. Rest in bed as much as possible

Answer: 2

Rationale: Treatment for irritable bowel syndrome includes stress-reduction measures such as biofeedback, progressive relaxation, and regular exercise. The client should also learn to limit his or her own responsibilities. Other measures include increased fluid and fiber in the diet and antispasmodic or sedative medications as needed.

Test-Taking Strategy: Begin to answer this question by eliminating options 3 and 4. Remember that options that are similar are not likely to be correct. Next eliminate option 1, because the word "every" makes the option implausible. If you had difficulty with this question, take time to review appropriate stress-management techniques for the client with irritable bowel syndrome!

Level of Cognitive Ability: Application
Phase of Nursing Process: Planning
Client Needs: Psychosocial Integrity
Content Area: Adult Health/Gastrointestinal

Reference

Black, J., & Matassarin-Jacobs, E. (1997). *Medical-surgical nursing: Clinical management for continuity of care* (5th ed.). Philadelphia: W. B. Saunders, pp. 1824–1825.

30. A postmenopausal client's doctor has proposed hormone replacement therapy (HRT). Which of the following statements, if made by the client, would indicate that the nurse should plan to give additional emotional support?

1. "I'm not sure that I want to start these medications and get my period again."
2. "This medication will take care of my depression, and I'll be like I used to be."
3. "With my family history of heart disease, I should really, seriously consider this therapy."
4. "My friend is doing so well on HRT, I think I'll try it, too."

Answer: 2

Rationale: Option 1 indicates a teaching opportunity and not specifically the need for emotional support. Options 3 and 4 are realistic client responses to a newly prescribed therapy. Option 2 is unrealistic. A medication does not eliminate depression on its own, and this is not a proven therapeutic indication for HRT.

Test-Taking Strategy: Note the key phrase "give additional emotional support." From this point, use the process of elimination. The only option that specifically addresses the need for emotional support is option 2!

Level of Cognitive Ability: Application
Phase of Nursing Process: Planning
Client Needs: Psychosocial Integrity
Content Area: Adult Health/Endocrine

Reference

Black, J., & Matassarin-Jacobs, E. (1997). *Medical-surgical nursing: Clinical management for continuity of care* (5th ed.). Philadelphia W. B. Saunders, pp. 2393–2395.

---

31. A client is to be discharged to the home and will continue with intermittent infusions of antibiotics via a peripherally inserted central catheter (PICC line). The nurse plans to include which of the following instructions to be done on a daily basis?

1. Keep the affected arm immobilized with an arm board or other splint
2. Assess the insertion site and length of the arm for signs of infection
3. Aspirate a small amount of blood from the catheter to determine patency
4. Maintain continuous infusion of fluids in between doses of antibiotics

Answer: 2

Rationale: A PICC is designed to be a long-term indwelling catheter, usually inserted into the median cubital vein. The tip of the catheter should lie in the superior vena cava. A PICC does not require the affected arm to be immobilized (a major advantage of a PICC) and can be used for intermittent or continuous infusions of fluids. Although the risk of infection is less with a PICC than with a subclavian or other central line, it is possible for phlebitis or infection to develop. Clients must be aware of the need for daily inspection and report any discharge, redness, or pain immediately to the nurse or physician. Although a PICC can be used for obtaining blood specimens, it is not recommended for routine aspiration of blood to determine patency.

Test-Taking Strategy: It is essential that you understand the placement and purposes of a PICC as well as the differences between a PICC and other types of indwelling venous catheters. Option 1 may be appropriate for a short-length peripheral intravenous catheter, if it is placed in a mobile and vulnerable spot such as the wrist. Option 3 is incorrect, because aspiration of blood from the catheter is not recommended as a routine means of determining placement. Because the nature of a PICC allows for either continuous or intermittent infusions, option 4 is also incorrect. Basic principles of infection control dictate that when there is any break in skin integrity that could lead to infection, signs of infection must be carefully assessed and symptoms must be reported immediately. In addition, option 2 addresses the first step of the nursing process: Assessment!

Level of Cognitive Ability: Application
Phase of Nursing Process: Planning
Client Needs: Physiological Integrity
Content Area: Fundamental Skills

Reference

Lewis, S., Collier, I., & Heitkemper, M. (1996). *Medical-surgical nursing: Assessment and management of clinical problems* (4th ed.). St. Louis: Mosby–Year Book, pp. 292–293.

32. To successfully and appropriately work with a woman victimized by physical abuse, the nurse would plan to first

1. Agree with the woman that it is possible she might have acted in a manner that provoked the abuse.
2. Carefully examine own personal attitudes toward the abused and abusers before working with the client.
3. Establish firm time lines for the woman to make the necessary changes in her life situation.
4. Reinforce that dealing with the psychological and physical aspects is of the highest priority.

Answer: 2

Rationale: The nurse must work through her or his personal fears and prejudices in order to be an advocate for the client and to effectively identify and interact therapeutically with victims of physical violence. Option 1 fosters the notion of the client as being at fault. In options 3 and 4, the nurse may be making unreasonable demands, which could cause further distress for the client. Both of these are inconsistent with the right of the client to self-determination and competent nursing care.

Test-Taking Strategy: Determine what the question is asking you to identify. The focus is the nurse's accountability in providing competent care to an emotionally vulnerable client. Carefully note any potential responses that decrease or eliminate the client's part in decision making. These kinds of responses (such as options 3 and 4) are almost universally incorrect choices. To discriminate between options 1 and 2, note that option 1 places blame on the client. This is again a universally incorrect choice. In addition, option 2 addresses the first step of the nursing process: Assessment!

Level of Cognitive Ability: Application
Phase of Nursing Process: Planning
Client Needs: Psychosocial Integrity
Content Area: Mental Health

Reference

Clark, M. (1996). *Nursing in the community* (2nd ed.). Stamford, CT: Appleton & Lange, pp. 485–486.

---

33. The nurse is administering amphotericin B (Fungizone) to a client intravenously. The nurse plans to monitor the results of which of the following electrolyte studies during therapy with this medication?

1. Sodium
2. Potassium
3. Calcium
4. Chloride

Answer: 2

Rationale: Life-threatening hypokalemia can occur after each dose of amphotericin B. To minimize this occurrence, the nurse monitors the results of serum potassium levels, which should be measured at least biweekly. Magnesium levels should also be monitored.

Test-Taking Strategy: Specific knowledge of amphotericin B is needed to answer this question correctly. Take time now to review this medication if you had difficulty with this question!

Level of Cognitive Ability: Application
Phase of Nursing Process: Planning
Client Needs: Physiological Integrity
Content Area: Pharmacology

Reference

Hodgson, B., & Kizior, R. (1998). *Saunders nursing drug handbook 1998*. Philadelphia: W. B. Saunders, pp. 58–59.

34. A pregnant client is admitted to the obstetrical unit during an exacerbation of a heart condition. When planning for the nutritional requirements of the client, the nurse would consult with the dietitian to ensure which of the following?

1 A low-calorie diet to ensure absence of weight gain
2 A diet low in fluids and fiber to decrease blood volume
3 A diet high in fluids and fiber to decrease constipation
4 Unlimited sodium intake to increase circulating blood volume

Answer: 3

Rationale: Constipation causes the client to use the Valsalva maneuver. This causes blood to rush to the heart and overload the cardiac system. Absence of weight gain is not recommended during pregnancy. Diets low in fluid and fiber would cause a decrease in blood volume, which in turn deprives the fetus of nutrients. Too much sodium could cause an overload to the circulating blood volume and contribute to the cardiac condition.

Test-Taking Strategy: Use the process of elimination to answer the question, remembering that there are two clients that need to be considered: both the mother and fetus. This should assist you in eliminating options 1, 2, and 4 because low-calorie, low-fluid, and unlimited-sodium intake can be harmful to the mother and/or fetus. If you had difficulty with this question, take time now to review the care of the pregnant client with cardiac disease!

Level of Cognitive Ability: Application
Phase of Nursing Process: Planning
Client Needs: Physiological Integrity
Content Area: Maternity

Reference

Lowdermilk, D., Perry, S., & Bobak, I. (1997). *Maternity & women's health care* (6th ed.). St. Louis: Mosby–Year Book, p. 835.

---

35. When caring for the obstetric client with human immunodeficiency virus (HIV), which of the following goals would be most appropriate?

1 The client will not have sexual relations during the remainder of pregnancy
2 The client will not develop an opportunistic infection during the remainder of pregnancy
3 The client is advised of an HIV support group
4 The client is assisted with the grief process

Answer: 2

Rationale: Acquired immunodeficiency syndrome (AIDS) is caused by a retrovirus (HIV) that invades T lymphocytes. This disables the body's ability to fight infection. Nursing goals are directed at the prevention of infections. Sexual relations are not contraindicated if protective devices are properly used. Options 3 and 4 are the focus of interventions, not goals.

Test-Taking Strategy: The stem asks for a goal. Options 3 and 4 refer to the effects of interventions; therefore eliminate these options. Option 1 may be a forced goal that the client may not want to adhere to. Knowledge regarding the infectious nature of HIV is the priority!

Level of Cognitive Ability: Application
Phase of Nursing Process: Planning
Client Needs: Physiological Integrity
Content Area: Maternity

Reference

Pillitteri, A. (1995). *Maternal and child health nursing: Care of the childbearing and childrearing family* (2nd ed.). Philadelphia: Lippincott-Raven, pp. 334–335.

36. An appropriate intervention for the nurse to incorporate into an HIV-positive pregnant client's care plan during the antenatal period would be to

1 Minimize contact with other HIV-positive childbearing women.
2 Avoid discussing potential fetal complications with client.
3 Encourage the client to discuss her fears, concerns, and feelings with counselors and support people after the baby is delivered.
4 Refer client to community support groups to reduce anxiety and fear and to enhance coping during pregnancy.

Answer: 4

Rationale: The HIV-positive pregnant woman frequently possesses a knowledge deficit related to HIV, the AIDS disease process, and potential treatment options. In addition, she may express fears and anxiety related to her own well-being and that of her developing fetus. Nursing interventions are aimed at providing accurate information, enhancing the client's self-perception, and introducing the childbearing woman to potential support services and community resources.

Test-Taking Strategy: Use the process of elimination. The correct response to this question is based on the nurse's use of appropriate therapeutic communication skills to promote the client's positive adaptation both during the pregnancy and after birth, thus meeting the psychosocial needs of the childbearing woman with HIV. Options 1 and 2 distance the woman from other potential sources of support. Option 3 addresses only postdelivery issues.

Level of Cognitive Ability: Application
Phase of Nursing Process: Planning
Client Needs: Psychosocial Integrity
Content Area: Maternity

Reference

Reeder, S., Martin, L., & Koniak-Griffin, D. (1997). *Maternity nursing: Family, newborn and women's health care* (18th ed.). Philadelphia: Lippincott-Raven, pp. 289–290.

37. The nurse is planning care for a child recently admitted with meningitis. What goal would best provide a safe environment for the child and the child's contacts?

1 Maintain respiratory isolation for 24 hours after antibiotic therapy is started
2 Provide a quiet room away from the nurses' station and elevators
3 Permit only soft washable toys in the child's room
4 Maintain complete bed rest until recovery

Answer: 1

Rationale: The correct answer is the only option that reduces risk of infection for both the child and the contacts through the use of isolation. This time period is recommended because most antibiotics achieve a therapeutic blood level in 24 hours, therefore reducing communicability. Option 2 reduces stimuli, but the acutely ill child requires closer observation initially. In option 3, washable items are important for isolation and soft items may be indicated if the child is experiencing seizures. Option 4 is seldom an appropriate goal because long-term inactivity increases the risk of complications.

Test-Taking Strategy: Because all the options could provide a safe environment, it is important to carefully read the question. The child has a potentially communicable disease, so isolation is the best choice. Because early ambulation is always encouraged to prevent complications, option 4 wouldn't be correct unless another factor necessitated immobility. Option 3 is an appropriate option, but the presence of the key word "best" in the stem should direct you to choose option 1 as the priority answer.

Level of Cognitive Ability: Application
Phase of Nursing Process: Planning
Client Needs: Safe, Effective Care Environment
Content Area: Child Health

Reference

Wong, D. (1997). *Whaley and Wong's Essentials of pediatric nursing* (5th ed.). St. Louis: Mosby–Year Book, pp. 1012–1013.

38. The nurse is developing a teaching plan for the client who has undergone laryngectomy and radical neck dissection. Which of the following points would not be included by the nurse in developing the plan?

1. The shoulder is expected to droop on the affected side
2. Range-of-motion exercises should be done with the affected shoulder
3. Exercises such as walking the fingers up the wall are beneficial
4. Swimming provides good exercise, especially if done three times per week

Answer: 4

Rationale: After radical neck dissection and laryngectomy, the affected shoulder is expected to droop, as a result of interruption of the spinal accessory nerve. Range-of-motion exercises of the head, neck, and shoulder are beneficial to this client, as well as exercises such as walking the fingers up the wall. Swimming is contraindicated for the client with laryngectomy, because the water would enter the client's airway.

Test-Taking Strategy: The question is worded to elicit a response that is an incorrect statement. Remember that options that are similar are not likely to be correct. In this question, options 2 and 3 are similar and are therefore discarded. From the remaining two options, option 4 is contraindicated, considering concepts related to airway protection.

Level of Cognitive Ability: Application
Phase of Nursing Process: Planning
Client Needs: Health Promotion and Maintenance
Content Area: Adult Health/Respiratory

Reference

Burrell, P., Gerlach, M., & Pless, B. (1997). *Adult nursing: Acute and community care* (2nd ed.). Stamford, CT: Appleton & Lange, p. 753.

---

39. The nurse is caring for the client at risk for acute renal tubular necrosis after a crushing injury to the leg. The nurse plans which of the following measures to minimize this particular risk for the client?

1. Use of sheepskin and bed cradle
2. Frequent position changes in bed
3. Administration of antibiotics in a timely manner
4. Careful monitoring of IV fluids to ensure sufficient intake

Answer: 4

Rationale: After a crushing injury, myoglobin released from damaged muscle cells circulates in the blood stream and can clog renal tubules. It is important to maintain an increased fluid intake to "flush" the kidneys and minimize this occurrence. The other options may be part of the management of this client but do not specifically relate to this potential complication.

Test-Taking Strategy: The key words in the stem of this question include "renal tubular necrosis" and "minimize." Use the process of elimination and select the option that is directly related to this complication. The only option that is directly related is option 4.

Level of Cognitive Ability: Application
Phase of Nursing Process: Planning
Client Needs: Physiological Integrity
Content Area: Adult Health/Renal

Reference

Burrell, P., Gerlach, M., & Pless, B. (1997). *Adult nursing: Acute and community care* (2nd ed.). Stamford, CT: Appleton & Lange, p. 1251.

40. During a routine prenatal visit the client states, "I have not been able to get my wedding ring off for the past 2 days. I guess the heat is making my fingers swell." The nurse plans to further assess the client for

1 Blood pressure changes and protein in her urine.
2 Height of the fundus in comparison to the date of her last menstrual period.
3 Blood glucose level.
4 Any vaginal discharge.

Answer: 1

Rationale: Option 1 contains assessments for pregnancy-induced hypertension (PIH). Finger edema is a frequent forerunner of PIH and should be investigated further. Options 2, 3, and 4 are all assessments of other problems such as diabetes, infections, and molar pregnancy.

Test-Taking Strategy: Knowledge regarding the significance of the symptoms presented in the question will assist in directing you to the correct option. Use the ABCs—airway, breathing and circulation—to answer the question if you are having difficulty. This should direct you to select the option that addresses blood pressure. Take time now to review the signs and symptoms associated with PIH if you had difficulty with this question!

Level of Cognitive Ability: Application
Phase of Nursing Process: Planning
Client Needs: Physiological Integrity
Content Area: Maternity

Reference

Reeder, S., Martin, L., & Koniak-Griffin, D. (1997). *Maternity nursing: Family, newborn and women's health care* (18th ed.). Philadelphia: Lippincott-Raven, p. 837.

---

41. The nurse prepares a teaching plan for a pregnant client with newly diagnosed diabetes. Which of the following should not be included in the teaching plan?

1 Effects of diabetes on the pregnancy and fetus
2 Nutritional requirements for pregnancy and diabetic control
3 Avoidance of exercise because of the negative effects on insulin production
4 Awareness of any infections and reporting these immediately to the health care provider

Answer: 3

Rationale: Options 1, 2, and 4 are all important points to include in the teaching plan for the patient with newly diagnosed diabetes. Exercise is necessary for the pregnant diabetic. Concepts related to the timing of exercise, control of food intake, and insulin around the time of exercise should be included in the plan.

Test-Taking Strategy: Note that the stem of the question includes the key word "not." Use the process of elimination. Note the word "avoidance" in option 3, the correct option for this question as it is stated. Take time now to review client teaching points for the pregnant client with newly diagnosed diabetes if you had difficulty with this question.

Level of Cognitive Ability: Application
Phase of Nursing Process: Planning
Client Needs: Health Promotion and Maintenance
Content Area: Maternity

Reference

Reeder, S., Martin, L., & Koniak-Griffin, D. (1997). *Maternity nursing: Family, newborn and women's health care* (18th ed.). Philadelphia: Lippincott-Raven, p. 86.

42. A newborn male infant with respiratory distress syndrome (RDS) is admitted to intensive care unit for intubation and mechanical ventilation. The parents are entering the nursery to see the infant for the first time after delivery. A plan of care is developed by the nurse to help the parents cope. Which of the following interventions is least likely to help them during this initial, critical phase?

1. Giving a complete, honest report of their infant's status
2. Explaining the purpose of various pumps, monitors, and equipment in simple terms
3. Encouraging the discussion of difficult topics with the nurse practitioner
4. Referring to the infant by name

Answer: 3

Rationale: Parents need complete and honest information about their infant. A basic knowledge of all equipment and monitors is helpful for the parents to understand why they are being used on their baby. Referring to their baby by name gives the baby a personal identity. The intervention least likely to help the parents cope during this initial, critical phase is to encourage the discussion of difficult topics with another individual—in this case, the nurse practitioner.

Test-Taking Strategy: This question asks for the intervention least likely to help the parents. Options 1, 2, and 4 address issues surrounding the infant. Option 3 places the parents' concerns and issues on hold. Avoid communication blocks!

Level of Cognitive Ability: Application
Phase of Nursing Process: Planning
Client Needs: Psychosocial Integrity
Content Area: Maternity

References

Ashwill, J., & Droske, S. (1997). *Nursing care of children: Principles and practice.* Philadelphia: W. B. Saunders, pp. 550–556.
Nichols, F., & Zwelling, E. (1997). *Maternal-newborn nursing: Theory and practice.* Philadelphia: W. B. Saunders, pp. 580, 1340–1345.

---

43. A nurse assesses a 3-hour-old infant and finds that the infant has not eaten since birth, is jittery, and has a weak cry. The mother states that she can't get the baby to eat. Which of the following actions should the nurse plan to take first?

1. Let the baby sleep
2. Check blood glucose level
3. Call the doctor
4. Feed the baby

Answer: 2

Rationale: The nurse's role is pivotal in the prompt recognition of the signs and symptoms of hypoglycemia. This infant has classic symptoms of hypoglycemia. The nurse is responsible to screen the infant's blood glucose level to determine the extent of hypoglycemia, if any, and then to take action by calling the doctor or feeding the infant as per the policy of the unit. To let the baby sleep may cause the hypoglycemia to remain untreated and result in neurological damage.

Test-Taking Strategy: Identify the key word in the question—"first"—that indicates the need for you to prioritize. In this case, hypoglycemia is the suspected problem, and the nurse needs to understand the proper steps to take when an infant is suspected of hypoglycemia. Use the nursing process to prioritize. Option 2 addresses the first step in the nursing process: Assessment!

Level of Cognitive Ability: Application
Phase of Nursing Process: Planning
Client Needs: Safe, Effective Care Environment
Content Area: Maternity

References

Ashwill, J., & Droske, S. (1997). *Nursing care of children: Principles and practice.* Philadelphia: W. B. Saunders, pp. 562–564.
Nichols, F., & Zwelling, E. (1997). *Maternal-newborn nursing: Theory and practice.* Philadelphia: W. B. Saunders, pp. 1187–1188.

44. A client with a fractured femur with possible knee injuries is being admitted to the nursing unit before surgery. The nurse should plan to have which type of traction set up as the most suitable one for this client?

1 Halo
2 Russell's
3 Pelvic
4 Buck's

Answer: 2

Rationale: The purpose of Russell's traction is to stabilize a fractured femur before surgery and may be used for some knee injuries. Halo traction or a halo vest is indicated to stabilize fractures of dislocated cervical vertebrae. Pelvic traction is used for certain lumbar and sacral disorders. Buck's traction immobilizes a fractured hip and relieves muscle spasms before hip surgery.

Test-Taking Strategy: Knowledge of the use of traction is essential when answering this question. Using the inappropriate type of traction may consequently lead to further damage to the joints. Take time now to review the different types of traction if you had difficulty with this question!

Level of Cognitive Ability: Application
Phase of Nursing Process: Planning
Client Needs: Health Promotion and Maintenance
Content Area: Adult Health/Musculoskeletal

References
Ashwill, J., & Droske, S. (1997). *Nursing care of children: Principles and practice.* Philadelphia: W. B. Saunders, p. 1101.
Black, J., & Matassarin-Jacobs, E. (1997). *Medical-surgical nursing: Clinical management for continuity of care* (5th ed.). Philadelphia: W. B. Saunders, pp. 2138–2139.

---

45. The emergency room nurse admits a client with an obvious deformity, severe pain, and restricted movement of the upper right extremity caused by a fall. The initial nursing plan includes which of the following?

1 Obtain an x-ray of the right shoulder
2 Assist with the relocation of the right shoulder
3 Place the client's right arm in a sling and arrange for an orthopedic consultation
4 Check for distal pulses and assess neurovascular status

Answer: 4

Rationale: The immediate intervention is to examine the extremity and obtain a history. Details of the actual history are helpful to determine what type of fracture may have occurred. A physician is responsible for obtaining an x-ray and relocating or reducing a fracture. It is appropriate to splint and immobilize the extremity, but first the nurse should assess the extremity.

Test-Taking Strategy: The question asks for the "initial" plan. Use both the steps of the nursing process and the ABCs—airway, breathing, and circulation—to answer the question. Option 4 addresses Assessment and circulation!

Level of Cognitive Ability: Application
Phase of Nursing Process: Implementation
Client Needs: Physiological Integrity
Content Area: Adult Health/Musculoskeletal

Reference
Sheehy, S., & Lombardi, J. (1995). *Manual of emergency care* (4th ed.). St. Louis: Mosby–Year Book, p. 551.

46. The depressed client has been admitted as a result of a suicide attempt. The client was accidentally found by a neighbor when the neighbor entered the garage. The client had the car on and the door closed. The client is quite upset about being rescued and has been admitted to the hospital by an emergency court order. In planning care for the client's safety, the nurse knows that this client

1 Is at high risk for trying again.
2 Does not have the means to do it now.
3 Should be placed in a private room.
4 May be embarrassed to discuss it.

Answer: 1

Rationale: The client who has chosen a highly lethal method, has been discovered by accident, and is quite upset by the discovery may look for a way to carry out the act in the hospital. Any depressed client who has suicidal thoughts can find a means for carrying out the act and should be observed closely. A private room may encourage too much isolation, and this client needs involvement with others right now. The client may be relieved to discuss reasons for the suicide attempt. Group therapy could encourage discussion, particularly if there are other clients there who have had a similar experience.

Test-Taking Strategy: The highest priority is to keep the client safe, and option 1 most clearly addresses that issue. Review care of the hospitalized client after a suicide attempt now if you had difficulty with this question!

Level of Cognitive Ability: Application
Phase of Nursing Process: Planning
Client Needs: Safe, Effective Care Environment
Content Area: Mental Health

Reference

Johnson, B. (1997). *Psychiatric–mental health nursing: Adaptation and growth* (4th ed.). Philadelphia: Lippincott-Raven, p. 867.

---

47. The lithium level for the bipolar client is 1.8 mEq/liter. The nurse should plan to take which of the following actions?

1 Withhold the lithium until the physician is contacted
2 Report to the client that this is in the therapeutic range
3 Give the medication as prescribed
4 No action is indicated at the present time

Answer: 1

Rationale: The acceptable range for lithium is 0.6–1.2 mEq/liter. A level of 1.8 mEq/liter is approaching toxic levels, and the physician must be notified for instructions regarding further dosing. If the nurse were to give the medication as prescribed, the safety of the client would be jeopardized. Lack of action by the nurse would indicate inadequate knowledge of the medication precautions.

Test-Taking Strategy: Knowledge regarding the therapeutic lithium level is necessary to answer the question. Remember that if a level is approaching toxicity, the medication needs to be withheld and the physician needs to be contacted. Take time now to review this therapeutic level if you had difficulty with this question!

Level of Cognitive Ability: Application
Phase of Nursing Process: Planning
Client Needs: Physiological Integrity
Content Area: Mental Health

Reference

Hodgson, B., & Kizior, R. (1998). *Saunders nursing drug handbook 1998.* Philadelphia: W. B. Saunders, pp. 598–600.

48. The client has just been found in the room with a hanger around the neck. Breathing is shallow, and pulse is present. Which of the following actions should the nurse plan to take as the highest priority at this time?

1 Call the doctor immediately
2 Check vital signs and level of consciousness
3 Have another health team member call a Code Blue
4 Ask the unit clerk to call family immediately

Answer: 2

Rationale: The client is breathing and has a pulse. Further assessment is needed before the nurse takes any other action. Level of consciousness and vital signs should be assessed. Once that assessment is made, the physician does need to be notified, as does the family. Code Blue is not indicated at the present time. Further assessment might warrant that later.

Test-Taking Strategy: In view of the fact that the client is breathing and has a pulse, the first priority in the nurse's emergency plan of care is to assess further. Use the steps of the nursing process. The only option that addresses Assessment is option 2!

Level of Cognitive Ability: Application
Phase of Nursing Process: Planning
Client Needs: Physiological Integrity
Content Area: Mental Health

Reference

Black, J., & Matassarin-Jacobs, E. (1997). *Medical-surgical nursing: Clinical management for continuity of care* (5th ed.). Philadelphia: W. B. Saunders, pp. 2519–2520.

---

49. When preparing to teach a parent prevention of dietary causes of diarrhea in a 6-month-old infant, which of these instructions should a nurse include?

1 Ask the pediatrician before changing formula brands
2 Keep uneaten food in the same jar in the refrigerator
3 Add only a small amount of corn syrup to the formula
4 Plan to give only 8 ounces of formula six times a day

Answer: 1

Rationale: Another brand may have a different formula composition that might cause diarrhea. Also, adding new foods to the diet may precipitate diarrhea. Option 2 is incorrect because uneaten food should be refrigerated in a new jar to prevent further food breakdown and bacterial growth. Option 3 is incorrect because excessive sugar can cause an osmotic diarrhea, and it is not necessary to add sugar to the formula. Option 4 is incorrect because a 6-month-old infant should receive 6 ounces of formula four to five times a day to prevent overfeeding.

Test-Taking Strategy: Knowledge regarding the causes of diarrhea is helpful in answering the question. A key word in the stem that the reader should focus on is "prevention." Option 1 prevents diarrhea, whereas options 2, 3, and 4 are dietary causes of diarrhea. In addition, option 1 addresses the first step of the nursing process: Assessment!

Level of Cognitive Ability: Application
Phase of Nursing Process: Planning
Client Needs: Health Promotion and Maintenance
Content Area: Child Health

Reference

Wong, D. (1997). *Whaley and Wong's Nursing care of infants and children* (5th ed.). St. Louis: Mosby–Year Book, pp. 542, 544, 1234.

50. A child is receiving famotidine (Pepcid) as a part of the treatment for chalasia. A nurse should plan to teach the mother to give the medication to the child as prescribed to prevent

1 Regurgitation.
2 Constipation.
3 Esophageal irritation.
4 Increased peristalsis.

Answer: 3

Rationale: Pepcid is an H_2 blocker that decreases the production of gastric acid in the stomach. When gastric acid is decreased, there is less likelihood that esophageal irritation will occur as a result of reflux. Options 1 and 4 are incorrect because Pepcid does not affect motility of the gastrointestinal tract. Option 2 is incorrect because constipation is a side effect of Pepcid.

Test-Taking Strategy: Knowledge regarding the pharmacological action of Pepcid and why this medication is used for a client with chalasia is necessary to answer the question. If this question was difficult, review these concepts now!

Level of Cognitive Ability: Application
Phase of Nursing Process: Planning
Client Needs: Health Promotion and Maintenance
Content Area: Child Health

References

Hodgson, B., & Kizior, R. (1998). *Saunders nursing drug handbook 1998.* Philadelphia: W. B. Saunders, pp. 401–402.
Wong, D. (1997). *Whaley and Wong's Nursing care of infants and children* (5th ed.). St. Louis: Mosby–Year Book, p. 1461.

51. In planning care for a client who is to undergo cardiac catheterization, it is most important that the nurse include client's history of

1 Allergy to shellfish.
2 Hypertension.
3 Atrial fibrillation.
4 Cigarette smoking.

Answer: 1

Rationale: Allergy to seafood, iodine, or iodine contrast media in the preprocedure period may necessitate a skin test for allergy severity and the use of prophylactic antihistamines to prevent allergic response to the contrast medium. The other options are important parts of the client's history but are not specific to the issue of the question.

Test-Taking Strategy: Identify the key phrase "most important." Examine each option for relevance to the key issue: cardiac catheterization. Remember that the contrast medium used for cardiac catheterization usually has an iodine base and that the allergen in shellfish is usually iodine. Remember also that determining allergies is a key component of the initial assessment!

Level of Cognitive Ability: Application
Phase of Nursing Process: Planning
Client Needs: Safe, Effective Care Environment
Content Area: Adult Health/Cardiovascular

Reference

Chernecky, C., & Berger, B. (1997). *Laboratory tests and diagnostic procedures* (2nd ed.). Philadelphia: W. B. Saunders, pp. 322–324.

52. The plan of care for a client with acute myocardial infarction (MI) contains the nursing diagnosis Risk for Activity Intolerance. The nurse plans to

1 Provide positive reinforcement and encouragement during physical activity.
2 Provide adequate fluid intake before and after physical activity.
3 Provide assistance with self-care and provide frequent rest periods.
4 Administer oxygen as needed during activity.

Answer: 3

Rationale: The issue of the question is "activity intolerance." Progressive, gradual increases in activity should be done after MI. Gradual increases in activity prevent or minimize overtaxing of the heart. The nurse's role is to monitor and adjust client's activity level according to individual tolerance. Providing positive reinforcement and encouragement during physical activity and providing adequate fluid intake will not prevent or minimize the activity intolerance. Although administering oxygen seems to be an appropriate option, it is not the best choice in terms of the issue, activity intolerance.

Test-Taking Strategy: The issue of the question is the selection of the option that reflects the best plan for preventing or minimizing activity intolerance. Each of the incorrect options refers to specific ways to assist the client before, during, or after exercise. The correct answer is the option that is also the most global response.

Level of Cognitive Ability: Application
Phase of Nursing Process: Planning
Client Needs: Physiological Integrity
Content Area: Adult Health/Cardiovascular

Reference

Black, J., & Matassarin-Jacobs, E. (1997). *Medical-surgical nursing: Clinical management for continuity of care* (5th ed.). Philadelphia: W. B. Saunders, pp. 1264, 1273.

53. The client has polycystic kidney disease. Which nursing intervention would be included in developing a plan of care for this client?

1 Restrict fluid and sodium intake
2 Increase fluid and sodium intake
3 Insert an indwelling catheter
4 Monitor bladder for distention

Answer: 2

Rationale: Clients with polycystic kidney disease seem to waste, rather than retain, sodium. Thus they need an increased sodium intake and fluid intake of 1500–2000 mL per day.

Test-Taking Strategy: Knowledge of significant laboratory values in polycystic disease is required. Use the process of elimination. The client with polycystic disease would not necessarily demonstrate alterations in urinary elimination, which would eliminate options 3 and 4. In addition, option 3 presents the potential for infection. Restricting fluids is an unlikely intervention. If you had difficulty with this question, take time now to review therapeutic management in polycystic disease!

Level of Cognitive Ability: Application
Phase of Nursing Process: Planning
Client Needs: Physiological Integrity
Content Area: Adult Health/Renal

Reference

Black, J., & Matassarin-Jacobs, E. (1997). *Medical-surgical nursing: Clinical management for continuity of care* (5th ed.). Philadelphia: W. B. Saunders, p. 1679.

54. The nurse is caring for a full-term infant who is small for gestational age (SGA) immediately after delivery. The nurse's initial care plan in the delivery room to prevent heat loss would include

1. Placing the infant in a prewarmed transport unit.
2. Drying the infant with a warm blanket.
3. Submerging the infant's body into a warm water bath.
4. Allowing the mother to hold the infant immediately after delivery.

Answer: 2

Rationale: Immediately after delivery, the infant is extremely prone to heat loss by evaporation of amniotic fluid and needs to be thoroughly dried. The infant may then be placed in a prewarmed radiant warmer. If the infant does not need resuscitation, the infant may be wrapped in a warm blanket and given to the mother to hold. SGA infants are at higher risk for hypothermia and therefore should not be placed in a warm water bath, which could cause a decrease in body temperature. The infant is placed in a prewarmed transport unit in preparation for transfer to the nursery.

Test-Taking Strategy: The question asks you to identify the initial plan of care for the SGA newborn. Knowledge of the primary course of heat loss in the delivery room must be applied to select the correct answer. You should be able to eliminate options 1 and 3. For the remaining two options, remember that the infant needs to be dried first. If you had difficulty with this question, take time now to review the immediate care of the infant in the delivery room!

Level of Cognitive Ability: Application
Phase of Nursing Process: Planning
Client Needs: Safe, Effective Care Environment
Content Area: Maternity

Reference

Olds, S., London, M., & Ladewig, P. (1996). *Clinical handbook for maternal-newborn nursing: A family-centered approach* (5th ed.). Menlo Park, CA: Addison-Wesley, pp. 797, 863, 927.

---

55. The nurse is planning for the initial visit of the parents of a 26-week newborn with respiratory distress syndrome. Which of the following should the nurse plan to best facilitate bonding during the initial visit?

1. Explain the equipment used and how it functions to assist their newborn
2. Encourage the parents to touch their newborn
3. Identify specific caretaking tasks that may be assumed by the parents
4. Give the parents pamphlets that will help them understand their infant's condition

Answer: 2

Rationale: The best initial action that begins the attachment process and promotes bonding is to encourage the parents to touch their infant. The parents' initial need is to become acquainted with their newborn. Option 1 is important but should not overshadow the parent-infant bonding activities. Option 3 would be too frightening because of the condition of the newborn and the unfamiliarity of high-risk infant care practices. This option will be appropriate as the infant becomes stable. Option 4 is inappropriate initially; requiring parents to refocus on pamphlets or literature does not enhance the parent-infant bond.

Test-Taking Strategy: The issue of the question is the intervention that will "facilitate bonding." Use the process of elimination. All of the options are correct, but the priority or best choice is option 2 because this is the only option that addresses touch, which is directly related to bonding!

Level of Cognitive Ability: Application
Phase of Nursing Process: Planning
Client Needs: Psychosocial Integrity
Content Area: Maternity

Reference

Reeder, S., Martin, L., & Koniak-Griffin, D. (1997). *Maternity nursing: Family, newborn, and women's health care* (18th ed.). Philadelphia: Lippincott-Raven, p. 1148.

56. A Latino client has been diagnosed with myasthenia gravis. The client is unfamiliar with Western nursing practices, and neostigmine bromide (Prostigmin), 200 mg PO every 3–4 hours, has been prescribed. The nurse is concerned that the client will not comply with the medication regimen as prescribed. The most effective nursing plan of instruction should include

1 Having the client answer simply "Yes" or "No."
2 Avoiding slang to explain a medical term.
3 Touching the client while speaking.
4 Using a fluent translator.

Answer: 4

Rationale: The most effective plan is to use a translator (someone of the same language or culture) to explain the medication regimen. Options 1 and 2 do not ensure client understanding of the medical regimen. Touch is an unacceptable practice in many cultures.

Test-Taking Strategy: Use the process of elimination noting the key phrase "most effective." Eliminate options 1 and 2 first because these interventions do not ensure understanding. Remember that for a client from a different culture, touch may not be an acceptable practice and can adversely affect the nurse-client relationship.

Level of Cognitive Ability: Application
Phase of Nursing Process: Planning
Client Needs: Health Promotion and Maintenance
Content Area: Fundamental Skills

Reference

Hodgson, B., & Kizior, R. (1998). *Saunders nursing drug handbook 1998.* Philadelphia: W. B. Saunders, pp. 732–735.

---

57. The client has an occipital lobe infarct with homonymous hemianopsia and requires safe surroundings when ambulating. The nurse's care plan would include

1 Use of a hand-held magnifier for reading and close work.
2 Routine visual field examinations.
3 Color-contrasted doors and hallways.
4 Eye patch to affected eye.

Answer: 3

Rationale: Ambulatory clients with visual field deficits do not distinguish between colors very well and therefore require bright (not pastel) colored doors, doorknobs, hallway corners, and other environmental landmarks. Visual acuity, addressed in option 1, is important but is not directly related to this client's specific problem. Option 2 is important but not related to the question. Option 4 would be inappropriate because the medical condition, homonymous hemianopsia, involves half vision of both eyes.

Test-Taking Strategy: Knowledge regarding the physiological manifestations associated with homonymous hemianopsia is necessary to answer the question. This condition and safety are the issues of the question. Take time now to review interventions specifically appropriate to this condition if you had difficulty with this question. You are likely to find a question related to this condition on NCLEX-RN!

Level of Cognitive Ability: Application
Phase of Nursing Process: Planning
Client Needs: Safe, Effective Care Environment
Content Area: Adult Health/Neurological

Reference

Black, J., & Matassarin-Jacobs, E. (1997). *Medical-surgical nursing: Clinical management for continuity of care* (5th ed.). Philadelphia: W. B. Saunders, pp. 712–713.

58. The nurse plans the care of an elderly client admitted with osteoporosis. The physician has scheduled a diagnostic technique, photon absorptiometry, for the morning. The nurse recognizes a vital step in the development of this plan of care to be

1 Protect client from high-dose radiation.
2 Prepare the area to be injected aseptically.
3 Ensure that the client has no metal on clothing.
4 Inform the client that the procedure is painless.

Answer: 4

Rationale: Photon absorptiometry uses two sources of radiation of different energies to measure the density of the bone with a low dose of radiation. This diagnostic test requires no invasive technique such as an injection or placement of a scope. The test does not use a magnetic field so there is no danger with metal.

Test-Taking Strategy: To answer the question, an adequate knowledge of the common diagnostic tests that measure the density of bone with osteoporosis is required. Take time now to review this diagnostic test if you are unfamiliar with it!

Level of Cognitive Ability: Application
Phase of Nursing Process: Planning
Client Needs: Safe, Effective Care Environment
Content Area: Adult Health/Musculoskeletal

Reference

Lewis, S., Collier, I., & Heitkemper, M. (1996). *Medical-surgical nursing: Assessment and management of clinical problems* (4th ed.). St. Louis: Mosby–Year Book, pp. 1834–1835.

---

59. The nurse prepares a nursing care plan for the client with inflamed joints. In the planning stage, the essential tool/tools identified to maintain proper positions of rest for inflamed joints is/are

1 Large pillows.
2 Foot boards.
3 Small pillows.
4 Soft mattress.

Answer: 3

Rationale: Small pillows, trochanter rolls, and splints will properly and safely maintain proper positions for rest of inflamed joints. Large pillows may cause positions of more flexion than indicated. A soft mattress and foot boards should be avoided.

Test-Taking Strategy: Knowledge regarding appropriate modalities will aid in answering the question. Read each response and eliminate answers that are not beneficial to properly maintain inflamed joints. Eliminate option 2 first, because there is no direct relationship to resting joints. In general, soft mattresses are not beneficial. For the remaining two options, try to visualize the use of each. Soft pillows will be most effective in positioning inflamed joints. If you had difficulty with this question, take time now to review care of the client with inflamed joints!

Level of Cognitive Ability: Application
Phase of Nursing Process: Planning
Client Needs: Safe, Effective Care Environment
Content Area: Adult Health/Musculoskeletal

Reference

Burrell, P., Gerlach, M., & Pless, B. (1997). *Adult nursing: Acute and community care* (2nd ed.). Stamford, CT: Appleton & Lange, p. 1648.

---

60. A client with active tuberculosis is admitted to the medical-surgical unit for treatment of pneumonia. When a bed assignment is planned, proper acid-fast bacteria isolation precautions are followed when the nurse

1 Transfers the client to the intensive care unit (ICU).
2 Assigns the client to a double room, because intravenous antibiotics will be administered.
3 Assigns the client to a double room and places a "strict handwashing" sign outside the door.
4 Places the client in a private, well-ventilated room.

Answer: 4

Rationale: According to category-specific (respiratory) isolation precautions, acid-fast bacteria isolation always necessitates a private room. The room is well-ventilated and should have at least six exchanges of fresh air per hour and should be ventilated to the outside if possible. Therefore, option 4 is the only appropriate answer.

Test-Taking Strategy: Note that the question states "active tuberculosis." Knowledge of acid-fast bacteria (respiratory) isolation will assist you in answering this question. Option 4 is the only correct response. Options 2 and 3 are similar in that they involve a double room. Remember that options that are similar are not likely to be correct. Review care of the client with active tuberculosis now if you had difficulty with this question!

Level of Cognitive Ability: Application
Phase of Nursing Process: Planning
Client Needs: Safe, Effective Care Environment
Content Area: Adult Health/Respiratory

Reference

Ignatavicius, D. D., Workman, M. L., & Mishler, M. A. (1995). *Medical-surgical nursing: A nursing process approach* (2nd ed.). Philadelphia: W. B. Saunders, pp. 595, 720.

---

61. The client with acquired immunodeficiency syndrome (AIDS) is experiencing shortness of breath related to *Pneumocystis carinii* pneumonia. Which of the following measures does the nurse include in the plan of care to assist the client in performing activities of daily living?

1 Provide supportive care
2 Provide meals and snacks with high protein, high calorie, and high nutritional value
3 Provide small frequent meals
4 Offer food with low microbial content

Answer: 1

Rationale: Providing supportive care as needed reduces the client's physical and emotional energy demands and conserves energy resources for other functions, such as breathing. Options 2, 3, and 4 are important interventions for the client with AIDS, but they do not answer the question. Option 2 will assist the client in maintaining appropriate weight and proper nutrition. Option 3 will assist the client in tolerating meals better. Option 4 will decrease the client's risk of infection.

Test-Taking Strategy: Identify the issue of the question. Options 2, 3, and 4 are all important interventions for the client with AIDS, but they do not address the question. Option 1 is the only response that answers the question. Also, if you look at the other options, you will notice a similarity in that they are all dietary interventions. Option 1 is the option that is different.

Level of Cognitive Ability: Application
Phase of Nursing Process: Planning
Client Needs: Physiological Integrity
Content Area: Adult Health/Respiratory

Reference

Ignatavicius, D. D., Workman, M. L., & Mishler, M. A. (1995). *Medical-surgical nursing: A nursing process approach* (2nd ed.). Philadelphia: W. B. Saunders, pp. 516–517.

---

62. While doing discharge planning for a female teenager with anorexia nervosa, the nurse suggests that the client attend a meeting of the local chapter of Anorexia Nervosa and Associated Disorders. Which of the following responses by the teen indicates that she will most likely be compliant with this plan?

1 "I'll go once but if I don't like it I won't go back."
2 "I'll think about it."
3 "I'll do whatever I have to do to get out of this place."
4 "I'm going to do whatever it takes to get better."

Answer: 4

Rationale: Self-help groups have grown in numbers and credibility in recent years and serve to reduce the possibilities of further emotional distress that leads to pathology and necessary treatment. Option 1 indicates that the client already has doubts about participation and has given herself permission to terminate it before giving it a try. Option 2 could be correct at first glance but displays an ambivalent attitude that promises nothing. Option 3 indicates that the client's thinking is limited to short-term goals. Option 4 shows that the client is a proactive participant in her plan of care.

Test-Taking Strategy: Identify the key word "most" in the question. Use the process of elimination in answering this question, selecting the option that demonstrates the most positive client response in terms of participation!

Level of Cognitive Ability: Application
Phase of Nursing Process: Planning
Client Needs: Psychosocial Integrity
Content Area: Mental Health

Reference

Townsend, M. (1996). *Psychiatric–mental health nursing: Concepts of care* (2nd ed.). Philadelphia: F. A. Davis, p. 141.

63. The client is scheduled to have electroconvulsive therapy (ECT). The nurse plans to teach the client that

1 There are no expected side effects associated with ECT.
2 Amnesia of events occurring near the period of the treatment is common.
3 Many clients suffer long-term memory loss.
4 The client will receive no medications during the procedure.

Answer: 2

Rationale: The most common side effects of ECT include amnesia of events occurring near the period of the treatment and the potential for transient confusion as a result of the seizure and barbiturate anesthetic. Option 1 is clearly incorrect. Option 3 is incorrect because in most cases clients suffer little long-term memory loss. Option 4 is a false statement because general anesthesia and a muscle relaxant (often succinylcholine) are the usual clinical standards.

Test-Taking Strategy: This question is testing knowledge of the specific teaching necessary to prepare the client for ECT therapy. The nurse needs to know expected side effects and associated medication therapy to correctly apply this knowledge when planning a teaching session. Review the side effects related to ECT now if you had difficulty with this question!

Level of Cognitive Ability: Application
Phase of Nursing Process: Planning
Client Needs: Safe, Effective Care Environment
Content Area: Mental Health

Reference

Carson, V., & Arnold, E. (1996). *Mental health nursing: The nurse-patient journey.* Philadelphia: W. B. Saunders, p. 785.

64. A 4-year-old child is reluctant to take deep breaths after abdominal surgery. An effective plan to encourage deep breathing is to

1 Have the child pretend that he or she is the big, bad wolf blowing the little pig's house down.
2 Give the child colorful balloons to blow up.
3 Tell the child to exhale forcefully through the peak flow meter.
4 Administer chest percussion in several postural drainage positions.

Answer: 1

Rationale: The preschooler has a vivid imagination and loves to pretend. Engaging the child in therapeutic play appropriate to age is considered the most effective way to intervene. Balloons are unsafe because of the potential for aspiration of latex. The peak flow meter is used to assess vital capacity rather than to encourage breathing. Chest percussion and postural drainage will not affect depth of respiration.

Test-Taking Strategy: With careful reading of the situation for age, option 2 can be eliminated for safety reasons, and option 3 because of language too advanced for the child's age. Option 4 does not relate directly to the outcome of deep breathing and can be eliminated. Incorporating play into interventions for children often is an indication of a correct response. Review the stages of growth and development and the relationship to the hospitalized child now if you had difficulty with this question!

Level of Cognitive Ability: Application
Phase of Nursing Process: Planning
Client Needs: Physiological Integrity
Content Area: Child Health

Reference

Wong, D. (1997). *Whaley and Wong's Essentials of pediatric nursing* (5th ed.). St. Louis: Mosby–Year Book, p. 644.

65. The nurse's teaching plan for the client with a family history of breast cancer should include

1 Teaching breast self-examination technique, to be done every month.
2 Teaching the importance of weight-bearing exercises.
3 Assessing for grief reactions.
4 Implementing measures to prevent breast cancer.

Answer: 1

Rationale: Monthly breast self-examination is recommended for all adult women. It is especially important for those with a familial history of breast cancer. Although a healthy lifestyle, including diet and exercise, decreases the risk for cancer, weight-bearing exercises are important specifically in preventing osteoporosis. Assessing for grief does not relate to the issue of the question. There are no specific measures that can be implemented by the client that will prevent breast cancer.

Test-Taking Strategy: This question focuses on teaching, which allows you to eliminate options 3 and 4 first. Of the remaining two options, option 1 directly relates to the issue of the question. If this question was difficult, take a few moments to review cancer prevention and detection techniques for major cancer sites!

Level of Cognitive Ability: Application
Phase of Nursing Process: Planning
Client Needs: Health Promotion and Maintenance
Content Area: Adult Health/Oncology

Reference

Black, J., & Matassarin-Jacobs, E. (1997). *Medical-surgical nursing: Clinical management for continuity of care* (5th ed.). Philadelphia: W. B. Saunders, p. 2432.

---

66. A client is being treated with levothyroxine sodium (Synthroid). A nurse should plan to teach the client that possible side effects of this medication would include

1 Constipation.
2 Weight gain.
3 Chest pain.
4 Sleepiness.

Answer: 3

Rationale: Thyroid preparations increase metabolic rate, oxygen demands, and demands on the heart. This can result in angina pectoris. Options 1, 2, and 4 result from a deficit of thyroid hormone.

Test-Taking Strategy: Knowledge of the effects of thyroid hormone secretion will assist you in selecting the correct answer. A review of this medication may be helpful if this question was difficult. Take time now to review!

Level of Cognitive Ability: Application
Phase of Nursing Process: Planning
Client Needs: Health Promotion and Maintenance
Content Area: Adult Health/Endocrine

Reference

LeMone, P., & Burke, K. M. (1996). *Medical-surgical nursing: Critical thinking in client care.* Menlo Park, CA: Addison-Wesley, pp. 683, 685.

---

67. Which of these measures planned by the nurse would be most effective in preventing complications for a client with Addison's disease?

1 Restricting fluid intake
2 Offering foods high in potassium
3 Assessing family support system
4 Monitoring blood glucose

Answer: 4

Rationale: The decrease in cortisol secretion that characterizes Addison's disease can result in hypoglycemia. Fluid intake should be encouraged to compensate for dehydration. Potassium intake should be restricted due to hyperkalemia. Option 3 is not a priority for this client in the question as stated.

Test-Taking Strategy: Knowledge regarding the manifestations associated with Addison's disease is necessary to answer this question. Use the steps of the nursing process which will assist in eliminating options 1 and 2. Options 3 and 4 both address assessment; however, option 4 addresses the physiological need. According to Maslow's hierarchy of needs theory, physiological needs come first!

Level of Cognitive Ability: Application
Phase of Nursing Process: Planning
Client Needs: Physiological Integrity
Content Area: Adult Health/Endocrine

Reference

LeMone, P., & Burke, K. M. (1996). *Medical-surgical nursing: Critical thinking in client care.* Menlo Park, CA: Addison-Wesley, pp. 696, 698.

68. What equipment should the nurse plan to have at the bedside when initiating a clear liquid diet in a postoperative client who has had general anesthesia?

1 Oxygen via nasal cannula
2 Suction equipment
3 Cardiac monitor
4 A straw

Answer: 2

Rationale: General anesthesia depresses the gag reflex, which in turn increases the risk for aspiration. Suction equipment must be available in the event the client aspirates. Oxygen may be administered postoperatively and a cardiac monitor may be present, but they have nothing to do with initiation of postoperative diet intake. A straw may help the client sip fluids but is not necessary.

Test-Taking Strategy: Identify the issue of the question, which is the risk for aspiration and airway clearance. Options 3 and 4 can be easily eliminated. For the remaining two options, remember the issue. Option 2 maintains airway clearance.

Level of Cognitive Ability: Application
Phase of Nursing Process: Planning
Client Needs: Safe, Effective Care Environment
Content Area: Fundamental Skills

Reference

Craven, R. F., & Hirnle, C. J. (1996). *Fundamentals of nursing: Human health and function* (2nd ed.). Philadelphia: Lippincott-Raven, pp. 674–675.

---

69. The client is scheduled for endoscopic retrograde cholangiopancreatography (ERCP). In order to care for the client undergoing this procedure, the nurse would include which of the following in the plan of care?

1 Administer enemas the evening before and the morning of the procedure
2 After the procedure, keep client NPO until the gag reflex returns
3 Keep the client on clear liquids for 24 hours before the procedure
4 Tell the client that substances used contain only traces of radioactivity

Answer: 2

Rationale: ERCP requires that a client is on NPO status 8 hours before the procedure. Because an endoscope is inserted through the oral cavity, the throat will be sprayed with an anesthetic and the client will be kept NPO until the gag reflex returns. A client will be on clear liquids 1–3 days before a colonoscopy. Enemas are used the evening before and morning of a proctosigmoidoscopy procedure. Nuclear imaging scans use tracer doses of radioactive isotopes.

Test-Taking Strategy: Knowledge of the care of a client undergoing common diagnostic procedures is needed to answer this question. In addition, if you know that ERCP involves endoscopic insertion through the throat with no bowel preparation needed, you will determine that option 2 is the right answer by the process of elimination.

Level of Cognitive Ability: Application
Phase of Nursing Process: Planning
Client Needs: Safe, Effective Care Environment
Content Area: Adult Health/Gastrointestinal

Reference

Lewis, S., Collier, I., & Heitkemper, M. (1996). *Medical-surgical nursing: Assessment and management of clinical problems* (4th ed.) St. Louis: Mosby–Year Book, p. 1093.

---

70. The anticipated therapeutic effect of fludrocortisone acetate (Florinef) for the treatment of Addison's disease is to

1 Stimulate the immune response.
2 Promote electrolyte balance.
3 Stimulate thyroid production.
4 Stimulate thyrotropin production.

Answer: 2

Rationale: Florinef is a long-acting oral medication with mineralocorticoid and moderate glucocorticoid activity that is used for long-term management of Addison's disease. Mineralocorticoids act on the renal distal tubules to enhance the reabsorption of sodium and chloride ions and the excretion of potassium and hydrogen ions. In small doses, fludrocortisone acetate causes sodium retention and increased urinary potassium excretion. Hypotension and fluid and electrolyte imbalance can develop rapidly if the medication is discontinued abruptly.

Test-Taking Strategy: Remember that Addison's disease produces deficiencies of glucocorticoids, mineralocorticoids, and androgens. Eliminate options 3 and 4 because they are similar. For the remaining two options, knowledge that Addison's disease is not related to the immune system will assist in directing you to the correct option, option 2.

Level of Cognitive Ability: Application
Phase of Nursing Process: Planning
Client Needs: Physiological Integrity
Content Area: Adult Health/Endocrine

Reference

Pinnell, N. (1996). *Nursing pharmacology.* Philadelphia: W. B. Saunders, p. 535.

---

71. The client diagnosed with paranoid schizophrenia has been exceedingly agitated, threatening and shouting at everyone and refusing to participate in therapy. Projection and denial are evident in these behaviors. The nursing action most important to the plan of care would be to

1 Collect information to develop a database.
2 Explore past experiences of acting out.
3 Explain that nothing is wrong and accept the behavior.
4 Recognize the level of client anxiety and set limits.

Answer: 4

Rationale: Denial is a failure of the client to recognize what is occurring in a situation and may result in inappropriate behavior. Projection is the disowning and attributing process that enables a person to remain blind to aspects of self and to distant perceptions of others. Setting firm limits on unacceptable and inappropriate behaviors in a nondefensive manner is part of the nursing role.

Test-Taking Strategy: Note the client behaviors identified in the question. Behaviors as such necessitate intervention by the nurse. This should direct you to option 4 because it is the only option that specifically provides client intervention. Limit setting is clarifying appropriate, expected behavior in lieu of potential or actual inappropriate behaviors.

Level of Cognitive Ability: Application
Phase of Nursing Process: Planning
Client Needs: Safe, Effective Care Environment
Content Area: Mental Health

Reference

Haber, J. (1997). *Comprehensive psychiatric nursing* (5th ed.). St. Louis: Mosby–Year Book, pp. 389, 391, 471, 473.

---

72. A client experiencing delusions of being poisoned is admitted to the hospital after not eating or drinking for several days. The client shows no evidence of dehydration and malnutrition at this time. The nurse should immediately prepare a nursing care plan for the client's need for

1 Physiological care.
2 Safety and security.
3 Self-esteem.
4 Love and belonging.

Answer: 2

Rationale: An important consideration when working with clients who have delusions is the maintenance of safety. There are no data to indicate that options 1, 3, and 4 require immediate attention.

Test-Taking Strategy: Knowledge of unsafe behaviors and delusions is necessary to assist you in answering this question. A key phrase is that the client "shows no evidence of dehydration and malnutrition." Use Maslow's hierarchy of needs. If a physiological need does not exist, safety takes precedence.

Level of Cognitive Ability: Application
Phase of Nursing Process: Planning
Client Needs: Safe, Effective Care Environment
Content Area: Mental Health

Reference

Haber, J. (1997). *Comprehensive psychiatric nursing* (5th ed.). St. Louis: Mosby–Year Book, pp. 595, 597.

73. The nurse is developing a nursing care plan for an elderly client with diabetic retinopathy secondary to Type II (non–insulin-dependent) diabetes. Which of the following nursing diagnoses would the nurse plan to address first as the highest priority for this client?

1 Body Image Disturbance related to perceived negative effect of visual changes
2 Pain related to degeneration of retina
3 Self-Concept Disturbance related to perceived loss of independence
4 High Risk for Injury related to decreased visual acuity

Answer: 4

Rationale: The individual with retinopathy suffers from varying degrees of visual impairment. Thus falls are a major concern, especially for the elderly client. According to Maslow's hierarchy of needs theory, safety would take precedence over self-concept and body image, thus eliminating options 1 and 3. Retinopathy is a painless pathological condition of diabetes, so option 2 is incorrect.

Test-Taking Strategy: The key concept inherent in this question is visual impairment, because the client has retinopathy. Knowing that retinopathy is a painless condition, eliminate option 2. Then select the option that addresses the most serious consequence of impaired vision: the risk for injury!

Level of Cognitive Ability: Application
Phase of Nursing Process: Planning
Client Needs: Safe, Effective Care Environment
Content Area: Adult Health/Endocrine

Reference

Ignatavicius, D. D., Workman, M. L., & Mishler, M. A. (1995). *Medical-surgical nursing: A nursing process approach* (2nd ed.). Philadelphia: W. B. Saunders, p. 1898.

---

74. After a home visit, a community health nurse is completing a plan of care for an elderly client who has hyperparathyroidism with severe osteoporosis. Which of the following high-risk nursing diagnoses would be the highest priority for this client?

1 Risk for Injury related to demineralization of bone, resulting in pathological fractures
2 Risk for Alteration in Nutrition: Less than Body Requirements related to anorexia and nausea
3 Risk for Constipation related to adverse effects of hypercalcemia on gastrointestinal tract
4 Risk for Ineffective Management of Therapeutic Regimen related to medication

Answer: 1

Rationale: The individual with hyperparathyroidism and severe osteoporosis would be at great risk for pathological fractures because of bone demineralization (option 1). Thus home safety would be a priority. Although options 2, 3, and 4 could be problematic for the client, the question does not specifically address these issues. Nursing diagnoses are prioritized by urgency of the problem and the degree of harm to the client if untreated.

Test-Taking Strategy: Use principles of prioritizing to answer this question. In addition, the question specifies that the client has severe osteoporosis as part of the hyperthyroidism. Select the response that has a similar concept (option 1): demineralization of bone, resulting in pathological fractures.

Level of Cognitive Ability: Application
Phase of Nursing Process: Planning
Client Needs: Safe, Effective Care Environment
Content Area: Adult Health/Endocrine

Reference

Black, J., & Matassarin-Jacobs, E. (1997). *Medical-surgical nursing: Clinical management for continuity of care* (5th ed.). Philadelphia: W. B. Saunders, p. 2033.

---

75. The nurse is developing a nursing care plan for a client with myxedema. The diagnosis identified is Alteration in Nutrition. Which of the following food sources would be most appropriate to include in the plan?

1 Peanut butter, avocado, and red meat
2 Skim milk, apples, whole-grain bread, and cereal
3 Organ meat, carrots, and skim milk
4 Seafood, spinach, and cream cheese

Answer: 2

Rationale: The nursing diagnosis for clients with hypothyroidism is Alteration in Nutrition: More than Body Requirements related to their decreased metabolic need. They should consume foods from all food groups, which will provide them with the necessary nutrients; however, the foods should be low in calories. Option 2 is the only one in which all the food choices are low in calories.

Test-Taking Strategy: Be careful with your selection of an answer when the options contain the word "and." Remember that the entire option must be correct. Therefore, carefully read the content before and after the "and." In options 1, 3, and 4, at least one of the food sources is high in fat content. All foods listed in option 2 are low in fat.

Level of Cognitive Ability: Application
Phases of Nursing Process: Planning
Client Needs: Health Promotion and Maintenance
Content Area: Adult Health/Endocrine

Reference

Ignatavicius, D. D., Workman, M. L., & Mishler, M. A. (1995). *Medical-surgical nursing: A nursing process approach* (2nd ed.). Philadelphia: W. B. Saunders, pp. 1778, 1847.

---

76. A client with Parkinson's disease "freezes" while ambulating, which increases the risk for falls. Which of the following suggestions might the nurse include in this client's plan of care to alleviate this problem?

1 Stand erect and use a cane to ambulate
2 Keep your feet close together while ambulating and use a walker
3 Consciously think about walking over imaginary lines on the floor
4 Use a wheelchair to move around

Answer: 3

Rationale: Clients with Parkinson's disease can develop bradykinesia (slow movement) or akinesia (freezing or no movement). Having these individuals imagine lines on the floor to step over can keep them moving forward. Although standing erect and using a cane can help prevent falls, these measures will not help a person with akinesia move forward. Clients with Parkinson's disease should walk with a wide gait, not with the feet close together. A wheelchair should be used only when the client can no longer ambulate with assistive devices such as canes or walkers.

Test-Taking Strategy: Knowledge regarding the manifestations of Parkinson's disease is necessary to answer the question. The stem asks for a plan for a client who "freezes" while ambulating. Option 3 encourages forward movement while ambulating. Take time now to review ambulation measures associated with Parkinson's disease if you had difficulty with this question!

Level of Cognitive Ability: Application
Phase of Nursing Process: Planning
Client Needs: Safe, Effective Care Environment
Content Area: Adult Health/Neurological

Reference

Polaski, A., & Tatro, S. (1996). *Luckmann's Core principles and practice of medical-surgical nursing.* Philadelphia: W. B. Saunders, p. 1177.

---

77. The nurse is caring for a client with adult respiratory distress syndrome (ARDS) who is mechanically ventilated. To which of the following client outcomes would the nurse assign the highest priority?

1 Having no occurrence of aspiration
2 Having pink, moist, intact, mucous membranes
3 Having an effective method of communication
4 Having no evidence of infection

Answer: 1

Rationale: Aspiration, mucous membrane lesions, ineffective communication, and infection are all possible complications for clients on mechanical ventilation. Aspiration takes the highest priority as it is the complication associated with maintaining a patent airway.

Test-Taking Strategy: Use the principles associated with prioritizing when answering this question. Remember the ABCs: airway, breathing, and circulation. Aspiration would jeopardize airway patency.

Level of Cognitive Ability: Application
Phase of Nursing Process: Planning
Client Needs: Safe, Effective Care Environment
Content Area: Adult Health/Respiratory

Reference

Burrell, P., Gerlach, M., & Pless, B. (1997). *Adult nursing: Acute and community care* (2nd ed.). Stamford, CT: Appleton & Lange, pp. 1967–1969.

78. The nurse is caring for a client with pneumonia who is to receive oxygen via nasal cannula. The nurse plans to provide a safe and effective delivery of the oxygen. Which of the following will not be a part of the nursing care plan?

1. Secure the oxygen tubing to the client's bottom sheet
2. Keep the humidification jar filled at all times with distilled water
3. Observe the client's nares frequently for skin breakdown
4. Check the oxygen flow rate and physician's orders every shift

Answer: 1

Rationale: If the tubing is attached to the client's bed linen, it could become dislodged from the nares whenever the client moves. The tubing should have sufficient slack and be secured to the client's clothes. Keeping the humidification jar filled will help prevent the client from breathing dehumidified oxygen. The nares should be checked frequently because oxygen will dry the nasal mucosa. Oxygen is a medication and should be verified every shift to ensure the correct rate.

Test-Taking Strategy: All of the answers with the exception of option 1 will promote the safe delivery of oxygen. Option 1, if implemented, could clearly disrupt the flow of oxygen for the client. Use the process of elimination in answering the question. If you had difficulty with this question, take time now to review the safety procedures associated with the administration of oxygen!

Level of Cognitive Ability: Application
Phase of Nursing Process: Planning
Client Needs: Safe, Effective Care Environment
Content Area: Fundamental Skills

Reference

Potter, P., & Perry, A. (1997). *Fundamentals of nursing: Concepts, process and practice* (4th ed.). St. Louis: Mosby–Year Book, pp. 1234–1235.

---

79. Which of these outcomes would be most appropriate for a client with dementia who has a nursing diagnosis of Self-Care Deficit?

1. Client will be oriented to place by the time of discharge
2. Client will correctly identify objects in his or her room by the time of discharge
3. Client will be free of hallucinations by the time of discharge
4. Client feeds self with cueing within 24 hours

Answer: 4

Rationale: Option 4 identifies an outcome directly related to the client's ability to care for self. Options 1, 2, and 3 are not related to the nursing diagnosis of Self-Care Deficit.

Test-Taking Strategy: Based on Maslow's hierarchy of needs theory, physiological needs take precedence. Option 4 is the only option that addresses a physiological need.

Level of Cognitive Ability: Application
Phase of Nursing Process: Planning
Client Needs: Physiological Integrity
Content Area: Mental Health

Reference

Luckmann, J. (1997). *Saunders manual of nursing care.* Philadelphia: W. B. Saunders, p. 167.

---

80. Which of the following goals would be planned by the emergency room nurse when a client comes in with rape-trauma syndrome?

1. Client will accept the trauma that has happened
2. Client will begin the healthy grief process
3. Client will not experience psychological trauma
4. Client will not use defense mechanisms

Answer: 2

Rationale: The client who has been raped is in the beginning stages of the grieving process. No one can be in the acceptance phase immediately after the rape. The goal that the individual will not experience psychological trauma is negated by the fact that the victim has been raped. Clients use defense mechanisms to help with the anxiety and some defense mechanisms, such as denial, have been described to be helpful to the client, especially in the immediate post-traumatic period.

Testing Taking Strategy: Use the process of elimination. Eliminate options 3 and 4 first, because the client is experiencing psychological trauma and because the use of defense mechanisms is helpful to clients in traumatic situations. Eliminate option 1 because the immediate period is too early to accept the trauma.

Level of Cognitive Ability: Application
Phase of Nursing Process: Planning
Client Needs: Psychosocial Integrity
Content Area: Mental Health

Reference

Townsend, M. (1996). *Psychiatric–mental health nursing: Concepts of care* (2nd ed.). Philadelphia: F. A. Davis, p. 770.

---

81. The client was admitted with 40% TBSA (total body surface area) burn wounds, primarily second-degree. Treatment consists of daily hydrotherapy and dressing changes. Before each hydrotherapy session, 10 mg of morphine is given IV. The client gets very agitated before the procedure and is having trouble sleeping at night because of nightmares about the previous procedures and worrying about future procedures. The nursing diagnosis is Anxiety related to the hydrotherapy and dressing changes. You should plan to speak with the physician about

1. Increasing the preprocedure dose of IV morphine.
2. Changing the preprocedure medication to meperidine (Demerol) 100 mg intramuscularly (IM).
3. Adding a benzodiazepine, such as midazolam (Versed), to the preprocedure medications.
4. Giving the client a sedative such as chloral hydrate prior to the procedure.

Answer: 3

Rationale: Midazolam (Versed) is commonly given before procedures to decrease the client's anxiety before the procedure. Midazolam also produces temporary amnesia during the procedure. The amnesia can help decrease insomnia because the client does not ruminate about the procedure after it. In addition, anxiety is further decreased before the procedure as a result of amnesia because there is less pain anticipation.

Test-Taking Strategy: Eliminate option 1 first because the client is already getting a moderate dose of morphine. Anxiety is likely to be a major factor in the perception of pain, and so at this time, the more appropriate intervention would be to decrease the anxiety. Option 2 is incorrect; IM injections are avoided in burn care because of the erratic fluid shifts that occur. Option 4 is eliminated next because this medication is used to treat insomnia and is administered at bedtime.

Level of Cognitive Ability: Application
Phase of Nursing Process: Planning
Client Needs: Psychosocial Integrity
Content Area: Adult Health/Integumentary

Reference

Richard, R., & Staley, M. (1994). *Burn care and rehabilitation: Principles and practice*. Philadelphia: F. A. Davis, pp. 490–496.

---

82. In planning a diet for the client with hypoparathyroidism, which of the following foods would be most suitable for the nurse to include?

1. Those high in calcium and low in phosphorus
2. Those low in vitamins A, D, E, and K
3. Those high in sodium with no fluid restriction
4. Those low in water-insoluble fiber

Answer: 1

Rationale: Hypocalcemia is the end result of hypoparathyroidism due to either a lack of parathyroid hormone (PTH) secretion or ineffective PTH on tissue. Calcium is the major controlling factor of PTH secretion. Dietary intervention therefore mandates ingestion of foods that are high in calcium but low in phosphorus, because these two electrolytes must exist in inverse proportions in the body. The other options are not even considered for dietary intervention with hypoparathyroidism.

Test-Taking Strategy: Knowledge of hypoparathyroidism and the associated hypocalcemia will assist you in selecting the correct answer. Options 2, 3, and 4 do not correct hypocalcemia. Take time now to review these concepts related to hypoparathyroidism if you had difficulty with this question!

Level of Cognitive Ability: Application
Phase of Nursing Process: Planning
Client Needs: Health Promotion and Maintenance
Content Area: Adult Health/Endocrine

Reference
Ignatavicius, D. D., Workman, M. L., & Mishler, M. A. (1995). *Medical-surgical nursing: A nursing process approach* (2nd ed.). Philadelphia: W. B. Saunders, pp. 1793, 1854.

---

83. The nurse is planning care for a client with Bell's palsy. Which of the following measures should be included?

1 Apply cold pack to the affected side QID
2 Have the client avoid wearing dark glasses
3 Instill artificial tears and patch or tape the affected eye at night
4 Have the client avoid touching the affected side

Answer: 3

Rationale: Instilling artificial tears and patching or taping the affected eye at night protects the eye from corneal abrasions. Warm, not cold, packs should be used. Dark glasses are recommended, as is gentle massage of the affected side.

Test-Taking Strategy: Knowledge regarding the pathophysiology and care of a client with Bell's palsy is necessary to answer the question. If this question was difficult, take a few moments to review this disorder and the nursing care now!

Level of Cognitive Ability: Application
Phase of Nursing Process: Planning
Client Needs: Safe, Effective Care Environment
Content Area: Adult Health/Neurological

Reference
Lewis, S., Collier, I., & Heitkemper, M. (1996). *Medical-surgical nursing: Assessment and management of clinical problems* (4th ed.). St. Louis: Mosby–Year Book, p. 1796.

---

84. A client with Guillain Barré syndrome has been asking many questions about the condition. The staff feels that the client is very discouraged. When planning care for this client, it is important for the nurse to include which of the following information?

1 Maximum paralysis is reached within 48 hours
2 Paralysis occurs proximally to distally
3 With maximum rehabilitation, function is regained within 3 months
4 In general, 85%–90% of people recover from this condition

Answer: 4

Rationale: Most clients with Guillain Barré syndrome recover from the paralysis because it affects peripheral nerves, which have the capacity to remyelinate. Maximum paralysis can take up to 4 weeks to develop. Paralysis progresses distally to proximally. Rehabilitation can take from 6 months to 2 years.

Test-Taking Strategy: Options 1 and 3 present very restricted time frames. Disease progression and rehabilitation are generally individualized. The correct response allows more latitude. Remember that if one option includes qualifiers such as usually or generally (option 4), and the other options do not, select that option. One way to remember the progression of paralysis with *G*uillain *B*arré is that it moves from the "*G*round to the *B*rain."

Level of Cognitive Ability: Application
Phase of Nursing Process: Planning
Client Needs: Psychosocial Integrity
Content Area: Adult Health/Neurological

References
Black, J., & Matassarin-Jacobs, E. (1997). *Medical-surgical nursing: Clinical management for continuity of care* (5th ed.). Philadelphia: W. B. Saunders, p. 877.
Polaski, A., & Tatro, S. (1996). *Luckmann's Core principles and practice of medical-surgical nursing*. Philadelphia: W. B. Saunders, p. 385.

85. A client with myasthenia gravis is being discharged with a prescription of pyridostigmine bromide (Mestinon). The nurse planning discharge teaching should include which of the following information?

1 Take this medication on an empty stomach
2 Take the medication before activities such as eating, activities of daily living (ADLs), or work
3 Tonic water with quinine and antacids, such as Maalox, improve the effect of Mestinon
4 It is not important when you take the medication, as long as you take exact amount prescribed

Answer: 2

Rationale: Taking this medication before activities helps lessen fatigue and dysphagia and improves muscle strength. The medication should be taken with food. Clients should avoid quinine, magnesium, and morphine and its derivatives, because these medications can reverse the action of the Mestinon and increase weakness. The medication should be taken regularly and on time to prevent fluctuating blood levels, which can cause weakness.

Test-Taking Strategy: Knowledge of the medication and its nursing implications is necessary to answer this question. However, you might safely assume that because muscle weakness is a major problem with the disease, the medication would work best if taken before activities. Take time now to review this medication of you had difficulty with this question!

Level of Cognitive Ability: Application
Phase of Nursing Process: Planning
Client Needs: Health Promotion and Maintenance
Content Area: Pharmacology

Reference

Ignatavicius, D. D., Workman, M. L., & Mishler, M. A. (1995). *Medical-surgical nursing: A nursing process approach* (2nd ed.). Philadelphia: W. B. Saunders, p. 1228.

---

86. Discharge plans are being made for a client newly diagnosed with type II diabetes. Which of the following outcomes would be most important for this client?

1 Maintains health at optimum level
2 Achieves and maintains ideal body weight
3 Adjusts insulin to capillary blood glucose
4 Avoids all strenuous activities

Answer: 2

Rationale: Approximately 80% of all clients with non–insulin-dependent diabetes mellitus (NIDDM, or type II diabetes) are obese (more than 20% above ideal body weight). Overweight clients require more insulin to metabolize the food they eat. Circulating insulin, levels of which are increased with obesity, causes insulin resistance. Therefore, the best control of blood glucose levels occurs when the client is at ideal body weight.

Test-Taking Strategy: Use the process of elimination. The key words in this question are "most important." Because weight control is a crucial factor in achieving a goal of normoglycemia, option 2 is the correct answer. Option 1 is too vague. Option 3 is incorrect because most clients with newly discovered type II diabetes are placed on a regimen of diet, exercise, and possible oral hypoglycemic agents. Insulin is usually not given at this time.

Level of Cognitive Ability: Application
Phase of Nursing Process: Planning
Client Needs: Health Promotion and Maintenance
Content Area: Adult Health/Endocrine

Reference

Black, J., & Matassarin-Jacobs, E. (1997). *Medical-surgical nursing: Clinical management for continuity of care* (5th ed.). Philadelphia: W. B. Saunders, p. 1965.

87. When planning care for a woman with pregnancy-induced hypertension (PIH), which one of the following behaviors should be encouraged?

1. Expression of hope for a positive outcome
2. Delaying preparations for the nursery
3. Walking 1–2 miles daily
4. Anticipatory grieving

Answer: 1

Rationale: Hoping for a positive outcome is an appropriate coping mechanism. It is important to support an expression of hope by a client with a high-risk pregnancy as long as the hope is realistic (e.g., fetus is viable). Anticipatory grieving is no longer considered a positive adaptation. Grieving should begin when a loss occurs. Delaying nursery preparations reflects expectation of the worst and anticipatory grieving. Walking 1–2 miles is contraindicated for a woman with PIH.

Test-Taking Strategy: Knowledge of appropriate coping mechanisms and behaviors is necessary to answer this question. If you do not know the answer, try looking for similar distracters. Options 2 and 4 include the same idea of "preparing for the worst," and therefore neither of these options can be the correct answer. Eliminate option 3 because walking 1–2 miles daily is much too strenuous. Take time now to review the plan of care for a client with PIH if you had difficulty with this question!

Level of Cognitive Ability: Application
Phase of Nursing Process: Planning
Client Needs: Psychosocial Integrity
Content Area: Maternity

Reference

Nichols, F., & Zwelling, E. (1997). *Maternal-newborn nursing: Theory and practice.* Philadelphia: W. B. Saunders, pp. 650–652.

88. A woman with insulin-dependent diabetes is in labor. On the basis of the knowledge about insulin-dependent diabetes and pregnancy, the nurse will be prepared for a baby who is most likely to have which one of the following complications?

1. Macrosomia
2. Hyperglycemia
3. Postmaturity syndrome
4. Anemia

Answer: 1

Rationale: Typically, infants of diabetic mothers are large for gestational age. Maternal glucose crosses over the placenta to the fetus. The fetus is able to produce its own insulin; therefore excessive body growth (macrosomia) results from high maternal glucose. After birth, hypoglycemia may be a problem because the infant's pancreas continues to produce large amounts of insulin (hyperinsulinemia), which quickly depletes the infant's glucose supply. Infants of diabetic mothers are usually delivered just before or at term because of an increased risk of ketoacidosis and intrauterine fetal death after 36 weeks. Polycythemia, not anemia, is common in infants of diabetic women.

Test-Taking Strategy: This question is asking you to apply knowledge about diabetes and pregnancy in order to anticipate the needs of the infant after birth. If terms are unfamiliar, try to figure out the meaning by breaking the word down (e.g., "macro" = large; "soma" = body). Take time now to review diabetes and pregnancy if you had difficulty with this question!

Level of Cognitive Ability: Application
Phase of Nursing Process: Planning
Client Needs: Health Promotion and Maintenance
Content Area: Maternity

Reference

Nichols, F., & Zwelling, E. (1997). *Maternal-newborn nursing: Theory and practice.* Philadelphia: W. B. Saunders, p. 669.

89. In planning care for a client with impaired renal function who is receiving ergonovine maleate (Ergotrate) in the postpartum period, the nurse should plan care with the knowledge that

1. The medication may be given orally or by intramuscular injection.
2. The medication is eliminated mainly by hepatic metabolism and biliary excretion.
3. The medication is eliminated by hepatic metabolism and renal excretion.
4. The uterine stimulation effects persist for about 3 hours.

Answer: 2

Rationale: A client with impaired renal function is at less risk for medication side effects if given a uterine stimulating agent excreted mainly by hepatic metabolism. Route of administration and duration of effect are not major factors in the specific strategies used to produce uterine stimulation in the client with impaired renal function.

Test-Taking Strategy: Use knowledge of this medication and concepts related to renal disease to answer this question. Eliminate options 1 and 4 first. Of the remaining options, select option 2 because it is unlikely that this medication would be administered to a client with renal impairment if the medication is eliminated via renal excretion. If the question was difficult, take a few moments now to review the medication!

Level of Cognitive Ability: Application
Phase of Nursing Process: Planning
Client Needs: Safe, Effective Care Environment
Content Area: Maternity

Reference

Hodgson, B., & Kizior, R. (1998). *Saunders nursing drug handbook 1998*. Philadelphia: W. B. Saunders, p. 374.

---

90. What should the nurse know about erythromycin base (Ilotycin) ophthalmic ointment when planning newborn care immediately after delivery?

1. Ilotycin is more irritating to the newborn's eyes than are silver nitrate drops
2. It must be administered at room temperature to prevent side effects
3. It stains the infant's skin and must be wiped off immediately
4. Ilotycin is useful to protect the newborn from both neisserial gonorrhea and chlamydia

Answer: 4

Rationale: Erythromycin (Ilotycin) is effective against both neisserial gonorrhea and chlamydia. It is less irritating to the newborn's eyes than silver nitrate, does not stain, and may be administered safely at any temperature.

Test-Taking Strategy: Specific medication knowledge is needed to answer this question. If it is necessary, take a few moments now to review this medication!

Level of Cognitive Ability: Application
Phase of Nursing Process: Planning
Client Needs: Physiological Integrity
Content Area: Maternity

Reference

Hodgson, B., & Kizior, R. (1998). *Saunders nursing drug handbook 1998*. Philadelphia: W. B. Saunders, p. 377.

91. An antenatal client who has experienced two episodes of bleeding caused by a borderline placenta previa will be discharged to home care tomorrow. The nurse is planning the discharge instructions. The nurse is aware that there is a potential for fetal distress should the bleeding recur. Which of the following should be included in the nurse's plan in order to assist the client to identify whether the baby may be distressed?

1 Arrange for a Doppler study at home and teach the father to listen to the fetal heart tones daily
2 Make a referral to a home health agency for weekly ultrasound examinations for a biophysical profile
3 Give the mother instructions for daily fetal movement count sheets with instructions and assist her to practice today
4 Teach the father to measure the abdominal girth and fundal height of the client each morning

Answer: 3

Rationale: Regular fetal movements have been determined to be reliable indicators of fetal health. Maternal assessment of fetal movements has been reported to be at least 90% accurate as verified by ultrasonography. The procedure is easy to learn and noninvasive. It also allows self-care and reporting, which are major goals of health maintenance.

Test-Taking Strategy: Use teaching and learning principles when answering a health promotion or maintenance question. These include determining what can be done by the client and what needs professional intervention. Simplicity of the task and convenience should also be considered. Eliminate options that would not meet the educational goal. Option 4 addresses the father. Options 1 and 2 address professional intervention. Option 3 specifically addresses a task that the mother can perform and monitor.

Level of Cognitive Ability: Application
Phase of Nursing Process: Planning
Client Needs: Health Promotion and Maintenance
Content Area: Maternity

Reference

Lowdermilk, D., Perry, M., & Bobak, I. (1997). *Maternity and women's health care* (6th ed.). St. Louis: Mosby–Year Book, pp. 235, 773.

92. The client who was tested for human immunodeficiency virus (HIV) after a recent exposure had a negative test result. Which of the following items should the nurse plan to include in post-test counseling?

1 The test should be repeated in 6 months
2 This ensures that the client is not infected with HIV
3 The client no longer needs to protect sexual partners
4 The client probably has immunity to the acquired immunodeficiency syndrome (AIDS) virus

Answer: 1

Rationale: A negative test result indicates that no HIV antibodies were detected in the blood sample. A repeat test in 6 months is recommended because false-negative results have been obtained early in the course of infection.

Test-Taking Strategy: Begin to answer this question by eliminating options 3 and 4 because they are false statements. Even without specific knowledge of the implications of test results, you would choose option 1 over option 2 because the word "ensures" in that option is absolute and is therefore not likely to be correct.

Level of Cognitive Ability: Application
Phase of Nursing Process: Planning
Client Needs: Safe, Effective Care Environment
Content Area: Adult Health/Respiratory

Reference

Ignatavicius, D. D., Workman, M. L., & Mishler, M. A. (1995). *Medical-surgical nursing: A nursing process approach* (2nd ed.). Philadelphia: W. B. Saunders, p. 508.

93. A 15-year-old female seeks treatment for a sexually transmitted disease at a local clinic. The nurse plans to do which of the following to uphold the law regarding informed consent?

1 Immediately telephone the client's parents
2 Obtain her signature of informed consent
3 Withhold treatment pending approval of court order for treatment
4 Mail a copy of the consent to the parents by registered mail

Answer: 2

Rationale: Parents must give informed consent for treatment of a minor with three exceptions. The first is to give emergency treatment. The second is when the consent of the minor is sufficient, such as for treatment of a sexually transmitted disease. The third is when a court order or other legal authorization has been made.

Test-Taking Strategy: Look for key words or phrases, which in this question are "15-year-old," "sexually transmitted disease," and "law." Remember also that options that are similar are more likely to be incorrect; thus eliminate options 1 and 4. To discriminate correctly between options 2 and 3, it is necessary to know the law regarding consent for treatment of minors. Review these laws now if you had difficulty with this question!

Level of Cognitive Ability: Application
Phase of Nursing Process: Planning
Client Needs: Safe, Effective Care Environment
Content Area: Fundamental Skills

Reference

DeLaune, S., & Ladner, P. (1998). *Fundamentals of nursing: Standards and practice.* Albany, NY: Delmar, p. 238.

---

94. The nurse is teaching a series of classes on maintaining a healthy pregnancy. The goal for tonight's class is "The pregnant woman will verbalize measures which may prevent traumatic conditions distressing to the fetus." Which of the following is a part of the teaching plan for this class?

1 Travel precautions and use of shoulder seat belts
2 Use of over-the-counter medications
3 Fetotoxic substances in the work place
4 Effects of primary and secondary cigarette smoke on the fetus

Answer: 1

Rationale: Placental separation as a result of uterine distortion can result from trauma, such as in car accidents. Placental separation decreases or shuts off uteroplacental circulation. Partial separation results in fetal distress; the distress increases in accordance with the degree of separation. Complete separation leads to sudden severe fetal distress, followed by fetal death. Use of the shoulder seat belt decreases the risk of placental separation by preventing the traumatic flexion of the woman's body that results from sharp braking or impact.

Test-Taking Strategy: Note the issue of the question "traumatic conditions." Option 1 specifically addresses trauma related to such injuries as a car or other vehicle accident. Options 2, 3, and 4 are also important teaching points but are not directly related to the issue of the question!

Level of Cognitive Ability: Application
Phase of Nursing Process: Planning
Client Needs: Health Promotion and Maintenance
Content Area: Maternity

Reference

Olds, S., London, M., & Ladewig, P. (1996). *Clinical handbook for maternal-newborn nursing: A family-centered approach* (5th ed.). Menlo Park, CA: Addison-Wesley, p. 138.

---

95. A client with a history of preterm labor is being managed at home on oral terbutaline sulfate (Brethine). The home care nurse develops a care plan that includes instructing the client taking this medication to

1 Watch for the side effects of nausea and vomiting.
2 Check her pulse before taking each dose.
3 Expect to feel chills during the course of treatment.
4 Realize it is normal to feel lethargic while taking this medication.

Answer: 2

Rationale: A major side effect of terbutaline (Brethine) is tachycardia. Other side effects include hyperglycemia, flushing, diaphoresis, tremors, and restlessness.

Test-Taking Strategy: Knowledge of this medication and its side effects is needed. By the process of elimination, note that option 2 involves an action on the part of the client rather than simple knowledge of the side effects. If you are unfamiliar with this medication, take time now to review this medication and its associated side effects!

Level of Cognitive Ability: Application
Phase of Nursing Process: Planning
Client Needs: Physiological Integrity
Content Area: Pharmacology

Reference

Hodgson, B., & Kizior, R. (1998). *Saunders nursing drug handbook 1998.* Philadelphia: W. B. Saunders, pp. 968–970.

96. Risk factors for placental abruption include lifestyle situations. In planning client education to prevent this complication, the nurse includes discussion of risks associated with use of

1 Cocaine.
2 Artificial sweeteners.
3 Salt.
4 Aspirin.

Answer: 1

Rationale: Identified risk factors for placental abruption include substances that decrease blood flow to the placenta or increase intrauterine pressure. Cocaine is a potent vasoconstrictor that has been associated with an increased risk for abruption. The other options have no known effect on decreasing circulation or increasing intrauterine pressure.

Test-Taking Strategy: By the process of elimination, look at the option that is known to be a high-risk substance. Knowledge of cocaine's effects and contributing factors to the development of placental abruption is needed. The phrase "lifestyle situations" in the question should assist in directing you to the correct option. Review this content now if you had difficulty answering the question!

Level of Cognitive Ability: Application
Phase of Nursing Process: Planning
Client Needs: Health Promotion and Maintenance
Content Area: Maternity

Reference

Nichols, F., & Zwelling, E. (1997). *Maternal-newborn nursing: Theory and practice.* Philadelphia: W. B. Saunders, p. 874.

97. The child with spina bifida (meningomyelocele) is found to have a neurogenic bladder with hydronephrosis. The nurse prepares a nursing care plan for this child with the understanding that hydronephrosis is a condition that

1 Results from urinary vesicoureteral reflux.
2 Causes blood in the urine.
3 Is not a curable condition.
4 Is manifested by decreased bowel sounds.

Answer: 1

Rationale: Vesicoureteral reflux results from enlargement of the ureters and incomplete emptying of the neurogenic bladder. Urine flows back up into the ureters and eventually into the kidneys. This causes hydronephrosis (enlarged kidneys). Protein, not blood, would be found in the urine at this time. Intermittent catheterization technique carried out around the clock and ureteral reimplant surgery are methods of treatment used. Bowel sounds are not related to the urinary system.

Test-Taking Strategy: Knowledge regarding hydronephrosis is necessary to answer the question. Eliminate option 4 first because the condition is not bowel related. Eliminate option 3 next because of the use of the absolute term "not." From this point, the term "hydronephrosis" does not indicate blood; therefore, the best option is option 1.

Level of Cognitive Ability: Analysis
Phase of Nursing Process: Planning
Client Needs: Physiological Integrity
Content Area: Child Health

Reference

Ashwill, J., & Droske, S. (1997). *Nursing care of children: Principles and practice.* Philadelphia: W. B. Saunders, p. 1234.

98. For a client with a T4 spinal cord injury, the nurse would develop which plan that would most likely prevent autonomic dysreflexia?

1 The client performs self-catheterization every 6 hours
2 The client turns, coughs, and deep breathes every 2 hours
3 The client takes anticoagulant as ordered daily
4 The client wears elastic stockings while upright

Answer: 1

Rationale: Autonomic dysreflexia (hyperreflexia) often results from a full bladder. Clients are taught to perform self-catheterization regularly to prevent the problem.

Test-Taking Strategy: Both options 3 and 4 are measures to prevent thromboembolism. Because they are similar, neither is correct. Dysreflexia is not caused by respiratory complications; therefore, eliminate option 2. Take time now to review the precipitating factors of autonomic dysreflexia if you had difficulty with this question!

Level of Cognitive Ability: Application
Phase of Nursing Process: Planning
Client Needs: Physiological Integrity
Content Area: Adult Health/Neurological

Reference

Ignatavicius, D. D., Workman, M. L., & Mishler, M. A. (1995). *Medical-surgical nursing: A nursing process approach* (2nd ed.). Philadelphia: W. B. Saunders, p. 1186.

---

99. Which of the following activities would the nurse include in the care plan to maximize the safety of the client when positioning?

1 Position upper extremities at a zero to 20 degree angle to the body only
2 Position bony prominences such as the heels and elbows on a firm surface
3 Position the safety strap directly above the knees
4 Position body for weight to be distributed as evenly as possible

Answer: 4

Rationale: To minimize the complications in client positioning, the body weight should be distributed as evenly as possible to decrease pressure on bony prominences. Upper extremities should not be positioned at an angle greater than 90 degrees because this could crush the brachial plexus between the first rib and scapula. Bony prominences such as the heels, elbows, and sacrum are vulnerable pressure points and should be well padded. The safety strap should be applied 2 inches above the knees to avoid pressure on the popliteal nerve.

Test-Taking Strategy: All of the answers include concepts necessary for the provision of a safe environment. Note the key word "maximize." There is only one correct statement. Through the process of elimination, determine that option 4 is the only correct statement. The correct angle in option 1 should be 90 degrees or less. In option 2, the bony prominences should be padded to prevent pressure. The safety strap in option 3 should be placed 2 inches above the knees.

Level of Cognitive Ability: Application
Phase of Nursing Process: Planning
Client Needs: Safe, Effective Care Environment
Content Area: Fundamental Skills

Reference

Black, J., & Matassarin-Jacobs, E. (1997). *Medical-surgical nursing: Clinical management for continuity of care* (5th ed.). Philadelphia: W. B. Saunders, p. 477.

---

100. The physician has ordered digoxin (Lanoxin), 0.25 mg PO daily, for a client who has a myocardial infarction. Currently the client is in normal sinus rhythm (NSR) with a pulse rate of 96. In preparing the care plan, the nurse knows that Lanoxin will

1 Not affect cardiac conduction.
2 Slow the cardiac rate.
3 Maintain a constant cardiac rate.
4 Increase the cardiac rate.

Answer: 2

Rationale: Lanoxin improves cardiac contraction, slows the heart rate, promotes diuresis, and increases cardiac output.

Test-Taking Strategy: This question requires knowledge of the actions and uses of this medication, a cardiac glycoside. If you had difficulty with this question, take the time now to review this important medication!

Level of Cognitive Ability: Application
Phase of Nursing Process: Planning
Client Needs: Safe, Effective Care Environment
Content Area: Pharmacology

Reference

Hodgson, B., & Kizior, R. (1998). *Saunders nursing drug handbook 1998*. Philadelphia: W. B. Saunders, pp. 324–326.

101. The client is concerned about the electrocardiographic (ECG) rhythm displayed on the monitor. The nurse plans to discuss with the client basic information about the ECG wave form. Which of the following should the nurse plan to ask at the beginning of the education session?

1 "Are you concerned about the ECG rhythm?"
2 "What do you understand about the ECG rhythm?"
3 "Do you think there is a problem with your heart?"
4 "Do you know how to interpret an ECG rhythm strip?"

Answer: 2

Rationale: During the planning stage for client teaching, the nurse should plan for expected outcomes that identify the expected behavioral response of the client. In this case, plan to determine the client's knowledge and understanding of the ECG rhythm.

Test-Taking Strategy: Client-initiated teaching sessions begin with what the client already knows. Use the process of elimination. Option 4 can easily be eliminated because of the word "interpret." Options 1 and 3 focus on a problem with the client's heart. Option 2 allows the nurse to assess what has been taught and to determine what needs to be reinforced or what needs to change if further teaching is needed. Option 2 is also the only open-ended question of all the responses. Review teaching learning principles now if you had difficulty with this question!

Level of Cognitive Ability: Application
Phase of Nursing Process: Planning
Client Needs: Psychosocial Integrity
Content Area: Fundamental Skills

Reference

Smeltzer, S., & Bare, B. (1996). *Brunner and Suddarth's Textbook of medical-surgical nursing* (8th ed.). Philadelphia: Lippincott-Raven, p. 45.

102. The physician has prescribed propranolol (Inderal) for the client with frequent symptomatic premature ventricular contractions (PVCs). The nurse collects material to conduct an education session with the client and the client's family. Which of the following should the nurse plan to include in the teaching session?

1 Information about side effects
2 A description of other effective medications
3 Material about the cellular effect of the medication
4 Data regarding various dysrhythmias

Answer: 1

Rationale: This medication has side effects that could be disturbing to the client. These include hypotension, insomnia, lethargy, nightmares, and heart failure. The client should be alert to these so that appropriate follow-through can be sought.

Test-Taking Strategy: With this type of question, look carefully at the options. All of the options are related to the question; however, consider which options are inappropriate for client teaching, and eliminate those options. Option 2 is not directly related to Inderal. Option 3 addresses "cellular" effects, which may not be understood by the client. Option 4 addresses dysrhythmias, which is not directly related to the Inderal and may not be understood by the client.

Level of Cognitive Ability: Application
Phase of Nursing Process: Planning
Client Needs: Health Promotion and Maintenance
Content Area: Pharmacology

Reference

Hartshorn, J. C., Sole, M. L., & Lamborn, M. L. (1997). *Introduction to critical care nursing* (2nd ed.). Philadelphia: W. B. Saunders, p. 253.

103. The physician writes a prescription for digoxin (Lanoxin), 0.25 mg QD. The nurse plans to conduct an education session about the medication. Which of the following should the nurse stress in this teaching session?

1 Take the medication at the same time each day
2 Take both the radial and carotid pulses
3 Call the physician if the pulse is below 60 beats per minute
4 Stop taking the medication if the pulse is higher than 100

Answer: 3

Rationale: An important part of taking this medication is the pulse rate. Although it is important to take the medication at the same time each day, of greater importance is knowing the pulse rate. The pulse rate will guide the client in either taking the medication or calling the physician.

Test-Taking Strategy: Option 4 is inappropriate because the client should be taught never to stop taking a medication unless it has been discussed with the physician. Options 1, 2, and 3 are all appropriate; however, you must prioritize which is the most appropriate. Because the medication affects the pulse rate, knowing the pulse is essential in determining which action to take next—that is, to take the medication or to notify the physician. Option 3 is specific to digoxin and is the best option. Review this medication now if you had difficulty answering this question. This is an important medication, and you should be familiar with it!

Level of Cognitive Ability: Application
Phase of Nursing Process: Planning
Client Needs: Safe, Effective Care Environment
Content Area: Pharmacology

Reference

Kee, J., & Hayes, E. (1997). *Pharmacology: A nursing process approach* (2nd ed.). Philadelphia: W. B. Saunders, p. 474.

---

104. The client recovering from cardiogenic shock has experienced episodes of postural hypotension. Which action should the nurse plan to ensure safety while transferring the client from bed to chair?

1. Perform transfer only while using a hydraulic lift
2. Put client's shoes on, in order to avoid slipping on floor during transfer
3. Arrange for a transfer board to be used
4. Allow the client to dangle legs in a sitting position on the bed before transfer with nurse's assistance to chair

Answer: 4

Rationale: In cardiogenic shock, the nurse must take an active role in ensuring the client's safety and physical comfort. A major role of the nurse is monitoring the client's hemodynamic and cardiac status and then planning care to maximize cardiac function and provide safety. Allowing the client to sit on the side of the bed before transfer enables the body's baroreceptors to adjust vital centers to position changes and stabilize, thereby avoiding a fall as a result of postural hypotension. The nurse should remain with the client and assist in transfer to the chair.

Test-Taking Strategy: The issue of the question is "postural hypotension." Option 1 does not address the cause of hypotension or method of adjusting activity in client; a hydraulic lift would not be feasible or available in many cases. Option 2 may keep the client's feet from sliding but does not address adjustments needed in activity to avoid postural hypotension. Option 3 does not address the problem of hemodynamic adjustment to the client's position change.

Level of Cognitive Ability: Application
Phase of Nursing Process: Planning
Client Needs: Safe, Effective Care Environment
Content Area: Adult Health/Cardiovascular

Reference

Smeltzer, S., & Bare, B. (1996). *Brunner and Suddarth's Textbook of medical-surgical nursing* (8th ed.). Philadelphia: Lippincott-Raven, p. 259.

---

105. The client has a history of seizures. The physician ordered amitriptyline (Elavil), 25 mg three times daily. The nurse develops a plan of care for the priority nursing diagnosis for this client, which is High Risk for Injury related to

1. Decreased platelet aggregation.
2. Decreased seizure threshold.
3. Decreased mental acuity.
4. Depressed immunological system.

Answer: 2

Rationale: Elavil, a tricyclic antidepressant, lowers the seizure threshold, increasing the risk of seizures. This may not be the medication of choice for a client who is already at risk for seizure activity.

Test-Taking Strategy: The issue of the question relates to seizures and the use of the medication Elavil. Knowledge regarding this medication is necessary to answer the question. Use the process of elimination, noting that option 2 is the only option that is directly related to the issue of the question. Take time now to review the use and contraindications of Elavil if you had difficulty with this question!

Level of Cognitive Ability: Analysis
Phase of Nursing Process: Planning
Client Needs: Physiological Integrity
Content Area: Mental Health

Reference

Hodgson, B., & Kizior, R. (1998). *Saunders nursing drug handbook 1998*. Philadelphia: W. B. Saunders, p. 1103.

106. What is an appropriate nursing goal for a client with a nursing diagnosis of Alteration in Nutrition: More than Body Requirements related to uncontrolled eating?

1. Obtain a list of the client's food preferences
2. Daily weight measurement, using the same scale
3. Client will lose 2 pounds each week while hospitalized
4. Client is able to correctly identify nutritional value of selected foods

Answer: 3

Rationale: The case situation identifies the need for a behavioral outcome, which is written in very defined terms: they are specific and measurable, and they identify a time frame. Options 1, 2, and 4 can easily be eliminated if these criteria are used.

Test-Taking Strategy: Use the principles applied to the planning stage of the nursing process to answer this question. Options 1 and 2 are nursing orders. Option 4 is an evaluative statement. Goal statements are written in the future tense and identify a measurable outcome.

Level of Cognitive Ability: Application
Phase of Nursing Process: Planning
Client Needs: Physiological Integrity
Content Area: Adult Health/Gastrointestinal

Reference

Carpenito, L. (1995). *Nursing diagnosis: Application to clinical practice* (6th ed.). Philadelphia: Lippincott-Raven, pp. 644–645.

---

107. After assessing the client's acute anginal chest discomfort, the nurse should next plan to administer

1. Intravenous morphine sulfate.
2. Intravenous nitroglycerin (Tridil).
3. Sublingual nifedipine (Procardia).
4. Sublingual nitroglycerin (Nitrostat).

Answer: 4

Rationale: Angina usually responds to sublingual nitroglycerin. Pain relief usually begins within 1 or 2 minutes after the administration of sublingual nitroglycerin. Morphine sulfate and IV nitroglycerin are usually administered after the sublingual route has failed. Nifedipine is often used in the maintenance treatment of angina rather than for acute episodes.

Test-Taking Strategy: The question involves prioritizing of the plan of care. A key to the question is the client's problem, acute angina chest discomfort. Knowledge of the medication nitroglycerin and its roles in the treatment of angina is needed. Whereas all options are used in treating angina pectoris, only options 1, 2, and 4 are used for chest discomfort. From this point, remember that IV morphine sulfate and IV nitroglycerin are generally used after sublingual nitroglycerin has failed to relieve symptoms. Review these medications now if you had difficulty with this question!

Level of Cognitive Ability: Application
Phase of Nursing Process: Planning
Client Needs: Physiological Integrity
Content Area: Adult Health/Cardiovascular

Reference

Ignatavicius, D. D., Workman, M. L., & Mishler, M. A. (1995). *Medical-surgical nursing: A nursing process approach* (2nd ed.). Philadelphia: W. B. Saunders, p. 992.

---

108. A pregnant client at 28 weeks' gestation is scheduled by the nurse for a routine 1-hour oral glucose tolerance test (OGTT). The nurse should plan to teach the client to do which of the following for 3 days before the test?

1. Eat a diet with at least 150 g of carbohydrate
2. Eat a diet with at least 60 g of fat
3. Refrain from physical activity
4. Push fluids to 3000 mL per day

Answer: 1

Rationale: Client preparation for an OGTT includes ingestion of a diet with at least 150 g of carbohydrate per day for 3 days before the test. It is not necessary to recommended to increase fat intake for this test. Normal physical activity should be encouraged, not discontinued. Adjustment of fluid intake before the test is unnecessary.

Test-Taking Strategy: Begin to answer this question by recalling that an OGTT measures the ability of the body to handle carbohydrate. The carbohydrate is administered as a bolus, usually in a flavored beverage. Look for key words in the stem of the question such as "routine" and "3 days before." Combining your knowledge of the nature of the test with the knowledge that this is preparation for a routine screening, you would then eliminate each of the incorrect options, as they would not affect (options 2 and 4) or interfere with (option 3) test results.

Level of Cognitive Ability: Application
Phase of Nursing Process: Planning
Client Needs: Safe, Effective Care Environment
Content Area: Maternity

References

Black, J., & Matassarin-Jacobs, E. (1997). *Medical-surgical nursing: Clinical management for continuity of care* (5th ed.). Philadelphia: W. B. Saunders, pp. 1962–1963.

Wong, D., & Perry, S. (1998). *Maternal-child nursing care.* St. Louis: Mosby–Year Book, pp. 131, 265–266.

---

109. The adult client just admitted with heart failure also has a history of diabetes mellitus. The nurse would plan to call the physician to verify an order for which of the following medications that the client was also taking before admission?

1 NPH Insulin
2 Chlorpropamide (Diabinese)
3 Regular Insulin
4 Acarbose (Precose)

Answer: 2

Rationale: Chlorpropamide is an oral hypoglycemic agent that exerts an antidiuretic effect and should be administered cautiously or avoided in the client with cardiac impairment or fluid retention. It is a first-generation sulfonylurea. Insulin does not cause or aggravate fluid retention. Acarbose is a miscellaneous oral hypoglycemic agent.

Test-Taking Strategy: To answer this question correctly, it is necessary to know that chlorpropamide causes fluid retention. The key words in this question include "heart failure," "diabetes," and "verify." Taken together, these words imply that there is either an additive or adverse effect from one of the medications listed in the options. If you are unfamiliar with these medications, take a few moments now to review them!

Level of Cognitive Ability: Application
Phase of Nursing Process: Planning
Client Needs: Physiological Integrity
Content Area: Adult Health/Endocrine

Reference

McKenry, L., & Salerno, E. (1998). *Mosby's pharmacology in nursing* (20th ed.). St. Louis: Mosby–Year Book, pp. 804–805.

---

110. The nurse is planning a teaching session with the client with newly diagnosed diabetes who is taking NPH insulin at 7:00 A.M. The nurse would include self-monitoring for which of the following signs and symptoms in the late afternoon?

1 Nausea; vomiting; and abdominal pain
2 Drowsiness; red, dry skin; and fruity breath odor
3 Hunger; shakiness; and cool, clammy skin
4 Increased urination; thirst; and rapid, deep breathing

Answer: 3

Rationale: The client taking NPH insulin would experience peak effects of the medication from 6–12 hours after administration. At the time that the medication peaks, the client is at risk of hypoglycemia if food intake is insufficient. The nurse would teach the client to watch for signs and symptoms of hypoglycemia during this time frame. These signs and symptoms include anxiety, confusion, difficulty concentrating, blurred vision, cold sweating, headache, increased pulse, shakiness, and hunger. The other options list assorted signs and symptoms of hyperglycemia.

Test-Taking Strategy: Look for the key words in the stem, which include "NPH insulin," "self-monitoring," and "late afternoon." Using your knowledge of NPH insulin therapy, recall that this medication's effects peak during the afternoon, putting the client at risk for hypoglycemia. Knowledge of these signs and symptoms is needed to choose the correct option. It may be helpful to use the following rhyme to help remember hypoglycemia: "Cool and clammy, need some candy." Take a few moments to review the signs and symptoms of hypoglycemia now if you had difficulty with this question!

Level of Cognitive Ability: Application
Phase of Nursing Process: Planning
Client Needs: Health Promotion and Maintenance
Content Area: Adult Health/Endocrine

Reference

Black, J., & Matassarin-Jacobs, E. (1997). *Medical-surgical nursing: Clinical management for continuity of care* (5th ed.). Philadelphia: W. B. Saunders, p. 1989.

111. The nurse is planning to teach the diabetic client to perform blood glucose self-monitoring. The nurse should incorporate which of the following strategies to best help the client obtain an adequate capillary sample?

1 Cleanse the hands beforehand, using cool water
2 Let the arm hang dependently, and milk the digit
3 Puncture the center of the finger pad
4 Puncture the finger as deeply as possible

Answer: 2

Rationale: To stimulate circulation, which aids in an adequate capillary sample, the client should first wash the hands with warm water. The arm should be allowed to hang dependently, and the finger may be milked to promote obtaining a good-sized blood drop. The finger should be punctured near the side, not the center, because there are fewer nerve endings along the side of the finger. The puncture is only as deep as needed to obtain an adequate blood drop. Excessively deep punctures may lead to pain and bruising.

Test-Taking Strategy: Note the keys words in the stem, which are "best help." This implies that more than one option may be partially or totally correct. Begin to answer this question by eliminating options 3 and 4, because these are completely incorrect. Recall that vasodilation is stimulated by warmth, not cold. Therefore, option 2 is more correct than option 1. The hands should be cleansed before puncture, but warm water is better than cool.

Level of Cognitive Ability: Application
Phase of Nursing Process: Planning
Client Needs: Health Promotion and Maintenance
Content Area: Fundamental Skills

Reference
Lewis, S., Collier, I., & Heitkemper, M. (1996). *Medical-surgical nursing: Assessment and management of clinical problems* (4th ed.). St. Louis: Mosby–Year Book, p. 1455.

112. The nurse is planning to instruct the diabetic client with hypertension about "sick day management." Which of the following would the nurse avoid putting on a list of easily consumed carbohydrate containing beverages, for use when the client cannot tolerate food orally?

1 Ginger ale
2 Apple juice
3 Regular cola
4 Tomato juice

Answer: 4

Rationale: Diabetic clients should take in approximately 15 g of carbohydrate (CHO) every 1–2 hours when unable to tolerate food because of illness. Each of the beverages listed in options 1, 2, and 3 provide approximately 13–15 g of CHO in a 1/2-cup serving. Tomato juice is incorrect for two reasons: first, it is high in sodium and should not be used by the client with hypertension; second, it is a lesser source of CHO, providing only 5 g of CHO per 1/2 cup.

Test-Taking Strategy: Note the key words in the stem, which include "diabetic," "hypertension," and "avoid." This tells you that the question is looking for an item that should not be used by the hypertensive client. Because hypertension is aggravated by excess sodium intake, use the process of elimination and seek the option that is highest in sodium to be the correct answer to the question as stated.

Level of Cognitive Ability: Application
Phase of Nursing Process: Planning
Client Needs: Health Promotion and Maintenance
Content Area: Adult Health/Endocrine

Reference
Lutz, C., & Przytulski, K. (1997). *Nutrition and diet therapy* (2nd ed.). Philadelphia: F. A. Davis, p. 354.

113. The elderly diabetic client has difficulty viewing the calibration marks on a syringe and cannot accurately draw up the daily NPH insulin dose. The client is expressing doubt about self-management of this disorder, and the client's only close relative lives 30 minutes away. The nurse in the acute care facility should plan to investigate which of the following options before the client's discharge?

1. Obtaining a referral to a home health agency for prefilling syringes and ongoing support
2. Having the relative give the daily dose of insulin before going to work
3. Increasing the dose of the oral agent instead
4. Obtaining a large magnifying glass for the client's use at home

Answer: 1

Rationale: The key information in the stem of this question includes the client's physical inability to draw up the medication, the self-doubt regarding ability to manage the diabetes, and the unavailability of the family member. Combining these three factors would lead you to choose option 1 as the only option that considers each of these three variables in the client's situation.

Test-Taking Strategy: Read the stem of the question carefully. Evaluate each of the options as it relates to the stem. Options 2 and 4 are eliminated because they focus on the insulin therapy and do not consider the client's ability to self-manage the disease independently at home. Option 3 is blatantly incorrect. This leaves option 1 as the only choice that addresses all of the issues presented in the question.

Level of Cognitive Ability: Application
Phase of Nursing Process: Planning
Client Needs: Safe, Effective Care Environment
Content Area: Adult Health/Endocrine

Reference

Black, J., & Matassarin-Jacobs, E. (1997). *Medical-surgical nursing: Clinical management for continuity of care* (5th ed.). Philadelphia: W. B. Saunders, pp. 1978–1980.

---

114. The nurse has admitted a client with diabetic ketoacidosis (DKA) who has been placed on an insulin drip. The nurse plans to monitor which of the following serial laboratory results as they become available?

1. Calcium level
2. Sodium level
3. Potassium level
4. Serum osmolality

Answer: 3

Rationale: The client with DKA initially becomes hyperkalemic as potassium leaves the cells in response to lowered pH. Once the client is treated with fluid replacement and insulin therapy, the potassium level drops quickly. This is because potassium is carried into the cells along with glucose and insulin and also because potassium is excreted in the urine once rehydration has occurred. Thus the nurse must plan to carefully monitor the results of serum potassium levels and report hypokalemia promptly.

Test-Taking Strategy: To answer this question correctly, it is necessary to understand the relationship among glucose, insulin, and potassium in the treatment of DKA. Simply remembering that a relationship exists among these three components may assist in directing you to the correct option. This is an important concept and should be reviewed at this time if you had difficulty with this question!

Level of Cognitive Ability: Application
Phase of Nursing Process: Planning
Client Needs: Physiological Integrity
Content Area: Adult Health/Endocrine

Reference

Black, J., & Matassarin-Jacobs, E. (1997). *Medical-surgical nursing: Clinical management for continuity of care* (5th ed.). Philadelphia: W. B. Saunders, pp. 1983–1984.

115. The nurse enters the room of a diabetic client, and finds the client difficult to arouse, with warm, flushed skin. The pulse and respiratory rate are elevated from the client's baseline. Which of the following should the nurse plan to do first?

1. Prepare an insulin drip
2. Give the client a glass of orange juice
3. Administer a bolus dose of 50% dextrose
4. Check the client's capillary blood glucose

Answer: 4

Rationale: The client's signs and symptoms are consistent with hyperglycemia. The nurse must first obtain a blood glucose reading, which would then be reported to the physician for subsequent orders. Options 2 and 3 would be used as needed in the treatment of hypoglycemia.

Test-Taking Strategy: Determine that the signs and symptoms presented in the question are indicative of hyperglycemia. Note the key word "first" in the question. This tells you that more than one option may be partially or totally correct. In this question, options 2 and 3 are incorrect because they relate to treatment of hypoglycemia. You would choose option 4 over option 1 because insulin therapy is guided by blood glucose measurement. In addition, option 4 provides some firm data, which can then be reported to the physician as needed.

Level of Cognitive Ability: Application
Phase of Nursing Process: Planning
Client Needs: Safe, Effective Care Environment
Content Area: Adult Health/Endocrine

Reference

Black, J., & Matassarin-Jacobs, E. (1997). *Medical-surgical nursing: Clinical management for continuity of care* (5th ed.). Philadelphia: W. B. Saunders, p. 1991.

116. The client with recently diagnosed insulin-dependent diabetes mellitus (IDDM) tells the clinic nurse that he or she is anxious about proper diabetic self-management during an upcoming 6-hour airplane flight. Which of the following pieces of information should the nurse give the client to help allay the anxiety about traveling with diabetes?

1. Keep snacks in carry-on luggage to prevent hypoglycemia during the flight
2. Store insulin and syringes in a padded compartment of stowed luggage to prevent breakage
3. Check the blood glucose hourly during the flight
4. Obtain a referral to a physician in the destination city

Answer: 1

Rationale: One of the biggest concerns for diabetics during air travel, especially for long-distance flights, is the availability of food at times that correspond with the timing and peak action of the client's insulin. For this reason, the nurse may suggest that the client have carbohydrate snacks on hand for use as needed. Insulin equipment and supplies should always be placed in carry-on luggage (not stowed). This provides ready access to treat hyperglycemia, if needed, and also prevents loss of equipment if luggage is lost. Options 3 and 4 are not necessary.

Test-Taking Strategy: Note the key information in the stem. The key elements are "IDDM" and "air travel." Recall that either hyperglycemia or hypoglycemia can occur if meal times are disrupted for the client with IDDM. This is likely to occur during a lengthy air flight. Therefore, you would look for the option that indicates a strategy for preventing or managing these complications. Correct information will help alleviate the client's stress during this situation. Options 2 and 4 are incorrect and do not help the client during the flight. You would choose option 1 over option 3 by knowing that option 1 is correct or by recognizing that option 3 is excessive in time frame.

Level of Cognitive Ability: Application
Phase of Nursing Process: Planning
Client Needs: Psychosocial Integrity
Content Area: Adult Health/Endocrine

Reference

Lewis, S., Collier, I., & Heitkemper, M. (1996). *Medical-surgical nursing: Assessment and management of clinical problems* (4th ed.). St. Louis: Mosby–Year Book, pp. 1460–1461.

117. The diabetic client who is performing self-monitoring of blood glucose at home asks the clinic nurse why a glycosylated hemoglobin level needs to be drawn. The nurse should plan to incorporate which of the following into a response?

1 This laboratory test is done yearly to predict likelihood of long-term complications
2 This laboratory test gives an indication of glycemic control over the past 3 months
3 It is done as a method of verifying the accuracy of the meter used at home
4 It is done to predict risk of hypoglycemia with current diet and medication regimen

Answer: 2

Rationale: The normal value for glycosylated hemoglobin is 6%–7% and gives an indication of glycemic control over the past 3 months. With elevations in blood glucose, some of the glucose molecules attach to the red blood cell (RBC) and remain there for the life of the RBC. Therefore, high values in this test correlate with high blood glucose levels, indicating poor long-term control of blood glucose. Poor control of blood glucose is thought to be related to the development of complications in the client with IDDM.

Test-Taking Strategy: Specific knowledge of this test is needed to answer this question accurately. If needed, take a few moments now to review this test and its use in the clinical management of diabetes!

Level of Cognitive Ability: Application
Phase of Nursing Process: Planning
Client Needs: Physiological Integrity
Content Area: Adult Health/Endocrine

Reference

Black, J., & Matassarin-Jacobs, E. (1997). *Medical-surgical nursing: Clinical management for continuity of care* (5th ed.). Philadelphia: W. B. Saunders, p. 1962.

---

118. The nurse is preparing for intershift report when a nurse's aide pulls an emergency call light in a client's room. Upon answering the light, the nurse finds a new postoperative client with tachycardia and tachypnea. Blood pressure is 88/60. The nurse should plan to do which of the following first?

1 Check the hourly urine output
2 Check the IV site for infiltration
3 Place the client in modified Trendelenburg position
4 Call the physician

Answer: 3

Rationale: The client is exhibiting signs of shock, and requires emergency intervention. Placing the client in modified Trendelenburg position increases blood return from the legs, which increases venous return and subsequently blood pressure. The nurse can then verify the client's volume status by assessing the urine output and whether the IV line is running. The nurse should obtain all this information quickly before calling the physician, which is also done rapidly.

Test-Taking Strategy: Note that the key word in this question is "first." This implies that more than one or all of the options are partially or totally correct, and you must prioritize your choices. After analyzing that this is an emergency situation, you would look for a response that supports the ABCs: airway, breathing, circulation. Because option 3 is the only option that supports the client's immediate physiological needs, this is action that the nurse should take first. The others may follow in rapid sequence.

Level of Cognitive Ability: Application
Phase of Nursing Process: Planning
Client Needs: Safe, Effective Care Environment
Content Area: Adult Health/Cardiovascular

Reference

Luckmann, J. (1997). *Saunders manual of nursing care*. Philadelphia: W. B. Saunders, p. 373.

---

119. The client who is in the first trimester of pregnancy complains of morning sickness. Which of the following suggestions would the nurse avoid when counseling this client about this problem?

1 Eat crackers or dry toast before arising
2 Eat small, frequent meals
3 Avoid spicy or fatty foods
4 Postpone eating until the supper hour

Answer: 4

Rationale: Standard measures for control of morning sickness include eating crackers or toast before arising from bed in the morning, eating small frequent meals, avoiding fatty and spicy foods, and arising slowly to avoid orthostatic hypotension. Delaying eating until suppertime does not promote proper nutrition for the pregnant woman and fetus. It is also true that morning sickness can occur at any time of the day or night, which also makes option 4 incorrect.

Test-Taking Strategy: The wording of the question guides you to look for an option that is incorrect. Using the principles of nutrition and management of nausea and vomiting, you should be able to systematically eliminate each of the correct options. If this question was difficult, take a few moments to review the management of this problem, which is common during pregnancy!

Level of Cognitive Ability: Application
Phase of Nursing Process: Planning
Client Needs: Health Promotion and Maintenance
Content Area: Maternity

Reference

Luckmann, J. (1997). *Saunders manual of nursing care.* Philadelphia: W. B. Saunders, p. 431.

---

120. The client with cancer has a nursing diagnosis of Risk for Injury related to thrombocytopenia secondary to side effects of chemotherapy. The nurse would plan to monitor the results of which of the following laboratory studies closely?

1 Platelet count
2 White blood cell (WBC) count
3 Erythrocyte sedimentation rate (ESR)
4 Antinuclear antibody (ANA) titer

Answer: 1

Rationale: The client who is at risk for injury related to thrombocytopenia has an insufficient number of platelets. This puts the client at risk for bleeding. Other related studies that should be monitored include hemoglobin, hematocrit, and coagulation studies. The WBC count indicates infection; the ESR is a nonspecific test indicating inflammation. The ANA titer is a test of immune function and can indicate the presence of certain autoimmune disorders.

Test-Taking Strategy: Knowledge of effects of chemotherapy and diagnostic tests is useful in answering this question. However, the correct answer can be logically deduced by knowing the definition of thrombocytopenia. Briefly review common side effects of chemotherapy now if you had difficulty with this question!

Level of Cognitive Ability: Application
Phase of Nursing Process: Planning
Client Needs: Physiological Integrity
Content Area: Adult Health/Oncology

Reference

Luckmann, J. (1997). *Saunders manual of nursing care.* Philadelphia: W. B. Saunders, p. 619.

---

121. The nurse is preparing the client for upcoming radiation therapy for cancer. The nurse would plan to teach the client to avoid which of the following actions as part of skin care of the affected site?

1 Patting the skin dry
2 Wearing loose clothing
3 Using mild soap
4 Removing skin markings

Answer: 4

Rationale: Proper skin care during radiation therapy is extremely important. The nurse teaches the client to wash the skin gently, using only lukewarm water and patting the skin dry. The skin should not be rubbed; nor should that area of the skin be shaved. The client should use only mild soaps for cleansing to avoid chemical irritation of the skin and should avoid lotions, creams, powders, and perfumes in the affected area. Finally, the client should not remove any skin markings placed by the radiologist to guide the radiation therapy.

Test-Taking Strategy: The wording of the question guides you to look for an item that is contraindicated during radiation therapy. Options 1, 2, and 3 are similar in that they protect the skin. Remember, options that are similar are not likely to be correct. This leaves option 4 as the correct choice. Skin markings should never be removed by the client. Review skin care measures for the client receiving radiation therapy now if you had difficulty with this question!

Level of Cognitive Ability: Application
Phase of Nursing Process: Planning
Client Needs: Safe, Effective Care Environment
Content Area: Adult Health/Oncology

Reference

Luckmann, J. (1997). *Saunders manual of nursing care.* Philadelphia: W. B. Saunders, p. 626.

122. The nurse applies oxygen via nasal cannula at 4 liters/minute to a client having multiple premature ventricular contractions (PVCs). Which nursing action would not be appropriate to include in a plan of care for this client?

1 Provide water soluble lubricant to nares
2 Instruct the family that there is no smoking in the room
3 Humidify the oxygen if the client complains of dry nose
4 Instruct the client to breath through the nose only

Answer: 4

Rationale: The nasal cannula provides for lower concentrations of oxygen and can even be used with mouth breathers because movement of air through the oropharynx creates the Bernoulli effect, pulling oxygen from the nasopharynx. It is not necessary to instruct a client to breathe only through the nose.

Test-Taking Strategy: The word "not" in the stem of this question indicates a negative polarity and the question being asked is concerned with what is false. Absolute terminology such as "only" in option 4 tends to make a statement false. Review nursing measures for a client receiving oxygen now if you had difficulty with this question!

Level of Cognitive Ability: Application
Phase of Nursing Process: Planning
Client Needs: Safe, Effective Care Environment
Content Area: Fundamental Skills

Reference
Hudak, C., & Gallo, B. (1994). *Critical care nursing: A holistic approach* (6th ed.). Philadelphia: Lippincott-Raven, pp. 450–451, 453.

---

123. The nurse is caring for a client who is scheduled for radiation therapy. The nurse prepares a nursing care plan for the client, and in the planning, the nurse expects that the most common response by the client would be

1 "I'm certain that this will do the trick."
2 "Will I be radioactive afterwards?"
3 "This is just one of several options I have for treatment."
4 "This treatment is great because it is invisible and very effective."

Answer: 2

Rationale: Radiation therapy is often a source of fear and misconceptions for clients and their families. Education by the nurse can erase much of the anxiety and support the client. Some of the most common fears and misconceptions include fear of being burned, the radioactive treatment, treatment failure, and the adverse effects.

Test-Taking Strategy: This question assesses your knowledge of the common fears and misconceptions about radiation therapy. Use the process of elimination. Option 1 is an overcompensation and the opposite of the common fear usually observed. Options 3 and 4 are the opposites of the most common fears and are false reassurances.

Level of Cognitive Ability: Analysis
Phase of Nursing Process: Planning
Client Needs: Psychosocial Integrity
Content Area: Adult Health/Oncology

Reference
Black, J., & Matassarin-Jacobs, E. (1997). *Medical-surgical nursing: Clinical management for continuity of care* (5th ed.). Philadelphia: W. B. Saunders, pp. 533–561.

---

124. The client has newly diagnosed hypertension. The nurse would plan to do which of the following as the first step in teaching the client about the disorder?

1 Gather all available resource materials
2 Plan for the evaluation of the session
3 Assess the client's knowledge and needs
4 Decide on the teaching approach

Answer: 3

Rationale: Determining what to teach a client begins with an assessment of the client's own knowledge and learning needs. Once these have been determined, the nurse can effectively plan a teaching approach, the actual content, and resource materials that may be needed. The evaluation is done after teaching is completed.

Test-Taking Strategy: Note the key word "first" in the stem of the question. This implies that more than one or all of the options may be correct. It also implies that there is a correct sequencing of the activity. To correctly answer this question, recall that effective client teaching is individualized. An assessment of the client's individual learning needs is prerequisite to developing an effective teaching plan. Remember that Assessment is the first step of the nursing process!

Level of Cognitive Ability: Application
Phase of Nursing Process: Planning
Client Needs: Health Promotion and Maintenance
Content Area: Fundamental Skills

Reference

DeLaune, S., & Ladner, P. (1998). *Fundamentals of nursing: Standards and practice.* Albany, NY: Delmar, pp. 570–571.

---

125. A client's medication is available for injection in an ampule. Which of the following should the nurse plan to do when drawing up this medication?

1 Shake the ampule gently to mix the contents
2 Place an alcohol wipe around the neck of the ampule
3 Snap the top of the ampule backward away from the nurse
4 Wipe the neck of the ampule after snapping it open

Answer: 2

Rationale: Basic procedure for drawing up medication from an ampule involves tapping the top chamber until the medication lies in the lower area, placing an alcohol wipe around the neck of the ampule, snapping the top toward the nurse so it opens away from the nurse, and withdrawing the medication without injecting air into the ampule. Snapping the ampule so that it opens away from the nurse prevents injury from possible shattered glass fragments. The neck is not wiped with the gauze, because first, it is unnecessary and, second, it could cause injury to the nurse's fingers from sharp glass edges.

Test-Taking Strategy: Note that the question is worded in a positive manner. This tells you that you are looking for a correct statement. Review each of the options systematically. Knowledge of basic medication administration principles allows you to eliminate each of the incorrect options. Try to visualize the information in each of the options when selecting an answer. Review medication preparation from an ampule now if you had difficulty with this question!

Level of Cognitive Ability: Application
Phase of Nursing Process: Planning
Client Needs: Safe, Effective Care Environment
Content Area: Fundamental Skills

Reference

DeLaune, S., & Ladner, P. (1998). *Fundamentals of nursing: Standards and practice.* Albany, NY: Delmar, pp. 898–899.

---

126. The client has a nursing diagnosis of Ineffective Airway Clearance. The nurse would plan to use which of the following indicators as the best guide to determine when the client needs suctioning?

1 Oxygen saturation measurement
2 Respiratory rate
3 Breath sounds
4 Arterial blood gas results

Answer: 3

Rationale: Suctioning is indicated when the client cannot expectorate mucus by using a variety of other assistive methods. The need for suctioning is best determined by listening for coarse gurgling or bubbling respirations or by hearing adventitious breath sounds during auscultation. The other options are indirect indicators; that is, they could be affected by factors other than accumulation of secretions.

Test-Taking Strategy: The key word in the question is "best." Although arterial blood gas results, oxygen saturation, and respiratory rate may change as a result of mucus accumulation, it is the presence of noisy respirations or adventitious breath sounds that actually indicates the presence of secretions that require removal. Remember also that options that are similar are also likely to be incorrect. Therefore, you may immediately eliminate options 1 and 4, because both refer to oxygen levels in the blood stream.

Level of Cognitive Ability: Application
Phase of Nursing Process: Planning
Client Needs: Physiological Integrity
Content Area: Fundamental Skills

Reference

DeLaune, S., & Ladner, P. (1998). *Fundamentals of nursing: Standards and practice.* Albany, NY: Delmar, p. 805.

127. The postoperative client has pneumatic compression boots in place. The nurse plans to remove the compression sleeves at which of the following intervals?

1 Every hour for 5 minutes
2 Every 4 hours for 30 minutes
3 Three times a day for 20–30 minutes
4 Once a day for 1 hour

Answer: 3

Rationale: The sleeves of the pneumatic compression device are removed by the nurse three times a day for 20–30 minutes so that hygiene may be performed. The circulation to the extremities and the placement of the sleeves should be checked every 2–3 hours for client safety.

Test-Taking Strategy: Think about the purpose for the compression sleeves and the possible rationales for their removal. Also, look at the time frames presented in each of the options. This line of reasoning will help you eliminate each of the incorrect options, as the time frames listed are either too broad or too narrow. Take time now to review nursing care of the client with pneumatic compression boots if you had difficulty with this question!

Level of Cognitive Ability: Application
Phase of Nursing Process: Planning
Client Needs: Physiological Integrity
Content Area: Fundamental Skills

Reference
DeLaune, S., & Ladner, P. (1998). *Fundamentals of nursing: Standards and practice.* Albany, NY: Delmar, p. 660.

---

128. The nurse is assigned to the care of a client who is dying. In developing a plan of care, which of the following items would be least helpful to this client?

1 Provide extremely thorough answers to each question asked by client or family
2 Make referrals to other disciplines based on client's stated needs
3 Plan to balance the client's need for assistance with the need for independence
4 Offer to contact clergy to support the spiritual needs of the client

Answer: 1

Rationale: In planning care for the dying client, the nurse provides information and answers questions to the extent that is most helpful to the client. This may include responses that are either brief or lengthy, depending on the situation. The nurse does make referrals to other disciplines and clergy on the basis of an assessment of need and tries to balance the client's need for assistance with the need to maintain some measure of independence. Another item that is very helpful to the dying client is to plan time to spend with the client.

Test-Taking Strategy: Note that the question asks for the item that is "least helpful" to the client. This guides you to look for an incorrect response. Eliminate options 2 and 4 first, because they are similar in nature. Knowledge of basic human needs will help you choose option 1 over option 3 as the answer to the question as stated. In addition, note the phrase "extremely thorough" in option 1. The exaggerated detail of response implied in this option makes it likely to be the least helpful item.

Level of Cognitive Ability: Application
Phase of Nursing Process: Planning
Client Needs: Psychosocial Integrity
Content Area: Fundamental Skills

Reference
DeLaune, S., & Ladner, P. (1998). *Fundamentals of nursing: Standards and practice.* Albany, NY: Delmar, pp. 548–549.

---

129. The nurse is preparing the client for surgery who will have spinal anesthesia. The nurse would place highest priority on reporting which of the following items?

1 Blood pressure of 126/78
2 Pulse rate of 78
3 Voided 300 mL just after admission
4 Presence of weakness in left lower extremity

Answer: 4

Rationale: It is important to report any preoperative weakness or impaired movement of a lower extremity in the client who is to have spinal anesthesia. This is because spinal anesthesia causes temporary paralysis of the lower extremities. When the client's function returns, the preoperative weakness or impairment will not be misinterpreted as a complication of anesthesia.

Test-Taking Strategy: The key words in the stem are "spinal anesthesia" and "highest priority." The term "highest priority" implies that more than one or all of the responses may be partially or totally correct. You would arrive at the correct choice either by knowing that impaired function in the lower extremities needs to be reported or by knowing that each of the other options contains normal data and therefore is not of highest priority.

Level of Cognitive Ability: Application
Phase of Nursing Process: Planning
Client Needs: Physiological Integrity
Content Area: Fundamental Skills

Reference

DeLaune, S., & Ladner, P. (1998). *Fundamentals of nursing: Standards and practice.* Albany, NY: Delmar, p. 649.

---

130. The client has an order for a wound culture to be done with the next wound irrigation and dressing change. The nurse would plan to use which of the following solutions for irrigation before this particular procedure?

1 Povidone iodine (Betadine)
2 Half-strength hydrogen peroxide
3 Normal saline
4 Acetic acid

Answer: 3

Rationale: Wound irrigation with normal saline is done before obtaining a wound culture because it can remove substances such as proteins or exudate. It is important to avoid irrigation with an antiseptic solution, which could destroy wound bacteria and invalidate the culture results.

Test-Taking Strategy: Remember that options that are similar are not likely to be correct. In each of the options listed, the only one that is not considered an antiseptic solution is normal saline. Thus each of the incorrect responses may be eliminated systematically. If this question was difficult, take a few moments to review basic concepts related to wound care and obtaining wound cultures now!

Level of Cognitive Ability: Application
Phase of Nursing Process: Planning
Client Needs: Physiological Integrity
Content Area: Fundamental Skills

Reference

DeLaune, S., & Ladner, P. (1998). *Fundamentals of nursing: Standards and practice.* Albany, NY: Delmar, pp. 982–983.

---

131. The nurse is caring for a pediatric client with an IV infusion running. Which of the following items would the nurse plan to use as the safest means of preventing fluid overload for this client?

1 Armboard
2 Macrodrip infusion set
3 Large-bore intravenous catheter
4 Infusion pump

Answer: 4

Rationale: The most effective means of preventing irregularities in volume infusion for the pediatric client is the use of an infusion pump. This prevents both overhydration and underhydration. A small-bore catheter is used in the pediatric client because of vein size, and a microdrip infusion set is used, rather than a macrodrip set. An armboard may be helpful in certain instances to minimize movement of the extremity with the catheter, but it is not the most effective means for regulating IV flow.

Test-Taking Strategy: Note that the question asks for the "safest means" of preventing fluid overload. Begin to answer this question by eliminating options 2 and 3, because they are totally incorrect. You would next eliminate option 1, the armboard, because although this would help prevent catheter kinking, infiltration, or removal, it would not be as useful as an infusion pump in preventing fluid overload.

Level of Cognitive Ability: Application
Phase of Nursing Process: Planning
Client Needs: Physiological Integrity
Content Area: Child Health

Reference

DeLaune, S., & Ladner, P. (1998). *Fundamentals of nursing: Standards and practice.* Albany, NY: Delmar, p. 1060.

132. The nurse prepares a medication teaching plan for the depressed client who has just been placed on phenelzine (Nardil), 15 mg PO TID. Which of the statements contains the most vital nursing instruction?

1. "Report severe, sudden, or unusual headache to your physician immediately."
2. "Limit the same food and medications for 10 days after the medication is discontinued."
3. "Drink 8 glasses of fluid each day."
4. "Eat green vegetables and bran every day."

Answer: 1

Rationale: The onset of a headache that is sudden, severe, or unusual may be the beginning of hypertensive crisis. In addition, stiff neck, vomiting, and sharply increased blood pressure are observed in hypertensive crisis. This condition leads to intracranial bleeding and is one of the most threatening side effects of monoamine oxidase inhibitors (MAOIs). Hypertensive crisis can be caused by the ingestion of foods containing the amino acid tyramine and by the ingestion of sympathomimetic medications.

Test-Taking Strategy: Note the key word "vital" in the question and key phrase "severe, sudden" in the correct option. Although all of the statements are valid instructions, option 1 is the most vital instruction because it refers to the presence of a severe side effect of an MAOI, such as Nardil. Option 2 teaches the client to restrict tyramine-containing foods and sympathomimetic agents, which can cause hypertensive crisis. Options 3 and 4 teach the client measures to prevent constipation, which can be another side effect of MAOIs. Review the MAOIs now if you had difficulty with this question!

Level of Cognitive Ability: Application
Phase of Nursing Process: Planning
Client Needs: Safe, Effective Care Environment
Content Area: Pharmacology

Reference

Antai-Otong, D., & Kongale, G. (1995). *Psychiatric nursing: Biological and behavioral concepts.* Philadelphia: W. B. Saunders, pp. 554–556.

---

133. The client has begun medication therapy with colchicine. The nurse would plan to monitor for which of the following expected effects of this medication?

1. Reduction in joint pain
2. Reduction of temperature
3. Increase in blood pressure
4. Increase in urine output

Answer: 1

Rationale: Colchicine is classified as an antigout agent. Its expected effects include reduced joint swelling and pain and prevention of acute gouty attacks. It is not an antipyretic, antihypertensive, or diuretic.

Test-Taking Strategy: Note the key phrase "expected effects" in the stem of the question. Basic knowledge of this medication is needed to answer this question correctly. Take a few moments now to review this medication if you have the need!

Level of Cognitive Ability: Application
Phase of Nursing Process: Planning
Client Needs: Physiological Integrity
Content Area: Pharmacology

Reference

Hodgson, B., & Kizior, R. (1998). *Saunders nursing drug handbook 1998.* Philadelphia: W. B. Saunders, p. 252.

---

134. The client is receiving diflunisal (Dolobid) in the treatment of rheumatoid arthritis. The nurse would plan to monitor for which of the following most frequent side effects of this medication?

1. Gastrointestinal (GI) discomfort
2. Joint swelling
3. Elevated temperature
4. Dizziness

Answer: 1

Rationale: Diflunisal is a nonsteroidal anti-inflammatory drug (NSAID). The most common side effects include GI complaints, including nausea, vomiting, discomfort, and diarrhea. Joint swelling should be relieved, not enhanced, by the medication. Elevated temperature is not a side effect. Dizziness can occur but is not frequent.

Test-Taking Strategy: To answer this question correctly, it is necessary to know both that this medication is an NSAID and that this type of medication commonly causes GI side effects. This will allow you to eliminate each of the other incorrect responses systematically. Take time now to review this medication if you had difficulty with this question!

Level of Cognitive Ability: Application
Phase of Nursing Process: Planning
Client Needs: Physiological Integrity
Content Area: Pharmacology

Reference

Hodgson, B., & Kizior, R. (1998). *Saunders nursing drug handbook 1998.* Philadelphia: W. B. Saunders, pp. 322–324.

---

135. The nurse is assigned to care for a client receiving filgrastim (Neupogen). The nurse would plan to administer the medication by which of the following routes?

1 Oral
2 Intradermal
3 Intramuscular
4 Subcutaneous

Answer: 4

Rationale: Filgrastim (Neupogen) is a granulocyte colony–stimulating factor used to increase the white blood cell count in clients after bone marrow transplantation and in clients who have received chemotherapeutic agents that suppress bone marrow production. It is administered by the intravenous or subcutaneous route.

Test-Taking Strategy: Specific knowledge of this medication and the accepted routes of administration is needed to answer this question correctly. Take time now to review this medication if the question was difficult for you!

Level of Cognitive Ability: Application
Phase of Nursing Process: Planning
Client Needs: Physiological Integrity
Content Area: Pharmacology

Reference

Hodgson, B., & Kizior, R. (1998). *Saunders nursing drug handbook 1998.* Philadelphia: W. B. Saunders, pp. 411–421.

---

136. The client has received a loading dose of lidocaine (Xylocaine), 100 mg IV, for the treatment of ventricular tachycardia. The nurse would plan to do which of the following as follow-up treatment for this dysrhythmia?

1 Hang a continuous IV infusion at 1–4 mg/minute
2 Repeat the dose every 10 minutes, PRN, for 1 hour
3 Begin oral procainamide (Pronestyl) therapy
4 Prepare for pacemaker insertion to override the dysrhythmia

Answer: 1

Rationale: Lidocaine is given by the IV push route in doses of 50–100 mg (1 mg/kg) to suppress ventricular dysrhythmias. The initial loading dose is followed by continuous IV infusion at a rate of 1–4 mg/minute. The dose may be repeated once in 5 minutes, but the client should not receive more than 200–300 mg in one hour. Options 3 and 4 are not part of routine follow-up therapy.

Test-Taking Strategy: To answer this question correctly, it is necessary to know that this medication is an antidysrhythmic and maintenance of a therapeutic blood level is required for proper effectiveness. This would guide you to eliminate each of the incorrect responses systematically. Take time now to review this medication if you had difficulty with this question!

Level of Cognitive Ability: Application
Phase of Nursing Process: Planning
Client Needs: Physiological Integrity
Content Area: Pharmacology

Reference

Deglin, J., & Vallerand, A. (1997). *Davis's drug guide for nurses* (5th ed.). Philadelphia: F. A. Davis, p. 697.

---

137. The client has been prescribed metolazone (Zaroxolyn). The nurse would plan to teach the client to avoid which of the following foods while taking this medication?

1 Spinach
2 Pickles
3 Broccoli

Answer: 2

Rationale: Metolazone is classified as a thiazide-like diuretic and an antihypertensive agent. Because of the risk of hypokalemia, clients are encouraged to eat foods rich in potassium, such as spinach, broccoli, and bananas. The client is taught to avoid foods high in sodium, such as pickles.

Test-Taking Strategy: Note the key word "avoid" in the stem of the question. To answer this question accurately, it is necessary to know

4 Bananas

that this medication acts as an antihypertensive and is potassium wasting. It is also necessary to know which foods are high in sodium and potassium. Of the four options presented, note that option 2 is highest in sodium content. If necessary, review this medication and the foods to avoid now!

Level of Cognitive Ability: Application
Phase of Nursing Process: Planning
Client Needs: Health Promotion and Maintenance
Content Area: Pharmacology

Reference

Deglin, J., & Vallerand, A. (1997). *Davis's drug guide for nurses* (5th ed.). Philadelphia: F. A. Davis, pp. 784–785, 1285.

---

138. The client receiving lithium carbonate (Eskalith) begins to exhibit slurred speech, drowsiness, muscle twitching, and muscle incoordination. The nurse should plan to do which of the following before administering the next dose?

1 Encourage intake of a stimulant such as coffee or tea
2 Obtain an order for an electroencephalogram (EEG)
3 Restrict fluids
4 Call the physician

Answer: 4

Rationale: The nurse recognizes these symptoms as signs of lithium toxicity and notifies the physician before administering the next scheduled dose. Fluid intake, up to a level of 2000–3000 mL/day, should be encouraged in conjunction with this therapy unless contraindicated. Excessive amounts of coffee, tea, or colas are restricted because of their diuretic effect. The nurse does not routinely order diagnostic tests such as an EEG.

Test-Taking Strategy: To answer this question correctly, it is necessary to know the signs of lithium toxicity and the appropriate action to take. This would cause you to eliminate each of the incorrect responses systematically. When toxicity occurs, it is necessary to notify the physician. If you had difficulty with this question, take time now to review the signs of toxicity. You are likely to find a question related to this medication on NCLEX-RN!

Level of Cognitive Ability: Application
Phase of Nursing Process: Planning
Client Needs: Physiological Integrity
Content Area: Pharmacology

Reference

Hodgson, B., & Kizior, R. (1998). *Saunders nursing drug handbook 1998.* Philadelphia: W. B. Saunders, pp. 598–600.

---

139. The nurse is teaching the hypertensive client about strategies to prevent episodes of lightheadedness after taking antihypertensive medication. The nurse would plan to include which of the following points in the discussion?

1 "Standing motionless during the first hour after the dose is helpful."
2 "Move quickly when rising from sitting to standing position."
3 "Take warm baths to enhance medication effects."
4 "Limit or avoid alcohol intake after taking medication."

Answer: 4

Rationale: The client taking antihypertensive medications should be taught to avoid situations that promote lightheadedness and dizziness. These include warm baths, excessive alcohol intake, and standing motionless for long periods of time. The client should rise slowly from sitting to standing positions and should wiggle the toes or do leg muscle-setting exercises when standing to avoid lightheadedness.

Test-Taking Strategy: The issue of the question is to prevent lightheadedness. The wording of the question guides you to look for a positive or correct response. Knowing that lightheadedness results from a drop in blood pressure, you would choose the answer that does not aggravate or trigger vasodilatation.

Level of Cognitive Ability: Application
Phase of Nursing Process: Planning
Client Needs: Health Promotion and Maintenance
Content Area: Adult Health/Cardiovascular

Reference

Burrell, P., Gerlach, M., & Pless, B. (1997). *Adult nursing: Acute and community care* (2nd ed.). Stamford, CT: Appleton & Lange, p. 505.

140. The client being treated for hypertension is also taking tranylcypromine (Parnate). The nurse would plan to teach the client to avoid eating which of the following foods?

1. Baked potatoes
2. Cottage cheese
3. Steak
4. Bananas

Answer: 4

Rationale: Tranylcypromine (Parnate) is a monoamine oxidase inhibitor (MAOI). Hypertensive clients who are taking MAOIs should avoid ingesting foods that are high in tyramine, which can result in hypertension and chest pain. Foods that interact with MAOIs include aged cheese, yeast, chocolate, sherry, beer and red wine, smoked meats, ripe bananas, smoked fish, soy sauce, ripe avocadoes, yogurt, and yeast extract.

Test-Taking Strategy: Specific knowledge of the interactive effects of MAOIs and tyramine-containing foods is needed to answer this question. If you know that this medication is an MAOI, you will be able, by the process of elimination, to select the correct answer. If this question was difficult, take time to review this medication and the foods high in tyramine!

Level of Cognitive Ability: Application
Phase of Nursing Process: Planning
Client Needs: Health Promotion and Maintenance
Content Area: Adult Health/Cardiovascular

Reference

Pinnell, N. (1996). *Nursing pharmacology.* Philadelphia: W. B. Saunders, pp. 202–203.

---

141. The nurse is developing a teaching plan for the client with peripheral arterial insufficiency. The nurse would not include which of the following points when developing the plan?

1. "Refrain from walking, to avoid triggering claudication pain."
2. "Discontinue the use of products containing nicotine."
3. "Lose excess weight."
4. "Inspect the feet daily for injury."

Answer: 1

Rationale: Standard teaching points for the client with arterial insufficiency include abstinence from smoking, weight loss as appropriate, regular exercise, daily foot care, and the importance of taking prescribed medications. The client should exercise, preferably by walking, to increase collateral circulation to the legs, which ultimately reduces pain.

Test-Taking Strategy: Note the key word "not" in the stem of the question. This guides you to look for an incorrect response. Knowledge of concepts related to atherosclerosis and therapeutic measures helps you to readily eliminate each of the incorrect options. Take time now to review these teaching points if you had difficulty with this question!

Level of Cognitive Ability: Application
Phase of Nursing Process: Planning
Client Needs: Health Promotion and Maintenance
Content Area: Adult Health/Cardiovascular

Reference

Burrell, P., Gerlach, M., & Pless, B. (1997). *Adult nursing: Acute and community care* (2nd ed.). Stamford, CT: Appleton & Lange, p. 512.

---

142. The client has experienced a sudden arterial embolus to the left lower leg. The nurse would plan to do which of the following in the management of this problem?

1. Elevate the foot of the bed 6 inches
2. Put sheepskin and bed cradle in place
3. Place a warm heating pad on the left leg
4. Wrap the extremity tightly with an Ace wrap.

Answer: 2

Rationale: With sudden arterial occlusion, the nurse plans actions that will protect the extremity from further harm. These would include use of sheepskin and bed cradle to protect leg tissue from injury and wrapping the extremity loosely to promote warmth. Ace wraps would be harmful because the compression could injure tissues already at risk. The use of local heat is contraindicated because it increases the metabolic needs of tissues that are already deprived of oxygen and nutrients as a result of blockage of blood flow. Elevation of the leg is harmful because gravity further limits circulation to the leg.

Test-Taking Strategy: The key phrases in this question are "sudden arterial embolus" and "plan to do." This guides you to look for an action that is expected by the nurse. Eliminate option 4 because of the word "tightly." Eliminate option 3 because of the word "warm." Eliminate option 1 because of the word "elevate." Basic knowledge of principles of care for clients with impaired circulation guides you to eliminate each of the incorrect options as being potentially harmful to the client. Review these now if you had difficulty with this question!

Level of Cognitive Ability: Application
Phase of Nursing Process: Planning
Client Needs: Physiological Integrity
Content Area: Adult Health/Cardiovascular

Reference
Burrell, P., Gerlach, M., & Pless, B. (1997). *Adult nursing: Acute and community care* (2nd ed.). Stamford, CT: Appleton & Lange, p. 523.

---

143. The nurse is caring for a postoperative client. The nurse plans to diligently carry out which of the following to best prevent the development of deep vein thrombosis (DVT) in this client?

1 Incisional splinting
2 Coughing and deep breathing
3 Frequent ambulation
4 Regular removal of antiembolism stockings

Answer: 3

Rationale: Several measures are instituted postoperatively to prevent the development of complications. Prevention of DVT is best accomplished by early and frequent ambulation of the client. Other helpful measures are the use of compression sleeves or stockings and teaching the client to do leg and foot exercises while in bed.

Test-Taking Strategy: The question asks for the "best" method of preventing DVT in the client. Begin to answer this question by eliminating options 1 and 2, because they prevent atelectasis and pneumonia. You would then choose option 3 over option 4 on the basis of fundamental nursing knowledge and because removal of antiembolism stockings will not prevent DVT!

Level of Cognitive Ability: Application
Phase of Nursing Process: Planning
Client Needs: Physiological Integrity
Content Area: Fundamental Skills

Reference
Burrell, P., Gerlach, M., & Pless, B. (1997). *Adult nursing: Acute and community care* (2nd ed.). Stamford, CT: Appleton & Lange, p. 534.

---

144. The client has a platelet count of 60,000/mm^3. The nurse would plan to use which of the following measures in the care of this client whenever possible?

1 Straight razor for shaving
2 Firm-bristle toothbrush
3 Use of oral or IV route for medications
4 Vigorous skin care

Answer: 3

Rationale: The client with a low platelet count is at risk for bleeding. Therefore, the nurse institutes measures that will minimize the risk of injury or bleeding. The nurse would administer medications whenever possible by the oral or IV route to minimize tissue trauma from needlesticks. The nurse would avoid vigorous washing or rubbing of the skin, to avoid causing ecchymoses. The nurse would also avoid the use of straight razors or firm-bristle toothbrushes, which could also cause bleeding.

Test-Taking Strategy: To answer this question correctly, you need to know that the platelet count is low and that the client is therefore at risk for bleeding. This knowledge allows you to eliminate each of the incorrect responses easily. If you had difficulty with this question, take time now to review the precautions needed for clients at risk for bleeding!

Level of Cognitive Ability: Application
Phase of Nursing Process: Planning
Client Needs: Safe, Effective Care Environment
Content Area: Adult Health/Cardiovascular

Reference
Burrell, P., Gerlach, M., & Pless, B. (1997). *Adult nursing: Acute and community care* (2nd ed.). Stamford, CT: Appleton & Lange, p. 565.

145. The client who has experienced myocardial infarction is at risk for bradycardia. The nurse plans to teach the client that which of the following activities is allowed?

1 Breathing in and out during activities
2 Routine use of suppositories
3 Isometric leg exercises
4 Lifting small-weight barbells

Answer: 1

Rationale: It is important for the post–myocardial infarction client to breathe in and out during activities. This will prevent vagal stimulation and subsequent bradycardia. The client is taught to avoid activities that tense the body, such as resistive exercise (isometrics, weight lifting). Although the client is taught to avoid constipation, which could lead to vagal stimulation during straining at stool, the choice of laxative should be a bulk-forming laxative or a stool softener. Use of suppositories can also cause vagal stimulation.

Test-Taking Strategy: To answer this question accurately, you need to know that bradycardia is caused or aggravated by activities that provide vagal stimulation. Analysis of each of the options as they relate to the likelihood of vagal stimulation leads you to eliminate each of the incorrect choices. Take time now to review the activities that should be avoided if you had difficulty with this question!

Level of Cognitive Ability: Application
Phase of Nursing Process: Planning
Client Needs: Physiological Integrity
Content Area: Adult Health/Cardiovascular

Reference

Burrell, P., Gerlach, M., & Pless, B. (1997). *Adult nursing: Acute and community care* (2nd ed.). Stamford, CT: Appleton & Lange, p. 442.

146. The client with heart failure is taking furosemide (Lasix) and digoxin (Lanoxin). The client complains of anorexia and nausea as the nurse brings the breakfast tray into the room. The nurse should plan to take which of the following actions first?

1 Withhold the morning dose of Lasix
2 Check the result of the potassium level drawn at 5 A.M.
3 Administer the daily dose of digoxin
4 Call the dietary department for a banana for the client

Answer: 2

Rationale: Anorexia and nausea are two of the common symptoms associated with digitalis toxicity. Digitalis toxicity is compounded by hypokalemia. The nurse should first check the results of the morning potassium level. This provides additional data to report to the physician, which is a key follow-up nursing action. The nurse would not withhold the Lasix without an order, in view of the information provided. The nurse *would* withhold the digoxin until the physician has been consulted. If the client does have hypokalemia, additional sources of potassium such as bananas would be helpful as a follow-up action.

Test-Taking Strategy: Note that the question contains the key word "first." This implies that more than one or all of the responses may be partially or totally correct. Options 1 and 3 are incorrect and are eliminated first. You would choose option 2 over option 4 because the information that will be gained in option 2 tells you whether option 4 is necessary.

Level of Cognitive Ability: Application
Phase of Nursing Process: Planning
Client Needs: Physiological Integrity
Content Area: Adult Health/Cardiovascular

Reference

Burrell, P., Gerlach, M., & Pless, B. (1997). *Adult nursing: Acute and community care* (2nd ed.). Stamford, CT: Appleton & Lange, p. 421.

147. The nurse is caring for the client with urinary incontinence. The nurse should plan to avoid which of the following measures in the care of this client?

1 Maintenance of fluid restriction
2 Encouragement of Kegel exercises
3 Avoidance of constipation
4 Instructions about weight control

Answer: 1

Rationale: A fluid intake of 1500–2000 mL/day is encouraged for the client with incontinence. This allows for adequate bladder filling and stretching, which aids in bladder retraining. Straining from constipation and excess weight causes excess sphincter pressure or decreased sphincter tone, both of which aggravate the problem. Kegel exercises are beneficial and are a classic exercise for use in treating this problem.

Test-Taking Strategy: Note the key word "avoid" in the question. The wording of the question guides you to look for an option that will not be helpful in controlling incontinence. Remember that fluids are important unless they are contraindicated. Knowledge of these specific techniques allows you to eliminate each of the incorrect options systematically. Review these techniques now if you had difficulty with this question!

Level of Cognitive Ability: Application
Phase of Nursing Process: Planning
Client Needs: Physiological Integrity
Content Area: Adult Health/Renal

Reference
Burrell, P., Gerlach, M., & Pless, B. (1997). *Adult nursing: Acute and community care* (2nd ed.). Stamford, CT: Appleton & Lange, p. 1237.

---

148. The nurse is planning a medication teaching session for a client who is being treated with carbamazepine (Tegretol) for bipolar disorder. Which of the following statements by the nurse would best ensure health maintenance?

1 "Your illness is marked by mood swings that cycle very quickly and need a stronger medication."
2 "You will need to have your blood drawn frequently at the beginning and every 3 months or so afterwards."
3 "This mood stabilizer works by causing the nerve impulses to increase the flow of sodium ions across the cell membrane in the pons."
4 "Unlike other atypical mood stabilizers, this medication acts like a birth control pill."

Answer: 2

Rationale: While lithium is an effective mood stabilizer for 80% of the clients with bipolar disorder, it has high failure rates for the other 20% who have bipolar disorder that is characterized by rapid cycling mood swings. Carbamazepine (Tegretol), one treatment alternative to lithium, seems to inhibit nerve impulses, causing the limitation of sodium ions across the cell membrane in the motor cortex. When treatment is started, it is important to obtain blood level of the medication frequently and every 3 months or so thereafter.

Test-Taking Strategy: This question draws upon your ability to apply your knowledge of the medication management that is required for health maintenance and promotion in the treatment of bipolar disorder. In option 1, although it is true that carbamazepine is often successfully used in clients with mood swings that cycle very quickly, it is not true that such medication has stronger potency than lithium. Option 3 contains incorrect information; Tegretol inhibits nerve impulses to limit the flow of sodium ions across the cell membrane in the motor cortex, not the pons. Option 3 also contains wording that is too technical to be useful for most clients. Option 4 is also untrue; Tegretol interferes with the contraceptive ability of the birth control pill. Review this medication now if you had difficulty with this question!

Level of Cognitive Ability: Application
Phase of Nursing Process: Planning
Client Needs: Health Promotion and Maintenance
Content Area: Pharmacology

Reference
Antai-Otong, D., & Kongale, G. (1995). *Psychiatric nursing: Biological and behavioral concepts*. Philadelphia: W. B. Saunders, pp. 172–173.

---

149. The client undergoing peritoneal dialysis complains of shoulder pain. The nurse should plan to

1 Obtain an order for a narcotic analgesic.
2 Infuse the dialysate more slowly.
3 Stop the dialysis and drain the abdomen.
4 Elevate the head of the bed.

Answer: 4

Rationale: The occurrence of shoulder pain during peritoneal dialysis is called Kehr's sign and is caused by irritation of the diaphragm by the dialysate. The appropriate nursing action is to raise the head of the bed. This will cause gravity to move the dialysate away from the diaphragm.

Test-Taking Strategy: To answer this question accurately, it is necessary to know that the shoulder pain results from diaphragmatic irritation. Combining this knowledge with the principle of gravity will lead you to choose the correct option. Review the complications associated with peritoneal dialysis and the appropriate nursing interventions now if you had difficulty with this question!

Level of Cognitive Ability: Application
Phase of Nursing Process: Planning
Client Needs: Safe, Effective Care Environment
Content Area: Adult Health/Renal
Reference

Burrell, P., Gerlach, M., & Pless, B. (1997). *Adult nursing: Acute and community care* (2nd ed.). Stamford, CT: Appleton & Lange, p. 1271.

---

150. The nurse is obtaining a urine sample from a client with an indwelling Foley catheter. In order to prevent bladder distention and possible subsequent hydronephrosis, the nurse plans to

1 Clamp the tubing 3 inches below the catheter connection point.
2 Use a small-gauge needle to aspirate the sample.
3 Release the clamp immediately after the sample is obtained.
4 Angle the needle toward the drainage bag.

Answer: 3

Rationale: Bladder distention and hydronephrosis in the client with an indwelling Foley catheter can result from kinking or obstruction of the catheter. To prevent this occurrence, the nurse releases the clamp immediately after obtaining the sample. Each of the other options represents correct procedure but they do not prevent bladder distention and hydronephrosis. Option 1 aids in obtaining the sample. Option 2 prevents subsequent leakage from the port. Option 4 prevents puncture of the balloon inflation port.

Test-Taking Strategy: The key words in the question are "bladder distention" and "hydronephrosis." Knowing that these result from obstruction, you can easily eliminate each of the incorrect options. Try to visualize the process of collecting a urine sample from a Foley catheter as you read each option. Take time now to review this procedure if you had difficulty with this question!

Level of Cognitive Ability: Application
Phase of Nursing Process: Planning
Client Needs: Safe, Effective Care Environment
Content Area: Fundamental Skills

Reference

Burrell, P., Gerlach, M., & Pless, B. (1997). *Adult nursing: Acute and community care* (2nd ed.). Stamford, CT: Appleton & Lange, p. 1214.

---

151. The nurse is planning care for the client with renal insufficiency. Which of the following strategies by the nurse would be the least helpful in managing the client's fluid volume status?

1 Weigh the client daily at the same time and on the same scale
2 Avoid placing a water pitcher at the bedside
3 Give IV medications in the largest acceptable volume
4 Determine the client's preferences for beverages to drink

Answer: 3

Rationale: The client with renal insufficiency is prone to fluid retention and may have fluid restrictions imposed. To maintain control over fluid intake and prevent the development of edema, the nurse should avoid placing a water pitcher at the client's bedside. Because fluid intake is limited, the client should be served beverages that he or she enjoys. IV medications should be placed in the smallest allowable volume to allow the client more intake by the oral route. Daily weight measurement is beneficial in tracking the client's fluid volume status.

Test-Taking Strategy: Note the phrase "least helpful" in the stem of the question. The wording of the question guides you to look for an option that represents an incorrect action. To answer this question accurately, it is necessary to know that fluid intake in this client will be limited. This knowledge will help you to eliminate each of the incorrect options. Review these nursing measures now if you had difficulty with this question!

Level of Cognitive Ability: Application
Phase of Nursing Process: Planning
Client Needs: Physiological Integrity
Content Area: Adult Health/Renal

Reference

Burrell, P., Gerlach, M., & Pless, B. (1997). *Adult nursing: Acute and community care* (2nd ed.). Stamford, CT: Appleton & Lange, p. 1223.

152. The nurse is caring for the client with a renal transplant who is receiving immunosuppressant therapy, including corticosteroids. The nurse would plan to carefully monitor which of the following laboratory results for this client?

1 Serum albumin
2 Blood glucose
3 Magnesium
4 Potassium

Answer: 2

Rationale: Corticosteroid therapy can result in glucose intolerance, leading to elevated blood glucose levels. The nurse monitors these levels to detect this side effect of therapy. With successful transplantation, the client's serum electrolyte levels should be better regulated, although corticosteroids could also cause sodium retention.

Test-Taking Strategy: To answer this question accurately, specific knowledge about the side effects of corticosteroid therapy is needed. Remembering that corticosteroids affect blood glucose will assist in directing you to the correct option. If this question was difficult, take a few moments now to review this important type of medication!

Level of Cognitive Ability: Application
Phase of Nursing Process: Planning
Client Needs: Physiological Integrity
Content Area: Adult Health/Renal

Reference

Burrell, P., Gerlach, M., & Pless, B. (1997). *Adult nursing: Acute and community care* (2nd ed.). Stamford, CT: Appleton & Lange, p. 1129.

---

153. The client with end-stage renal disease (ESRD) has a nursing diagnosis of Ineffective Individual Coping related to terminal disease. The nurse plans to avoid using which of the following approaches in working with this client?

1 Set limits on mood swings and expressions of hostility
2 Assess the individual and family coping patterns
3 Explore meaning of the illness for this particular client
4 Give the client information when the client is ready to listen

Answer: 1

Rationale: Clients with ESRD may likely have mood swings, hostility, anger, and depression, among other responses. The nurse acknowledges the client's feelings and is supportive. The responses in options 2, 3, and 4 are also helpful to the client.

Test-Taking Strategy: Note the key word "avoid" in the stem of the question. Note that the wording of the question guides you to look for an incorrect response. Therefore, the answer to the question is something that the nurse would not do in the situation. Knowledge of basic communication strategies and psychological support allows you to eliminate each of the incorrect responses. Setting limits would not be helpful in this client situation.

Level of Cognitive Ability: Application
Phase of Nursing Process: Planning
Client Needs: Psychosocial Integrity
Content Area: Adult Health/Renal

Reference

Burrell, P., Gerlach, M., & Pless, B. (1997). *Adult nursing: Acute and community care* (2nd ed.). Stamford, CT: Appleton & Lange, p. 1264.

---

154. The nurse would plan to avoid which of the following actions in the management of the client with ascites?

1 Record abdominal girth daily at the level of the umbilicus
2 Encourage frequent exercise to prevent atelectasis
3 Elevate the legs while in bed
4 Carefully maintain a limit on sodium intake

Answer: 2

Rationale: Clients with ascites commonly have restrictions placed on sodium intake and possibly on fluid intake. It is common practice to monitor the extent of ascites by measuring the abdominal girth daily at the level of the umbilicus. The legs are also commonly edematous and are therefore elevated while the client is in bed. The nurse maintains rest as prescribed. The client may often be on bed rest, which has the effect of decreasing sodium retention and increasing renal clearance of sodium.

Test-Taking Strategy: The wording of this question guides you to look for an incorrect response. To answer this question correctly, you must use concepts related to fluid retention, edema, and sodium retention. Remembering that bed rest is a component of care will assist in directing you to the correct option. If this question was difficult, take a few moments to review nursing care related to this disorder!

Level of Cognitive Ability: Application
Phase of Nursing Process: Planning
Client Needs: Physiological Integrity
Content Area: Adult Health/Renal

Reference

Burrell, P., Gerlach, M., & Pless, B. (1997). *Adult nursing: Acute and community care* (2nd ed.). Stamford, CT: Appleton & Lange, p. 1497.

---

155. The nurse is preparing to administer medications to the client with hepatic encephalopathy. The nurse plans to administer which of the following medications to the client as prescribed?

1 Magnesium hydroxide (Milk of Magnesia)
2 Phenolphthalein (Ex-Lax)
3 Psyllium hydrophilic mucilloid (Metamucil)
4 Lactulose syrup (Chronulac)

Answer: 4

Rationale: Lactulose syrup is a hyperosmotic laxative agent that has the adjunct benefit of lowering serum ammonia levels. This occurs because the medication lowers bowel pH, which aids the conversion of ammonia in the gut to the ammonium ion, which is poorly absorbed. Magnesium hydroxide is a saline laxative, whereas phenolphthalein is a stimulant laxative. Metamucil is a bulk laxative.

Test-Taking Strategy: To answer this question accurately, it is necessary to know specific effects of this medication and the benefits of use in the client with impaired liver function. If this question was difficult, take a few moments to review the action and purpose of this medication!

Level of Cognitive Ability: Application
Phase of Nursing Process: Planning
Client Needs: Physiological Integrity
Content Area: Pharmacology

Reference

Burrell, P., Gerlach, M., & Pless, B. (1997). *Adult nursing: Acute and community care* (2nd ed.). Stamford, CT: Appleton & Lange, p. 1501.

---

156. The nurse is developing a teaching plan for the client with viral hepatitis. The nurse should plan to incorporate which of the following information in the teaching session?

1 "Activity should be limited to prevent fatigue."
2 "The diet should be low in calories."
3 "Meals should be few and large to conserve energy."
4 "Alcohol intake should be limited to 2 oz per day."

Answer: 1

Rationale: The client with viral hepatitis should limit activity to avoid fatigue during the recuperation period. The diet should be optimal in calories, protein, and carbohydrate. The client should take in several small meals per day. Alcohol is strictly forbidden.

Test-Taking Strategy: Knowledge regarding the components of care in the client with hepatitis will assist in answering this question. Use the process of elimination noting that the key phrase in the correct option is "prevent fatigue." Take time now to review care of the client with hepatitis if you had difficulty with this question!

Level of Cognitive Ability: Application
Phase of Nursing Process: Planning
Client Needs: Physiological Integrity
Content Area: Adult Health/Gastrointestinal

Reference

Black, J., & Matassarin-Jacobs, E. (1997). *Medical-surgical nursing: Clinical management for continuity of care* (5th ed.). Philadelphia: W. B. Saunders, pp. 1870–1871.

157. The nurse is preparing to teach colostomy irrigation to a client with a new colostomy. Which of the following points would the nurse include when developing the teaching plan?

1. "Use 500–1000 mL of warm tap water."
2. "Suspend irrigant 36 inches above the stoma."
3. "Insert the irrigation cone 1/2 inch into the stoma."
4. "If cramping occurs, open the irrigation clamp further."

Answer: 1

Rationale: The usual procedure for colostomy irrigation includes using 500–1000 mL of warm tap water. The solution is suspended 18 inches above the stoma. The cone is inserted 2 to 4 inches into the stoma but should never be forced. If cramping occurs, the client should decrease the flow rate of the irrigant as needed by closing the irrigation clamp.

Test-Taking Strategy: The wording of the question guides you to look for a correct statement. Basic knowledge of colostomy care then guides you to eliminate each of the incorrect responses. You can easily eliminate option 4. Eliminate option 2 next, knowing that 36 inches is much too high, followed by option 3 because a 1/2-inch insertion would not be effective. If you have had limited experience with ostomy care, take a few moments now to review this material.

Level of Cognitive Ability: Application
Phase of Nursing Process: Planning
Client Needs: Health Promotion and Maintenance
Content Area: Adult Health/Gastrointestinal

Reference

Black, J., & Matassarin-Jacobs, E. (1997). *Medical-surgical nursing: Clinical management for continuity of care* (5th ed.). Philadelphia: W. B. Saunders, p. 1815.

---

158. The client is being prepared for electroconvulsive therapy (ECT). The nurse's plan of care for the night before ECT treatment includes ensuring that the client

1. Is placed on nothing by mouth (NPO) status for 12 to 16 hours.
2. Receives no visitors and participates in limited unit activities.
3. Shampoos and dries hair, freeing it of all hair spray and creams.
4. Does not smoke cigarettes.

Answer: 3

Rationale: The client is instructed to shampoo and dry hair the night before ECT treatment. In addition, the client is instructed not to use hair sprays or creams before ECT, in order to reduce the risk of burns. The client is on NPO status for 6 to 8 hours before treatment; the 12 to 16 hours prescribed in option 1 is excessive. Some hospitals place inpatient clients on NPO status at midnight before ECT in the morning. Some clients who are on cardiovascular medication may be instructed to take their medicine with sips of water several hours before ECT. Option 2 is incorrect, as is option 4.

Test-Taking Strategy: Knowledge of the pretreatment preparation for ECT is essential for the nurse. In addition to informed consent and minimization of anxiety and fears concerning the procedure for client and family, keeping the client free from injury is a key treatment goal for the client undergoing ECT. Use the process of elimination to answer the question. Review the preprocedure preparation now if you had difficulty with this question!

Level of Cognitive Ability: Application
Phase of Nursing Process: Planning
Client Needs: Safe, Effective Care Environment
Content Area: Mental Health

Reference

Antai-Otong, D., & Kongale, G. (1995). *Psychiatric nursing: Biological and behavioral concepts*. Philadelphia: W. B. Saunders, pp. 584–589.

159. The client who has undergone neck dissection for a tumor has a nursing diagnosis of Ineffective Airway Clearance related to obstruction secondary to postoperative edema, drainage, and secretions. The nurse would plan to promote adequate respiratory function by avoiding which of the following activities?

1. Placing the bed in low Fowler's position
2. Supporting the neck incision while the patient coughs
3. Suctioning the client on a PRN basis
4. Encouraging coughing every 2 hours

Answer: 1

Rationale: The client's respiratory status is promoted by the use of high Fowler's position after this surgery. Low Fowler's position is avoided because it could result in increased venous pressure on the graft and increases risk of regurgitation and aspiration. It is also helpful to encourage the client to cough and deep breathe every 2 hours, to splint the neck incision while the client coughs, and to suction periodically as needed by the client.

Test-Taking Strategy: Note the key word "avoid" in the question. Identify the issue of the question as promoting adequate respiratory function. Knowledge of basic airway management principles allows you to eliminate each of the incorrect options systematically. Remember that the head of the bed needs to be elevated. Review the basic principles of promoting adequate respiratory function now if you had difficulty with this question!

Level of Cognitive Ability: Application
Phase of Nursing Process: Planning
Client Needs: Physiological Integrity
Content Area: Adult Health/Respiratory

Reference

Smeltzer, S., & Bare, B. (1996). *Brunner and Suddarth's Textbook of medical-surgical nursing* (8th ed.). Philadelphia: Lippincott-Raven, p. 847.

---

160. The client who has undergone radical neck dissection has a nursing diagnosis of Impaired Communication related to postoperative hoarseness. The nurse would formulate which of the following as the most appropriate goal for this nursing diagnosis?

1. Using nonverbal communication only
2. Incorporating nonverbal forms of communication as needed
3. Describing the hoarseness as permanent
4. Initiating communication only when necessary

Answer: 2

Rationale: The client may experience temporary hoarseness after neck dissection. Goals for the client include using nonverbal forms of communication as needed, expressing willingness to ring call bell for assistance, and using services of a speech pathologist if prescribed.

Test-Taking Strategy: Begin to answer this question by eliminating options 1 and 4. The use of the word "only" in these options makes them unsuitable, as they are too limiting to be useful. Because hoarseness is a temporary postoperative situation, option 2 is the best answer to the question. Review communication strategies for the client with impaired communication if you had difficulty with this question!

Level of Cognitive Ability: Application
Phase of Nursing Process: Planning
Client Needs: Psychosocial Integrity
Content Area: Fundamental Skills

Reference

Smeltzer, S., & Bare, B. (1996). *Brunner and Suddarth's Textbook of medical-surgical nursing* (8th ed.). Philadelphia: Lippincott-Raven, p. 849.

---

161. The client has suffered chemical burns to the esophagus after ingestion of lye. The nurse would plan to question an order for which of the following by the physician?

1. NPO status
2. Gastric lavage
3. Intravenous fluid therapy
4. Preparation for barium swallow

Answer: 2

Rationale: The client who has suffered chemical burns to the esophagus is placed on NPO status, is given IV fluids for replacement and treatment of possible shock, and is prepared for esophagoscopy and barium swallow to determine the extent of damage. A nasogastric tube may be inserted, but gastric lavage and emesis are avoided, to prevent further erosion of the mucosa by the irritating substances.

Test-Taking Strategy: The client who has suffered chemical burns to the esophagus is at risk for going into shock; thus options 1 and 3 are plausible and are therefore not the answers to the question as stated. You would choose option 2 over option 4 either by knowing that this diagnostic test is appropriate or by knowing that lavage or emesis is contraindicated after ingestion of a corrosive substance. Review care of the client after burns caused by the ingestion of chemicals if you had difficulty with this question!

Level of Cognitive Ability: Application
Phase of Nursing Process: Planning
Client Needs: Physiological Integrity
Content Area: Adult Health/Integumentary

Reference

Smeltzer, S., & Bare, B. (1996). *Brunner and Suddarth's Textbook of medical-surgical nursing* (8th ed.). Philadelphia: Lippincott-Raven, p. 854.

---

162. The nurse has inserted a Keofeed tube into the client's stomach in preparation for enteral feedings. The nurse would plan to have the client lie in which position to help the tube pass from the stomach into the small intestine?

1 High Fowler's
2 Low Fowler's
3 Left side
4 Right side

Answer: 4

Rationale: The client is placed lying on the right side to help a Dobbhoff or Keofeed tube pass from the stomach into the small intestine, which usually takes about 24 hours. Once feedings have begun, keeping the head of the bed elevated will help to prevent aspiration.

Test-Taking Strategy: To answer this question accurately, it is necessary to know which position aids in the passage of contents from the stomach into the small intestine. Remembering the anatomical location of the stomach in relation to the small intestine may help you eliminate each of the incorrect options. Review this now if you had difficulty with this question!

Level of Cognitive Ability: Application
Phase of Nursing Process: Planning
Client Needs: Physiological Integrity
Content Area: Adult Health/Gastrointestinal

Reference

Smeltzer, S., & Bare, B. (1996). *Brunner and Suddarth's Textbook of medical-surgical nursing* (8th ed.). Philadelphia: Lippincott-Raven, p. 862.

---

163. The nurse makes rounds after receiving report and assesses that the stoma of a client with a new colostomy is a dark, dusky color. The nurse should plan to take which of the following actions?

1 Change the ostomy bag
2 Irrigate the colostomy
3 Order a larger size bag
4 Notify the surgeon

Answer: 4

Rationale: The color of a stoma should be a moist, beefy red. A dark, dusky stoma indicates ischemia, necessitating that the physician be notified. All of the other responses are incorrect nursing actions.

Test-Taking Strategy: To answer this question accurately, be aware of the characteristics of a viable stoma. The question is worded in the affirmative, so there is only one correct answer. Basic knowledge of ostomy assessment and care helps you eliminate each of the incorrect responses. The key phrase to guide you to the correct option is "dark, dusky color." Review ostomy assessment now if you had difficulty with this question!

Level of Cognitive Ability: Application
Phase of Nursing Process: Planning
Client Needs: Physiological Integrity
Content Area: Adult Health/Gastrointestinal

Reference

Ignatavicius, D. D., Workman, M. L., & Mishler, M. A. (1995). *Medical-surgical nursing: A nursing process approach* (2nd ed.). Philadelphia: W. B. Saunders, p. 1606.

164. The nurse is participating in a health fair and is teaching ways to decrease dietary risk factors for cancer. The nurse would plan to include which of the following pieces of information?

1. "Avoid excess fat intake."
2. "Limit intake of cruciferous vegetables."
3. "Increase intake of smoked and processed meats."
4. "Limit intake of dietary fiber."

Answer: 1

Rationale: Current dietary guidelines to reduce cancer risk include limiting intake of foods known to have a carcinogenic effect, as well as increasing intake of foods known to have a protective effect. Foods that should be limited include those with high fat content, red meat, and foods containing nitrites (smoked or processed meats). Foods that should be increased are cruciferous vegetables (e.g., broccoli, cauliflower), foods that have high vitamins A and C content, and foods with high fiber content.

Test-Taking Strategy: The question is worded positively, so you are looking for a single correct answer. Begin to answer this question by eliminating option 3, because highly processed meats have a high content of added chemicals. Knowing that fiber, fruits, and vegetables are also healthy diet choices helps you to eliminate options 2 and 4 next. Option 1, the correct answer, is a generally accepted recommendation for all clients and reduces risk of developing a wide variety of disorders.

Level of Cognitive Ability: Application
Phase of Nursing Process: Planning
Client Needs: Health Promotion and Maintenance
Content Area: Adult Health/Oncology

Reference

Ignatavicius, D. D., Workman, M. L., & Mishler, M. A. (1995). *Medical-surgical nursing: A nursing process approach* (2nd ed.). Philadelphia: W. B. Saunders, p. 557.

---

165. The nurse notices that the client has a pigmented mole and determines through further assessment that the mole has recently undergone color changes and has become larger. The nurse should plan to take which of the following most important steps?

1. Tell the client to keep a small bandage over the site
2. Instruct the client to buy an over-the-counter wart removal product
3. Relay the information to the client's primary care provider
4. Advise the client to use skin products with sunscreen

Answer: 3

Rationale: This information should be reported to the client's primary care provider. One of the seven warning signs of cancer is "An obvious change in a wart or mole." Pigmented moles are also considered to be precancerous lesions, which could undergo malignant degeneration at any time. Clients who have these should monitor them regularly for changes and report them if changes are found.

Test-Taking Strategy: The question asks for the most important step. This implies that more than one or all of the options may be partially or totally correct. Eliminate options 1 and 2 first because they are incorrect. You would choose option 3 over option 4 (which is also correct) by recognizing that changes described in the mole could indicate that the growth has become malignant.

Level of Cognitive Ability: Application
Phase of Nursing Process: Planning
Client Needs: Physiological Integrity
Content Area: Adult Health/Oncology

Reference

Ignatavicius, D. D., Workman, M. L., & Mishler, M. A. (1995). *Medical-surgical nursing: A nursing process approach* (2nd ed.). Philadelphia: W. B. Saunders, p. 557.

---

166. The client experienced acetylsalicylic acid (ASA) overdose 24 hours before being admitted. The nurse would plan to monitor the client for signs and symptoms of which of the following acid-base imbalances?

1. Respiratory acidosis
2. Respiratory alkalosis
3. Metabolic acidosis
4. Metabolic alkalosis

Answer: 3

Rationale: Acetylsalicylic acid is aspirin, overdose of which leads to metabolic acidosis as a later complication. In the early phase after aspirin overdose, the client may experience respiratory alkalosis as a compensatory mechanism as the body is trying the combat the developing metabolic acidosis.

Test-Taking Strategy: To answer this question accurately, you must know that an excess of ingested acids, such as aspirin, can lead to metabolic acidosis. Note that the question tells you that the overdose occurred 24 hours earlier. This helps you eliminate the compensatory mechanism, respiratory alkalosis, as a possible answer. Review the causes of metabolic acidosis now if you had difficulty with this question!

Level of Cognitive Ability: Application
Phase of Nursing Process: Planning
Client Needs: Physiological Integrity
Content Area: Adult Health/Endocrine

Reference

Ignatavicius, D. D., Workman, M. L., & Mishler, M. A. (1995). *Medical-surgical nursing: A nursing process approach* (2nd ed.). Philadelphia: W. B. Saunders, pp. 333–334.

---

167. The client has chronic respiratory acidosis. The nurse would plan to use which of the following most appropriate means for administering oxygen to the client?

1 Partial rebreather mask
2 100% oxygen non-rebreather mask
3 High-flow 60% oxygen via face mask
4 Low-flow oxygen via nasal prongs at 2 L/minute

Answer: 4

Rationale: The client with chronic respiratory acidosis has chronically high circulating carbon dioxide levels. For this reason, the body becomes insensitive to carbon dioxide levels in the blood stream in regulating ventilation and uses arterial oxygen levels instead. The client must receive low-flow oxygen, or respiratory failure could result.

Test-Taking Strategy: Note the key word "chronic" in the question. To answer this question accurately, recall that chronic respiratory acidosis is usually associated with chronic respiratory disease, such as chronic obstructive pulmonary disease (COPD). Knowing that this client must receive low-flow oxygen, you would then eliminate options 2 and 3. You would next eliminate option 1 because a client with this condition should not rebreathe his or her own exhaled carbon dioxide. Review the treatment measures for chronic respiratory acidosis now if you had difficulty with this question!

Level of Cognitive Ability: Application
Phase of Nursing Process: Planning
Client Needs: Safe, Effective Care Environment
Content Area: Adult Health/Respiratory

Reference

Ignatavicius, D. D., Workman, M. L., & Mishler, M. A. (1995). *Medical-surgical nursing: A nursing process approach* (2nd ed.). Philadelphia: W. B. Saunders, pp. 339, 692.

---

168. The client admitted with peptic ulcer has been taking large amounts of antacids for the condition. The nurse would plan to monitor the client for which of the following acid-base imbalances?

1 Respiratory acidosis
2 Respiratory alkalosis
3 Metabolic acidosis
4 Metabolic alkalosis

Answer: 4

Rationale: Ingestion of large amounts of antacids places the client at risk for metabolic alkalosis because antacids neutralize the hydrochloric acid in the stomach and decrease the number of hydrogen ions available to the body. The nurse would therefore monitor this client for signs of metabolic alkalosis.

Test-Taking Strategy: Begin to answer this question by examining the key word "antacid." This would lead you to conclude that overuse of this product would result in alkalosis. You would then discriminate between respiratory and metabolic by realizing that the alkaline substance was ingested and that the respiratory system is not a prime trigger for this event. Review the causes of metabolic alkalosis now if you had difficulty with this question!

Level of Cognitive Ability: Application
Phase of Nursing Process: Planning
Client Needs: Physiological Integrity
Content Area: Adult Health/Gastrointestinal

Reference

Ignatavicius, D. D., Workman, M. L., & Mishler, M. A. (1995). *Medical-surgical nursing: A nursing process approach* (2nd ed.). Philadelphia: W. B. Saunders, p. 342.

169. The preoperative client complains of anxiety, accompanied by tingling in the fingers and toes. The client has a pulse of 100, respiratory rate of 30, and blood pressure of 138/86. The nurse should plan to do which of the following as an initial measure?

1 Obtain an order for midazolam (Versed)
2 Instruct the client to concentrate on breathing more slowly
3 Obtain an electrocardiogram
4 Institute seizure precautions

Answer: 2

Rationale: The tingling in fingers and toes is a classic symptom of alkalosis. Clients who are anxious and have a high respiratory rate are likely to have respiratory, not metabolic, alkalosis. The indicated initial treatment is to have the client breathe more slowly. Breathing into a paper bag may also be useful. If the condition continues, the client may benefit from a preoperative sedative medication, such as midazolam.

Test-Taking Strategy: The key words and phrases in this question are "anxiety," "tingling in fingers and toes," "respiratory rate 30," and "initial." To answer this question correctly, it is helpful to know that tingling in the fingers and toes is associated with alkalosis. The high respiratory rate would then guide you to conclude that the client has respiratory alkalosis. You would then eliminate options 3 and 4 because they are of no benefit in this situation. You would then choose option 2 over option 1 as the best "initial" measure. Review treatment measures for the client with respiratory alkalosis now if you had difficulty with this question!

Level of Cognitive Ability: Application
Phase of Nursing Process: Planning
Client Needs: Physiological Integrity
Content Area: Adult Health/Respiratory

Reference

Ignatavicius, D. D., Workman, M. L., & Mishler, M. A. (1995). *Medical-surgical nursing: A nursing process approach* (2nd ed.). Philadelphia: W. B. Saunders, pp. 342, 343.

170. The client is admitted with diabetic ketoacidosis (DKA). The nurse plans to monitor the client for respirations that are

1 Shallow and labored.
2 Shallow and nonlabored.
3 Deep and nonlabored.
4 Deep and labored.

Answer: 3

Rationale: The client with DKA exhibits Kussmaul respirations. These are respirations that are deep and nonlabored and occur because the body tries to eliminate carbon dioxide to compensate for acidosis. As ketoacidosis improves, this pattern of respiration resolves. The nurse monitors the client's respiratory status as part of the entire clinical picture.

Test-Taking Strategy: The key words in the stem are "ketoacidosis" and "respirations." In order to answer this question correctly, recall that the body compensates for metabolic acidosis through respiratory alkalosis. If the primary problem is not respiratory in origin, the respirations are not likely to be labored. Thus options 1 and 4 may be eliminated first. You would choose option 3 over option 2 by knowing that deep respirations are more likely to aid excretion of carbon dioxide and other volatile body acids.

Level of Cognitive Ability: Application
Phase of Nursing Process: Planning
Client Needs: Physiological Integrity
Content Area: Adult Health/Endocrine

Reference

Ignatavicius, D. D., Workman, M. L., & Mishler, M. A. (1995). *Medical-surgical nursing: A nursing process approach* (2nd ed.). Philadelphia: W. B. Saunders, pp. 336–337.

171. The client is scheduled to have an arterial blood gas measurement, with the sample drawn from the radial artery. The nurse plans to determine which of the following before the sample is drawn?

1. Patency of the brachial artery
2. Patency of the ulnar artery
3. Whether the client is allergic to heparin
4. Whether the client has weakness in that extremity

Answer: 2

Rationale: Before drawing an arterial sample from the radial artery, or before insertion of an intra-arterial catheter at that site, Allen's test should be performed. This involves compression of the radial and ulnar arteries and then releasing either vessel to determine its patency. Both arteries are tested, one at a time. The vessel being tested is patent if the hand becomes pale when both arteries are occluded and then becomes pink when that artery is released.

Test-Taking Strategy: Specific knowledge of this maneuver is needed to answer this question correctly. Option 1 can be eliminated first because the brachial artery is not involved. Eliminate option 3 next because heparin is not administered. For the remaining two options, use the ABCs: airway, breathing, and circulation. You should be directed to option 2 as it relates to circulation. If necessary, take a few moments now to review this simple but important test!

Level of Cognitive Ability: Application
Phase of Nursing Process: Planning
Client Needs: Safe, Effective Care Environment
Content Area: Adult Health/Cardiovascular

Reference

Luckmann, J. (1997). *Saunders manual of nursing care.* Philadelphia: W. B. Saunders, p. 918.

---

172. The nurse is planning a health fair at a local college. Information about testicular cancer is to be included. Which of the following pieces of information would the nurse plan to provide about the early signs of testicular cancer?

1. "It is accompanied by sharp pain and scrotal heaviness."
2. "There is the presence of a palpable, painful lump."
3. "There is a sensation of heaviness and an enlarged, painful scrotum."
4. "There is a palpable, painless lump with possible scrotal enlargement."

Answer: 4

Rationale: An early sign of testicular cancer is a painless, palpable, often pea-sized lump in the testicular area, which may be accompanied by a sensation of scrotal heaviness and swelling. This type of cancer has excellent cure rates if detected early. The nurse teaches about the signs of testicular cancer, which may be detected with monthly testicular self-examination.

Test-Taking Strategy: Remember that options that are similar are not likely to be correct. In this question, each of the incorrect responses includes the presence of pain. The correct answer is the response that does not include pain as a symptom. Review the signs of testicular cancer now if you had difficulty with this question!

Level of Cognitive Ability: Application
Phase of Nursing Process: Planning
Client Needs: Health Promotion and Maintenance
Content Area: Adult Health/Oncology

Reference

Luckmann, J. (1997). *Saunders manual of nursing care.* Philadelphia: W. B. Saunders, p. 1435.

---

173. A client has cirrhosis complicated by ascites. The nurse would plan to monitor for which of the following expected but adverse laboratory results?

1. Low serum albumin
2. Low urine specific gravity
3. High serum calcium
4. High urine sodium

Answer: 1

Rationale: The client with ascites as a complication of cirrhosis loses plasma proteins into the ascitic fluid. Over time this causes the client's serum albumin and total protein levels to decrease. This problem is also aggravated by decreased protein synthesis by the cirrhotic liver.

Test-Taking Strategy: To answer this question accurately, recall the normal functions of the liver and the makeup of fluid that is lost in the abdominal cavity. Knowledge of either of these allows you to eliminate each of the incorrect responses systematically. Review the physiological processes associated with cirrhosis now if you had difficulty with this question!

Level of Cognitive Ability: Application
Phase of Nursing Process: Planning
Client Needs: Physiological Integrity
Content Area: Adult Health/Gastrointestinal

Reference

Ignatavicius, D. D., Workman, M. L., & Mishler, M. A. (1995). *Medical-surgical nursing: A nursing process approach* (2nd ed.). Philadelphia: W. B. Saunders, p. 1672.

---

174. The client with ascites is being discharged to home. The nurse would plan to encourage the client to eat which of the following foods that the client enjoys?

1 Canned vegetables
2 Fresh apples
3 Potato chips
4 Corned beef

Answer: 2

Rationale: The client with ascites is generally encouraged to avoid foods that are high in sodium, which could aggravate fluid retention. The diet should be high in protein (unless specifically advised otherwise) and high in calories.

Test-Taking Strategy: To answer this question accurately, it is necessary to know that high-sodium foods are to be avoided by the client with ascites. Remember that responses that are similar are not likely to be correct. In this question, all of the incorrect responses are examples of foods that are high in sodium. Take time now to review the diet recommended for the client with ascites if you had difficulty with this question!

Level of Cognitive Ability: Application
Phase of Nursing Process: Planning
Client Needs: Health Promotion and Maintenance
Content Area: Adult Health/Gastrointestinal

Reference

Ignatavicius, D. D., Workman, M. L., & Mishler, M. A. (1995). *Medical-surgical nursing: A nursing process approach* (2nd ed.). Philadelphia: W. B. Saunders, p. 1682.

---

175. The client admitted with Laënnec's cirrhosis is ready for discharge and expresses the motivation to prevent this condition from worsening. The nurse would plan to teach the client and family about which of the following resources to assist the client?

1 Public library
2 American Cancer Society
3 Overeaters Anonymous
4 Alcoholics Anonymous

Answer: 4

Rationale: Laënnec's cirrhosis results from chronic alcoholism. This client may benefit from a support group that concentrates on the source of the medical problem: alcoholism. Referrals to agencies for psychosocial support are best provided when the client is motivated.

Test-Taking Strategy: To answer this question accurately, it is necessary to know that Laënnec's cirrhosis results from excessive intake of alcohol. This knowledge would allow you to eliminate each of the incorrect responses easily. Review this type of cirrhosis now if you had difficulty with this question!

Level of Cognitive Ability: Application
Phase of Nursing Process: Planning
Client Needs: Psychosocial Integrity
Content Area: Adult Health/Gastrointestinal

Reference

Ignatavicius, D. D., Workman, M. L., & Mishler, M. A. (1995). *Medical-surgical nursing: A nursing process approach* (2nd ed.). Philadelphia: W. B. Saunders, pp. 1666, 1683.

176. The nurse is planning discharge teaching for the client with viral hepatitis. Which of the following dietary considerations should the nurse include in the instructions?

1 Small, frequent meals
2 Fluid restriction
3 Diet high in fat
4 Diet low in carbohydrate

Answer: 1

Rationale: The diet for the client recovering from viral hepatitis should be high in carbohydrates and calories. Protein and fat intake should be moderate, and some providers prescribe a diet that is low in fat. The client should have smaller, more frequent meals. Fluid restriction is not indicated.

Test-Taking Strategy: To answer this question accurately, it is necessary to understand the nature of the diet needed in recovery from viral hepatitis. Remembering that fatigue is a problem with these clients may assist in directing you to the correct option. If needed, take time now to review this content!

Level of Cognitive Ability: Application
Phase of Nursing Process: Planning
Client Needs: Health Promotion and Maintenance
Content Area: Adult Health/Gastrointestinal

Reference

Luckmann, J. (1997). *Saunders manual of nursing care.* Philadelphia: W. B. Saunders, p. 1316.

---

177. The client hospitalized with hepatitis complains of fatigue and feelings of depression. The nurse plans which of the following strategies to help the client cope effectively during recuperation?

1 Encourage lengthy visits by the family
2 Have the client remain in the unit lounge during the day
3 Encourage restful diversional activities per client preference
4 Concentrate all activities requiring exertion early in the day

Answer: 3

Rationale: The client with hepatitis suffers from fatigue as an expected part of the clinical picture. However, fatigue may lead to feelings of frustration and depression by the client. The nurse plans daily client activities to carefully achieve a balance of rest and activity. The nurse also encourages short visits from family and quiet diversional activities to help the client cope during the recuperative period.

Test-Taking Strategy: To answer this question accurately, recall that fatigue is an important consequence of the disease process and that it has an effect on the client's psychosocial status. With these concepts in mind, you can systematically eliminate each of the incorrect responses. Options 1, 2, and 4 would not provide the required rest and would cause additional fatigue in the client.

Level of Cognitive Ability: Application
Phase of Nursing Process: Planning
Client Needs: Psychosocial Integrity
Content Area: Adult Health/Gastrointestinal

Reference

Ignatavicius, D. D., Workman, M. L., & Mishler, M. A. (1995). *Medical-surgical nursing: A nursing process approach* (2nd ed.). Philadelphia: W. B. Saunders, pp. 1692–1693.

---

178. The client requires insertion of an oropharyngeal airway. The nurse would plan to use which of the following correct insertion procedures?

1 Leave any dentures in place
2 Flex the client's neck
3 Insert the airway with the tip pointed upward
4 Suction the client's mouth once per shift

Answer: 3

Rationale: Before insertion of an oropharyngeal airway, any dentures or partial plates should be removed from the client's mouth. An airway that is an appropriate size should be selected. The client should be positioned supine, with the neck hyperextended if possible. The airway is inserted with the tip facing upward and is then rotated downward once the flange has reached the client's teeth. After insertion, the client's mouth is suctioned every hour or as necessary. The airway is removed for inspection of the mouth every 2 to 4 hours.

Test-Taking Strategy: The key words in this question are "correct insertion procedure." Begin to answer this question by eliminating option 4, because this is not part of the insertion procedure. Next eliminate option 2, because the neck is hyperextended (unless contraindicated) to open the airway. To discriminate between the remaining two options, you must be familiar with insertion technique. It may be helpful to reason that dentures should be removed, as they are a potential source of airway obstruction. Review this procedure now if you had difficulty with this question!

Level of Cognitive Ability: Application
Phase of Nursing Process: Planning
Client Needs: Safe, Effective Care Environment
Content Area: Adult Health/Respiratory

Reference

Burrell, P., Gerlach, M., & Pless, B. (1997). *Adult nursing: Acute and community care* (2nd ed.). Stamford, CT: Appleton & Lange, p. 675.

---

179. The nurse is assisting the physician with insertion of an endotracheal tube (ETT). The nurse should plan to assure that which of the following is done as a final measure to determine correct tube placement?

1 Hyperoxygenate the client
2 Listen for bilateral breath sounds
3 Tape the tube securely in place
4 Verify by the chest x-ray

Answer: 4

Rationale: The issue of the question is to identify the last action needed to verify ETT placement. The final measure to determine ETT placement is to verify by chest x-ray. The chest x-ray shows the exact placement of the tube in the trachea, which should be above the bifurcation of the right and left mainstem bronchi. The other options are incorrect because they are completed initially after tube placement.

Test-Taking Strategy: The key words in the question are "final measure" and "correct." These words tell you that you are looking for a correct item and also imply a time sequence. Knowing that the client is hyperoxygenated before and immediately after insertion, you would eliminate option 1. Option 2 is eliminated next because it is the initial means used to verify placement, not the final one. Option 3 is done before option 4 to avoid tube displacement before or during the x-ray.

Level of Cognitive Ability: Application
Phase of Nursing Process: Planning
Client Needs: Safe, Effective Care Environment
Content Area: Adult Health/Respiratory

Reference

Burrell, P., Gerlach, M., & Pless, B. (1997). *Adult nursing: Acute and community care* (2nd ed.). Stamford, CT: Appleton & Lange, p. 678.

---

180. The client has an endotracheal tube (ETT) in place and is also receiving enteral tube feedings by nasogastric tube. The nurse is suctioning cream-colored secretions from the ETT. Which of the following measures should the nurse plan to determine whether the secretions are sputum or tube feeding?

1 Stop the feeding and see whether the secretions diminish
2 Place methylene blue coloring in the feeding bag
3 Obtain an order to decrease the tube feeding rate
4 Obtain an order to change from continuous to intermittent feedings

Answer: 2

Rationale: Because sputum characteristics sometimes resemble the characteristics of tube feedings, it may be difficult for the nurse to determine whether sputum or feedings are being removed during the suctioning procedure. Tube feeding may be present in the trachea if the client regurgitates and then aspirates or if the client develops a tracheoesophageal fistula. A green or blue food coloring (such as methylene blue) may be added to the feeding. If a blue (or green) coloration appears in the sputum, the client has aspirated feeding into the trachea. If the sputum remains unchanged, then the client has not aspirated the tube feeding.

Test-Taking Strategy: The key words in the question are "determine," "sputum," and "tube feeding." This guides you to look for an option that will help discriminate one event from the other. Eliminate options 3 and 4 first, because they will not help diagnose the problem. You would choose option 2 over option 1 because it does not impair the client's nutritional status and it is a more effective procedure.

Level of Cognitive Ability: Application
Phase of Nursing Process: Planning
Client Needs: Safe, Effective Care Environment
Content Area: Adult Health/Respiratory

Reference

Burrell, P., Gerlach, M., & Pless, B. (1997). *Adult nursing: Acute and community care* (2nd ed.). Stamford, CT: Appleton & Lange, p. 680.

181. The nurse is caring for the client being discharged to home with a tracheostomy. Which of the following approaches should the nurse take to best help the client adjust to caring for the tracheostomy at home?

1. Give thorough, detailed explanations of the procedure
2. Keep the focus of teaching on the client, but not the family
3. Provide sufficient practice time for skill development before discharge
4. Provide a written list of all the equipment needed in the home setting

Answer: 3

Rationale: It is reassuring to the client to feel comfortable with the actual tracheostomy care procedure before the time of discharge. The amount and depth of information that is given depends on the client's individual learning needs. The family is included in the teaching, because it is beneficial for the family to know these procedures. A list of equipment needed may be a useful adjunct to the client.

Test-Taking Strategy: Note the key phrases and word in the question, which are "best help," "adjust," and "tracheostomy care." The presence of the word "best" implies that more than one or all of the options may be partially or totally correct. You must determine which option will be most beneficial to the client. Options 1 and 2 are eliminated first because they are not the most helpful approaches. You would choose option 3 over option 4 because comfort with a skill is more important than having a list in hand.

Level of Cognitive Ability: Application
Phase of Nursing Process: Planning
Client Needs: Psychosocial Integrity
Content Area: Adult Health/Respiratory

Reference

Burrell, P., Gerlach, M., & Pless, B. (1997). *Adult nursing: Acute and community care* (2nd ed.). Stamford, CT: Appleton & Lange, p. 740.

---

182. The nurse is caring for a woman with a twin pregnancy. Which of the following nursing diagnoses would the nurse plan to formulate to address an issue related to the twin pregnancy?

1. Ineffective Individual Coping related to infection process
2. Altered Nutrition: More than Body Requirements, related to hyperglycemia
3. Risk for Altered Growth and Development related to preterm labor
4. Decreased Cardiac Output related to increased blood volume

Answer: 3

Rationale: A client with a twin pregnancy is at increased risk for preterm labor. Preterm delivery has negative implications for the infants' growth and development. With increased blood volume, cardiac output normally increases 30%–50% in the second trimester.

Test-Taking Strategy: This question can be answered by eliminating distracting information in the options. Hyperglycemia and infection are not mentioned in the stem of the question and are not special consequences of a twin pregnancy; thus options 1 and 2 can be eliminated. Increased cardiac output is a normal symptom of pregnancy and is not significantly affected by a multiple pregnancy. Thus option 4 is not an appropriate choice, either.

Level of Cognitive Ability: Analysis
Phase of Nursing Process: Planning
Client Needs: Physiological Integrity
Content Area: Maternity

Reference

Nichols, F., & Zwelling, E. (1997). *Maternal-newborn nursing: Theory and practice.* Philadelphia: W. B. Saunders, pp. 564, 641–685.

---

183. A manic client is admitted to the unit with a recent history of weight loss and sleep deprivation. In planning care to meet the nutritional needs of the client, the nurse

1. Orders a high-protein diet.
2. Requests an order for an IV infusion.
3. Asks the client to eat meals in the dayroom.
4. Offers frequent high-calorie snacks and finger foods.

Answer: 4

Rationale: Manic clients may receive insufficient nutrition as they are too involved mentally to attend to physiological signals. Offering frequent high-calorie snacks and finger foods will assist best in providing adequate nutrition during this period.

Test-Taking Strategy: Use the process of elimination considering the client's diagnosis. Options 2 and 3 are incorrect because both are restrictive measures. Option 1 is less correct than option 4, because the client does not have the attention span to sit and eat a meal and because there is no clinical indication for increasing protein intake.

Level of Cognitive Ability: Application
Phase of Nursing Process: Planning
Client Needs: Health Promotion and Maintenance
Content Area: Mental Health

Reference
Wilson, H., & Kneisl, C. (1996). *Psychiatric nursing* (5th ed.). Menlo Park, CA: Addison-Wesley, p. 350.

---

184. An elderly man is admitted to the acute psychiatric unit with a diagnosis of depression. He is unclean, unshaven, and inappropriately dressed. He is accompanied by his adult daughter, who is very upset about her father's lack of interest in his appearance. In planning care for this client, it is most important for the client and his daughter to understand that

1 Hygiene is not important to those who socially isolate themselves.
2 The nurse will assist the client in meeting hygiene needs until the client is able to resume self-care.
3 Client self-esteem needs take priority over appearances.
4 Group peer pressure on the unit will soon have the client attending to his hygiene needs.

Answer: 2

Rationale: Both the client and his family need to know that the nurse will assist the client until he can resume self-care activities. The client is experiencing psychomotor retardation and decreased energy at this time and requires assistance.

Test-Taking Strategy: The question is asking what is most important in planning care for this client. Both the client and family member need to see the nurse as a supportive professional in the setting. Option 2 is the only option that addresses the specific needs of the client in a supportive manner.

Level of Cognitive Ability: Application
Phase of Nursing Process: Planning
Client Needs: Safe, Effective Care Environment
Content Area: Mental Health

Reference
Wilson, H., & Kneisl, C. (1996). *Psychiatric nursing* (5th ed.). Menlo Park, CA: Addison-Wesley, p. 325.

---

185. The depressed client tells the nurse that he or she is powerless and unworthy of having friends and that on occasion has taken too many pills. The nurse's priority in planning care for this client is to

1 Continuously assess for suicidal ideation.
2 Provide structured activities with other clients.
3 Monitor the effects of the prescribed tricyclic antidepressant.
4 Acknowledge the client's accomplishments to build self-esteem.

Answer: 1

Rationale: Client safety always takes priority over other nursing care concerns. The other options are correct nursing measures to take with a depressed client, but they are not the priority in planning care.

Test-Taking Strategy: Note the key phrase "has taken too many pills." Note that the stem of the question asks for the priority in planning care. The potential for suicide is of highest priority and takes precedence over other planned nursing actions.

Level of Cognitive Ability: Application
Phase of Nursing Process: Planning
Client Needs: Safe, Effective Care Environment
Content Area: Mental Health

Reference
Wilson, H., & Kneisl, C. (1996). *Psychiatric nursing* (5th ed.). Menlo Park, CA: Addison-Wesley, p. 332.

---

186. In collaboratively planning care, the suicidal client has signed a no self-harm/no suicide contract. On the basis of this plan, which of the following is not an appropriate nursing action?

1 Using the contract as a way of connecting with and staying with the client
2 Placing more trust in the contract than in her or his clinical judgment
3 Specifying in the contract time intervals for reevaluation
4 Including alternatives in the contract, such as "If I feel like hurting myself, I will call the nurse."

Answer: 2

Rationale: Clients who are acutely suicidal may agree to the contract even though they have no intention of adhering to it. A contract is a helpful therapeutic tool but in itself does not replace clinical judgment.

Test-Taking Strategy: Read the stem carefully. Note that the stem states "not an appropriate nursing action." This should assist in directing you to the correct option, which in this case is an incorrect nursing action. If you had difficulty with this question, take time now to review nurse-client contracts!

Level of Cognitive Ability: Application
Phase of Nursing Process: Planning
Client Needs: Safe, Effective Care Environment
Content Area: Mental Health

Reference
Wilson, H., & Kneisl, C. (1996). *Psychiatric nursing* (5th ed.) Menlo Park, CA: Addison-Wesley, p. 598.

187. The nurse formulates a nursing diagnosis of Activity Intolerance related to underlying cardiovascular disease as evidenced by exertional fatigue and increased blood pressure. The nurse would write which of the following goal statements to best evaluate client progress in this area?

1. "Engages in progressive self-care activities."
2. "Ambulates 10 feet further each day."
3. "Understands the importance of physical conditioning."
4. "Selects an appropriate diet to meet metabolic needs."

Answer: 2

Rationale: The question asks you to select a response that can "best evaluate." The general concept inherent in each of the goals is good. However, goal statements must be clear and measurable to be most effective. Option 2 meets all criteria for goal statements.

Test-Taking Strategy: The verb "understands" in option 3 makes that an incorrect response, as it cannot be measured. The adjectives "progressive" and "appropriate" in options 1 and 4 are vague. Option 2 is the clearest and most measurable of all the choices.

Level of Cognitive Ability: Application
Phase of Nursing Process: Planning
Client Needs: Health Promotion and Maintenance
Content Area: Adult Health/Cardiovascular

Reference

Cox, H., Hinz, M., Lubno, M., et al. (1997). *Clinical applications of nursing diagnosis* (3rd ed.). Philadelphia: F. A. Davis, p. 252.

---

188. An elderly client with ischemic heart disease is admitted to the medical nursing unit after experiencing an episode of dizziness and shortness of breath. The nurse formulates a nursing diagnosis of Decreased Cardiac Output related to possible dysrhythmias as evidenced by dyspnea and syncopal episode. The nurse would plan to take which most important action in the care of the client?

1. Measure blood pressure every 4 hours
2. Monitor oxygen saturation levels continuously
3. Check capillary refill at least once per shift
4. Place the client on a cardiac monitor

Answer: 4

Rationale: The client with decreased cardiac output and possible dysrhythmias should be placed on continuous cardiac monitoring so myocardial perfusion can be most accurately assessed. Other cardiovascular assessments should be made at least every 2 hours initially.

Test-Taking Strategy: The phrase "most important action" limits the viable choices to options 2 and 4. Because option 4 is a more direct measurement about cardiovascular status, it is chosen over option 2 (which in the absence of cardiac monitoring would be a reasonable choice).

Level of Cognitive Ability: Application
Phase of Nursing Process: Planning
Client Needs: Safe, Effective Care Environment
Content Area: Adult Health/Cardiovascular

Reference

Cox, H., Hinz, M., Lubno, M., et al. (1997). *Clinical applications of nursing diagnosis* (3rd ed.). Philadelphia: F. A. Davis, p. 278.

---

189. The home care nurse is planning adaptations needed for activities of daily living for the client with a nursing diagnosis of Decreased Cardiac Output. The nurse would incorporate which of the following suggestions in discussions with the client?

1. Consume 1–2 oz of liquor each night to promote vasodilatation
2. Try to engage in vigorous activity to strengthen cardiac reserve
3. Take in adequate daily fiber to prevent straining at stool
4. Force fluids to 3000 mL/day to promote renal perfusion

Answer: 3

Rationale: Standard home care instructions for a client with this nursing diagnosis include, among others, lifestyle changes such as decreasing alcohol intake, avoiding activities that increase the demands on the heart, instituting a bowel regimen to prevent straining and constipation, and maintaining fluid and electrolyte balance.

Test-Taking Strategy: The question asks "which of the following" with no modifiers, which tells you that three answers are incorrect. Read the words in each option carefully examining the impact of each of those options on the heart. This should help you eliminate each of the incorrect options systematically and direct you toward the correct option.

Level of Cognitive Ability: Application
Phase of Nursing Process: Planning
Client Needs: Physiological Integrity
Content Area: Adult Health/Cardiovascular

Reference

Cox, H., Hinz, M., Lubno, M., et al. (1997). *Clinical applications of nursing diagnosis* (3rd ed.). Philadelphia: F. A. Davis, p. 284.

190. In planning care for the suicidal client, the nurse meets with family members and identifies community resources that may be of help to the client after discharge. The nurse takes these actions because the nurse is aware that suicidal clients

1 Demonstrate delusions of grandeur.
2 Have limited social support systems.
3 Tend to be noncompliant.
4 Rarely can return to their occupations.

Answer: 2

Rationale: The nurse mobilizes social supports for the suicidal client because these clients have very limited internal and external resources.

Test-Taking Strategy: Options 1 and 4 can be ruled out as being incorrect. Option 3 may be true of some clients, but option 2 is true of all suicidal clients. Note the relationship between "community resources" in the question and "support systems" in the correct option!

Level of Cognitive Ability: Application
Phase of Nursing Process: Planning
Client Needs: Psychosocial Integrity
Content Area: Mental Health

Reference
Stuart, G., & Sundeen, S. (1995). *Principles and practice of psychiatric nursing* (5th ed.). St. Louis: C. V. Mosby, p. 468.

---

191. To reduce the anxiety of a client who is going to have a plaster cast applied, the nurse plans to teach the client about the procedure. The nurse would not include which of the following items in the discussion?

1 A stockinette will be placed over the leg area to be casted
2 The cast edges may be trimmed with a cast knife
3 The cast will give off heat as it dries
4 The client may bear weight on the cast in half an hour

Answer: 4

Rationale: The procedure for casting involves washing and drying the skin and placing a stockinette material over the area to be casted. A roll of padding is then applied smoothly and evenly. The plaster is rolled onto the padding, and the edges are trimmed or smoothed as needed. A plaster cast gives off heat as it dries. A plaster cast can tolerate weight bearing once it is dry, which varies from 24 to 72 hours, depending on the nature and thickness of the cast.

Test-Taking Strategy: Familiarity with the different types of casting materials and their differences helps you to answer this question with ease. Options 1, 2, and 3 are all true for plaster casts. Option 4 is true for nonplaster casts. Because of this, the nurse would not include option 4 in the discussion, and so it is the answer to this question as stated.

Level of Cognitive Ability: Application
Phase of Nursing Process: Planning
Client Needs: Psychosocial Integrity
Content Area: Adult Health/Musculoskeletal

Reference
Smeltzer, S., & Bare, B. (1996). *Brunner and Suddarth's Textbook of medical-surgical nursing* (8th ed.). Philadelphia: Lippincott-Raven, p. 1851.

---

192. The nurse is planning to teach the client with a left arm cast about measures to keep the left shoulder from becoming stiff and "frozen." Which of the following suggestions would the nurse include in the teaching plan?

1 "Lift the left arm up over the head."
2 "Lift the right arm up over the head."
3 "Make a fist with the hand of the casted arm."
4 "Use a sling on the left arm."

Answer: 1

Rationale: Immobility and the weight of a casted arm may cause the shoulder above an arm fracture to become stiff. The shoulder of a casted arm should be lifted over the head periodically as a preventive measure. The use of slings further immobilizes the shoulder and may be contraindicated. Making a fist with the left hand is an isometric exercise that benefits the hand but not the shoulder. Range of motion of the affected fingers is also a useful general measure. Lifting the right arm is of no particular value.

Test-Taking Strategy: Imagine each of the movements and think about the muscle groups that are moved with each. Options 2 and 4 provide for no movement of the left arm and are eliminated first. Making a fist with the hand on the casted arm provides good isometric exercise to the muscles surrounding the fracture, but again, does nothing for the shoulder. The only viable option is raising the arm over the head, which provides some range of motion for the shoulder joint.

Level of Cognitive Ability: Application
Phase of Nursing Process: Planning
Client Needs: Health Promotion and Maintenance
Content Area: Adult Health/Musculoskeletal

Reference

Black, J., & Matassarin-Jacobs, E. (1997). *Medical-surgical nursing: Clinical management for continuity of care* (5th ed.). Philadelphia: W. B. Saunders, p. 2151.

---

193. The nurse is one of several people who witness a vehicle hit a pedestrian at fairly low speed on a small street. The pedestrian is dazed and tries to get up. One leg appears fractured. The nurse would plan to

1 Stay with the person and coax the person to remain still.
2 Assist the person to get up and walk to the sidewalk.
3 Leave the person for a few moments to call an ambulance.
4 Try to manually reduce the fracture.

Answer: 1

Rationale: With a suspected fracture, the client is not moved unless it is dangerous to remain in that spot. The nurse should remain with the client and have someone else call for emergency help. A fracture is not reduced at the scene. Before the client is moved, the site of fracture is immobilized to prevent further injury.

Test-Taking Strategy: Options 2 and 4 are the worst choices and should be eliminated first. Either of these options could result in further injury to the client. Of the two remaining choices, the more prudent action would be for the nurse to remain with the client and have someone else call for emergency assistance.

Level of Cognitive Ability: Application
Phase of Nursing Process: Planning
Client Needs: Physiological Integrity
Content Area: Adult Health/Musculoskeletal

Reference

Black, J., & Matassarin-Jacobs, E. (1997). *Medical-surgical nursing: Clinical management for continuity of care* (5th ed.). Philadelphia: W. B. Saunders, p. 2134.

---

194. The home health nurse is planning to teach the client with osteoporosis about home modifications to reduce the risk of falls. Which of the following recommendations would be unnecessary to include in the teaching plan?

1 Use of staircase railings
2 Use of nightlights
3 Removing wall-to-wall carpeting
4 Placing handrails in the bathroom

Answer: 3

Rationale: Home modifications to reduce the risk for falls includes use of railings on all staircases, ample lighting, removing scatter rugs, and placing hand rails in the bathroom. Removal of wall-to-wall carpeting is not warranted.

Test-Taking Strategy: Begin to answer this question by eliminating options 1 and 4. Both of these items provide physical support to the client and are needed. Nightlights will enhance vision for the client getting up at night to use the bathroom, and their use is also warranted. The only remaining option, which is the correct answer, involves the wall-to-wall carpeting. This does not pose a risk to the client and does not need to be removed.

Level of Cognitive Ability: Application
Phase of Nursing Process: Planning
Client Needs: Health Promotion and Maintenance
Content Area: Adult Health/Musculoskeletal

Reference

Black, J., & Matassarin-Jacobs, E. (1997). *Medical-surgical nursing: Clinical management for continuity of care* (5th ed.). Philadelphia: W. B. Saunders, p. 2103.

195. The nurse is teaching the client about ofloxacin (Floxin), which has been ordered for the treatment of prostatitis. The nurse would plan to include which of the following in the instructions to prevent crystalluria from developing?

1. Drink at least 1500–2000 mL of fluid per day
2. Drink at least 6 glasses of milk per day
3. Avoid beverages that contain salts, such as mineral water
4. Avoid beverages that are carbonated

Answer: 1

Rationale: To prevent crystalluria, the client should consume at least 1500–2000 mL of fluid per day. Milk interferes with the absorption of the medication, and six glasses per day is excessive. Carbonated beverages and mineral water are not contraindicated.

Test-Taking Strategy: To answer this question correctly, recall the principles involved in crystal formation. There must be sufficient solute load to precipitate crystal formation. According to this line of reasoning, if there is sufficient solvent (fluids), crystal formation is minimized. This would allow you to eliminate each of the incorrect options systematically. Review prevention measures if you had difficulty with this question!

Level of Cognitive Ability: Application
Phase of Nursing Process: Planning
Client Needs: Health Promotion and Maintenance
Content Area: Adult Health/Renal

Reference

Hodgson, B., & Kizior, R. (1998). *Saunders nursing drug handbook 1998.* Philadelphia: W. B. Saunders, pp. 766–768.

---

196. The nurse caring for a client undergoing peritoneal dialysis notes drainage of cloudy dialysate. The nurse should plan to first

1. Stop peritoneal dialysis.
2. Obtain a culture and sensitivity test of the peritoneal outflow.
3. Institute emergency hemodialysis.
4. Add antibiotics to the next several dialysate bags.

Answer: 2

Rationale: When the dialysate becomes cloudy, peritonitis is suspected. A culture is obtained, and broad-spectrum antibiotics are added to the dialysis solution pending results of culture and sensitivity tests. The dialysate may also be heparinized to prevent catheter occlusion. Some clients must switch to hemodialysis if peritonitis is severe or recurring, but it is not done on an emergency basis with this situation.

Test-Taking Strategy: To begin to answer this question, recall that cloudy dialysate indicates infection—in this case, peritonitis. Note that the question contains the key word "first." This implies that more than one or all of the options may be correct. You must prioritize the necessary actions to arrive at the correct answer. In this case, knowing that a culture should be obtained before antibiotic therapy is instituted would guide you to the correct answer.

Level of Cognitive Ability: Application
Phase of Nursing Process: Planning
Client Needs: Physiological Integrity
Content Area: Adult Health/Renal

Reference

Luckmann, J. (1997). *Saunders manual of nursing care.* Philadelphia: W. B. Saunders, p. 1193.

---

197. The nurse is caring for the client who is having a peritoneal dialysis catheter inserted at the bedside. The nurse plans to enhance the client's comfort during the procedure by

1. Telling the client not to speak during catheter insertion.
2. Assisting the client to a side-lying position.
3. Encouraging the client to hold the breath while the catheter is introduced.
4. Obtaining an order for premedication.

Answer: 4

Rationale: The client's comfort is enhanced during insertion of the peritoneal dialysis catheter by premedication with a narcotic analgesic and a local anesthetic before introducing the catheter. The client is not placed in a side-lying position for insertion. Holding the breath will not promote comfort, and in fact would increase tension on the abdominal wall, which is counterproductive. The client should be encouraged to speak as needed during the procedure.

Test-Taking Strategy: The question is asking for a method of increasing client comfort during a painful procedure. Eliminate options 1 and 3 first because they are not helpful in promoting comfort. You would choose option 4 over option 2 if you knew that the client should receive medication before the procedure or if you knew the proper positioning for catheter introduction. Review client preparation for this procedure now if you had difficulty with this question!

Level of Cognitive Ability: Application
Phase of Nursing Process: Planning
Client Needs: Safe, Effective Care Environment
Content Area: Adult Health/Renal

Reference

Black, J., & Matassarin-Jacobs, E. (1997). *Medical-surgical nursing: Clinical management for continuity of care* (5th ed.). Philadelphia: W. B. Saunders, p. 1649.

---

198. The nurse is assisting the physician who will insert a peritoneal dialysis catheter into a client's abdomen at the bedside. To prevent complications of catheter insertion, the nurse should plan to

1 Assist the client to a standing position.
2 Ensure that the client's bladder is empty before catheter insertion.
3 Administer a narcotic analgesic before catheter placement.
4 Obtain a baseline temperature for the client's record.

Answer: 2

Rationale: To prevent bladder perforation during peritoneal dialysis catheter insertion, the client's bladder should be emptied before the procedure. The client is positioned lying in bed, not standing. A narcotic analgesic may be ordered, and a local anesthetic is used before catheter insertion; however, these may not prevent complications of insertion. A baseline temperature is useful, but it also does not prevent complications.

Test-Taking Strategy: Note that the question asks for an action to prevent a complication. Thus the correct answer cannot be an observation. This eliminates option 4 as the correct answer. To discriminate among the other choices correctly, it is necessary to be familiar with the insertion procedure for peritoneal dialysis catheters. If you are not familiar with the procedure, take a few moments to review it briefly. You might have also arrived at the correct answer by reasoning that perforation is a potential complication. This would also guide you to choose option 2 as the correct choice.

Level of Cognitive Ability: Application
Phase of Nursing Process: Planning
Client Needs: Safe, Effective Care Environment
Content Area: Adult Health/Renal

Reference

Black, J., & Matassarin-Jacobs, E. (1997). *Medical-surgical nursing: Clinical management for continuity of care* (5th ed.). Philadelphia: W. B. Saunders, p. 1650.

---

199. The nurse is about to begin peritoneal dialysis for a client. The nurse would plan to do which of the following before infusing the dialysate solution?

1 Shake the dialysate bag vigorously
2 Chill the dialysate solution
3 Ensure that the dialysate is at room temperature
4 Warm the dialysate slightly

Answer: 4

Rationale: The dialysate solution is warmed slightly before it is infused into the client. This prevents the client from becoming chilled and also helps to dilate the peritoneal blood vessels for better excretion of waste metabolites. It is unnecessary to shake the bag vigorously. The other options are incorrect.

Test-Taking Strategy: To answer this question correctly, it is necessary to understand the effects of heat and cold on the body. This knowledge would enable you to eliminate each of the incorrect responses readily. Eliminate option 1 because of the word "vigorously." Remember that warmth dilates. If this question was difficult, take a few moments to review peritoneal dialysis procedures at this time!

Level of Cognitive Ability: Application
Phase of Nursing Process: Planning
Client Needs: Safe, Effective Care Environment
Content Area: Adult Health/Renal

Reference

Black, J., & Matassarin-Jacobs, E. (1997). *Medical-surgical nursing: Clinical management for continuity of care* (5th ed.). Philadelphia: W. B. Saunders, p. 1649.

200. A client is admitted to the day hospital in a community mental health center because his or her ritualistic behavior is so time consuming that the client is unable to keep a job. The initial priority in the nursing plan of care is to

1 Provide the client with day hospital rules.
2 Allow the client time to perform rituals.
3 Confront the client about his or her poor use of time.
4 Assist the client in carrying out rituals.

Answer: 2

Rationale: Compulsive rituals control the client's anxiety. It is usually not fruitful to interfere prematurely with a ritual, unless it threatens the client's health.

Test-Taking Strategy: The question asks for the initial action in the plan of care. Options 1, 3, and 4 are not therapeutic. Options 1 and 3 would increase the client's anxiety, and option 4 would reinforce the client's behavior. Initially, allow the client to perform rituals that are necessary to control anxiety. If you are unfamiliar with obsessive-compulsive disorders, review the content now!

Level of Cognitive Ability: Application
Phase of Nursing Process: Planning
Client Needs: Psychosocial Integrity
Content Area: Mental Health

Reference

Wilson, H., & Kneisl, C. (1996). *Psychiatric nursing* (5th ed.). Menlo Park, CA: Addison-Wesley, p. 381.

---

201. When planning postprocedure care for a client who is having a barium enema, the nurse is most careful to include

1 Bed rest for 8 hours after procedure.
2 Monitoring urinary output.
3 Administration of a laxative or enema after the procedure.
4 Reordering the client's diet.

Answer: 3

Rationale: A client is at high risk for a barium impaction after a barium enema. To prevent this, the nurse should obtain a physician's order for laxative or enema to follow the procedure; force fluids; and monitor bowel movements.

Test-Taking Strategy: Use the process of elimination. Both options 2 and 4 are components of assessing and implementing care of the client's hydration and nutrition status, but the priority related to the barium enema is to avoid the barium impaction. Option 1 is incorrect because bed rest is not usually a part of postprocedure care for a barium enema. Review postprocedure care after a barium enema if you had difficulty with this question!

Level of Cognitive Ability: Application
Phase of Nursing Process: Planning
Client Needs: Safe, Effective Care Environment
Content Area: Adult Health/Gastrointestinal

Reference

Black, J., & Matassarin-Jacobs, E. (1997). *Medical-surgical nursing: Clinical management for continuity of care* (5th ed.). Philadelphia: W. B. Saunders, p. 251

---

202. To prevent tracheal aspiration by the client with a hiatal hernia, the nurse should plan to

1 Administer antacids PRN.
2 Instruct the client to not smoke.
3 Instruct the client to lose weight.
4 Elevate the head of bed on 4–6 inch blocks.

Answer: 4

Rationale: Regurgitation with tracheal aspiration is a major complication of a hiatal hernia. Although antacids, avoidance of smoking, and losing weight will assist in alleviating the discomfort that can occur, these measures will not prevent aspiration.

Test-Taking Strategy: Note the issue of the question, to prevent tracheal aspiration. Options 1, 2, and 3 are all interventions that may be used with the client with a hiatal hernia, but they do not prevent regurgitation and aspiration. Option 4 is the only option that will prevent them.

Level of Cognitive Ability: Application
Phase of Nursing Process: Planning
Client Needs: Safe, Effective Care Environment
Content Area: Adult Health/Gastrointestinal

Reference

Lewis, S., Collier, I., & Heitkemper, M. (1996). *Medical-surgical nursing: Assessment and management of clinical problems* (4th ed.). St. Louis: Mosby–Year Book, p. 1157.

203. To try to stop bleeding in a client with esophageal varices, a Sengstaken-Blakemore tube is inserted to apply pressure against the varices (tamponade). The nurse plans to implement postprocedure safety measures, which include

1. Elevating the head of bed 90 degrees.
2. Having suction available and scissors at bedside.
3. Monitoring intake and output.
4. Checking level of consciousness every hour.

Answer: 2

Rationale: Balloon tamponade is one method used to stop bleeding from esophageal varices, but the pressure may cause tissue necrosis. Scissors should be at the bedside in order to remove the tube in an emergency. Also, saliva and secretions may accumulate above the tube, so to prevent aspiration, suction may be used.

Test-Taking Strategy: The key phrase is "safety measures." Option 1 is incorrect because it is not necessary to elevate the bed a full 90 degrees. Options 3 and 4 are important assessment areas to monitor in bleeding clients but are not specific safety factors in the client with the balloon tamponade. Take time now to review post-procedure care after insertion of a Sengstaken-Blakemore tube if you had difficulty with this question!

Level of Cognitive Ability: Application
Phase of Nursing Process: Planning
Client Needs: Safe, Effective Care Environment
Content Area: Adult Health/Gastrointestinal

Reference

Black, J., & Matassarin-Jacobs, E. (1997). *Medical-surgical nursing: Clinical management for continuity of care* (5th ed.). Philadelphia: W. B. Saunders, p. 1885.

---

204. The nursing diagnosis for the client with an identified duodenal ulcer is Pain related to decreased mucosal protection, increased gastric secretions, and burning, cramping, and abdominal pain 2–4 hours after meals. The nurse plans to instruct the client that when this occurs, he or she should

1. Drink a cup of tea.
2. Take an enteric-coated aspirin.
3. Take an antacid.
4. Drink a cup of hot milk.

Answer: 3

Rationale: Antacids are the initial medications of choice in the relief of symptoms of duodenal ulcers because they decrease gastric acidity and acid content of chyme reaching the duodenum. In addition, some antacids bind to bile salts and decrease the harmful effects on gastric mucosa. Because of its antiplatelet properties, enteric-coated aspirin is contraindicated in duodenal ulcer disease (option 2). Tea and other caffeinated drinks should be avoided (option 1), and hot drinks and food should be avoided (option 4).

Test-Taking Strategy: Use the process of elimination to answer the question, considering the effect each identified option may have on the gastric mucosa. Option 2 can easily be eliminated. Options 1 and 4 are similar in that both are warm drinks. This leaves option 3 as the correct option. Review dietary measures associated with duodenal ulcers if you had difficulty with this question!

Level of Cognitive Ability: Application
Phase of Nursing Process: Planning
Client Needs: Psychosocial Integrity
Content Area: Adult Health/Gastrointestinal

Reference

Lewis, S., Collier, I., & Heitkemper, M. (1996). *Medical-surgical nursing: Assessment and management of clinical problems* (4th ed.). St. Louis: Mosby–Year Book, p. 1190.

205. A client is being discharged from the hospital after a gastrectomy for cancer of the stomach. The prognosis is good if chemotherapy is successful. Daily wound care will be needed. In planning for discharge, the nurse determines that the appropriate agency for referral for the client is

1 Hospice.
2 American Cancer Society.
3 Home health agency.
4 Parish nurse registry.

Answer: 3

Rationale: Although the client may use the services of all the agencies at some point, a home health agency is the one needed now. Hospice is usually for the terminally ill (Option 1). The American Cancer Society (Option 2) has some client services available but not direct care. Parish nurse services vary regionally, but if direct care is provided, the home health nurse would probably provide the information and instruction for care. The client will probably need direct care for the wound and/or instructions on how to care for the wound. This is a role of the home health nurse.

Test-Taking Strategy: Note the key phrase "daily wound care will be needed." This should assist in eliminating options 1, 2, and 4. If you had difficulty with this question, take time now to review the services provided by the agencies presented in the options!

Level of Cognitive Ability: Application
Phase of Nursing Process: Planning
Client Needs: Health Promotion and Maintenance
Content Area: Adult Health/Oncology

Reference
Lewis, S., Collier, I., & Heitkemper, M. (1996). *Medical-surgical nursing: Assessment and management of clinical problems* (4th ed.). St. Louis: Mosby–Year Book, p. 1204.

206. The client states, "I feel like I am losing my mind. I keep hearing the gunshots and seeing my friend lying on the ground." The nurse plans strategies to begin to formulate a therapeutic alliance, which will include

1 Asking the psychiatrist to order an antianxiety medication.
2 Encouraging the client to talk about the event and feelings related to it.
3 Encouraging the client to think about how lucky he or she is to be alive.
4 Teaching the client relaxation techniques.

Answer: 2

Rationale: In developing a therapeutic alliance, it is important to acknowledge and validate the client's feelings. Although teaching the client relaxation techniques may be helpful at some point, it is not related to the issue of the question. Options 1 and 3 are nontherapeutic techniques that do not promote a therapeutic alliance.

Test-Taking Strategy: Use therapeutic communication techniques to answer the question. Neither option 1 nor option 3 allows for further discussion about the client's feelings. Teaching the client how to relax will be helpful later on but not in the beginning of the therapeutic relationship. Remember to address client's feelings!

Level of Cognitive Ability: Application
Phase of Nursing Process: Planning
Client Needs: Psychosocial Integrity
Content Area: Mental Health

Reference
Carson, V., & Arnold, E. (1996). *Mental health nursing: The nurse-patient journey.* Philadelphia: W. B. Saunders, pp. 207–208.

207. The client has a compulsive bed-making ritual in which the client remakes the bed numerous times. The client often misses breakfast and some of the morning activities because of the ritual. Which of the following plans might be helpful?

1. Verbalize tactful, mild disapproval of the behavior
2. Help the client to make the bed so that the task can be finished quicker
3. Discuss the ridiculousness of the behavior
4. Offer reflective feedback, such as "I see you have made your bed several times. You must be exhausted."

Answer: 4

Rationale: Reflective feedback lets the client know that the nurse acknowledges the behavior and understands that it can be very tiring. Verbalizing minimal disapproval would increase the client's anxiety and reinforce the need to perform the ritual. Helping with the ritual is nontherapeutic and reinforces the behavior. The client is usually aware of the irrationality (or ridiculousness) of the behavior.

Test-Taking Strategy: Use the process of elimination to answer the question. Knowing that the purpose of the ritual is to relieve anxiety would lead the test taker to eliminate options 1 and 3 because they would increase the anxiety. Eliminate option 2 because there is no therapeutic value in participating in the ritual.

Level of Cognitive Ability: Application
Phase of Nursing Process: Planning
Client Needs: Psychological Integrity
Content Area: Mental Health

Reference

Carson, V., & Arnold, E. (1996). *Mental health nursing: The nurse-patient journey.* Philadelphia: W. B. Saunders, p. 703.

208. The nurse is preparing to admit a client with AIDS who has *Pneumocystis carinii* pneumonia. In planning for infection control for this client, which would be the most appropriate form of isolation to institute to prevent the spread of HIV to others?

1. Strict isolation
2. Respiratory isolation
3. Enteric precautions
4. Blood and body fluid precautions

Answer: 4

Rationale: HIV is transmitted through anal or oral sexual contact with infected semen or vaginal secretion, contact with blood or blood products, and transmission of the virus from mother to fetus during childbirth or via breast-feeding. *P. carinii* is an organism that causes opportunistic infection in clients with compromised immune function. Blood and body fluid precautions will prevent contact with infectious matter. Strict isolation is not needed and may contribute to the client's feelings of isolation. A majority of people by the age of 4 have antibodies against pneumocystic pneumonia. Enteric precautions alone are insufficient to protect from transmission of HIV.

Test-Taking Strategy: An understanding of HIV transmission is essential to answer this question. Option 4 provides the most global response. If you are unfamiliar with the transmission of HIV and isolation techniques, it is important to review this information!

Level of Cognitive Ability: Application
Phase of Nursing Process: Planning
Client Needs: Safe, Effective Care Environment
Content Area: Fundamental Skills

Reference

Ignatavicius, D. D., Workman, M. L., & Mishler, M. A. (1995). *Medical-surgical nursing: A nursing process approach.* (2nd ed.). Philadelphia: W. B. Saunders, pp. 524–526, 595.

209. The nurse assists the client with hepatitis C in planning and developing goals to maintain a safe environment. Which of the following statements identifies an accurate and most appropriate goal?

1 The client will describe at least three practices that reduce the transmission of hepatitis C before discharge
2 The client will maintain nutritional intake to optimize immunological status throughout hospitalization
3 The nurse will instruct on methods to control sexually transmitted disease before client discharge
4 The client will maintain interaction with family members on a daily basis to prevent depression and feelings of isolation

Answer: 1

Rationale: An accurate goal must be client-centered, not nurse-centered. Goals must contain target dates. Goals must be specific and measurable. The question asks for a goal to maintain a safe environment. Although nutrition is important to optimize immunological status, this does not relate to the environment. Option 4 addresses the environment in relation to psychosocial issues but does not address safety.

Test-Taking Strategy: Be sure to identify critical elements of the question. This question addresses a safety need. This eliminates options 2 and 4 because they do not address safety. Option 3 must be eliminated because it is not a client goal.

Level of Cognitive Ability: Application
Phase of Nursing Process: Planning
Client Needs: Safe, Effective Care Environment
Content Area: Adult Health/Gastrointestinal

Reference
Ignatavicius, D. D., Workman, M. L., & Mishler, M. A. (1995). *Medical-surgical nursing: A nursing process approach* (2nd ed.). Philadelphia: W. B. Saunders, pp. 1691–1693.

210. The nurse plans interventions for the client with tuberculosis (TB) in an acute care setting to maintain a safe environment. Which of the following guidelines would the nurse use to best promote a safe environment for this client?

1 Place the client in strict isolation and instruct health care workers to use a high-efficiency particulate air (HEPA) respirator
2 Place the client in respiratory isolation and instruct health care workers to use a HEPA respirator
3 Place the client in strict isolation and instruct health care workers to use a simple disposable mask
4 Place the client in respiratory isolation and instruct health care workers to use a simple disposable mask.

Answer: 2

Rationale: TB is spread by droplet nuclei. It is not carried on fomites. Therefore, strict isolation is not required. A well-ventilated room with fresh air exchange is important. The HEPA respirator is used in the care of clients with actual or suspected TB infection.

Test-Taking Strategy: Knowledge that TB is spread by droplet nuclei will assist in eliminating options 1 and 3. Eliminate option 4 because it states "simple" mask. If you are unfamiliar with the method of transmission of TB, take time now to review this important disease!

Level of Cognitive Ability: Application
Phase of Nursing Process: Planning
Client Needs: Safe, Effective Care Environment
Content Area: Adult Health/Respiratory

Reference
Ignatavicius, D. D., Workman, M. L., & Mishler, M. A. (1995). *Medical-surgical nursing: A nursing process approach* (2nd ed.). Philadelphia: W. B. Saunders, p. 722.

211. The client is scheduled for removal of a chest tube in the morning. Of the following outcome criteria, which would be an appropriate indicator that the nurse's plan has minimized fear of pain during the procedure?

1 Client expresses satisfaction with pain control
2 Client expresses contentment with physical surroundings
3 Client seeks information to reduce anxiety
4 Client verbalizes increase in psychological comfort

Answer: 4

Rationale: A decrease in fear would mean the client has an increase in psychological comfort. Although the presence of fear is known to increase pain levels, a person can be pain free and continue to experience fear. Contentment with physical surroundings will help reduce stress levels, but clients can continue to experience fear in comfortable surroundings. A client may seek information about anxiety reduction. Receiving information does not necessarily mean there is a change in behavior.

Test-Taking Strategy: Be sure to address the issue of the question. In this case, the focus of the question is minimized fear in the client. Do not be distracted by other options that are not directly related to what the question is asking. Note the key phrase "psychological comfort" in the correct option.

Level of Cognitive Ability: Application
Phase of Nursing Process: Planning
Client Needs: Psychosocial Integrity
Content Area: Adult Health/Respiratory

Reference

Ignatavicius, D. D., Workman, M. L., & Mishler, M. A. (1995). *Medical-surgical nursing: A nursing process approach.* (2nd ed.). Philadelphia: W. B. Saunders, pp. 744–747.

---

212. The nurse has an order to suction the postoperative client. The client is visibly anxious about the procedure. The nurse would plan to avoid which of the following actions to make the experience as tolerable to the client as possible?

1 Putting the head of bed in semi-Fowler's position
2 Explaining the procedure to the client calmly
3 Ensuring that the client has received recent pain medication
4 Using the largest catheter available so only one pass is made into the trachea

Answer: 4

Rationale: The client being suctioned who is awake is placed in semi-Fowler's position to increase ease of breathing. The nurse should explain the procedure to alleviate some of the client's anxiety. The postoperative client benefits from recent pain medication to minimize pain that could occur with coughing during the procedure. The catheter size should be large enough to obtain secretions but small enough to prevent inducing hypoxia in the client.

Test-Taking Strategy: The wording of the question guides you to look for an item that will not help the client tolerate the suctioning procedure. Options 1 and 2 are consistent with standard nursing practice and are therefore eliminated. Premedicating the postoperative client before a procedure that induces coughing (and therefore possible pain) is also correct and is eliminated. This leaves option 4, which is potentially harmful to the client. Because too large a catheter could induce hypoxia, it is not helpful to the client's tolerance of the procedure (or safety). Because of this, it is the answer to the question as stated.

Level of Cognitive Ability: Application
Phase of Nursing Process: Planning
Client Needs: Psychosocial Integrity
Content Area: Adult Health/Respiratory

Reference

Taylor, C., Lillis, C., & LeMone, P. (1997). *Fundamentals of nursing: The art and science of nursing care* (3rd ed.). Philadelphia: Lippincott-Raven, pp. 1348–1349.

---

213. The nurse is preparing to transport a client with a portable oxygen cylinder. The nurse would plan to avoid doing which of the following while preparing the client and oxygen equipment?

1 Turning the cylinder key counterclockwise to check the amount of oxygen available.
2 Attaching the humidifier bottle to the flowmeter adapter and client's oxygen cannula.
3 Coiling excess tubing to place under the client's pillow on the stretcher.
4 Placing the cylinder between the client's legs on the stretcher.

Answer: 4

Rationale: Proper procedure includes checking the amount of oxygen in the cylinder by turning the key counterclockwise and reading the pressure gauge, and attaching a humidifier bottle between the flowmeter adapter and the cannula. Any excess tubing is coiled and placed under the pillow or secured to the client's gown. The nurse avoids putting the cylinder between the client's legs or anywhere else on the stretcher, so that the client does not experience injury. The cylinder is always secured in the proper holder.

Test-Taking Strategy: Knowledge of the basic practices involved in oxygen therapy is needed to answer this question quickly and accurately. The question asks you to select an item to avoid, which calls to mind the concept of safety. When you reevaluate the client in terms of safe practice, option 4 is the most plausible option. A cylinder that is not secured could harm the client, and this is the answer to this question.

Level of Cognitive Ability: Application
Phase of Nursing Process: Planning
Client Needs: Safe, Effective Care Environment
Content Area: Adult Health/Respiratory
Reference

Taylor, C., Lillis, C., & LeMone, P. (1997). *Fundamentals of nursing: The art and science of nursing care* (3rd ed.). Philadelphia: Lippincott-Raven, pp. 1339.

214. The nurse is planning to teach the client with multiple allergies about measures to reduce allergens in the home. Which of the following items is unnecessary to include in this teaching plan?

1 Clean air conditioners periodically
2 Use a humidifier year round
3 Use a damp cloth for dusting
4 Avoid having pets with hair

Answer: 2

Rationale: Common allergens in the home include animal dander, dust, smoke, fumes, and mold. Animal dander can be eliminated by not having pets with hair. Use of a damp cloth will prevent dust from being dispersed in the air with dusting. Air conditioners and furnace humidifiers are sources of mold that could be allergenic, and these appliances should be cleaned periodically. Use of a humidifier year round is of no particular benefit. In fact, it could be contraindicated during summer months, when a dehumidifier is needed to reduce environmental moisture (and subsequent mold growth).

Test-Taking Strategy: Begin to answer this question by eliminating options 3 and 4 first. Environmental dust and pet dander are obvious allergens, and these interventions are quite useful in limiting exposure to these substances. To distinguish between the remaining two options, note that option 1 addresses "cleaning" an air conditioner unit, which would remove potentially allergenic substances. Option 2 advocates year-round humidification, which could result in overhumidification of air, leading to growth of mold and fungus. Thus option 2 is the item to be left out the teaching plan.

Level of Cognitive Ability: Application
Phase of Nursing Process: Planning
Client Needs: Health Promotion and Maintenance
Content Area: Adult Health/Respiratory

Reference

Black, J., & Matassarin-Jacobs, E. (1997). *Medical-surgical nursing: Clinical management for continuity of care* (5th ed.). Philadelphia: W. B. Saunders, p. 1039.

215. The nurse is monitoring the respiratory status of a client who also has expressive aphasia. The nurse would plan to use a visual analog scale to measure which of the client's respiratory signs and symptoms?

1 Cough
2 Hemoptysis
3 Dyspnea
4 Wheezing

Answer: 3

Rationale: Dyspnea is difficult to measure, as it tends to be subjective in nature. The client using a visual analog scale points to the description of dyspnea felt when questioned about breathlessness experienced with certain activities. Cough, hemoptysis, and wheezing are all measurable by the nurse without a need for further description by the client.

Test-Taking Strategy: Recall that a visual analog scale is useful in helping to quantify "something" experienced by the client. This is usually an item that is subjective in nature and not readily or directly measurable by the nurse. (Pain is the other symptom that commonly involves use of an analog scale). Because the nurse can directly assess cough, wheezing, and hemoptysis through her or his own vision and hearing, it is unnecessary to use an analog scale to rate these items.

Level of Cognitive Ability: Application
Phase of Nursing Process: Planning
Client Needs: Physiological Integrity
Content Area: Adult Health/Respiratory

Reference

Black, J., & Matassarin-Jacobs, E. (1997). *Medical-surgical nursing: Clinical management for continuity of care* (5th ed.). Philadelphia: W. B. Saunders, p. 1036.

216. An initial planning goal for a newly admitted client with schizophrenia would be to

1. Improve self-care.
2. Decrease bizarre behavior.
3. Develop a trusting relationship.
4. Encourage verbalization of feelings.

Answer: 3

Rationale: Clients with schizophrenia exhibit isolation from others as a result of mistrust. Trust must be established before therapeutic intervention can occur, and it lays the foundation of the nurse-client relationship.

Test-Taking Strategy: Knowledge of the psychodynamics associated with schizophrenia as well as of the nurse-client relationship is necessary to assist you in answering this question. Patterns of problems with trusting are a primary feature of schizophrenia. Option 1 occurs after trust is established. Option 2 may not change until medication becomes fully effective (4 to 8 weeks). Option 4 is a long-term goal.

Level of Cognitive Ability: Application
Phase of Nursing Process: Planning
Client Needs: Psychosocial Integrity
Content Area: Mental Health

Reference

Carson, V., & Arnold, E. (1996). *Mental health nursing: The nurse-patient journey.* Philadelphia: W. B. Saunders, p. 244.

---

217. On the basis of an understanding of defense-oriented behavior, the nurse plans that the first nursing action for a client using defense mechanisms is to

1. Get an order for medication.
2. Call the physician.
3. Intervene in anxiety.
4. Take the client to seclusion.

Answer: 3

Rationale: Defense-oriented behavior is using mental mechanisms to lessen uncomfortable feelings of anxiety and to prevent pain, regardless of cost. The person has little awareness of what is happening and even less control over events. Initially, these reactions may help control anxiety, but they interfere with the ability to grow or cope successfully. The nurse must decrease the threat so that more constructive behavior occurs.

Test-Taking Strategy: Use the process of elimination. Options 1 and 2 are similar. There is no need for option 4. This leaves option 3 as the best response.

Level of Cognitive Ability: Application
Phase of Nursing Process: Planning
Client Needs: Safe, Effective Care Environment
Content Area: Mental Health

Reference

Wilson, H., & Kneisl, C. (1996). *Psychiatric nursing* (5th ed.). Menlo Park, CA: Addison-Wesley, pp. 76–77, 378.

---

218. An adult client has a halo vest traction because of a cervical dislocation. Which of the following measures should the nurse include in the client's plan of care to prevent injury?

1. Tape the pliers to the vest so the client can remove the lower part of the vest for hygiene
2. Teach the client to turn his or her head slowly to maintain alignment
3. Perform ongoing cranial nerve assessment to identify nerve damage
4. Ensure that the weights hang freely and that the head of the bed is flat to maintain traction

Answer: 3

Rationale: Neurapraxia can occur if the nerves have been stretched by the traction forces, and their location at the base of the skull makes them more susceptible to damage by the force of the traction. If identified early, the paralysis can be reversed. An Allen wrench, not pliers, is needed for vest removal for emergencies only, not for hygiene needs. The release screws need to be brightly marked. Clients in halo vest traction cannot turn their heads. Halo vest traction does not involve the use of weights, although cervical skin traction and use of Crutchfield tongs do involve weights.

Test-Taking Strategy: Knowledge of halo vest traction equipment, application, potential complications, and applicable client care is extremely helpful for answering this question. Remembering that halo vest traction is a type of skeletal traction that should never be removed without a physician's order or emergency would assist in eliminating option 1. Also remembering that dislocations are treated with immobilization would assist in eliminating option 2. Weights are not used;

therefore, eliminate option 4. Remember that Assessment is the first step of the nursing process; therefore, select option 3!

Level of Cognitive Ability: Application
Phase of Nursing Process: Planning
Client Needs: Safe, Effective Care Environment
Content Area: Adult Health/Neurological

Reference

Ignatavicius, D. D., Workman, M. L., & Mishler, M. A. (1995). *Medical-surgical nursing: A nursing process approach* (2nd ed.). Philadelphia: W. B. Saunders, pp. 1188, 1193.

---

219. In the emergency room, a client has a newly applied plaster short arm cast for a fractured wrist. In order to prevent complications associated with the cast, the nurse should plan to include which of the following instructions before discharge?

1 "Perform range-of-motion exercise of all joints routinely."
2 "Wrap a towel around the cast before showering."
3 "Pad any object before inserting it under the cast."
4 "Use a hair dryer on low setting to dry the cast."

Answer: 4

Rationale: Because neither the arm cast nor the injury will immobilize the client, range of motion of all joints is unnecessary. The client does need to be reminded to flex and extend the elbow of the affected extremity. Because water weakens a plaster cast, the client needs plastic around the cast while bathing, so option 2 is incorrect. Nothing should ever be inserted under the cast because of the danger of skin injury and subsequent infection, so option 3 is incorrect. Because the client is to be discharged from the emergency room and because it takes 24–72 hours for the cast to dry, the client needs to be taught how to decrease drying time to prevent possible cast damage or breakage.

Test-Taking Strategy: Knowledge of cast care and types of casting materials would be helpful in answering this question. Plaster casts differ from synthetic casts in that they must not be gotten wet and they require a longer drying time. Use the process of elimination and principles related to cast care in answering the question. Review these principles now if you had difficulty with this question!

Level of Cognitive Ability: Application
Phase of Nursing Process: Planning
Client Needs: Safe, Effective Care Environment
Content Area: Adult Health/Musculoskeletal

Reference

Black, J., & Matassarin-Jacobs, E. (1997). *Medical-surgical nursing: Clinical management for continuity of care* (5th ed.). Philadelphia: W. B. Saunders, pp. 2147–2148.

220. At a rehabilitation facility, a stable elderly client with left-sided weakness after a cerebrovascular accident will begin ambulating with a cane. To promote client safety while ambulating with a cane, the nurse should plan to stand

1. Slightly behind the client's left side and have the client move the cane forward about 1 foot, move the left leg forward, and then move the right leg forward ahead of the cane and the left leg.
2. Slightly ahead of the client's right side and have the client move the cane forward about 1 foot, move the right leg forward, and then move the left leg forward ahead of the cane and the right leg.
3. About 1 foot directly in front of the client and have the client move the right leg forward about 1 foot, move the left leg forward, and then move the cane slightly ahead of the right leg.
4. Next to the client to the right and have the client move the right leg forward about 1 foot, move the cane, then move the right leg forward ahead of the cane.

Answer: 1

Rationale: Option 1 is correct because the nurse needs to stand slightly behind the client on the client's weaker side. The gait described in option 1 provides at least two points of support continuously. Option 2 is incorrect because the nurse is ahead of the client, on the client's strong side, and allows only one point of support (the cane), when the strong (right) leg is lifted. Standing directly in front of a client is unsafe because the client may fall backwards and the nurse cannot catch or support the client as he or she falls, so option 3 is incorrect. Also, the gait described in option 3 does not maintain maximum support or body alignment. Option 4 is incorrect because the nurse is away from the client's weak side, and the gait is incorrect because the client's left side is unsupported by the cane.

Test-Taking Strategy: Recognition that the cane would be held in the right hand and that the nurse needs to be positioned slightly behind the stable client's weaker side is helpful in answering the question. Remember basic safety needs of the client while promoting independent ambulation with a cane. Also, remember that at least two points of support are necessary while ambulating with an assistive device. Review ambulation with a cane if you had difficulty with this question!

Level of Cognitive Ability: Application
Phase of Nursing Process: Planning
Client Needs: Health Promotion and Maintenance
Content Area: Adult Health/Musculoskeletal

Reference

Lammon, C. B., Foote, A. W., Leli, P. G., et al. (1995). *Clinical nursing skills.* Philadelphia: W. B. Saunders, pp. 238–239.

221. A female client with a long leg cast has been using crutches to assist ambulation for 1 week. She comes to the clinic with complaints of pain, fatigue, and frustration with crutch walking and a "crippled leg." In planning the client's nursing care, which of the following responses by the nurse is most appropriate?

1. "I know how you feel; I had to use crutches before, too."
2. "Just remember, you'll be done with the crutches in another month."
3. "Why don't you take a couple of days off work and rest."
4. "Tell me what is more bothersome for you."

Answer: 4

Rationale: Option 4 is correct because it is a therapeutic communication technique of clarification and validation and indicates that the nurse is dealing with current client problems from the client's perspective. Option 1 is devaluating and thus blocks communication. Option 2 gives false reassurances because the client may not be done with the crutches in a month and it does not focus on the current problem. Option 3 gives advice and is a communication blocker.

Test-Taking Strategy: Knowledge of therapeutic communication techniques is essential to answer this question. Also note that option 4 is the only statement that invites a client response and thus encourages communication. Female clients tend to have less upper body strength than do male clients and therefore have more difficulty initially with crutch walking.

Level of Cognitive Ability: Application
Phase of Nursing Process: Planning
Client Needs: Psychosocial Integrity
Content Area: Adult Health/Musculoskeletal

Reference

Potter, P., & Perry, A. (1997). *Fundamentals of nursing: Concepts, process, and practice* (4th ed.). St. Louis: Mosby–Year Book, p. 242.

222. A nurse is asked to go to a community school and talk to high school students about sexually transmitted diseases (STDs). The nurse plans the discussion to address which of the following?

1. Birth control pills as the only way to prevent sexually transmitted diseases
2. The diaphragm to provide a barrier to prevent STDs
3. The use of condoms, which do not provide any protection at all
4. The use of condoms and avoiding casual sex with multiple partners

Answer: 4

Rationale: The use of condoms and avoiding casual sex with multiple partners should be the focus of discussion. The use of condoms does provide some protection against STDs. Birth control pills and the diaphragm help to prevent pregnancy but offer little protection from STDs.

Test-Taking Strategy: The issue of the question relates to STDs, not pregnancy. Eliminate the options that do not supply correct information about STDs: options 1, 2, and 3. Review the methods of protection against STDs now if you had difficulty with this question!

Level of Cognitive Ability: Application
Phase of Nursing Process: Planning
Client Needs: Safe, Effective Care Environment
Content Area: Child Health

Reference

Wong, D. (1997). *Whaley and Wong's Essentials of pediatric nursing* (5th ed.). St. Louis: Mosby–Year Book, pp. 499–501.

---

223. In planning care for a child with an infectious disease, the primary goal is to plan so that

1. The child will experience minor complications.
2. The child will not spread the infection to others.
3. The public health department will be notified.
4. The child will experience mild discomfort.

Answer: 2

Rationale: The primary goal is to prevent spreading of the disease to others. The child should experience no complications. Although the health department may need to be notified at some point, it is not the most important primary goal. The goal is to promote comfort, preventing discomfort as much as possible.

Test-Taking Strategy: Note the key phrase "primary goal." This indicates that one or more options may be correct. Eliminate options 1 and 4 first. For the remaining two options, remember the key phrase and that physiological needs are primary. This should direct you to the correct option, option 2.

Level of Cognitive Ability: Application
Phase of Nursing Process: Planning
Client Needs: Health Promotion and Maintenance
Content Area: Child Health

Reference

Wong, D., & Perry, S. (1998). *Maternal-child nursing care*. St. Louis: Mosby–Year Book, p. 1028.

---

224. In planning care for an infant with pertussis, which of the following nursing diagnoses is the most critical?

1. Ineffective Airway Clearance
2. Fluid Volume Excess
3. Sleep Pattern Disturbance
4. High Risk for Infection

Answer: 1

Rationale: The most important nursing diagnosis relates to adequate air exchange. Because of the copious, thick secretions that occur with pertussis and because the airway of an infant is small, air exchange is critical. Fluid volume would be possibly less than body requirements because of the thick secretions and vomiting they cause. Sleep patterns may be disturbed because of the coughing, but it is not the most critical issue. High-risk problems are addressed after actual problems.

Test-Taking Strategy: Eliminate option 4 because this is a potential, not an actual, problem. For the remaining three options, use the ABCs: airway, breathing, and circulation. Airway is always the most critical. This should direct you to option 1!

Level of Cognitive Ability: Application
Phase of Nursing Process: Planning
Client Needs: Physiological Integrity
Content Area: Child Health

Reference
Wong, D., & Perry, S. (1998). *Maternal-child nursing care.* St. Louis: Mosby–Year Book, p. 1034.

---

225. The community health nurse plans a visit to the client who has just been discharged from the hospital after receiving a permanent pacemaker. Immediately after discharge, the priority nursing action to maintain a safe environment for the client would be to check the client's home for

1 Hair dryers and electric blankets, which can cause electromagnetic interference.
2 Electric toothbrushes, which, even if used by other family members, can cause microshock to occur.
3 Electric items that have strong electrical currents or magnetic fields.
4 Electric items such as a personal computer or security device, which can cause failure to pace.

Answer: 3

Rationale: This question tests your knowledge of a safe, effective care environment for the client with a permanent pacemaker. The pacemaker is shielded from interference from most electric devices. Radio, TV, electric blankets, toaster, microwave ovens, heating pads, and hair dryers are considered safe. Devices to be forewarned about include antitheft devices in stores, metal detectors used in airports, and radiation therapy (if applicable, and which might require relocation of the pacemaker).

Test-Taking Strategy: This question assesses knowledge of strategies to provide a safe environment for the client with a permanent pacemaker. Use the process of elimination, noting that option 3 is the most global option, addressing items with strong electrical currents or magnetic fields.

Level of Cognitive Ability: Application
Phase of Nursing Process: Planning
Client Needs: Safe, Effective Care Environment
Content Area: Adult Health/Cardiovascular

Reference
Luckmann, J. (1997). *Saunders manual of nursing care.* Philadelphia: W. B. Saunders, p. 1019.

---

226. The client is diagnosed with deep vein thrombosis. The nurse prepares a nursing care plan for the client, including which of the following goals in nursing management?

1 Promoting bed rest for 1 week, using an overbed trapeze, heel protectors, a pressure-reduction mattress, stool softener, coughing, and deep breathing
2 Maintaining both legs in direct alignment with the heart
3 Using elastic wraps on the affected leg from toe to groin, which remain on during bed rest
4 Using cold packs to the affected area to relieve discomfort

Answer: 1

Rationale: The goals of nursing management are to prevent existing thrombi from becoming emboli and to prevent new thrombi from forming. Bed rest for 5 to 7 days is usually ordered to prevent emboli. Both legs are elevated to decrease venous pressure and increase blood flow by elevating the foot of the bed 6 inches (Trendelenburg's position) with slight bending of the knees (to prevent popliteal pressure). Elastic wraps from toe to groin are used to promote venous return and are rewrapped every 4 to 8 hours. Warm packs are used to relieve discomfort.

Test-Taking Strategy: Use knowledge regarding the treatment plan for deep vein thrombosis to assist in answering the question. Eliminate incorrect options and note that option 1, the correct option, is most thorough and includes the correct components of care. If you had difficulty with this question, take time now to review care of the client with deep vein thrombosis!

Level of Cognitive Ability: Application
Phase of Nursing Process: Planning
Client Needs: Safe, Effective Care Environment
Content Area: Adult Health/Cardiovascular

Reference
Luckmann, J. (1997). *Saunders manual of nursing care.* Philadelphia: W. B. Saunders, p. 1019.

227. The physician orders support stockings for the client with varicose veins. The nurse prepares a teaching plan that addresses the correct application of support stockings. Which of the following would be included in the plan of care?

1 Applying the stockings every night before going to bed
2 Applying the stockings every morning before getting up
3 Applying the stockings every day at noon during lunch break
4 Removing the stockings every morning when getting up

Answer: 2

Rationale: Teaching the correct procedure and use of support stockings is a crucial part of the medical management of varicose veins. The procedure is as follows: application every morning (before presence of edema), application while lying down if the client is able to perform this, application from foot to ankle to calf, checking for proper fit and comfort, and removal if cyanosis or discomfort occurs.

Test-Taking Strategy: This question tests your ability to apply the scientific principles for the application of support stockings with varicosities. Options 1, 3, and 4 are incorrect because stockings should be applied before edema occurs. Although in some situations support stockings might be ordered at night the application process above is the most commonly prescribed for varicose veins. Review the procedure if you had difficulty with this question!

Level of Cognitive Ability: Application
Phase of Nursing Process: Planning
Client Needs: Health Promotion and Maintenance
Content Area: Adult Health/Cardiovascular

Reference

Luckmann, J. (1997). *Saunders manual of nursing care.* Philadelphia: W. B. Saunders, p. 1019.

228. The nurse is planning care for the client with Buerger's disease, who says, "I'm worried that I'll get a gangrenous foot like my father did with this disease." After facilitating the client's communication, the nurse plans to include teaching the client

1 Acceptance of the disease's poor prognosis.
2 About the new treatments that have been developed to eliminate the disease.
3 Lifestyle measures to slow the disease's progression.
4 To move to a warmer climate to arrest the disease.

Answer: 3

Rationale: Treatment of Buerger's disease is aimed toward slowing the progress of the disease, controlling the pain, protecting the extremity from extremes in temperature, elimination of tobacco, performing foot care daily, and performing Buerger-Allen exercises. The disorder occurs most often in men between 20 and 40 years of age and is seen more frequently in the Orient, India, and Israel than in America. Although not well understood in terms of the disease's process, risk factors include family history of the disease and cigarette smoking.

Test-Taking Strategy: Use the process of elimination. Eliminate option 1, "poor prognosis"; option 2, "eliminate the disease"; and option 4, "arrest the disease." Knowledge that lifestyle measures are important in management will assist in directing you to the correct option. If you had difficulty with this question, take time now to review Buerger's disease!

Level of Cognitive Ability: Application
Phase of Nursing Process: Planning
Client Needs: Psychosocial Integrity
Content Area: Adult Health/Cardiovascular

Reference

Luckmann, J. (1997). *Saunders manual of nursing care.* Philadelphia: W. B. Saunders, pp. 1102–1115.

229. The community health nurse plans to visit a client with Raynaud's disease. The nurse prepares a nursing care plan for the client and in the planning, the nurse understands that Raynaud's disease is a condition that

1. Causes vasospasm and pain in the digits when exposed to cold, vibration, or stress.
2. Is more common in men between the ages of 40 and 60 years.
3. Causes connective tissue to collect in the veins.
4. Produces a slow, irregular peripheral pulse rate.

Answer: 1

Rationale: Raynaud's disease produces closure of the small arteries in the distal extremities in response to cold, vibration, or stress. Its incidence is highest in women between the ages of 11 and 45. Palpation for diminished or absent peripheral pulse is a way of checking for interruption of circulation.

Test-Taking Strategy: This question assesses your ability to identify the pathophysiology, incidence, and clinical manifestations of Raynaud's disease. The incidence of the disease is highest among females between the ages of 11 and 45 years, making option 2 incorrect. The etiology is unknown, so option 3 is incorrect. Peripheral pulses are diminished or absent, and thus option 4 is incorrect. Review the manifestations of Raynaud's disease now if you had difficulty with this question!

Level of Cognitive Ability: Application
Phase of Nursing Process: Planning
Client Needs: Health Promotion and Maintenance
Content Area: Adult Health/Cardiovascular

Reference

Luckmann, J. (1997). *Saunders manual of nursing care.* Philadelphia: W. B. Saunders, pp. 1115–1116.

230. The client is diagnosed with HIV in the middle stage. The nurse prepares a nursing care plan for the client and family. The priority nursing care goal to reduce stress for the family and/or significant others is to be able to

1. Stop smoking, because it will predispose the client to respiratory infections.
2. Use only cooked vegetables and fruit because raw or improperly washed foods can produce microbes.
3. Discuss their feelings and make rational decisions for caring for their loved one on the basis of knowledge of the disease and community resources.
4. Avoid becoming pregnant, because the fetus would be at risk for AIDS or HIV infection.

Answer: 3

Rationale: The family and significant others with a loved one who has HIV/AIDS need to communicate their feelings regarding the client's diagnosis and prognosis, identify precautions for the prevention of transmission of HIV to themselves or others, and solve problems effectively to make rational decisions about the care of their loved one by using appropriate community resources.

Test-Taking Strategy: The issue of the question involves a care plan to reduce stress for the HIV-infected client's family and significant others. Note the key word "priority." This can indicate that more than one option is correct. Option 1 is correct for the client and certainly correct for family members when they are in the client's environment, but it does not relate to stress reduction. Option 2 is also correct, but it is more directly related to the client and whoever does the food preparation. Option 4 is correct only if the individuals have been exposed to HIV (or are not using safe sex practices). Finally, option 3 is the correct answer because it encompasses all the outcomes that the nurse would plan for in the care of families and significant others in general.

Level of Cognitive Ability: Application
Phase of Nursing Process: Planning
Client Needs: Psychosocial Integrity
Content Area: Adult Health/Respiratory

Reference

Black, J., & Matassarin-Jacobs, E. (1997). *Medical-surgical nursing: Clinical management for continuity of care* (5th ed.). Philadelphia: W. B. Saunders, pp. 614–651.

231. The client is diagnosed with HIV infection. The nurse prepares a nursing care plan for the client. In the planning phase, the nurse understands that HIV/AIDS is a lethal clinical condition in which

1 Immunosuppression is indicated by a T4 lymphocyte count of less than 200/mm^3.
2 Bacterial infection causes weak extremities, cognitive impairments, headache, visual disturbances, ataxia, and hemiparesis.
3 Immunosuppression is indicated by a T4 lymphocyte count of less than 800/mm^3.
4 Protozoan infection causes fever, exertional dyspnea, and nonproductive cough.

Answer: 1

Rationale: HIV infection is characterized by immunosuppression, indicated by a T4 lymphocyte count of less than 200/mm^3.

Test-Taking Strategy: Eliminate options 2 and 4 first because the infection is caused by a virus, not by bacteria or protozoa. Because immunosuppression is severe in HIV infection, the best selection from the remaining two options is option 1. Take time now to review HIV infection if you had difficulty with this question!

Level of Cognitive Ability: Analysis
Phase of Nursing Process: Planning
Client Needs: Physiological Integrity
Content Area: Adult Health/Respiratory

Reference

Black, J., & Matassarin-Jacobs, E. (1997). *Medical-surgical nursing: Clinical management for continuity of care* (5th ed.). Philadelphia: W. B. Saunders, pp. 614–651.

---

232. A child is sent home from school by the school nurse with rubeola (measles). The mother asks how to care for the child. The nurse tells the mother that she should

1 Allow the child to play in the sunlight to help bring the rash out.
2 Give the child aspirin for the fever.
3 Give the child warm baths to help prevent itching.
4 Keep the child in a room with dim lights to protect the child's eyes.

Answer: 4

Rationale: A nursing consideration for rubeola is eye care. The child usually has photophobia, so in planning for care, the nurse should suggest to the parent to keep the child out of brightly lit areas. Children with viral infections are not to be given aspirin, because of the risk of Reye's syndrome. Warm baths will aggravate itching.

Test-Taking Strategy: Use the process of elimination. Options 1 and 3 suggest warmth, which will aggravate the condition. Eliminate option 2 because aspirin is not to be administered. Children with rubeola develop eye problems, so option 4 is the best answer. Review nursing care of the child with rubeola now if you had difficulty with this question!

Level of Cognitive Ability: Application
Phase of Nursing Process: Planning
Client Needs: Safe, Effective Care Environment
Content Area: Child Health

Reference

Wong, D. (1997). *Whaley and Wong's Nursing care of infants and children* (5th ed.). St. Louis: Mosby–Year Book, pp. 672–673.

233. A 6-month-old child has a history of severe local reactions to previous diphtheria, tetanus, and pertussis (DTP) immunizations. When planning for future DTP immunization administration, what technique could the nurse use that would be most effective in reducing local irritation?

1 Warm the vaccine to increase speed of absorption
2 Use at least a 1-inch needle to deposit the vaccine deep into muscle tissue
3 Divide the dose and give on two separate visits
4 Apply a topical anesthetic to the injection site for 24 hours

Answer: 2

Rationale: Depositing the DTP deep into the muscle can reduce the irritating effect. Warming the vaccine may alter its chemical makeup. Adhering strictly to manufacturer's temperature requirements is very important. Divided doses and a topical anesthetic may be used with physician orders.

Test-Taking Strategy: Unless physician orders are indicated in the question, eliminate options 3 and 4 and focus on independent nursing interventions. The key word in the stem is "technique." Think about the typical steps in giving any injection, such as choosing needle size. Of the remaining two options, option 2 refers to technique!

Level of Cognitive Ability: Application
Phase of Nursing Process: Planning
Client Needs: Safe, Effective Care Environment
Content Area: Child Health

Reference

Wong, D. (1997). *Whaley and Wong's Essentials of pediatric nursing* (5th ed.). St. Louis: Mosby–Year Book, pp. 319, 322.

---

234. The client is prescribed aspirin (acetylsalicylic acid, or ASA), 325 mg PO daily. The nurse prepares a nursing care plan for the client and in the planning, the nurse understands that aspirin is effective in

1 Adding vitamin K to the clotting factors.
2 Women who have experienced a transient ischemic attack (TIA).
3 Men who have experienced a transient ischemic attack (TIA).
4 Neutralizing the thrombin-fibrinogen syndrome.

Answer: 3

Rationale: Aspirin, an antiplatelet agent, works by inhibiting the formation of thromboxane A by platelets. Aspirin provides effective treatment for clients who are over 50 years and at risk for atherosclerotic heart disease from smoking, high blood pressure, and high cholesterol levels. It is also effective for men who have experienced ministrokes and TIAs. There is a dramatic effect in the provision of prevention for men, but this effect has not been shown in women. Most studies have also been performed in men, but researchers believe that the medication's effects may not apply for women.

Test-Taking Strategy: This question tests your knowledge of aspirin's mechanism of action and its uses as an antiplatelet agent. Aspirin is prescribed for clients with angina, after myocardial infarction, with prosthetic heart valves, and after coronary artery bypass surgery. Options 1 and 4 do not describe the antiplatelet mechanism of action. Option 2 is incorrect as the discussion in the rationale points out. Review the action and therapeutic use of aspirin now if you had difficulty with this question!

Level of Cognitive Ability: Knowledge
Phase of Nursing Process: Planning
Client Needs: Physiological Integrity
Content Area: Pharmacology

Reference

Hodgson, B., & Kizior, R. (1998). *Saunders nursing drug handbook 1998.* Philadelphia: W. B. Saunders, pp. 75–77.

235. In order to most effectively meet the preoperative needs of an infant who has pyloric stenosis, the nurse would plan to

1 Strictly monitor IV infusion, monitor intake and output, and weigh diapers.
2 Provide small frequent feedings of glucose, water, and electrolytes.
3 Administer enemas until returns are clear.
4 Provide the mother privacy to breast-feed every 2 hours.

Answer: 1

Rationale: Preoperatively, important nursing responsibilities include careful monitoring of the intravenous infusion, strict monitoring of intake and output, and measurements of urine specific gravity. Weighing the infant's diapers provides information regarding output. Preoperatively, the infant is allowed nothing by mouth. Enemas would further compromise the fluid volume status and would not be an option for an infant who has a fluid volume deficit.

Test-Taking Strategy: The issue of the question addresses the infant's needs during the preoperative period. Eliminate options 2 and 4 because the infant needs to be NPO in the preoperative period. Eliminate option 3 because enemas would further compromise the fluid balance status. Review preoperative care of the infant with pyloric stenosis now if you had difficulty with this question!

Level of Cognitive Ability: Application
Phase of Nursing Process: Planning
Client Needs: Physiological Integrity
Content Area: Child Health

Reference

Wong, D. (1997). *Whaley and Wong's Nursing care of infants and children* (5th ed.). St. Louis: Mosby–Year Book, p. 1476.

---

236. The nurse is preparing to give the client a dose of iron dextran (Infed) by the intramuscular route. The nurse should plan to

1 Use a 5/8-inch, 25-gauge needle.
2 Administer into the deltoid muscle in the arm.
3 Inject deeply, using a Z-track technique.
4 Avoid changing the needle between medication aspiration and injection.

Answer: 3

Rationale: Iron dextran may permanently stain subcutaneous tissue. For this reason, the medication is administered by use of Z-track technique deep into the upper outer quadrant of the buttock. It is never given in the arm or in other exposed areas. A 2- to 3-inch, 19- or 20-gauge needle is used. The needle is changed after the medication is drawn up and before administration, to minimize subcutaneous staining.

Test-Taking Strategy: Specific information about this medication is needed to answer this question correctly. A key phrase is "intramuscular route." This should assist in eliminating options 1 and 2. Remembering that iron stains will assist in eliminating option 4. If needed, take time now to review the important administration points about this medication!

Level of Cognitive Ability: Application
Phase of Nursing Process: Planning
Client Needs: Safe, Effective Care Environment
Content Area: Pharmacology

Reference

Deglin J., & Vallerand, A. (1997). *Davis's drug guide for nurses* (5th ed.). Philadelphia: F. A. Davis, p. 661.

---

237. The nurse is preparing to give the client a first dose of cyclosporine (Sandimmune). The nurse should plan to have which of the following available at the bedside?

1 Cardiac monitor
2 Oxygen saturation monitor
3 Oxygen and epinephrine
4 Foley catheter insertion kit

Answer: 3

Rationale: During early therapy with cyclosporine, the client is most at risk for hypersensitivity reactions (wheezing, dyspnea, and flushing of the face and neck) and anaphylaxis. The nurse should be ready to manage these emergencies by having oxygen and epinephrine readily available. A code cart should also be in close proximity.

Test-Taking Strategy: To answer this question accurately, first read the information in the stem carefully. Note that the question tells you that it is the client's first dose. This warns you that the nurse should plan for an untoward reaction to the medication. If you know that the medication carries a risk of allergic reaction, then you will easily eliminate each of the incorrect responses.

Level of Cognitive Ability: Application
Phase of Nursing Process: Planning
Client Needs: Safe, Effective Care Environment
Content Area: Pharmacology

Reference

Deglin, J., & Vallerand, A. (1997). *Davis's drug guide for nurses* (5th ed.). Philadelphia: F. A. Davis, p. 310.

---

238. The nurse is planning to teach the client about therapy with cyclosporine (Sandimmune). The nurse would not plan to include which of the following items in the information given to the client?

1 Need to obtain yearly influenza vaccine
2 How to self-monitor blood pressure at home
3 Need to call the physician if urine volume decreases or becomes cloudy
4 Need to have dental checkups every 3 months

Answer: 1

Rationale: Cyclosporine is an immunosuppressant medication. Because of the effects of the medication, the client should not receive any vaccinations without first consulting the physician. The client should report decreased or cloudy urine, which could indicate either kidney rejection or infection, respectively. The client must be able to self-monitor blood pressure to check for the side effect of hypertension. The client needs meticulous oral care and dental cleaning every 3 months to help prevent gingival hyperplasia.

Test-Taking Strategy: Note the key phrase "would not plan to include." Specific knowledge of this medication as an immunosuppressive will assist in directing you to the correct option. Take time now to review this important medication if this question was difficult!

Level of Cognitive Ability: Application
Phase of Nursing Process: Planning
Client Needs: Health Promotion and Maintenance
Content Area: Pharmacology

Reference

Hodgson, B., & Kizior, R. (1998). *Saunders nursing drug handbook 1998*. Philadelphia: W. B. Saunders, pp. 272–274.

---

239. The client with a renal transplant is taking azathioprine (Imuran). In developing a teaching plan about this medication, the nurse would avoid including which of the following pieces of information?

1 "Monitor self daily for signs of infection."
2 "Discontinue the medication after 14 days of use."
3 "Call the physician if more than one dose is missed."
4 "Take with meals to minimize nausea."

Answer: 2

Rationale: Azathioprine is an immunosuppressant medication which is taken for life. Because of the effects of the medication, the client must monitor self for signs of infection, which are reported immediately to the health care provider. The client should also call the provider if more than one dose is missed. The medication may be taken with meals to minimize nausea.

Test-Taking Strategy: Note the key word "avoid" in the stem. This tells you that the correct answer will be an inaccurate piece of information. Knowing that the nurse would not instruct the client to discontinue medication, this becomes the option of choice. Take time now to review this medication if you had difficulty with this question!

Level of Cognitive Ability: Application
Phase of Nursing Process: Planning
Client Needs: Health Promotion and Maintenance
Content Area: Pharmacology

Reference

Deglin, J., & Vallerand, A. (1997). *Davis's drug guide for nurses* (5th ed.). Philadelphia: F. A. Davis, p. 120.

240. The client has been prescribed phenazopyridine hydrochloride (Pyridium) after a urological procedure. Which of the following would the nurse plan to include in the medication instructions to the client?

1 "The medication exerts an antimicrobial effect."
2 "The urine may have a reddish-orange discoloration, which may stain clothing."
3 "The medication provides an antibacterial effect."
4 "The medication should be taken on an empty stomach."

Answer: 2

Rationale: Phenazopyridine is a urinary tract analgesic with no antimicrobial or antibacterial properties. It relieves frequency, burning sensation, or dysuria that follows urological procedures or accompanies infection. The medication is usually taken for 2 days or until symptoms have resolved, and then it is discontinued. Any accompanying antibiotics are continued until finished. It stains clothing and bedclothes an orange-red color, which is permanent. For this reason, clients are advised to wear sanitary napkins to protect undergarments. The medication is best taken with food to avoid gastrointestinal upset.

Test-Taking Strategy: Eliminate options 1 and 3 first because they are similar. It is also helpful to know that phenazopyridine is not an antibiotic and that it discolors urine, possibly staining clothing with an orange-red color. Take time now to review this medication if you are not familiar with it!

Level of Cognitive Ability: Application
Phase of Nursing Process: Planning
Client Needs: Physiological Integrity
Content Area: Pharmacology

Reference

Hodgson, B., & Kizior, R. (1998). *Saunders nursing drug handbook 1998.* Philadelphia: W. B. Saunders, pp. 812–813.

---

241. The client has a cuffed tracheostomy tube and is being weaned from its use. The nurse would plan to make which of the following critical observations before plugging the client's tracheostomy?

1 The airway is totally free of secretions
2 The cuff is fully deflated
3 The oxygen saturation is at least 99%
4 The chest x-ray shows no abnormalities

Answer: 2

Rationale: Before a cuffed tracheostomy tube is plugged, the cuff must be deflated. Otherwise, the client cannot ventilate around the tube and could suffer respiratory arrest. Other correct nursing actions include suctioning the airway to promote ventilation and monitoring adequacy of oxygen saturation (baseline may vary slightly, depending on client). The client may have some residual abnormality on chest x-ray, depending on the underlying pathology.

Test-Taking Strategy: The question asks for a "critical observation" before the tracheostomy is plugged. Options 3 and 4 indicate good respiratory status, but these values or results may not be realistic for every client and are certainly not "critical." Also, it is hard to ensure that the airway is "totally" free of secretions. The best answer is option 2: the tracheostomy cuff should be totally deflated.

Level of Cognitive Ability: Application
Phase of Nursing Process: Planning
Client Needs: Safe, Effective Care Environment
Content Area: Adult Health/Respiratory

Reference

Black, J., & Matassarin-Jacobs, E. (1997). *Medical-surgical nursing: Clinical management for continuity of care* (5th ed.). Philadelphia: W. B. Saunders, p. 1071.

242. The client with an oral endotracheal tube (ETT) in place has the nursing diagnosis Risk for Altered Oral Mucous Membrane. Which of the following interventions would not be included by the nurse in developing the plan of care for this client?

1. Provide frequent oral suction above the ETT cuff
2. Move the ETT from one corner of the mouth to the other every 6 hours
3. Avoid using products with alcohol or lemon in cleaning the client's teeth and gums
4. Apply a lubricant to the client's lips as needed

Answer: 2

Rationale: The ETT is moved from one corner of the mouth to the other at least every day to minimize the risk of necrosis of the mouth and pharynx that results from pressure. Doing this every 6 hours is excessive. The nurse does suction the oropharynx above the ETT frequently to prevent accumulation of secretions above the ETT cuff. Products with lemon or alcohol are not used because they cause drying of oral mucosa. For the same reason, the lips are lubricated as needed.

Test-Taking Strategy: The wording of the question guides you to select an incorrect nursing intervention. Eliminate option 1 first as an obviously correct option. Options 3 and 4 are also beneficial to the client and may thus be eliminated. This leaves option 2 as the answer; the endotracheal tube does not need to be repositioned that frequently.

Level of Cognitive Ability: Application
Phase of Nursing Process: Planning
Client Needs: Health Promotion and Maintenance
Content Area: Adult Health/Respiratory

Reference

Black, J., & Matassarin-Jacobs, E. (1997). *Medical-surgical nursing: Clinical management for continuity of care* (5th ed.). Philadelphia: W. B. Saunders, pp. 1175–1176.

---

243. The female client states she was just raped while sleeping in her bed at home. In preparing a nursing care plan, one of the most immediate goals the nurse will set, in addition to medical attention, will include

1. Providing instructions for medical follow-up.
2. Obtaining counseling for the victim.
3. Providing anticipatory guidance for police investigations, medical questions, and court proceedings.
4. Exploring safety concerns by obtaining permission to notify significant others who can provide shelter and by guiding them in responding to the victim.

Answer: 4

Rationale: After the provision of medical treatment, the nurse's next priority would be obtaining support and planning for safety. Option 4 provides the priority nursing interventions. Options 2 and 3 seek to satisfy emotional needs related to the rape and emotional readiness for the process of discovery and legal action. Option 1 is long term in that it is concerned with ensuring that the victim understands the importance of and commits to the need for medical follow-up.

Test-Taking Strategy: This question assesses your ability to determine the victim's immediate needs. If you consider Maslow's hierarchy of needs theory, you can readily see that after physical care must come safety and support. Although options 2 and 3 seek to satisfy emotional needs, this does not take priority over the establishment of physical safety.

Level of Cognitive Ability: Analysis
Phase of Nursing Process: Planning
Client Needs: Physiological Integrity
Content Area: Mental Health

Reference

Antai-Otong, D., & Kongale, G. (1995). *Psychiatric nursing: Biological and behavioral concepts*. Philadelphia: W. B. Saunders, pp. 407–426.

244. The client is diagnosed as experiencing unresolved sexual trauma. In preparing a nursing care plan for the client, the nurse understands that this is a condition in which the client

1 Experiences complete recovery on the surface but feels badly internally.
2 Remembers the event every year at the same time with decreasing feelings of trauma.
3 Experiences a persistent phobia such as a prolonged fear of being alone.
4 Uses the family, friends, and other support systems to combat the fears and anxieties that are part of the recovery process.

Answer: 3

Rationale: Unresolved sexual trauma occurs when the following conditions are present: development of a persistent phobia such as that of being alone or going out; retreat from sexual themes and possession of low self-esteem and guilt feelings; recurrence of the symptoms of rape trauma triggered by seemingly minor events; recurrence of the symptoms of rape trauma triggered by the anniversary date of the rape trauma; avoidance of contact with members of the opposite sex; and negatively altered relationships with family and friends, such as withdrawal, unusual anger, or silence (negativity may be displacement of feelings of assailant).

Test-Taking Strategy: Knowledge regarding unresolved sexual trauma is necessary to answer the question. Use the process of elimination, noting that options 1, 2, and 4 identify some sort of resolution. Option 3 identifies a persistent phobia. Take time now to review this disorder if you had difficulty with the question!

Level of Cognitive Ability: Analysis
Phase of Nursing Process: Planning
Client Needs: Psychosocial Integrity
Content Area: Mental Health

Reference

Antai-Otong, D., & Kongale, G. (1995). *Psychiatric nursing: Biological and behavioral concepts*. Philadelphia: W. B. Saunders, pp. 407–426.

245. The male client is diagnosed as a power rapist. The nurse prepares a nursing care plan for the client, and in the planning, the nurse understands that the power rapist is one who

1 Seeks to use sexual assault to express and discharge feelings of intense anger, frustration, and contempt.
2 Finds pleasure in bondage and torture because of intense anger and the need to control becoming sexualized.
3 Wants to place a woman in a helpless controlled situation in which she cannot resist or refuse him.
4 Is motivated by something that arouses his sexual interest.

Answer: 3

Rationale: The power rapist wants to place a woman in a helpless controlled situation in which she cannot resist or refuse him. In this situation, the power rapist is provided with a reassuring sense of strength, mastery, security, and control. He uses these feelings to compensate for his feelings of inadequacy. Although the offender usually does not consciously intend to hurt his victim, he does aim to have complete control over her. As the offender's behavior becomes repetitive and compulsive, his need to achieve feelings of power, control, and adequacy may lead him to increase the aggression over time.

Test-Taking Strategy: Note that the issue of the question is the power rapist. With this in mind, seek the option that best identifies the description of this type of rapist. Option 3, "place a woman in a helpless controlled situation," suggests the act of "power." If you had difficulty with this question, take time now to review the characteristics of rapists!

Level of Cognitive Ability: Analysis
Phase of Nursing Process: Planning
Client Needs: Psychosocial Integrity
Content Area: Mental Health

Reference

Antai-Otong, D., & Kongale, G. (1995). *Psychiatric nursing: Biological and behavioral concepts*. Philadelphia: W. B. Saunders, pp. 407–426.

246. The nurse is planning care for a newly admitted suicidal client. In order to provide a caring, therapeutic environment, which of the following is included in the nursing care plan?

1. Placing the client in a private room to ensure privacy and confidentiality
2. Establishing a therapeutic relationship and conveying unconditional positive regard
3. Placing the person in charge of a meaningful unit activity such as the morning chess tournament
4. Maintaining a distance of 12 inches at all times to ensure the client that control will be provided

Answer: 2

Rationale: The establishment of a therapeutic relationship with the suicidal client increases feelings of acceptance. Although the suicidal behavior and thinking of the client is unacceptable, the use of unconditional positive regard acknowledges the client in a human-to-human context and increases the client's sense of self-worth. The only time that a client may be isolated is when the client's condition is extremely acute because this action would intensify the client's feelings of worthlessness. Placing the client in charge of the morning chess game is a premature intervention that can overwhelm and cause the client to fail. This can reinforce the client's feelings of worthlessness. Distances of 18 inches or less between two individuals constitutes intimate space. Invasion of this space may be misinterpreted by the client and increase the client's tension and feelings of helplessness.

Test-Taking Strategy: This question asks you to be able to plan the nursing care for a suicidal client. Use the process of elimination. Eliminate option 1 because isolation is not the safe and therapeutic intervention. Option 3 may produce feelings of worthlessness. Eliminate option 4 because a distance of 12 inches is restrictive. Option 2 is the only option that addresses a therapeutic environment!

Level of Cognitive Ability: Application
Phase of Nursing Process: Planning
Client Needs: Safe, Effective Care Environment
Content Area: Mental Health

Reference

Townsend, M. (1996). *Psychiatric–mental health nursing: Concepts of care* (2nd ed.). Philadelphia: F. A. Davis, pp. 212, 254–255.

---

247. A mother of a 5-year-old with newly diagnosed diabetes is very concerned about her child's going to school and participating in social events. A nursing care goal for this family would be which of the following?

1. The child's normal growth and development will be maintained
2. The child and family will discuss all aspects of the illness and its treatments
3. The child will use effective coping mechanisms to manage anxiety
4. The child and family will integrate diabetes care into patterns of daily living

Answer: 4

Rationale: In order to effectively manage social events in the child's life, the family and the child need to integrate the care and management of diabetes into their daily living.

Test-Taking Strategy: The issue of the question is social. From the options presented, integrating diabetes into the life of the family is the only way to deal with social issues. The other options are all goals for the family; however, they do not deal with social issues.

Level of Cognitive Ability: Application
Phase of Nursing Process: Planning
Client Needs: Psychosocial Integrity
Content Area: Child Health

Reference

Ashwill, J., & Droske, S. (1997). *Nursing care of children: Principles and practice.* Philadelphia: W. B. Saunders, p. 1205.

248. When care is planned for a child in cervical traction with Crutchfield tongs, the most appropriate nursing goals include

1 Assess neurological status and maintain strict input and output.
2 Monitor neurovascular status and provide emotional support.
3 Promote mobility and maintain skin integrity.
4 Maintain proper alignment and prevent infection.

Answer: 4

Rationale: Caring for a child in traction includes ensuring the equipment is in proper position and the child's body is in proper alignment. Cervical traction with Crutchfield tongs is a type of skeletal traction that requires pin site assessment and pin care to prevent infection. Neurological status and fluid balance (input and output) should not be affected by cervical traction. Immobilization until bone healing occurs is the essential goal of cervical traction.

Test-Taking Strategy: Eliminate options 1 and 2 because they are similar. Knowledge that immobilization is required until healing occurs will assist in eliminating option 3. Take time now to review the care of the child in cervical traction with Crutchfield tongs if you had difficulty with this question!

Level of Cognitive Ability: Application
Phase of Nursing Process: Planning
Client Needs: Safe, Effective Care Environment
Content Area: Child Health

Reference

Wong, D. (1997). *Whaley and Wong's Essentials of pediatric nursing* (5th ed.). St. Louis: Mosby–Year Book, pp. 1134–1135.

---

249. When planning care for an adolescent with juvenile rheumatoid arthritis (JRA), it is important to include which of the following strategies to address the problem of Body Image Disturbance?

1 Encourage child to use coping mechanisms
2 Use age-appropriate support groups to assist the child in identifying concerns
3 Assess child's perception of chronic illness
4 Maintain a calm and consistent environment

Answer: 2

Rationale: Age-appropriate support groups will assist the child in identifying areas of concern related to esteem and body image. Options 1 and 4 do not address the issue of altered body image. Assessment of the child's perception of the chronic illness will be done before the planning phase of the nursing process.

Test-Taking Strategy: The question asks for a strategy for an adolescent who has a Body Image Disturbance. Options 1 and 4 do not address the issues of the question. Option 3 is done prior to the planning phase.

Level of Cognitive Ability: Application
Phase of Nursing Process: Planning
Client Needs: Psychosocial Integrity
Content Area: Child Health

Reference

Ashwill, J., & Droske, S. (1997). *Nursing care of children: Principles and practice.* Philadelphia: W. B. Saunders, p. 1131.

---

250. An 8-month-old is admitted to the orthopedic unit in Bryant's traction for treatment of congenital hip dysplasia. Which of the following will be included in the plan of care?

1 Use restraints as needed to maintain the child in supine position
2 Cleanse pin sites every shift
3 Elevate head of bed 20 to 30 degrees for correct alignment
4 Check sling placement to prevent peroneal nerve damage

Answer: 1

Rationale: Restraints would most likely be necessary for an 8-month-old to maintain supine position and maintain safe and proper countertraction with child's weight. Bryant's traction is skin traction, so there are no pin sites to clean. Head of bed elevation, which is used with cervical traction, would affect countertraction with Bryant's traction and is therefore inappropriate. Sling placement is checked frequently to prevent peroneal nerve damage with Russell's traction.

Test-Taking Strategy: Knowledge that Bryant's traction is a type of skin traction usually for children less than 2 years old will assist in answering the question. This visual image of Bryant's traction should help you eliminate option 2 (skeletal traction), option 3 (cervical traction), and option 4 (Russell traction). If you had difficulty with this question, take time now to review this type of traction!

Level of Cognitive Ability: Application
Phase of Nursing Process: Planning
Client Needs: Safe, Effective Care Environment
Content Area: Child Health

Reference

Ashwill, J., & Droske, S. (1997). *Nursing care of children: Principles and practice.* Philadelphia: W. B. Saunders, pp. 1100–1101.

---

251. What information should the nurse include in a teaching plan for the parents of a newborn who has just received a diagnosis of bilateral clubfoot?

1 "Genetic testing is wise for future pregnancies, because other children may also be affected."
2 "If casting is needed, it will begin at birth and continue for 12 weeks, when the condition will be reevaluated."
3 "Surgery performed immediately after birth has been found to be most effective in achieving a complete recovery."
4 "The regimen of manipulation and casting is effective in 95% of cases of bilateral clubfoot."

Answer: 2

Rationale: Casting should begin at birth and continue for at least 12 weeks until maximum correction is achieved. At this time, corrective shoes may provide support to maintain alignment, or surgery can be performed. Surgery is usually delayed until the child is 4–12 months of age.

Test-Taking Strategy: Knowledge regarding the treatment plan for the child with bilateral clubfoot is necessary to answer the question. Although option 1 is correct, this is not the time to discuss the future. Option 3 is incorrect in that surgery is always delayed to allow for maximum restoration. Option 4 contains inaccurate information. Option 2 provides accurate information in the most matter-of-fact manner. Review the treatment plan for bilateral clubfoot now if you had difficulty with this question!

Level of Cognitive Ability: Application
Phase of Nursing Process: Planning
Client Needs: Health Promotion and Maintenance
Content Area: Child Health

Reference

Ball, J., & Bindler, R. (1995). *Pediatric nursing: Caring for children.* Stamford, CT: Appleton & Lange, p. 588.

---

252. The nurse is preparing to discharge an infant with newly diagnosed hemophilia. Which of the following should be included in the teaching plan for home care for this child?

1 "Use a soft toothbrush for dental hygiene."
2 "Pad crib rails and table corners."
3 "Use a generous amount of lubricant when taking a rectal temperature."
4 "Include instructions regarding the appropriate dose of aspirin to give for pain relief."

Answer: 2

Rationale: Establishment of an age-appropriate safe environment is of paramount importance for hemophiliacs. A safe environment for infants includes padding table corners and crib rails, providing extra "joint" padding on clothes, observing a mobile child at all times, and keeping items that can be pulled down onto the child out of reach. Use of a soft toothbrush is an appropriate measure for an older child with hemophilia but is not typically necessary for an infant. Rectal temperature measurements and the use of aspirin are contraindicated for hemophiliacs.

Test-Taking Strategy: The question seeks "discharge information" for an "infant" with "hemophilia." Eliminate option 1 because a toothbrush would not be indicated for an infant. Next eliminate option 4 because aspirin would not be administered. Option 3 can be eliminated because rectal temperature measurements are contraindicated with hemophilia. In addition, the phrase "generous amount" should be a clue that this is an incorrect option. Review discharge teaching points for an infant with hemophilia now if you had difficulty with this question!

Level of Cognitive Ability: Application
Phase of Nursing Process: Planning
Client Needs: Health Promotion and Maintenance
Content Area: Child Health

Reference

Ashwill, J., & Droske, S. (1997). *Nursing care of children: Principles and practice.* Philadelphia: W. B. Saunders, p. 981.

253. The client is diagnosed with rape trauma syndrome. The nursing care plan for the client is based on the nurse's understanding that rape trauma syndrome is a condition that involves

1 More than one assault.
2 Imagining use of force in a sexual situation.
3 Actively initiating situations in which sex is forced.
4 Reexperiencing recollections of the trauma.

Answer: 4

Rationale: The major trauma involved in rape or sexual assault involves the victim's emotional reaction to being physically forced to do something against his or her will. The life-threatening nature of the crime, which is accompanied by feelings of helplessness, loss of control, and the experiencing of self as an object of the perpetrator's rage, combine to produce the victim's overpowering fear and stress. This syndrome has been called rape trauma syndrome and the client reexperiences the trauma, evidenced by recurrent recollections of the event. Some diagnosticians feel that this syndrome is part of posttraumatic stress disorder (PTSD).

Test-Taking Strategy: The issue of the question is rape trauma syndrome. Note the key word "trauma" in the question. Attempt to use knowledge regarding this syndrome to answer the question, but if you are unable to, note the relationship between this key word and option 4. Review rape trauma syndrome now if you had difficulty with this question!

Level of Cognitive Ability: Analysis
Phase of Nursing Process: Planning
Client Needs: Physiological Integrity
Content Area: Mental Health

Reference

Antai-Otong, D., & Kongale, G. (1995). *Psychiatric nursing: Biological and behavioral concepts*. Philadelphia: W. B. Saunders, pp. 407–426.

254. The client has just returned to the nursing unit after thoracic surgery and has two chest tubes in place. The nurse plans to monitor the drainage from each chest tube

1 Hourly.
2 Every 2 hours.
3 Every 4 hours.
4 Every 8 hours.

Answer: 1

Rationale: In the first 24 hours after thoracic surgery, the nurse notes and records the amount of drainage hourly. After the first 24 hours, the frequency of measurement usually decreases to once every 8 hours. Individual surgeon preference may dictate the frequency of observation and measurement.

Test-Taking Strategy: Knowledge of the complications of thoracic surgery and nursing management are needed to answer this question. However, if you are unfamiliar with the specifics and are given a question in which the postoperative client has just returned to the nursing unit, you should select the hourly parameter as the safest educated guess. Review postoperative procedures now if you had difficulty with this question!

Level of Cognitive Ability: Application
Phase of Nursing Process: Planning
Client Needs: Safe, Effective Care Environment
Content Area: Adult Health/Respiratory

Reference

Ignatavicius, D. D., Workman, M. L., & Mishler, M. A. (1995). *Medical-surgical nursing: A nursing process approach* (2nd ed.). Philadelphia: W. B. Saunders, p. 748.

255. The client has an order for continuous monitoring of oxygen saturation (SaO_2). The nurse would plan to do which of the following to ensure accurate readings on the oximeter?

1. Apply the sensor to a finger that is cool to the touch
2. Place the sensor distal to an IV site with a continuous infusion
3. Apply the sensor on a finger with dark nail polish
4. Ask the client not to frequently move the hand that is attached to the pulse oximeter

Answer: 4

Rationale: Despite advances in technology, several factors can still interfere with accurate SaO_2 levels on a pulse oximeter. To ensure accurate readings, the nurse should ask the client to limit motion of the area attached to the sensor. The nurse should apply the device to a warm area, because hypotension, hypothermia, and vasoconstriction interfere with blood flow to the area. The nurse should avoid placing the sensor distal to any invasive arterial or venous catheters, pressure dressings, or blood pressure cuffs. The nurse needs to know that very dark nail polish (black, brown-red, blue, green) interferes with accurate measurement, whereas red nail polish and artificial nails do not.

Test-Taking Strategy: This question is worded to elicit a correct nursing action on the part of the nurse. Options 2 and 3 may be eliminated first as the least plausible choices. Of the two remaining, knowing that motion and decreased circulation to the extremity interfere with the readings helps you to choose option 4 over option 1. Review pulse oximetry now if you had difficulty with this question!

Level of Cognitive Ability: Application
Phase of Nursing Process: Planning
Client Needs: Safe, Effective Care Environment
Content Area: Adult Health/Respiratory

Reference

Black, J., & Matassarin-Jacobs, E. (1997). *Medical-surgical nursing: Clinical management for continuity of care* (5th ed.). Philadelphia: W. B. Saunders, p. 1053.

---

256. The nurse has an order to collect a sputum sample from a client for Gram stain and for culture and sensitivity testing. Which of the following would the nurse avoid, to ensure that an optimal specimen is sent to the laboratory?

1. Having the client brush the teeth and rinse the mouth before the sample is obtained
2. Having the client take a few deep breaths before coughing
3. Utilizing a clean container from the supply area
4. Sending the specimen immediately to the laboratory

Answer: 3

Rationale: Because of the nature of the test, the sputum must be collected in a sterile (not a clean) container. The client should brush the teeth and rinse the mouth to decrease contaminating organisms. The client should take a few deep breaths and then cough forcefully, not spit, into the container. The specimen is sent directly to the laboratory and is not allowed to sit for long periods of time at room temperature. This measure also prevents overgrowth of contaminating organisms.

Test-Taking Strategy: Knowledge of specimen handling is helpful in beginning to answer this question. This would help you eliminate option 4 first, because this is indicated, and the question asks for an item to avoid. Knowing that a specimen for culture must be placed in a sterile container helps you to choose correctly among the three remaining options. Review this procedure now if you had difficulty with this question!

Level of Cognitive Ability: Application
Phase of Nursing Process: Planning
Client Needs: Safe, Effective Care Environment
Content Area: Adult Health/Respiratory

Reference

Black, J., & Matassarin-Jacobs, E. (1997). *Medical-surgical nursing: Clinical management for continuity of care* (5th ed.). Philadelphia: W. B. Saunders, p. 1063.

257. The client has had a set of arterial blood gases measured. The results are as follows: pH of 7.34, carbon dioxide tension ($PaCO_2$) of 37, oxygen tension (PaO_2) of 79, and bicarbonate level (HCO_3) of 19. The nurse interprets these findings to mean that the client is experiencing

1 Respiratory acidosis.
2 Respiratory alkalosis.
3 Metabolic acidosis.
4 Metabolic alkalosis.

Answer: 3

Rationale: Metabolic acidosis occurs when the pH falls below 7.35 and the bicarbonate level falls below 22 mEq/liter. With respiratory acidosis, the pH drops below 7.35 and the carbon dioxide level rises above 45 mmHg. With respiratory alkalosis, the pH rises above 7.45 and the carbon dioxide level falls below 35 mmHg. With metabolic alkalosis, the pH rises above 7.45 and the bicarbonate level rises above 26 mEq/liter.

Test-Taking Strategy: Knowing that a pH of 7.34 is acidotic allows you to eliminate options 2 and 4 first. To discriminate between the remaining two options, knowing that a metabolic condition exists when the bicarbonate follows the same up-or-down pattern as the pH helps you choose option 3 over option 1.

Level of Cognitive Ability: Analysis
Phase of Nursing Process: Analysis
Client Needs: Physiological Integrity
Content Area: Adult Health/Respiratory

Reference

Black, J., & Matassarin-Jacobs, E. (1997). *Medical-surgical nursing: Clinical management for continuity of care* (5th ed.). Philadelphia: W. B. Saunders, pp. 1056–1057.

---

258. The nurse is planning to assist with obtaining a set of arterial blood gas measurements on a client. In addition to sending the specimen to the laboratory immediately, the nurse would plan to do which of the following to optimally maintain the integrity of the specimen?

1 Use a syringe containing a preservative
2 Use a syringe containing a preservative and send the specimen on ice
3 Use a heparinized syringe
4 Use a heparinized syringe and send the specimen on ice

Answer: 4

Rationale: The arterial blood gas sample is obtained with a heparinized syringe. The completed sample is placed on ice and sent to the laboratory immediately.

Test-Taking Strategy: Knowing that the syringe is heparinized helps you to eliminate options 1 and 2 first. Knowing that the specimen must be placed on ice helps you to discriminate between the remaining two options. If you are unfamiliar with this procedure, take a few moments to memorize these two details now.

Level of Cognitive Ability: Application
Phase of Nursing Process: Planning
Client Needs: Safe, Effective Care Environment
Content Area: Adult Health/Respiratory

Reference

Black, J., & Matassarin-Jacobs, E. (1997). *Medical-surgical nursing: Clinical management for continuity of care* (5th ed.). Philadelphia: W. B. Saunders, p. 1055.

259. The nurse is caring for the hospitalized client with chronic airflow limitation. The room next to the client's is being thoroughly cleaned by environmental services personnel. The client complains that fumes from the chemicals used for cleaning are causing difficulty breathing. Which of the following represents the best action plan by the nurse?

1 Move the client to another area until the cleaning is done
2 Close the door to the client's room
3 Use air freshener in the client's room to mask the smell
4 Place a fan in the client's room venting toward the door

Answer: 1

Rationale: The client with chronic airflow limitation should avoid exposure to toxic or irritating chemicals, such as aerosols, harsh chemicals, and smoke. Removing the client to another area prevents the client from breathing in irritants that are airborne in and around the client's room.

Test-Taking Strategy: The question asks for the best plan on the part of the nurse. Eliminate option 3 first as the least effective method, because air fresheners do not remove chemicals; they only mask the odor. Closing the door and placing a fan in the room may reduce the client's contact with the chemicals but are not likely to completely eliminate them. For this reason, these options are also eliminated. This leaves option 1 as the best choice to protect the client from inhalation of irritating chemicals.

Level of Cognitive Ability: Application
Phase of Nursing Process: Planning
Client Needs: Safe, Effective Care Environment
Content Area: Adult Health/Respiratory

Reference
Ignatavicius, D. D., Workman, M. L., & Mishler, M. A. (1995). *Medical-surgical nursing: A nursing process approach* (2nd ed.). Philadelphia: W. B. Saunders, p. 683.

---

260. The client is to undergo renal arteriography to rule out renal pathology. As an essential element of care, the nurse would plan to ask the client about a history of

1 Frequent antibiotic use.
2 Long-term diuretic therapy.
3 Allergy to shellfish or iodine.
4 Familial renal disease.

Answer: 3

Rationale: The client undergoing any type of arteriography should be questioned about allergy to shellfish, seafood, or iodine. This is essential for identifying potential allergic reaction to contrast dye, which may be used in some diagnostic tests. The other items are also useful as part of the health history but are not as critical as the allergy determination.

Test-Taking Strategy: Note that the stem of the question includes the phrase "essential element of care." This implies that more than one or all options may be correct. However, one of them is of highest priority. Option 4 can be eliminated first as the least pertinent to current care. Because the stem indicates that arteriography is planned, the items are evaluated against their potential connection to this test. Thus you would eliminate all options except the third, which is directly related to the test.

Level of Cognitive Ability: Application
Phase of Nursing Process: Planning
Client Needs: Safe, Effective Care Environment
Content Area: Adult Health/Renal

Reference
Black, J., & Matassarin-Jacobs, E. (1997). *Medical-surgical nursing: Clinical management for continuity of care* (5th ed.). Philadelphia: W. B. Saunders, p. 1550.

261. The nurse is planning to implement a bladder retraining program for the client who has incontinence. Which of the following interventions would be contraindicated as the nurse develops this plan?

1 Limit the oral fluid intake of the client
2 Teach pelvic muscle–strengthening exercises
3 Ensure accessibility to a toilet
4 Adhere strictly to scheduled toileting times

Answer: 1

Rationale: In order for a bladder retraining program to be successful, several components must be in place. The client should learn and practice pelvic muscle–strengthening exercises to promote bladder emptying. The nurse should ensure accessibility to bathroom facilities and strict adherence to the toileting schedule. Limiting fluid intake is contraindicated; adequate fluid intake is necessary to produce enough urine to stimulate micturition.

Test-Taking Strategy: The wording of the statement guides you to look for an incorrect response. Because options 3 and 4 are most obviously correct, these are eliminated as answers according to the wording of the question. To discriminate between the last two options, it is necessary to know that sufficient fluid is necessary to cause bladder filling and proper stimulation of the micturition reflex. Knowing this would allow you to select option 1.

Level of Cognitive Ability: Application
Phase of Nursing Process: Planning
Client Needs: Safe, Effective Care Environment
Content Area: Adult Health/Renal

Reference
Black, J., & Matassarin-Jacobs, E. (1997). *Medical-surgical nursing: Clinical management for continuity of care* (5th ed.). Philadelphia: W. B. Saunders, p. 1610.

262. Acute bronchitis has been diagnosed in the client. The nurse would plan to teach the client about which of the following items that aggravate the symptoms?

1 Moving from an area of warm air to cold
2 Using a humidifier in the home
3 Ingesting large amounts of fluids
4 Ingesting warm liquids

Answer: 1

Rationale: Moving from an area of warm air to cold irritates the respiratory passages, triggering cough and perhaps bronchospasm. Humidification of air is a high priority to keep the airways from becoming dry and irritated. Warmth is soothing and may be used as steam inhalations, warm beverages, and warm, moist heat applications to the chest.

Test-Taking Strategy: Remember that options that are similar are not likely to be correct. In this question, options 2, 3, and 4 involve moisture. Option 1 is different from the others and is the answer to the question as stated. Review treatment measures for acute bronchitis now if you had difficulty with this question!

Level of Cognitive Ability: Application
Phase of Nursing Process: Planning
Client Needs: Health Promotion and Maintenance
Content Area: Adult Health/Respiratory

Reference
Burrell, P., Gerlach, M., & Pless, B. (1997). *Adult nursing: Acute and community care* (2nd ed.). Stamford, CT: Appleton & Lange, p. 754.

263. The client has undergone intermaxillary fixation (jaw wiring). The nurse would plan to avoid which of the following immediately after the client returns to the surgical nursing unit?

1. Elevating the head of bed to a 45-degree angle
2. Applying moist heat to the jaws for comfort
3. Keeping wire cutters or scissors at the bedside
4. Performing oral suctioning

Answer: 2

Rationale: The client who has had intermaxillary fixation has limited movement of the mouth and is at risk of aspiration. Performing oral suctioning and elevating the head of the bed after recovery from anesthesia promotes maintenance of a patent airway. The presence of wire cutters or scissors at the bedside is also indicated in case the client experiences respiratory obstruction from vomiting or other causes. When the client is admitted to the unit, the nurse verifies with the physician the circumstances under which the wires may be cut. Ice is applied to the jaws for 30 minutes out of every hour for the first 12 hours postoperatively in an effort to reduce swelling.

Test-Taking Strategy: Examine this question from the viewpoint of airway maintenance. The question is basically asking you for an action that is contraindicated. Knowing that heat promotes swelling, you would choose this as the option that could compromise the airway. You would arrive at the same conclusion by reasoning that each of the other options promotes airway maintenance. Review postoperative care after intermaxillary fixation if you had difficulty with this question!

Level of Cognitive Ability: Application
Phase of Nursing Process: Planning
Client Needs: Physiological Integrity
Content Area: Adult Health/Respiratory

Reference

Burrell, P., Gerlach, M., & Pless, B. (1997). *Adult nursing: Acute and community care* (2nd ed.). Stamford, CT: Appleton & Lange, p. 722.

---

264. The client with chronic obstructive pulmonary disease (COPD) asks the nurse about ways to minimize exposure to environmental pollutants. The nurse would plan to incorporate which of the following items when addressing this client's concern?

1. "Use Venetian blinds rather than curtains."
2. "Use wood-burning stove only if soft wood is used."
3. "Remove carpeting whenever possible."
4. "Keep indoor plants with strong scents watered very well."

Answer: 3

Rationale: To decrease environmental pollution which can aggravate COPD, the client's home should be cleaned regularly, and dusting should be done with a damp cloth. Washable curtains are preferred to Venetian blinds, which can gather dust. Wood-burning stoves should not be used. Carpets should also be removed when it is possible, because they also harbor dust. Plants that have strong scents should be removed from the home.

Test-Taking Strategy: To answer this question accurately, you should know where the sources of dust in the home are and ways to minimize them. It is also necessary to know that strong odors are aggravating factors and should be eliminated. From this point, use the process of elimination to answer the question.

Level of Cognitive Ability: Application
Phase of Nursing Process: Planning
Client Needs: Health Promotion and Maintenance
Content Area: Adult Health/Respiratory

Reference

Burrell, P., Gerlach, M., & Pless, B. (1997). *Adult nursing: Acute and community care* (2nd ed.). Stamford, CT: Appleton & Lange, p. 775.

265. The client is being discharged to the home but requires ongoing chest physiotherapy (CPT). The nurse would plan to incorporate which of the following items in teaching the family how to correctly perform this procedure?

1 Perform the procedure within 1 hour after a meal
2 Position the client so the head and chest are elevated
3 Expect the respiratory status to worsen during the procedure
4 Continue the therapy up to the prescribed ideal time if tolerated

Answer: 4

Rationale: CPT should be avoided for 2 hours after meals, to avoid vomiting after mealtime. The head and chest are placed in the proper position prescribed for the client, and the head and chest should be lower than the rest of the body, if tolerated. The client's respiratory status should be monitored and the procedure modified if the respiratory status worsens. The therapy is performed to the ideal time, usually 15 minutes, as long as it is tolerated by the client.

Test-Taking Strategy: Note that the key words in this question are "teaching" and "correctly." This tells you that the correct response will also be consistent with the correct method of carrying out this procedure. Recalling that CPT uses principles of gravity, you would eliminate options 1 and 2. Option 3 does not offer protection for the client's airway and is therefore eliminated next. Review the procedure for CPT now if you had difficulty with this question!

Level of Cognitive Ability: Application
Phase of Nursing Process: Planning
Client Needs: Safe, Effective Care Environment
Content Area: Adult Health/Respiratory

Reference

Burrell, P., Gerlach, M., & Pless, B. (1997). *Adult nursing: Acute and community care* (2nd ed.). Stamford, CT: Appleton & Lange, p. 665.

---

266. The client presents to the Emergency Room with status asthmaticus. The nurse would plan to do which of the following first?

1 Place the client in high Fowler's position
2 Obtain a set of vital signs
3 Start an IV line
4 Administer oxygen at 21%

Answer: 1

Rationale: The initial nursing action is to place the client in a position that aids in respiration, which would be sitting bolt upright or in high Fowler's. Other nursing actions follow in rapid sequence and include monitoring vital signs, administering bronchodilators and oxygen (but at levels of 2–5 liters/minute, or 24%–28% by Ventimask). Insertion of an IV line and ongoing monitoring of respiratory status are also indicated.

Test-Taking Strategy: Note that the key word in this question is the word "first." Eliminate option 4 first, because oxygen at 21% is ambient air, not supplemental oxygen. Option 2 is an assessment and is not the best first choice when a client is in respiratory distress. The correct option protects the client's airway, which guides you to choose option 1 over option 3.

Level of Cognitive Ability: Application
Phase of Nursing Process: Planning
Client Needs: Physiological Integrity
Content Area: Adult Health/Respiratory

Reference

Burrell, P., Gerlach, M., & Pless, B. (1997). *Adult nursing: Acute and community care* (2nd ed.). Stamford, CT: Appleton & Lange, p. 761.

---

267. The client is experiencing diabetes insipidus secondary to cranial surgery. The nurse plans to institute which of these anticipated therapies?

1 Fluid restriction
2 IV replacement of fluid losses
3 Increased sodium intake
4 Vasodilators

Answer: 2

Rationale: The client with diabetes insipidus excretes large amounts of extremely dilute urine. This usually occurs as a result of decreased synthesis or release of antidiuretic hormone (ADH) from conditions such as head injury, surgery near the hypothalamus, or increased intracranial pressure. Corrective measures include allowing ample oral fluid intake, administering IV fluid as needed to replace sensible and insensible losses, and administering vasopressin (Pitressin). Sodium is not administered because the serum sodium level is usually high, as is the serum osmolality.

Test-Taking Strategy: In order to answer this question correctly, you must understand that large fluid loss is the problem in this client. The wording of the question guides you to choose an option that will restore fluids to the client. Using this rationale, eliminate options 1 and 4 first. You would choose option 2 over option 3 by knowing either that the serum sodium level is already high in this disorder, or by knowing that fluid replacement is the most direct form of therapy for fluid loss. Review treatment for diabetes insipidus now if you had difficulty with this question!

Level of Cognitive Ability: Application
Phase of Nursing Process: Planning
Client Needs: Physiological Integrity
Content Area: Adult Health/Neurological

Reference

Burrell, P., Gerlach, M., & Pless, B. (1997). *Adult nursing: Acute and community care* (2nd ed.). Stamford, CT: Appleton & Lange, p. 919.

---

268. The client inquires about foods that are low in tyramine to help lessen the frequency of migraine headaches. The nurse would plan to teach the client to avoid which of the following items in the diet?

1 Cherries
2 Whole wheat bread
3 Aged cheeses
4 Chicken

Answer: 3

Rationale: Some foods that are naturally high in tyramine include aged cheeses, yogurt, canned meats, beef or chicken liver, sausage, dried fish, beer and some wines, and chocolate. These should be eliminated in the diet of a client prone to migraine headaches. The client may consume any bread and cereal products, as well as most fruits and vegetables. The fruits and vegetables that should be avoided are bananas, figs, broad-leaf beans and pea pods, eggplant, and mixed Chinese vegetables.

Test-Taking Strategy: To answer this question correctly, it is necessary to know which types of foods are high in tyramine. Take a few moments to review this material if the question was difficult!

Level of Cognitive Ability: Application
Phase of Nursing Process: Planning
Client Needs: Health Promotion and Maintenance
Content Area: Adult Health/Neurological

References

Burrell, P., Gerlach, M., & Pless, B. (1997). *Adult nursing: Acute and community care* (2nd ed.). Stamford, CT: Appleton & Lange, p. 914.
Lutz, C., & Przytulski, K. (1997). *Nutrition and diet therapy* (2nd ed.). Philadelphia: F. A. Davis, p. 304.

---

269. The nurse is called by a physical therapist to the room of a client experiencing a seizure. The nurse would plan to do which of the following to ensure the client's safety?

1 Wiggle a bite stick between the client's clenched teeth
2 Restrain the client to prevent bruising
3 Draw the curtain around the bedside area
4 Turn the client to the side if possible

Answer: 4

Rationale: Nursing management during a seizure includes easing the client to the floor if out of bed and loosening clothing such as a belt, tie, or collar. The client is rolled to the side whenever possible to allow drainage of secretions from the mouth. An airway is never forced between the teeth of a client during a seizure; this could damage the teeth and gums. The client is not restrained, because the strong muscle contractions during seizure activity could cause injury to the restrained client. The curtain should be drawn, but it is done for privacy, not to prevent injury.

Test-Taking Strategy: The key words in the question are "ensure" and "safety." With this in mind, eliminate options 1 and 2 because they could harm the client. Discriminate between options 3 and 4 by keeping the focus on a safety-oriented action. Option 4 addresses safety!

Level of Cognitive Ability: Application
Phase of Nursing Process: Planning
Client Needs: Safe, Effective Care Environment
Content Area: Adult Health/Neurological

Reference

Burrell, P., Gerlach, M., & Pless, B. (1997). *Adult nursing: Acute and community care* (2nd ed.). Stamford, CT: Appleton & Lange, p. 912.

---

270. The client with a head injury and a feeding tube continuously tries to remove the tube. Which of the following methods should the nurse plan to use in restraining the client?

1 Mitten splints
2 Wrist restraints
3 Waist restraint
4 Vest restraint

Answer: 1

Rationale: Mitten splints are useful for this client because the client cannot pull against them, which would create resistance that could lead to increased intracranial pressure (ICP). Wrist restraints do provide resistance. Vest and waist restraints prevent the client from getting up or falling out of bed but do nothing to limit hand movement.

Test-Taking Strategy: The question guides you to look for an option that safely limits hand movement. Begin to answer this question by eliminating options 3 and 4, because they do not address the problem stated in the stem. You would choose option 1 over option 2 by understanding the mechanisms and danger of ICP.

Level of Cognitive Ability: Application
Phase of Nursing Process: Planning
Client Needs: Physiological Integrity
Content Area: Adult Health/Neurological

Reference

Burrell, P., Gerlach, M., & Pless, B. (1997). *Adult nursing: Acute and community care* (2nd ed.). Stamford, CT: Appleton & Lange, p. 897.

---

271. The client has undergone intracranial surgery and has a decreasing pulse rate with increasing blood pressure. The nurse plans to avoid which of the following activities until the client is stabilized?

1 Elevating head of bed to 30 degrees
2 Suctioning
3 Keeping the neck midline
4 Administering the current order for mannitol

Answer: 2

Rationale: The client is showing signs of increasing intracranial pressure (ICP). The nurse avoids activities that further increase the ICP, such as suctioning the client. The nurse positions the head of bed at 30 degrees and keeps the neck midline to promote venous drainage from the cranium. The nurse administers osmotic diuretics as ordered and carefully monitors fluid intake to prevent fluid overload.

Test-Taking Strategy: To answer this question correctly, you must recognize the signs of increased intracranial pressure and recall preventative measures. The key word in the question is "avoid." Therefore, you would choose the response that aggravates rising intracranial pressure. There is only one correct response, in view of the wording of this question. Review care of the client after intracranial surgery now if you had difficulty with this question!

Level of Cognitive Ability: Application
Phase of Nursing Process: Planning
Client Needs: Physiological Integrity
Content Area: Adult Health/Neurological

Reference

Burrell, P., Gerlach, M., & Pless, B. (1997). *Adult nursing: Acute and community care* (2nd ed.). Stamford, CT: Appleton & Lange, p. 901.

272. The client has an order for seizure precautions. The nurse would plan to avoid doing which of the following when planning care for the client?

1. Remain in the bathroom while the client is showering
2. Push the lock-out button on the electric bed to keep in lowest position
3. Keep the overhead lights on in the room at night
4. Assist the client to ambulate in the hallway

Answer: 3

Rationale: A quiet, restful environment is provided as part of seizure precautions. This includes undisturbed times for sleep, with the use of a nightlight for safety. The client should be accompanied during activities such as bathing and walking, so that assistance is readily available and injury is minimized if a seizure begins. Maintain the bed in low position for safety.

Test-Taking Strategy: Note that the wording of the question includes the word "avoid." This guides you to look for a response that represents incorrect planning on the part of the nurse. Knowing that options 1 and 4 indicate safe planning, you eliminate these choices easily. You would next eliminate option 2, because it also represents an item that plans for client safety.

Level of Cognitive Ability: Application
Phase of Nursing Process: Planning
Client Needs: Safe, Effective Care Environment
Content Area: Adult Health/Neurological

Reference

Burrell, P., Gerlach, M., & Pless, B. (1997). *Adult nursing: Acute and community care* (2nd ed.). Stamford, CT: Appleton & Lange, p. 911.

---

273. The nurse is preparing to feed the client with dysphagia. The nurse should plan to do which of the following to assist the client with swallowing?

1. Place the equivalent of 30 mL of food on the fork
2. Place food on the tip of the tongue
3. Use water to help client swallow food in the mouth
4. Provide foods that have a soft consistency

Answer: 4

Rationale: No more than a standard amount of food should be placed on the feeding utensil, which is roughly the equivalent of 15 mL. Food should be placed on the posterior part of the tongue to aid in swallowing. Foods that have a soft consistency are provided. Liquids are thickened and are given separately from solid foods to prevent choking.

Test-Taking Strategy: Knowledge of the effects of dysphagia is needed to answer this question accurately. If this question was difficult, take a few moments now to review this key area of nursing practice!

Level of Cognitive Ability: Application
Phase of Nursing Process: Planning
Client Needs: Physiological Integrity
Content Area: Adult Health/Neurological

Reference

Burrell, P., Gerlach, M., & Pless, B. (1997). *Adult nursing: Acute and community care* (2nd ed.). Stamford, CT: Appleton & Lange, pp. 923–924.

---

274. The client suffers from Sleep Pattern Disturbance. The nurse plans to do which of the following to best help the client obtain sufficient rest?

1. Adjust the number of pillows, lights, and noise according to client preference
2. Institute a rigid time frame for delivery of nursing care
3. Use maximum doses of sedative medication at bedtime
4. Allow at least 60 minutes of uninterrupted sleep at a time

Answer: 1

Rationale: An environment that is conducive to sleep is one that simulates the client's natural environment, including number of pillows, bedcovers, light, temperature, and noise. The nurse should plan to be flexible in care delivery times to allow the client rest periods as needed. Sedative medications are used as necessary and ideally are limited to three times per week. The client needs at least 90 minutes without interruption to complete one sleep cycle.

Test-Taking Strategy: The key words in the question are "best help" and "sufficient rest." Eliminate options 2 and 3 first because they contain the words "rigid" and "maximum," respectively. Knowing that a full sleep cycle is 90 minutes long helps you to choose option 1 over option 4.

Level of Cognitive Ability: Application
Phase of Nursing Process: Planning
Client Needs: Physiological Integrity
Content Area: Fundamental Skills

Reference

Burrell, P., Gerlach, M., & Pless, B. (1997). *Adult nursing: Acute and community care* (2nd ed.). Stamford, CT: Appleton & Lange, p. 925.

---

275. The client with a closed-head injury has fluid leaking from the ear. The nurse should first plan to

1 Irrigate the ear canal gently.
2 Test the drainage for glucose.
3 Test the drainage for pH.
4 Notify the physician.

Answer: 2

Rationale: The client with a closed-head injury may have leakage of cerebrospinal fluid (CSF) from the nose or ear. The nurse first determines whether glucose is present in the fluid, indicating that the fluid is indeed CSF. The nurse would then notify the physician if drainage of CSF is found. The ear is not irrigated, because of the risk of infection. Testing of pH is not indicated.

Test-Taking Strategy: To answer this question correctly, you must know that this client is at risk for CSF leakage, and you must know the appropriate method of determining the type of fluid. With these concepts in mind, you would eliminate options 1 and 3. You would choose option 2 over 4 because of the key word "first" in the stem.

Level of Cognitive Ability: Application
Phase of Nursing Process: Planning
Client Needs: Physiological Integrity
Content Area: Adult Health/Neurological

Reference

Burrell, P., Gerlach, M., & Pless, B. (1997). *Adult nursing: Acute and community care* (2nd ed.). Stamford, CT: Appleton & Lange, p. 933.

---

276. The nurse is accepting a post-craniectomy client in transfer from the post-anesthesia care unit. The client's incision is supratentorial. How should the nurse plan to position the client's head?

1 Head of bed flat
2 Head of bed elevated 90 degrees
3 Head of bed elevated 30 degrees
4 Lying on the operative side

Answer: 3

Rationale: Craniectomy involves removal of a portion of the client's cranium, and lying on the operative side is therefore contraindicated, because the bony protection of the skull has been removed. The head of bed should be raised to 30 degrees to promote optimal venous drainage while maintaining arterial perfusion to the brain.

Test-Taking Strategy: To answer this question correctly, it is necessary to understand the impact of craniectomy on client positioning, as well as concepts related to the general positioning of the client with a neurological problem. Remember that "supra" means "up"! This will assist in eliminating options 1 and 4. Visualize the positions in the remaining two options. Option 3 would provide more client comfort than option 2. Option 3 also does not potentially interfere with arterial circulation to the brain. If this question was difficult, take a few moments now to review this topic!

Level of Cognitive Ability: Application
Phase of Nursing Process: Planning
Client Needs: Physiological Integrity
Content Area: Adult Health/Neurological

Reference

Burrell, P., Gerlach, M., & Pless, B. (1997). *Adult nursing: Acute and community care* (2nd ed.). Stamford, CT: Appleton & Lange, p. 932.

277. The previously healthy client with a long leg cast is on prescribed bed rest. The nurse plans to institute which of the following general measures in client care?

1 Assess neurovascular status every 8 hours
2 Reposition every 4–6 hours
3 Request a low-fiber diet
4 Increase fluids to 3 liters per day

Answer: 4

Rationale: Routine measures for the immobile client who has had application of a long leg cast include assessing neurovascular status every 1–4 hours (depending on time since application), repositioning every 2–4 hours, and providing a diet high in fiber and fluids (to prevent constipation).

Test-Taking Strategy: The key word and phrases in this question are "previously healthy," "cast," and "bed rest." Knowledge of basic care measures for the immobile client will lead you to eliminate options 2 and 3. Knowledge of concepts related to cast care, assessment, and time frames would cause you to eliminate option 1. Review nursing measures for cast care now if you had difficulty with this question!

Level of Cognitive Ability: Application
Phase of Nursing Process: Planning
Client Needs: Physiological Integrity
Content Area: Adult Health/Musculoskeletal

Reference
Burrell, P., Gerlach, M., & Pless, B. (1997). *Adult nursing: Acute and community care* (2nd ed.). Stamford, CT: Appleton & Lange, pp. 1594–1595.

---

278. The client with a long leg cast is afraid of wetting the top of the cast while urinating. The nurse would best plan to keep the cast dry by doing which of the following?

1 Requesting an order for a Foley catheter
2 Petaling the edges of the cast
3 Using a trapeze when placing the client on a bedpan
4 Tucking a plastic material (such as food wrap) around the area before toileting

Answer: 4

Rationale: A water-proof material such as plastic food wrap is very useful in preventing cast material from becoming wet during voiding. Using a trapeze aids in proper positioning but does not necessarily prevent spillage or wetting during urination. Petaling cast edges prevents skin irritation but does not affect wetting. Foley catheter insertion carries a risk of infection and is not recommended unless needed for other reasons.

Test-Taking Strategy: Note that the key phrase and words in the question are "best plan," "cast," and "dry." Focus on the issue of the question. Eliminate option 1 first by using principles of infection control. Eliminate option 2 next because it does not address the problem stated in the question. You would choose option 4 over option 3 because it most directly prevents the problem of getting the cast wet.

Level of Cognitive Ability: Application
Phase of Nursing Process: Planning
Client Needs: Physiological Integrity
Content Area: Adult Health/Musculoskeletal

Reference
Burrell, P., Gerlach, M., & Pless, B. (1997). *Adult nursing: Acute and community care* (2nd ed.). Stamford, CT: Appleton & Lange, p. 1595.

279. The nurse is caring for the client with skeletal traction who requires pin care and has moderate amounts of crusty drainage at the pin sites. The nurse would plan to avoid doing which of the following during the procedure?

1 Using sterile solution and applicators
2 Pouring the solution into a sterile bowl
3 Using one cotton-tipped applicator per pin site
4 Moistening any 2 × 2 inch sponges stuck to the site before removal

Answer: 3

Rationale: The use of sterile supplies and technique is critical for preventing infection in the client with skeletal pins in place. The solution (water or saline), swabs, and containers all must be checked for sterility. Each applicator is swabbed on the site once and thrown away. Pin sites with sufficient drainage may require the use of several individual swabs. Any gauze sponges that are stuck to the site are moistened with sterile saline or water before removal. This prevents the sponges from having a local débriding effect.

Test-Taking Strategy: Note the key phrases and word in the question: "pin care," "crusty drainage," and "avoid." The wording of the question guides you to look for an incorrect statement. Eliminate options 1 and 2 first, because they are obviously consistent with correct practice. Knowledge of wound care and sterile technique will help you discriminate between options 3 and 4.

Level of Cognitive Ability: Application
Phase of Nursing Process: Planning
Client Needs: Safe, Effective Care Environment
Content Area: Adult Health/Musculoskeletal

Reference

Burrell, P., Gerlach, M., & Pless, B. (1997). *Adult nursing: Acute and community care* (2nd ed.). Stamford, CT: Appleton & Lange, p. 1602.

280. The client has been placed in skeletal leg traction. The nurse would plan to avoid which of the following as part of routine care?

1 Keeping all ropes in the center of the pulley track
2 Repositioning the client from side to side
3 Having client push up in bed, using unaffected foot
4 Inspecting bony prominences

Answer: 2

Rationale: The client in skeletal traction is kept in the supine position. Minor position changes are made only briefly to expedite delivery of basic nursing care. All parts of the traction setup are regularly assessed for integrity. Bony prominences are inspected as part of diligent, ongoing skin care. The client is allowed to push with the unaffected foot to aid in repositioning.

Test-Taking Strategy: The wording of the question guides you to look for an incorrect response. Knowledge of the principles of traction and basic nursing care allow you to eliminate each of the incorrect responses systematically. Try to visualize providing care to this client. This may assist in directing you to the correct option. Take time now to review the principles of care related to traction if you had difficulty with this question!

Level of Cognitive Ability: Application
Phase of Nursing Process: Planning
Client Needs: Physiological Integrity
Content Area: Adult Health/Musculoskeletal

Reference

Burrell, P., Gerlach, M., & Pless, B. (1997). *Adult nursing: Acute and community care* (2nd ed.). Stamford, CT: Appleton & Lange, p. 1604.

281. The nurse is teaching the client about how to use cold therapy at home after suffering a sprained ankle. The nurse would plan to teach the client to

1 Immerse the leg in a cold bath once an hour for 10 minutes.
2 Let the injured part rest on the cold pack continuously.
3 Place ice cubes inside a washcloth and apply this directly to the skin.
4 Place ice cubes in a plastic bag and cover with a small towel before applying to skin.

Answer: 4

Rationale: Cold therapy should be used for 20–30 minutes two to three times a day. The injured tissue should not rest directly on the source of cold, as the combination of pressure and cold could produce tissue ischemia. Placing ice cubes in a plastic bag and then wrapping them in a small towel also prevents injury from ischemia and frostbite.

Test-Taking Strategy: This question requires use of concepts related to pressure and cold. Eliminate options 2 and 3 because they are similar. Eliminate option 1 because of the time frame presented. Option 4 provides safety because the plastic bag provides a measure of insulation against excessive cold. If this question was difficult, take a few moments to review cold therapy at this time!

Level of Cognitive Ability: Application
Phase of Nursing Process: Planning
Client Needs: Physiological Integrity
Content Area: Adult Health/Musculoskeletal

Reference

Burrell, P., Gerlach, M., & Pless, B. (1997). *Adult nursing: Acute and community care* (2nd ed.). Stamford, CT: Appleton & Lange, pp. 1608–1609.

---

282. The client who has had application of a right long arm cast for a fractured humerus complains of pain at the wrist when the arm is passively moved. The nurse should plan to first

1 Check for paresthesias and paralysis of the right arm.
2 Check for similar symptoms on the left arm.
3 Medicate with an additional dose of narcotic.
4 Call the physician.

Answer: 1

Rationale: Compartment syndrome is a complication for the client who has trauma to the extremities and application of a cast. Pain in the compartment may occur with passive movement, rather than at the site of injury. Additional symptoms to assess for include paresthesias, paralysis, and excessive edema. Medication at this time without further assessment is not a safe nursing action. Calling the physician without additional data is not warranted.

Test-Taking Strategy: Note the key words and phrase in the question: "humerus," "pain at the wrist," and "first." Eliminate option 3 first as unsafe. Eliminate option 2 next as irrelevant. Discriminate between options 1 and 4 by reasoning that a single piece of data is not usually reported to the physician without additional data.

Level of Cognitive Ability: Application
Phase of Nursing Process: Planning
Client Needs: Physiological Integrity
Content Area: Adult Health/Musculoskeletal

Reference

Burrell, P., Gerlach, M., & Pless, B. (1997). *Adult nursing: Acute and community care* (2nd ed.). Stamford, CT: Appleton & Lange, p. 1621.

---

283. The elderly client who has undergone internal fixation after fractured left hip has a reddened left heel. The nurse would plan to obtain which of the following as a priority item?

1 Bed cradle
2 Sheepskin
3 Trapeze
4 Drawsheet

Answer: 2

Rationale: The reddened heel results from pressure of the foot against the mattress. The nurse should obtain a sheepskin, heel protectors, or an alternating-pressure mattress. The bed cradle is unnecessary in managing this problem. A drawsheet and a trapeze are of general use for this client.

Test-Taking Strategy: Note the issue of the question: a reddened left heel. Eliminate option 1 first as an unnecessary measure. Eliminate options 3 and 4 next, because although they are generally helpful in aiding the client's mobility, they are not the "priority." The correct answer is the one that addresses the problem stated in the stem of the question.

Level of Cognitive Ability: Application
Phase of Nursing Process: Planning
Client Needs: Physiological Integrity
Content Area: Adult Health/Musculoskeletal

Reference

Burrell, P., Gerlach, M., & Pless, B. (1997). *Adult nursing: Acute and community care* (2nd ed.). Stamford, CT: Appleton & Lange, p. 1629.

---

284. The client with a diagnosis of cholelithiasis is experiencing severe pain. The nurse would anticipate an order for which of the following narcotic analgesics?

1 Oxycodone (Percocet)
2 Hydromorphone (Dilaudid)
3 Meperidine (Demerol)
4 Morphine sulfate

Answer: 3

Rationale: Meperidine is a synthetic opiate and does not produce spasm of the biliary tract and sphincter of Oddi, as do other opiate medications. For this reason, it is a commonly used medication for clients experiencing pain with cholelithiasis and pancreatitis.

Test-Taking Strategy: To answer this question correctly, it is necessary to know that meperidine does not induce spasm of the biliary tract and adjacent structures. If this question was difficult, review the actions of these medications and treatment of cholelithiasis now!

Level of Cognitive Ability: Application
Phase of Nursing Process: Planning
Client Needs: Safe, Effective Care Environment
Content Area: Adult Health/Gastrointestinal

Reference

Luckmann, J. (1997). *Saunders manual of nursing care.* Philadelphia: W. B. Saunders, pp. 1337, 1882.

---

285. The client with low back pain asks the nurse which type of sports will best strengthen the lower back muscles. The nurse would plan to incorporate which of the following exercises in a response?

1 Tennis
2 Diving
3 Canoeing
4 Swimming

Answer: 4

Rationale: Walking and swimming are very beneficial in strengthening back muscles for the client with low back pain. The other options involve twisting and pulling of the back muscles, which is not helpful to the client experiencing back pain.

Test-Taking Strategy: Knowing that low back pain is aggravated by any activity that twists or turns the spine, evaluate each of the responses according to this guideline. This will enable you to systematically eliminate options 1, 2, and 3.

Level of Cognitive Ability: Application
Phase of Nursing Process: Planning
Client Needs: Health Promotion and Maintenance
Content Area: Adult Health/Neurological

Reference

Ignatavicius, D. D., Workman, M. L., & Mishler, M. A. (1995). *Medical-surgical nursing: A nursing process approach* (2nd ed.). Philadelphia: W. B. Saunders, p. 1171.

---

286. When the nurse is changing the back dressing of a client who has had a lumbar laminectomy, the nurse observes bulging at the incision site. The nurse should plan to take which of the following most important actions?

1 Notify the surgeon
2 Place a soft, multilayer absorbent dressing
3 Try to express fluid from the incision site
4 Apply a clear, transparent dressing

Answer: 1

Rationale: After laminectomy or diskectomy, bulging at the incision site could indicate hematoma formation or cerebrospinal fluid leakage. This must be reported to the surgeon. The nurse should not try to express the fluid, because this could disrupt the incision and possibly introduce pathogens. A dressing should be replaced as part of routine nursing practice, but the most important action is notification of the surgeon about this complication.

Test-Taking Strategy: Note the key phrase in the question, which is "most important." This implies that more than one or all of the responses are partially or totally correct. As a nurse, you must prioritize your answer. Knowing that bulging at the incisional site indicates a complication of surgery, you would then eliminate each of the incorrect options and notify the surgeon.

Level of Cognitive Ability: Application
Phase of Nursing Process: Planning
Client Needs: Physiological Integrity
Content Area: Adult Health/Neurological

Reference

Ignatavicius, D. D., Workman, M. L., & Mishler, M. A. (1995). *Medical-surgical nursing: A nursing process approach* (2nd ed.). Philadelphia: W. B. Saunders, p. 1180.

---

287. The client who has had a spinal cord injury is wheelchair-bound. The nurse would plan to obtain which of the following most effective pressure relief devices to place in the seat of the client's wheelchair?

1 Egg crate pad
2 Gel pad
3 Soft pillow
4 Air ring

Answer: 2

Rationale: The client who is wheelchair-bound is acutely at risk for skin breakdown over bony prominences and benefits greatly from special pressure-relief devices such as gel pads. The other items are useful for some clients in selected situations but do not disperse pressure the way that gel pads do.

Test-Taking Strategy: The key phrase in the stem of the question is "most effective." To select the correct answer, you must be familiar with these various items and their intended uses. Review them now if you had difficulty with this question!

Level of Cognitive Ability: Application
Phase of Nursing Process: Planning
Client Needs: Health Promotion and Maintenance
Content Area: Adult Health/Neurological

Reference

Ignatavicius, D. D., Workman, M. L., & Mishler, M. A. (1995). *Medical-surgical nursing: A nursing process approach* (2nd ed.). Philadelphia: W. B. Saunders, pp. 1189–1190.

---

288. The client is seen in the ambulatory care clinic with a complaint of "feeling something in my eye." The nurse prepares for ocular irrigation by obtaining which of the following solutions to be used as an irrigant?

1 Proparacaine hydrochloride (Ophthaine)
2 Fluorescein
3 Sterile normal saline (0.9%)
4 Sterile water

Answer: 3

Rationale: Ocular irrigation is performed with sterile normal saline because it is an isotonic solution. Fluorescein is used to visualize a corneal abrasion secondary to injury. Proparacaine hydrochloride is used as a topical anesthetic before the irrigation is performed.

Test-Taking Strategy: Begin to answer this question by eliminating options 1 and 2 because they are the least plausible options. The question specifically asks for an irrigating solution. To discriminate between sterile saline and water, knowledge of isotonic solutions will assist in directing you to the correct option.

Level of Cognitive Ability: Application
Phase of Nursing Process: Planning
Client Needs: Physiological Integrity
Content Area: Adult Health/Eye

Reference

Ignatavicius, D. D., Workman, M. L., & Mishler, M. A. (1995). *Medical-surgical nursing: A nursing process approach* (2nd ed.). Philadelphia: W. B. Saunders, p. 1343.

289. The nurse is admitting to the clinical unit a client who is legally blind. Which of the following should the nurse plan to do to best help the client become oriented to the unfamiliar environment?

1 Attach the call bell to the right side rail
2 Keep the bed in the lowest position
3 Keep a light on in the bathroom
4 Describe the arrangement of the room in relation to the bed

Answer: 4

Rationale: The client who is blind benefits from orientation to surroundings by using one object, such as a bed, as the focal point of the room. The nurse then describes the position of other objects in the room as they relate to that focal point. The call bell should be placed in whatever location the client prefers. Keeping the bed in lowest position and keeping the bathroom lit are good general safety measures, but they do not provide orientation to the surroundings.

Test-Taking Strategy: Note the key phrases and word in the question are "best help," "oriented," and "unfamiliar environment." Eliminate options 2 and 3 first because they are least helpful in answering the question as stated. You would choose option 4 over option 1 by knowing that the visually impaired client should have a choice in determining where objects are placed. You would also choose correctly by reasoning that the client needs to know the setup of the room as a whole to be able to function most effectively.

Level of Cognitive Ability: Application
Phase of Nursing Process: Planning
Client Needs: Safe, Effective Care Environment
Content Area: Adult Health/Eye

Reference
Ignatavicius, D. D., Workman, M. L., & Mishler, M. A. (1995). *Medical-surgical nursing: A nursing process approach* (2nd ed.). Philadelphia: W. B. Saunders, p. 1348.

---

290. The elderly client has a prescription for zolpidem tartrate (Ambien) to aid in sleep. The nurse would plan to teach the client which of the following information about this medication?

1 Elderly clients are more sensitive to the effects of the medication
2 The medication is used for long-term management of insomnia
3 The client should take the medication with the supper meal
4 The medication has no central nervous system (CNS) side effects

Answer: 1

Rationale: Ambien is a sedative-hypnotic medication used in the short-term management of insomnia. The elderly are more sensitive to the effects of the medication. Taking the medication with food will delay the onset of sleep. The client should be cautioned that dizziness and drowsiness may occur during use. Because of the CNS effects of the medication, concurrent use of other CNS depressants such as alcohol should be avoided.

Test-Taking Strategy: Knowledge about the general effects of sedative medications, and about this one in particular, is needed to answer this question accurately. If needed, take a few moments to review this medication!

Level of Cognitive Ability: Application
Phase of Nursing Process: Planning
Client Needs: Health Promotion and Maintenance
Content Area: Pharmacology

Reference
Kuhn, M. (1998). *Pharmacotherapeutics: A nursing process approach* (4th ed.). Philadelphia: F. A. Davis, p. 365.

---

291. The client is taking ticlopidine hydrochloride (Ticlid). The nurse would plan to teach the client to avoid taking which of the following medications while taking Ticlid?

1 Acetaminophen (Tylenol)
2 Acetylsalicylic acid (aspirin)
3 Vitamin C
4 Vitamin D

Answer: 2

Rationale: Ticlid is a platelet aggregation inhibitor. It is used to lower the risk of thrombotic strokes in clients who display precursor symptoms. Because it is an antiplatelet agent, other medications that precipitate or aggravate bleeding should be avoided during its use. Thus aspirin and any aspirin-containing products should be avoided.

Test-Taking Strategy: To answer this question accurately, it is necessary to know the nature of this medication and its associated risks. Take time now to review this medication if you had difficulty with this question!

Level of Cognitive Ability: Application
Phase of Nursing Process: Planning
Client Needs: Health Promotion and Maintenance
Content Area: Pharmacology

Reference

Kuhn, M. (1998). *Pharmacotherapeutics: A nursing process approach* (4th ed.). Philadelphia: F. A. Davis, pp. 525–526.

---

292. The client who has episodes of bronchospasm also has a history of tachydysrhythmias. The nurse would plan to teach the client to avoid taking which of the following bronchodilators?

1 Metaproterenol (Alupent)
2 Albuterol (Proventil)
3 Epinephrine (Primatene Mist)
4 Salmeterol (Serevent)

Answer: 3

Rationale: A client with a history of tachydysrhythmias should avoid using bronchodilators that contain catecholamines, such as epinephrine and isoproterenol. Other sympathomimetics that are noncatecholamines should be used instead. These include metaproterenol, albuterol, and salmeterol.

Test-Taking Strategy: To answer this question correctly, you must know that epinephrine is a catecholamine, which should be avoided with tachydysrhythmias. Because this is such an important concept, take the time to learn it now if this question was difficult.

Level of Cognitive Ability: Application
Phase of Nursing Process: Planning
Client Needs: Physiological Integrity
Content Area: Pharmacology

Reference

Kuhn, M. (1998). *Pharmacotherapeutics: A nursing process approach* (4th ed.). Philadelphia: F. A. Davis, p. 589.

---

293. The client is being given prednisone as part of anticancer therapy. The nurse would plan to avoid giving the client which of the following analgesics to minimize side effects of prednisone?

1 Oxycodone (OxyContin)
2 Propoxyphene (Darvon)
3 Acetaminophen (Tylenol)
4 Acetylsalicylic acid (aspirin)

Answer: 4

Rationale: Prednisone is irritating to the gastrointestinal (GI) tract, which could be worsened by use of other products that have the same side effect. Therefore, products such as aspirin and nonsteroidal anti-inflammatory drugs are not used during steroid therapy.

Test-Taking Strategy: To answer this question accurately, it is necessary to know the side effects of prednisone therapy and how to avoid them. Remembering that aspirin is irritating to the GI tract will assist in answering the question. If this question was difficult, take a few moments now to review this important medication!

Level of Cognitive Ability: Application
Phase of Nursing Process: Planning
Client Needs: Physiological Integrity
Content Area: Pharmacology

References

Deglin, J., & Vallerand, A. (1997). *Davis's drug guide for nurses* (5th ed.). Philadelphia: F. A. Davis, pp. 546, 897, 1027.
Kuhn, M. (1998). *Pharmacotherapeutics: A nursing process approach* (4th ed.). Philadelphia: F. A. Davis, p. 818.

294. The client with advanced cirrhosis of the liver is not tolerating protein well, as evidenced by abnormal laboratory values. The nurse anticipates that which of the following medications will be instituted?

1 Lactulose (Chronulac)
2 Ethacrynic acid (Edecrin)
3 Folic acid (Folvite)
4 Thiamine (vitamin B_1)

Answer: 1

Rationale: The client with cirrhosis has impaired ability to metabolize protein as a result of liver dysfunction. Administration of lactulose aids in the clearance of ammonia by using the GI tract. Ethacrynic acid is a diuretic. Folic acid and thiamine are vitamins, which may be used in clients with liver disease as supplemental therapy.

Test-Taking Strategy: To answer this question correctly, it is necessary to know that ammonia levels are elevated with advanced liver disease and that lactulose is a standard form of medication therapy for this condition. Take time now to review the purpose of this medication if you had difficulty with this question!

Level of Cognitive Ability: Application
Phase of Nursing Process: Planning
Client Needs: Physiological Integrity
Content Area: Pharmacology

References

Hodgson, B., & Kizior, R. (1998). *Saunders nursing drug handbook 1998.* Philadelphia: W. B. Saunders, pp. 573–574.
Kuhn, M. (1998). *Pharmacotherapeutics: A nursing process approach* (4th ed.). Philadelphia: F. A. Davis, pp. 786–787.

295. The nurse is caring for the client in cardiogenic shock who is receiving dopamine (Intropin) by continuous IV infusion. The nurse would plan to have which of the following medications available if the IV line infiltrates?

1 Phenobarbital (Luminol)
2 Phentolamine mesylate (Regitine)
3 Phenelzine (Nardil)
4 Phenytoin (Dilantin)

Answer: 2

Rationale: Regitine is the agent used if infiltration of dopamine occurs. It is a vasodilator whose other use is the management of severe hypertension associated with pheochromocytoma. Phenobarbital is a barbiturate. Phenelzine is a monoamine oxidase inhibitor (MAOI). Phenytoin is an anticonvulsant.

Test-Taking Strategy: To answer this question correctly, it is necessary to be familiar with these different medications and their uses. Take a few moments to review them now if you had difficulty with this question!

Level of Cognitive Ability: Application
Phase of Nursing Process: Planning
Client Needs: Safe, Effective Care Environment
Content Area: Pharmacology

Reference

Hodgson, B., & Kizior, R. (1998). *Saunders nursing drug handbook 1998.* Philadelphia: W. B. Saunders, pp. 819–820.

296. The nurse is caring for the client with pericardial tamponade. The nurse notes that the client's systolic blood pressure has dropped by more than 30 mmHg. The nurse prepares for which of the following anticipated interventions?

1 Administration of high-dose salicylates
2 Administration of indomethacin
3 Continuous cardiac monitoring
4 Pericardiocentesis

Answer: 4

Rationale: Pericardiocentesis is indicated in the client with cardiac tamponade if the systolic blood pressure drops by more than 30 mmHg. The client should already be on a continuous cardiac monitor if tamponade is suspected. Administration of salicylates and indomethacin is part of standard therapy and is not reserved for emergency treatment only.

Test-Taking Strategy: To answer this question correctly, it is necessary to know that pericardial tamponade is an accumulation of blood around the heart in the pericardial sac, causing pressure on the heart and interfering with cardiac output. This would lead you to select the option that involves removal of the fluid, which is pericardiocentesis. Review this procedure now if you are unfamiliar with it!

Level of Cognitive Ability: Application
Phase of Nursing Process: Planning
Client Needs: Safe, Effective Care Environment
Content Area: Adult Health/Cardiovascular

Reference

Lewis, S., Collier, I., & Heitkemper, M. (1996). *Medical-surgical nursing: Assessment and management of clinical problems* (4th ed.). St. Louis: Mosby–Year Book, pp. 1014–1015.

---

297. The client has undergone repair of an abdominal aortic aneurysm (AAA). The nurse would place highest priority on which of the following nursing activities immediately after surgery?

1 Assessment of peripheral pulses
2 Administration of oral narcotic analgesics
3 Pulmonary hygiene measures
4 Application of pneumatic boots

Answer: 1

Rationale: Assessment of peripheral pulses is the highest priority of the nurse immediately after repair of AAA. This indicates whether the graft is patent and perfusing the lower extremities. The client would receive parenteral narcotics immediately after surgery. Prevention of respiratory and circulatory complications is also important but does not supersede determining graft patency.

Test-Taking Strategy: The key phrase and word in this question are "highest priority" and "AAA." Knowing that the surgical procedure is vascular in nature, you would look for the option that most directly addresses prevention or treatment of a vascular complication.

Level of Cognitive Ability: Application
Phase of Nursing Process: Planning
Client Needs: Physiological Integrity
Content Area: Adult Health/Cardiovascular

Reference

Lewis, S., Collier, I., & Heitkemper, M. (1996). *Medical-surgical nursing: Assessment and management of clinical problems* (4th ed.). St. Louis: Mosby–Year Book, pp. 1040–1041.

---

298. The client scheduled for annuloplasty asks the nurse to explain again what the surgical procedure entails. In planning a response, the nurse would incorporate which of the following points?

1 The stenotic valve leaflets are separated, and any calcium deposits are removed
2 The valve leaflets are repaired with possible implantation of a prosthetic ring
3 The valve is replaced with a mechanical valve
4 The valve is replaced with a biological valve

Answer: 2

Rationale: Annuloplasty is used for mitral or tricuspid regurgitation and involves reconstruction of the annulus and the valve leaflets. Annulus repair may or may not involve insertion of a prosthetic ring. Option 1 describes commissurotomy, whereas options 3 and 4 are types of valve replacement.

Test-Taking Strategy: It is necessary to be familiar with the different types of cardiac valvular surgery to answer this question correctly. The word "possible" in the correct option indicates that it may be the correct answer. Take a few moments to review the differences in the procedures if you are unfamiliar with them!

Level of Cognitive Ability: Application
Phase of Nursing Process: Planning
Client Needs: Physiological Integrity
Content Area: Adult Health/Cardiovascular

Reference

Lewis, S., Collier, I., & Heitkemper, M. (1996). *Medical-surgical nursing: Assessment and management of clinical problems* (4th ed.). St. Louis: Mosby–Year Book, pp. 1028–1030.

299. The nurse has been assigned to the care of a client in the diuretic phase of renal failure. The nurse would plan to monitor for which of the following findings in serum laboratory studies?

1 Hypocalcemia and hyperkalemia
2 Hypermagnesemia and hyperkalemia
3 Hypernatremia and hypokalemia
4 Hyponatremia and hypokalemia

Answer: 4

Rationale: In the diuretic phase of acute renal failure, the client loses large amounts of fluid, accompanied by losses of sodium and potassium. This is due to the kidney's inability to properly concentrate urine. The nurse monitors for these electrolyte imbalances, as well as for signs of dehydration.

Test-Taking Strategy: To answer this question accurately, it is necessary to understand the phases of renal failure and their effect on the function of the kidney. In a diuretic phase, you would expect losses of both fluids and electrolytes. The only option that addresses "hypo" in the entire option is option 4. Take a few moments to review this important content area if this question was difficult!

Level of Cognitive Ability: Application
Phase of Nursing Process: Planning
Client Needs: Physiological Integrity
Content Area: Adult Health/Renal

Reference

Lewis, S., Collier, I., & Heitkemper, M. (1996). *Medical-surgical nursing: Assessment and management of clinical problems* (4th ed.). St. Louis: Mosby–Year Book, p. 1374.

---

300. The nurse is caring for a client who underwent cardiac surgery complicated by acute renal failure, and the client is hemodynamically unstable. The physician has told the family that the client will be treated with continuous arteriovenous hemofiltration (CAVH). The nurse plans to allay the family's anxieties about this procedure by telling them that the procedure

1 Is safest because there is less risk that the client's blood pressure will drop.
2 Is the quickest solution to the acute renal failure.
3 Will raise the client's hospital bill the least.
4 Is less painful than any other form of dialysis.

Answer: 1

Rationale: CAVH, also called ultrafiltration, is a continuous treatment for acute renal failure that causes minimal or no changes in the client's blood pressure. It is therefore an ideal form of dialysis for the client who is hemodynamically unstable. This is reassuring to the family of a client whose illness has been compounded by complications.

Test-Taking Strategy: The key phrase in this question is "allay the family's anxieties." Begin to answer this question by eliminating options 2 and 3 first. These statements are not necessarily true and are not likely to address the real cause of the family's anxiety. Familiarity with the procedure would help you to choose option 1 over option 4. Option 1 also addresses the phrase "is safest"!

Level of Cognitive Ability: Application
Phase of Nursing Process: Planning
Client Needs: Psychosocial Integrity
Content Area: Adult Health/Renal

Reference

Lewis, S., Collier, I., & Heitkemper, M. (1996). *Medical-surgical nursing: Assessment and management of clinical problems* (4th ed.). St. Louis: Mosby–Year Book, pp. 1402–1403.

REFERENCES

Antai-Otong, D., & Kongale, G. (1995). *Psychiatric nursing: Biological and behavioral concepts*. Philadelphia: W. B. Saunders.

Ashwill, J., & Droske, S. (1997). *Nursing care of children: Principles and practices*. Philadelphia: W. B. Saunders.

Ball, J., & Bindler, R. (1995). *Pediatric nursing: Caring for children*. Stamford, CT: Appleton & Lange.

Bandman, E., & Bandman, B. (1995). *Nursing ethics through the life span*. Stamford, CT: Appleton & Lange.

Black, J., & Matassarin-Jacobs, E. (1997). *Medical-surgical nursing: Clinical management for continuity of care* (5th ed.). Philadelphia: W. B. Saunders.

Brent, N. (1997). *Nurses and the law*. Philadelphia: W. B. Saunders.

Burrell, P., Gerlach, M., & Pless, B. (1997). *Adult nursing: Acute and community care* (2nd ed.). Stamford, CT: Appleton & Lange.

Carpenito, L. (1995). *Nursing diagnosis: Application to clinical practice* (6th ed.). Philadelphia: Lippincott-Raven.

Carpenito, L. (1995). *Handbook of nursing diagnosis* (6th ed.). Philadelphia: Lippincott-Raven.

Carson, V., & Arnold, E. (1996). *Mental health nursing: The nurse-patient journey*. Philadelphia: W. B. Saunders.

Chernecky, C., & Berger, B. (1997). *Laboratory tests and diagnostic procedures* (2nd ed.). Philadelphia: W. B. Saunders.

Clark, M. (1996). *Nursing in the community* (2nd ed.). Stamford, CT: Appleton & Lange.

Como, N. (1995). *Home health nursing pocket consultant*. St. Louis: Mosby–Year Book.

Cox, H., Hinz, M., Lubno, M., et al. (1997). *Clinical applications of nursing diagnosis* (3rd ed.). Philadelphia: F. A. Davis.

Craven, R. F., & Hirnle, C. J. (1996). *Fundamentals of nursing: Human health and function* (2nd ed.). Philadelphia: Lippincott-Raven.

Deglin, J., & Vallerand, A. (1997). *Davis's drug guide for nurses* (5th ed.). Philadelphia: F. A. Davis.

DeLaune, S., & Ladner, P. (1998). *Fundamentals of nursing: Standards and practice*. Albany, NY: Delmar.

Haber, J. (1997). *Comprehensive psychiatric nursing* (5th ed.). St. Louis: Mosby–Year Book.

Hartshorn, J. C., Sole, M. L., & Lamborn, M. L. (1997). *Introduction to critical care nursing* (2nd ed.). Philadelphia: W. B. Saunders.

Hodgson, B., & Kizior, R. (1998). *Saunders nursing drug handbook 1998*. Philadelphia: W. B. Saunders.

Hudak, C., & Gallo, B. (1994). *Critical care nursing: A holistic approach* (6th ed.). Philadelphia: Lippincott-Raven.

Ignatavicius D. D., Workman, M. L., & Mishler, M. A. (1995). *Medical-surgical nursing: A nursing process approach* (2nd ed.). Philadelphia: W. B. Saunders.

Johnson, B. (1997). *Psychiatric–mental health nursing: Adaptation and growth* (4th ed.). Philadelphia: Lippincott-Raven.

Kee, J., & Hayes, E. (1997). *Pharmacology: A nursing process approach* (2nd ed.). Philadelphia: W. B. Saunders.

Kuhn, M. (1998). *Pharmacotherapeutics: A nursing process approach* (4th ed.). Philadelphia: F. A. Davis.

Lammon, C. B., Foote, A. W., Leli, P. G., et al. (1995). *Clinical nursing skills*. Philadelphia: W. B. Saunders.

LeMone, P., & Burke, K. M. (1996). *Medical-surgical nursing: Critical thinking in client care*. Menlo Park, CA: Addison-Wesley.

Lewis, S., Collier, I., & Heitkemper, M. (1996). *Medical-surgical nursing: Assessment and management of clinical problems* (4th ed.). Philadelphia: Mosby–Year Book.

Lowdermilk, D., Perry, M., & Bobak, I. (1997). *Maternity & women's health care* (6th ed.). St. Louis: Mosby–Year Book.

Luckmann, J. (1997). *Saunders manual of nursing care*. Philadelphia: W. B. Saunders.

Lutz, C., & Przytulski, K. (1997). *Nutrition and diet therapy* (2nd ed.). Philadelphia: F. A. Davis.

McKenry, L., & Salerno, E. (1998). *Mosby's pharmacology in nursing* (20th ed.). St. Louis: C. V. Mosby.

National Council of State Boards of Nursing. (1997). *Plan for the National Council Licensure Examination for Registered Nurses*. Chicago: National Council of State Boards of Nursing Inc.

Nichols, F., & Zwelling, E. (1997). *Maternal-newborn nursing: Theory and practice*. Philadelphia: W. B. Saunders.

Olds, S., London, M., & Ladewig, P. (1996). *Clinical handbook for maternal-newborn nursing: A family-centered approach* (5th ed.). Menlo Park, CA: Addison-Wesley.

O'Toole, M. (1997). *Miller-Keane Encyclopedia & dictionary of medicine, nursing, & allied health* (6th ed.). Philadelphia: W. B. Saunders.

Pillitteri, A. (1995). *Maternal and child health nursing: Care of the childbearing & childrearing family* (2nd ed.). Philadelphia: J. B. Lippincott.

Pinnell, N. (1996). *Nursing pharmacology*. Philadelphia: W. B. Saunders.

Polaski, A., & Tatro, S. (1996). *Luckmann's Core principles and practice of medical-surgical nursing*. Philadelphia: W. B. Saunders.

Potter, P., & Perry, A. (1997). *Fundamentals of nursing: Concepts, process, and practice* (4th ed.). Philadelphia: Mosby–Year Book.

Reeder, S., Martin, L., & Koniak-Griffin, D. (1997). *Maternity nursing* (18th ed.). Philadelphia: Lippincott-Raven.

Richard, R., & Staley, M. (1994). *Burn care and rehabilitation: Principles and practice*. Philadelphia: F. A. Davis.

Sheehy, S., & Lombardi, J. (1995). *Manual of emergency care* (4th ed.). St. Louis: Mosby–Year Book.

Smeltzer, S., & Bare, B. (1996). *Brunner and Suddarth's Textbook of medical-surgical nursing* (8th ed.). Philadelphia: Lippincott-Raven.

Stuart, G., & Sundeen, S. (1995). *Principles and practice of psychiatric nursing* (5th ed.). St. Louis: C. V. Mosby.

Taylor, C., Lillis, C., & LeMone, P. (1997). *Fundamentals of nursing: The art and science of nursing care* (3rd ed.). Philadelphia: Lippincott-Raven.

Townsend, M. (1996). *Psychiatric–mental health nursing: Concepts of care* (2nd ed.). Philadelphia: F. A. Davis.

Varcarolis, E. M. (1998). *Foundations of psychiatric–mental health nursing* (3rd ed.). Philadelphia: W. B. Saunders.

Wilson, H., & Kneisl, C. (1996). *Psychiatric nursing* (5th ed.). Menlo Park, CA: Addison-Wesley.

Wong, D. (1997). *Whaley and Wong's Essentials of pediatric nursing* (5th ed.). St. Louis: Mosby–Year Book.

Wong, D. (1997). *Whaley & Wong's Nursing care of infants & children* (5th ed.,). St. Louis: Mosby–Year Book.

Wong, D., & Perry, S. (1998). *Maternal-child nursing care*. St. Louis: Mosby–Year Book.

CHAPTER 8

The Process of Implementation

Implementation is the fourth step of the Nursing Process; it includes initiating and completing nursing actions required to accomplish the defined goals. This step is the action phase that involves counseling, teaching, organizing and managing client care, providing care to achieve established goals, supervising and coordinating the delivery of client care, and communicating and documenting the nursing interventions and client responses.

During implementation, the nurse uses intellectual skills, interpersonal skills, and technical skills. Intellectual skills involve critical thinking, problem solving, and making judgments. Interpersonal skills involve the ability to communicate, listen, and convey compassion. Technical skills relate to the performance of treatments, performance of procedures, and the use of necessary equipment when providing care to the client.

The nurse independently implements actions that include activities that do not require a physician's order. The nurse also implements actions collaboratively on the basis of the physician's orders. Sound nursing judgment and working with other health care members are incorporated in the process of implementation.

The implementation step concludes when the nurse's actions are completed and these actions, including their effects and the client's response, are communicated and documented.

PRACTICE TEST

1. All clients who undergo surgery have the potential to acquire an infection. Which of the following actions by the operative nurse is most appropriate for preventing a postoperative wound infection?

   1 Adhere to meticulous aseptic techniques
   2 Keep the temperature warm to prevent chilling the client
   3 Keep the doors to the suite open to improve ventilation
   4 Scrub the incision site vigorously to remove all bacteria

Answer: 1

Rationale: Surgical intervention breaks some of the body's primary defenses against infection. Infection can endanger the life of a client. The most important measure in preventing postoperative wound infection is adherence to meticulous aseptic techniques. The temperature in the surgical suite is kept cool to deter bacterial growth. Most pathogenic bacteria metabolize and reproduce at or near normal body temperature. Keeping the room temperature below body temperature may inhibit bacterial growth. Keeping air currents and movement to a minimum can control airborne contamination; therefore, doors to the surgical suite must remain closed at all times. The skin preparation is performed to free the operative site as much as possible from dirt, skin oils, and transient microbes. This should be accomplished with the least amount of tissue irritation.

Test-Taking Strategy: Identify the key word in the question that indicates the choice that you need to make. The words "most appropriate" suggest that three of the choices are incorrect. Options 2, 3, and 4 specify activities that would increase the potential for wound infection.

Level of Cognitive Ability: Application
Phase of Nursing Process: Implementation
Client Needs: Physiological Integrity
Content Area: Fundamental Skills

Reference

Phipps, W., Cassmeyer, V., Sands, J., et al. (1995). *Medical-surgical nursing: Concepts and clinical practice* (5th ed.). St. Louis: Mosby–Year Book, pp. 608–611, 623–624.

---

2. The nurse is called by a group of neighbors to the scene of a rural house fire, where a person fell down the stairs headfirst trying to escape the fire. The house is rapidly filling with smoke. After ensuring that the fire department has been called, which action is most appropriate for the nurse to take?

1 Place a wet towel over the victim's face and wait with the victim for the arrival of the fire department
2 Move the victim by assigning four people to slide the victim onto a hard board while the nurse maintains the head and neck in a neutral position
3 Move the victim by log-rolling the victim to a face-down position on a blanket and assign six people to carry the victim to safety
4 Move the victim to safety by pulling the victim's legs with the victim's back flat on the floor

Answer: 2

Rationale: In this situation, several helpers are available. The setting is rural, and smoke is rapidly accumulating, so both victim and rescuers may be endangered by remaining in the house until help arrives. Direct head blows are assumed to result in spinal cord injury until proven otherwise, making it imperative to maintain the head, neck, and trunk in a controlled neutral position on a hard surface.

Test-Taking Strategy: Key words in the question that enable you to rule out option 1 are "rural" (help may not be available immediately) and "rapidly" (smoke inhalation injury is likely). Covering the victim's face with a wet cloth helps to prevent smoke inhalation but does not protect the rescuer and is not a substitute for evacuation. Remember the RACE (*r*escue, *a*ctivate fire alarm, *c*ontain the fire, *e*xtinguish) formula: rescue first. Once the decision to move has been made, the question requires visualization of a technique that keeps the head and spine straight. Option 3 is attractive, because nurses often use log-rolling with spinal injury, but the transfer technique would bend the spine. Option 4 provides no stabilization of either the head or the spine.

Level of Cognitive Ability: Application
Phase of Nursing Process: Implementation
Client Needs: Safe, Effective Care Environment
Content Area: Adult Health/Neurological

Reference

Taylor, C., Lillis, C., & LeMone, P. (1997). *Fundamentals of nursing: The art and science of nursing care* (3rd ed.). Philadelphia: Lippincott-Raven, p. 493.

---

3. When giving an intramuscular injection to a 4-year-old child, it is most important to

1 Use the vastus lateralis muscle only.
2 Allow the child to choose between lying down and standing.
3 Have sufficient help to restrain the child.
4 Distract the child with conversation or a toy.

Answer: 3

Rationale: Preschoolers are often fearful and likely to move during an injection; thus it is most important to have assistance to safely restrain a child. Gluteal muscles may be used in preschoolers in addition to the vastus lateralis. The choice of standing is unacceptable because it is difficult for the nurse to locate landmarks and restrain the child. Distraction is helpful but not the highest priority.

Test-Taking Strategy: The key words "most important" identify the need for prioritizing. According to Maslow's hierarchy of needs theory, the safety intervention of restraint takes priority over the psychosocial options of offering choice or distraction. The term "only" in option 1 makes it unlikely to be correct because it is exclusive and limiting.

Level of Cognitive Ability: Application
Phase of Nursing Process: Implementation
Client Needs: Physiological Integrity
Content Area: Child Health

Reference

Wong, D. (1997). *Whaley and Wong's Essentials of pediatric nursing* (5th ed.). St. Louis: Mosby–Year Book, p. 718.

4. The nurse is caring for a client with a diagnosis of "stroke in progress." The client is anxious. In order to minimize the extent of the stroke, the nurse would

1 Focus on adequate hydration.
2 Report an increased blood pressure of 158/92.
3 Protect client from hypothermia.
4 Instruct in seizure precautions.

Answer: 1

Rationale: Hypotension from hypovolemia can cause further cerebral infarct. Blood pressure must be maintained sufficiently high to perfuse the brain. Only severe hypertension would be treated during the immediate phase of stroke. Preventing hypothermia will not necessarily minimize the extent of a stroke. Instructing the client in seizure precautions will not minimize the extent of a stroke.

Test-Taking Strategy: Use the process of elimination, noting the key phrase "minimize the extent." Option 1 is the best choice. Options 2, 3, and 4 are not relevant to the case.

Level of Cognitive Ability: Application
Phase of Nursing Process: Implementation
Client Needs: Physiological Integrity
Content Area: Adult Health/Neurological

Reference
Black, J., & Matassarin-Jacobs, E. (1997). *Medical-surgical nursing: Clinical management for continuity of care* (5th ed.). Philadelphia: W. B. Saunders, p. 716.

5. Excessive maternal blood loss and decreased tissue perfusion are risks with placental abruption. Nursing assessments for these risks include monitoring for

1 Bounding pulses.
2 Lethargy.
3 Decreased respirations.
4 Urinary output less than 30 mL/hour.

Answer: 4

Rationale: Urinary output will be decreased as a result of decreased renal perfusion. Other signs and symptoms of hypovolemic shock include decreased peripheral pulses, resulting from decreased circulating blood volume; restlessness or agitation, resulting from decreased cerebral perfusion; and increased respiratory rate, resulting from decreased circulating oxygen.

Test-Taking Strategy: Knowledge of signs and of the pathophysiological processes of hypovolemic shock is needed. This is the condition described in the case situation. Determine which option is the result of decreased tissue perfusion and excessive blood loss. A urinary output of less than 30 mL/hour is a cause for concern in any client!

Level of Cognitive Ability: Application
Phase of Nursing Process: Implementation
Client Needs: Physiological Integrity
Content Area: Maternity

Reference
Gorrie, T. M., McKinney, E. S., & Murray, S. S. (1998). *Foundations of maternal newborn nursing* (2nd ed.). Philadelphia: W. B. Saunders, p. 688.

6. A client is being treated for Tourette's syndrome. The physician orders a medication that controls tics and vocal utterances. The nurse would expect to administer which of the following prescribed medications?

1 Paroxetine (Paxil)
2 Amitriptyline (Elavil)
3 Haloperidol (Haldol)
4 Phenelzine sulfate (Nardil)

Answer: 3

Rationale: Haldol is the antipsychotic agent of choice used to control the tics and vocal utterances characteristic of Tourette's syndrome. The medication produces a tranquilizing effect. Paxil, Elavil, and Nardil are antidepressants. Their actions would not produce the desired effect.

Test-Taking Strategy: Eliminate similar distracters—options 1, 2, and 4—because these medications are antidepressants. Option 3 is different from the others and is therefore most probably the correct answer. Take time now to review these medications if you had difficulty with this question!

Level of Cognitive Ability: Analysis
Phase of Nursing Process: Implementation
Client Needs: Physiological Integrity
Content Area: Mental Health

Reference
Wilson, H., & Kneisl, C. (1996). *Psychiatric nursing* (5th ed.). Menlo Park, CA: Addison-Wesley, p. 929.

7. In caring for a client who is at risk for suicide, which of these nursing interventions should be given priority?

   1 Communicating the risk for suicide to all team members
   2 Developing a plan of activities for the client
   3 Providing the client with the cultural norms regarding suicide for his or her ethnic group
   4 Communicating the statistics for suicide to all team members

Answer: 1

Rationale: The priority intervention for the suicidal individual is to communicate the risk for suicide to all team members. The plan of activities would provide the suicidal client with something to do, but the communication of the risk is a priority intervention. The cultural norms regarding suicide are not a priority item. The statistics of suicidal incidents are also not the priority.

Test-Taking Strategy: Use the process of elimination in answering the question. Although all of the options are factors related to suicide, the priority item is the communication to other members of the health care team. If you had difficulty with this question, take time now to review nursing care required for a client at risk for suicide!

Level of Cognitive Ability: Application
Phase of Nursing Process: Implementation
Client Needs: Safe, Effective Care Environment
Content Area: Mental Health

Reference
Townsend, M. (1996). *Psychiatric-mental health nursing: Concepts of care* (2nd ed.). Philadelphia: F. A. Davis, p. 255.

---

8. The health care team has initiated a refeeding program for the client. After breakfast, the client complains of fullness and bloating. The most appropriate nursing response is

   1 "Don't worry about it."
   2 "These are normal feelings and they are temporary."
   3 "Focusing on your stomach will only make you feel worse."
   4 "I am so proud that you were able to eat all your breakfast."

Answer: 2

Rationale: The gastrointestinal tract takes time to adjust to unaccustomed intake. Option 4 focuses on the nurse's feelings and ignores the client's concern. Options 1 and 3 also ignore the client's concern. Option 2 directly addresses the client's feelings.

Test-Taking Strategy: Use therapeutic communication skills. Options 1 and 3 may block further communication with your client. Any form of communication block would constitute an incorrect response. Option 4 also blocks communication by avoiding focus on the client's concern. Option 2 addresses the client's complaints.

Level of Cognitive Ability: Application
Phase of Nursing Process: Implementation
Client Needs: Psychosocial Integrity
Content Area: Fundamental Skills

Reference
Wilson, H., & Kneisl, C. (1996). *Psychiatric nursing* (5th ed.). Menlo Park, CA: Addison-Wesley, pp. 433–434.

---

9. A client with a ruptured cerebral aneurysm who also has a history of essential hypertension exhibits a sudden elevation in blood pressure. Which of the following medications would the nurse expect to administer?

   1 Epinephrine (Adrenaline)
   2 Dobutamine (Dobutrex)
   3 Sodium nitroprusside (Nipride)
   4 Dopamine (Intropin)

Answer: 3

Rationale: Sodium nitroprusside decreases blood pressure by vasodilation, thus reducing pressure in the aneurysm. The other medications increase blood pressure, which may disrupt the clot and precipitate bleeding.

Test-Taking Strategy: The stem asks you to identify a medication that will produce an antihypertensive effect. If you had to guess, the correct medication has "nitro" as part of the name. Nitroglycerin compounds are vasodilators. Options 2 and 4 have similar names, with the suffix "-amine," which is similar to the adrenergic medication aminophylline. Both cannot be correct, so they can be eliminated. Adrenergics elevate blood pressure. If you had difficulty with this question, take time now to review the actions of these medications!

Level of Cognitive Ability: Analysis
Phase of Nursing Process: Implementation
Client Needs: Physiological Integrity
Content Area: Adult Health/Neurological

Reference

Smeltzer, S., & Bare, B. (1996). *Brunner and Suddarth's Textbook of medical-surgical nursing* (8th ed.). Philadelphia: Lippincott-Raven, pp. 754, 1765.

---

10. A child with Hirschsprung's disease has a nursing diagnosis of Fluid Volume Deficit. Which of the following nursing interventions would be most effective to stabilize the child's hydration status before surgery?

1 Daily weights
2 Measurement of intake and output (I&O)
3 Administration of intravenous (IV) fluids and electrolytes as prescribed
4 Repeated administration of tap water enemas to achieve bowel emptying

Answer: 3

Rationale: A child is stabilized with fluid and electrolyte therapy before surgical management of the aganglionic portion of the bowel. Daily weight and I&O measurements are important assessments with regard to hydration status, but they are not the actions most effective in stabilizing hydration status. Administration of prescribed IV fluids and electrolytes is most effective in stabilizing hydration status before surgery. Option 4 is incorrect; tap water enemas will further stress the child's hydration status.

Test-Taking Strategy: The key phrase to focus on is "most effective in stabilizing hydration status." Use the process of elimination. The only option that addresses stabilization is option 3. Also note the phrase "as prescribed" in this correct option.

Level of Cognitive Ability: Application
Phase of Nursing Process: Implementation
Client Needs: Physiological Integrity
Content Area: Child Health

Reference

Wong, D., & Perry, S. (1998). *Maternal-child nursing care.* St. Louis: Mosby–Year Book, pp. 1399–1401.

---

11. The client has received electroconvulsive therapy (ECT). In the post-treatment area and upon the client's awakening, the nurse will first engage in which of the following activities?

1 Discuss the treatment and monitor client's vital signs
2 Offer the client frequent reassurance and repeat orientation statements
3 Assist the client from the stretcher to a wheelchair
4 Assess the return of the gag reflex and then encourage the client in eating breakfast and resuming activity

Answer: 1

Rationale: The nurse would first monitor vital signs and review with the client that the client had just received an ECT treatment. The post-treatment area should include accessibility to the anesthesia staff, oxygen, suction, pulse oximeter, vital sign monitoring, and emergency equipment. The nursing interventions outlined in options 2, 3, and 4 will follow accordingly.

Test-Taking Strategy: Remember the ABCs (airway, breathing, and circulation) when selecting an answer addressing physiological integrity. Note also the key word "first," which tells you that more than one or all of the options may be correct. You must prioritize in selecting your answer.

Level of Cognitive Ability: Application
Phase of Nursing Process: Implementation
Client Needs: Physiological Integrity
Content Area: Mental Health

Reference

Stuart, G., & Sundeen, S. (1995). *Principles and practice of psychiatric nursing.* St. Louis: Mosby–Year Book, p. 710.

12. The physician ordered chlorpromazine (Thorazine) for the treatment of intractable hiccoughs. The client is also on a daily dose of 50 mg of atenolol (Tenormin). Concern for the client's safety leads the nurse to

1. Restrain the client.
2. Limit the client's fluid intake.
3. Monitor the client's blood pressure before administering the medication.
4. Request a sedative at bedtime for the client.

Answer: 3

Rationale: Atenolol is a beta-blocker with antihypertensive effects. Chlorpromazine can also lower blood pressure. Potential for falls related to orthostatic hypotension and sedation is of concern to the nurse administering Thorazine. This risk is greatly increased when an antihypertensive agent is added. There is no reason to restrain the client. A sedative will increase the risk for a fall. Limiting fluid intake is unrelated to the issue of the question. Teaching about side effects of the medication, monitoring blood pressure, and evaluating the client's ability to maintain equilibrium with position changes are appropriate interventions.

Test-Taking Strategy: Use the nursing process to correctly answer this question. Option 3 addresses the first stage of the nursing process, assessment, whereas the other choices address subsequent stages. Option 3 also addresses the ABCs: airway, breathing, and circulation!

Level of Cognitive Ability: Application
Phase of Nursing Process: Implementation
Client Needs: Physiological Integrity
Content Area: Pharmacology

Reference

Wilson, H., & Kneisl, C. (1996). *Psychiatric nursing* (5th ed.). Menlo Park, CA: Addison-Wesley, p. 926.

---

13. The nurse is leading a community support group for chronically mentally ill clients. The discussion topic relates to a risperidone (Risperdal) medication protocol. One client in the group asks the nurse about the client's need to have frequent blood tests. The nurse would respond best by

1. Referring the client's question to the group and encouraging the other clients to respond.
2. Highlighting that taking risperidone does not require the client to have blood testing and that it does not affect blood cells.
3. Asking the client whether the client has read the handouts on risperidone, which were already distributed in the group.
4. Reviewing the entire risperidone medication protocol again with the group.

Answer: 2

Rationale: The focus of the group session relates to risperidone medication teaching. Because it is an educationally oriented session, the nurse intervenes directly by answering the client's question and communicating clarification regarding client knowledge. The nurse would respond in a factual, nonjudgmental manner to encourage further questions and verbal expressions by group members. Such verbal implementation by the nurse would enhance clarification, understanding, and growth experience in the group. The nurse's educational/health counseling approach would enhance the group's knowledge.

Test-Taking Strategy: The nurse would review content in a factual manner during an educationally oriented group session. If the nurse perceived a concern related to specific content, the nurse would then explore further with the client for validation and/or clarification. Option 1 places the responsibility of teaching on the clients. Option 3 may embarrass the client and inhibit further questions from other clients. Option 4 would not be a time-managed approach to implementation of teaching/counseling for the group.

Level of Cognitive Ability: Application
Phase of Nursing Process: Implementation
Client Needs: Health Promotion and Maintenance
Content Area: Mental Health

Reference

Johnson, B. (1997). *Psychiatric-mental health nursing: Adaptation and growth* (4th ed.). Philadelphia: Lippincott-Raven, p. 268.

14. A client with trigeminal neuralgia undergoes intracranial surgery for pain relief. In the postoperative period, which nursing intervention best prevents an episode of facial pain?

1 Instructing the client to brush teeth thoroughly after meals
2 Bringing the client room-temperature water for washing
3 Teaching the client to chew on the affected side
4 Offering the client ice chips between meals

Answer: 2

Rationale: Temperature and touch are important factors to consider in caring for this postoperative client. Foods or liquids that are too hot or cold may trigger a bout of pain. Room-temperature food is recommended, as is room-temperature water for bathing. Rinsing the mouth with water is recommended, rather than tooth brushing. Chewing on the unaffected side is recommended for preventing a painful episode.

Test-Taking Strategy: Brushing or chewing in an affected area is not likely to prevent pain; therefore, you could eliminate options 1 and 3. Remembering that extremes in temperature can trigger an attack will assist in eliminating option 4. If you had difficulty with this question, take time now to review the precipitating factors of pain in the client with trigeminal neuralgia!

Level of Cognitive Ability: Application
Phase of Nursing Process: Implementation
Client Needs: Physiological Integrity
Content Area: Adult Health/Neurological

Reference
Black, J., & Matassarin-Jacobs, E. (1997). *Medical-surgical nursing: Clinical management for continuity of care* (5th ed.). Philadelphia: W. B. Saunders, p. 930.

15. During a neurological assessment, the client does not respond when the nurse walks into the room in front of the client. What action should the nurse take next to assess the client's level of consciousness?

1 Press a pen over the client's fingernail bed
2 Shake the client's shoulders
3 Rub the midsternal area firmly
4 Speak in a loud voice to the client

Answer: 4

Rationale: Cues used to assess level of consciousness are used in a particular order: visual, verbal, tactile, and noxious (painful). Because a visual cue was used in the question, the nurse would use option 4 next. If the client still did not respond, option 2 and then option 3 would be used. Use a sternal rub cautiously in clients with brittle bones or who bruise easily. Option 1 is a peripheral stimulus, not a central stimulus (which is often preferred), but it is sometimes used because little tissue trauma occurs.

Test-Taking Strategy: The basic neurological check is a common assessment performed by the nurse. Using the most minimal stimuli aids in preventing tissue trauma to the client and enables the nurse to determine sooner whether a decrease in level of consciousness has occurred. Learn the order of assessing neurological status—visual, verbal, tactile, and noxious (painful)—to assist in answering questions!

Level of Cognitive Ability: Application
Phase of Nursing Process: Implementation
Client Needs: Physiological Integrity
Content Area: Adult Health/Neurological

Reference
Black, J., & Matassarin-Jacobs, E. (1997). *Medical-surgical nursing: Clinical management for continuity of care* (5th ed.). Philadelphia: W. B. Saunders, pp. 715, 716, 747.

16. The nurse would administer magnesium sulfate by intramuscular injection to a pregnant client to

1 Control seizures caused by low magnesium levels.
2 Increase the amount of water in feces.
3 Increase sinoatrial (SA) node impulse formation.
4 Increase conduction time in the myocardium.

Answer: 1

Rationale: Magnesium sulfate is administered to pregnant women to suppress seizures resulting from hypomagnesemia (as in eclampsia) as a primary priority. A secondary effect of magnesium sulfate is that it acts as a laxative by increasing the water content of feces. Magnesium sulfate decreases SA node impulse formation and decreases myocardial conduction time.

Test-Taking Strategy: It is necessary to have an understanding of eclampsia and its treatment with magnesium sulfate to answer this question correctly. Use the process of elimination. Administering magnesium sulfate would most likely be required if the level were low. This would direct you to the correct option. Take a few moments now to review this material if the question was difficult.

Level of Cognitive Ability: Application
Phase of Nursing Process: Implementation
Client Needs: Physiological Integrity
Content Area: Pharmacology

Reference

Hodgson, B., & Kizior, R. (1998). *Saunders nursing drug handbook 1998.* Philadelphia: W. B. Saunders, pp. 617–620.

---

17. The nurse is caring for a client with cardiomyopathy. The client is scheduled for heart transplantation. The nurse would best meet the psychosocial needs of the client by

1 Giving the family time to be alone.
2 Making sure the client has seen a member of the clergy.
3 Giving the client information about the surgery.
4 Exploring the meaning of the surgery.

Answer: 4

Rationale: The nurse must understand, from the client's perspective, the meaning of the surgery in terms of pain, body image changes, and fear of surgery and dying. Then it is possible for the nurse to work effectively with the client and family.

Test-Taking Strategy: The stem indicates that the nurse should interact with the client. Option 1 does not involve the nurse. Option 2 does not directly involve the nurse with the client. Option 3 simply provides information. Option 4 is a direct action by the nurse that can best meet the client's need because it addresses the client's feelings. In questions relating to psychosocial needs, always address the client's feelings first!

Level of Cognitive Ability: Application
Phase of Nursing Process: Implementation
Client Needs: Psychosocial Integrity
Content Area: Adult Health/Cardiovascular

Reference

Black, J., & Matassarin-Jacobs, E. (1997). *Medical-surgical nursing: Clinical management for continuity of care* (5th ed.). Philadelphia: W. B. Saunders, pp. 1355–1356.

18. The nurse is caring for a client with cardiac disease. The client is scheduled for a treadmill test. Before the procedure, the nurse obtains a rhythm strip. The client was in sinus bradycardia. A fellow nurse asks what this means. The best response would be that

1. The atrioventricular (AV) node is firing as the pacemaker.
2. The Purkinje fibers are the primary source of this rhythm.
3. Conduction is slowed in the bundle of His.
4. The SA node is firing as the pacemaker.

Answer: 4

Rationale: All characteristics of sinus bradycardia are the same as those of normal sinus rhythm (NSR), except that the rate is slower.

Test-Taking Strategy: This question requires knowledge of the basics of an electrocardiogram (ECG) and understanding that if the word "sinus" is used in reference to an ECG, it refers to the sinoatrial (SA) node. Remembering this concept will assist in answering these types of questions!

Level of Cognitive Ability: Application
Phase of Nursing Process: Implementation
Client Needs: Physiological Integrity
Content Area: Adult Health/Cardiovascular

Reference
Smeltzer, S., & Bare, B. (1996). *Brunner and Suddarth's Textbook of medical-surgical nursing* (8th ed.). Philadelphia: Lippincott-Raven, p. 619.

---

19. The charge nurse observes that a nurses' aide did not wash hands after emptying a catheter bag. The nurse implements a staff development plan incorporating which of the following principles?

1. Learning involves a change of behavior
2. Adults need close supervision during the learning process
3. Negative rewards reduce undesirable behavior and support learning
4. Learning is a cognitive, passive process

Answer: 1

Rationale: The charge nurse assumes leadership for improving client care by implementing a staff development program that has the potential for changing behavior. Persons who change their behavior have internalized information and apply it to their actions. Options 2 and 3 use negative strategies to change behavior, and these are not usually successful. Option 4 views the learner as not being actively involved in translating the learning into actions.

Test-Taking Strategy: Use the process of elimination and the principles related to teaching and learning to answer the question. Option 1 identifies the desired outcome of learning: a change in behavior. Options 2 and 3 do not present a positive view of learners. Learning should be an active, not passive, process. Review teaching/learning principles if you had difficulty with this question!

Level of Cognitive Ability: Application
Phase of Nursing Process: Implementation
Client Needs: Safe, Effective Care Environment
Content Area: Fundamental Skills

Reference
Potter, P., & Perry, A. (1997). *Fundamentals of nursing: Concepts, process, and practice* (4th ed.). St. Louis: Mosby–Year Book, p. 265.

20. On the basis of a complete assessment, the nurse has just instituted measures related to an occult prolapsed cord on a client just entering second-stage labor. The sudden change of the labor plan has alarmed the client and her husband. They are anxiously asking what is happening and whether the baby is "OK." To reduce the fear and stress to the couple, the nurse would

1. Assure the couple that the obstetrician will explain everything upon arrival.
2. Explain to the couple what is happening, how it is being managed, and what they can do to help.
3. Ask the couple what they mean by "OK."
4. Reply, "Don't worry, we are taking good care of you and the baby."

Answer: 2

Rationale: Giving information that explains the situation clearly empowers the couple, reducing fear and fostering willingness to cooperate in a positive way. It also enhances the couple's feeling that the nurse is supportive and in control of the situation. Stressing what they can do to help will prevent or decrease any feelings of helplessness.

Test-Taking Strategy: For a question dealing with feelings, read the question carefully to identify what has triggered the emotional response. In this case, it is a situational crisis: the prolapsed cord. Recall that the goal of psychosocial nursing is to promote adaptation and coping by the client. Therapeutic communication tools are used in any question requiring a verbal response. These include being silent, offering assistance, being empathic, focusing, restatement, validation, giving information, and dealing with the here and now. Giving information about the here and now will maintain the trusting relationship between client and nurse as well as encourage the client to cooperate. Incorrect answers to communication questions can often be determined by ruling out answers that include communication blocks. In this case, placing the client's issues on "hold" (until the doctor arrives; option 1), requesting an unnecessary explanation (option 3), and using a nursing cliché that subtly devalues the client's feelings (option 4) all are "blockers" in the incorrect responses.

Level of Cognitive Ability: Application
Phase of Nursing Process: Implementation
Client Needs: Psychosocial Integrity
Content Area: Maternity

Reference

Lowdermilk, D., Perry, S., & Bobak, I. (1997). *Maternity and women's health care* (6th ed.). St. Louis: Mosby–Year Book, p. 360.

---

21. The nurse in the prenatal clinic has just completed an assessment and client education of a client who is 32 weeks pregnant. The client has positioned herself supine on the examination table to await the obstetrician. The client says, "I'm feeling a little lightheaded and sick to my stomach. Do you suppose I'm hypoglycemic? I just ate a little lunch." The nurse notes that the client is also pale and recognizes that she may be experiencing vena cava syndrome (hypotensive syndrome). What will be the next action of the nurse?

1. Take another set of vital signs
2. Give the client a glass of orange juice
3. Place a folded towel or sheet under the right hip
4. Call the obstetrician to see the client immediately

Answer: 3

Rationale: Lying supine (on the back) applies additional gravity pressure on the abdominal blood vessels (iliac vessels, inferior vena cava, and ascending aorta), increasing compression and impeding blood flow and cardiac output. This results in hypotension, dizziness, nausea, pallor, clammy (cool, damp) skin, and sweating. Raising one hip higher than the other reduces the pressure on the vena cava, restoring the circulation and relieving the symptoms.

Test-Taking Strategy: Use the process of elimination and knowledge regarding interventions related to vena cava syndrome to answer the question. The only option that addresses the issue of the question is option 3. If you had difficulty with this question, take time now to review this important syndrome!

Level of Cognitive Ability: Application
Phase of Nursing Process: Implementation
Client Needs: Physiological Integrity
Content Area: Maternity

Reference

Lowdermilk, D., Perry, S., & Bobak, I. (1997). *Maternity and women's health care* (6th ed.). St. Louis: Mosby–Year Book, p. 232.

22. The physician places a Miller-Abbott tube in a client. Six hours later the nurse measures the length of the tube outside the nares and finds that the tube has advanced 6 cm since it was first placed. Which of the following actions should the nurse take?

1 Notify the physician immediately
2 Pull the tube out 6 cm and secure the tube to the nose with tape
3 Document the assessment in the client's record
4 Initiate the tube feeding

Answer: 3

Rationale: The Miller-Abbott tube is a nasoenteric tube, which is used to decompress the intestine and correct a bowel obstruction. Initial insertion of the tube is a physician's responsibility. The tube is mercury weighted and advances by gravity or is sometimes ordered to be advanced manually. Advancement of the tube can be monitored by measuring the tube and by x-ray.

Test-Taking Strategy: The issue of the question is specific content regarding assessment of a client with a Miller-Abbott tube. Remembering that tube advancement by gravity is expected will assist in directing you to the correct option. If you had difficulty with this question, take time now to review the function of this tube and the nursing care involved. You are likely to see questions related to this tube on NCLEX-RN!

Level of Cognitive Ability: Application
Phase of Nursing Process: Implementation
Client Needs: Physiological Integrity
Content Area: Adult Health/Gastrointestinal

Reference

Black, J., & Matassarin-Jacobs, E. (1997). *Medical-surgical nursing: Clinical management for continuity of care* (5th ed.). Philadelphia: W. B. Saunders, pp. 1749–1752.

23. A pregnant client has just been admitted with severe preeclampsia. The nurse knows it is important to assess for other complications at this time. As part of the plan of care for this client, the nurse regularly observes for

1 Any bleeding, such as in the gums, and petechiae and purpura.
2 Enlargement of the breasts.
3 Periods of fetal movement followed by quiet periods.
4 Complaints of feeling hot when the room is cool.

Answer: 1

Rationale: Bleeding is an early sign of disseminated intravascular coagulation (DIC) and should be reported. Options 2, 3, and 4 all are normal occurrences in the last trimester of pregnancy.

Test-Taking Strategy: Looking for similarities in the answer may help eliminate incorrect options. In this question, options 2, 3, and 4 are similar in that all are normal occurrences in pregnancy. Therefore, the correct answer is the one that is not a normal occurrence. Bleeding does not normally occur with pregnancy.

Level of Cognitive Ability: Application
Phase of Nursing Process: Implementation
Client Needs: Physiological Integrity
Content Area: Maternity

Reference

Reeder, S., Martin, L., & Koniak-Griffin, D. (1997). *Maternity nursing: Family, newborn, and women's health care* (18th ed.). Philadelphia: Lippincott-Raven, p. 830.

24. The client recovering from cardiogenic shock is anxious about the condition and being alone. What action should the nurse take in order to give the client some control over the condition and the fear of being left alone?

1. Turn on the television to provide a means of distraction for the client
2. Open the blinds over the window so the client can remain oriented to day/night cycle
3. Demonstrate to the client the use of the call button and place it in easy reach of the client at all times
4. Place a clock in easy view of the client to assist in time orientation

Answer: 3

Rationale: By placing the call button in easy reach of the client, the client has immediate access to the health care team. The client can be reassured that a member of the health care team is available and will come if the client calls. It is hoped that this will decrease the client's perception of being alone and give the client some sense of control.

Test-Taking Strategy: Use the process of elimination. Option 1 offers only a means of distraction; it does not offer the client any control over the situation. Options 2 and 4 are techniques to assist in keeping the client oriented to time and do not offer the client any control or provide a means to lessen the fear of being left alone. Option 3 provides control and will lessen the fear of being left alone.

Level of Cognitive Ability: Application
Phase of Nursing Process: Implementation
Client Needs: Psychosocial Integrity
Content Area: Fundamental Skills

Reference

Kozier, B., Glenora, E., & Blais, K. (1995). *Fundamentals of nursing* (5th ed.). Menlo Park, CA: Addison-Wesley, p. 257.

---

25. An adult client is ordered to receive 500 mL of Intralipid 20%, a fat emulsion, intravenously over 10 hours. The nurse takes care to infuse the lipids at the correct rate because

1. The solution is a hypertonic solution.
2. There will be a minimized risk of allergic reaction.
3. The fat must clear from the circulation.
4. The solution cannot be filtered.

Answer: 3

Rationale: Intralipid 20% is a brand of intravenous fat emulsion. Fat administered intravenously is converted to triglycerides and then to free fatty acids and glycerol by the lipoprotein lipase. The free fatty acids are transported to the tissues, where they are used for energy or stored. It is important that lipids be infused at the recommended rate to reduce the risk of hyperlipidemia, which will occur if the fat is not cleared from the circulating blood.

Test-Taking Strategy: Knowledge regarding the administration of fat emulsions is necessary to answer the question. If you must guess, option 3 is the only option that addresses fat. Review the concepts of fat emulsion now if you are unfamiliar with the content!

Level of Cognitive Ability: Analysis
Phase of Nursing Process: Implementation
Client Needs: Physiological Integrity
Content Area: Pharmacology

Reference

Lehne, R. A. (1998). *Pharmacology for nursing care* (3rd ed.). Philadelphia: W. B. Saunders, p. 832.

---

26. Home care nurses often use the expertise of the home health care rehabilitation team, such as therapists, in caring for clients with physical limitations at home. The home care nurse assigned to a client with cognitive-perceptual difficulties and difficulties with fine motor coordination would request consultation with the

1. Physical therapist.
2. Occupational therapist.
3. Speech pathologist.
4. Recreational therapist.

Answer: 2

Rationale: One of the primary roles of the home health care nurse is to make referrals to rehabilitation team members, usually upon the approval of the primary physician. The occupational therapist focuses on the development of fine motor skills. Speech pathologists and recreational therapists do not play a role in this aspect of care.

Test-Taking Strategy: Begin to answer this question by eliminating the speech pathologist and recreational therapist immediately. Physical therapists work on gross motor coordination, leaving fine-motor skills, retraining, and cognitive-perceptual skill development to the occupational therapists. If you are unfamiliar with the roles of the health care members identified in the options, take time now to review this information!

Level of Cognitive Ability: Application
Phase of Nursing Process: Implementation
Client Needs: Physiological Integrity
Content Area: Adult Health/Neurological

Reference

Rice, R. (1996). *Home health nursing practice: Concepts and application* (2nd ed.). St. Louis: Mosby–Year Book, p. 298.

---

27. The home care nurse who is implementing standard precautions in the home routinely and carefully

1 Conducts handwashing only before donning gloves.
2 Uses protective equipment, such as masks and gowns, when completing all physical assessments.
3 Disposes of sharps, needles, and syringes in the client's regular garbage.
4 Institutes protective measures whenever the potential for exposure to body fluids or blood exists.

Answer: 4

Rationale: Handwashing must be done before and after all procedures and client contact, regardless of the use of gloves. Protective equipment is necessary only when exposure is likely or anticipated, not for all client contact or for each client assessment. Sharps, needles, and syringes must be disposed of in puncture-resistant containers. Waste regulations may vary from state to state, but the sharp items must nonetheless be in separate containers.

Test-Taking Strategy: Option 1 is eliminated because of the word "only." Knowledge of standard precaution measures will assist in eliminating option 2. Options 3 and 4 require discrimination. You would choose option 4 by recognizing that protective measures are used for potential to exposure. Option 4 is also more inclusive than option 3, because waste regulations may vary from state to state. Remember that sharps should not be disposed of in the client's regular garbage.

Level of Cognitive Ability: Application
Phase of Nursing Process: Implementation
Client Needs: Safe, Effective Care Environment
Content Area: Fundamental Skills

Reference

Zang, S., & Bailey, N. (1997). *Home care manual: Making the transition.* Philadelphia: Lippincott-Raven, p. 141.

---

28. The nurse is preparing to defibrillate a client in ventricular tachycardia. Which nursing action provides for the safest environment during a defibrillation attempt?

1 Hand the charged paddles one at a time to the nurse defibrillating
2 Place no lubricant on the paddles
3 Apply light pressure on the chest to prevent burns
4 Perform a visual and verbal check of "all clear"

Answer: 4

Rationale: Safety during defibrillation is essential for preventing injury to the client and to the personnel assisting with the procedure. The person performing the defibrillation ensures that all personnel are standing clear of the bed by a verbal and visual check of "all clear." Charged paddles should never be handed to other personnel. For the shock to be effective, some type of conductive medium (lubricant, gel) must be placed between the paddles and the skin. Firm pressure is needed to reduce the chances of arcing and to reduce impedance to the flow of current.

Test-Taking Strategy: This question requires the identification of safe principles of defibrillation. In finding the nursing action that provides the safest environment during defibrillation, the nurse must look not only at the nurse and the client but also at all the personnel involved in the defibrillation attempt. Option 1 involves the safety of the nurses, and options 2 and 3 deal with the safety of the client. Option 4 involves a verbal and visual check of "all clear," providing for the safety of all involved.

Level of Cognitive Ability: Application
Phase of Nursing Process: Implementation
Client Needs: Safe, Effective Care Environment
Content Area: Adult Health/Cardiovascular

Reference

Hartshorn, J., Sole, M., & Lamborn, M. (1997). *Introduction to critical care nursing* (2nd ed.). Philadelphia: W. B. Saunders, pp. 181–183.

29. A client with an increasing number of premature ventricular contractions (PVCs) is scheduled for 24-hour Holter monitoring. The nurse instructs the client to

1 Remain on nothing by mouth (NPO) status after midnight for the procedure.
2 Disconnect the electrodes only to bathe.
3 Keep an accurate record of activity during the day.
4 Restrict the amount of movement and activity to limit mechanical interference.

Answer: 3

Rationale: Continuous ambulatory monitoring or Holter monitoring can be used to evaluate pacemaker function and the effectiveness of antianginal or antidysrhythmic medications; it is also helpful in correlating symptoms of syncope, lightheadedness, chest pain, and dyspnea with dysrhythmias. In order to evaluate cardiac function, an accurate record of the client's normal activities throughout the day must be recorded along with any signs and symptoms. No special preparation is necessary before the procedure; however, the client must understand that this is a continuous monitoring process and that the electrodes must remain intact for the entire period.

Test-Taking Strategy: This is a client-oriented question that involves the education of a client undergoing Holter monitoring. Understanding that this procedure is noninvasive and that there is no need for NPO status will assist in eliminating option 1. Options 2 and 4 defeat the purpose of the Holter monitoring and thus can be eliminated. Option 3 is the remaining correct choice. Review client instructions for Holter monitoring now if you had difficulty with this question!

Level of Cognitive Ability: Application
Phase of Nursing Process: Implementation
Client Needs: Safe, Effective Care Environment
Content Area: Adult Health/Cardiovascular

Reference

VanRiper, S., & VanRiper, J. (1997). *Cardiac diagnostic tests: A guide for nurses.* Philadelphia: W. B. Saunders, pp. 91–93.

---

30. The parents of an infant with pyloric stenosis ask the nurse why their child developed pyloric stenosis. An appropriate response by the nurse would be

1 "Infants do best when they are on a set feeding schedule."
2 "No one really knows why this problem develops, but it is most common in boys."
3 "In 'failure to thrive' cases such as this, a physiological cause is usually found."
4 "Pyloric stenosis is caused by a structural problem, and there really isn't anything you could have done to prevent it."

Answer: 4

Rationale: Most parents need support and reassurance that this condition is caused by a structural problem and is not a reflection of their parenting skills and capabilities. Option 2 is inaccurate. Although pyloric stenosis is caused by a structural problem, there is no indication that the infant's feeding schedule is related in any way. The use of terms such as "failure to thrive" in addressing parents is not recommended.

Test-Taking Strategy: Knowledge regarding the cause of pyloric stenosis is necessary to answer the question. If you were not exactly sure of the correct answer, select the response that addresses providing support and reassurance to the parents!

Level of Cognitive Ability: Application
Phase of Nursing Process: Implementation
Client Needs: Psychosocial Integrity
Content Area: Child Health

Reference

Wong, D., & Perry, S. (1998). *Maternal-child nursing care.* St. Louis: Mosby–Year Book, pp. 971–974.

31. Which of the following orders should the nurse question for a client in the acute phase of an uncomplicated myocardial infarction (MI)?

1 Digoxin, 0.25 mg PO daily
2 Heparin, 5000 U subcutaneously (SC) every 12 hours
3 Morphine, 6 mg intravenous (IV) push every 3 hours PRN
4 Nitroglycerin, 0.4 mg sublingually (SL) every 5 minutes × 3 PRN

Answer: 1

Rationale: The goal of pharmacotherapy with the client after an MI is to increase oxygen supply to the myocardium, provide anticoagulation, and provide analgesia. Heparin, morphine, and nitroglycerin will accomplish this. Digoxin, which is a positive inotropic agent, increases cardiac output by improving the contractile force of the heart. This is contraindicated in the acute phase of MI. Digoxin will be used if heart failure develops.

Test-Taking Strategy: This question requires an understanding of the physiological response to a myocardial infarction. Note the key phrase "should the nurse question." Use the process of elimination, remembering that the goal of therapy is to increase myocardial oxygen supply. If you had difficulty with this question, take time now to review treatment of an MI and the specific actions of these medications!

Level of Cognitive Ability: Analysis
Phase of Nursing Process: Implementation
Client Needs: Safe, Effective Care Environment
Content Area: Adult Health/Cardiovascular

Reference

Smeltzer, S., & Bare, B. (1996). *Brunner and Suddarth's Textbook of medical-surgical nursing* (8th ed.). Philadelphia: Lippincott-Raven, p. 650.

---

32. The client with hypertension is being treated with captopril (Capoten). The nurse should teach the client that which of the following common side effects are related to this medication?

1 Blurred vision
2 Drowsiness
3 Palpitations
4. Swelling of the face and hands

Answer: 4

Rationale: Clients taking captopril should be instructed to report sore throat, fever, chest pain, edema, or swelling of face, hands, and feet. Swelling of face, lips, hands, or feet may be indicative of angioedema (an acute, painless dermal swelling). Angioedema is a common side effect of captopril.

Test-Taking Strategy: Knowledge regarding this medication is necessary to answer this question. Angioedema is unusual as a side effect in general, but it can occur with the use of captopril. Review the side effects of this medication now if you had difficulty with this question!

Level of Cognitive Ability: Analysis
Phase of Nursing Process: Implementation
Client Needs: Health Promotion and Maintenance
Content Area: Pharmacology

Reference

Hodgson, B., & Kizior, R. (1998). *Saunders nursing drug handbook 1998.* Philadelphia: W. B. Saunders, pp. 142–144.

---

33. The client is being treated for hypertension with spironolactone (Aldactone). Which of the following orders should the nurse question?

1 Atenolol (Tenormin), 50 mg PO QD
2 Digoxin (Lanoxin), 0.25 mg PO QD
3 Potassium chloride (Slow-K), 20 mEq PO QD
4 Furosemide (Lasix), 20 mg PO QD

Answer: 3

Rationale: Aldactone is a potassium-sparing diuretic. The client taking a potassium-sparing diuretic is at risk for hyperkalemia. If a potassium supplement were prescribed, the nurse would question the order.

Test-Taking Strategy: To answer this question correctly, you must know that Aldactone is a potassium-sparing diuretic. This enables you to eliminate each of the other incorrect options systematically. If you had difficulty with this question, take time now to review the potassium-sparing diuretics!

Level of Cognitive Ability: Analysis
Phase of Nursing Process: Implementation
Client Needs: Safe, Effective Care Environment
Content Area: Pharmacology

Reference

Hodgson, B., & Kizior, R. (1998). *Saunders nursing drug handbook 1998.* Philadelphia: W. B. Saunders, pp. 942–944.

---

34. When working with the client with cardiomyopathy, the nurse is careful to instruct the client not to bear down when having a bowel movement. The nurse explains to the client that avoiding this action is required to prevent

1 Exercise tolerance.
2 Tachycardia.
3 Increased cardiac output.
4 Decreased cardiac output.

Answer: 4

Rationale: Bearing down while defecating causes a Valsalva effect, which decreases cardiac output and venous return and puts the client at risk for syncope and dysrhythmias. Option 2 is incorrect because a Valsalva effect will cause bradycardia. Option 3 is the opposite of the correct answer. Option 1 does not occur with the Valsalva maneuver.

Test-Taking Strategy: This question requires that you identify the Valsalva maneuver as the issue of the question. Knowledge that the Valsalva maneuver will decrease cardiac output is necessary to answer the question correctly. Review the physiological principles related to the Valsalva maneuver now, if you have the need!

Level of Cognitive Ability: Application
Phase of Nursing Process: Implementation
Client Needs: Physiological Integrity
Content Area: Adult Health/Cardiovascular

Reference

Black, J., & Matassarin-Jacobs, E. (1997). *Medical-surgical nursing: Clinical management for continuity of care* (5th ed.). Philadelphia: W. B. Saunders, p. 1343.

---

35. A client has surgery for valve prolapse. The client states "If I can't do anything, I might as well be dead." The nurse's best response to this statement would be

1 "You aren't better off dead."
2 "It is normal to be depressed after surgery."
3 "Let's talk more about the way you feel."
4 "You should be more positive."

Answer: 3

Rationale: Option 3 encourages the client to share his or her fears. Options 1, 2, and 4 limit conversation and make the client defensive.

Test-Taking Strategy: Applying the rules of interpersonal communication helps you to answer this question. Use the process of elimination in selecting the option that addresses the client's feelings. Option 3 is nonjudgmental and allows conversation to continue. Remember that the client's feelings are the priority!

Level of Cognitive Ability: Analysis
Phase of Nursing Process: Implementation
Client Needs: Psychosocial Integrity
Content Area: Fundamental Skills

Reference

Ignatavicius, D. D., Workman, M. L., & Mishler, M. A. (1995). *Medical-surgical nursing: A nursing process approach* (2nd ed.). Philadelphia: W. B. Saunders, p. 910.

36. The nurse is examining a pregnant woman with acquired immunodeficiency syndrome (AIDS) who is exhibiting nonspecific symptoms such as fever, weight loss, and persistent candidiasis. Which of the following nursing interventions is of highest priority for the nurse to implement?

1 Provide emotional support
2 Assess history for AIDS risk factors
3 Provide clear information about AIDS and its implications for the woman and child
4 Use disposable latex gloves when in contact with nonintact skin

Answer: 4

Rationale: Progression of human immunodeficiency virus (HIV)–positive symptoms in asymptomatic women may be accelerated by pregnancy. Standard precautions (e.g., latex gloves) should be used during direct interventions throughout pregnancy and delivery care.

Test-Taking Strategy: Identify the critical case elements, which are HIV status and the "highest priority" intervention. When dealing with questions involving priority setting, more than one option may be partially or totally correct. Use Maslow's hierarchy of needs theory, remembering that physiological needs are to be addressed first, followed by safety needs and then psychosocial needs!

Level of Cognitive Ability: Application
Phase of Nursing Process: Implementation
Client Needs: Safe, Effective Care Environment
Content Area: Maternity

Reference
Olds, S., London, M., & Ladewig, P. (1996). *Clinical handbook for maternal-newborn nursing: A family-centered approach* (5th ed.). Menlo Park, CA: Addison-Wesley, pp. 54–55.

---

37. After birth, the nurse allows ample bonding time with the mother and family before administering silver nitrate ophthalmic drops to the newborn. The nurse takes this sequence of action in order to

1 Prevent *Neisseria gonorrhoeae* infections acquired during the birth process.
2 Protect the infant from external environmental stimuli acting on the eye.
3 Allow maternal-child interaction before instillation of drops that may temporarily diminish the infant's vision and attention span.
4 Promote maternal awareness of health promotion issues with her newborn.

Answer: 3

Rationale: Silver nitrate ophthalmic drops may irritate the infant's eyes, cause discomfort, and interrupt the quality of the initial bonding interaction. Administration of the drops, which provide the newborn protection from *N. gonorrhoeae* infection, can be safely postponed until after the maternal-child interaction.

Test-Taking Strategy: This question uses the key phrase "sequence of action" and addresses the issue of promoting bonding. Identifying the issue and the key words will assist in directing you to the correct option!

Level of Cognitive Ability: Application
Phase of Nursing Process: Implementation
Client Needs: Psychosocial Integrity
Content Area: Maternity

Reference
Olds, S., London, M., & Ladewig, P. (1996). *Clinical handbook for maternal-newborn nursing: A family-centered approach* (5th ed.). Menlo Park, CA: Addison-Wesley, p. 138.

---

38. The nurse wears gloves in accordance with the current guidelines of the Centers for Disease Control and Prevention (CDC), which require the use of standard precautions for contact with body fluids of neonates. This means that the nurse wears gloves and a gown when touching a baby from the time of birth until the baby's first bath is completed. The nurse also dons gloves when

1 Discharging the infant.
2 Feeding the infant.
3 Providing cord care.
4 Changing the infant's clothes.

Answer: 3

Rationale: The CDC's standard precautions state that nonsterile, clean gloves should be worn when touching nonintact skin.

Test-Taking Strategy: Remembering the principle of wearing gloves when in contact with nonintact skin will assist in the process of elimination and selection of the correct response. The nurse should wear gloves when changing the baby's diaper and providing cord care. If you are unfamiliar with standard precautions, review these principles now!

Level of Cognitive Ability: Application
Phase of Nursing Process: Implementation
Client Needs: Safe, Effective Care Environment
Content Area: Maternity

Reference
Nichols, F., & Zwelling, E. (1997). *Maternal-newborn nursing: Theory and practice.* Philadelphia: W. B. Saunders, p. 1580.

39. A client is admitted to the emergency department with complaints of severe, radiating chest pain. The client is extremely restless, frightened, and dyspneic. Immediate admission orders include oxygen by nasal cannula at 4 liters per minute, stat creatine phosphokinase (CPK) and isoenzymes, a chest x-ray, a 12-lead ECG, and 2 mg of morphine sulfate IV. Which initial action should the nurse take?

1 Obtain the 12-lead ECG
2 Call the laboratory to order the stat blood work
3 Call radiology to order the chest x-ray
4 Administer the morphine intravenously

Answer: 4

Rationale: Pain control is a priority because the chest pain indicates cardiac ischemia. Pain also stimulates the autonomic nervous system and increases preload, increasing myocardial demands. The ECG in option 1 can provide evidence of cardiac damage and the location of myocardial ischemia. However, pain control is the priority to prevent further cardiac damage. The stat blood work is not a priority. The cardiac isoenzymes can help in determining the choice of treatment. However, they don't begin to rise until 1–2 hours after the onset of a myocardial infarction. Although the chest x-ray can show cardiac enlargement, having the chest x-ray would not influence immediate treatment.

Test-Taking Strategy: The key word is "initial." Remember the immediate goal of therapy: to prevent myocardial ischemia. The only option that will achieve that goal is option 4. If you had difficulty with this question, take time now to review care of the client with a myocardial infarction!

Level of Cognitive Ability: Application
Phase of Nursing Process: Implementation
Client Needs: Physiological Integrity
Content Area: Adult Health/Cardiovascular

Reference

Black, J., & Matassarin-Jacobs, E. (1997). *Medical-surgical nursing: Clinical management for continuity of care* (5th ed.). Philadelphia: W. B. Saunders, pp. 1264–1270.

---

40. A client with Addison's disease has developed melanosis and says to the nurse, "I hate these dark areas in my skin." The most appropriate response by the nurse is

1 "Tell me more about what you are thinking."
2 "Don't think about them, they are not that bad."
3 "These skin changes are upsetting to you?"
4 "You need to ask the doctor about your skin changes."

Answer: 3

Rationale: Option 3 uses the therapeutic communication technique of reflection. It clarifies and encourages further expression of client's feelings. Option 1 does not encourage expression of feelings. Options 2 and 4 deny the client's concerns.

Test-Taking Strategy: Remember to identify the use of communication blocks, such as the use of cliché and false reassurance (option 2), placing the client's issues on "hold" (option 4), or requesting an explanation at the cognitive level (option 1). Look for an answer that reflects or facilitates the client's expression of feelings.

Level of Cognitive Ability: Application
Phase of Nursing Process: Implementation
Client Needs: Psychosocial Integrity
Content Area: Adult Health/Endocrine

Reference

Taylor, C., Lillis, C., & LeMone, P. (1997). *Fundamentals of nursing: The art and science of nursing care* (3rd ed.). Philadelphia: Lippincott-Raven, pp. 371, 374.

---

41. A toddler who is dehydrated from vomiting after receiving weekly chemotherapy asks a nurse for something to drink. Which of these beverages is most appropriate for a nurse to offer this child?

1 Pedialyte
2 Ginger ale
3 Apple juice
4 Chicken broth

Answer: 1

Rationale: Pedialyte is an oral rehydration solution (ORS) that replenishes lost electrolytes. ORS is not contraindicated in a child who is vomiting. Options 2 and 3 are incorrect because these beverages, although they contain calories, contain few electrolytes. Option 4 is incorrect because this beverage contains few calories and too much salt.

Test-Taking Strategy: Focus on the words "most appropriate." You should know that electrolytes are lost with dehydration and that they must be replenished. Pedialyte is the only solution that contains the required amount of electrolytes.

Level of Cognitive Ability: Application
Phase of Nursing Process: Implementation
Client Needs: Physiological Integrity
Content Area: Child Health

Reference

Wong, D. (1995). *Whaley and Wong's Nursing care of infants and children* (5th ed.). St. Louis: Mosby–Year Book, pp. 1238–1240.

---

42. A client is admitted to the hospital with a diagnosis of aldosteronism. When providing care, which of the following nursing actions is most appropriate based on the client's medical condition?

1 Monitoring color of the stools
2 Preventing hypoglycemia
3 Recording intake and output
4 Restricting foods rich in potassium

Answer: 3

Rationale: Aldosterone plays a major role in fluid and electrolyte balance. The nurse maintains an accurate intake and output record to monitor this function. Options 1 and 2 are not related to the clinical manifestations of this medical condition. An important goal of medical treatment is to correct hypokalemia, making option 4 incorrect.

Test-Taking Strategy: This is a difficult question, and an understanding of the nature of the disorder is needed in order to select the correct option. If you had difficulty with the question or are unfamiliar with the disorder, take time now to review!

Level of Cognitive Ability: Application
Phase of Nursing Process: Implementation
Client Needs: Physiological Integrity
Content Area: Adult Health/Endocrine

Reference

Black, J., & Matassarin-Jacobs, E. (1997). *Medical-surgical nursing: Clinical management for continuity of care* (5th ed.). Philadelphia: W. B. Saunders, pp. 2055–2056.

---

43. The intake status for an adult client with heart failure has changed from NPO to clear liquids. An order is written to change digoxin (Lanoxin), 0.25 mg IV every morning, to digoxin (Lanoxin), 0.25 mg orally QID. The nurse's first action should be to

1 Check the client's potassium level.
2 Call the doctor to question the order.
3 Check the client's apical pulse.
4 Check the client's serum digoxin level.

Answer: 2

Rationale: The usual maintenance dose of Lanoxin is 0.125–0.5 mg daily. The doctor should be called since the order is written for four times daily, which would exceed the usual daily dose. This action is the highest priority, even though all of the other options are accurate in nature. It is true that digitalis toxicity is more prevalent when serum potassium is less than 3.0 mEq/liter (option 1). The apical pulse should be at least 60 beats/minute and should be taken immediately before administration (option 3). Option 4 is accurate because the Lanoxin dose is adjusted to the client's clinical condition. Clients with advanced heart disease are more prone to digitalis toxicity.

Test-Taking Strategy: The issue of the question relates to an inaccurate medication dosage prescribed for the client. Note the change from "daily" to "QID" in the question. In addition, note the phrase "first action." What the nurse does first is based on the information provided in the question. Remember also that all or more than one option may be correct in questions dealing with priorities of action. Review this very important medication now if you had difficulty with this question!

Level of Cognitive Ability: Application
Phase of Nursing Process: Implementation
Client Needs: Safe, Effective Care Environment
Content Area: Adult Health/Cardiovascular

Reference

Black, J., & Matassarin-Jacobs, E. (1997). *Medical-surgical nursing: Clinical management for continuity of care* (5th ed.). Philadelphia: W. B. Saunders, pp. 1283–1284.

44. A client is admitted with severe bone pain associated with multiple myeloma. Which of the following medical treatments would the nurse carry out as a part of the treatment plan?

1. Radiation therapy
2. Hydration with normal saline
3. Bed rest
4. NPO except medication

Answer: 1

Rationale: Clients with multiple myeloma suffer severe bone pain resulting from destructive bone lesions that are visible on x-ray. Radiation is very useful in relieving bone pain and reducing the size of plasma cell tumors. Fluids should be encouraged, and hydration is important, but hydration should not be limited to normal saline. Bed rest is contraindicated because of hypercalcemia.

Test-Taking Strategy: The stem tells you the client has bone pain associated with multiple myeloma. Knowledge regarding this disorder would assist in the process of elimination and in answering the question. Note the key phrase "medical treatments." This may assist in directing you to the correct option. If you had difficulty with this question, take time now to review nursing care for clients with this disorder!

Level of Cognitive Ability: Application
Phase of Nursing Process: Implementation
Client Needs: Physiological Integrity
Content Area: Adult Health/Oncology

Reference

Smeltzer, S., & Bare, B. (1996). *Brunner and Suddarth's Textbook of medical-surgical nursing* (8th ed.). Philadelphia: Lippincott-Raven, p. 798.

---

45. An automobile accident victim is admitted to the intensive care unit (ICU) with a medical diagnosis of increased intracranial pressure. To maintain the client's rights, the nurse would

1. Incorporate available and appropriate material resources.
2. Reinforce the consideration of individual's dignity.
3. Keep accurate and current data and daily information.
4. Collaborate with other health care team members on discharge planning.

Answer: 2

Rationale: Option 2 reflects the Client's Bill of Rights, numbers 1 and 5. Option 1 reflects safety issues and state-of-the-art technology. Option 3 reflects documentation and record keeping. Option 4 reflects case management functions for discharge planning. Although each of these are appropriate nursing interventions, they are not directly referred to in the Client's Bill of Rights.

Test-Taking Strategy: Read the question carefully to determine what the question is asking. The key words in the stem are "maintain the client's rights." Use the process of elimination in selecting the option that impacts on the client's rights. Review Client's Bill of Rights now if you had difficulty with this question!

Level of Cognitive Ability: Application
Phase of Nursing Process: Implementation
Client Needs: Safe, Effective Care Environment
Content Area: Fundamental Skills

Reference

Potter, P., & Perry, A. (1997). *Fundamentals of nursing: Concepts, process, and practice* (4th ed.). St. Louis: Mosby–Year Book, pp. 66–67.

46. The nurse notices that a client with Guillain-Barré syndrome has a positive gag reflex but tends to drool excessively. Which of the following interventions is most important to implement for this client?

1 Administering oxygen via nasal cannula at 2 liters per minute
2 Offering frequent mouth care
3 Having the client sit in high Fowler's position and use a "chin tuck" with swallowing
4 Placing an emesis basin and tissues within easy reach

Answer: 3

Rationale: Excessive drooling is an indicator of a client's inability to handle secretions and of risk for aspiration. Because clients with Guillain-Barré syndrome have dysphagia, sitting in high Fowler's position and using a "chin tuck" while swallowing help decrease the risk of aspiration. Although all of the responses may be appropriate, the greatest risk to client safety is aspiration; thus option 3 is most important.

Test-Taking Strategy: Note the key phrase "most important" and the issue of the question: "excessive drooling." Use the process of elimination. Oxygen will not alleviate drooling. Options 2 and 4 are appropriate interventions; however, the most important intervention is to prevent aspiration!

Level of Cognitive Ability: Application
Phase of Nursing Process: Implementation
Client Needs: Physiological Integrity
Content Area: Adult Health/Neurological

Reference

Lewis, S., Collier, I., & Heitkemper, M. (1996). *Medical-surgical nursing: Assessment and management of clinical problems* (4th ed.). St. Louis: Mosby–Year Book, p. 1798.

---

47. Chemical cardioversion is prescribed for the client with atrial fibrillation. The nurse prepares which of the following medications specific for chemical cardioversion?

1 Verapamil (Calan)
2 Nifedipine (Procardia)
3 Quinidine (Quinidex)
4 Bretylium (Bretylol)

Answer: 3

Rationale: Quinidine is an antidysrhythmic. Verapamil is generally used to control heart rate. Nifedipine is a vasodilator. Bretylium is generally used for control of ventricular dysrhythmia.

Test-Taking Strategy: Note the key phrase "chemical cardioversion." Answering this question requires an understanding of the action of these medications and the preprocedure care of a client preparing for chemical cardioversion. If you are unfamiliar with these medications or with preprocedure care, review now!

Level of Cognitive Ability: Application
Phase of Nursing Process: Implementation
Client Needs: Physiological Integrity
Content Area: Adult Health/Cardiovascular

Reference

Black, J., & Matassarin-Jacobs, E. (1997). *Medical-surgical nursing: Clinical management for continuity of care* (5th ed.). Philadelphia: W. B. Saunders, p. 1302.

---

48. At the beginning of the shift, a client with diabetic ketoacidosis (DKA) has orders to receive 1 liter of 0.9% normal saline the first hour, followed by a decrease to 300 mL/hour for 7 hours. How much 0.9% normal saline will this client receive during the 8-hour shift?

1 1000 mL
2 3.1 liters
3 2.1 liters
4 12,100 mL

Answer: 2

Rationale: 1000 mL in first hour + 300 mL/hour × 7 hours equals 1000 mL + 2,100 mL, which equals 3100 mL. Convert 3100 mL to liters (divide by 1000 mL) to obtain 3.1 liters.

Test-Taking Strategy: Answering this question requires addition and multiplication, followed by conversion to liters. Do the math calculations on scratch paper. Check your calculations before selection of the correct option!

Level of Cognitive Ability: Application
Phase of Nursing Process: Implementation
Client Needs: Physiological Integrity
Content Area: Fundamental Skills

Reference

Tierney, L., McPhee, S., & Papadakis, M. (1997). *Current medical diagnosis and treatment* (36th ed.). Stamford, CT: Appleton & Lange, p. 1101.

49. Which of the following interventions would best assist the nurse to maintain a safe environment for a client with severe hypoparathyroidism?

1. Applying chest and limb restraints
2. Instituting seizure precautions
3. Assessing skin temperature and adjusting heat control accordingly
4. Adjusting the bed to a modified Trendelenburg position

Answer: 2

Rationale: Hypoparathyroidism is a problem in which parathyroid hormone is lacking and its absence causes low serum calcium levels. Hypocalcemia can cause tetany, which, if untreated, can lead to seizures. It would be prudent for the nurse to anticipate such a complication and institute seizure precautions in order to maintain a safe environment. Option 1 is inappropriate. In addition, if tetany and seizures develop, limbs should not be restrained. Likewise, options 3 and 4 are not appropriate.

Test-Taking Strategy: The key phrases in this question are "best assist" and "maintain a safe environment" for the client with "hypoparathyroidism." Option 1 is safety oriented; however, it is not appropriate because limbs should not be restrained. Option 3 is not acceptable because clients with this disorder do not have problems with temperature regulation. Likewise, a modified Trendelenburg position would be of no benefit to this client because hypotension is not a problem. This leaves option 2, which is correct because if the condition is severe and if calcium levels are very low, tetany can eventually lead to seizures.

Level of Cognitive Ability: Application
Phase of Nursing Process: Implementation
Client Needs: Safe, Effective Care Environment
Content Area: Adult Health/Endocrine

Reference

Ignatavicius, D. D., Workman, M. L., & Mishler, M. A. (1995). *Medical-surgical nursing: A nursing process approach* (2nd ed.). Philadelphia: W. B. Saunders, p. 1854.

---

50. The nurse suspects that the female client is a victim of physical abuse. Which of the following statements is most likely to encourage the client to confide in the nurse?

1. "You've got a huge bruise on your face. Did your husband hit you?"
2. "If your boyfriend has hit you, you can take him to court or get a restraining order for that."
3. "I sometimes see women who have been hurt by their boyfriends or husbands. Did anyone hit you?"
4. "That looks very sore. I don't know how people can do that to one another."

Answer: 3

Rationale: Women must be asked in a caring and nonthreatening manner about violence in their lives. Options 1 and 2 are confrontational, and option 2 is based on the nurse's assumption that the client wants a restraining order. Option 4 is incorrect because it is a highly judgmental statement on the nurse's part. The nurse must avoid judgment of the victim/suspected victim's situation. It can take a great deal of time for a woman to admit that there is in fact abuse, and the nurse must avoid becoming another controller in the woman's life. Only option 3 allows the client the option of rejecting or accepting further intervention on the part of the nurse, inasmuch as the nurse is making an indirect, general statement to which the client can answer "yes" or "no."

Test-Taking Strategy: Use principles of effective interpersonal communication in answering this question. The question indicates that the client may be a victim of violence. By carefully considering the potential impact of each statement on the client who is in an abusive situation, the nurse determines that options 1, 2, and 4 each are potentially confrontational and judgmental. The nurse must not impose personal will upon the client. Note also the key word "most" in the stem. This will help you differentiate any possible answers from the one best option.

Level of Cognitive Ability: Application
Phase of Nursing Process: Implementation
Client Needs: Psychosocial Integrity
Content Area: Mental Health

Reference

Clark, M. (1996). *Nursing in the community* (2nd ed.). Stamford, CT: Appleton & Lange, pp. 471–472, 485–486.

51. A client with hyperaldosteronism is being discharged from the hospital. Dietary discharge instructions by the nurse include decreasing dietary

1 Sodium.
2 Potassium.
3 Carbohydrates.
4 Protein.

Answer: 1

Rationale: Clients with hyperaldosteronism are maintained on a low-sodium diet as an adjunct to medical management in order to lower the serum sodium levels. They are encouraged to follow a diet with adequate protein, carbohydrates, and fats that enables them to maintain a normal body weight. Potassium intake needs to be maintained because the client is at risk for hypokalemia.

Test-Taking Strategy: This question is asking you to identify client teaching related to dietary management of hyperaldosteronism. Begin to answer this question by recalling the effect that hyperaldosteronism has on the body, particularly in relation to metabolic processes. Recalling that aldosterone is a mineralocorticoid that helps to regulate sodium and potassium levels should narrow your choices to either option 1 or 2. It is essential to understand the physiological action of aldosterone to select the correct option. Review this action now if you had difficulty with this question!

Level of Cognitive Ability: Application
Phase of Nursing Process: Implementation
Client Needs: Health Promotion and Maintenance
Content Area: Adult Health/Endocrine

Reference
Luckmann, J. (1997). *Saunders manual of nursing care.* Philadelphia: W. B. Saunders, p. 1407.

---

52. The nurse is caring for a client requiring body cast therapy. The client asks for a snack. The nurse would encourage which of the following snacks as the most appropriate choice to meet nutritional needs?

1 Crackers with cheese
2 Apple slices with peanut butter
3 Toast with jelly
4 Milk and graham crackers

Answer: 2

Rationale: Most clients in body casts are nonambulatory and are likely to develop constipation. The use of fruits, fruit juices, and high-fiber foods will promote normal bowel elimination habits. The option that provides the high-fiber food is option 2.

Test-Taking Strategy: Use caution when selecting an answer that contains the words "and" or "with." Remember that the entire option needs to be correct. Therefore, carefully read the content before and after the "and" or "with." Consider the client condition; in this case the issue relates to a nonambulatory status and the potential for constipation. Using the process of elimination, you should be directed toward option 2!

Level of Cognitive Ability: Application
Phase of Nursing Process: Implementation
Client Needs: Physiological Integrity
Content Area: Adult Health/Musculoskeletal

Reference
Burrell, P., Gerlach, M., & Pless, B. (1997). *Adult nursing: Acute and community care* (2nd ed.). Stamford, CT: Appleton & Lange, p. 1595.

53. During an office visit, a prenatal client with mitral stenosis states that she has been under a lot of stress lately. During the examination, the client questions everything the nurse does and behaves in an anxious manner. The best nursing response at this time would be to

1 Tell her not to worry.
2 Ignore her unfounded concerns and continue.
3 Explain the purpose of the nurse's actions and answer all questions.
4 Refer her to a counselor.

Answer: 3

Rationale: For the prenatal cardiac client, stress should be reduced as much as possible. Be certain that the woman understands the purpose of any test or assessments so that she does not worry unnecessarily. Options 1, 2, and 4 are nontherapeutic methods of communication at this time. Explaining the purpose of nursing actions will assist in decreasing the stress level of the client.

Test-Taking Strategy: Remember that therapeutic communication techniques are used to answer questions regarding responses to a client. Therapeutic communication techniques enhance communication. Always select the answer that will enhance communication. Avoid selecting responses that will block communication. Always address the client's concerns and feelings!

Level of Cognitive Ability: Application
Phase of Nursing Process: Implementation
Client Needs: Psychosocial Integrity
Content Area: Maternity

Reference
Gorrie, T. M., McKinney, E. S., & Murray, S. S. (1998). *Foundations of maternal newborn nursing* (2nd ed.). Philadelphia: W. B. Saunders, pp. 24–25.

54. The nurse is instructing a postpartum client with endometritis about preventing the spread of infection to the newborn. Which of the following statements would the nurse make to the client?

1 Hands should be washed thoroughly before holding the infant
2 The infant will not be allowed in the room at all
3 There is no danger of the newborn's contracting the disease
4 Visitors are not allowed to hold the baby

Answer: 1

Rationale: Transmission of infectious diseases can occur through contaminated items such as hands and bed linens of clients with endometritis. An important method of preventing infection is to break the chain of infection. Infectious processes occur most readily in the very young and the very old. Handwashing is one of the most effective methods of preventing the transmission of infectious diseases.

Test-Taking Strategy: Avoid extreme answers and absolutes such as those used in options 2, 3, and 4. These use the words "all," "not," and "no." Knowledge of the transmission of infection and how to break the chain of infection is necessary to answer the question. Handwashing is the key!

Level of Cognitive Ability: Application
Phase of Nursing Process: Implementation
Client Needs: Safe, Effective Care Environment
Content Area: Maternity

Reference
Pillitteri, A. (1995). *Maternal and child health nursing: Care of the childbearing and childrearing family* (2nd ed.). Philadelphia: Lippincott-Raven, pp. 714–715, 1305–1306.

55. The nurse teaches the parents and a 10-year-old with newly diagnosed diabetes type I about exercise. Which of the following instructions should the nurse include for preventing hypoglycemic reactions while participating in team sports?

1 Avoid all contact sports
2 Seek immediate medical care for all cuts
3 Eat a snack half an hour before the activities and every hour during play
4 Omit the insulin dose before the activity

Answer: 3

Rationale: Age-appropriate activity is encouraged for normal growth and development. Exercise increases calorie needs and also increases sensitivity to insulin; therefore a dietary increase is needed to maintain a normal blood glucose level. No sport needs to be avoided because of diabetes. In option 2, cuts should be monitored for signs of infection before care is sought. Trauma and infection usually increase blood glucose as a result of the release of catecholamines. Omitting insulin is never recommended, but adjustment of dosage may be needed.

Test-Taking Strategy: Absolute terms such as "all" (options 1 and 2) often make a statement false. Eliminate option 4 because medication adjustments are not within the scope of nursing practice. Because of the increased metabolism from both growth and exercise, adding calories is an appropriate way to maintain normal blood glucose level for 10-year-olds. When in doubt, use normal growth and development guidelines to help you answer the question.

Level of Cognitive Ability: Application
Phase of Nursing Process: Implementation
Client Needs: Health Promotion and Maintenance
Content Area: Child Health

Reference

Wong, D. (1995). *Whaley and Wong's Nursing care of infants and children* (5th ed.). St. Louis: Mosby–Year Book, pp. 1770–1771, 1783–1784.

---

56. The nurse provides guidance to the client after an emergency cesarean section. The nurse's first priority would be to

1 Provide as much information about recovery and child care needs as time allows.
2 Assess the mother's information needs and provide information accordingly.
3 Determine the woman's ability to take in and process information at this time.
4 Make referrals to community agencies and support groups.

Answer: 3

Rationale: Anxiety and/or effects of medication and anesthesia given during an emergency cesarean section interfere with the client's ability to concentrate and function cognitively. Therefore, the nurse's first priority would be to determine the client's anxiety level, extent of recovery from anesthesia, and ability to take in and process information. Information given before anxiety reduction or recovery would be ineffective and wasted effort.

Test-Taking Strategy: Use the phases of the nursing process to answer each question. Assessment is the first step in the nursing process. From this point, eliminate options 1 and 4. In selecting from the remaining two options, use teaching and learning theory. Remember that the first priority is assessing client motivation and client readiness to learn. This should direct you to option 3.

Level of Cognitive Ability: Application
Phase of Nursing Process: Implementation
Client Needs: Psychosocial Integrity
Content Area: Maternity

Reference

Nichols, F., & Zwelling, E. (1997). *Maternal-newborn nursing: Theory and practice.* Philadelphia: W. B. Saunders, pp. 921-923.

---

57. In the event of a precipitous delivery in which the nurse has no assistance, the nurse would place the client into which of the following suggested positions?

1 Lithotomy position
2 Lateral Sims' position
3 Hands-and-knees position
4 Semirecumbent position

Answer: 2

Rationale: When a woman is in a lateral Sims' position, less stress is placed on the perineum and the perineum can be better visualized as the upper leg is supported. The lateral Sims' position increases the space needed for delivery. In addition, the lateral Sims' reduces the pressure of the gravid uterus on the mother's great vessels, thus improving circulation to the fetus.

Test-Taking Strategy: Specific knowledge of the various positions used during labor is needed to answer this question. Note that the stem tells you that the nurse is unassisted. This guides you to select option 2 as the correct answer. Review the appropriate nursing intervention in precipitous delivery if you had difficulty with this question!

Level of Cognitive Ability: Application
Phase of Nursing Process: Implementation
Client Needs: Physiological Integrity
Content Area: Maternity

Reference

Lowdermilk, D., Perry, S., & Bobak, I. (1997). *Maternity and women's health care* (6th ed.). St. Louis: Mosby–Year Book, pp. 410–411.

58. In completing diet counseling for a client with heart failure, the home health care nurse should emphasize

1. Eliminating all alcohol intake, replacing it with mineral water or fruit juices.
2. Eliminating high-calorie snacks, replacing them with high-fiber breads and granola cereals.
3. Avoiding foods high in salt, replacing them with fresh fruits and vegetables.
4. Avoiding fast-food restaurants, carrying a cold lunch of yogurt and lunch meat sandwiches.

Answer: 3

Rationale: Fresh fruits and vegetables are lowest in calories, sodium, and cholesterol. Option 1 is incorrect because mineral water is high in sodium. The commercial granola in option 2 is high in sodium. In a low-sodium diet, milk products are limited to 2 cups daily; lunch meat is high in sodium (option 4).

Test-Taking Strategy: Knowledge of low- and high-sodium diets and that the client with heart failure requires a low-sodium diet is needed to answer this question. The first portions of each of the options have plausible answers. The second portions of the options for the three incorrect answers contain incorrect information. Remember that for an option to be correct, all its parts must be correct. Review foods low in sodium now if you had difficulty with this question!

Level of Cognitive Ability: Application
Phase of Nursing Process: Implementation
Client Needs: Health Promotion and Maintenance
Content Area: Adult Health/Cardiovascular

Reference

Black, J., & Matassarin-Jacobs, E. (1997). *Medical-surgical nursing: Clinical management for continuity of care* (5th ed.). Philadelphia: W. B. Saunders, p. 1286.

---

59. A client with an intrapartum uterine fetal demise asks, "When can we have another child?" Which of the following would be the best response by the nurse?

1. "How does your husband feel about having more children?"
2. "You should wait for the genetic test results before becoming pregnant again."
3. "We can discuss planning for your next pregnancy, but first tell me how you are feeling about this pregnancy."
4. "You are young; you can try to get pregnant after your 6-week check-up."

Answer: 3

Rationale: Another pregnancy soon after the loss of this child may interrupt the grieving process, which may then continue after the birth of the next child. Parents need to feel free to express their emotions and to know that someone will listen to them. This response encourages the client to explore feelings about this pregnancy and loss.

Test-Taking Strategy: Remember that therapeutic communication techniques enhance communication. Try to address the client's feelings or concerns. Option 3 addresses the client's feelings!

Level of Cognitive Ability: Application
Phase of Nursing Process: Implementation
Client Needs: Psychosocial Integrity
Content Area: Maternity

Reference

Nichols, F., & Zwelling, E. (1997). *Maternal-newborn nursing: Theory and practice.* Philadelphia: W. B. Saunders, pp. 902–903, 635.

---

60. The nurse encourages a woman in labor to void every 2 hours. The client asks the nurse why this is necessary. The nurse's best response would be to tell the client that the voiding is done primarily to prevent

1. Fluid volume excess.
2. Constipation and hemorrhoids.
3. Confusion between urine and amniotic fluid.
4. Prolonged labor and trauma of the bladder.

Answer: 4

Rationale: The woman in labor may be unaware of a full bladder because of the sensations of pain and pressure she experiences with contractions. A distended bladder can increase the woman's discomfort with contractions, impede descent of the fetus, and result in decreased bladder tone after birth.

Test-Taking Strategy: Use the process of elimination. Option 4 is the option that specifically addresses the issue of the question: labor. If you had difficulty with this question, take time now to review care during labor!

Level of Cognitive Ability: Application
Phase of Nursing Process: Implementation
Client Needs: Physiological Integrity
Content Area: Maternity

Reference

Nichols, F., & Zwelling, E. (1997). *Maternal-newborn nursing: Theory and practice.* Philadelphia: W. B. Saunders, pp. 772, 805.

---

61. A client with a spinal deformity has been admitted for a work-up before the implantation of a Harrington rod system. The nurse informs the client that postoperative care will include bed rest in which of the following positions?

1 High Fowler's
2 Side-lying
3 Supine
4 Prone

Answer: 3

Rationale: After Harrington rod implantation, the client is required to be on bed rest for an extended period of time in the supine position, but may be log-rolled every 2 hours. When turning the client, the nurse should be aware of the fact that the client's proper body alignment must be maintained.

Test-Taking Strategy: Knowledge of the proper positioning after Harrington rod implantation is necessary to answer this question. Knowledge that the client must be kept in proper body alignment will assist in eliminating options 1, 2, and 4. If you had difficulty with this question, take time now to review postoperative positioning after this procedure!

Level of Cognitive Ability: Application
Phase of Nursing Process: Implementation
Client Needs: Physiological Integrity
Content Area: Adult Health/Musculoskeletal

Reference

Black, J., & Matassarin-Jacobs, E. (1997). *Medical-surgical nursing: Clinical management for continuity of care* (5th ed.). Philadelphia W. B. Saunders, pp. 2120–2121.

---

62. The postpartum client with gestational diabetes is scheduled for discharge. During the discharge teaching, she asks the nurse, "Do I have to worry about this diabetes anymore?" The best response by the nurse would be

1 "Your blood glucose level is within normal limits now; you will be all right."
2 "You will have to worry about the diabetes only if you become pregnant again."
3 "You will be at risk for developing gestational diabetes with your next pregnancy and developing overt diabetes mellitus."
4 "Once you have gestational diabetes, you have overt diabetes and must be treated with medication for the rest of your life."

Answer: 3

Rationale: The client is at risk for developing gestational diabetes with each pregnancy. She also has an increased risk of developing overt diabetes and needs to have follow-up assessments. She also needs to be taught techniques to lower her risk for developing diabetes, such as weight control. The diagnosis of gestational diabetes indicates that this client has an increased risk for development of overt diabetes; however, with proper care, it may not develop.

Test-Taking Strategy: Identify the issue of the question, which is the long-term effects of gestational diabetes. Knowledge regarding the long-term effects of diabetes is necessary to answer the question. Take time now to review this information if you had difficulty with this question!

Level of Cognitive Ability: Application
Phase of Nursing Process: Implementation
Client Needs: Physiological Integrity
Content Area: Maternity

Reference

Lowdermilk, D., Perry, S., & Bobak, I. (1997). *Maternity and women's health care* (6th ed.). St. Louis: Mosby–Year Book, p. 818.

63. During electroconvulsive therapy (ECT), the client is mechanically ventilated. The nurse assists with this procedure, knowing that this may be necessary because

1 Grand mal seizure activity depresses respiration.
2 Muscle relaxants given to prevent injury during seizure activity depress respirations.
3 Anesthesia is administered during the procedure.
4 Decreased oxygen to the brain increases confusion and disorientation.

Answer: 2

Rationale: A short-acting skeletal muscle relaxant such as succinylcholine (Anectine) is administered to prevent injuries during the seizure. The client must be ventilated until the muscle relaxant is metabolized, usually for 2–3 minutes.

Test-Taking Strategy: Knowledge regarding grand mal seizures, ECT, and medications administered is necessary to answer the question. With this knowledge, you can use the process of elimination. If you are unfamiliar with this content, review it now. You are likely to find questions related to ECT on NCLEX-RN!

Level of Cognitive Ability: Application
Phase of Nursing Process: Implementation
Client Needs: Physiological Integrity
Content Area: Mental Health

Reference
Carson, V., & Arnold, E. (1996). *Mental health nursing: The nurse-patient journey.* Philadelphia: W. B. Saunders, p. 785.

---

64. The client says to the nurse, "My obstetrician has just told me I'm going to deliver several babies—it looks like there are five of them!" The most therapeutic response by the nurse is

1 "Congratulations! You and your husband must be very excited!"
2 " 'Way to go, girl!' You and your husband better get some 'R and R' now!"
3 "Oh, how wonderful! You must be on cloud nine!"
4 "Oh, my. How are you, your husband, and families feeling?"

Answer: 4

Rationale: The client has just been informed that she is expecting not one but five babies. In option 1, the nurse gives a response that conforms to social norms but also gives approval, which might prevent the client from vocalizing negative responses. In option 2, the nurse gives another response that confers approval and again might prevent the client from verbalizing negative responses. In addition, the humor of the second remark is fairly inappropriate. Option 3 again uses social responses that would not enable the client to express feelings, concerns, or anxieties.

Test-Taking Strategy: This question tests your knowledge of the appropriate therapeutic communication technique to employ to allow clients to ventilate feelings. Remember that both positive and negative life events create anxiety. In option 4, the nurse employs an empathetic stance and asks a question that will allow the client to verbalize feelings without fear of being judged.

Level of Cognitive Ability: Application
Phase of Nursing Process: Implementation
Client Needs: Psychosocial Integrity
Content Area: Maternity

Reference
Antai-Otong, D. (1995). *Psychiatric nursing: Biological and behavioral concepts.* Philadelphia: W. B. Saunders, pp. 543–576.

---

65. A drug-addicted male newborn client needs a pharmacological agent to help control the withdrawal symptoms. His diarrhea, vomiting, fever, and tachypnea are severe. The selection of a medication is based on its ability to control both the central nervous system (CNS) and gastrointestinal (GI) symptoms. The nurse prepares to administer which of the following medications?

1 Diazepam (Valium)
2 Cimetidine (Tagamet)
3 Oral morphine solution
4 Paregoric

Answer: 3

Rationale: Oral morphine solution controls both the CNS and GI symptoms. Valium significantly decreases the infant's sucking ability. Cimetidine works only for the GI symptoms, and paregoric contains camphor, a CNS stimulant.

Test-Taking Strategy: Knowledge of the actions and uses of these medications is necessary to correctly answer this question. The question asks about control of the CNS and GI symptoms that result from drug withdrawal, both of which are controlled by the oral morphine solution. If you are unfamiliar with the medications addressed in this question, it is important to review them!

Level of Cognitive Ability: Application
Phase of Nursing Process: Implementation
Client Needs: Physiological Integrity
Content Area: Maternity

Reference

Ashwill, J., & Droske, S. (1997). *Nursing care of children: Principles and practice.* Philadelphia: W. B. Saunders, pp. 575–576.

---

66. The nurse is observing a newly licensed R.N. auscultate the breath sounds of a client on the nursing unit. The nurse would intervene if the second R.N. were observed performing which of the following incorrect actions?

1 Placing the stethoscope directly on the client's skin
2 Using the bell of the stethoscope
3 Asking the client to sit upright
4 Asking the client to breathe slowly and deeply through the mouth

Answer: 2

Rationale: The nurse assesses the breath sounds of the client by asking the client to sit up and breathe slowly and deeply through the mouth. Breath sounds are auscultated by using the diaphragm of the stethoscope, which is warmed before use. The stethoscope is always placed directly on the client's skin and not over a gown or clothing.

Test-Taking Strategy: This question is straightforward in wording and tests a fundamental concept of basic nursing assessment. Use the process of elimination. If this question was problematic, take a few moments to review auscultation as a physical assessment technique!

Level of Cognitive Ability: Application
Phase of Nursing Process: Implementation
Client Needs: Health Promotion and Maintenance
Content Area: Adult Health/Respiratory

Reference

Taylor, C., Lillis, C., & LeMone, P. (1997). *Fundamentals of nursing: The art and science of nursing care* (3rd ed.). Philadelphia: Lippincott-Raven, pp. 496–497.

---

67. Realizing that postpartum diabetic clients are prone to infection, the nurse quickly reports the following signs to the physician: scant lochia with a foul odor and a temperature of 101°F on the second postpartum day. Of the following orders written, which one should the nurse complete first?

1 Place client on complete bed rest in a supine position
2 Increase fluid intake
3 Obtain culture and sensitivity tests of lochia and urine
4 Administer cefoperazone sodium (Cefobid) IV

Answer: 3

Rationale: The client should be placed in a semi-Fowler's position. Options 2 and 4 are important in the treatment of postpartum infection. However, they are not the top priority. The culture and sensitivity tests need to be obtained before any antibiotic therapy is started so as not to mask the microorganism.

Test-Taking Strategy: Note the key word "first." The focus then should be on prioritizing care. Eliminate option 1 because the client should be placed in semi-Fowler's to assist in drainage. Based on the signs presented in the question, the first action then should be to obtain the culture and sensitivity tests.

Level of Cognitive Ability: Application
Phase of Nursing Process: Implementation
Client Needs: Physiological Integrity
Content Area: Maternity

Reference

Hodgson, B., & Kizior, R. (1998). *Saunders nursing drug handbook 1998.* Philadelphia: W. B. Saunders, pp. 173–174.

68. A full-term infant is admitted to the neonatal intensive care unit with a diagnosis of possible sepsis. The nurse would immediately report which of the following findings to the perinatal medical team?

1 Oxygen partial tension (PO_2), 94%
2 Diastolic blood pressure (BP), 32 mmHg
3 Temperature, 98.2°F
4 Respiratory rate, 62 breaths/minute

Answer: 2

Rationale: The normal values for the term neonate being monitored for sepsis include PO_2 of 92%–96%, temperature of 97.8°–99.0°F, and respiratory rate of less than 70 breaths/minute. A blood pressure with a mean of less than 40 mm/Hg may be indicative of impending circulatory failure and should be reported immediately.

Test-Taking Strategy: An accurate knowledge of the normal physiological parameters of the neonate is needed to answer this question. Use the process of elimination, selecting the sign that is abnormal in the neonate. Take time now to review normal vital signs in the neonate if you had difficulty with this question!

Level of Cognitive Ability: Application
Phase of Nursing Process: Implementation
Client Needs: Physiological Integrity
Content Area: Maternity

Reference
Nichols, F., & Zwelling, E. (1997). *Maternal-newborn nursing: Theory and practice.* Philadelphia: W. B. Saunders, pp. 1547–1551.

69. The depressed client tells the nurse that sleep is more important today than attending the scheduled program and says to the nurse, "Just go away and leave me alone." The nurse's best response is

1 "It is okay for you to sleep today."
2 "I will go with you in 15 minutes."
3 "You know you don't really mean that."
4 "Your roommate is depending on you."

Answer: 2

Rationale: The depressed client must be encouraged to attend the programming; otherwise withdrawal will only increase. Option 1 does not encourage attendance. Option 2 lets the client know that he or she is expected to attend and that he or she is worthy of the nurse's time. Option 3 is not effective, and it negates the client's verbalization. Option 4 uses guilt, and the depressed client feels guilty already. It does not improve the client's psychosocial integrity.

Test-Taking Strategy: Use the process of elimination. With communication questions, the nurse must always keep the client's feelings in mind. Communication should be direct, and it should always relay to the client a sense of worthiness. Clearly, then, option 2 is the best response.

Level of Cognitive Ability: Application
Phase of Nursing Process: Implementation
Client Needs: Psychosocial Integrity
Content Area: Mental Health

Reference
Johnson, B. (1997). *Psychiatric-mental health nursing: Adaptation and growth:* (4th ed.). Philadelphia: Lippincott-Raven, p. 548.

70. The elderly depressed client complains that eating is just too difficult. The client says "I will just drink the milk . . . It doesn't matter anyway." The appropriate action by the nurse is

1 Wait until the client is feeling better to stress the intake of food.
2 Sit with the client and feed the meal slowly.
3 Encourage the client to sit with the other clients during the meal.
4 Tell the client that low energy is understandable right now.

Answer: 2

Rationale: When a client is unable to meet needs of feeding, dressing, and grooming, the nurse must meet those needs. To neglect those needs only reinforces the idea that the client is unworthy. In this situation, food is important for physiological integrity.

Test-Taking Strategy: Options 1 and 4 are very similar and do not modify the situation at all. Sitting with other clients is a good response, but not the best. It does not change the fact that the client is unable to eat. With these considerations in mind, option 2 is the only correct choice.

Level of Cognitive Ability: Application
Phase of Nursing Process: Implementation
Client Needs: Physiological Integrity
Content Area: Fundamental Skills

Reference
Johnson, B. (1997). *Psychiatric-mental health nursing: Adaptation and growth* (4th ed.). Philadelphia: Lippincott-Raven, pp. 556–557.

71. A preschool child with infectious diarrhea is to be placed in isolation. Which of these nursing actions is most appropriate when admitting the child to the room?

1 Identify yourself after putting on protective equipment
2 Provide gown and gloves for therapeutic play
3 Explain that isolation is needed to protect other kids
4 Ask the mother to bring a favorite stuffed animal

Answer: 2

Rationale: Children in isolation will experience loss of control and fear bodily harm. Allowing the child to see, touch, and play with protective equipment will relieve some of the anxiety associated with isolation. Option 1 is incorrect because a nurse should identify herself or himself before putting on protective equipment. Option 3 is incorrect because preschool children have trouble understanding cause-and-effect relationships. Therefore, it does not matter to this child that other children are protected. Option 4 is incorrect because a stuffed animal is hard to clean and can harbor infectious pathogens. An easily cleaned toy is a better choice.

Test-Taking Strategy: The reader should focus on the words "most appropriate." This gives a clue to the reader that more than one option may be correct. This question is testing your knowledge of growth and development and principles of isolation. On the basis of these principles, use the process of elimination!

Level of Cognitive Ability: Application
Phase of Nursing Process: Implementation
Client Needs: Psychosocial Integrity
Content Area: Child Health

Reference
Wong, D. (1995). *Whaley and Wong's Nursing care of infants and children* (5th ed.). St. Louis: Mosby–Year Book, p. 1120.

72. After feeding a child who has gastroesophageal reflux (GER), a nurse should place the child in which of the following positions?

1 High Fowler's
2 Prone, head elevated
3 Right side–lying
4 Left side–lying

Answer: 2

Rationale: The infant who has GER should be placed in a prone position with the head of the bed elevated 30 degrees. Options 1, 3, and 4 are incorrect. A nurse must place the child with GER in a position to reduce gastric reflux and prevent aspiration of stomach contents.

Test-Taking Strategy: This question requires knowledge of how to reduce gastric reflux and prevent aspiration of gastric contents in a child with GER. Options 3 and 4 can be easily eliminated. From this point, use knowledge regarding positioning to answer the question. If you had difficulty with this question, take time now to review care of the child with GER!

Level of Cognitive Ability: Application
Phase of Nursing Process: Implementation
Client Needs: Physiological Integrity
Content Area: Child Health

Reference

Ashwill, J., & Droske, S. (1997). *Nursing care of children: Principles and practice.* Philadelphia: W. B. Saunders, p. 714.

---

73. After the client undergoes cardiac catheterization, the nurse encourages the client's fluid intake by explaining that it

1 Prevents postprocedure hyperthermia.
2 Expands the vascular volume for possible angioplasty.
3 Increases the quality of peripheral pulses.
4 Promotes renal excretion of contrast material.

Answer: 4

Rationale: Fluid intake is encouraged after cardiac catheterization (if there are no contraindications) for adequate fluid replacement and renal elimination of the contrast material.

Test-Taking Strategy: Identify the issue of the question as a specific nursing action encouraging fluid intake. Eliminate option 1 because hyperthermia is unrelated to the issue. Eliminate option 2 because there is no mention of angioplasty or the need for it. For the remaining two options, remembering that contrast material is used will assist in directing you to the correct option.

Level of Cognitive Ability: Application
Phase of Nursing Process: Implementation
Client Needs: Physiological Integrity
Content Area: Adult Health/Cardiovascular

Reference

Black, J., & Matassarin-Jacobs, E. (1997). *Medical-surgical nursing: Clinical management for continuity of care* (5th ed.). Philadelphia: W. B. Saunders, p. 1232.

---

74. After cardiac catheterization of a client with angina pectoris, the nurse observes for nausea, vomiting, flushing, and rash and is prepared to take action for

1 Impending myocardial infarction.
2 Normal side effects of contrast material.
3 Hematoma formation.
4 Hypersensitivity to contrast material.

Answer: 4

Rationale: On occasion, clients have an allergic reaction to the iodine-based contrast medium. In the period after cardiac catheterization, the nurse should observe for nausea, vomiting, flushing, rash, and other signs of hypersensitivity to the contrast material.

Test-Taking Strategy: Note the signs presented in the question: nausea, vomiting, flushing, and rash. Remembering that these signs are indicative of hypersensitivity should assist in directing you to the correct option!

Level of Cognitive Ability: Application
Phase of Nursing Process: Implementation
Client Needs: Physiological Integrity
Content Area: Adult Health/Cardiovascular

Reference

Black, J., & Matassarin-Jacobs, E. (1997). *Medical-surgical nursing: Clinical management for continuity of care* (5th ed.). Philadelphia: W. B. Saunders, pp. 1231, 1232.

75. The client with polycystic kidney disease says to the nurse, "My father had this disease, and now me. I'm not sure about having children." The most appropriate response by the nurse would be which of the following?

1 "There is no reason to worry."
2 "I think you are making the right decision."
3 "You should ask your doctor about your decision."
4 "You are not sure about having children?"

Answer: 4

Rationale: Option 4 involves reflecting/repeating the client's message and serves to encourage the client to elaborate on thoughts and feelings. Option 4 uses the therapeutic communication technique of paraphrasing. In option 1, the nurse is offering false reassurance. In option 2, the nurse is expressing approval, which can be harmful to a nurse-client relationship. Option 3 places the client's feelings on hold.

Test-Taking Strategy: Therapeutic communication techniques are the answers to questions regarding responses to clients. Always select answers that will enhance communication. Always address the client's concerns and feelings!

Level of Cognitive Ability: Application
Phase of Nursing Process: Implementation
Client Needs: Psychosocial Integrity
Content Area: Adult Health/Renal

Reference
Black, J., & Matassarin-Jacobs, E. (1997). *Medical-surgical nursing: Clinical management for continuity of care* (5th ed.). Philadelphia: W. B. Saunders, pp. 1678–1679.

---

76. The mother of an infant born at 42 weeks' gestation arrives to the neonatal intensive care unit to visit her infant. The mother observes that her infant is on a ventilator and responds, "I don't understand. I thought my baby would be fine. Why is my baby on this machine?" The nurse responds

1 "Babies who are born post-term all need artificial ventilation."
2 "Your baby aspirated meconium, and the ventilator helps the baby breathe easier."
3 "If the doctor had delivered your baby a little earlier, the baby probably would not need this machine."
4 "Your baby will need this machine until the lungs are fully developed."

Answer: 2

Rationale: Post-term infants may experience meconium aspiration syndrome from the effects of anoxia in utero. Infants suffering from meconium aspiration may require ventilator support. Option 1 is absolute and incorrect and does not specifically respond to the mother's question. Option 3 places blame on the doctor, which is inappropriate therapeutic communication. Option 4 refers to the preterm infant who has immature lungs, which is not the issue in this question.

Test-Taking Strategy: This question asks you to respond to the mother's question in a therapeutic manner. It is also important that the response is accurate in content. Option 1 contains an absolute "all," thereby making it incorrect. Option 2 provides information with correct terminology. Option 3 focuses on inappropriate issues and places blame, which is a communication block. Option 4 provides inaccurate information.

Level of Cognitive Ability: Application
Phase of Nursing Process: Implementation
Client Needs: Psychosocial Integrity
Content Area: Maternity

Reference
Pillitteri, A. (1995). *Maternal and child health nursing: Care of the childbearing and childrearing family* (2nd ed.). Philadelphia: Lippincott-Raven, pp. 760–761.

---

77. The client has developed generalized convulsive status epilepticus. In preparing to care for the client, the nurse would first

1 Obtain the crash cart from the next room.
2 Start an IV infusion of 10% dextrose in water (D10W).
3 Administer parenteral diazepam (Valium).
4 Administer parenteral ethosuximide (Zarontin).

Answer: 3

Rationale: Diazepam is the medication of choice for the condition described. Although the brain does use large amounts of glucose during a seizure, option 2 is contraindicated. Option 4 is also not the best choice for this situation. Furthermore, in this situation, the nurse would not leave the client to obtain the crash cart. Rather, the nurse would instruct another person to obtain the crash cart.

Test-Taking Strategy: Use the process of elimination. Eliminate option 1 first because the nurse would not leave the client. For the remaining options, remember that the seizures need to be controlled. Review the purpose and action of Valium and care of the client with seizures if you had difficulty with this question!

Level of Cognitive Ability: Application
Phase of Nursing Process: Implementation
Client Needs: Physiological Integrity
Content Area: Adult Health/Neurological

Reference

Lehne, R. A. (1998). *Pharmacology for nursing care* (3rd ed.). Philadelphia: W. B. Saunders, p. 208.

---

78. The nurse is caring for a client with a diagnosis of complete placenta previa who is having contractions. In preparing the client for delivery, which procedure would the nurse need to perform?

1 Administer a soap suds enema
2 Insert a Foley catheter
3 Apply a fetal scalp electrode
4 Perform a perineal shave prep

Answer: 2

Rationale: With complete placenta previa, cesarean delivery is indicated because the placenta covers the entire internal cervical os. A Foley catheter is indicated to keep the bladder empty and less vulnerable to trauma during the surgery. Enemas are contraindicated because of their stimulatory effect on contractions, which can contribute to maternal-fetal hemorrhage as the cervix dilates and pulls away from the back of the placenta. An abdominal, not perineal, shave prep is done in preparation for abdominal surgery. Applying a fetal scalp electrode is not normal procedure for a cesarean delivery.

Test-Taking Strategy: Knowledge regarding the pathophysiological processes and treatment of placenta previa is necessary. The key phrases in the case presentation include "complete placenta previa" and "preparation for delivery." Knowing that a cesarean delivery is indicated, pick the option that is a preoperative procedure for this type of delivery. Options 1, 3, and 4 are not routine preoperative procedures for a cesarean delivery. Review this now if you had difficulty with the question!

Level of Cognitive Ability: Application
Phase of Nursing Process: Implementation
Client Needs: Physiological Integrity
Content Area: Maternity

Reference

Nichols, F., & Zwelling, E. (1997). *Maternal-newborn nursing: Theory and practice.* Philadelphia: W. B. Saunders, p. 874.

---

79. The client with myasthenia gravis asks the nurse about two prescribed medications: pyridostigmine bromide (Mestinon) and prednisone. The client has a history of hyperthyroidism. The nurse instructs the client most safely when stating

1 "Mestinon is intended to improve endurance, but expect some fatigue."
2 "Prednisone may make you feel weak for a time, but symptoms may improve."
3 "Mestinon is intended to restore muscle strength; the dose is highly individualized."
4 "Prednisone is to be taken after meals."

Answer: 3

Rationale: Note the key phrase "the dose is highly individualized" in the correct option. Mestinon is intended to improve both muscle strength and endurance. A history of hyperthyroidism complicates therapy because the danger of cardiac dysrhythmia exists; therefore, any symptom such as fatigue should be reported to the physician. Prednisone is given to clients with myasthenia gravis for decreasing effect on the acetylcholine antibody titer and/or for its ability to reduce symptoms of the disease. Prednisone is given without regard to food unless gastrointestinal upset occurs.

Test-Taking Strategy: The medications used to treat myasthenia gravis are appropriate. What are vague are the closing phrases of options 1 and 2. With regard to option 1, fatigue is reportable because of the possibility of cardiac involvement. With regard to option 2, prednisone is specifically intended to effect the restoration of muscle strength. Option 4 is incorrect. Only option 3 addresses all the information presented in the question, gives true information about restoration of muscle strength, and addresses the client's medical history of hyperthyroidism.

Level of Cognitive Ability: Application
Phase of Nursing Process: Implementation
Client Needs: Physiological Integrity
Content Area: Adult Health/Neurological

Reference

Hodgson, B., & Kizior, R. (1998). *Saunders nursing drug handbook 1998.* Philadelphia: W. B. Saunders, pp. 888–890.

---

80. The physician has prescribed warm hydrotherapy to ease joint motion and pain. The client says to the nurse, "I'm not sure this procedure is the best treatment for me." The nurse's most appropriate response is

1 "Don't worry, your doctor treats all clients this way."
2 "I know you are making the right decision."
3 "The joint pain has made you very sick."
4 "You have concerns about the treatment for your joints?"

Answer: 4

Rationale: Option 4, paraphrasing, is a restatement of the client's message in the nurse's own words; it is therapeutic communication. In option 2, the nurse is offering false reassurance and thus blocks communication. In option 1, the nurse is expressing the lack of client's right to an option, which represents a block to communication. There are no data in the question to support option 3.

Test-Taking Strategy: Therapeutic communication techniques enhance communication. Always select the answers which will enhance communication. Avoid responses that will block communication. Remember to always address the client's concerns and feelings!

Level of Cognitive Ability: Application
Phase of Nursing Process: Implementation
Client Needs: Psychosocial Integrity
Content Area: Fundamental Skills

Reference

Potter, P., & Perry, A. (1997). *Fundamentals of nursing: Concepts, process, and practice* (4th ed.). St. Louis: Mosby–Year Book, pp. 240–246.

---

81. The nurse is caring for a client with osteosarcoma. The alkaline phosphatase test yields a significantly increased value. The nurse should

1 Call the physician immediately.
2 Carefully assess neurological status.
3 Administer antibiotic therapy as prescribed.
4 Gently perform routines that cause movement.

Answer: 4

Rationale: Alkaline phosphatase is an enzyme found in osteoblasts that reflects osteoblastic activity. The alkaline phosphatase level is expected to be significantly increased with osteosarcoma. An elevated level is also seen in clients with Paget's disease, rickets, hyperparathyroidism, myeloma, and sarcoidosis. Care should be taken to decrease risk of fractures and to reduce pressure and skin breakdown.

Test-Taking Strategy: Knowledge of alkaline phosphatase is necessary to answer this question. Remembering that osteosarcoma relates to a bone disorder may assist in directing you to the correct option. Use the principles associated with reducing the risk of fractures and preventing skin breakdown.

Level of Cognitive Ability: Application
Phase of Nursing Process: Implementation
Client Needs: Physiological Integrity
Content Area: Adult Health/Oncology

Reference

Burrell, P., Gerlach, M., & Pless, B. (1997). *Adult nursing: Acute and community care* (2nd ed.). Stamford, CT: Appleton & Lange, pp. 1578, 1659.

82. A nurse provides a review session about suicide with the staff members on the nursing unit. Which of these accurate statements would the nurse share with the staff members?

1 "Suicide runs in the family, so there is nothing we can do about it."
2 "The suicidal attempts are just attention-seeking behaviors."
3 "Eighty percent of individuals who really do kill themselves have talked about their suicidal intentions."
4 "Only psychotic individuals commit suicide."

Answer: 3

Rationale: Of every 10 people who do commit suicide, 8 have given definite clues or warnings about their intentions. Suicidal tendency is not an inherited condition; it is an individual condition. An attempt is not an attention-seeking behavior, and each act should be taken very seriously. The individual who is suicidal is not necessarily psychotic or even mentally ill.

Test-Taking Strategy: Options 1, 2, and 4 are considered myths about suicide. Eliminate option 1 because of the statement "there is nothing we can do about it." Eliminate option 2 because of the statement "just attention-seeking behaviors." Eliminate option 4 because of the word "only." Review concepts related to suicide now if you had difficulty with this question!

Level of Cognitive Ability: Application
Phase of Nursing Process: Implementation
Client Needs: Safe, Effective Care Environment
Content Area: Mental Health

Reference

Townsend, M. (1996). *Psychiatric-mental health nursing: Concepts of care* (2nd ed.). Philadelphia: F. A. Davis, p. 251.

---

83. The nurse is instructing the client with tuberculosis on the medication regimen. The client says to the nurse, "I'm really frightened about the fatigue; do you think the medication will take it away?" The most appropriate response by the nurse is which of the following?

1 "Don't worry, everything will work out."
2 "The fatigue will be easier to deal with when you get used to it."
3 "As long as you take the medication as directed, you will notice the fatigue diminishing as treatment progresses."
4 "You must do what the doctor ordered even if you are tired."

Answer: 3

Rationale: Fatigue can be frightening to the client. The nurse is realistic in offering a positive outlook for the client as long as he or she complies with the medication regimen and in suggesting that fatigue will diminish as treatment progresses. The client's feelings are minimized in option 1. The statement in option 2 is incorrect because the fatigue will diminish as treatment progresses. Option 4 blocks communication and does not take the client's feelings into consideration.

Test-Taking Strategy: It is important for the nurse to address client concerns and offer a positive outlook as long as the client complies with the medication regimen. Options 1, 2, and 4 do not address the client's concerns and must be eliminated. In addition, options 1, 2, and 4 are not supportive responses. Address client feelings!

Level of Cognitive Ability: Application
Phase of Nursing Process: Implementation
Client Needs: Psychosocial Integrity
Content Area: Adult Health/Respiratory

Reference

Ignatavicius, D. D., Workman, M. L., & Mishler, M. A. (1995). *Medical-surgical nursing: A nursing process approach* (2nd ed.). Philadelphia: W. B. Saunders, pp. 720, 722.

84. The nurse is caring for a client with acquired immunodeficiency syndrome (AIDS) who is being treated with trimethoprim and sulfamethoxazole (Bactrim, Septra) for *Pneumocystis carinii* pneumonia. Which of the following nursing interventions is performed in regard to this medication?

1 Monitor intake and output and encourage fluids
2 Monitor blood pressure, heart rate, and rhythm and administer while the client is lying down
3 Monitor for hypoglycemia and administer IV over 1 hour
4 Advise the client to avoid sun and alcohol for at least 3 weeks after treatment

Answer: 1

Rationale: Intake and output are monitored and fluid intake is encouraged because Bactrim is nephrotoxic. The interventions in options 2 and 3 are appropriate for the medication pentamidine isethionate (pentamidine), which is also used to treat *P. carinii* pneumonia. Pentamidine causes hypotension, when administered rapidly, and severe hypoglycemia, which may be fatal. Option 4 is not an appropriate intervention with regard to this medication.

Test-Taking Strategy: Knowledge regarding specific nursing interventions related to Bactrim is necessary to answer this question. Side effects related to another medication used to treat *P. carinii* pneumonia, pentamidine isethionate, were included in options 2 and 3 as distracters. Review nursing implications related to both of these medications now if you had difficulty with this question!

Level of Cognitive Ability: Application
Phase of Nursing Process: Implementation
Client Needs: Physiological Integrity
Content Area: Pharmacology

Reference

Ignatavicius, D. D., Workman, M. L., & Mishler, M. A. (1995). *Medical-surgical nursing: A nursing process approach* (2nd ed.). Philadelphia: W. B. Saunders, p. 510.

---

85. The client with obesity says to the clinic nurse, "I'm not sure that attending my Weight Watchers support group is the best thing for me to do." The best response by the nurse is which of the following?

1 "Weight Watchers has been successful for many of our clients in the past."
2 "Your doctor has decided that you should give Weight Watchers a chance."
3 "I feel certain that you have made the right decision by giving Weight Watchers a try."
4 "You have concerns about attending the Weight Watchers support group?"

Answer: 4

Rationale: In option 4, the nurse has restated the client's message in an open-ended question. Option 1 represents a block to communication and is impersonal. Option 2 devalues the client, implying that the doctor knows best. In Option 3, the nurse is expressing approval, which can be detrimental to the nurse-client relationship. Option 4 represents the therapeutic communication technique of paraphrasing.

Test-Taking Strategy: In questions requiring a response to a client, avoid options that contain blocks to communication. Always select the answer that includes a therapeutic communication technique such as, in this question, the technique of paraphrasing. Address client feelings!

Level of Cognitive Ability: Application
Phase of Nursing Process: Implementation
Client Needs: Psychosocial Integrity
Content Area: Fundamental Skills

Reference

Sieh, A., & Brentin, L. (1997). *The nurse communicates.* Philadelphia: W. B. Saunders, p. 16.

86. A client is scheduled for an electroconvulsive therapy (ECT) treatment and says to the nurse, "I've seen this in a movie and I'm scared that it will hurt." The most appropriate response by the nurse is which of the following?

1. "Don't be afraid. Your doctor has done this procedure hundreds of times and you needn't worry."
2. "You have a very serious psychiatric problem that can be helped by this procedure."
3. "Tell me what you know about the procedure."
4. "Everything will be okay. All clients undergoing ECT have the same fears."

Answer: 3

Rationale: Option 3 is a therapeutic communication technique that explores the client's feelings and will establish a baseline for further teaching needs. Option 1 diminishes the client's feelings by directing attention away from the client and to the doctor's importance. Option 2 does not address the client's fears, and the use of the phrase "a very serious psychiatric problem" may further alarm the client and escalate anxiety. Option 4 offers false reassurance and does not provide individualized nursing care.

Test-Taking Strategy: In questions requiring a response to a client, be alert to options that contain blocks to communication. Always select the answer that includes a therapeutic communication technique. Focus on the client's feelings!

Level of Cognitive Ability: Application
Phase of Nursing Process: Implementation
Client Needs: Psychosocial Integrity
Content Area: Mental Health

Reference

Sieh, A., & Brentin, L. (1997). *The nurse communicates.* Philadelphia: W. B. Saunders, pp. 16–17.

---

87. Which intervention would the nurse carry out to promote safety for a 2-month-old hospitalized child?

1. Place the infant in a supine position for sleep
2. Remove the pacifier from the mouth as soon as sleep begins
3. Place netting over crib when the infant is unsupervised
4. Use only plastic bottles and toys

Answer: 1

Rationale: The American Academy of Pediatrics recommends the supine position for sleep to reduce the risk of sudden infant death syndrome (SIDS). Safety netting is not necessary for 2-month-olds because they are unable to roll over or stand alone. Plastic bottles are not necessary because the caregiver will hold the bottle for the 2-month-old. Cloth toys that can easily be cleaned are acceptable. Pacifiers are considered safe and appropriate at this age.

Test-Taking Strategy: Read the situation carefully, identifying the client's age to help you eliminate distracters that are not safety issues for that developmental stage. Knowledge of teaching points to reduce the risk of SIDS is necessary to recognize the correct response. Review SIDS and developmental milestones for a 2-month-old now if you had difficulty with this question!

Level of Cognitive Ability: Application
Phase of Nursing Process: Implementation
Client Needs: Safe, Effective Care Environment
Content Area: Child Health

Reference

Wong, D. (1997). *Whaley and Wong's Essentials of pediatric nursing* (5th ed.). St. Louis: Mosby–Year Book, p. 353.

---

88. As the nurse prepares to change an abdominal dressing on a 15-year-old, the client refuses to allow the nurse to proceed and says, "Leave me alone. The dressing is fine." The best response is

1. "You can refuse if you want to, but I'll have to do it later anyway."
2. "Why are you upset with me? I am here to help you."
3. "This will only take a few minutes, then you can be alone."
4. "I'll close the door and expose only the incision for the dressing. Can I do that now?"

Answer: 4

Rationale: The correct response shows respect for the primary concerns of the hospitalized adolescent by assuring privacy, modesty, and control. The other options do not respond to these issues and show lack of respect.

Test-Taking Strategy: In communication questions, the correct response focuses on client's feelings and needs. Responses with communication blocks can be eliminated, such as those of options 1, 2, and 3. Remember the issues related to the developmental stages of adolescence in answering the question, and review these issues now if you had difficulty with this question!

Level of Cognitive Ability: Application
Phase of Nursing Process: Implementation
Client Needs: Psychosocial Integrity
Content Area: Child Health

Reference

Ball, J., & Bindler, R. (1995). *Pediatric nursing: Caring for children.* Stamford, CT: Appleton & Lange, p. 153.

---

89. The nurse enters the room of a client who begins to discuss anger toward the spouse after an argument on the telephone. Which of the following statements by the nurse would be a barrier to effective communication with the client?

1 "You seem quite upset."
2 "Do you and your wife have frequent arguments?"
3 "Every couple has their share of arguments."
4 "Would you like to talk about this incident?"

Answer: 3

Rationale: Option 3 is a stereotypical comment. Such comments imply a lack of understanding of a client's uniqueness and create or maintain distance between the nurse and the client. Option 1 acknowledges the client's distress; option 2 attempts to obtain further information; and option 4 provides an opportunity for the client to discuss feelings.

Test-Taking Strategy: Therapeutic communication techniques address the client's concerns, feelings, or seek to elicit further information. Note the word "barrier" in the question. You can easily eliminate options 1 and 4. From the remaining two options, although option 2 may not be the best statement, option 3 is definitely a stereotypical comment and therefore is the answer to the question as stated. Avoid responding to clients in ways that will block communication, such as stereotypical responses.

Level of Cognitive Ability: Application
Phase of Nursing Process: Implementation
Client Needs: Psychosocial Integrity
Content Area: Fundamental Skills

Reference

Haber, J. (1997). *Comprehensive psychiatric nursing* (5th ed.). St. Louis: Mosby–Year Book, p. 139.

---

90. A client is admitted with a diagnosis of anxiety disorder. The client says to the nurse, "I came in to get away from the pressure at home." Which of the following nursing responses would be best to use in this introductory meeting with the client?

1 "I'm glad you came into the hospital at this time."
2 "Can you tell me what made you feel overwhelmed at home?"
3 "We will be able to help you here in the hospital."
4 "What are your feelings about being hospitalized?"

Answer: 2

Rationale: Option 2 seeks to obtain further specific information from the client regarding stresses that led to the client's hospitalization by offering a general lead. Obtaining information is an important aspect of the nursing assessment when the client is initially hospitalized. Options 3 and 4 introduce an unrelated topic. Option 1 is giving approval or praise, which may hinder the client's learning because the client may seek to gain the nurse's approval rather than focus on learning.

Test-Taking Strategy: When answering communication questions, use of therapeutic communication techniques must be used. You can easily eliminate options 1 and 3. For the remaining two options, in this question, it is important to recognize that this is an introductory meeting, when assessment of the client's reasons for admission is indicated. Option 2 specifically addresses the issue of the question.

Level of Cognitive Ability: Application
Phase of Nursing Process: Implementation
Client Needs: Psychosocial Integrity
Content Area: Mental Health

Reference

Carson, V., & Arnold, E. (1996). *Mental health nursing: The nurse-patient journey.* Philadelphia: W. B. Saunders, p. 696.

91. The nurse is teaching a mother about follow-up care for her 6-month-old, who just received a third diphtheria, tetanus, and pertussis (DTP) immunization. The nurse should stress that

1 Mild reactions may occur 1 week after the injection.
2 Aspirin should be used prophylactically for discomfort.
3 Any unusual side effects should be reported immediately to the physician.
4 The child should avoid contact with immunosuppressed individuals.

Answer: 3

Rationale: Although unusual side effects are rare, they are potentially serious and need immediate attention. All the other options are incorrect. Mild reactions occur between the first few hours and the first few days. Aspirin is not given to children because of the risk of Reye's syndrome. Option 4 is applicable only when live viruses are administered.

Test-Taking Strategy: Use the process of elimination. Eliminate option 2 first because aspirin should not be administered. Eliminate option 4 because this statement is applicable only when live viruses are administered. For the remaining two options, note the phrase "occur 1 week after" in option 1. This is an unlikely time for a reaction to occur. Thus option 3 is the best response!

Level of Cognitive Ability: Application
Phase of Nursing Process: Implementation
Client Needs: Physiological Integrity
Content Area: Child Health

Reference

Wong, D. (1997). *Whaley and Wong's Essentials of pediatric nursing* (5th ed.). St. Louis: Mosby–Year Book, p. 318.

---

92. When teaching the postmenopausal client breast self-examination (BSE), the nurse teaches the client to

1 Always begin BSE on the right breast first.
2 Palpate the breasts before inspection.
3 Perform BSE on the same day every month.
4 Call the physician if breasts are not the same size.

Answer: 3

Rationale: From 5–10 days after the first day of menses is the best time for BSE. After menopause, BSE needs to continue once a month and should be done on the same day of the month for ease in remembering to do so. BSE may begin on either breast but is usually performed on the left breast first. As with nursing assessments, inspection is the first step in BSE. Breasts of unequal size are common; changes in size or contour are findings that should be reported to the practitioner.

Test-Taking Strategy: Eliminate option 1 because of the word "always." Eliminate option 2, remembering that of the steps of assessment, inspection is first! Eliminate option 4 because it is not abnormal for breasts to be unequal in size. Review the process of BSE now if you had difficulty with this question!

Level of Cognitive Ability: Application
Phase of Nursing Process: Implementation
Client Needs: Health Promotion and Maintenance
Content Area: Adult Health/Oncology

Reference

Black, J., & Matassarin-Jacobs, E. (1997). *Medical-surgical nursing: Clinical management for continuity of care* (5th ed.). Philadelphia: W. B. Saunders, pp. 2314–2315.

---

93. The nurse is caring for a client who has recently undergone bilateral adrenalectomy. Which of the following actions by the nurse represents appropriate care for this client?

1 Restricting fluid intake
2 Monitoring blood glucose
3 Encouraging calcium intake
4 Observing color of the stools

Answer: 2

Rationale: Adrenal insufficiency can result in hypoglycemia. Aldosterone insufficiency can result in hypovolemia. Options 3 and 4 are unrelated to adrenal insufficiency.

Test-Taking Strategy: Knowledge of the function of adrenocortical hormones will assist you in selecting the correct option. Take time now to review the care of a client after adrenalectomy if you had difficulty with this question!

Level of Cognitive Ability: Application
Phase of Nursing Process: Implementation
Client Needs: Physiological Integrity
Content Area: Adult Health/Endocrine

Reference

LeMone, P., & Burke, K. (1996). *Medical-surgical nursing: Critical thinking in client care.* Menlo Park, CA: Addison-Wesley, pp. 696, 697.

---

94. A client with hypothyroidism asks the nurse why it is necessary to take levothyroxine sodium (Synthroid). The best response is that this medication

1 Increases energy level.
2 Promotes weight gain.
3 Decreases body temperature.
4 Inhibits acid production.

Answer: 1

Rationale: Synthroid is a synthetically prepared thyroid hormone that increases body metabolism. It also promotes weight loss and increases body temperature. It does not affect acid production.

Test-Taking Strategy: Use the process of elimination. Remember the concepts related to *hypo*thyroidism. Medication is administered because of the "hypo" effects that this disorder causes. If you are unfamiliar with the clinical manifestations associated with hypothyroidism and the effects of levothyroxine sodium (Synthroid), review now. You are likely to find a question related to this medication on NCLEX-RN!

Level of Cognitive Ability: Application
Phase of Nursing Process: Implementation
Client Needs: Physiological Integrity
Content Area: Adult Health/Endocrine

Reference

Wilson, B., Shannon, M., & Stang, C. (1997). *Nurses drug guide.* Stamford, CT: Appleton & Lange, pp. 774, 775.

---

95. When assisting a client who has had a cerebrovascular accident (CVA) to eat, the nurse can promote independence by which of the following actions?

1 Offer only pureed foods
2 Sit the client in high Fowler's position
3 Allow the client to participate in feeding self as much as possible in eating
4 Encourage the client to eat with other clients who have had a CVA

Answer: 3

Rationale: Independence is promoted by allowing the client to have control in a given situation. Options 1, 2, and 4 do not offer the client control. Option 3 promotes a self-care activity.

Test-Taking Strategy: Note the key phrase "promote independence." "Independence" means freedom from the help of others. Promoting independence is similar to allowing the client to participate. Option 3 is the only option focusing on client action and promoting independence!

Level of Cognitive Ability: Application
Phase of Nursing Process: Implementation
Client Needs: Psychosocial Integrity
Content Area: Fundamental Skills

Reference

Black, J., & Matassarin-Jacobs, E. (1997). *Medical-surgical nursing: Clinical management for continuity of care* (5th ed.). Philadelphia: W. B. Saunders, p. 796.

---

96. Which of the following is the priority action by the nurse when initiating an intermittent enteral feeding?

1 Measuring intake and output
2 Weighing the client
3 Adding blue food coloring to the formula to aid in diagnosing aspiration
4 Determining tube placement

Answer: 4

Rationale: Initiating a tube feeding without checking tube placement can lead to serious complications such as aspiration. Options 1 and 2 are part of the total plan of care for a client on enteral feedings but are not priorities. Option 3 is instituted for a client who has been identified as being at high risk for aspiration.

Test-Taking Strategy: The question is directed toward client safety. Options 3 and 4 address safety issues. In the steps of the nursing process, assessment is done before action; thus option 4 is the correct answer because it is the only option that addresses an assessment. Review content on enteral feedings now if you had difficulty answering this question!

Level of Cognitive Ability: Application
Phase of Nursing Process: Implementation
Client Needs: Safe, Effective Care Environment
Content Area: Fundamental Skills

References

Burrell, P., Gerlach, M., & Pless, B. (1997). *Adult nursing: Acute and community care* (2nd ed.). Stamford, CT: Appleton & Lange, p. 1346.

---

97. The client with chronic pancreatitis is preparing for discharge from the hospital. While reviewing the discharge order with the nurse, the client says, "I hope I can handle all this at home. It's a lot to remember." The nurse's best response would be

1 "I'm sure you can do it. You're a very smart person."
2 "Maybe we should arrange for you to stay in the hospital one more day."
3 "Oh, your sister can take care of it for you."
4 "You seem to be nervous about going home."

Answer: 4

Rationale: Option 4 uses the technique of attempting to reflect the client's feelings in words that encourage the client to verbalize feelings. Options 1 and 3 devalue the client's feelings, and option 2 attempts to give advice.

Test-Taking Strategy: Always select the answer that not only acknowledges the client's feelings but also further explores and encourages the client to ventilate feelings. Always address the client's feelings and concerns!

Level of Cognitive Ability: Application
Phase of Nursing Process: Implementation
Client Needs: Psychosocial Integrity
Content Area: Fundamental Skills

Reference

Townsend, M. (1996). *Psychiatric mental health nursing: Concepts of care* (2nd ed.). Philadelphia: F. A. Davis, p. 107.

---

98. Clients experiencing negative symptoms of schizophrenia may exhibit retarded motor processes. When helping such a client with personal hygiene and grooming, the nurse should

1 Suggest that the client bathe and dress in a hospital gown.
2 Encourage the client to bathe and dress quickly.
3 Allow the client time to choose attractive clothing after bathing.
4 Assist the client with personal hygiene and dress needs.

Answer: 4

Rationale: Negative symptoms denote a lessening or complete loss of normal functions such as grooming. Clients often respond slowly to nursing interactions. Nurses need to design interventions that address the specific self-care problem. Option 1 is degrading and not reality based. Option 2 ignores the increased time needed for action after processing information. Option 3 does not recognize that clients with schizophrenia experience decreased decision-making ability.

Test-Taking Strategy: Knowledge of abnormal motor behaviors involved in schizophrenia with negative symptoms is necessary in order for you to answer this question. The key phrase in the question is "retarded motor processes." This should provide you with the guidance to selecting option 4, which contains the key word "assist." Take time now to review nursing interventions specific to the client with schizophrenia if you had difficulty with this question!

Level of Cognitive Ability: Application
Phase of Nursing Process: Implementation
Client Needs: Physiological Integrity
Content Area: Mental Health

Reference

Haber, J. (1997). *Comprehensive psychiatric nursing* (5th ed.). St. Louis: Mosby–Year Book, pp. 573, 593, 597.

99. A hospitalized 19-year-old female pianist wanders in and out of other client rooms, taking their possessions while singing to herself, and then giggles for no apparent reason. The nurse, recognizing the severe regression of the client and the difficulty with limit setting, chooses which of the following actions?

1 Putting her arms around the client saying, "You're okay. You just need a hug."
2 Taking the client to seclusion until she cooperates with unit rules.
3 Saying, "I can see you are very anxious today. Let's go and play the piano."
4 Taking her to the lounge saying, "Sit here and behave yourself."

Answer: 3

Rationale: Regression allows the threatened client to move backward developmentally to a stage at which more security is felt. The recognition of regression is a signal that the client feels anxious. The first category of response is to help the client feel less anxious. Severe anxiety allows decompensation of ego functions so that the client is overwhelmed and thus should not be left alone. Option 3 does not isolate the client and directs the client's focus to a nonthreatening activity.

Test-Taking Strategy: To answer this question accurately, you must know the role of defense mechanisms in altering anxiety. Their use permits a person to avoid the painful experience of anxiety or to transform it into a more tolerable symptom such as regression. Because anxiety consumes energy, it can be redirected into a healthier task. Note the relationship of the word "pianist" in the question and the phrase "Let's go and play the piano" in the correct response!

Level of Cognitive Ability: Application
Phase of Nursing Process: Implementation
Client Needs: Psychosocial Integrity
Content Area: Mental Health

Reference

Carson, V., & Arnold, E. (1996). *Mental health nursing: The nurse-patient journey.* Philadelphia: W. B. Saunders, pp. 696–97.

---

100. The client with hyperparathyroidism has just finished speaking with the physician about surgery. The client says to the nurse, "I'm not sure that I want my neck cut open!" The most appropriate response by the nurse is which of the following?

1 "There is no reason to worry. The surgeon is a wonderful doctor!"
2 "You are very ill. Your doctor has made the right decision."
3 "I think you will feel much healthier postoperatively."
4 "Can you tell me more about what you are thinking?"

Answer: 4

Rationale: Focusing on the client helps promote effective communication within a therapeutic relationship. Option 4 is paraphrasing the client's message in the nurse's own words and allows the client and nurse to continue the discussion. The other options are blocks to communication and are not therapeutic.

Test-Taking Strategy: Therapeutic communication techniques enhance the nurse-client relationship to effect a positive outcome. Options 1, 2, and 3 do not provide opportunities for the client to discuss concerns but rather "dead-end" the discussion. Option 4 promotes the conversation. Always select the option that addresses clients' concerns and feelings!

Level of Cognitive Ability: Application
Phase of Nursing Process: Implementation
Client Needs: Psychosocial Integrity
Content Area: Adult Health/Endocrine

Reference

Potter, P., & Perry, A. (1997). *Fundamentals of nursing: Concepts, process, and practice* (4th ed.). St. Louis: Mosby–Year Book, pp. 242, 244–245.

---

101. An insulin-dependent diabetic client notifies the nurse that he or she is having a hypoglycemic reaction. Which of the following foods would the nurse select as the best treatment choice for this problem?

1 4 oz of diet cola
2 8 oz of black coffee with 1 teaspoon of sugar
3 4 oz of orange juice
4 Peanut butter crackers

Answer: 3

Rationale: Reversal of hypoglycemia requires a 10- to 15-g simple carbohydrate load to work quickly to increase the blood glucose levels. Options 1, 2, and 4 do not provide sufficient simple carbohydrates and thus cannot produce a quick rise in the glucose levels.

Test-Taking Strategy: Remember that in treatment of hypoglycemia, the goal is to raise the glucose levels in the blood. Three of the four options are liquids; thus you could eliminate option 4 simply because it would take too long to work. Diet cola doesn't contain sugar, so option 1 can be eliminated next. The question asks what is the "best" treatment. Option 3 has more sugar than option 2, and therefore it is the best selection.

Level of Cognitive Ability: Application
Phase of Nursing Process: Implementation
Client Needs: Physiological Integrity
Content Area: Adult Health/Endocrine

Reference

Black, J., & Matassarin-Jacobs, E. (1997). *Medical-surgical nursing: Clinical management for continuity of care* (5th ed.). Philadelphia: W. B. Saunders, p. 1989.

---

102. The family of a client with myxedema is extremely distressed about how the disease is affecting the client's intellectual functions, with manifestations such as impaired memory, inattentiveness, and lethargy. Which of the following statements would be most appropriate for the nurse to make?

1. "It sounds as though the disease is in the advanced stage, and unfortunately the symptoms are irreversible."
2. "Don't worry! I've taken care of similar clients before. All will be fine."
3. "I can see that you are concerned, but these symptoms are normal with myxedema and should improve with therapy."
4. "Would you like me to let the physician know about this so a tranquilizer can be prescribed?"

Answer: 3

Rationale: The nurse acknowledges the family's concerns and relates that the behaviors presented by the client are classical neurological manifestations of myxedema. With thyroid hormone therapy, these symptoms should decrease, and mentation usually returns to normal within 2 weeks. There is no indication that the myxedema has advanced to a crisis stage. Option 2 offers false reassurance and ignores the concerns of the family, thereby blocking further communication. Option 4 doesn't address their concerns but instead requires the family to make a decision. This option is not appropriate and indicates that the nurse does not understand the disease.

Test-Taking Strategy: Remember that therapeutic communication techniques are the answers to questions regarding responses to a client or family. Therapeutic communication techniques enhance communication because they address the concerns of the client or family as presented in option 3. Also, remember that in myxedema, neurological symptoms are reversible with the appropriate therapy.

Level of Cognitive Ability: Application
Phase of Nursing Process: Implementation
Client Needs: Psychosocial Integrity
Content Area: Adult Health/Endocrine

Reference

Ignatavicius, D. D., Workman, M. L., & Mishler, M. A. (1995). *Medical-surgical nursing: A nursing process approach* (2nd ed.). Philadelphia: W. B. Saunders, pp. 1847–1848.

---

103. The client with a goiter has a subtotal thyroidectomy. Which of the following interventions would best enable the nurse to assess the incision for bleeding?

1. Applying Montgomery straps at the incision area
2. Redressing the incision every 2 hours, using strict aseptic technique
3. Loosening the tapes at both ends of the dressing if the client complains of "tightness" at the incision
4. Slipping a hand behind the client's neck and depressing the mattress to inspect for blood on the neck or linens

Answer: 4

Rationale: Because of the anatomical location of the gland and the effects of gravity, the nurse should inspect for bleeding around the back of the client's neck. If the client is hemorrhaging, blood will usually leak down the sides of the incision and saturate the bed linens, whereas the anterior dressing will remain clean and dry. The application of Montgomery straps simply decreases tissue irritation caused by frequent removal of the tape. Redressing the incision every 2 hours, even under aseptic technique, is not of value when trying to assess whether the client is hemorrhaging. Complaints of "tightness" may indicate swelling.

Test-Taking Strategy: Focus on key words such as "best enable the nurse." Recalling principles of postoperative incision care will assist you when answering this question. The type of dressing or how it is applied does not help the nurse to assess for bleeding. Instead, recall that because of the location of the incision and in the presence of bleeding, it will flow to the back of the neck and "pool" on the mattress, whereas the anterior portion of the dressing will remain dry and intact.

Level of Cognitive Ability: Application
Phase of Nursing Process: Implementation
Client Needs: Physiological Integrity
Content Area: Adult Health/Endocrine

Reference

Ignatavicius, D. D., Workman, M. L., & Mishler, M. A. (1995). *Medical-surgical nursing: A nursing process approach* (2nd ed.). Philadelphia: W. B. Saunders, pp. 1840–1842.

---

104. Which of the following nursing activities would most likely prevent the occurrence of respiratory infection?

1 Encouraging chronically ill clients to obtain both influenza and pneumococcal vaccines
2 Placing clients with altered consciousness in side-lying positions
3 Repositioning immobile clients every 2 hours
4 Using strict asepsis while performing endotracheal suctioning

Answer: 4

Rationale: Strict surgical asepsis must be adhered to while the nurse performs endotracheal suctioning, in order to prevent the introduction of pathogens into the lung field. Influenza often progresses to pneumonia in chronically ill clients, so both vaccines are highly recommended. Repositioning immobile clients at least every 2 hours will help prevent orthostatic pneumonia. Clients who are unconscious need to be placed in positions (side-lying, Fowler's) that will help minimize the possibility of aspiration pneumonia.

Test-Taking Strategy: Note the key phrase "most likely." This indicates that more than one option may be correct and that you need to prioritize in order to select the correct option. Options 1, 2, and 3 all are basic nursing strategies used for preventing pneumonia. It is important to remember that when a body cavity is entered, strict asepsis is of paramount importance in order to prevent the possibility of infection. Option 4 is the only option that addresses an invasive procedure.

Level of Cognitive Ability: Application
Phase of Nursing Process: Implementation
Client Needs: Physiological Integrity
Content Area: Adult Health/Respiratory

Reference

Lewis, S., Collier, I., & Heitkemper, M. (1996). *Medical-surgical nursing: Assessment and management of clinical problems* (4th ed.). St. Louis: Mosby–Year Book, pp. 631–633.

---

105. The nurse is caring for a client with acute respiratory distress syndrome (ARDS) who is being mechanically ventilated and is experiencing problems with communication. Which of the following actions by the nurse would be inappropriate in fostering effective communication for this client?

1 Telling the client that communication will be impossible until the tube is removed
2 Providing easy accessibility to a call light
3 Expressing empathy for the client
4 Learning to read the client's body language

Answer: 1

Rationale: Although verbal communication is impossible for the intubated client, alternative means of communication should be tried. Alternative means may include the use of an alphabet board or pencil and paper. The call light will at least enable the client to summon assistance. Expressing empathy acknowledges that it is frustrating not to be able to speak. Learning to read the client's body language will ease the client's efforts to communicate.

Test-Taking Strategy: Note the key phrase in the stem "would be inappropriate." This question is asking for an inappropriate or false response. Absolute terminology such as "impossible" tends to make a statement false. In addition, communication by some means is not "impossible"!

Level of Cognitive Ability: Application
Phase of Nursing Process: Implementation
Client Needs: Psychosocial Integrity
Content Area: Adult Health/Respiratory

Reference

Lewis, S., Collier, I., & Heitkemper, M. (1996). *Medical-surgical nursing: Assessment and management of clinical problems* (4th ed.). St. Louis: Mosby–Year Book, p. 1985.

106. The client is an electrician and has just sustained a high-voltage electrical injury. The nurse notes that the urine color is dark, and laboratory results show that the urine is positive for myoglobin. Which of the following interventions would be appropriate at this time?

1 Elevate the head of the bed, administer oxygen by 100% non-rebreather mask, and prepare to intubate the client
2 Administer 1 mg/kg IV of lidocaine and prepare a lidocaine drip
3 Increase the rate of IV lactated Ringer's solution to maintain a urine output of 100–150 mL/hour
4 Insert a nasogastric tube and prepare an iced-saline lavage

Answer: 3

Rationale: To prevent myoglobin from precipitating in the renal tubules, the IV rate is increased to maintain a urine output of 100–150 mL/hour until the urine is grossly clear of myoglobin. The other responses are incorrect because myoglobin does not affect the respiratory system, the cardiovascular system, or the gastrointestinal system.

Test-Taking Strategy: Myoglobinuria is a common finding after significant electrical injury or other significant muscular trauma. To answer this question accurately, it is necessary to know that a potential complication of myoglobinuria is acute tubular necrosis. IV rate is increased to clear myoglobin from the kidneys. Note the relationship of the issue "urine" in the question to "urine output" in the correct option!

Level of Cognitive Ability: Application
Phase of Nursing Process: Implementation
Client Needs: Physiological Integrity
Content Area: Adult Health/Integumentary

Reference

Black, J., & Matassarin-Jacobs, E. (1997). *Medical-surgical nursing: Clinical management for continuity of care* (5th ed.). Philadelphia: W. B. Saunders, p. 2236.

---

107. A client with Parkinson's disease expresses embarrassment because of tremors and drooling and states that he or she no longer wants to be seen in public. Which of the following responses by the nurse is most appropriate?

1 "You shouldn't feel that way; it's not that noticeable."
2 "You should just ignore the people who are staring at you."
3 "It must be difficult for you; would you like to talk about your concerns?"
4 "Don't worry; lots of people have disabilities."

Answer: 3

Rationale: The correct response shows empathy and offers assistance by the nurse. Options 1 and 4 devalue the client's feelings and offer false reassurance. Option 2 offers advice.

Test-Taking Strategy: Empathy and offering assistance are positive tools that encourage client communication. Devaluing feelings, giving advice, and offering false reassurance are blocks to effective communication. Always address clients' feelings first!

Level of Cognitive Ability: Application
Phase of Nursing Process: Implementation
Client Needs: Psychosocial Integrity
Content Area: Adult Health/Neurological

Reference

Lewis, S., Collier, I., & Heitkemper, M. (1996). *Medical-surgical nursing: Assessment and management of clinical problems* (4th ed.). St. Louis: Mosby–Year Book, pp. 1771–1774.

---

108. A client with Parkinson's disease is concerned because of tremors and asks the nurse what can be done to minimize them. Which of the following responses by the nurse would be most appropriate while implementing care for this client?

1 "There is nothing much that can be done to diminish them."
2 "Once the L-dopa is working, they will stop completely."
3 "Try sitting, with your hands resting on your lap or a table."
4 "Try grasping coins in your pocket or holding onto the arm of a chair."

Answer: 4

Rationale: Clients with Parkinson's disease generally have resting tremors, and the tremor diminishes with voluntary activity. Tremors also diminish with medications, and although they improve with L-dopa, they do not stop completely. Tremors are worse at rest.

Test-Taking Strategy: Options 1 and 2 contain absolute words ("nothing" and "completely"), which tend to make those responses incorrect. Options 3 and 4 are opposite of each other, which indicates that one of them may be correct. Remembering that tremors diminish with voluntary activities will assist in directing you to the correct option!

Level of Cognitive Ability: Application
Phase of Nursing Process: Implementation
Client Needs: Health Promotion and Maintenance
Content Area: Adult Health/Neurological

Reference

Polaski, A., & Tatro, S. (1996). *Luckmann's Core principles and practice of medical-surgical nursing.* Philadelphia: W. B. Saunders, p. 379.

109. Which of the following information is most important for the nurse to review with the male client who is about to undergo treatment for Hodgkin's disease?

1 Heat caps for alopecia
2 Sperm banking
3 Vital sign measurement
4 Mask use to prevent spread of infection

Answer: 2

Rationale: Permanent sterility for males is a side effect of radiation to the abdominopelvic region as a treatment for Hodgkin's disease. Because the incidence of Hodgkin's disease peaks in clients in their middle to late 20s, fertility is an important issue.

Test-Taking Strategy: Knowing that radiation is a treatment for Hodgkin's disease is essential to answer the question. Ice caps instead of heat caps are used for alopecia. Eliminate option 4 because masks in cancer clients are used to protect the client, not to prevent the client from spreading infection. Vital signs may be important but do not relate to the issue of the question. Noting the key word "male" in the question may assist in directing you to the correct option.

Level of Cognitive Ability: Application
Phase of Nursing Process: Implementation
Client Needs: Physiological Integrity
Content Area: Adult Health/Oncology

Reference

Ignatavicius, D. D., Workman, M. L., & Mishler, M. A. (1995). *Medical-surgical nursing: A nursing process approach* (2nd ed.). Philadelphia: W. B. Saunders, pp. 1069–1070.

110. Nursing management for a client with Bell's palsy includes which of the following?

1 Applying warm packs to the affected side
2 Vigorous massaging of the affected side
3 Encouraging the client to chew on the affected side
4 Instilling artificial tears only at bedtime

Answer: 1

Rationale: Warm packs have been found to be an effective measure in treating Bell's palsy. Vigorous massage can be harmful, whereas gentle massage can help. Clients should be encouraged to chew on the unaffected side. Artificial tears should be used frequently throughout the day and at bedtime.

Test-Taking Strategy: "Vigorous" (option 2) and "only" (option 4) are examples of extreme or absolute terms and are usually incorrect. For the remaining two options, note the phrase "chew on the affected side" in option 3. Because symptoms are worse on the affected side, the client should not chew on that side. Review nursing interventions for Bell's palsy now if you had difficulty with this question!

Level of Cognitive Ability: Application
Phase of Nursing Process: Implementation
Client Needs: Physiological Integrity
Content Area: Adult Health/Neurological

Reference

Polaski, A., & Tatro, S. (1996). *Luckmann's Core principles and practice of medical-surgical nursing.* Philadelphia: W. B. Saunders, p. 416.

111. A mother with insulin-dependent diabetes mellitus (IDDM) questions the nurse about the need to perform a heel puncture for the frequent blood glucose screening on her infant. The nurse's best response to the mother is which of the following?

1. "The doctor ordered them. It's only a little stick."
2. "Don't worry about them. They are covered by insurance."
3. "It bothers you to have the baby stuck so often. It is painful. However, it is necessary to see how the baby's blood glucose is doing."
4. "If you ask me, I would be much more concerned with your baby's breathing. Did you notice how the baby is breathing so fast?"

Answer: 3

Rationale: Most mothers are very concerned about any painful procedure performed on their infants. Option 3 is correct because the nurse reflects the perceived feelings of the mother, validates that the procedure is painful, and then provides the correct rationale for the procedure. Most infants of IDDM mothers are monitored regularly for several hours or until the glucose levels are stable. Responses that distract, devalue the client's feelings, or are defensive should be avoided.

Test-Taking Strategy: When you answer communication questions, the correct answer will include addressing the client's feelings and concerns, restatement, validation, and giving information. Communication blocks indicate an incorrect answer. These blocks include devaluing clients' feelings, placing the clients' issues on hold, or focusing on inappropriate issues. Always focus on the client's feelings first!

Level of Cognitive Ability: Application
Phase of Nursing Process: Implementation
Client Needs: Psychosocial Integrity
Content Area: Maternity

Reference

Nichols, F., & Zwelling, E. (1997). *Maternal-newborn nursing: Theory and practice.* Philadelphia: W. B. Saunders, pp. 1357–1359.

---

112. The nurse caring for a client with trigeminal neuralgia should implement which of the following activities?

1. Gently massaging the affected side
2. Applying cold packs to the affected side
3. Providing a water jet device for mouth care
4. Premedicating the client immediately before morning care

Answer: 3

Rationale: Tooth brushing can cause pain with trigeminal neuralgia, and a water pick and/or warm mouthwash should be used instead. Massage and exposure to cold can increase pain. Morning care should be carried out when effects of pain medication peak.

Test-Taking Strategy: Eliminate option 4, noting the phrase "immediately before." Extremes of temperature and touch can trigger pain in clients with trigeminal neuralgia. Also, note that options 1 and 2 address the "affected side." Take time now to review the interventions for trigeminal neuralgia if you had difficulty with this question!

Level of Cognitive Ability: Application
Phase of Nursing Process: Implementation
Client Needs: Physiological Integrity
Content Area: Adult Health/Neurological

Reference

Black, J., & Matassarin-Jacobs, E. (1997). *Medical-surgical nursing: Clinical management for continuity of care* (5th ed.). Philadelphia: W. B. Saunders, p. 930.

---

113. A client who has just undergone parathyroidectomy returns to the room. The nurse checks the client's blood pressure and finds it to be 90/60, with an apical pulse of 102. The nurse's first action would be to

1. Take the vital signs again.
2. Place the client in a Trendelenburg position.
3. Check the back of the dressing for bleeding.
4. Notify the physician of the findings.

Answer: 3

Rationale: A decrease in blood pressure and tachycardia could indicate postoperative bleeding. Bleeding is considered to be a complication of a parathyroidectomy. Often bleeding cannot be observed on the front of the dressing, because it trickles around the neck to the back. Therefore, it is important for the nurse to check the front, sides, and back of the dressing and the sheets underneath the neck.

Test-Taking Strategy: Always think of bleeding as a crisis and therefore a priority situation. Nursing interventions must be implemented in order of importance. Although the other options may be performed at some point, assessment of bleeding (a complication of parathyroidectomy) must be done first. The question asks you the first action after discovering hypotension and tachycardia. Further evaluation of the bleeding is the correct action. Option 3 addresses assessment, the first step of the nursing process!

Level of Cognitive Ability: Application
Phase of Nursing Process: Implementation
Client Needs: Physiological Integrity
Content Area: Adult Health/Endocrine

Reference

Ignatavicius, D. D., Workman, M. L., & Mishler, M. A. (1995). *Medical-surgical nursing: A nursing process approach* (2nd ed.). Philadelphia: W. B. Saunders, pp. 1840–1842.

---

114. A newborn is admitted to intensive care for respiratory distress syndrome (RDS). Which of the following nursing interventions is most effective in keeping the infant's oxygen consumption as low as possible?

1 Maintain a neutral thermal environment
2 Interpret blood gases
3 Assess for equal and bilateral breath sounds
4 Do heel sticks for blood glucose screening

Answer: 1

Rationale: Every effort should be made to maintain the infant in a neutral thermal environment. Oxygen consumption increases rapidly at temperatures above or below the neutral thermal range. Handling the newborn, which includes auscultation of breath sounds and heel sticks, stimulates movement and oxygen consumption. Interpretation of blood gases is diagnostic; they indicate the effectiveness of interventions that have been used.

Test-Taking Strategy: Identify the key phrase that indicates the need for you to prioritize, which is "most effective" in this question. Focusing on the issue of the question, keeping the infant's oxygen consumption as low as possible, will assist in directing you to the correct option!

Level of Cognitive Ability: Application
Phase of Nursing Process: Implementation
Client Needs: Physiological Integrity
Content Area: Maternity

References

Ashwill, J., & Droske, S. (1997). *Nursing care of children: Principles and practice.* Philadelphia: W. B. Saunders, pp. 550–556.
Nichols, F., & Zwelling, E. (1997). *Maternal-newborn nursing: Theory and practice.* Philadelphia: W. B. Saunders, pp. 1340–1345.

---

115. To help prevent the transmission of human immunodeficiency virus (HIV) from an HIV-positive woman to her baby during the intrapartum period, the nurse needs to initiate measures to avoid

1 Cesarean birth.
2 Intrauterine pressure catheter insertion.
3 Epidural anesthesia.
4 Direct (internal) fetal heart rate monitoring.

Answer: 4

Rationale: Health care professionals must use caution during the intrapartal period to reduce the risk of the transmission of HIV to the fetus. Any procedure that exposes blood or body fluids from the mother to the fetus should be avoided. It is important for nurses to guard against procedures that would result in a loss of skin integrity and expose the fetus to maternal blood or body fluids. Direct (internal) fetal monitoring is a procedure that may expose the fetus to maternal blood or body fluids and therefore should be avoided.

Test-Taking Strategy: Knowledge of how HIV is transmitted is necessary to answer this question. All the options address invasive procedures that may take place during the intrapartum period, but only option 4 is invasive with regard to the fetus. Knowing that transmission of HIV occurs primarily by the exchange of body fluids should assist you in selecting the correct option. If you do not know the answer, look for a similar word or phrase in the stem or case situation and in one of the options. In this question, the similarity of thought is preventing transmission of HIV to the fetus and direct (internal) fetal monitoring.

Level of Cognitive Ability: Application
Phase of Nursing Process: Implementation
Client Needs: Physiological Integrity
Content Area: Maternity

Reference

Nichols, F., & Zwelling, E. (1997). *Maternal-newborn nursing: Theory and practice.* Philadelphia: W. B. Saunders, p. 1500.

116. Which intervention should the nurse implement when caring for a client with pregnancy-induced hypertension (PIH) who is exhibiting the potential for grand mal seizures?

1 Teach the woman and her support person how to assess vital signs
2 Pad side rails and take seizure precautions
3 Assess breath sounds
4 Assess laboratory results

Answer: 2

Rationale: The nurse caring for a client with PIH who is demonstrating the potential for grand mal seizures should pad the side rails and take seizure precautions to provide a safe and effective care environment. Teaching is an intervention not directly related to the presenting symptoms (grand mal seizure). Options 3 and 4 do not relate specifically to the issue of the question!

Test-Taking Strategy: Identify the issue of the question which is the potential for grand mal seizures. The only option that relates specifically to this issue is option 2.

Level of Cognitive Ability: Application
Phase of Nursing Process: Implementation
Client Needs: Safe, Effective Care Environment
Content Area: Maternity

Reference
Olds, S., London, M., & Ladewig, P. (1996). *Clinical handbook for maternal-newborn nursing: A family-centered approach* (5th ed.). Menlo Park, CA: Addison-Wesley, pp. 40–47.

---

117. The nurse is caring for a child with increased intracranial pressure after a head trauma resulting from a motor vehicle accident. The child is scheduled for a craniotomy because of a depressed skull fracture. In the preoperative period, the primary nursing action would be to monitor

1 Pupillary responses to light.
2 Urine for protein and glucose.
3 Urinary specific gravity greater than 1.030.
4 Orthostatic blood pressures.

Answer: 1

Rationale: Pupil checks, with a flashlight, assess the pressure that is present. Urine is not positive for glucose and protein in the presence of cerebral trauma. Specific gravity is maintained between 1.002 and 1.030 for fluid balance in the body. Syndrome of inappropriate antidiuretic hormone (SIADH) is a complication of head trauma, and the specific gravity can drop to 1.000 with this complication, not rise. The best positioning for this child is to elevate the head at least 30 degrees to decrease the amount of cerebral edema. The nurse would monitor for an increase in pulse pressure.

Test-Taking Strategy: Focus on the option that specifically addresses neurological assessment. Option 1 specifically addresses a component of neurological assessment. Although monitoring blood pressure is important, monitoring for an increase in pulse pressure, not orthostatic pressure, is the focus.

Level of Cognitive Ability: Application
Phase of Nursing Process: Implementation
Client Needs: Physiological Integrity
Content Area: Child Health

Reference
Ashwill, J., & Droske, S. (1997). *Nursing care of children: Principles and practice.* Philadelphia: W. B. Saunders, pp. 1260–1262.

---

118. A client with Parkinson's disease has a nursing diagnosis of Self Care Deficit: Feeding related to tremor, rigidity, and bradykinesia. Which of the following medications should the nurse administer as prescribed to control these symptoms?

1 Phenytoin (Dilantin)
2 Carbidopa-levodopa (Sinemet)
3 Pyridostigmine (Mestinon)
4 Warfarin (Coumadin)

Answer: 2

Rationale: Tremor, rigidity, and bradykinesia are three classic manifestations of Parkinson's disease. One of the medications frequently used for treatment is Sinemet. Dilantin is an anticonvulsant and antidysrhythmic. Mestinon is a cholinergic often used to treat myasthenia gravis. Coumadin is an anticoagulant.

Test-Taking Strategy: In Parkinson's disease, the underlying interference is a lack of dopamine in the brain. Sinemet is a combination medication. Levodopa is a precursor of dopamine, and carbidopa prevents large amounts of levodopa breakdown before it passes the blood-brain barrier. The other medications are of other classifications but can be used for clients with different neurological difficulties. Take time now to review this action of this medication if you had difficulty with this question!

Level of Cognitive Ability: Application
Phase of Nursing Process: Implementation
Client Needs: Physiological Integrity
Content Area: Adult Health/Neurological

Reference

Black, J., & Matassarin-Jacobs, E. (1997). *Medical-surgical nursing: Clinical management for continuity of care* (5th ed.). Philadelphia: W. B. Saunders, p. 880.

---

119. The client is in a coma of unknown cause. The physician has just intubated the client. Which of the following procedures would the nurse withhold until the client was properly intubated?

1 Gastric lavage
2 Fingerstick for blood glucose level
3 Urethral catheterization
4 Venipuncture for complete blood cell (CBC) count

Answer: 1

Rationale: Intubation should always precede gastric lavage to prevent pulmonary aspiration. All other selections, although not priorities related to an effective and patent airway, could be initiated before intubation of client.

Test-Taking Strategy: The question addresses ability to identify priorities in caring for a client in a coma. Option 1 is the only test that could directly jeopardize client safety. Options 2, 3, and 4 are pertinent to early care of a comatose client. Use the process of elimination, considering the ABCs: airway, breathing, and circulation!

Level of Cognitive Ability: Application
Phase of Nursing Process: Implementation
Client Needs: Physiological Integrity
Content Area: Adult Health/Neurological

Reference

Ignatavicius, D. D., Workman, M. L., & Mishler, M. A. (1995). *Medical-surgical nursing: A nursing process approach* (2nd ed.). Philadelphia: W. B. Saunders, pp. 756–757.

---

120. Fetal/infant exposure to HIV from an HIV-positive mother can be decreased by use of certain procedures during the labor and delivery of the baby, assuming that the baby has not already contracted the virus. Which of the following procedures, if performed by the nurse, places the infant at risk for exposure to the virus?

1 Avoiding the use of forceps or vacuum extraction
2 Prompt bath of the newborn
3 Immediate administration of vitamin K
4 Discouraging breast-feeding

Answer: 3

Rationale: Vitamin K is routinely given to every newborn as an injection. However, any injection would need to wait until after the bath of the infant, when the skin is thoroughly cleansed. Newborns are covered with amniotic fluid, vernix, mucus, and maternal blood. Any of these fluids could contain the virus. An injection would take the virus directly into the host system. Avoiding the use of forceps and vacuum extractions helps avoid lacerations to the infant's scalp. A prompt bath removes the body fluids, and breast-feeding is discouraged because the virus can be transmitted through the breast milk to the baby.

Test-Taking Strategy: Carefully read the stem of the question, seeking the procedure, if performed by the nurse, that places the infant at risk for exposure to the virus. Remember that invasive procedures and exposure to body fluids place the infant at risk. With this concept in mind, select the invasive option, option 3!

Level of Cognitive Ability: Application
Phase of Nursing Process: Implementation
Client Needs: Safe, Effective Care Environment
Content Area: Maternity

Reference

Nichols, F., & Zwelling, E. (1997). *Maternal-newborn nursing: Theory and practice.* Philadelphia: W. B. Saunders, pp. 1187–1188.

121. A client is diagnosed with terminal carcinoma of the lung. The nurse is assisting the client to plan for the end-of-life issues. The most appropriate nursing intervention is to assist the client to

1 Describe all futile treatments before death.
2 Gain control over the end-of-life issues through advance directives.
3 Engage an attorney to sue the hospital upon death.
4 Direct the insurance company to pay all expenses upon death.

Answer: 2

Rationale: Option 2 is client centered and allows the client to have control of treatment. The word "all" indicates that option 1 may be incorrect. It is also a nontherapeutic intervention. There is no evidence that an attorney is necessary (option 3) because the stem gives no evidence of malpractice. Option 4 is incorrect because insurance companies have guidelines that provide for payment of death expenses.

Test-Taking Strategy: The key phrase in the stem is "plan for end-of-life issues." With this in mind, you may eliminate each of the incorrect options systematically and you should be easily directed toward option 2.

Level of Cognitive Ability: Application
Phase of Nursing Process: Implementation
Client Needs: Safe, Effective Care Environment
Content Area: Adult Health/Oncology

Reference
Ellis, J., & Hartley, C. (1995). *Nursing in today's world: Challenges, issues, and trends* (5th ed.). Philadelphia: Lippincott-Raven, p. 255.

---

122. A client receives a diagnosis of non–insulin-dependent diabetes mellitus (NIDDM) and is started on glyburide (Micronase), 2.5 mg PO QD. The client smiles and says, "Oh good, as long as I take this pill, I can eat whatever I want." In this situation, the nurse's intervention is focused to address which coping mechanism?

1 Denial
2 Anger
3 Depression
4 Acceptance

Answer: 1

Rationale: The client is denying the experience of a chronic illness that will require the client to make lifestyle changes. There is no evidence of anger or depression in the statement made by the client. The client has not accepted the disease if expectations are unrealistic.

Test-Taking Strategy: Use the process of elimination, focusing on the behaviors and client statement as identified in the question. This will assist in identifying the maladaptive coping mechanism being exhibited by the client. If you had difficulty with this question, take time now to review the definitions of these coping mechanism!

Level of Cognitive Ability: Application
Phase of Nursing Process: Implementation
Client Needs: Psychosocial Integrity
Content Area: Adult Health/Endocrine

Reference
Ignatavicius, D. D., Workman, M. L., & Mishler, M. A. (1995). *Medical-surgical nursing: A nursing process approach* (2nd ed.). Philadelphia: W. B. Saunders, pp. 1868–1869.

---

123. A manic client is placed in a seclusion room after an outburst of violent behavior that included physical assault on another client. As the client is being secluded, the nurse should

1 Remain silent because verbal interaction would be too stimulating.
2 Tell the client that he or she will be allowed to rejoin the others when he or she can behave.
3 Ask the client whether he or she understands why the seclusion is necessary.
4 Inform the client that he or she is being secluded to help regain control of self.

Answer: 4

Rationale: The client is removed to a nonstimulating environment as a result of behavior. Options 1, 2, and 3 are nontherapeutic. In addition, option 2 implies punishment. It is best to directly inform the client of the purpose of the seclusion.

Test-Taking Strategy: When answering a question as described, look for the response that presents reality most clearly to the client. Option 4 is the only option that provides a clear and direct purpose of the seclusion.

Level of Cognitive Ability: Application
Phase of Nursing Process: Implementation
Client Needs: Psychosocial Integrity
Content Area: Mental Health

Reference
Wilson, H., & Kneisl, C. (1996). *Psychiatric nursing* (5th ed.). Menlo Park, CA: Addison-Wesley, p. 831.

124. The nurse provides the manic client and family with instruction regarding lithium carbonate. The nurse tells the client and family that there is a narrow margin between therapeutic and toxic levels of lithium carbonate. The nurse alerts the client and family to which of the following as early signs of lithium toxicity?

1 Sore throat, runny nose, nonproductive cough, and neck pain
2 Night sweats, insomnia, restlessness, and itching
3 Vomiting, diarrhea, lethargy, and muscle twitching
4 Raised pink rash, fever, vomiting, and abnormal tongue movement

Answer: 3

Rationale: Early signs of lithium toxicity include vomiting, diarrhea, lethargy, and muscle twitching. Moderate toxicity results in ataxia, giddiness, tinnitus, blurred vision, clonic movements, and severe hypotension. Acute toxicity is characterized by seizures, oliguria, circulatory failure, and death.

Test-Taking Strategy: Knowledge of the signs characteristic of lithium toxicity is necessary to answer the question. If you had difficulty with this question, take time now to review these signs. You are likely to find a question related to the signs of lithium toxicity on NCLEX-RN!

Level of Cognitive Ability: Application
Phase of Nursing Process: Implementation
Client Needs: Physiological Integrity
Content Area: Mental Health

Reference
Wilson, H., & Kneisl, C. (1996). *Psychiatric nursing* (5th ed.). Menlo Park, CA: Addison-Wesley, p. 354.

---

125. In the second week of hospitalization, a depressed client comes to the dayroom dressed neatly in slacks and a blouse with hair combed back in a ponytail. The nurse's best response to this behavior is

1 "Wow, you look terrific!"
2 "You must be feeling better today."
3 "This is a first-time event!"
4 "I notice that you are dressed and that your hair is combed."

Answer: 4

Rationale: Accomplishments of depressed clients should be recognized appropriately without flattery or excessive praise. Appropriate recognition (rather than overly enthusiastic insincerity) increases the likelihood that the client will continue positive behavior. Insincerity can be perceived as ridicule.

Test-Taking Strategy: Note that the stem asks for the best response. The nurse's best response states the actual client behavior, which recognizes the client's accomplishment. Option 4 specifically states the nurse's observations!

Level of Cognitive Ability: Application
Phase of Nursing Process: Implementation
Client Needs: Psychosocial Integrity
Content Area: Mental Health

Reference
Carson, V., & Arnold, E. (1996). *Mental health nursing: The nurse-patient journey.* Philadelphia: W. B. Saunders, p. 218.

---

126. As the depressed client is feeling better—as demonstrated by increased interaction, increased energy levels, and more attention to personal hygiene—the nurse spends more one-to-one time with the client and is careful to check on the client frequently. The nurse takes these actions because the client

1 Is an elopement risk.
2 Needs the interpersonal support at this time.
3 Now has the energy to carry out a suicide plan.
4 Needs reinforcement of positive behaviors.

Answer: 3

Rationale: The client now has the energy to act on a suicide plan. Suicidal clients may appear to be feeling better immediately before making an attempt. This is attributed to a feeling of relief experienced when the decision has been made and plans have been finalized.

Test-Taking Strategy: Knowledge about depression and the risks associated with the act of suicide is necessary to answer the question. Think in terms of meeting the client's basic safety needs, using Maslow's hierarchy of needs theory. If you had difficulty with this question, review nursing content regarding suicide now. You are likely to find a question related to suicide on NCLEX-RN!

Level of Cognitive Ability: Application
Phase of Nursing Process: Implementation
Client Needs: Safe, Effective Care Environment
Content Area: Mental Health

Reference
Wilson, H., & Kneisl, C. (1996). *Psychiatric nursing* (5th ed.). Menlo Park, CA: Addison-Wesley, p. 467.

127. The client is to receive enoxaparin (Lovenox) SC every 12 hours for 10 days after hip surgery. The nurse implements a medication teaching plan that is based on the nurse's understanding that enoxaparin is

1 Shorter lasting than heparin.
2 Used to prevent postoperative deep vein thrombosis.
3 A new high-molecular-weight version of heparin.
4 Used to dissolve thromboemboli.

Answer: 2

Rationale: Enoxaparin (Lovenox) is used to prevent deep vein thrombosis after hip replacement surgery. It is administered by deep SC injection, which is started just after surgery and repeated every 12 hours for 7–10 days.

Test-Taking Strategy: This question assesses your knowledge of enoxaparin (Lovenox). Enoxaparin is longer lasting, not shorter lasting, than heparin; it is a new low-, not high-, molecular-weight version of heparin; and both heparin and enoxaparin are used to prevent the further formation of clots but cannot dissolve clots that have already formed. Review the purpose of this medication now if you had difficulty with this question!

Level of Cognitive Ability: Application
Phase of Nursing Process: Implementation
Client Needs: Physiological Integrity
Content Area: Pharmacology

Reference

Clark, J., Queener, S., & Karb, V. (1997). *Pharmacologic basis of nursing practice* (5th ed.). St. Louis: Mosby–Year Book, pp. 255–256.

128. A client has just had a Steinmann pin inserted to place skeletal traction to the fractured femur. Which of the following actions should the nurse take first?

1 Check the client's blood pressure
2 Assess the client's neurovascular status
3 Administer pain medication
4 Clean the pin sites

Answer: 2

Rationale: The neurovascular status of the injured extremity needs to be assessed before and after pin insertion and every 2 hours for the first 24 hours. Although cleaning the pin sites of bloody drainage would be appropriate, assessment of circulation and sensation of the injured extremity after manipulation would take top priority. Pain medication may be administered after the extremity assessment, because the client needs to be alert in order to answer questions about sensation. Although vital signs are assessed in clients after emergency procedures, it is not the priority assessment after Steinmann pin insertion.

Test-Taking Strategy: Answering this question requires knowing the nursing care for a client with a Steinmann pin. The first step of the nursing process is assessment, so options 3 and 4 can be eliminated. Assessment of the neurovascular status is more specific to the client situation than is vital signs assessment, so option 1 can be eliminated.

Level of Cognitive Ability: Application
Phase of Nursing Process: Implementation
Client Needs: Physiological Integrity
Content Area: Adult Health/Musculoskeletal

Reference

Ignatavicius, D. D., Workman, M. L., & Mishler, M. A. (1995). *Medical-surgical nursing: A nursing process approach* (2nd ed.). Philadelphia: W. B. Saunders, p. 1463.

129. The nurse is caring for a client with deep vein thrombosis and is monitoring for pulmonary emboli. The client is receiving IV heparin (Liquaemin). The nurse would anticipate that as treatment progresses over a couple of days, the most likely anticoagulant medication to be prescribed would be

1 Warfarin (Coumadin).
2 Imipramine (Tofranil).
3 Protamine sulfate.
4 Vitamin K (Mephyton).

Answer: 1

Rationale: In the event of a pulmonary embolism, anticoagulant therapy is initiated, usually with heparin, which is rapid acting. Because the warfarin derivatives require 24–48 hours to take effect, the more rapidly acting heparin is administered concurrently and then discontinued when the warfarin takes effect.

Test-Taking Strategy: This question assesses your knowledge of the anticoagulant therapy that is used to treat and prevent deep vein thrombosis and development of pulmonary embolism. Option 2 refers to a tricyclic antidepressant. Option 3 is a rapid-acting antidote for heparin, which takes effect immediately and lasts for 2 hours. Option 4 is the antidote for the warfarin derivatives.

Level of Cognitive Ability: Application
Phase of Nursing Process: Implementation
Client Needs: Physiological Integrity
Content Area: Pharmacology

References
Hodgson, B., & Kizior, R. (1998). *Saunders nursing drug handbook 1998.* Philadelphia: W. B. Saunders, pp. 489–491.
Luckmann, J. (1997). *Saunders manual of nursing care.* Philadelphia: W. B. Saunders, pp. 1117–1119.

130. A suspicious client tells the nurse that he or she will not attend the group therapy session because a student nurse has been sent to spy on him or her. The nurse's best response is

1 "If you attend group therapy, I'll take you for a walk."
2 "What makes you think the student is spying on you?"
3 "Student nurses attend group therapy as part of their education."
4 "Come to therapy with me, I'll protect you."

Answer: 3

Rationale: Option 3 gives the client a clear statement of reality. Options 1, 2, and 4 are nontherapeutic as they imply that there is something to be suspicious of, and this reinforces the client's delusion.

Test-Taking Strategy: The key to answering this question is to focus on reality. Option 3 is the only option that focuses on reality. Review the principles of caring for a paranoid client now if you had difficulty with this question!

Level of Cognitive Ability: Application
Phase of Nursing Process: Implementation
Client Needs: Psychosocial Integrity
Content Area: Mental Health

Reference
Wilson, H., & Kneisl, C. (1996). *Psychiatric nursing* (5th ed.). Menlo Park, CA: Addison-Wesley, p. 318.

131. After 5 days in the psychiatric unit, a manic client is able to tolerate short periods of time in the dayroom. The primary nurse overhears the client telling another client that he or she is a journalist posing as a client in order to write an article for a magazine. The nurse's best action is to

1 Ignore the delusion.
2 Confront the client with reality.
3 Take the client to a quiet room.
4 Support the client's denial of illness.

Answer: 2

Rationale: When dealing with a delusional client, clearly state that you do not share his or her perceptions. Options 1, 3, and 4 do not focus on reality and ignore the issue. Option 2 focuses on reality orientation.

Test-Taking Strategy: Use the process of elimination with the knowledge that reality orientation is the priority. Options 1 and 4 are nontherapeutic and can be eliminated. Option 3 takes the client out of the setting. Option 2, the correct answer, focuses on reality orientation.

Level of Cognitive Ability: Application
Phase of Nursing Process: Implementation
Client Needs: Psychosocial Integrity
Content Area: Mental Health

Reference
Wilson, H., & Kneisl, C. (1996). *Psychiatric nursing* (5th ed.). Menlo Park, CA: Addison-Wesley, p. 349.

132. Several months after a subtotal gastrectomy, a client presents with complaints of vertigo, tachycardia, pallor, and sweating soon after eating. The physician determines the client has dumping syndrome; therefore, the nurse teaches the client to

1 Lie down after meals.
2 Decrease fat intake.
3 Drink plenty of fluids with meals.
4 Follow a high-carbohydrate diet.

Answer: 1

Rationale: Dumping syndrome may occur because ingested food enters the jejunum too quickly before proper mixing and processing occurs. Management involves trying to delay gastric emptying, and one intervention for this is to lie down after meals. Fluids should be omitted as much as possible during meals; carbohydrates should be decreased; and fats should be increased.

Test-Taking Strategy: The goal of treating dumping syndrome is to delay gastric emptying. With this in mind, use the process of elimination and select the option that will prevent rapid gastric emptying. Lying down after meals will accomplish this goal. If you had difficulty with this question, take time now to review the interventions for dumping syndrome!

Level of Cognitive Ability: Application
Phase of Nursing Process: Implementation
Client Needs: Physiological Integrity
Content Area: Adult Health/Gastrointestinal

Reference
Black, J., & Matassarin-Jacobs, E. (1997). *Medical-surgical nursing: Clinical management for continuity of care* (5th ed.). Philadelphia: W. B. Saunders, p. 1779.

133. When the diagnostic clinic nurse enters the examining room, the client is crying and says, "I know I have stomach cancer and I know there's nothing that can be done for me." The nurse's best action is to

1 Quietly hold the client's hand.
2 Call the physician about the client's depression.
3 Ask the client, "What makes you think you have cancer?"
4 Inform the client that stomach cancer has a high survival rate.

Answer: 3

Rationale: Clarifying and focusing on the client's actions are two methods of therapeutic communication skills. Open-ended questions also often allow the nurse to assess several factors, including emotions, vocabulary, understanding of health, and any discrepancies in the client's responses. Option 1 may validate client fears. Options 2 and 4 are inappropriate.

Test-Taking Strategy: Although silence (option 1) is often an appropriate communication tool, in this case it may validate the client's fears. The client may believe that the nurse "knows something." It is important to have a better understanding of the basis of the client's fear before calling the physician (option 2). Option 4 may give the client false reassurance.

Level of Cognitive Ability: Application
Phase of Nursing Process: Implementation
Client Needs: Psychosocial Integrity
Content Area: Adult Health/Oncology

Reference
Potter, P., & Perry, A. (1997). *Fundamentals of nursing: Concepts, process, and practice* (4th ed.). St. Louis: Mosby–Year Book, pp. 241–245.

134. A client with severe manifestations of reflux caused by hiatal hernia is started on bethanechol (Urecholine). The order reads "Urecholine, 0.2 mg/kg/day in 2 divided doses." The client weighs 110 pounds. Urecholine is available in 5-mg tablets. The nurse will administer

1 1 tablet per dose.
2 2 tablets per dose.
3 3 tablets per day.
4 4 tablets per day.

Answer: 1

Rationale: First, determine the number of kilograms that the client weighs: 110 pounds ÷ 2.2 = 50 kg. Next, determine the total daily dose: 50 kg × 0.2 mg = 10 mg/day. Then determine the amount per dose: 10 mg/day ÷ 2 doses per day = 5 mg/dose. Finally, determine tablets per dose: 5 mg (desired) ÷ 5 mg/tablet (available) = 1 tablet per dose.

Test-Taking Strategy: Identify the figures required to calculate the appropriate dosage. Use the formula required, and label all calculations. Place decimals in the correct places. Make sure that the answer makes sense. If you had difficulty with this question, take time now to review the process of medication calculations!

Level of Cognitive Ability: Application
Phase of Nursing Process: Implementation
Client Needs: Physiological Integrity
Content Area: Pharmacology

Reference

Black, J., & Matassarin-Jacobs, E. (1997). *Medical-surgical nursing: Clinical management for continuity of care* (5th ed.). Philadelphia: W. B. Saunders, p. 1738.

---

135. The client's nursing diagnosis is High Risk for Hemorrhage related to esophageal varices secondary to portal hypertension. The nurse frequently should assess the client for

1 Complaints of nausea and vomiting.
2 Signs of pain or discomfort.
3 Changes in blood pressure and peripheral pulses.
4 Core body temperature.

Answer: 3

Rationale: Hemorrhage results in decreased cardiac output, which will be reflected in oxygenation status. Oxygenation assessments should include blood pressure readings, skin color, peripheral pulses, dyspnea, and level of consciousness. Options 1, 2, and 4 are not specific indicators of hemorrhage.

Test-Taking Strategy: The issue of the question relates to the indicators of hemorrhage. Nausea, vomiting, and temperature elevations are ordinarily not early signs of hemorrhage. Although the client may complain of chest pain as a result of decreased cardiac output, the earliest signs of hemorrhage will be low blood pressure and weakened peripheral pulses.

Level of Cognitive Ability: Application
Phase of Nursing Process: Implementation
Client Needs: Physiological Integrity
Content Area: Adult Health/Gastrointestinal

Reference

Black, J., & Matassarin-Jacobs, E. (1997). *Medical-surgical nursing: Clinical management for continuity of care* (5th ed.). Philadelphia: W. B. Saunders, p. 1886.

---

136. The physician prescribes metronidazole (Flagyl), 500 mg PO BID. The medication is diluted in 50 mL of normal saline, and pharmacy instructions are to infuse in 30 minutes. The infusion pump calibrates infusions via mL per hour. The nurse will set the IV infusion pump at

1 25 mL/hour.
2 50 mL/hour.
3 100 mL/hour.
4 200 mL/hour.

Answer: 3

Rationale: If the infusion pump calibrates infusions via mL per hour, then to infuse 50 mL in 30 minutes, the pump will be set at 100 mL/hour.

Test-Taking Strategy: Knowledge that the infusion pump can be calibrated by identifying the amount of milliliters in 1 hour is necessary to answer this question. If you set the pump at 50 mL, then it will take 1 hour for 50 mL to infuse. Therefore, to infuse 50 mL in 30 minutes, the pump needs to be set at 100 mL per hour!

Level of Cognitive Ability: Application
Phase of Nursing Process: Implementation
Client Needs: Physiological Integrity
Content Area: Pharmacology

Reference

Kee, J., & Marshall, S. (1996). *Clinical calculation with applications to general and specialty areas* (3rd ed.). Philadelphia: W. B. Saunders, p. 175.

---

137. What nursing intervention would be helpful in reducing a child's fear of going to school?

1 Group therapy
2 Biofeedback
3 Systematic desensitization
4 Medication referral

Answer: 3

Rationale: A child needs to be gradually exposed to what is causing the fear. Having the child attend school for short periods and gradually stay longer will help reduce the fear of school. With systematic desensitization, the child would be taken to school for a short period and be rewarded for staying. The length of time the child would be expected to stay would be increased gradually until the child is able to stay the full day.

Test-Taking Strategy: The key phrase in the question is "reducing the fear." Use the process of elimination, identifying the components of each type of therapy presented in the options. Focus on the issue of reducing fear. Review these types of therapy now if you had difficulty with this question!

Level of Cognitive Ability: Application
Nursing Process: Implementation
Client Needs: Psychosocial Integrity
Content Area: Child Health

Reference

Carson, V., & Arnold, E. (1996). *Mental health nursing: The nurse-patient journey.* Philadelphia: W. B. Saunders, p. 437.

---

138. Which of the following medications is effective in the treatment of obsessive-compulsive disorders?

1 Amitriptyline (Elavil)
2 Fluoxetine (Prozac)
3 Sertraline (Zoloft)
4 Clomipramine (Anafranil)

Answer: 4

Rationale: Clomipramine (Anafranil), a tricyclic antidepressant, is used in the treatment of obsessive-compulsive disorders. Amitriptyline (Elavil), a tricyclic antidepressant, is used to treat depression. Fluoxetine (Prozac), an antidepressant, is also used to treat depression. Sertraline (Zoloft), another antidepressant, is used to treat major depressive disorders and panic disorders.

Test-Taking Strategy: Knowledge regarding the actions and uses of the medications presented in the options is necessary to answer the question. Take time now to review these important medications if you had difficulty with this question!

Level of Cognitive Ability: Application
Phase of Nursing Process: Implementation
Client Needs: Physiological Integrity
Content Area: Mental Health

Reference

Hodgson, B., & Kizior, R. (1998). *Saunders nursing drug handbook 1998.* Philadelphia: W. B. Saunders, pp. 237–238.

---

139. The behavioral technique of "exposure" is an effective technique for treatment of many clients with phobias. When implementing this form of therapy, the nurse knows that the treatment includes

1 Frequent verbal reminders that the fear is irrational.
2 Encouraging the use of anxiolytics before going out in social situations that have previously caused the fear and anxiety.
3 Presenting increasingly anxiety-producing situations as discomfort dissipates at each level.
4 Having family members remind the client how the client's refusal to join them in social situations has affected them.

Answer: 3

Rationale: The use of exposure is a form of systematic desensitization and has been used in long- and short-term treatment of clients with phobias. This therapy has been found to have the greatest likelihood of effectiveness and is recommended before using medication therapy. Options 1 and 4 are incorrect because the client is well aware that the fear is irrational, and reminders will only serve to increase the client's anxiety.

Test-Taking Strategy: Use the process of elimination to answer the question. Note the key word "exposure" in the question. Note its relationship to the phrase "presenting increasingly anxiety-producing situations" in the correct option. Take time now to review this form of therapy if you had difficulty with this question!

Level of Cognitive Ability: Application
Phase of Nursing Process: Implementation
Client Needs: Psychosocial Integrity
Content Area: Mental Health

Reference

Carson, V., & Arnold, E. (1996). *Mental health nursing: The nurse-patient journey.* Philadelphia: W. B. Saunders, p. 437.

140. The client who had a right lobectomy for lung cancer is to be discharged to home the following day. The nurse prepares to initiate discharge teaching. Upon entering the room, the client complains of pain from the surgical incision. Of the following, which is the most appropriate nursing action?

1 Start discharge instructions because the pain is probably just mild at this time
2 Assess the client's pain level, medicate as prescribed, and delay discharge teaching
3 Medicate the client for pain as prescribed and initiate discharge teaching as planned
4 Medicate for pain and cancel discharge teaching because the client is too unstable to go home

Answer: 2

Rationale: A person in pain has a decreased ability to learn and assimilate new knowledge. The nurse should medicate the client and begin discharge teaching at a later time. Remember that persons receiving narcotics for acute pain control may experience a decreased ability to concentrate on instructions. Continued complaints of pain at this time do not indicate physiological instability to a degree that would delay discharge.

Test-Taking Strategy: Remember that physiological needs take precedence, according to Maslow's hierarchy of needs theory. The client does need medication first. Remember the first step of the nursing process, assessment. The only option that addresses assessment is option 2!

Level of Cognitive Ability: Application
Phase of Nursing Process: Implementation
Client Needs: Physiological Integrity
Content Area: Fundamental Skills

Reference
Ignatavicius, D. D., Workman, M. L., & Mishler, M. A. (1995). *Medical-surgical nursing: A nursing process approach* (2nd ed.). Philadelphia: W. B. Saunders, pp. 746–747.

---

141. The nurse is caring for the client with AIDS. The nurse best promotes trust and reduces the client's fear of social isolation by making which of the following statements?

1 "Don't worry about telling your friend about the AIDS virus; I'm sure it will be OK."
2 "If I were in your position, I would make out a Durable Power of Attorney for Health Care."
3 "Can you tell me who you have to help you?"
4 "I need to give you your medication and then I'll give you some privacy."

Answer: 3

Rationale: It is important to ask the client with AIDS about support persons. Many clients are reluctant to share the AIDS diagnosis because of the social stigma of the disease. Lack of social support may contribute to depression and risk for suicide. Option 1 is incorrect because the nurse should not give false reassurance. Option 2 is incorrect because the nurse should not give advice. Option 4 is incorrect because a focus on tasks does not promote communication and trust or reduce fear.

Test-Taking Strategy: Use therapeutic communication techniques. By the process of elimination, you should be directed to option 3, which is the only option that reflects a therapeutic response!

Level of Cognitive Ability: Application
Phase of Nursing Process: Implementation
Client Needs: Psychosocial Integrity
Content Area: Fundamental Skills

Reference
Ignatavicius, D. D., Workman, M. L., & Mishler, M. A. (1995). *Medical-surgical nursing: A nursing process approach* (2nd ed.). Philadelphia: W. B. Saunders, p. 522.

142. The nurse caring for the client with hepatitis implements care to optimize physiological integrity. Which of the following nursing interventions would best meet this client's needs?

1 Administer prochlorperazine maleate (Compazine) to relieve nausea
2 Provide a diet containing three standard-size meals to provide optimal nutrient intake
3 Assist with progressive increase in activity level with rest periods to promote healing
4 Administer acetaminophen (Tylenol) for general malaise

Answer: 3

Rationale: In clients with hepatitis, it is important to provide adequate rest throughout the course of illness. Bed rest during the acute stage of illness is encouraged. Compazine and Tylenol are known to have hepatotoxic effects. It is important to maintain optimal nutritional intake. A diet high in carbohydrates and proteins and low in fried and fatty foods is recommended. Small, frequent feedings are easier to digest than three standard-size meals.

Test-Taking Strategy: Remember that hepatitis involves the liver. Use the process of elimination and eliminate options 1 and 4 first because of the hepatotoxic effects of these medications. For the remaining two options, knowledge that rest is a key component of therapy will direct you to the correct option. If you are unfamiliar with the pathophysiological processes and treatment of hepatitis, take time now to review. You are likely to find questions related to this disorder on NCLEX-RN!

Level of Cognitive Ability: Application
Phase of Nursing Process: Implementation
Client Needs: Physiological Integrity
Content Area: Adult Health/Gastrointestinal

Reference

Ignatavicius, D. D., Workman, M. L., & Mishler, M. A. (1995). *Medical-surgical nursing: A nursing process approach* (2nd ed.). Philadelphia: W. B. Saunders, pp. 1691–1693.

---

143. The client with tuberculosis has been placed on rifampin (Rifadin). The nurse is going to instruct the client about the medication. Which of the following items would the nurse avoid teaching the client?

1 It is normal for secretions to turn orange
2 Oral contraceptives have decreased efficacy when taken with rifampin (Rifadin)
3 The client should report any jaundice, dark urine, or decreased appetite
4 Laboratory blood tests will be done every 3 months

Answer: 4

Rationale: Rifampin (Rifadin) is known to be hepatotoxic. Weekly analysis of liver function tests are necessary to maintain client safety. Jaundice, dark urine, and decreased appetite may be signs of liver toxicity. Urine, feces, saliva, sputum, sweat, and tears may take on an orange coloration. Oral contraceptives are not as effective when used in combination with rifampin (Rifadin).

Test-Taking Strategy: Note the key phrase in the stem of the question: "avoid teaching." Knowledge regarding this medication will then assist in directing you to the correct option. If you are unfamiliar with this medication, it is important to take time now to review. You are likely to find a question related to this medication on NCLEX-RN!

Level of Cognitive Ability: Application
Phase of Nursing Process: Implementation
Client Needs: Physiological Integrity
Content Area: Pharmacology

Reference

Hodgson, B., & Kizior, R. (1998). *Saunders nursing drug handbook 1998*. Philadelphia: W. B. Saunders, pp. 906–908.

---

144. The water seal chamber of a chest drainage system breaks. As an initial nursing action, the nurse uses which of the following items on hand?

1 Tape
2 Stethoscope
3 Bottle of sterile water
4 Pair of clamps

Answer: 3

Rationale: If the water seal chamber becomes broken, the nurse takes immediate action to prevent collapse of the lung. A temporary water seal can be made by placing the end of the chest tube tubing in water 2 cm below the surface. If sterile water is not available, the chest tube can be double clamped. However, clamping a chest tube enhances the risk that a tension pneumothorax will develop. Tape is useful in securing tubes but is not the first priority. A stethoscope is necessary to auscultate lung sounds but is also not the first priority.

Test-Taking Strategy: Note the key word "initial." Also, visualize the effectiveness of each of the items in the options in terms of the issue: a chest drainage system that breaks. If you are unfamiliar with care of a client with a closed chest drainage system, review now! You are likely to find questions related to these tubes on NCLEX-RN!

Level of Cognitive Ability: Application
Phase of Nursing Process: Implementation
Client Needs: Physiological Integrity
Content Area: Adult Health/Respiratory

Reference

Polaski, A., & Tatro, S. (1996). *Luckmann's Core principles and practice of medical-surgical nursing*. Philadelphia: W. B. Saunders, pp. 610–612.

---

145. The client has a synthetic cast on the right arm for a fractured ulna. The client asks if it would be possible to take a shower and wash hair. The nurse should respond by saying

1. "The cast padding may take a long time to dry."
2. "It is not safe for you to shower alone with a cast on."
3. "Hot water may soften the synthetic cast."
4. "It may lead to a serious infection."

Answer: 1

Rationale: Water does not damage the synthetic cast; however, the client should know that it may take a while for the cast padding to dry. It may be unsafe for the client to shower alone because the client may slip and fall, but not because of the cast. Water may soften a plaster cast but has no effect on a synthetic cast. A shower will not cause an infection.

Test-Taking Strategy: Knowledge regarding the differences between synthetic and plaster casts is pertinent to answering this question correctly. From this point, use the process of elimination. Take time now to review the differences between synthetic and plaster casts and the care appropriate for each if you had difficulty with this question!

Level of Cognitive Ability: Analysis
Phase of Nursing Process: Implementation
Client Needs: Health Promotion and Maintenance
Content Area: Adult Health/Musculoskeletal

Reference

Black, J., & Matassarin-Jacobs, E. (1997). *Medical-surgical nursing: Clinical management for continuity of care* (5th ed.). Philadelphia W. B. Saunders, p. 2147.

---

146. Which of the following interventions would the nurse carry out when performing pin care for a client with skeletal traction?

1. Remove crusted serous drainage
2. Apply continuous warm, sterile compresses
3. Apply antibiotic ointment and cover site with a dressing
4. Use a heat lamp three times a day

Answer: 1

Rationale: The purpose of pin care is to maintain free drainage of serous fluid from the pin site. Crusts should be gently removed and the skin around the area cleansed. Warm, sterile compresses may be therapeutic if there is infection at the pin site, but they are not part of routine skin care. Antibiotic ointment may be part of the protocol for pin care; however, the pin sites are usually cleansed with sterile saline or peroxide and not covered. A heat lamp is not part of routine pin site care and may heat the pin and cause injury and discomfort; therefore, it is not indicated.

Test-Taking Strategy: Knowledge of pin care is essential for answering this question. Use the process of elimination, considering how each option will affect the pin site. Eliminate option 4 because heat can injure the tissues. Compresses and antibiotics are indicated for infection, but there is no indication in the question that an infection exists. Therefore, eliminate options 2 and 3. If you are unfamiliar with routine pin cleansing, take time now to review!

Level of Cognitive Ability: Application
Phase of Nursing Process: Implementation
Client Needs: Physiological Integrity
Content Area: Adult Health/Musculoskeletal

Reference

LeMone, P., & Burke, K. (1996). *Medical-surgical nursing: Critical thinking in client care*. Menlo Park, CA: Addison-Wesley, p. 1566.

147. The nurse is caring for a client with paranoid schizophrenia who believes that the medications are poisoned. The client is scheduled to take medications. In preparing the client to take medications, the priority nursing action would be to discuss the client's level of

1 Isolation.
2 Anger.
3 Suspiciousness/fear.
4 Helplessness.

Answer: 3

Rationale: Delusions of persecution are most frequent and are the key symptom of paranoid schizophrenia. A more subtle form of delusions of persecution is suspiciousness and fear of being controlled. Accept the client by letting the client know you respect feelings, as this promotes unconditional acceptance that will be helpful in developing basic trust and compliance with therapy. General approaches to dealing with a suspicious person highlight reliability and consistency in interactions. Delusions often reflect client's fears and defense against the client's own aggressive feelings.

Test-Taking Strategy: An understanding of the feeling states underlying schizophrenic subtypes and delusions is necessary in order for you to answer this question. Note the issue of the question: that the client believes that the medications are poisoned. The only option that relates to this issue is option 3. Take time now to review the characteristics of delusions and the appropriate nursing interventions if you had difficulty with this question!

Level of Cognitive Ability: Application
Phase of Nursing Process: Implementation
Client Needs: Psychosocial Integrity
Content Area: Mental Health

Reference

Carson, V., & Arnold, E. (1996). *Mental health nursing: The nurse-patient journey.* Philadelphia: W. B. Saunders, p. 738.

---

148. Upon being discharged, a client with recurrent schizophrenic exacerbations tells the nurse, "I know I get sick when I don't take my medications, but I don't like the way they make me feel." The best response by the nurse would be

1 "Tell me what you plan to do."
2 "You're being stupid. You know you'll end up coming right back here."
3 "Take care of yourself and stay well."
4 "Why don't you like the medications?"

Answer: 1

Rationale: Focusing involves keeping the flow of communication goal directed, specific, and concrete. It also keeps the discussion concentrated. Options 2, 3, and 4 are nontherapeutic techniques that block communication or ignore feelings or plan of action and are therefore less helpful.

Test-Taking Strategy: Use the process of elimination, focusing on therapeutic and nontherapeutic communication techniques. Option 2 is degrading. Option 3 avoids the client's concerns. Avoid options that begin a statement with the word "Why." Such statements tend to produce defensiveness in the client. Focus on the client's issue and concerns!

Level of Cognitive Ability: Application
Phase of Nursing Process: Implementation
Client Needs: Psychosocial Integrity
Content Area: Mental Health

Reference

Haber, J. (1997). *Comprehensive psychiatric nursing* (5th ed.). St. Louis: Mosby–Year Book, p. 133.

149. A visitor brings a suicidal client a brightly packaged gift. The nurse goes with the visitor to the client's room. Which action should the nurse take now?

1. Let the visitor spend time alone with the client
2. Tell the client what a beautiful package this is
3. Suggest that the client open the gift now
4. Reinforce the safety policies with the client

Answer: 3

Rationale: The nurse must be concerned with the safety of the client. The visitor may or may not be aware of the client's suicidal thoughts or the hospital safety policies. The client should open the gift in the presence of the nurse so that sharp or unsafe objects could be locked in the client's safety box. Leaving the package unattended in the room with the client is hazardous.

Test-Taking Strategy: The issue in the stem of the question is that the client is suicidal. Use the process of elimination, keeping the issue of the question in mind. Because the client's safety is at stake, the only option that ensures that the gift is not dangerous for the suicidal client is for the nurse to ask the client to open it in the nurse's presence.

Level of Cognitive Ability: Application
Phase of Nursing Process: Implementation
Client Needs: Safe, Effective Care Environment
Content Area: Mental Health

Reference

Johnson, B. (1997). *Psychiatric-mental health nursing: Adaptation and growth* (4th ed.). Philadelphia: Lippincott-Raven, pp. 870–871.

150. A client with degenerative disk disease of the cervical spine has been receiving intermittent cervical traction for several weeks at the outpatient clinic. The client now states that the pain has spread to the jaw, especially during eating, and complains of ringing in the ears. Which action should the nurse take?

1. Assess the client's aspirin consumption
2. Discontinue the traction and notify the physician
3. Decrease the length of time the client is in the traction
4. Explain that the symptoms are expected with degenerative disk disease

Answer: 2

Rationale: The head halter worn during cervical traction puts pressure on the occiput and the chin and can cause temporomandibular joint syndrome, which is what the client is experiencing. Although aspirin use can cause ringing in the ears, there is no indication that the client is taking aspirin. Decreasing the length of time in the traction will not solve the problem. Jaw pain and tinnitus are not symptoms of degenerative disk disease.

Test-Taking Strategy: Use the process of elimination, noting the client symptoms. Pain that increases with chewing and the presence of tinnitus point to the temporomandibular joint. The history of use of cervical traction suggests joint stress. Discontinuing the traction will alleviate the stress, and because the traction is ordered by the physician, the physician should be notified so that treatment of the disk disease (pain management) can be altered. Review the complications of cervical traction now if you had difficulty with this question!

Level of Cognitive Ability: Application
Phase of Nursing Process: Implementation
Client Needs: Physiological Integrity
Content Area: Adult Health/Musculoskeletal

Reference

Black, J., & Matassarin-Jacobs, E. (1997). *Medical-surgical nursing: Clinical management for continuity of care* (5th ed.). Philadelphia: W. B. Saunders, p. 2137.

151. A client with a severely sprained left ankle needs to use crutch walking for ambulation. Which of the following nursing actions is essential before crutch use by the client?

1. Measure the client from the anterior fold of the axilla to the foot and add 2.5 cm (1 inch)
2. Have the client stand erect with the crutches positioned 1 finger width (1/2 inch) below the axilla to adjust the hand bar
3. Have the client flex and extend the arms repeatedly in multiple directions
4. Measure the client's arm length from the axilla to fingertip to determine hand bar length

Answer: 1

Rationale: To prevent complications, such as falls, crutch palsy, unsteady gait, and malalignment, associated with crutches that are too long or too short, it is essential that the nurse obtain the correct length. Option 1 is correct. Option 2 is incorrect because the crutches will be too long and could cause injury. Although exercises are recommended before crutch use, they are not essential, so option 3 is incorrect. Option 4 is incorrect because hand bar placement is determined by having a client stand upright with the top of the crutch resting 2.5–5 cm below the axilla and by measuring the degree of elbow flexion (it should be about 30 degrees).

Test-Taking Strategy: Correct placement of the crutches 2.5–5 cm below the axilla is essential to prevent nerve injury. Review this procedure now if you had difficulty with this question. You are likely to find a question related to measuring for crutches on NCLEX-RN!

Level of Cognitive Ability: Application
Phase of Nursing Process: Implementation
Client Needs: Physiological Integrity
Content Area: Adult Health/Musculoskeletal

Reference

Lammon, C. B., Foote, A. W., Leli, P. G., et al. (1995). *Clinical nursing skills.* Philadelphia: W. B. Saunders, p. 240.

---

152. Ambulation with a cane is prescribed for a client 4 weeks after total right knee replacement. The nurse would be correct in teaching the client to position the cane by holding the cane in the

1. Right hand, about 2 inches to the side and about 3 inches behind the right foot.
2. Right hand, about 4 inches to the side and ahead of the left foot.
3. Left hand, about 6 inches to the side and ahead of the left foot.
4. Left hand, about 1 inch to the side and 2 inches behind the left foot.

Answer: 3

Rationale: Option 3 is correct because canes should be held on the stronger side of the body; thus options 1 and 2 are incorrect. Option 4 is incorrect because the cane needs to be positioned about 6 inches to the side and ahead of the foot, not behind it.

Test-Taking Strategy: Choose the option that would provide the best alignment and support while ambulating. If you knew that the cane is positioned on the strong side of the body, you could eliminate options 1 and 2. Try to visualize the procedure. Positioning a device behind the foot does not support the affected extremity when the body is in forward motion or standing still.

Level of Cognitive Ability: Application
Phase of Nursing Process: Implementation
Client Needs: Safe, Effective Care Environment
Content Area: Adult Health/Musculoskeletal

Reference

Lammon, C. B., Foote, A. W., Leli, P. G., et al. (1995). *Clinical nursing skills.* Philadelphia: W. B. Saunders, pp. 238–239.

153. The client is being admitted with fractured ribs and pneumonia. The client's breathing is shallow and fast. On the basis of these findings, the nurse suspects hyperventilation. Which of the following should the nurse do first to promote optimal breathing?

1 Check the arterial blood gases (ABGs) to see whether the client is in respiratory alkalosis
2 Give pain medication and help the client to splint that side and deep breathe
3 Instruct the client to cough
4 Check for diminished breath sounds

Answer: 2

Rationale: The client is hyperventilating in response to the pain of the rib fractures. Giving pain medication and helping the client splint the area and deep breathe may help offset atelectasis and slow the respirations.

Test-Taking Strategy: Remember the ABCs: airway, breathing, and circulation. Option 2 reflects breathing and is the first priority!

Level of Cognitive Ability: Application
Phase of Nursing Process: Implementation
Client Needs: Physiological Integrity
Content Area: Adult Health/Respiratory

Reference

Black, J., & Matassarin-Jacobs, E. (1997). *Medical-surgical nursing: Clinical management for continuity of care* (5th ed.). Philadelphia: W. B. Saunders, p. 2526.

154. Health care professionals have an important role in management of children with tuberculosis (TB). What is the best method of obtaining a sputum culture from a young child?

1 Assist the child in coughing into a sputum cup after a meal
2 Explain procedure to parents, so that they can assist the child with the sputum specimen
3 Obtain a gastric washing per NG tube after breakfast
4 Obtain a gastric washing per NG tube before breakfast

Answer: 4

Rationale: It is very difficult to obtain sputum specimens from children because secretions are swallowed instead of expectorated. The aspiration or washing needs to be obtained early in the morning from contents of a fasting stomach. A young child will have difficulty coughing up sputum. Explaining the procedure to the parents will not ensure that the child will be able to expectorate a sputum specimen. A gastric washing obtained on a full stomach will be inaccurate and cause the child to vomit.

Test-Taking Strategy: The question asks for the best method of obtaining a sputum specimen from a young child. Note the phrase "young child." The young child will have difficulty understanding the directions for coughing up a specimen. Options 3 and 4 are similar except for the time frame. Remember that it is better to obtain the specimen if the child has an empty stomach. Review this procedure now if you had difficulty with this question!

Level of Cognitive Ability: Application
Phase of Nursing Process: Implementation
Client Needs: Physiological Integrity
Content Area: Child Health

Reference

Wong, D. (1997). *Whaley and Wong's Essentials of pediatric nursing* (5th ed.). St. Louis: Mosby–Year Book, p. 772

155. The recommended test for determining whether a child has been infected with tubercular bacillus is

1 The tine prong skin test.
2 An accurate history.
3 The Mantoux skin test (purified protein derivative [PPD]).
4 A complete blood cell (CBC) count.

Answer: 3

Rationale: The tine prong skin test can yield a false-positive result. An accurate history is not a test. A CBC count may show the presence of an infection but will not identify the tubercular bacillus. The Mantoux skin test is the recommended diagnostic test.

Test-Taking Strategy: Note the key phrase "test for determining." Eliminate option 2 because it is not a test. Eliminate option 4 because the CBC will not determine the presence of TB. From this point, remembering that the Mantoux skin test is the recommended test will direct you to the correct option.

Level of Cognitive Ability: Analysis
Phase of Nursing Process: Implementation
Client Needs: Physiological Integrity
Content Area: Child Health

Reference

Wong, D. (1997). *Whaley and Wong's Essentials of pediatric nursing* (5th ed.). St. Louis: Mosby–Year Book, pp. 769–770.

---

156. Hepatitis is a major cause of morbidity in children. The best preventive measure to institute in the pediatric unit is

1 Isolation of anyone suspected of having hepatitis.
2 Testing all admitted children for hepatitis.
3 Immunization of all children against hepatitis E.
4 Thorough handwashing.

Answer: 4

Rationale: Handwashing is the most critical measure in reducing the risk of hepatitis. Testing all children is impractical. No liver function test is specific for hepatitis. There is no immunization against hepatitis E. Children have vague, generalized symptoms that may not be specific for hepatitis. Precautions are instituted when the illness is diagnosed and a client is known to be infectious.

Test-Taking Strategy: Note the key phrase "best preventive measure." Remember that handwashing is the best measure to prevent the spread of infection. Review preventive measures in hepatitis now if you had difficulty with this question!

Level of Cognitive Ability: Application
Phase of Nursing Process: Implementation
Client Needs: Safe, Effective Care Environment
Content Area: Child Health

Reference

Wong, D., & Perry, S. (1998). *Maternal-child nursing care.* St. Louis: Mosby–Year Book, pp. 1414–1416.

---

157. A 7-year-old comes to the diabetic clinic with the parents. The child wants to play soccer with friends. The most appropriate nursing intervention is

1 Ask the child why he or she wants to play soccer and not baseball.
2 Support the child's desire to play soccer and explain to the parents that exercise is an important component of treatment.
3 Check the child's blood glucose level to see how soccer affects the levels.
4 Explain to the client that activities must be restricted because of the nature of the child's illness.

Answer: 2

Rationale: Exercise is important in the lowering of the client's glucose levels. It is included as a component of diabetic management and is planned around the child's interests and capabilities. The child needs to exercise. Whether the child plays soccer or baseball is not the important issue.

Test-Taking Strategy: Use the process of elimination. Option 4 can be easily eliminated. Option 3 can be eliminated because the child has not yet played soccer. Option 1 is not an appropriate question for the child. Review the components of diabetic management now if you had difficulty with this question!

Level of Cognitive Ability: Application
Phase of Nursing Process: Implementation
Client Needs: Psychosocial Integrity
Content Area: Child Health

Reference

Wong, D. (1997). *Whaley and Wong's Essentials of pediatric nursing* (5th ed.). St. Louis: Mosby–Year Book, p. 1053.

158. The nurse is caring for a neonate in the nursery. The most appropriate route and site for administering the hepatitis B vaccine are

1 Intramuscularly in the vastus lateralis muscle.
2 Intramuscularly in the dorsal gluteal muscle.
3 Subcutaneously in the abdomen.
4 Subcutaneously in the upper arm.

Answer: 1

Rationale: Intramuscularly is the appropriate mode of administration of hepatitis B vaccine. The vastus lateralis muscle is the preferred muscle. Administration in the dorsal gluteal muscle is associated with low antibody seroconversion rate, indicating a reduced immune response. This muscle is not well developed until the infant is walking.

Test-Taking Strategy: The issue of the question is neonate injection sites. Focus on the phrase "most appropriate route and site." Eliminate options 3 and 4 because hepatitis B vaccine is given intramuscularly. From this point, eliminate option 2 because the dorsal gluteal muscle is not a well-developed muscle in a neonate and is very close to the sciatic nerve. Review procedures regarding injection sites in a neonate now if you had difficulty with question!

Level of Cognitive Ability: Application
Phase of Nursing Process: Implementation
Client Needs: Physiological Integrity
Content Area: Child Health

Reference
Wong, D. (1997). *Whaley and Wong's Essentials of pediatric nursing* (5th ed.). St. Louis: Mosby–Year Book, p. 316.

---

159. Adolescents with up-to-date immunizations will need to be reimmunized as preventive care for which of the following communicable diseases?

1 Varicella (chickenpox)
2 *Haemophilus influenzae* (type B)
3 Polio
4 Tetanus

Answer: 4

Rationale: As part of preventive care, tetanus immunization boosters are needed every 5–10 years. Varicella (chickenpox), *H. influenzae* (type B), and polio reimmunizations are not necessary.

Test-Taking Strategy: Knowledge regarding immunizations and their schedules is necessary to answer this question. Note the key word "reimmunized." Use the process of elimination, identifying those that do not require reimmunization. Take time now to review the immunization schedule if you had difficulty with this question!

Level of Cognitive Ability: Application
Phase of Nursing Process: Implementation
Client Needs: Health Promotion and Maintenance
Content Area: Child Health

Reference
Wong, D. (1997). *Whaley and Wong's Essentials of pediatric nursing* (5th ed.). St. Louis: Mosby–Year Book, pp. 314–315, 479.

---

160. A 7-year-old child is admitted with acute lymphocytic leukemia (ALL). It is extremely busy in the pediatric unit when the admission office calls to send the child to the room in the pediatric unit. The most important nursing intervention would be

1 Have the blood work drawn in the central laboratory before admission to the unit.
2 Have the child come immediately to the unit and place the child in a clean, private room.
3 Have the child wait in the radiology department until the chest x-ray can be done.
4 Have the child wait in the admissions office until the unit is less hectic.

Answer: 2

Rationale: The priority action in the child with ALL is to prevent infection. Allowing the child to come to the pediatric unit and placing the child in a clean, private room decreases the risk of the child's contracting infections from the other hospital employees and other hospital clients. Going to the radiology department, going to the laboratory, or staying in the admissions office increases the child's exposure to potential infectious clients and health care workers.

Test-Taking Strategy: Use the process of elimination, focusing on the issue of the question: preventing infection. The only option that prevents the child from infection is option 2.

Level of Cognitive Ability: Application
Phase of Nursing Process: Implementation
Client Needs: Physiological Integrity
Content Area: Child Health

Reference
Wong, D. (1997). *Whaley and Wong's Essentials of pediatric nursing* (5th ed.). St. Louis: Mosby–Year Book, p. 925.

161. The nurse is caring for a client with Raynaud's disease. In caring for the client, the most appropriate nursing intervention would be to teach the client to

1 Avoid smoking because it causes cutaneous vasospasm.
2 Always wear warm clothing even in warm climates to prevent vasoconstriction.
3 Use nail polish to protect the nailbeds from injury.
4 Wear gloves for all activities involving use of both hands.

Answer: 1

Rationale: Smoking cessation is one of the most important lifestyle changes that the nurse can influence with teaching. The nurse should emphasize the effects of tobacco on the blood vessels. Options 2 and 3 are incorrect. Option 4 is not the priority.

Test-Taking Strategy: Use the process of elimination. Option 2 is incorrect because the client is advised to wear warm clothing but only in temperatures reflective of the need. Option 3 is incorrect because nail polish would not prevent injury to the nailbeds. In fact, if a cuticle were cut, the nailbed could become infected and the nail polish could mask an infected nailbed. Although wearing gloves for all activities involving use of both hands might not be a bad idea, it is not the priority. Take time now to review client teaching points for Raynaud's disease if you had difficulty with this question!

Level of Cognitive Ability: Application
Phase of Nursing Process: Implementation
Client Needs: Physiological Integrity
Content Area: Adult Health/Cardiovascular

Reference
Luckmann, J. (1997). *Saunders manual of nursing care.* Philadelphia: W. B. Saunders, pp. 1115–1116.

162. Children with leukemia have a potential for inadequate nutrition, less than body requirements, because of loss of appetite, nausea, and vomiting. What nursing intervention would best promote adequate nutrition?

1 Allow child any food tolerated
2 Serve a large selection of big portions of food at a meal in hopes that the child will eat some
3 Encourage parents to continue the same practices that they use with the other children
4 Restrict food brought from home because you don't know how it was prepared

Answer: 1

Rationale: Allowing any food the child can tolerate gives the child some control over what is eaten and helps the child to be involved in his or her own care. Large portions increase nausea; the goal is to maintain adequate nutrition. Food brought from home is familiar to the child and may increase the appetite. How the food from home is prepared is not the concern at this time.

Test-Taking Strategy: The key phrase is "best promote." Eliminate option 4 because of the word "restrict." Eliminate option 2 because of the phrase "big portions." For the remaining two options, consider the key phrase. Practices that are used with the other children are not the best method of promoting adequate nutrition because the child may not like those practices. Allow the child to select any food "tolerated."

Level of Cognitive Ability: Application
Phase of Nursing Process: Implementation
Client Needs: Physiological Integrity
Content Area: Child Health

Reference
Wong, D. (1997). *Whaley and Wong's Essentials of pediatric nursing* (5th ed.). St. Louis: Mosby–Year Book, p. 935.

163. The client is scheduled for surgical insertion of a permanent pacemaker and says to the nurse, "I'm afraid I'll be electrocuted when they put this thing in my heart." The most appropriate response by the nurse is which of the following?

1 "You seem to be concerned about having a pacemaker inserted."
2 "Don't worry, there's not a chance in the world of being electrocuted."
3 "You have a serious heart condition that needs to be monitored. This is simply a way to prevent further heart attacks, not cause them."
4 "I'm canceling the surgery until you feel more positive about it. The surgeon doesn't want you to go in unprepared."

Answer: 1

Rationale: Option 1 enables the client to express anxiety and fears and to work through the situation. Option 2 is incorrect because false reassurance is used. Option 4 is also incorrect; although the nurse may notify the surgeon of the client's seeming unreadiness, the nurse would not cancel the surgery. Option 3 provides the client with correct information but is not as appropriate a response as option 1.

Test-Taking Strategy: By using the therapeutic communication technique of reflection (repeating the client's verbal and nonverbal message for the client's benefit), the nurse reflects the content of the client's message to the client, thus providing the client an opportunity to hear and analyze what the nurse said. Option 1 is the only option that addresses the client's concerns. Remember to address the client's feelings first!

Level of Cognitive Ability: Application
Phase of Nursing Process: Implementation
Client Needs: Psychosocial Integrity
Content Area: Adult Health/Cardiovascular

Reference

Luckmann, J. (1997). *Saunders manual of nursing care*. Philadelphia: W. B. Saunders, pp. 1019–1020.

---

164. The nurse is caring for a client with varicose veins who has suffered skin breakdown related to venous disease and secondary infection. During care, the therapeutic nursing intervention would be to

1 Keep the legs aligned with the heart.
2 Pull the client onto the side every 2 hours.
3 Clean the skin with alcohol every hour.
4 Elevate the legs higher than the heart.

Answer: 4

Rationale: For the client with alterations in tissue perfusion related to skin breakdown caused by venous disease and secondary infection, nursing interventions include taking daily pedal pulses; monitoring vital signs and obtaining daily weights; cleaning the skin and providing wound care to protect it until it heals; and maintaining proper body positioning while the client is in bed, which includes elevating the legs above the heart and avoiding friction rubbing of the skin.

Test-Taking Strategy: This question assesses your ability to apply the nursing process for clients with varicose veins who have complications such as skin breakdown. Option 1 is incorrect because the correct position of the legs in a venous condition is elevation above the level of the heart. In option 2, the term "pull" would alert you to causing friction rubs. Option 3 is incorrect; remember that alcohol is very drying to the skin. Review care of clients with venous disease now if you had difficulty with this question!

Level of Cognitive Ability: Application
Phase of Nursing Process: Implementation
Client Needs: Physiological Integrity
Content Area: Adult Health/Cardiovascular

Reference

Luckmann, J. (1997). *Saunders manual of nursing care*. Philadelphia: W. B. Saunders, p. 1019.

165. The 6-year-old client tells the school nurse, "I wish my father wouldn't lick me 'down there.' He's always doing it when he sleeps with me. He told me to keep it 'our secret,' but I don't want to do this anymore." Which of the following is the most appropriate response by the nurse?

1 "It is not good for your father to do this. Tell him to stop. You know you have a fine father who loves you very much."
2 "Tell me more about this. When did your father last do this? Have you been watching television movies about this recently?"
3 "I'm glad you've come to me with this problem. Your father will not 'lick you down there' again. Can you stay here with your teacher while I make some phone calls?"
4 "You should always obey your parents. What did your mother say when you told her this?"

Answer: 3

Rationale: The child who experiences sexual abuse by the father requires encouragement to express feelings about the abuse. This is often accomplished through play therapy with the use of puppets or dolls, role playing, or art work. Although giving approval is not usually the therapeutic response, in this case and in view of the age of the child, it is appropriate to provide permission for the child to break the commitment to silence that the father has tried to obtain from the child. It is the nurse's legal and ethical responsibility to report this incident to the police and to the children's protective services.

Test-Taking Strategy: This question assesses your ability to assess the sexually abused child who is a victim of incest by her father. Option 1 not only is incorrect but also delivers a "double-bind" message (father is doing things that are not good and should be stopped and yet father is a fine man) that would produce confusion and anger in the child. Option 2 is incorrect; although it begins with a facilitative response, it leads into specific data collection that may be premature and force the child to focus on a situation that is unpleasant at best. It then, quite confusingly, insinuates that the child's report is the result of the influence of television. Option 4 is incorrect; it is controlling and patronizing in its use of clichés, and it insinuates that the child should have told the mother, which is an action that may be impossible for the child to take for a myriad of reasons.

Level of Cognitive Ability: Application
Phase of Nursing Process: Implementation
Client Needs: Safe, Effective Care Environment
Content Area: Child Health

Reference
Antai-Otong, D. (1995). *Psychiatric nursing: Biological and behavioral concepts.* Philadelphia: W. B. Saunders, pp. 407–426.

---

166. The client is being treated for acute respiratory failure. The client complains bitterly of dyspnea, even though the pulse oximetry reading shows 94% saturation. Which of the following actions would be most appropriate for the nurse to take?

1 Put the client in bed, in high Fowler's position
2 Discuss the connection between anxiety and dyspnea with the client
3 Encourage the client to set feasible but increasing goals in daily activities
4 Discuss the limitations imposed on the client by the chronic respiratory problem and offer coping strategies

Answer: 3

Rationale: Providing care to achieve established goals by providing information, strategies, or nursing interventions is the basic issue here. Creating an awareness that there is a way that the client can "work" to improve the condition gives the client hope. The pulse oximetry is adequate; therefore, according to the information presented, physiological integrity is not the issue. Putting the client to bed in high Fowler's is not required and ignores the issue. There is no mention of anxiety in the question. Discussing limitations is important, but it is most important to encourage the client.

Test-Taking Strategy: Use the process of elimination, noting that the parameter related to pulse oximetry is normal. The issue is not a physiological one. Therefore, eliminate option 1. Next, eliminate option 2 because anxiety is not presented in the question. For the remaining two options, remember that in this situation, encouraging is more important than discussing. In addition, option 3 is the more global option.

Level of Cognitive Ability: Application
Phase of Nursing Process: Implementation
Client Needs: Psychosocial Integrity
Content Area: Adult Health/Respiratory

Reference
Black, J., & Matassarin-Jacobs, E. (1997). *Medical-surgical nursing: Clinical management for continuity of care* (5th ed.). Philadelphia: W. B. Saunders, pp. 1169–1170.

167. The physician orders warfarin (Coumadin) for a client with multifocal atrial fibrillation. The community health nurse visits the client at home and teaches the client about the medication and its administration. Which of the following instructions would not be provided to the client by the nurse?

1 The urine will be orange in color
2 This medication will necessitate frequent blood work to monitor its effects
3 This medicine will still be working 4–5 days after it is discontinued
4 Aspirin and any aspirin-containing medications cannot be taken while on this medication

Answer: 1

Rationale: Warfarin (Coumadin) is an anticoagulant. Bleeding is a concern while the client is taking this medication. Orange coloration of urine indicates blood in the urine, resulting from an overdose of the medication. Bleeding may also be identified by urine that turns red, smoky, or black. Options 2, 3, and 4 all are correct regarding this medication.

Test-Taking Strategy: Note the key word "not" in the stem of the question, which alerts you to find an incorrect statement. Option 2 is correct because prothrombin time is measured to monitor the clotting mechanism. Option 3 is correct because the half-life of the medication is 2 days, the peak effect occurs between 1 and 3 days, and the anticoagulation effect extends 4–5 days after discontinuation. Option 4 is correct because aspirin is an antiplatelet agent and would increase the risk of bleeding.

Level of Cognitive Ability: Application
Phase of Nursing Process: Implementation
Client Needs: Health Promotion and Maintenance
Content Area: Pharmacology

Reference
Chernecky, C., & Berger, B. J. (1997). *Laboratory tests and diagnostic procedures* (2nd ed.). Philadelphia: W. B. Saunders, pp. 847–850.

168. The nurse is employed in a long-term care facility and is caring for elderly clients. In which of the following situations would the nurse withhold food from an elderly resident?

1 Decrease in appetite
2 Adequate ability to swallow
3 Normal bowel sounds
4 Episodes of vomiting

Answer: 4

Rationale: Maintaining the appetite is particularly difficult when the client is nauseated or is prone to vomiting. The nurse should limit food and fluid intake when discomfort is serious; then small amounts of fluid (or food) should be offered as tolerated. Options 1, 2, and 3 are not reasons to withhold food or fluids.

Test-Taking Strategy: Use the process of elimination. There is only one reason for withholding food from a client. Options 1, 2, and 3 do not indicate that there is any alteration in the gastrointestinal tract. Therefore, the only correct option is option 4.

Level of Cognitive Ability: Application
Phase of Nursing Process: Implementation
Client Needs: Physiological Integrity
Content Area: Fundamental Skills

Reference
Bolander, V. (1994). *Sorensen and Luckmann's Basic nursing: A psychophysiologic approach* (3rd ed.). Philadelphia: W. B. Saunders, p. 1090.

169. The nurse is caring for the client with HIV/AIDS. The client asks for a snack. Which of the following would be the most appropriate choice for this client to meet nutritional needs?

1 An apple
2 Home-made yogurt
3 A fresh fruit salad
4 Poached pears

Answer: 4

Rationale: Nursing care, focusing on ensuring the nutritional needs of clients with HIV/AIDS, revolves around nursing interventions to provide protection from infection. The main considerations to be remembered include avoiding all milk and milk products and cooking (well) all foods, especially raw vegetables and fruits. Remember that these clients are immunocompromised. Foods that have the potential to harbor bacteria need to be avoided.

Test-Taking Strategy: Use the process of elimination, remembering that these clients are immunocompromised and that foods that have the potential to harbor bacteria need to be avoided. Eliminate options 1 and 3 first because they are similar in that both are fresh fruits, and fresh fruits tend to harbor bacteria. Eliminate option 2 because yogurt contains yeast. Note that in option 4, poached pears, the food item is cooked. Review nutrition related to the client with HIV/AIDS now if you had difficulty with this question!

Level of Cognitive Ability: Application
Phase of Nursing Process: Implementation
Client Needs: Physiological Integrity
Content Area: Fundamental Skills

Reference

Black, J., & Matassarin-Jacobs, E. (1997). *Medical-surgical nursing: Clinical management for continuity of care* (5th ed.). Philadelphia: W. B. Saunders, pp. 614–651.

---

170. The client with HIV says to the nurse, "I'm uptight all the time; the slightest little twinge and I immediately think, 'Here it comes—it's the bed for me!'" Which of the following is the most appropriate therapeutic nursing response by the nurse?

1. "What ways have you developed to deal with anxiety in the past?"
2. "It seems as if you are 'on edge' all the time."
3. "Sounds like you have probably always been a 'type A' personality."
4. "You need to practice your relaxation technique more."

Answer: 2

Rationale: Anxiety is the most common emotion experienced by clients with HIV/AIDS. They live with a lethal clinical illness that brings with it fears of the future and of the illness itself. Option 1 is a premature communication technique for the client's expression of fear. It closes off the ability for the client to express anxiety and the constant fear that was causing tension and worry. Option 3 also closes off the client's emotions and labels the client's responses in a sarcastic style. Option 4 does not acknowledge the client's emotions or facilitate an expression of feelings. It also uses the word "need," which has a controlling connotation. Option 2 uses a therapeutic communication skill to assess anxiety in the client.

Test-Taking Strategy: Use the process of elimination and note the relationship between the client's statement "I'm uptight" in the question and the phrase "on edge" in the correct option.

Level of Cognitive Ability: Application
Phase of Nursing Process: Implementation
Client Needs: Psychosocial Integrity
Content Area: Fundamental Skills

Reference

Black, J., & Matassarin-Jacobs, E. (1997. *Medical-surgical nursing: Clinical management for continuity of care* (5th ed.). Philadelphia: W. B. Saunders, pp. 614–651.

---

171. The nurse is caring for a client with HIV infection. As part of the nursing care plan, the nurse monitors for opportunistic infection. In the event that the opportunistic infection pneumonia (*Pneumocystis carinii*) occurs, the nurse would anticipate that the most likely medication to be prescribed would be

1. Pentamidine (Pentam).
2. Nystatin (Nilstat, Mycostatin).
3. Acyclovir (Zovirax).
4. Bleomycin (Blenoxane).

Answer: 1

Rationale: Pentamidine, an antiprotozoal, is used to treat *P. carinii* infection. Nystatin, an antifungal and anti-infective agent, is used to treat candidal stomatitis. Acyclovir, an antiviral agent, is used to treat herpes simplex. Bleomycin, an antineoplastic and antibiotic agent, is used to treat Kaposi's sarcoma (KS) and non-Hodgkin's lymphoma.

Test-Taking Strategy: Two of the medications, acyclovir and nystatin, are probably most familiar to you, and you may be able to eliminate these options fairly easily. Bleomycin is an antineoplastic/antibiotic that may be used to treat Kaposi's sarcoma. Therefore, eliminate this option. Take time now to review the actions and purposes of these medications if you had difficulty with this question!

Level of Cognitive Ability: Application
Phase of Nursing Process: Implementation
Client Needs: Physiological Integrity
Content Area: Pharmacology

Reference

Black, J., & Matassarin-Jacobs, E. (1997). *Medical-surgical nursing: Clinical management for continuity of care* (5th ed.). Philadelphia: W. B. Saunders, pp. 614–651.

172. The client who is to begin oxygen therapy has a need for precise amounts of oxygen to be delivered to the lungs. The physician asks the nurse to bring "respiratory equipment" to the bedside. The nurse would select which of the following oxygen masks to bring to the client's bedside?

1 Venturi mask
2 Partial rebreather mask
3 Non-rebreather mask
4 Simple oxygen mask

Answer: 1

Rationale: An advantage of the Venturi mask is that it can deliver precise amounts of oxygen to the client. A partial rebreather mask is used to permit conservation of oxygen while allowing rebreathing of approximately one third of the client's exhaled air. The non-rebreather mask provides for the highest concentration of oxygen available. The simple oxygen mask is used for clients who need humidified oxygen by mask for short-term use (e.g., less than 12 hours) at rates of 6–10 liters/minute.

Test-Taking Strategy: To answer this question accurately, you need to be familiar with the different types of oxygen masks and their specific uses and advantages. If this question was difficult for you, take a few moments now to review these!

Level of Cognitive Ability: Application
Phase of Nursing Process: Implementation
Client Needs: Physiological Integrity
Content Area: Adult Health/Respiratory

Reference

Taylor, C., Lillis, C., & LeMone, P. (1997). *Fundamentals of nursing: The art and science of nursing care* (3rd ed.). Philadelphia: Lippincott-Raven, pp. 1341, 1343–1344.

173. The nurse is caring for the client with an endotracheal tube (ETT) in place. Which of the following methods of ETT cuff inflation selected by the nurse would indicate the safest nursing practice?

1 Inflating the cuff until it reaches 30 mmHg
2 Using exactly 5 mL of air to inflate the cuff
3 Inflating the cuff during inspiration until a leak is auscultated at the larynx
4 Inflating the cuff during inspiration until no sound is auscultated at the larynx

Answer: 4

Rationale: The most common and safest method of cuff inflation is to inflate the balloon during a positive pressure breath until no air can be heard with auscultation over the cuff area of the larynx. This provides an acceptable seal with the lowest amount of cuff pressure, and is referred to as the minimal occlusion volume technique. Cuff pressures should be maintained below 18–20 mmHg, as this is the venous pressure in the tracheal area. Using a preset amount of air as a guideline is dangerous because it provides no control over cuff pressure. Leaving a leak with an endotracheal tube is dangerous because the client may aspirate secretions that drop below the balloon. The client with an endotracheal tube cannot swallow.

Test-Taking Strategy: The question asks for the "safest" method of cuff inflation. Key concepts to recall to answer this question include full inflation and low pressure. Knowing that a leak does not indicate full inflation should prompt you to eliminate this option first. A preset volume of air (5 mL) does not give control over pressure, so this option is eliminated next. To discriminate between the last two options, you need to know that 30 mmHg of pressure is excessive. This would help you to choose option 4 over option 1 as the correct answer.

Level of Cognitive Ability: Application
Phase of Nursing Process: Implementation
Client Needs: Physiological Integrity
Content Area: Adult Health/Respiratory

Reference

Black, J., & Matassarin-Jacobs, E. (1997). *Medical-surgical nursing: Clinical management for continuity of care* (5th ed.). Philadelphia: W. B. Saunders, p. 1174.

174. The client who is intubated and receiving mechanical ventilation has a nursing diagnosis of Risk for Infection. The nurse would avoid doing which of the following in the care of this client?

1. Monitor the client's temperature at least once per shift
2. Monitor sputum characteristics and amounts
3. Use the closed-system method of suctioning
4. Drain water from the ventilator tubing into the humidifier bottle

Answer: 4

Rationale: Water in the ventilator tubing should be emptied, not drained back into the humidifier bottle. This puts the client at risk of acquiring infection, especially with *Pseudomonas* organisms. Monitoring temperature and sputum are indicated in the care of the client. A closed-system method of suctioning does not harm the client, although the extent of its advantages is still being researched.

Test-Taking Strategy: The wording of the question guides you to look for an option that puts the client more at risk for infection. Options 1, 2, and 3 all are indicators of safe, prudent nursing practice and do not put the client at risk for infection. The remaining option, drainage of water back into the humidifier bottle, is the only possible choice, even if you are relatively unfamiliar with concepts of ventilator care.

Level of Cognitive Ability: Application
Phase of Nursing Process: Implementation
Client Needs: Safe, Effective Care Environment
Content Area: Adult Health/Respiratory

Reference

Black, J., & Matassarin-Jacobs, E. (1997). *Medical-surgical nursing: Clinical management for continuity of care* (5th ed.). Philadelphia: W. B. Saunders, pp. 1175, 1181.

175. The physician tells the nurse that a client's chest tube is to be removed. The nurse would bring which of the following dressing materials to the bedside for the physician's use?

1. Telfa dressing and polymyxin/neomycin/bacitracin (Neosporin) ointment
2. Petrolatum gauze and sterile 4 × 4 gauze
3. Sterile 4 × 4 gauze and Elastoplast tape
4. Benzoin spray and a hydrocolloid dressing

Answer: 2

Rationale: Upon removal, the chest tube insertion site has a sterile petrolatum gauze applied, which is then covered with a sterile 4 × 4 gauze. The entire dressing is securely taped to ensure that it is occlusive. The petrolatum dressing is the key element in making an airtight seal at the former insertion site of the chest tube. The use of Telfa dressing, Neosporin ointment, hydrocolloid dressing, and benzoin spray is not indicated. Elastoplast tape could be used at the discretion of the physician as the tape of choice to make the dressing occlusive, but adhesive tape is most commonly used.

Test-Taking Strategy: Knowledge of the correct dressing material is needed to answer this question accurately. Remembering that an airtight seal is needed to cover the site after chest tube removal will assist in directing you to the correct option.

Level of Cognitive Ability: Application
Phase of Nursing Process: Implementation
Client Needs: Physiological Integrity
Content Area: Adult Health/Respiratory

Reference

Black, J., & Matassarin-Jacobs, E. (1997). *Medical-surgical nursing: Clinical management for continuity of care* (5th ed.). Philadelphia: W. B. Saunders, p. 1166.

176. The nurse enters the client's room with a pulse oximetry machine and tells the client that the physician has ordered continuous oxygen saturation readings. The client's facial expression changes to one of apprehension. The nurse would quickly and most effectively alleviate the client's anxiety by stating that pulse oximetry

1 Is painless and safe.
2 Causes only mild discomfort at the site.
3 Requires insertion of only a very small catheter.
4 Has an alarm to signal dangerous drops in oxygen saturation levels.

Answer: 1

Rationale: The nurse should reassure the client that pulse oximetry is a safe, painless, noninvasive method of monitoring oxygen saturation levels. There is no discomfort because the oximeter uses a sensor that is attached to a fingertip, toe, or earlobe. The machine does have an alarm that will ring if there is interference with monitoring or when the percentage of oxygen saturation moves below a preset level.

Test-Taking Strategy: Begin to answer this question by eliminating options 2 and 3, which are untrue statements. Of the two remaining, option 1 is a reassuring type of statement which would alleviate the client's anxiety, whereas option 4 is not (even though the factual information in option 4 is correct).

Level of Cognitive Ability: Application
Phase of Nursing Process: Implementation
Client Needs: Psychosocial Integrity
Content Area: Adult Health/Respiratory

Reference
Black, J., & Matassarin-Jacobs, E. (1997). *Medical-surgical nursing: Clinical management for continuity of care* (5th ed.). Philadelphia: W. B. Saunders, pp. 1051–1052.

---

177. The young adult client has never had a chest x-ray before, and expresses to the nurse a fear of experiencing some form of harm from the test. Which of the following responses by the nurse would provide the most reassurance to the client?

1 "You'll wear a lead shield to partially protect your organs from harm."
2 "The amount of x-ray exposure is not sufficient to cause DNA damage."
3 "The test isn't harmful at all. The most frustrating part is the long wait in radiology."
4 "The x-ray itself is painless, and a lead shield protects you from the minimal radiation."

Answer: 4

Rationale: Clients should be taught that the amount of exposure to radiation is minimal and that the test itself is painless. The wording in each of the other responses is partially true but provides no reassurance to the client.

Test-Taking Strategy: Eliminate options 1 and 2 first as the least reassuring to the client. Of the two remaining, option 4 is preferable to option 3. Option 4 is accurate and a therapeutic response.

Level of Cognitive Ability: Application
Phase of Nursing Process: Implementation
Client Needs: Psychosocial Integrity
Content Area: Adult Health/Respiratory

Reference
Black, J., & Matassarin-Jacobs, E. (1997). *Medical-surgical nursing: Clinical management for continuity of care* (5th ed.). Philadelphia: W. B. Saunders, p. 1060.

---

178. The client has had a sample for an arterial blood gas measurement drawn from the radial artery, and the nurse is asked to hold pressure on the site. The nurse would apply pressure for at least

1 1 minute.
2 2 minutes.
3 5 minutes.
4 10 minutes.

Answer: 3

Rationale: After drawing of samples for measuring arterial blood gases, continuous pressure must be applied to the site. The radial artery requires at least 5 minutes of pressure; the femoral artery requires 10. A small pressure dressing is often placed on the site afterward. The client receiving anticoagulant therapy may require pressure to be applied for a longer period of time.

Test-Taking Strategy: This question tests a fundamental concept related to the care of the client having samples drawn for arterial blood gas measurements. If you did not choose correctly, memorize this information as described in the rationale now, or review the procedure again briefly.

Level of Cognitive Ability: Application
Phase of Nursing Process: Implementation
Client Needs: Physiological Integrity
Content Area: Adult Health/Respiratory

Reference

Black, J., & Matassarin-Jacobs, E. (1997). *Medical-surgical nursing: Clinical management for continuity of care* (5th ed.). Philadelphia: W. B. Saunders, p. 1057.

---

179. The client experienced an open pneumothorax and a sucking chest wound, which has been covered with an occlusive dressing. The client begins to experience severe dyspnea, and the blood pressure begins to fall. The nurse should first

1. Remove the dressing.
2. Reinforce the dressing.
3. Call the physician.
4. Measure oxygen saturation by oximetry.

Answer: 1

Rationale: Placement of a dressing over a sucking chest wound could convert an open pneumothorax to a closed (tension) pneumothorax. This could result in a sudden decline in respiratory status, mediastinal shift, twisting of the great vessels, and circulatory compromise. If this occurs, the nurse removes the dressing immediately, allowing air to escape.

Test-Taking Strategy: To answer this question accurately, it is critical to understand that an open pneumothorax can be transformed into a tension pneumothorax with closure. The immediate action is to remove the dressing. All other responses are incorrect because the question asks for a "first" action. If this question was difficult, review this material again. You are likely to find a question related to this content on NCLEX-RN!

Level of Cognitive Ability: Application
Phase of Nursing Process: Implementation
Client Needs: Physiological Integrity
Content Area: Adult Health/Respiratory

Reference

Black, J., & Matassarin-Jacobs, E. (1997). *Medical-surgical nursing: Clinical management for continuity of care* (5th ed.). Philadelphia: W. B. Saunders, pp. 2524–2526.

---

180. The nurse is caring for a client who is to be treated with an anticholinesterase agent. As part of the medication teaching plan, the nurse plans to instruct the client regarding effects of this medication class. The nurse informs the client that which effects are likely to occur?

1. Digestive effects such as decreased motility and tone in the gut
2. Urinary effects such as urinary hesitation and retention
3. Cardiovascular effects such as tachycardia
4. Respiratory effects such as increased bronchial secretions

Answer: 4

Rationale: Anticholinesterase agents cause respiratory effects such as increased bronchial secretions, bronchoconstriction, weakness, and paralysis of respiratory muscles. Options 1, 2, and 3 are incorrect.

Test-Taking Strategy: Knowledge of the effects of the anticholinesterase agents is necessary to answer the question. Eliminate option 1 because digestive effects include increased motility and tone in the gut. Eliminate option 2 because urinary effects include urinary frequency and incontinence. Eliminate option 3 because cardiovascular effects include bradycardia. Review this medication class now if you had difficulty with this question!

Level of Cognitive Ability: Application
Phase of Nursing Process: Implementation
Client Needs: Physiological Integrity
Content Area: Pharmacology

Reference

Clark, J., Queener, S., & Karb, V. (1997). *Pharmacologic basis of nursing practice* (5th ed.). St. Louis: Mosby–Year Book, pp. 696–704.

181. A teenager diagnosed with active tuberculosis has been prescribed a combination of isoniazid (INH) PO and rifampin (Rifadin) PO for treatment. The nurse's teaching about effective medication therapy should include which of the following?

1. "Report any change in urine color."
2. "Take both medications together once a day."
3. "Both medications should be taken with food."
4. "Expect to take the medication for 2–3 weeks."

Answer: 2

Rationale: This combination taken together daily has proved effective in eliminating the tubercle bacilli from the sputum and improves clinical status faster than any other treatment. Rifampin in combination with INH prevents the emergence of medication-resistant organisms. Rifampin produces a harmless red-orange coloration in all body fluids and should be taken 1 hour before or 2 hours after eating, to maximize absorption. The treatment regimen is maintained for at least 6 months for effectiveness, although the therapeutic effect may be evident in 2–3 weeks.

Test-Taking Strategy: The word "effective" in the stem eliminates option 1 because this option is a side effect. The inclusive word "both" is used in two options. Knowledge regarding the length of treatment and the appropriate method of administration will easily direct you to option 2. Review these very important medications now if you had difficulty with this question!

Level of Cognitive Ability: Application
Phase of Nursing Process: Implementation
Client Needs: Physiological Integrity
Content Area: Pharmacology

Reference

Hodgson, B., & Kizior, R. (1998). *Saunders nursing drug handbook 1998*. Philadelphia: W. B. Saunders, pp. 550–552, 906–908.

---

182. After administration of the Mantoux tuberculin skin test, the nurse reads the results in

1. 24–36 hours.
2. 24–48 hours.
3. 36–48 hours.
4. 48–72 hours.

Answer: 4

Rationale: The Mantoux tuberculin skin test is the most accurate and reliable tuberculin skin test currently available. Interpretation of the Mantoux test is based on duration only, and reading should be done 48–72 hours after the injection of the tuberculin.

Test-Taking Strategy: Knowledge of the correct reading times after a tuberculin test is essential to answer this question. Take time now to review this test if you had difficulty with this question!

Level of Cognitive Ability: Application
Phase of Nursing Process: Implementation
Client Needs: Physiological Integrity
Content Area: Adult Health/Respiratory

Reference

Pinnell, N. L. (1996). *Nursing pharmacology*. Philadelphia: W. B. Saunders, p. 1065.

183. Which of the following should the nurse include in a postoperative teaching plan for a client with Harrington rod fusion who will be wearing a brace?

1. Instruct the client to tighten the brace during meals and loosen for the first 30 minutes after each meal
2. Tell the client to inspect the environment for safety hazards
3. Inform the client that lotions and body powders can be used for skin breakdown
4. Bed rest is required for one week

Answer: 2

Rationale: The client should be taught to loosen the brace during meals and for 30 minutes after each meal. Clients have difficulty eating if the brace is too tight. Loosening the brace after each meal will allow adequate digestion and promote comfort. The client needs to inspect the environment for safety hazards. Certain braces for spinal deviations do not allow the client to flex or bend the spinal column. The client should be encouraged to use handrails on stairways and to take precautions when walking. Powders and lotions should not be used because they may irritate the skin. As the client stabilizes postoperatively, mobility is quickly increased. Hospital discharge may occur by the fifth postoperative day.

Test-Taking Strategy: Be cautious with the selection of your answer when the choice contains the word "and." Keep in mind that the entire option needs to be correct. Use the process of elimination, noting that option 2 identifies safety measures and that it is the most global option. Review Harrington rod fusion and the use of a brace now if you had difficulty with this question!

Level of Cognitive Ability: Application
Phase of Nursing Process: Implementation
Client Needs: Physiological Integrity
Content Area: Adult Health/Neurological

Reference

Black, J., & Matassarin-Jacobs, E. (1997). *Medical-surgical nursing: Clinical management for continuity of care* (5th ed.). Philadelphia: W. B. Saunders, pp. 920, 2120–2121.

---

184. The nurse is caring for a client who is scheduled for arthroplasty (total joint replacement) of the hip. In the postoperative period, the priority nursing action would be to

1. Maintain the leg in an elevated position with the leg extended.
2. Limit exercises to bending at the waist to touch the toes three times daily.
3. Assess for circulation, sensation, and movement of the operative leg.
4. Maintain internal-external rotation of the operative leg and hip flexion.

Answer: 3

Rationale: Arthroplasty is the resurfacing of damaged or degenerative bones within a joint and replacement of damaged bone and cartilage with metal and plastic components. In total hip arthroplasty, the head of the femur is removed and replaced, and the acetabulum is resurfaced with a cup inserted. Arthroplasty of the hip requires postoperative assessing for circulation, sensation, and movement of the operative leg. The leg should be in the neutral position with the toes pointed upward. The legs are abducted with an abduction pillow or brace in place. The nurse should check with the surgeon to ascertain which side the client can turn toward.

Test-Taking Strategy: This question assesses your knowledge of arthroplasty (total hip or joint replacement). Option 1 is an incorrect position. Option 2 is completely incorrect. There may be a knee immobilizer on the leg to keep the knee straight, or the leg may be on a continuous passive motion exerciser. Option 4 states an inappropriate position. Use the ABCs: airway, breathing, and circulation. Option 3 addresses circulation!

Level of Cognitive Ability: Application
Phase of Nursing Process: Implementation
Client Needs: Physiological Integrity
Content Area: Adult Health/Musculoskeletal

Reference

Luckmann, J. (1997). *Saunders manual of nursing care.* Philadelphia: W. B. Saunders, pp. 1606–1609.

185. The nurse is caring for a client with a dermal ulcer just débrided by the physician. In caring for the client, the most appropriate nursing intervention would be to gently cleanse the wound with

1 Hypochlorite.
2 Povidone-iodine.
3 Dry cotton gauze.
4 Tepid normal saline.

Answer: 4

Rationale: After débridement, the nurse would gently cleanse the wound with tepid normal saline. Antiseptic solutions such as povidone-iodine and hypochlorite are cytotoxic to healthy tissue and not routinely used. The only exception might be for an infected wound, and the solutions are followed by a normal saline irrigation.

Test-Taking Strategy: This question assesses your knowledge of the medical management of dermal ulcers to promote their healing. Options 1 and 2 are incorrect. Option 3 is incorrect because débridement would remove necrotic tissue and leaves an ulcer pink with granulation tissue. Dry cotton gauze would irritate granulation tissue. Review care of ulcers now if you had difficulty with this question!

Level of Cognitive Ability: Application
Phase of Nursing Process: Implementation
Client Needs: Physiological Integrity
Content Area: Adult Health/Integumentary

Reference
Luckmann, J. (1997). *Saunders manual of nursing care.* Philadelphia: W. B. Saunders pp. 175–180.

186. The nurse is caring for a client who has suffered a cerebral vascular accident. It has been determined that the client experienced a hemorrhagic stroke. On the basis of this diagnosis, the nurse plans to place the client in which of the following positions?

1 Prone
2 Semi-Fowler's
3 Supine
4 Flat, side-lying

Answer: 2

Rationale: In a client with a hemorrhagic stroke, the head is elevated to 30 degrees to reduce intracranial pressure and to facilitate venous drainage. The head of the bed is kept flat for clients with ischemic strokes.

Test-Taking Strategy: Knowledge regarding the pathophysiological processes related to a hemorrhagic stroke is necessary to answer this question. Think about the principle of gravity. If hemorrhage is occurring in the brain, the head of the bed would be elevated to assist in the gravity drainage to prevent increased intracranial pressure.

Level of Cognitive Ability: Application
Phase of Nursing Process: Implementation
Client Needs: Physiological Integrity
Content Area: Adult Health/Neurological

Reference
Black, J., & Matassarin-Jacobs, E. (1997). *Medical-surgical nursing: Clinical management for continuity of care* (5th ed.). Philadelphia: W. B. Saunders, p. 793.

187. A newborn has just been delivered, and the nurse is following the steps of neonatal resuscitation. The nurse placed the newborn on a preheated surface, and the baby was dried, positioned in a "sniffing position," and provided tactile stimulation to initiate a cry. The nurse finds the infant to have gasping respirations and a heart rate below 100 beats/minute. What should the nurse do first?

1 Continue tactile stimulation until infant cries
2 Initiate bag and mask ventilation with 100% oxygen
3 Start chest compressions
4 Call the delivering doctor to help

Answer: 2

Rationale: The infant needs bag and mask ventilation because of the ineffective breathing, as evidenced by the lowered heart rate. Continuing tactile stimulation will not give the infant the oxygen needed. Starting chest compressions would not be recommended at this time, in view of the symptoms addressed in the question. The physician will need to be notified, but this is not the first action.

Test-Taking Strategy: Note the key word "first" in the stem of the question. Use the ABCs—airway, breathing, and circulation—to answer the question. This will direct you to the correct option. Concepts related to neonatal resuscitation should be reviewed if you had difficulty with this question!

Level of Cognitive Ability: Application
Phase of Nursing Process: Implementation
Client Needs: Physiological Integrity
Content Area: Maternity

References

Ashwill, J., & Droske, S. (1997). *Nursing care of children: Principles and practice.* Philadelphia: W. B. Saunders, pp. 550–556.
Nichols, F., & Zwelling, E. (1997). *Maternal-newborn nursing: Theory and practice.* Philadelphia: W. B. Saunders, pp. 1340–1345.

---

188. A family member of a client with HIV infection asks, "What can I dispose of in the toilet and do I need to use a separate bathroom?" Which of the following responses would the nurse not provide to the family?

1 "You can flush any blood or body fluids. Always be certain to wear gloves when you're handling this material, though."
2 "You will want to dispose of any organic material that is on the clothes or linens before you put them in the washing machine."
3 "I would certainly recommend that you create a separate bathroom just in case there is inadequate cleaning."
4 "All of the client's trash and soiled dressings must be tied securely in two plastic bags and thrown out with the family's trash."

Answer: 3

Rationale: HIV can be transmitted through intimate sexual contact with an HIV-seropositive person; by parenteral injection of blood or blood products infected with HIV; and through an HIV-infected mother to a fetus or newborn in utero, during labor or delivery, or in the early newborn period. AIDS cannot be contracted by sharing a bathroom. Because the AIDS virus dies quickly outside the body and requires living tissue to survive, it is killed by soap, disinfectants, cleansers, and hot water. Clothes can be laundered separately with bleach and other disinfectants. A 1:10 dilute bleach solution should be employed to clean the bathroom and kitchen surfaces.

Test-Taking Strategy: This question requires the application of knowledge of HIV/AIDS transmission. Use the process of elimination, noting the word "not" in the stem of the question. In addition, common sense must be your guide. Creating a separate bathroom can be a costly endeavor that makes both the client and family members feel an increased sense of isolation from each other.

Level of Cognitive Ability: Application
Phase of Nursing Process: Implementation
Client Needs: Health Promotion and Maintenance
Content Area: Fundamental Skills

Reference

Black, J., & Matassarin-Jacobs, E. (1997). *Medical-surgical nursing: Clinical management for continuity of care* (5th ed.). Philadelphia: W. B. Saunders, pp. 614–651.

189. The client with Bell's palsy says "I knew I'd had a stroke when I woke up like this!" Which of the following therapeutic communications would best reflect the nurse's understanding of the client's medical illness?

1. "It must be very frightening for you. Tell me more about how you plan to cope with the limitations of your illness."
2. "Everything is going to be all right. You really have no cause to worry about the stroke."
3. "It must be very difficult for you. How reassured you must be to learn that Bell's palsy is a temporary condition that resolves within a few weeks."
4. "Let's not discuss the consequences until you're feeling stronger and learn to live with the aftermath of Bell's palsy."

Answer: 3

Rationale: Many clients who first experience the temporary condition of facial paralysis that occurs in Bell's palsy think that they have had a stroke. It is important for the nurse to provide education about the illness and emotional support which results in the client's feeling reassured. In option 1, although the communication technique uses a response similar to the one in the correct answer, it does anticipate the client's own identification of feelings by labeling them "frightening." Option 2 falsely reassures the client and discourages the client from further expression of feelings. It also presents information the nurse cannot be certain of: that is, that the client has no need to worry. Option 4 refuses to consider and even somewhat devalues the client's behavior. In addition, the choice of the word "aftermath" infers that the illness is more serious than it is.

Test-Taking Strategy: Use therapeutic communication techniques, knowledge regarding Bell's palsy, and the process of elimination. Option 2 and 4 can be easily eliminated. Of the remaining options, option 3 addresses accurate information. Review Bell's palsy if you had difficulty with this question!

Level of Cognitive Ability: Application
Phase of Nursing Process: Implementation
Client Needs: Psychosocial Integrity
Content Area: Adult Health/Neurological

Reference

Black, J., & Matassarin-Jacobs, E. (1997). *Medical-surgical nursing: Clinical management for continuity of care* (5th ed.). Philadelphia: W. B. Saunders, pp. 915–932.

---

190. The nurse is caring for a client with Bell's palsy. As part of the nursing care plan, the nurse seeks to prevent complications and encourage nerve regeneration. To achieve these goals, the nurse's care plan will include

1. Patching the eye closed during the night to prevent corneal damage from inadequate eyelid closure during sleep.
2. Applying an ice bag to relieve pain and to support nerve regeneration.
3. Unpatching the eye during the night to prevent corneal damage from eyelid closure during sleep.
4. Patting the facial muscles gently, being careful not to increase circulation or to speed muscle tone.

Answer: 1

Rationale: In caring for clients with Bell's palsy, patching the eye closed during the night prevents corneal damage from inadequate eyelid closure during sleep. Methylcellulose eye drops several times a day will also prevent corneal damage from incomplete blinking. Massaging facial muscles promotes circulation and maintains muscle tone. Pain is relieved by warm, moist heat. Facial physical therapy exercises (grimacing, wrinkling the brow, forcing the eyes closed, whistling, and puffing the cheeks and blowing out air) for 5 minutes three times a day will increase nerve regeneration.

Test-Taking Strategy: This question not only assesses your knowledge of the nursing care required for clients with Bell's palsy, but it also assesses your grasp of the scientific principles underlying the nursing care for clients with cranial nerve disorders. Option 2 is incorrect because the use of ice will injure nerve regeneration, not support it. Option 3 is incorrect because leaving the eyelid unpatched at night can produce corneal damage from eyelid closure while sleeping. Option 4 is incorrect because light massage will promote circulation and speed muscle tone, which is needed for recovery. Review these principles now if you had difficulty with this question!

Level of Cognitive Ability: Application
Phase of Nursing Process: Implementation
Client Needs: Physiological Integrity
Content Area: Adult Health/Neurological

Reference

Luckmann, J. (1997). *Saunders manual of nursing care.* Philadelphia: W. B. Saunders, pp. 729–733.

191. The community health nurse visits a frail 80-year-old male client at home. The client has several bruises on his back, hips, and chest. The medication count and the client's mental status indicate that he's receiving too much sedation. Which of the following responses by the nurse would be appropriate when the client says, "My son gets tired having to tend me at night; I'm always wet, and it's all my fault. My son can't help being a little rough."

1 "You're saying that when you're incontinent at night, you feel that you're at fault and that your son can't help being rough?"
2 "Oh, he can't, can't he? I intend to report this abusive behavior to the police."
3 "Well, I know you feel that you're a bother, but you pay your way and then some. I'll talk with your son and clear this right up."
4 "Let's not dwell on this. After all, you are doing quite well and maybe we can arrange for you to go to a nursing home on the weekends."

Answer: 1

Rationale: The correct answer summarizes and focuses on the content of the client's message. In addition, it restates so the client can hear himself making excuses about his son's physical abuse. In option 2, the nurse is sarcastic and, without further investigation, moves to report the incident. In option 3, the nurse confirms the client's fear that he's a "bother" and then begins to insinuate that his son is using his money and that this will be cleared up just by the nurse's talking with the client's son. Option 4 is incorrect because it advocates avoiding the issue and then, incongruously, says things are proceeding well and yet that the client can go to "a nursing home on the weekends."

Test-Taking Strategy: This question assesses the nurse's ability to intervene in elder abuse and the use of therapeutic communication techniques. Use the process of elimination. Option 1 is the only option that reflects the use of therapeutic communication techniques.

Level of Cognitive Ability: Application
Phase of Nursing Process: Implementation
Client Needs: Psychosocial Integrity
Content Area: Mental Health

Reference

Antai-Otong, D. (1995). *Psychiatric nursing: Biological and behavioral concepts.* Philadelphia: W. B. Saunders, pp. 407–426.

192. The nurse is caring for a client who experienced blitz rape 2 hours ago. Which of the following statements by the nurse would best indicate an understanding of blitz rape?

1 "Of course you didn't close your bedroom window because it's so hot tonight. You ought to be able to open a window for fresh air."
2 "I am sorry this has happened to you. As a victim, you're not to blame. It's not your fault."
3 "It will be important to explore with your psychiatrist the meaning of the open window for you as you make your way back to normal."
4 "Why do you feel that this 'perp' wouldn't have gotten in if you had closed the window? They can get in many different ways."

Answer: 2

Rationale: Blitz rape, a type of sexual assault, occurs when the victim does not know who the rapist is and is unaware of vulnerability. Blitz rape occurs most often in the victim's home, or it might be a sudden attack in a parking lot, on the street, or in any place where the victim is alone or helpless. In a sexual assault, the woman fears for her life and must be reassured of her safety. Option 2 instills trust and validates self-worth for the victim who may be overcome with self-doubt and self-blame.

Test-Taking Strategy: The nurse's chief goal is to establish a therapeutic alliance with the victim. It is important for the nurse to use a nonjudgmental attitude. In option 1, the nurse's statement seems angry and vehement. In option 3, the nurse uses the term "normal." In view of the sensitive position of the victim, it can lead to self-blame and the thought that the victim is "abnormal." Moreover, the nurse's comment on the meaning of the window is premature. Option 4 would frighten the victim, and the use of the slang term "perp" would not be an appropriate therapeutic intervention for the client.

Level of Cognitive Ability: Application
Phase of Nursing Process: Implementation
Client Needs: Psychosocial Integrity
Content Area: Mental Health

Reference

Antai-Otong, D. (1995). *Psychiatric nursing: Biological and behavioral concepts.* Philadelphia: W. B. Saunders, pp. 407–426.

193. The client arrives at the emergency department, accompanied by her husband, seeking care for the seventh time for cuts around her left eye, two fractured ribs, and multiple contusions. The priority nursing intervention would be to

1 Take the client to a private area to perform the interview.
2 Confront the husband by reporting him to the police as a suspect of battering.
3 Say to the client, "When are you going to divorce this bully?"
4 Say to the husband, "What is your story this time?"

Answer: 1

Rationale: Taking the client to a private area is essential because the client is probably being battered by her husband, and she is unlikely to be truthful about her injuries. Some women are fearful that their partners will kill them, or they want to protect their partners. Client safety is the most important consideration of the nurse. If the victim gives permission, take pictures of all injuries. It is important to encourage the client to discuss the battering; also, in this case, remind her it has happened six times before. The nurse must not attempt rescue efforts but must offer support so that the final decision is the client's. If the client can make her own decision, it will give her a sense of control over her life.

Test-Taking Strategy: Option 2 is incorrect because it is the nurse's responsibility to support the client in making an appropriate decision, not to make it for her. This will increase the client's sense of control and self-worth, two feelings she is probably in need of at this time. In option 3, using the term "bully" to describe the husband may cause the client to defend him and become defensive with the nurse. In option 4, challenging the husband might cause him to take his wife away and then not bring her in when she needs care.

Level of Cognitive Ability: Application
Phase of Nursing Process: Implementation
Client Needs: Psychosocial Integrity
Content Area: Mental Health

Reference

Antai-Otong, D. (1995). *Psychiatric nursing: Biological and behavioral concepts.* Philadelphia: W. B. Saunders, pp. 407–426.

194. The nurse suspects that a 9-year-old client is a victim of child abuse. At the case conference, it is decided that the nurse will prepare a written report to the state authorities (child protective and law enforcement authorities). Which of the following would be included in the report?

1 Self-destructive acts, which include fire-setting, cruelty to animals, withdrawal, and avoidance behaviors
2 Demographics of child and family, detailed account of the nature and content of the injuries, and caretaker information
3 The child's sense of being different from other children and expressions of shame, embarrassment, and guilt
4 None, because this is the physician's and/or the advanced practice nurse's role; the generalist nurse must maintain confidentiality

Answer: 2

Rationale: The nurse is required by law to report child abuse in all states. The nurse must report child abuse to a variety of agencies, depending on the state in which the abuse occurs. In this case, the nurse has no responsibility to keep the abuse confidential because the child's rights take precedence over confidentiality as long as the reporter acts in good faith. In fact, failure to report may result in the nurse's liability for abuse that occurs later as a result of nonreporting. In essence, it is both a legal and an ethical responsibility for the nurse. The other situations in which the nurse may legally breach confidentiality include during emergencies, such as a client's expression of suicide or homicide (notifying potential victim); conforming to other legally reportable requirements, such as sexually transmitted diseases (STD); discussing a client with supervisors and others involved in caring for the client; and civil commitment situations by providing information without consent to document need for commitment. The documentation required in the written report is as stated in option 2, and the state's role is to initiate an investigation and perform a family assessment.

Test-Taking Strategy: Eliminate option 4 first because it is the nurse's responsibility to report abuse cases. Eliminate option 1 next because it is not related to the question. Of the remaining options, note that option 2 would provide concrete factual data, whereas option 3 would not!

Level of Cognitive Ability: Application
Phase of Nursing Process: Implementation
Client Needs: Psychosocial Integrity
Content Area: Child Health

Reference

Antai-Otong, D. (1995). *Psychiatric nursing: Biological and behavioral concepts.* Philadelphia: W. B. Saunders, pp. 88, 407–426.

195. The nurse is caring for a client after radiation therapy. Which of the following side effects would the nurse inform the client to expect?

1 Hair loss over the entire body
2 Weight gain
3 Anorexia and mild erythema
4 Multiple births in women of childbearing age

Answer: 3

Rationale: The skin may be burned (although this term is not used because it tends to frighten clients), and the manifestations range from a mild erythema to a moist desquamation (similar to a second-degree burn). In addition, nausea and anorexia can also be experienced.

Test-Taking Strategy: This question assesses your ability to apply knowledge of the side effects of radiation therapy. Option 1 is incorrect because the hair is usually lost only in the radiated area. Option 2 is incorrect and is exactly the opposite of the side effects usually experienced from radiation therapy. Option 4 is incorrect because in women of childbearing age, radiation therapy usually causes sterility.

Level of Cognitive Ability: Application
Phase of Nursing Process: Implementation
Client Needs: Physiological Integrity
Content Area: Adult Health/Oncology

Reference
Black, J., & Matassarin-Jacobs, E. (1997). *Medical-surgical nursing: Clinical management for continuity of care* (5th ed.). Philadelphia: W. B. Saunders, pp. 533–561.

---

196. The nurse is caring for a client with trigeminal neuralgia. As part of the nursing care plan, the nurse monitors for trigeminal pain. The nurse's goal is to provide relief from pain within 24–28 hours of beginning the medication. Which of the following medications, as prescribed, will the nurse administer?

1 Carbamazepine (Tegretol)
2 Sertraline (Zoloft)
3 Methylphenidate (Ritalin)
4 Fluoxetine (Prozac)

Answer: 1

Rationale: As stated in the stem, the goal of pharmacological intervention is to provide pain relief within 24–28 hours. The medications that are used include phenytoin (Dilantin), baclofen (Lioresal), and carbamazepine (Tegretol).

Test-Taking Strategy: This question assesses your knowledge of pharmacological agents that are used to treat trigeminal neuralgia. Options 2 and 4 are selective serotonin reuptake inhibitors used to treat depression. Option 3 is a stimulant that is used to treat hyperactivity and attention deficit disorder. Review these medications now if you had difficulty with this question!

Level of Cognitive Ability: Application
Phase of Nursing Process: Implementation
Client Needs: Physiological Integrity
Content Area: Adult Health/Neurological

Reference
Black, J., & Matassarin-Jacobs, E. (1997). *Medical-surgical nursing: Clinical management for continuity of care* (5th ed.). Philadelphia: W. B. Saunders, pp. 915–932.

197. The nurse is caring for a client scheduled for surgery for a large tumor on the skin. In the preoperative period, the client states to the nurse, "I don't think I'm going to make it through this surgery. I know it's worse than my surgeon is 'letting on.'" Which of the following is the most therapeutic communication by the nurse?

1 "Let's take this one step at a time. You have a good prognosis because the larger the tumor, the easier it is to surgically excise the lesion."
2 "Well, of course, it's as the surgeon stated: 'The larger they are, the easier they fall.'"
3 "You seem to be having some very fearful thoughts about your surgery."
4 "Remember that skin tumors usually grow rapidly, so the lesion may be more superficial than you fear."

Answer: 3

Rationale: The communication technique of exploration is the correct response because it facilitates expression of the client's feelings. The nurse also has an obligation to inform the surgeon and perhaps recommend postponement of the surgery until the client has a more optimistic view of the impending outcomes. Options 1, 2, and 4 are closed-ended responses and provide inaccurate information; option 4 also is incorrect in that skin tumors are usually slow-growing.

Test-Taking Strategy: Use the process of elimination and remember to select the option that addresses the client's feelings and concerns!

Level of Cognitive Ability: Application
Phase of Nursing Process: Implementation
Client Needs: Psychosocial Integrity
Content Area: Adult Health/Oncology

Reference

Black, J., & Matassarin-Jacobs, E. (1997). *Medical-surgical nursing: Clinical management for continuity of care* (5th ed.). Philadelphia: W. B. Saunders, pp. 533–561.

198. The client with pulmonary edema has orders for morphine sulfate to be administered intravenously. The nurse monitors which of these parameters with administration of this medication?

1 Respiratory rate and effort
2 Pulse rate
3 Peripheral tissue perfusion
4 Urine output

Answer: 1

Rationale: Morphine reduces anxiety and dyspnea in the client with pulmonary edema. It also decreases peripheral vascular resistance, and so blood pools in the periphery, decreasing pulmonary capillary pressure and fluid migration into alveoli. The client receiving morphine is monitored for signs and symptoms of respiratory depression, especially when morphine is administered intravenously.

Test-Taking Strategy: A critical concept with morphine administration is the side effect of respiratory depression. This basic concept could be tested in a number of different content areas, so make sure to know this one. Review this medication and the nursing implications associated with the medication now if you had difficulty with this question!

Level of Cognitive Ability: Application
Phase of Nursing Process: Implementation
Client Needs: Physiological Integrity
Content Area: Pharmacology

Reference

Smeltzer, S., & Bare, B. (1996). *Brunner and Suddarth's Textbook of medical-surgical nursing* (8th ed.). Philadelphia: Lippincott-Raven, p. 660.

199. The client in cardiogenic shock is scheduled to have insertion of an intra-aortic balloon pump (IABP). The client asks the nurse to explain how this is going to help. The nurse tells the client that this therapy will

1 Help measure right- and left-sided heart pressures.
2 Measure the arterial blood pressure constantly.
3 Detect changes in perfusion to the coronary arteries.
4 Help the heart circulate the blood more effectively.

Answer: 4

Rationale: The IABP is a type of left ventricular assist device. A catheter is inserted into the aorta, and a balloon on the catheter inflates during diastole, pushing blood forward into the circulation and backward through the coronary arteries. The overall effects are to decrease afterload and increase myocardial perfusion. The definitions in options 1 and 2 are for a multilumen pulmonary artery catheter and an intra-arterial line, respectively. There is no device that will directly detect perfusion to a coronary artery on an ongoing basis.

Test-Taking Strategy: Note the word "pump" in the name of the therapy, which implies motion or movement. Each of the incorrect options involves only a measurement. If you should get a question in which you are unsure of the topic, look for simple words or adjectives to help make sense of the question.

Level of Cognitive Ability: Application
Phase of Nursing Process: Implementation
Client Needs: Physiological Integrity
Content Area: Adult Health/Cardiovascular

Reference

Smeltzer, S., & Bare, B. (1996). *Brunner and Suddarth's Textbook of medical-surgical nursing* (8th ed.). Philadelphia: Lippincott-Raven, p. 672.

200. The nurse has removed the nasogastric tube (NGT) from a post–cardiac surgery client who has also been extubated. The nurse would not give the client sips of water if which of the following were present?

1 Lethargy and inability to stay awake
2 Hypoactive bowel sounds
3 Negative occult blood in the NGT drainage
4 Slight abdominal distention

Answer: 1

Rationale: The client may have sips of water 4 hours after extubation if the client is fully responsive, is not nauseated, and has bowel sounds.

Test-Taking Strategy: The question guides you to look for an item that would cause you to withhold fluids. Hypoactive bowel sounds and slight distention commonly occur postoperatively and are not of enough concern initially to withhold oral fluids. Negative occult blood drainage is normal. The correct response in this instance is the one that deals not with the gastrointestinal tract directly but with the neurological system. The client who is not awake and alert is at risk of aspiration.

Level of Cognitive Ability: Application
Phase of Nursing Process: Implementation
Client Needs: Physiological Integrity
Content Area: Adult Health/Cardiovascular

Reference

Black, J., & Matassarin-Jacobs, E. (1997). *Medical-surgical nursing: Clinical management for continuity of care* (5th ed.). Philadelphia: W. B. Saunders, p. 1361.

201. The nurse is implementing a bladder retraining program for the client who has incontinence. Which of the following interventions would be contraindicated as the nurse implements this plan?

1 Limiting the oral fluid intake of the client
2 Teaching pelvic muscle–strengthening exercises
3 Ensuring accessibility to a toilet
4 Adhering strictly to scheduled toileting times

Answer: 1

Rationale: In order for a bladder training program to be successful, several components must be in place. The client should learn and practice pelvic muscle–strengthening exercises to promote bladder emptying. The nurse should ensure accessibility to bathroom facilities and adhere strictly to the toileting schedule. Limiting fluid intake is contraindicated. Adequate fluid intake is necessary to produce enough urine to stimulate micturition.

Test-Taking Strategy: The wording of the statement guides you to look for an incorrect response. Because options 3 and 4 are most obviously correct actions, these are eliminated as answers according to the wording of the question. To discriminate between the last two options, it is necessary to know that sufficient fluid is necessary to cause bladder filling and proper stimulation of the micturition reflex. Knowing this would enable you to select option 1 as the correct answer.

Level of Cognitive Ability: Application
Phase of Nursing Process: Implementation
Client Needs: Physiological Integrity
Content Area: Adult Health/Renal

Reference

Black, J., & Matassarin-Jacobs, E. (1997). *Medical-surgical nursing: Clinical management for continuity of care* (5th ed.). Philadelphia: W. B. Saunders, p. 1610.

202. The client who has never been hospitalized before is having trouble initiating the stream of urine. Knowing that there is no pathological reason for this difficulty, the nurse avoids which of the following as the least helpful method of assisting the client?

1 Running tap water in the sink
2 Instructing the client to pour warm water over the perineal area
3 Assisting the client to a commode behind a closed curtain
4 Closing the bathroom door and instructing the client to pull the call bell when done

Answer: 3

Rationale: Lack of privacy is a key issue that may inhibit the ability of the client to void in the absence of known pathological processes. Ways to ensure privacy include placing locks on bathroom doors and having separate restrooms for men and women. Using a commode behind a thin curtain may inhibit voiding for some people. Use of a bathroom is preferable and may be supplemented with the use of running water or pouring water over the perineum as needed.

Test-Taking Strategy: This question is fairly straightforward in wording and tests a basic response of many clients to decreased privacy during voiding. Option 4 is most helpful and therefore is eliminated first, in view of the wording of the question. Knowing that options 1 and 2 are standard methods of assistance, you would then select option 3 as the least helpful method of assisting the client with elimination.

Level of Cognitive Ability: Application
Phase of Nursing Process: Implementation
Client Needs: Psychosocial Integrity
Content Area: Adult Health/Renal

Reference

Black, J., & Matassarin-Jacobs, E. (1997). *Medical-surgical nursing: Clinical management for continuity of care* (5th ed.). Philadelphia: W. B. Saunders, p. 1551.

203. The nurse has an order to obtain a 24-hour urine collection from a client with a renal disorder. The nurse would avoid which of the following to ensure proper collection of the 24-hour specimen?

1 Have the client void at the start time, and place this specimen in the container
2 Save all subsequent voidings in the 24-hour time period
3 Place the container on ice or in a refrigerator
4 Instruct the client to void at the end time, and put this specimen in the container

Answer: 1

Rationale: The nurse asks the client to void at the beginning of the collection period, and the nurse discards this urine sample. All subsequent voided urine is saved in a container, which is placed on ice or refrigerated. The client is asked to void at the finish time, and this sample is added to the collection. The container is labeled, placed on fresh ice, and sent to the laboratory immediately.

Test-Taking Strategy: Options 2 and 3 are the most obviously correct of all the actions, so these are eliminated, because the question asks for an item to avoid. To discriminate between the last two options, think about the process. Having the client void at the finish time makes sense, because this captures the urine that the bladder has stored between the last time of voiding and the finish time for the specimen. On the other hand, if you save the first specimen, you do not know how long that urine has been stored in the bladder. Therefore, you would not be getting a true "24-hour" collection. Thus you would decide that option 4 is correct, making option 1 the answer to the question as stated.

Level of Cognitive Ability: Application
Phase of Nursing Process: Implementation
Client Needs: Physiological Integrity
Content Area: Adult Health/Renal

Reference
Black, J., & Matassarin-Jacobs, E. (1997). *Medical-surgical nursing: Clinical management for continuity of care* (5th ed.). Philadelphia: W. B. Saunders, p. 1556.

---

204. The client with acute pyelonephritis who was started on antibiotic therapy 24 hours ago is still complaining of burning sensation with urination. The nurse would check the physician's orders to see whether which of the following medications is prescribed?

1 Oxybutynin chloride (Ditropan)
2 Bethanechol chloride (Urecholine)
3 Phenazopyridine (Pyridium)
4 Propantheline bromide (Pro-Banthine)

Answer: 3

Rationale: The pain experienced with pyelonephritis usually resolves as antibiotic therapy becomes effective. However, clients may be treated for urinary tract pain with phenazopyridine, which is a urinary analgesic. Bethanechol chloride is a cholinergic agent used for neurogenic bladder or for urinary retention. Oxybutynin and propantheline bromide are antispasmodics that are used to treat bladder spasm.

Test-Taking Strategy: Specific knowledge of the classifications of these medications is necessary to answer this question correctly. If this question was difficult, take a few moments to review these medications now!

Level of Cognitive Ability: Application
Phase of Nursing Process: Implementation
Client Needs: Physiological Integrity
Content Area: Pharmacology

Reference
Black, J., & Matassarin-Jacobs, E. (1997). *Medical-surgical nursing: Clinical management for continuity of care* (5th ed.). Philadelphia: W. B. Saunders, pp. 1576, 1629.

205. The nurse is teaching the client with nephrotic syndrome about managing the disorder. The nurse instructs the client to adjust which of the following upward or downward according to the amount of edema?

1 Water intake
2 Salt intake
3 Use of diuretics
4 Activity level

Answer: 4

Rationale: The client with nephrotic syndrome usually has a standard limit set on sodium intake, so this would not be adjusted. Fluids are not restricted unless the client is also hyponatremic. Diuretics are ordered on a specific schedule, and doses are not titrated according to the level of edema. The client is taught to adjust the activity level according to the amount of edema. As edema decreases, activity can increase. Correspondingly, as edema increases, the client should increase rest periods and limit activity. Bed rest is recommended during periods of severe edema.

Test-Taking Strategy: Knowing that sodium restrictions, if ordered, are not modified upward or downward allows you to discard option 2 first as obviously incorrect. Likewise, knowing that diuretics are not titrated allows you to eliminate option 3 next. To discriminate between options 1 and 4, it is necessary to know that fluids may or may not be restricted (depending on serum sodium level), whereas activity level is adjusted downward as edema increases.

Level of Cognitive Ability: Application
Phase of Nursing Process: Implementation
Client Needs: Physiological Integrity
Content Area: Adult Health/Renal

Reference

Black, J., & Matassarin-Jacobs, E. (1997). *Medical-surgical nursing: Clinical management for continuity of care* (5th ed.). Philadelphia: W. B. Saunders, p. 1635.

---

206. The nurse has an order to do intermittent bladder irrigation for the client after cystolitholapaxy. The client asks the nurse why this is being done. The nurse responds that this procedure will

1 Prevent postoperative stricture of the bladder neck.
2 Prevent any hemorrhage from occurring.
3 Ensure that postoperative infection does not occur.
4 Wash out any possible residual stone fragments.

Answer: 4

Rationale: Cystolitholapaxy is an endourological procedure in which a cystoscope is used to break up urinary stones with an instrument called a lithotrite. After this surgery, the nurse may have an order to perform intermittent bladder irrigations to wash out any residual stone fragments. After this procedure, the nurse also assesses for possible postoperative complications, which include hemorrhage, urinary retention, infection, and retained stone fragments.

Test-Taking Strategy: Begin to answer this question by eliminating option 3 first. It is unlikely that this nursing action can ensure that a complication, such as postoperative infection, does not occur. Next, eliminate option 1, because this is an implausible option. To discriminate between options 2 and 4, knowing that the purpose of this procedure is to break up urinary stones helps you to choose option 4 over option 2. Note the word fragment "lith," meaning stones, in the name of the procedure, and the word "stone" in the correct option!

Level of Cognitive Ability: Application
Phase of Nursing Process: Implementation
Client Needs: Physiological Integrity
Content Area: Adult Health/Renal

Reference

Black, J., & Matassarin-Jacobs, E. (1997). *Medical-surgical nursing: Clinical management for continuity of care* (5th ed.). Philadelphia: W. B. Saunders, p. 1597.

207. The nurse is providing care to the client after a bone biopsy of the femur. Which of the following actions by the nurse is not needed in the care of this client?

1 Monitoring site for swelling, bleeding, and hematoma
2 Administering intramuscular narcotic analgesics
3 Elevating the limb for 24 hours
4 Monitoring vital signs every 4 hours

Answer: 2

Rationale: Nursing care after a bone biopsy of the femur includes monitoring the site for swelling, bleeding, and hematoma formation. The biopsy site is elevated for 24 hours to reduce edema. The vital signs are monitored every 4 hours for 24 hours. The client usually requires mild analgesics. More severe pain usually indicates that complications are arising.

Test-Taking Strategy: One way to approach this question is to look at the method of anesthesia used for this procedure. If you know that this procedure is done under local anesthesia, it makes sense that monitoring vital signs every 4 hours is probably sufficient (option 4). The nurse would routinely monitor for complications (option 1). This narrows the choices to site elevation and narcotic analgesics. Of these two, site elevation makes sense to reduce edema, whereas narcotic administration by the intramuscular route seems excessive for a local procedure. Thus option 2 is the answer to the question as stated.

Level of Cognitive Ability: Application
Phase of Nursing Process: Implementation
Client Needs: Physiological Integrity
Content Area: Adult Health/Musculoskeletal

Reference

Black, J., & Matassarin-Jacobs, E. (1997). *Medical-surgical nursing: Clinical management for continuity of care* (5th ed.). Philadelphia: W. B. Saunders, p. 2095.

208. The nurse witnesses a client sustain a fall and suspects that one leg may be broken. Which of the following actions is the highest priority of the nurse?

1 Take a set of vital signs
2 Call the radiology department
3 Reassure the client that everything will be fine
4 Immobilize the leg before moving the client

Answer: 4

Rationale: When a fracture is suspected, it is imperative that the area is splinted before the client is moved. Emergency help should be called for if the client is outside a hospital, and a physician is called for the hospitalized client. The nurse should remain with the client and provide realistic reassurance.

Test-Taking Strategy: This question asks for the highest priority of the nurse, which tells you that more than one option may be correct. In this instance, eliminate option 2 because the nurse does not order x-rays. Option 3 is eliminated next because the nurse never tells a client that "everything will be fine." Of the remaining two choices, immobilizing the limb is imperative for the client's safety, which makes it a better choice than taking vital signs.

Level of Cognitive Ability: Application
Phase of Nursing Process: Implementation
Client Needs: Physiological Integrity
Content Area: Adult Health/Musculoskeletal

Reference

Black, J., & Matassarin-Jacobs, E. (1997). *Medical-surgical nursing: Clinical management for continuity of care* (5th ed.). Philadelphia: W. B. Saunders, p. 2134.

209. The nurse is admitting the client with multiple trauma to the nursing unit. The client has a leg fracture and had a plaster cast applied. In positioning the casted leg, the nurse should

1 Keep the leg in a level position.
2 Keep the leg level for 3 hours, and elevate it for 1 hour.
3 Elevate the leg on pillows continuously for 24–48 hours.
4 Elevate the leg for 3 hours, and lay it flat for 1 hour.

Answer: 3

Rationale: A casted extremity is elevated continuously for the first 24–48 hours to minimize swelling, and to promote venous drainage.

Test-Taking Strategy: To answer this question accurately, you should know that edema sets in after fracture and can be augmented by casting. For this reason, options 1 and 2 are the least helpful and can be eliminated first. There is no useful purpose for the timing in option 4. Thus option 3 is correct.

Level of Cognitive Ability: Application
Phase of Nursing Process: Implementation
Client Needs: Physiological Integrity
Content Area: Adult Health/Musculoskeletal

Reference

Black, J., & Matassarin-Jacobs, E. (1997). *Medical-surgical nursing: Clinical management for continuity of care* (5th ed.). Philadelphia: W. B. Saunders, p. 2150.

210. The nurse is giving the client with a left leg cast instructions on crutch walking with the use of the three-point gait. The client is allowed touch-down of the affected leg. The nurse tells the client to advance the

1 Left leg and right crutch, then right leg and left crutch.
2 Crutches and then both legs simultaneously.
3 Crutches and the right leg, then advance the left leg.
4 Crutches and the left leg, then advance the right leg.

Answer: 4

Rationale: A three-point gait requires good balance and arm strength. The crutches are advanced with the affected leg, and then the unaffected leg is moved forward. Option 1 describes a two-point gait. Option 2 describes a swing-to gait. Option 3 describes the three-point gait used for a right leg problem.

Test-Taking Strategy: Option 1 does not provide the support needed for the casted extremity described in the stem and should be eliminated as a possible answer. Option 2 is not necessary if the client is allowed to let the extremity touch the floor and is eliminated next. Of the two remaining options, option 4 provides support to the left leg and is the correct answer.

Level of Cognitive Ability: Application
Phase of Nursing Process: Implementation
Client Needs: Health Promotion and Maintenance
Content Area: Adult Health/Musculoskeletal

Reference

Potter, P., & Perry, A. (1997). *Fundamentals of nursing: Concepts, process, and practice* (4th ed.). St. Louis: Mosby–Year Book, p. 937.

211. The client with depression says to the nurse, "I'm divorced, my children are scattered over the country and hardly visit or phone me, and my job is a 'dead-end'! I wish I could just die!" The most therapeutic response by the nurse is

1 "Hmm [smiling], I guess I should just 'put you out of your misery'?"
2 "Things seem very bleak to you right now? Are you thinking of ending your life?"
3 "Try to take a more cheerful outlook. Remember, 'Behind every cloud there is a silver lining.'"
4 "You should mobilize your depression and find new interests."

Answer: 2

Rationale: Although humor can be therapeutic, it must be used with sensitivity to the client's current emotional status. Option 1 reinforces the client's fears of being useless and unwanted. Option 3 is directive and judgmental and contains a cliché. Option 4 takes a judgmental and belittling approach to the client's illness by implying that the client is directly able to control the depression and must want to be miserable. In the correct response, focusing and questioning are the therapeutic communication techniques which are used by the nurse.

Test-Taking Strategy: The first therapeutic communication technique employed by the nurse seeks to clarify among several issues within the content expressed by the client. In addition, it expresses empathy and respect for the client's feelings, two key elements in the therapeutic relationship. The second therapeutic communication technique used by the nurse is part of the lethality assessment of the suicidal ideation expressed by the client. The nurse is responsible for clarifying the client's statement even though dynamically it is a passive one with low potential for being acted upon.

Level of Cognitive Ability: Application
Phase of Nursing Process: Implementation
Client Needs: Psychosocial Integrity
Content Area: Mental Health

Reference

Antai-Otong, D. (1995). *Psychiatric nursing: Biological and behavioral concepts.* Philadelphia: W. B. Saunders, pp. 100–107.

---

212. The nurse is caring for a depressed client who has experienced a significant weight loss as a result of decreased appetite. When the nurse encourages eating, the client states, "I can't eat. It will only make me feel me feel worse." Which of the following statements is an example of a therapeutic nursing intervention that is based on cognitive-behavioral therapy?

1 "Yesterday we explored your denial of oral nutrition as a way of expressing your anger and punishing your mother. Do you feel you are doing this again?"
2 "Yesterday we talked about using negative automatic thoughts that prevent you from even trying. Do you identify your feelings as reinforcing negative self-perceptions?"
3 "If you do not even try to eat, I will 'feed' you intravenously."
4 "While you are feeling unable to eat at this time, your appetite will improve as the medication begins to work. In the meantime, do you think you could drink a protein supplement?"

Answer: 2

Rationale: Cognitive-behavioral therapy, a short-term therapy, involves didactic teaching in which the cognitive-behavioral view is explained to the client and followed by cognitive techniques, eliciting and testing negative automatic thoughts, and analyzing the basic maladaptation assumptions that cause the thinking. Behavioral techniques such as graded task assignments and role playing are also used to assist the client.

Test-Taking Strategy: Use the process of elimination. Option 1 sounds like rather pompous "psychobabble," and the communication technique contains a question that implies that the client's thinking is "wrong." Option 3 is a threatening response, which can lead to a regressive struggle between the nurse and the client. In option 4, the nurse's communication uses a medical-biological approach. Review the components of cognitive-behavioral therapy now if you had difficulty with this question!

Level of Cognitive Ability: Application
Phase of Nursing Process: Implementation
Client Needs: Psychosocial Integrity
Content Area: Mental Health

Reference

Antai-Otong, D. (1995). *Psychiatric nursing: Biological and behavioral concepts.* Philadelphia: W. B. Saunders, pp. 176–180; 100–107; 171.

---

213. The nurse is caring for client who is taking trimethadione (Tridione). What would the priority nursing action be if the nurse suspects that the client is experiencing side effects?

1 Check the complete blood cell (CBC) count, white blood cell (WBC) differential, hematocrit, hemoglobin, and platelet counts
2 Take the temperature by using a rectal thermometer
3 Bring client to sunporch three times a day to visit with other clients and visitors
4 Check the client's blood pressure for a sudden elevation

Answer: 1

Rationale: Trimethadione (Tridione) can produce serious allergic dermatitis, kidney and liver damage, agranulocytosis, and aplastic anemia. The nurse will want to check the CBC, WBC differential, hematocrit, hemoglobin, and platelet counts, as well as urinalysis. It is important to monitor these results for alterations (decreases) and to ensure frequent testing while the client is on the medication. Options 2, 3, and 4 are incorrect.

Test-Taking Strategy: Knowledge regarding the side effects associated with this medication is necessary to answer the question. If you are unfamiliar with this medication, take time now to review!

Level of Cognitive Ability: Application
Phase of Nursing Process: Implementation
Client Needs: Physiological Integrity
Content Area: Pharmacology

Reference

Clark, J., Queener, S., & Karb, V. (1997). *Pharmacologic basis of nursing practice* (5th ed.). St. Louis: Mosby–Year Book, pp. 584–588; 686–695.

214. The nurse is caring for client who is to take lamotrigine (Lamictal). What would the priority nursing action be if the client is a truck driver?

1 Caution client to take once a day early in the morning before getting out of bed

2 Stop the medication and notify the physician about the client's occupation

3 Nothing, because the physician has no other medication choices

4 Notify the physician about the client's occupation and instruct the client to take the medicine at bedtime

Answer: 4

Rationale: Lamotrigine (Lamictal), an anticonvulsant, may cause drowsiness and somnolence. Clients taking this medication are cautioned about operating heavy equipment and driving. Taking medication at bedtime or during the client's sleeping periods can mediate the sedative effects of the medication. The physician should be consulted.

Test-Taking Strategy: This question tests your knowledge of lamotrigine (Lamictal) and its side effects. Options 1, 2, and 3 all are incorrect answers. Although the physician may not know the client's occupation, letting the physician know about the client's occupation in view of the effect of the medication on the client is a sound nursing action. Stopping the medication abruptly could cause severe seizures.

Level of Cognitive Ability: Application
Phase of Nursing Process: Implementation
Client Needs: Health Promotion and Maintenance
Content Area: Pharmacology

Reference

Hodgson, B., & Kizior, R. (1998). *Saunders nursing drug handbook 1998.* Philadelphia: W. B. Saunders, pp. 576–577.

---

215. The community health nurse visits the family of a child with Lyme disease that is in the later stages. The client is being treated with IV penicillin G. Which of the following responses is the most therapeutic communication technique for instructing the client and family?

1 "I think you need to know that the arthritic symptoms may continue for a couple of years after treatment."

2 "I think that the rash will disappear now."

3 "I guarantee that the cardiac problems your child has had will clear up now."

4 "This treatment will cause your child to develop a temporary alopecia."

Answer: 1

Rationale: The nurse employs the therapeutic communication technique of information giving in order to allay anxieties and to instruct the child and family. Stage I Lyme disease is characterized by rash (occurs 2–30 days after exposure), which consists of erythematous papules that form concentric rings and resemble a bull's eye at the site of the tick bite and can grow to 50–60 cm, and 7–10 days of flu-like symptoms that can occur and recur. In stage II Lyme disease, if untreated (occurs in 1–6 months), temporary paralysis, cardiac problems (usually conduction defects), and neurological disorders may appear. In stage III Lyme disease, arthritic symptoms (occur in 1 to several months), such as arthralgia and enlarged or inflamed joints, can persist for several years after infection.

Test-Taking Strategy: This question tests your knowledge of Lyme disease and the appropriate therapeutic communication technique to use to impart information. The nurse identifies the intravenous antibiotic treatment that is being administered as being used only in the later stages of the disease. In option 2, the nurse's discussion of a rash indicates that the client is in stage I. In regard to option 3, cardiac problems can occur in stage II, but the nurse's use of the word "guarantee" is inappropriate, and such a guarantee may not be possible. In option 4, alopecia, which is partial or total hair loss caused by infectious processes, systemic disorders, or cutaneous disorders, is not a clinical manifestation of this disease.

Level of Cognitive Ability: Application
Phase of Nursing Process: Implementation
Client Needs: Psychosocial Integrity
Content Area: Child Health

Reference

Luckmann, J. (1997). *Saunders manual of nursing care.* Philadelphia: W. B. Saunders, pp. 1655–1657.

216. The community health nurse visits the family of a child with a recent diagnosis of hemophilia. The family expresses to the nurse concerns about the safety of the required blood transfusions. Which of the following responses would indicate that the nurse is using the most therapeutic communication technique to instruct the family?

1 "In the past, clients with hemophilia did have shorter life expectancies, but since then their life span is relatively the same as for any normal human being."
2 "There is a risk of contracting HIV and shortening life with transfusions."
3 "Your concerns are totally unfounded and serve only to increase anxiety for you and your child."
4 "It's a toss-up. Your decisions are frankly very limited because without transfusions, your child will die."

Answer: 1

Rationale: Hemophilia, a disease in which bleeding time is increased because of impairment of blood coagulability, can cause abnormal hemorrhaging if the blood fails to clot. In the past, blood products used in transfusions sometimes became infected with the human immunodeficiency virus. Since that time, this risk has diminished because of rigorous blood testing. The therapeutic communication technique of information giving is employed to instruct the client and family.

Test-Taking Strategy: This question tests your knowledge of the therapeutic communication technique of information giving and your knowledge of hemophilia. Eliminate option 2 because in the past, blood transfusions sometimes became infected with the human immunodeficiency virus, but this risk has diminished because of rigorous blood testing. Option 3 is incorrect information. Option 4 is a sarcastic comment and also trivializes a serious concern that the family has expressed.

Level of Cognitive Ability: Application
Phase of Nursing Process: Implementation
Client Needs: Psychosocial Integrity
Content Area: Child Health

Reference

Luckmann, J. (1997). *Saunders manual of nursing care.* Philadelphia: W. B. Saunders, pp. 1161–1164.

---

217. The nurse is implementing a teaching plan for a 72-year-old client with angina pectoris and the client's family. Which of the following points would the nurse include to individualize the plan for the elderly client?

1 Irregular pulse rate due to dysrhythmias is always serious and possibly life-threatening
2 Older adults can participate in exercise programs liberally because the decrease in muscle mass with age decreases tissue oxygen requirements
3 Chest pain in the older adult may not be apparent, but associated symptoms such as dyspnea or confusion may be evident
4 The client need not worry about medication side effects because low doses are usually ordered for elderly clients

Answer: 3

Rationale: The elderly client may have atypical manifestation of angina pectoris. Symptoms such as dyspnea or confusion may replace the classic chest pain. Exercise programs should be assumed gradually, with longer warm-up and cool-down times as well. Dysrhythmias are of concern if they cause associated symptoms, which should then be reported to the physician. Medication side effects are always of concern because medications may be metabolized more slowly with increasing age.

Test-Taking Strategy: Knowledge of the normal changes associated with aging are necessary to answer this question. The words or phrases "always," "liberally," and "need not worry" are extreme and make them less plausible choices. Therefore, eliminate options 1, 2, and 4.

Level of Cognitive Ability: Application
Phase of Nursing Process: Implementation
Client Needs: Health Promotion and Maintenance
Content Area: Adult Health/Cardiovascular

Reference

Ignatavicius, D. D., Workman, M. L., & Mishler, M. A. (1995). *Medical-surgical nursing: A nursing process approach* (2nd ed.). Philadelphia: W. B. Saunders, p. 998.

218. The nurse is caring for a client who is to receive anticoagulant therapy at home. As part of the nursing care plan, the nurse teaches the client and family about the side effects that may occur and need to be reported immediately. In the event that the client misses a dose, the nurse would instruct the client to

1 Wait until the next scheduled dose.
2 Take the dose unless it is too close to the time of the next dose, in which case it should be omitted.
3 Call the physician for blood work to determine the time and amount of the next dose.
4 Double the dose.

Answer: 2

Rationale: The correct procedure for handling a missed dose of anticoagulants is to take it immediately unless the next dose is imminent. If the missed dose is too close to the next dose, it is to be omitted, because doubling the dose may cause bleeding.

Test-Taking Strategy: This question tests your ability to identify the correct procedure for anticoagulant therapy administration. When considering principles of client education for anticoagulant or any medication therapy, you should remember that, unless specifically specified, it is never good policy to double any medication dose as suggested in option 4. In option 1, the nurse would be unnecessarily eliminating the dose even if it were missed by only a short time. In option 3, it would be unnecessary to consult the physician about one missed dose or to obtain blood work at this time.

Level of Cognitive Ability: Application
Phase of Nursing Process: Implementation
Client Needs: Physiological Integrity
Content Area: Pharmacology

Reference

Clark, J., Queener, S., & Karb, V. (1997). *Pharmacologic basis of nursing practice* (5th ed.). St. Louis: Mosby–Year Book, pp. 263–267.

219. The nurse is caring for a client on IV heparin therapy who is experiencing hemorrhaging. In the event that the hemorrhaging must be stopped immediately, the nurse would anticipate that the most likely medication to be administered would be

1 Protamine sulfate.
2 Vitamin K_4 (menadiol).
3 Phentolamine mesylate (Regitine).
4 Vitamin K_1 (phytonadione).

Answer: 1

Rationale: Protamine sulfate, an anticoagulant with a longer half-life than heparin, works because it is a highly positively charged molecule that complexes the negatively charged heparin and is used when immediate coagulation is needed.

Test-Taking Strategy: Although both vitamins K_4 and K_1 are forms of replacement therapy, only vitamin K_1 is an effective antidote for severe bleeding episodes caused by an overdose of "oral" anticoagulants. Thus eliminate options 2 and 4 because they are similar. In option 3, the medication Regitine is a vasodilator. Learn the antidote for heparin now if you had difficulty with this question!

Level of Cognitive Ability: Analysis
Phase of Nursing Process: Implementation
Client Needs: Physiological Integrity
Content Area: Pharmacology

Reference

Clark, J., Queener, S., & Karb, V. (1997). *Pharmacologic basis of nursing practice* (5th ed.). St. Louis: Mosby–Year Book, pp. 256–257, 261.

220. The client who has undergone mastectomy says to the nurse. "When I woke up and realized that the surgeon had to cut off both of my breasts, I realized I'm really very bad off [client laughs], sicker than I thought!" The most therapeutic response by the nurse is

1 "You're laughing, yet I feel that you aren't really 'laughing'?"
2 "How awful for you to wake up like that and find that the cancer had spread!"
3 "Well, you knew that could happen. You signed the informed consent which described the consequences in detail."
4 "I've been hearing about the number of needless mastectomies. Do you think that having a lumpectomy would have been sufficient?"

Answer: 1

Rationale: In the most therapeutic response, the nurse reflects the client's response back to the client. Sharing perceptions is a therapeutic communication technique that conveys the nurse's understanding to the client and "sets the stage" to clear up any skewed communication. Option 2 demonstrates the nurse's attempt at an empathic stance, which, however, ends with an insensitive approach by vocalizing the client's fears too early in the dynamic communication process. Option 3 provides a nontherapeutic communication technique that sets up a barrier and is defensive. Option 4 undermines the client's treatment and self-esteem.

Test-Taking Strategy: This question tests your knowledge of therapeutic communication techniques for a client who seems to be in crisis. Options 2, 3, and 4 are insensitive to the client's feelings. Remember to reflect and address the client's feelings and concerns!

Level of Cognitive Ability: Application
Phase of Nursing Process: Implementation
Client Needs: Psychosocial Integrity
Content Area: Adult Health/Oncology

References
Antai-Otong, D. (1995). *Psychiatric nursing: Biological and behavioral concepts.* Philadelphia: W. B. Saunders, pp. 543–546.

---

221. The nurse is caring for a client who has returned to a surgical unit from a critical care unit after undergoing pelvic exenteration. The client complains of pain in the calf. The nurse would

1 Administer PRN meperidine (Demerol) as ordered.
2 Observe calf for temperature, color, and size.
3 Lightly massage area to relieve muscle pain.
4 Ask client to walk, and observe the client's gait.

Answer: 2

Rationale: The nurse needs to monitor for postoperative complications such as deep vein thrombosis, pulmonary emboli, and wound infection. Change in color, temperature, or size of client's calf could indicate a deep vein thrombosis. Options 1, 3, and 4 are inappropriate actions.

Test-Taking Strategy: Use the steps of the nursing process, remembering that assessment is the first step. Option 2 addresses assessment!

Level of Cognitive Ability: Application
Phase of Nursing Process: Implementation
Client Needs: Physiological Integrity
Content Area: Adult Health/Oncology

Reference
Smeltzer, S., & Bare, B. (1996). *Brunner and Suddarth's Textbook of medical-surgical nursing* (8th ed.). Philadelphia: Lippincott-Raven, pp. 2250–2255.

222. A Native American client states, "I'm concerned because my 15-year-old son told me he wants to die and join his horse, who had to be 'put down' 3 weeks ago. I thought he was just sad at losing his horse, but he seems to be getting sadder even though I bought him a new horse. Do you feel that I'm just overreacting?" Which of the following would be the most therapeutic response by the nurse?

1. "No, the risk for suicide increases when young children experience serious distress and talk of dying. Suicide is also high among Native Americans."
2. "Yes, it is a natural reaction. Children, especially Indian children, are very attached to their horses."
3. "No, you have done the right thing. Native American children never show their feelings, so this response is extreme."
4. "Yes. You know that all children at this age exhibit hysterical responses to losing their pets. Death is not understandable at this age, so children are more likely to respond in this manner."

Answer: 1

Rationale: The expression of suicidal ideation by children is far more serious than when expressed by adults because they have immature egos and cognitive functions. Although girls contemplate suicide three times more frequently than boys, boys kill themselves four times more frequently than girls.

Test-Taking Strategy: In option 2, a stereotype of Native Americans is used in a somewhat disparaging communication style, and the notion that with loss, it is only "natural" to become suicidal is incorrect. Suicidal ideation and/or behavior is never natural or normal. Option 3 provides agreement and approval, which is nontherapeutic. In addition, it also provides another stereotype of Native Americans. Option 4 provides incorrect information and labels the client's behavior as "hysterical." Even if the child did not understand death, it does not follow that a lack of understanding would produce hysteria.

Level of Cognitive Ability: Application
Phase of Nursing Process: Implementation
Client Needs: Psychosocial Integrity
Content Area: Mental Health

Reference

Antai-Otong, D. (1995). *Psychiatric nursing: Biological and behavioral concepts.* Philadelphia: W. B. Saunders, pp. 343–347.

---

223. The client is to be treated with felbamate (Felbatol) for treatment of Lennox-Gastaut syndrome. Interventions for this client include monitoring which of the following laboratory values?

1. Alanine transaminase (ALT), aspartate transaminase (AST), and bilirubin
2. Bence-Jones proteins
3. TORCH (toxoplasmosis, other infections, rubella, cytomegalovirus, herpes simplex) test
4. Enzyme-linked immunosorbent assay (ELISA) test

Answer: 1

Rationale: Felbamate (Felbatol) is used alone or with other medications to treat children with Lennox-Gastaut syndrome, a severe epileptic encephalopathy. Felbamate can cause aplastic anemia and/or liver failure. ALT, AST, and bilirubin need to be monitored weekly. Bence-Jones proteins, synthesized by malignant plasma cells in bone marrow, are diagnostic of multiple myeloma. The TORCH test is a screening test used to detect toxoplasmosis (a systemic parasitic disease transmitted to humans by ingesting undercooked meat or handling contaminated cat litter), rubella (an acute viral communicable disease transmitted by droplet or direct contact), cytomegalovirus (CMV) and herpes simplex (both herpesviruses) in a mother or an infant. The ELISA test is used to diagnose HIV infection and to screen blood intended for transfusion.

Test-Taking Strategy: Knowledge of the medication Felbamate is necessary to answer this question. Take time now to review this medication if you had difficulty with this question!

Level of Cognitive Ability: Application
Phase of Nursing Process: Implementation
Client Needs: Physiological Integrity
Content Area: Pharmacology

Reference

Hodgson, B., & Kizior, R. (1998). *Saunders nursing drug handbook 1998.* Philadelphia: W. B. Saunders, p. 1101

224. A child is being admitted to the hospital with the tentative diagnosis of pertussis (whooping cough). What would the nurse do first as the child is admitted to the unit?

1. Attach a pulse oximeter to the child and place the child on a cardiorespiratory monitor
2. Weigh the child
3. Deep suction the airway to clear it of secretions
4. Send the child for a chest x-ray

Answer: 1

Rationale: To adequately evaluate the child to determine whether the child is getting enough oxygen, a pulse oximeter is attached to the child. The pulse oximeter will then provide ongoing information on the child's oxygen level. The child is placed on a cardiorespiratory monitor to provide close supervision and early identification if the child has periods of apnea and bradycardia.

Test-Taking Strategy: Use the principles associated with prioritizing when answering this question. Remember the ABCs: airway, breathing, and circulation. For this child, the concern is all three. To monitor all three, monitoring devices are necessary. A chest x-ray is medical management. A child's weight needs to be obtained sometime; however, it is not a priority for this child. Deep suctioning will affect oxygen levels.

Level of Cognitive Ability: Application
Phase of Nursing Process: Implementation
Client Needs: Physiological Integrity
Content Area: Child Health

Reference

Ashwill, J., & Droske, S. (1997). *Nursing care of children: Principles and practice.* Philadelphia: W. B. Saunders, p. 613.

225. The client who is taking ethosuximide (Zarontin) says to the nurse, "My doctor says I have absence epilepsy. If it's absent, why do I have to take this medication?" Which of the following would be the most appropriate response by the nurse?

1. "When you suffer from those flashes of light and numbness, you're really having a seizure. This medicine makes those episodes go away."
2. "When you experience those changes in temperament, get confused, and feel everything is unreal, you're having a seizure. This medicine helps to prevent them."
3. "When you had the test on your head, a pattern was found that tells your doctor that you probably think you're only daydreaming."
4. "When you can't control the turning of your head, this is a problem which this medicine helps to prevent."

Answer: 3

Rationale: Absence epilepsy (which used to be called petit mal) occurs mainly in children from 4 to 12 years of age. The client suddenly loses consciousness for a few seconds while body tone is retained, and the client regains consciousness without any confusion. Often, the client appears to be daydreaming or inattentive, and only a slight blinking or hand movement may be seen. It can be diagnosed by electroencephalography (EEG).

Test-Taking Strategy: Option 1 describes a simple partial seizure, which begins with a specific symptom that reflects the part of the brain being affected. Visual seizures, which include flashes of light, and/or tactile seizures, such as feelings of tingling or numbness, can occur. Although the client knows what's happening and there is no loss of consciousness, the client cannot control the symptoms. Option 2 describes automatism, which occurs in psychomotor epilepsy. Option 4 describes a focal motor seizure, which occurs with simple partial seizures.

Level of Cognitive Ability: Application
Phase of Nursing Process: Implementation
Client Needs: Psychosocial Integrity
Content Area: Adult Health/Neurological

Reference

Black, J., & Matassarin-Jacobs, E. (1997). *Medical-surgical nursing: Clinical management for continuity of care* (5th ed.). Philadelphia: W. B. Saunders, p. 837.

226. The client is to be treated with valproic acid (Depakene). The nurse monitors for the most serious side effect of this medication which is

1. Hand tremors.
2. Liver involvement.
3. Sedation.
4. Acne.

Answer: 2

Rationale: The most serious side effect of valproic acid is liver failure. Valproic acid is metabolized by the liver, and some metabolites are active or toxic; thus it is contraindicated in clients with liver disease. Although liver failure is rare, it is potentially fatal, and the nurse would want to carefully monitor for the adverse reaction for all clients on this medication. Hand tremors can occur with higher doses but are not life-threatening. Sedation is marked at the beginning of treatment unless the dosage is increased gradually. Acne is not usually a clinical manifestation.

Test-Taking Strategy: Knowledge regarding the toxic effects related to this medication is necessary to answer the question. Option 2 is the only option that identifies a body organ. This would be your best selection, Review the effects of this medication now if you had difficulty with this question!

Level of Cognitive Ability: Application
Phase of Nursing Process: Implementation
Client Needs: Physiological Integrity
Content Area: Pharmacology

Reference

Hodgson, B., & Kizior, R. (1998). *Saunders nursing drug handbook 1998.* Philadelphia: W. B. Saunders, pp. 1039–1041.

---

227. The nurse is preparing to perform tracheostomy care. The nurse would discard which of the following tracheostomy care items found at the bedside?

1. Sterile tracheostomy dressings
2. Bottle of sterile water, marked and dated 8 hours ago
3. Bottle of sterile saline, marked and dated 12 hours ago
4. Suction catheter package with an edge torn open

Answer: 4

Rationale: Proper aseptic technique must be followed by the nurse when caring for the client's tracheostomy. This includes diligent handwashing and correct use of sterile supplies such as water, saline, gloves, dressing materials, and suction catheters. A suction catheter package with an edge torn open is considered no longer sterile and is discarded. Solution bottles are changed every 24 hours.

Test-Taking Strategy: Knowledge of the basics of asepsis is needed to answer this question. Sterile dressings are obviously usable, and so option 1 is eliminated as a possible answer to this question. Liquids used for tracheostomy care are usable for 24 hours after opening, as long as the bottles are capped between uses. Thus options 2 and 3 are also eliminated. The remaining option (4) is the answer to the question. The nurse does not use any sterile product that has lost the integrity of its seal or packaging. Any such item should be discarded.

Level of Cognitive Ability: Application
Phase of Nursing Process: Implementation
Client Needs: Safe, Effective Care Environment
Content Area: Adult Health/Respiratory

Reference

Black, J., & Matassarin-Jacobs, E. (1997). *Medical-surgical nursing: Clinical management for continuity of care* (5th ed.). Philadelphia: W. B. Saunders, p. 1074.

---

228. The nurse is transporting the client with a chest tube by stretcher. In which of the following locations should the nurse place the Pleur-Evac chest drainage system that is attached to the chest tube?

1. Suspend it from the IV pole on the stretcher
2. Stand it upright on the stretcher
3. Lay it down next to the client on the stretcher
4. Attach it to the stretcher so that it hangs below the mattress

Answer: 4

Rationale: A chest tube drainage system must always be kept level and below the waist of the client (which keeps it lower than the level of the client's chest). Laying the system on its side would disrupt the water seal and the integrity of the system. Putting it higher than the level of the client's chest would allow fluid to drain back into the pleural space and is contraindicated.

Test-Taking Strategy: Begin to answer this question by recalling that the integrity of the water seal must be maintained for the system to function and to protect the client from complications such as pneumothorax. This would help you eliminate option 3 as a possible choice. Knowing that the drainage collection chamber must be below the level of the client's chest helps you eliminate options 1 and 2 as incorrect.

Level of Cognitive Ability: Application
Phase of Nursing Process: Implementation
Client Needs: Safe, Effective Care Environment
Content Area: Adult Health/Respiratory

Reference

Black, J., & Matassarin-Jacobs, E. (1997). *Medical-surgical nursing: Clinical management for continuity of care* (5th ed.). Philadelphia: W. B. Saunders, p. 1165.

---

229. The nurse is caring for a client who is to take phenobarbital (Luminal). The nurse monitors for an allergic reaction, which would include which of the following?

1 Butterfly (resembles systemic lupus) rash
2 A chickenpox-type rash
3 Scarlatiniform (resembling scarlet fever) rash
4 Megaloblastic anemia

Answer: 3

Rationale: Phenobarbital (Luminal) inhibits the spread of seizure activity by increasing the threshold for neuronal firing and may also enhance gamma-aminobutyric acid (GABA)–ergic inhibition. Its adverse reactions include rashes, which are considered to be allergic reactions. The rashes are scarlatiniform (resembling scarlet fever) or morbilliform and are usually treated by discontinuing the medication.

Test-Taking Strategy: This question, which may seem deceptively simple, actually tests you in two ways. It tests whether you understand the distinction between adverse reactions that are hematological in origin (e.g., megaloblastic anemia) and those that are allergic. If you selected option 4, you will want to review the definitions of hematological, allergic, and other adverse medication reactions. Options 1 and 2 are incorrect answers for this medication.

Level of Cognitive Ability: Application
Phase of Nursing Process: Implementation
Client Needs: Physiological Integrity
Content Area: Pharmacology

Reference

Hodgson, B., & Kizior, R. (1998). *Saunders nursing drug handbook 1998.* Philadelphia: W. B. Saunders, pp. 815–818.

---

230. The client with adult respiratory distress syndrome (ARDS) is being mechanically ventilated and has been ordered to begin tube feedings. The nurse checks the ingredients of the ordered feeding to ensure that there is not excessive

1 Fat.
2 Carbohydrate.
3 Protein.
4 Water.

Answer: 2

Rationale: The client being mechanically ventilated requires tube feeding or parenteral nutrition because he or she cannot eat for nourishment. It is important to give the client well-balanced nutrition without giving excessive carbohydrate loads. Excess carbohydrate increases production of carbon dioxide, which could result in hypercapnia. Products such as Pulmocare are specifically manufactured to meet this need.

Test-Taking Strategy: To answer this question correctly, it is necessary to understand that excess carbohydrate metabolism yields high levels of carbon dioxide, which is not helpful for the client with ARDS. With this in mind, each of the other incorrect options is eliminated systematically.

Level of Cognitive Ability: Application
Phase of Nursing Process: Implementation
Client Needs: Physiological Integrity
Content Area: Adult Health/Respiratory

Reference

Black, J., & Matassarin-Jacobs, E. (1997). *Medical-surgical nursing: Clinical management for continuity of care* (5th ed.). Philadelphia: W. B. Saunders, p. 1182.

231. The client with chronic airflow limitation (CAL) is admitted to the nursing unit with a diagnosis of exacerbation of the condition. A set of admission blood gases reveals an arterial oxygen level of 45 and a carbon dioxide level of 63. The nurse has an order to administer oxygen at 4 liters/minute. The nurse should

1 Attach a humidifier bottle to the oxygen setup.
2 Request a change to a non-rebreather mask.
3 Have a Venturi face mask available in case more oxygen is ordered.
4 Question the order.

Answer: 4

Rationale: The client with hypoxemia and chronic hypercarbia usually has lower oxygen delivery rates, such as 1–2 liters/minute. An order for 2–4 liters/minute is usually ordered for the average client. Administering excess oxygen to the client with chronic hypercarbia could result in respiratory distress and arrest. This occurs because the client's respiratory drive is based on hypoxia, rather than hypercarbia.

Test-Taking Strategy: To answer this question correctly, it is necessary to know the normal values for arterial oxygen and to understand the concept of the hypoxic drive. Knowing that the oxygen level is low helps you eliminate option 1 as an unrelated item. Understanding the concept of the hypoxic drive forces you to eliminate options 2 and 3 as nonhelpful. This leaves option 4 as the correct answer. The nurse questions the order, knowing that excess oxygen could cause the client to experience respiratory failure and arrest.

Level of Cognitive Ability: Application
Phase of Nursing Process: Implementation
Client Needs: Safe, Effective Care Environment
Content Area: Adult Health/Respiratory

Reference
Black, J., & Matassarin-Jacobs, E. (1997). *Medical-surgical nursing: Clinical management for continuity of care* (5th ed.). Philadelphia: W. B. Saunders, p. 1117.

---

232. The client who is being treated with warfarin sodium (Coumadin), 2 mg PO daily, to prevent postoperative thromboembolism, says to the nurse, "I'm not sure that I want to be on a medication that can cause so many side effects." Which of the following is the most appropriate response by the nurse?

1 "I understand that you have concerns, but the medication has been used for some time at this dosage and had very few, if any, problems. But I would like to hear all of your concerns. Let's discuss this some more."
2 "I understand that you have concerns, but the medication prevents you from having problems that can kill you, so the side effects are really a small price to pay."
3 "You make an excellent point, which I would urge you to discuss with your physician. It is, after all, your body and your decision, not your physician's. But I would like to hear all of your concerns. Let's discuss this some more."
4 "Your concerns are very real, but the physician must weigh the side effects against the seriousness of your illness. On balance, the side effects are little enough if they save your life."

Answer: 1

Rationale: Option 2 begins by acknowledging the client's concerns but is less appropriate in its use of the word "kill," which would only increase the client's anxiety. In addition, it patronizes the client's feelings and medical risks. This approach can be demeaning and demoralizing to clients. Option 3 makes a judgment (use of the word "excellent" suggests approval). It also contains language that undermines the physician's authority by making the innuendo that the physician is insensitive to the client's concerns and risk. Option 4 validates the client's concerns and then minimizes and negates them by placing the decision out the client's hands and into the physician's. In addition, it could frighten the client by stating that the illness is so serious that side effects are not a consideration.

Test-Taking Strategy: The client is vocalizing anxiety from worry as well as some misinformation. The communication techniques of paraphrasing, giving information, giving recognition, and offering assistance in option 1 are used to acknowledge the client's feelings, correct the client's thinking, and provide the client with the emotional support to further explore the problem.

Level of Cognitive Ability: Application
Phase of Nursing Process: Implementation
Client Needs: Psychosocial Integrity
Content Area: Pharmacology

Reference
Hodgson, B., & Kizior, R. (1998). *Saunders nursing drug handbook 1998.* Philadelphia: W. B. Saunders, pp. 1062–1064.

233. After an initial bolus dose of 5000 units of heparin IV, the physician orders heparin, 1000 units IV, continuously every hour. Which of the following instructions, if made by the nurse manager to the staff nurse, would indicate an understanding of the nursing implications of maintaining a safe environment for this client?

1. "Set up the tubing and make certain you check the stools for guaiac. Be certain to use well-padded wrist restraints to avoid any bruising."
2. "Flush the tubing with 1 mL of normal saline before and after administering 5000 units of IV heparin in the dextrose solution."
3. "Set up microdrip tubing via the infusion pump and monitor the partial thromboplastin time (PTT), platelet, and hematocrit levels."
4. "Observe for bruising and bleeding, and check the stools for guaiac biweekly."

Answer: 3

Rationale: Continuous infusion is used to prevent further growth of venous thrombi. Remember that heparin will not dissolve emboli or clots that are already formed. Continuous IV heparin infusion results in a lower risk for bleeding than does intermittent infusion, so it is most commonly used. It is important to use an infusion monitor and to carefully maintain the IV drip to prevent overdosing. The PTT, platelet, and hematocrit levels are monitored.

Test-Taking Strategy: Use the process of elimination. In option 1, no reference is made to the type of tubing and/or the need for an electronic infusion device. In addition, restraints are contraindicated except for extreme need and then only if well-padded to prevent easy bruising. In option 2, the procedure outlined partially describes the procedure for inserting IV medication via a heparin well or a heparin-primed infusion access device. Option 4 is incorrect because the nurse checks for the appearance of bruising and bleeding at least twice daily and preferably at least every shift. The stools are checked for guaiac as frequently as possible. Review this important medication now if you had difficulty with this question!

Level of Cognitive Ability: Application
Phase of Nursing Process: Implementation
Client Needs: Physiological Integrity
Content Area: Pharmacology

Reference

Clark, J., Queener, S., & Karb, V. (1997). *Pharmacologic basis of nursing practice* (5th ed.). St. Louis: Mosby–Year Book, pp. 64–65, 265.

---

234. The nurse is caring for a client who is receiving heparin and other IV medications via an intermittent IV device. The most appropriate nursing action before administering heparin or other medications would be to assess for pain, tenderness, swelling, or redness and

1. Flush the intermittent IV device with 1 or 2 mL of sterile water.
2. Gently flush the IV device with 1 to 2 mL of normal saline.
3. Prime the intermittent IV device with a solution of 1 mL of 1000 units of IV heparin per millimeter.
4. Gently aspirate 5 mL of blood and flush with 2 mL of sterile water.

Answer: 2

Rationale: Always check for patency and location of the intermittent IV device before administering heparin or other medications, and employ the appropriate procedure for caring for the device. Option 1 is incorrect because normal saline, not sterile water, is used to flush the intermittent IV device. In option 3, the solution of heparin is too high and should be measured per milliliter, not millimeter. Option 4 is incorrect because it is not necessary to aspirate 5 mL of blood, and normal saline, not sterile water, is used.

Test-Taking Strategy: This question tests your knowledge of the correct nursing interventions for caring for clients receiving heparin or other IV medications via an intermittent IV device. Eliminate options 1 and 4 first, knowing that normal saline, not sterile water, is used. For the remaining options, note the word "gently" in the correct option. Review this procedure now if you had difficulty with this question!

Level of Cognitive Ability: Application
Phase of Nursing Process: Implementation
Client Needs: Physiological Integrity
Content Area: Fundamental Skills

Reference

Clark, J., Queener, S., & Karb, V. (1997). *Pharmacologic basis of nursing practice* (5th ed.). St. Louis: Mosby–Year Book, pp. 64–65, 265.

235. A client is admitted to undergo an emergency cesarean section. In preparing the client, which datum requires physician notification?

1 Maternal temperature of 100.2°
2 Contractions present and occurring every 15 minutes
3 Mother has had no preparation for cesarean birth
4 Food has been ingested within the last 2 hours

Answer: 4

Rationale: General anesthesia may be an option considered for an emergency birth if time is an element. Of the complications occurring after a cesarean section, aspiration is one of the leading causes of death. This is because the gastric emptying time is slowed. Gastric contents are very acidic and can produce chemical pneumonitis if aspirated. A prophylactic nonparticulate oral antacid may be administered. Options 1, 2, and 3 do not require physician notification.

Test-Taking Strategy: The order of priority is based on the ABCs: airway, breathing, and circulation. The correct option pertains to maintaining an open airway and breathing. In order to answer this question correctly, it is necessary to know that aspiration is a major risk with an emergency cesarean section because the client has not been prepared with NPO status.

Level of Cognitive Ability: Analysis
Phase of Nursing Process: Implementation
Client Needs: Physiological Integrity
Content Area: Maternity

Reference
Olds, S., London, M., & Ladewig, P. (1996). *Clinical handbook for maternal-newborn nursing: A family-centered approach* (5th ed.). Menlo Park, CA: Addison-Wesley, pp. 694–695.

236. The nurse is counseling the client about smoking cessation. The client reports several attempts to quit independently and has not had any sustained success. The nurse suggests which of the following methods of smoking cessation to this particular client?

1 Nicotine patch
2 Nicorette gum
3 Trying a "smoke-out" day first
4 Joining the SmokEnders resource group

Answer: 4

Rationale: The client who is unable to stop smoking independently may benefit from a resource group such as SmokEnders or the American Cancer Society.

Test-Taking Strategy: The key information in the stem of this question is the client's lack of success with "independent" attempts to quit smoking. This implies that the client would benefit from some type of support. The only option that gives a measure of social support to the client is the SmokEnders resource group. Thus each of the other options is rapidly eliminated.

Level of Cognitive Ability: Application
Phase of Nursing Process: Implementation
Client Needs: Psychosocial Integrity
Content Area: Adult Health/Respiratory

Reference
Smeltzer, S., & Bare, B. (1996). *Brunner and Suddarth's Textbook of medical-surgical nursing* (8th ed.). Philadelphia: Lippincott-Raven, p. 516.

237. The nurse is communicating with a client with flail chest who is extremely anxious. The nurse would avoid doing which of the following when talking with this client?

1 Giving clear but simple explanations and directions
2 Speaking as little as possible
3 Talking in a low, soothing voice
4 Allowing ample time for client to respond to questions

Answer: 2

Rationale: The client with flail chest usually is extremely anxious. The nurse communicates most effectively by giving information in a clear but simple manner, speaking in a reassuring tone of voice, and giving the client time to speak and answer questions. This is especially important because the client also is dyspneic. The nurse would not speak as little as possible. The anxious client needs to have effective lines of communication with the nurse.

Test-Taking Strategy: This question is worded so that you will select an incorrect action. Options 1 and 4 are obviously correct and are therefore eliminated as possible answers to this question. Of the two remaining, option 3 enhances communication, whereas option 2 does not. Therefore, option 2 is the answer because the question asks for a behavior to be avoided.

Level of Cognitive Ability: Application
Phase of Nursing Process: Implementation
Client Needs: Psychosocial Integrity
Content Area: Adult Health/Respiratory

Reference

Ignatavicius, D. D., Workman, M. L., & Mishler, M. A. (1995). *Medical-surgical nursing: A nursing process approach* (2nd ed.). Philadelphia: W. B. Saunders, p. 768.

---

238. The client with pneumonia on oxygen at 2 liters/minute has an order for albuterol (Proventil) to be administered by nebulizer. The nurse avoids which of the following actions when preparing and administering this medication therapy?

1. Adding 3 mL of normal saline to the dose in the cup of the nebulizer
2. Attaching the nebulizer to the oxygen source
3. Instructing the client to breathe rhythmically in and out without pause
4. Rinsing the equipment in warm water and air drying on a clean towel after use

Answer: 3

Rationale: The client using a nebulizer is instructed to hold each breath for 5 or 10 seconds, or as long as possible with each breath. Proper use of a nebulizer includes placing the prescribed medication and diluent in the cup of the nebulizer. The cover is screwed onto the cup, which is then attached to the nebulizer. Tubing is used to connect the nebulizer to an oxygen or compressed air source, and the air or oxygen is then turned on. The client places the mouthpiece into the mouth and holds it securely with the teeth and lips. The client inhales slowly and holds each breath for 5–10 seconds. This is repeated until all the medication has been inhaled (usually about 15 minutes). The client may gargle with tap water after use. Equipment is cleaned in warm water and air dried before storage.

Test-Taking Strategy: This question tests fundamental concepts related to the administration of respiratory medications with a nebulizer. The wording of the question guides you to look for an incorrect procedure. Eliminate options 2 and 4 first, as the most obviously correct actions. For the two remaining, you would need to know that the breath should be held with each inhalation to make the correct choice.

Level of Cognitive Ability: Application
Phase of Nursing Process: Implementation
Client Needs: Physiological Integrity
Content Area: Adult Health/Respiratory

Reference

Ignatavicius, D. D., Workman, M. L., & Mishler, M. A. (1995). *Medical-surgical nursing: A nursing process approach* (2nd ed.). Philadelphia: W. B. Saunders, p. 717.

---

239. The nurse enters the room of a client after the physician has obtained consent for a voiding cystourethrogram. The client asks the nurse to explain the procedure again. The nurse tells the client that the client is asked to void after

1. Injection of a radioisotope into the blood stream.
2. Injection of contrast dye into the blood stream.
3. Injection of contrast dye into the bladder via a catheter.
4. Injection of a radioisotope into the bladder via a catheter.

Answer: 3

Rationale: A voiding cystourethrogram involves instillation of a radiopaque material into the bladder by means of a urethral catheter. The catheter is then removed and the client is asked to void while films are being taken. This helps visualize obstructions or lesions in the bladder or urethra. It may be embarrassing or difficult for the client to void in front of others, and emotional support from the nurse is required.

Test-Taking Strategy: A basic knowledge or acquaintance with this procedure is needed to answer this question. Knowing that a dye is instilled will assist in eliminating options 1 and 4. From this point, note the relationship between "cysto" in the name of the test and "bladder" in the correct option. If this question was difficult, take a few moments to read about this procedure now!

Level of Cognitive Ability: Application
Phase of Nursing Process: Implementation
Client Needs: Physiological Integrity
Content Area: Adult Health/Renal

Reference

Black, J., & Matassarin-Jacobs, E. (1997). *Medical-surgical nursing: Clinical management for continuity of care* (5th ed.). Philadelphia: W. B. Saunders, p. 1564.

240. The nurse is counseling the client who has developed renal failure and is exploring the client's feelings about dialysis. After determining that the client is active and is most upset about disruption in the daily routine, the nurse advises the client to explore which of the following treatment options with the physician?

1 Hemodialysis
2 Continuous ambulatory peritoneal dialysis (CAPD)
3 Continuous cyclic peritoneal dialysis (CCPD)
4 Intermittent peritoneal dialysis (IPD)

Answer: 2

Rationale: A key advantage to CAPD is that it does not interfere with the client's routine, in that it does not require machinery, electricity, or a water source. Another advantage, unrelated to this question, is that there are fewer dietary and fluid restrictions, because this mode of dialysis more closely resembles the (continuous) normal renal function. CCPD and IPD are two forms of automated peritoneal dialysis (APD). These require the use of an automatic cycling device, which limits the client's mobility and freedom. Hemodialysis is also disruptive to the client's normal routine because it usually involves a 3- to 4-hour hemodialysis session three times a week.

Test-Taking Strategy: This question is asking you which method of dialysis is the least disruptive to the client's lifestyle. A knowledge of the different types of dialysis is necessary to answer this question accurately. Note the word "active" in the question and "ambulatory" in the correct option. If this question was difficult, take a few moments to review these variations now!

Level of Cognitive Ability: Application
Phase of Nursing Process: Implementation
Client Needs: Psychosocial Integrity
Content Area: Adult Health/Renal

Reference

Black, J., & Matassarin-Jacobs, E. (1997). *Medical-surgical nursing: Clinical management for continuity of care* (5th ed.). Philadelphia: W. B. Saunders, pp. 1648–1649.

---

241. A client is scheduled for insertion of a soft peritoneal dialysis catheter. The client asks the nurse why the catheter must be tunneled under the skin. The nurse responds that this procedure will

1 Decrease dwell times and reduce the incidence of complications.
2 Allow for larger fluid infusions and for better fluid drainage.
3 Cause less discomfort and give longer catheter life.
4 Stabilize the catheter and reduce the risk of infection.

Answer: 4

Rationale: The reasons for tunneling the peritoneal dialysis catheter under the skin before inserting it into the peritoneal cavity are to stabilize the catheter and to reduce the likelihood of infection. These catheters have cuffs that allow ingrowth of fibroblasts and blood vessels, thereby preventing leakage of fluid and reducing bacterial invasion into the peritoneum.

Test-Taking Strategy: Note that each of the responses has two parts. In order for the option to be correct, both parts of that option must be correct. Knowing that dwell times and fluid volumes are not regulated by the type of catheter, you would eliminate options 1 and 2 first. Knowing that the type of catheter is not related to comfort, you would then eliminate option 3.

Level of Cognitive Ability: Application
Phase of Nursing Process: Implementation
Client Needs: Physiological Integrity
Content Area: Adult Health/Renal

Reference

Black, J., & Matassarin-Jacobs, E. (1997). *Medical-surgical nursing: Clinical management for continuity of care* (5th ed.). Philadelphia: W. B. Saunders, p. 1649.

242. The nurse is teaching the client to perform peritoneal dialysis in preparation for discharge to home. The nurse teaches the client to use which of the following to prevent infection when connecting and disconnecting the peritoneal dialysis system?

1 Gloves only
2 Gloves and mask
3 Gloves, mask, and goggles
4 Gloves, mask, and apron

Answer: 2

Rationale: Gloves and mask should be worn during connection and disconnection of peritoneal dialysis circuits. This prevents transmission of microorganisms by contact and via the airborne route. Goggles are unnecessary for preventing client infection, as is an apron.

Test-Taking Strategy: To answer this question correctly, a basic understanding of infection control principles is needed. If you realize that the hands are the only body parts that touch the dialysis tubing, then it is obvious that apron and goggles are unnecessary for adequate infection control. Knowledge of airborne transmission of microbes would guide you to choose option 2 over option 1 as the correct choice.

Level of Cognitive Ability: Application
Phase of Nursing Process: Implementation
Client Needs: Health Promotion and Maintenance
Content Area: Adult Health/Renal

Reference

Black, J., & Matassarin-Jacobs, E. (1997). *Medical-surgical nursing: Clinical management for continuity of care* (5th ed.). Philadelphia: W. B. Saunders, p. 1658.

---

243. The nurse is giving a client instructions about taking ciprofloxacin (Cipro). The nurse teaches the client that the medication is most effective when taken

1 With antacids.
2 With milk or yogurt.
3 During meals.
4 On an empty stomach.

Answer: 4

Rationale: Ciprofloxacin is one of a group of antibiotics called fluoroquinolones. These medications are most effective when taken on an empty stomach—that is, 1 hour before or 2 hours after a meal. If necessary, it may be taken with meals to avoid stomach upset. Antacids, milk, and yogurt interfere with absorption of the medication and should not be taken concurrently with the dose of ciprofloxacin.

Test-Taking Strategy: Note the key words "most effective" in the stem. This implies that more than one option may be partially or totally correct. Knowing that antacids and milk products interfere with the absorption of more than one type of antibiotic, you should eliminate options 1 and 2 first. To discriminate between options 3 and 4, it is necessary to know that the medication is best absorbed on an empty stomach.

Level of Cognitive Ability: Application
Phase of Nursing Process: Implementation
Client Needs: Physiological Integrity
Content Area: Pharmacology

Reference

Deglin, J., & Vallerand, A. (1997). *Davis's drug guide for nurses* (5th ed.). Philadelphia: F. A. Davis, pp. 501–502.

244. The client has been given a prescription for methenamine mandelate (Mandelamine). The nurse notes that the client also takes an antacid that contains magnesium. The nurse tells the client to

1 Take the antacid at the same time as Mandelamine.
2 Take the antacid between doses of Mandelamine.
3 Drink plenty of water while taking both these medications.
4 Avoid taking the antacid while taking Mandelamine.

Answer: 4

Rationale: Mandelamine exerts its effects by releasing acids and formaldehyde and is ineffective in alkaline urine. Medications that produce alkaline urine should be avoided while this medication is being taken. These include calcium- and magnesium-containing antacids, carbonic anhydrase inhibitors, thiazide diuretics, citrates, and sodium bicarbonate. Option 3 is unrelated to antacid administration.

Test-Taking Strategy: To answer this question correctly, it is necessary to know that Mandelamine acidifies the urine. It is also necessary to know that urinary alkalinizers are contraindicated. If this medication is unfamiliar to you, take a few moments to review this medication now!

Level of Cognitive Ability: Application
Phase of Nursing Process: Implementation
Client Needs: Physiological Integrity
Content Area: Pharmacology

Reference

Lehne, R. A. (1998). *Pharmacology for nursing care* (3rd ed.). Philadelphia: W. B. Saunders, p. 904.

245. The client has been prescribed nitrofurantoin (Macrodantin). Which of the following would the nurse not include in medication instructions for the client?

1 The medication discolors the urine to brownish, which is not significant
2 The medication may cause dizziness or drowsiness
3 If a dose is missed, double the dose at the next scheduled time
4 Rinse the mouth with water after taking the oral suspension, to avoid staining teeth

Answer: 3

Rationale: Doses should not be skipped or doubled. If a dose is missed, the client should take the dose as soon as remembered and should space the next dose 2–4 hours later. The medication does discolor the urine, which is not significant. The client should avoid driving until tolerance of the medication is known, because the medication causes dizziness and drowsiness. Because the oral suspension may stain teeth, it is recommended that the client rinse the mouth with water after a dose.

Test-Taking Strategy: Familiarity with this medication is needed to answer this question correctly. Remember that a general principle with medications is that doses should not be doubled if missed. If necessary, take a few moments to review this medication at this time!

Level of Cognitive Ability: Application
Phase of Nursing Process: Implementation
Client Needs: Health Promotion and Maintenance
Content Area: Pharmacology

Reference

Deglin, J., & Vallerand, A. (1997). *Davis's drug guide for nurses* (5th ed.). Philadelphia: F. A. Davis, p. 866.

246. A child with bilateral clubfoot is going home with corrective braces after having both casts removed. The nurse is completing discharge teaching for the parents, and a priority nursing action is to instruct them to

1. Increase the interval of time wearing the braces and eventually have the child wear them as much as possible.
2. Use lotion and then powder to prepare the skin before applying the corrective braces to the legs.
3. Keep the braces concealed under long pants to reduce any embarrassment the child might feel.
4. Remove the braces whenever the child is in public because the psychological impact may be harmful.

Answer: 1

Rationale: The child begins wearing the braces for periods of 1–2 hours and then progresses to keeping the braces on as much as tolerated. The child should have adequate mobility whenever wearing the brace as well. Lotion and powder can be irritating to the skin. Option 3 suggests that the condition be treated as something to be despised. Option 4 reflects a negative view regarding the use of braces. Neither option 3 nor 4 acknowledges the condition.

Test-Taking Strategy: Eliminate options 3 and 4 because they are similar. Remembering that lotions and powders can irritate the skin will assist in eliminating option 2. Review care of the child who requires braces if you had difficulty with this question!

Level of Cognitive Ability: Application
Phase of Nursing Process: Implementation
Client Needs: Physiological Integrity
Content Area: Child Health

Reference

Ball, J., & Bindler, R. (1995). *Pediatric nursing: Caring for children.* Stamford, CT: Appleton & Lange, p. 589.

---

247. The client admitted with chest pain did not experience relief after one dose of nitroglycerin sublingually. The nurse would check the client's vital signs and, if they are stable, would

1. Notify the physician.
2. Call to obtain an electrocardiogram (ECG).
3. Give another dose of nitroglycerin.
4. Add a dose of nitroglycerin paste.

Answer: 3

Rationale: Standard protocol is to administer up to three doses of nitroglycerin 5 minutes apart as long as the client has stable vital signs. After three doses, the physician is called if the client does not experience relief.

Test-Taking Strategy: The stem makes no reference to standing orders or other specific physician orders, so eliminate options 2 and 4. The stem also tells you that the client is physiologically stable after the first dose of nitroglycerin. This guides you to pick option 3 over option 1 because the physician is called if three doses of nitroglycerin do not provide relief or if the client's vital signs deteriorate.

Level of Cognitive Ability: Application
Phase of Nursing Process: Implementation
Client Needs: Physiological Integrity
Content Area: Adult Health/Cardiovascular

Reference

Ignatavicius, D. D., Workman, M. L., & Mishler, M. A. (1995). *Medical-surgical nursing: A nursing process approach* (2nd ed.). Philadelphia: W. B. Saunders, p. 992.

248. A home health nurse is visiting an elderly home-bound client who lives alone. The client complains of chest pain that is unrelieved by three sublingual nitroglycerin tablets. Which of the following actions should the nurse take first?

1. Call for an ambulance to transport the client to the emergency department
2. Drive the client to the physician's office
3. Notify a family member who is next of kin
4. Inform the home care agency supervisor that the visit may be prolonged

Answer: 1

Rationale: Chest pain that is unrelieved by rest and three doses of nitroglycerin given 5 minutes apart may not be typical anginal pain but may signal myocardial infarction (MI). Because the risk of sudden cardiac death is greatest in the first 24 hours after MI, it is imperative that the client receive emergency cardiac care.

Test-Taking Strategy: The question asks for the first nursing action, which makes you prioritize among plausible nursing actions. Because MI is a medical emergency, valuable treatment time could be lost by choosing option 2, 3, or 4 first. Option 2 is less plausible than option 1 because a physician's office does not have the optimal resources for administering emergency cardiac care.

Level of Cognitive Ability: Application
Phase of Nursing Process: Implementation
Client Needs: Physiological Integrity
Content Area: Adult Health/Cardiovascular

Reference

Smeltzer, S., & Bare, B. (1996). *Brunner and Suddarth's Textbook of medical-surgical nursing* (8th ed.). Philadelphia: Lippincott-Raven, p. 642.

---

249. A client admitted 12 hours ago to the coronary care unit (CCU) asks the nurse if he or she can go for a short walk in the hall. The nurse responds that during the first 24 hours after admission, the client has an activity order for

1. Bed rest only.
2. Bed rest with commode privileges.
3. Bed rest with bathroom privileges.
4. Bed rest with ambulation of 50 feet twice daily.

Answer: 2

Rationale: In the first 24–36 hours after myocardial infarction (MI), the client is maintained on bed rest with commode privileges or being allowed to stand to void. Options 3 and 4 are not allowable activities during this time period.

Test-Taking Strategy: The question asks you about activity within the first 12 hours after MI. Use concepts related to heart rest to answer this question. It may help to discriminate between options 1 and 2 by avoiding the option with the word "only." Review care of the client after MI if you had difficulty with this question!

Level of Cognitive Ability: Application
Phase of Nursing Process: Implementation
Client Needs: Physiological Integrity
Content Area: Adult Health/Cardiovascular

Reference

Ignatavicius, D. D., Workman, M. L., & Mishler, M. A. (1995). *Medical-surgical nursing: A nursing process approach* (2nd ed.). Philadelphia: W. B. Saunders, p. 998.

---

250. A client with myocardial infarction has received thrombolytic therapy with tissue plasminogen activator (t-PA). The nurse caring for this client monitors for signs of complications of this therapy, which would include

1. Decreased urine output.
2. Orange urine.
3. Tarry stools.
4. Nausea and vomiting.

Answer: 3

Rationale: Thrombolytic agents are used to dissolve existing thrombi, and the nurse must monitor the client for obvious or occult signs of bleeding.

Test-Taking Strategy: The word "thrombolytic," meaning to dissolve clots, focuses your attention on blood coagulation. Look for an item that has a hematological connection: in this case, option 3, which is occult bleeding from the gastrointestinal tract. Review this important medication now if you had difficulty with this question!

Level of Cognitive Ability: Application
Phase of Nursing Process: Implementation
Client Needs: Physiological Integrity
Content Area: Adult Health/Cardiovascular

Reference

Smeltzer, S., & Bare, B. (1996). *Brunner and Suddarth's Textbook of medical-surgical nursing* (8th ed.). Philadelphia: Lippincott-Raven, p. 996.

251. The ambulatory care nurse notes that a client has a pigmented mole. As a priority measure, the nurse teaches the client about the importance of limiting which of the following items before the end of the visit?

1 Alcohol intake
2 Exposure to sunlight
3 Exposure to secondary smoke
4 Foods that are high in vitamin C

Answer: 2

Rationale: A pigmented mole is a precancerous lesion that could undergo degenerative changes. The nurse should plan to teach the client about primary and secondary prevention measures, which include the use of sunscreen, avoiding excessive exposure to sunlight, and regular monitoring of the mole for changes. Options 1 and 3 are healthy measures but do not specifically relate to the stem of the question. Option 4 is incorrect.

Test-Taking Strategy: The key phrase and words in the stem of the question include "pigmented mole," "teach," and "priority." Option 2 is the only choice that addresses a problem that is related to the skin.

Level of Cognitive Ability: Application
Phase of Nursing Process: Implementation
Client Needs: Health Promotion and Maintenance
Content Area: Adult Health/Oncology

Reference

Black, J., & Matassarin-Jacobs, E. (1997). *Medical-surgical nursing: Clinical management for continuity of care* (5th ed.). Philadelphia: W. B. Saunders, p. 2224.

252. The client at risk for shock has been started on low-dose dopamine (Intropin) at 2.0 μg/kg/minute. The nurse measures which of the following parameters to determine the effectiveness of this therapy?

1 Urine output
2 Pulse rate
3 Respiratory rate
4 Blood pressure

Answer: 1

Rationale: Dopamine has different effects on the cardiovascular system, depending on the dose. Low-dose dopamine (administered at a rate of 0.5–3.0 μg/kg/minute) increases blood flow through the renal and mesenteric blood vessels. It improves urine output but does not improve cardiac output. Medium-dose dopamine (4–8 μg/kg/minute) improves cardiac output and slightly increases the pulse rate. High-dose dopamine (8–10 μg/kg/minute) causes vasoconstriction, increases afterload, and increases cardiac work. Therefore, the client's response to the dose must be carefully monitored.

Test-Taking Strategy: To answer this question accurately, you must be familiar with this medication and the expected effects at each dosage range. Note that option 1 relates to the renal system, whereas options 2, 3, and 4 relate to the cardiopulmonary system. If this medication is unfamiliar to you, take a few moments to review it now!

Level of Cognitive Ability: Application
Phase of Nursing Process: Implementation
Client Needs: Physiological Integrity
Content Area: Adult Health/Cardiovascular

Reference

Smeltzer, S., & Bare, B. (1996). *Brunner and Suddarth's Textbook of medical-surgical nursing* (8th ed.). Philadelphia: Lippincott-Raven, p. 258.

253. The nurse is caring for the client scheduled for surgery during the shift and has several tasks to complete. The nurse would do which of the following preoperative activities last?

1 Ensuring that the surgical consent form is signed
2 Asking the client to void in the bathroom
3 Administering preanesthetic medication
4 Assisting the client onto the stretcher

Answer: 3

Rationale: Of these options, the nurse first ensures that the surgical consent form has been signed. Just before sending the client to the operating room, the nurse asks the client to void, assists the client onto the stretcher, and finally administers any preanesthetic medications that may be ordered. Sedative medications are administered last, to maintain client safety. If the client has not been placed on the stretcher before these medications are administered, the client must remain in bed with the side rails up.

Test-Taking Strategy: The key word in the question is "last." Using client safety as your guide to the order of activities (because one of the options involves sedative medications), you would easily eliminate each of the incorrect options.

Level of Cognitive Ability: Application
Phase of Nursing Process: Implementation
Client Needs: Safe, Effective Care Environment
Content Area: Fundamental Skills

Reference

Smeltzer, S., & Bare, B. (1996). *Brunner and Suddarth's Textbook of medical-surgical nursing* (8th ed.). Philadelphia: Lippincott-Raven, p. 370.

---

254. The client returns to the nursing unit after surgery. The nurse notes that the client's urine output is 25 mL for this hour. The first action of the nurse is to

1. Check the client's overall intake and output record.
2. Increase the fluid rate of the IV.
3. Administer a 250-mL bolus of normal saline (0.9%).
4. Call the physician.

Answer: 1

Rationale: The nurse needs additional data to accurately interpret the meaning of this piece of data. Clients are at risk for becoming hypovolemic after surgery; often the first sign of hypovolemia is a decrease in urine output. To validate this information, the nurse looks for additional data. Options 2 and 3 are not done without an order. The physician is called once the nurse has gathered all necessary assessment data, including overall fluid status and vital signs.

Test-Taking Strategy: Note that the key word in the stem is "first." This tells you that more than one or all of the options may be partially or totally correct. Attempt to visualize the situation. Use your knowledge of basic skills and prioritizing to select the correct answer.

Level of Cognitive Ability: Application
Phase of Nursing Process: Implementation
Client Needs: Physiological Integrity
Content Area: Fundamental Skills

Reference

Smeltzer, S., & Bare, B. (1996). *Brunner and Suddarth's Textbook of medical-surgical nursing* (8th ed.). Philadelphia: Lippincott-Raven, p. 402.

---

255. The client has undergone surgery and is entering the postanesthesia care unit (PACU). The first action of the nurse receiving the client in transfer is to determine the

1. Status of the client's airway.
2. Pulse, blood pressure, and oxygen saturation level.
3. Appearance of the dressing.
4. Client's level of consciousness.

Answer: 1

Rationale: The PACU nurse follows the ABCs (airway, breathing, and circulation) when admitting a client from the operating room. After airway and breathing are assessed, the nurse checks circulation (pulse, blood pressure) and then the condition of the surgical dressing or site and the level of consciousness.

Test-Taking Strategy: The key word in the question is "first." This tells you that more than one or all of the options may be correct, and you must determine which action is most important. Following the ABCs, you will systematically eliminate each of the responses that have lower priority. In actual practice, all of these are assessed rapidly, but in a predetermined order.

Level of Cognitive Ability: Application
Phase of Nursing Process: Implementation
Client Needs: Physiological Integrity
Content Area: Fundamental Skills

Reference

Smeltzer, S., & Bare, B. (1996). *Brunner and Suddarth's Textbook of medical-surgical nursing* (8th ed.). Philadelphia: Lippincott-Raven, p. 394.

256. The nurse is ordering a diet for the client with a major burn who is beginning oral intake. The nurse orders a diet that is

1 High in calories and high in fat.
2 High in protein and high in carbohydrates.
3 High in carbohydrates and low in protein.
4 High in fat and low in carbohydrates.

Answer: 2

Rationale: The diet of the client with a major burn needs to be high in calories, protein, and carbohydrates for adequate wound healing. The client has increased metabolic needs and could easily become malnourished. This type of diet keeps the client in positive nitrogen balance.

Test-Taking Strategy: Use knowledge of principles related to nutrition to answer this question. You would choose the correct answer by reasoning that the body needs increased amounts of these nutrients to regenerate tissue lost from burns. In addition, knowledge that protein is required for tissue healing will assist in directing you to the correct option.

Level of Cognitive Ability: Application
Phase of Nursing Process: Implementation
Client Needs: Physiological Integrity
Content Area: Adult Health/Integumentary

Reference
Lewis, S., Collier, I., & Heitkemper, M. (1996). *Medical-surgical nursing: Assessment and management of clinical problems* (4th ed.). St. Louis: Mosby–Year Book, p. 544.

---

257. The nurse is getting the postoperative client out of bed for the first time since surgery. When the head of the bed is raised to about 60 degrees, the client complains of dizziness. Which of the following actions should the nurse take first?

1 Check the oxygen saturation
2 Check the blood pressure
3 Lower the head of bed slowly until dizziness is relieved
4 Have the client breathe in and out deeply five times

Answer: 3

Rationale: Dizziness or feeling faint is not uncommon when a postoperative client is positioned upright for the first time after surgery. If it occurs, the nurse relieves the feeling by lowering the head of the bed slowly until the client is comfortable again. The nurse may then check the pulse and blood pressure. Because the problem is circulatory, not respiratory, the other options have lesser value to the nurse in this instance.

Test-Taking Strategy: Note that the question contains the key word "first." Answer this question by examining which option will alleviate the client's distress. This would be the first nursing action. Eliminate options 1 and 2 first because they are assessments, not nursing actions. Choose option 3 over option 4 because it more directly addresses the cause of the dizziness.

Level of Cognitive Ability: Application
Phase of Nursing Process: Implementation
Client Needs: Physiological Integrity
Content Area: Fundamental Skills

Reference
Smeltzer, S., & Bare, B. (1996). *Brunner and Suddarth's Textbook of medical-surgical nursing* (8th ed.). Philadelphia: Lippincott-Raven, p. 401.

258. The nurse is changing the surgical dressing for a postoperative client. The nurse removes the old dressing

1 At a right angle to the skin surface and in the direction of hair growth.
2 At a right angle to the skin surface and in the opposite direction of hair growth.
3 Parallel to the skin surface and in the direction of hair growth.
4 Parallel to the skin surface and in the opposite direction of hair growth.

Answer: 3

Rationale: The nurse removes a dressing by holding the dressing material parallel to the skin surface and by pulling it in the direction of hair growth. This method is the most comfortable for the client and the least traumatic to the skin tissue.

Test-Taking Strategy: A quick review of the options tells you that there is only one correct response. Use your knowledge of basic wound care procedures to answer this question. Eliminate options 2 and 4 first because of the phrase "opposite direction of hair growth." It makes more sense to remove a dressing by pulling it parallel rather than at a right angle. Therefore, eliminate option 1.

Level of Cognitive Ability: Application
Phase of Nursing Process: Implementation
Client Needs: Physiological Integrity
Content Area: Fundamental Skills

Reference
Smeltzer, S., & Bare, B. (1996). *Brunner and Suddarth's Textbook of medical-surgical nursing* (8th ed.). Philadelphia: Lippincott-Raven, p. 417.

---

259. The nurse is reading the results of the client's Mantoux test. The client is not elderly or immunosuppressed. The nurse palpates a 2-mm area of induration. The nurse records that the result is

1 Negative.
2 Uncertain.
3 Positive.
4 Insignificant.

Answer: 1

Rationale: An area of 10 mm or more of induration is positive or significant in the client who is not immunosuppressed or elderly. An area that measures 2 mm of induration is a negative result. Options 2, 3, and 4 are incorrect.

Test-Taking Strategy: To answer this question accurately, it is necessary to be familiar with guidelines for interpreting tuberculin skin tests. If this question was difficult, review this material and become familiar with it. You are likely to find a question related to this content on NCLEX-RN!

Level of Cognitive Ability: Application
Phase of Nursing Process: Implementation
Client Needs: Physiological Integrity
Content Area: Adult Health/Respiratory

Reference
Smeltzer, S., & Bare, B. (1996). *Brunner and Suddarth's Textbook of medical-surgical nursing* (8th ed.). Philadelphia: Lippincott-Raven, p. 497.

---

260. The male client who has a new diagnosis of tuberculosis is visibly upset and tells the nurse that he is not sure how he will cope with having to stay away from people for the next 6 months. The nurse reassures the client by telling him that he will not be infectious after

1 1 week of medication therapy.
2 2–3 weeks of medication therapy.
3 6 weeks of medication therapy.
4 2 months of medication therapy.

Answer: 2

Rationale: The client being treated for tuberculosis is not considered infectious after 2–3 weeks of continuous medication therapy.

Test-Taking Strategy: Specific knowledge is needed to answer this question correctly. If this question was difficult, take the time to review this important content area now. You are likely to find test questions related to tuberculosis on NCLEX-RN!

Level of Cognitive Ability: Application
Phase of Nursing Process: Implementation
Client Needs: Psychosocial Integrity
Content Area: Adult Health/Respiratory

Reference
Smeltzer, S., & Bare, B. (1996). *Brunner and Suddarth's Textbook of medical-surgical nursing* (8th ed.). Philadelphia: Lippincott-Raven, p. 498.

261. The client with pleurisy of the right lung tells the home health nurse that it is difficult to sleep with the discomfort of breathing. The nurse suggests that the client try to sleep

1. Supine.
2. Prone.
3. On the right side.
4. On the left side.

Answer: 3

Rationale: The client with pleurisy should be encouraged to sleep on the affected side. This will splint the chest wall and lessen the amount of stretching of the pleura. This will then enable the client to get the rest that is needed to aid in healing.

Test-Taking Strategy: Read the entire question and review each of the options. The wording of the question indicates that there is only one correct response. Use principles related to splinting of painful areas to make your choice. These principles should direct you to the correct option. If you had difficulty with this question, take time now to review measures associated with the care of the client with pleurisy!

Level of Cognitive Ability: Application
Phase of Nursing Process: Implementation
Client Needs: Physiological Integrity
Content Area: Adult Health/Respiratory

Reference

Smeltzer, S., & Bare, B. (1996). *Brunner and Suddarth's Textbook of medical-surgical nursing* (8th ed.). Philadelphia: Lippincott-Raven, p. 502.

---

262. The client who returned to the nursing unit 4 hours ago after lung biopsy reports to the nurse the production of blood-streaked sputum. The nurse would

1. Call the physician.
2. Suction the client vigorously.
3. Ask the client to cough and deep breathe.
4. Reassure the client that this is expected at this time.

Answer: 4

Rationale: After lung biopsy, the production of sputum that has blood streaks is normal for several hours after the procedure. The nurse continues to monitor the client for signs of complications, which would include hemoptysis, dyspnea, stridor, hypotension, dysrhythmias, and tachycardia.

Test-Taking Strategy: To answer this question correctly, you must be familiar with the procedure and the expected effects in the immediate postoperative period. Note the phrase "blood-streaked." This should assist you in eliminating option 1. You should also be able to easily eliminate option 2. Coughing and deep breathing will not help the situation. The phrase "blood-streaked" should also provide you with a clue that this is an expected occurrence!

Level of Cognitive Ability: Application
Phase of Nursing Process: Implementation
Client Needs: Physiological Integrity
Content Area: Adult Health/Respiratory

Reference

Monahan, F., & Neighbors, M. (1998). *Medical-surgical nursing: Foundations for clinical practice* (2nd ed.). Philadelphia: W. B. Saunders, p. 549.

---

263. The client is awake and alert after bronchoscopy and complains of pain in the throat. The nurse would avoid using which of the following interventions to increase comfort?

1. Hydrocollator pack
2. Ice collar
3. Lozenges
4. Throat gargles

Answer: 1

Rationale: Interventions to ease throat pain or discomfort after bronchoscopy include the use of gargles, throat lozenges, and warm liquids that are soothing to the throat lining. These measures may be instituted once cough and swallow reflexes have returned. Application of an ice collar eases discomfort while preventing swelling in the area.

Test-Taking Strategy: The wording of the question guides you to look for an incorrect choice. Knowing that gargles and lozenges are helpful guides you to eliminate options 3 and 4. You would use principles of heat and cold applications to choose option 1 over option 2 as the correct answer to the question as it is stated.

Level of Cognitive Ability: Application
Phase of Nursing Process: Implementation
Client Needs: Physiological Integrity
Content Area: Adult Health/Respiratory

Reference

Monahan, F., & Neighbors, M. (1998). *Medical-surgical nursing: Foundations for clinical practice* (2nd ed.). Philadelphia: W. B. Saunders, p. 550.

264. An anxious client scheduled for laryngoscopy asks the nurse whether it would be possible to ask the physician to have general anesthesia for the procedure. The nurse would use which of the following pieces of information in a response?

1. Anxiety is usually an indication to use general anesthesia for the procedure
2. General anesthesia takes longer to reverse, but may be more beneficial for this client
3. There is a lower complication rate if local anesthesia is used
4. It should be done under local anesthesia so the client can phonate during the procedure

Answer: 4

Rationale: Laryngoscopy is usually performed under local anesthesia so that the client can vocalize or phonate during the procedure upon request. Vocal cord motility can be seen only when the client is awake and able to make these sounds.

Test-Taking Strategy: To answer this question accurately, it is necessary to be familiar with this procedure and associated client teaching. Knowledge regarding the principles and uses of general anesthesia may assist you in eliminating options 1, 2, and 3. Review this procedure briefly if you are not familiar with it!

Level of Cognitive Ability: Application
Phase of Nursing Process: Implementation
Client Needs: Physiological Integrity
Content Area: Adult Health/Respiratory

Reference
Monahan, F., & Neighbors, M. (1998). *Medical-surgical nursing: Foundations for clinical practice* (2nd ed.). Philadelphia: W. B. Saunders, p. 550.

---

265. The client expresses to the nurse anxiety about experiencing pain during a planned thoracentesis. The nurse most effectively reduces the client's anxiety during the procedure by

1. Giving closest attention to the status of the equipment being used.
2. Offering the client narcotic analgesia during the procedure.
3. Remaining with the client, using eye contact and touch for reassurance.
4. Explaining at length the different sensations that might be experienced.

Answer: 3

Rationale: Nursing responsibilities during thoracentesis are varied and include obtaining necessary equipment, assessing client status, and giving client support. The role of the nurse in this situation that is most anxiety-relieving for the client is the use of touch and eye contact to give reassurance during the procedure.

Test-Taking Strategy: Note that the question asks specifically about how the nurse will most effectively reduce anxiety. Knowledge of basic therapeutic communication skills allows you to eliminate each of the incorrect responses. Option 3 will most effectively reduce anxiety!

Level of Cognitive Ability: Application
Phase of Nursing Process: Implementation
Client Needs: Psychosocial Integrity
Content Area: Adult Health/Respiratory

Reference
Monahan, F., & Neighbors, M. (1998). *Medical-surgical nursing: Foundations for clinical practice* (2nd ed.). Philadelphia: W. B. Saunders, p. 552.

---

266. The nurse is giving the client instructions about pursed lip breathing to help the client adapt to chronic obstructive pulmonary disease (COPD). The nurse teaches the client correct procedure by telling the client to

1. Inhale through the mouth.
2. Tighten abdominal muscles with inhalation.
3. Contract the abdominal muscles with exhalation.
4. Make inhalation twice as long as exhalation.

Answer: 3

Rationale: Correct procedure for pursed-lip breathing includes having the client inhale slowly through the nose with abdominal muscles relaxed; exhale slowly through pursed lips while keeping the abdominal muscles contracted; and keep the exhalation phase twice as long as the inhalation phase. Pursed-lip breathing helps increase pressure in lower airways by prolonging exhalation, thus preventing bronchiolar collapse and air trapping.

Test-Taking Strategy: Familiarity with this particular breathing exercise is needed to answer this question accurately. Because this is an important exercise for clients with respiratory disorders, take a few moments to review the specific technique if you had difficulty with this question!

Level of Cognitive Ability: Application
Phase of Nursing Process: Implementation
Client Needs: Health Promotion and Maintenance
Content Area: Adult Health/Respiratory

Reference

Monahan, F., & Neighbors, M. (1998). *Medical-surgical nursing: Foundations for clinical practice* (2nd ed.). Philadelphia: W. B. Saunders, p. 553.

---

267. The nurse is preparing the client for insertion of a transtracheal catheter for oxygen therapy. The nurse would

1 Ensure the client has been on NPO status for 6–8 hours.
2 Add to the chart a permit for general anesthesia.
3 Sign out a preoperative narcotic analgesic.
4 Place the client on high-flow oxygen therapy.

Answer: 1

Rationale: A transtracheal oxygen catheter is inserted in some clients needing long-term home oxygen therapy. Client preparation for the procedure includes ensuring that the client maintains NPO status and administering a sedative and cough suppressant preoperatively. Informed consent is required, but the procedure is done under local anesthesia. Clients needing this type of catheter have chronic lung disease and should be limited to low-flow oxygen therapy. Narcotic analgesics could depress respiration.

Test-Taking Strategy: Begin to answer this question by eliminating option 4 because the client with respiratory disease should not receive high-flow oxygen therapy. Familiarity with the procedure allows you to choose correctly. Review this procedure now if you had difficulty with this question!

Level of Cognitive Ability: Application
Phase of Nursing Process: Implementation
Client Needs: Physiological Integrity
Content Area: Adult Health/Respiratory

Reference

Monahan, F., & Neighbors, M. (1998). *Medical-surgical nursing: Foundations for clinical practice* (2nd ed.). Philadelphia: W. B. Saunders, pp. 557–558.

---

268. The nurse is caring for the restless client who keeps biting down on an orotracheal tube. The nurse uses which of the following to prevent the client from obstructing this airway with the teeth?

1 Nasal airway
2 Oral airway
3 Bite stick
4 Padded tongue blade

Answer: 2

Rationale: An oral airway may be used to keep the client from biting down on and occluding an orotracheal tube. A nasal airway is not used in conjunction with an oral endotracheal tube. A padded tongue blade or a bite stick may be used initially to open the mouth for easier insertion of an oral airway.

Test-Taking Strategy: Visualize the equipment being described in this question. Use your knowledge of basic principles of airway management to eliminate each of the incorrect responses. Note the relationship between "orotracheal" in the question and "oral airway" in the correct option!

Level of Cognitive Ability: Application
Phase of Nursing Process: Implementation
Client Needs: Physiological Integrity
Content Area: Adult Health/Respiratory

Reference

Monahan, F., & Neighbors, M. (1998). *Medical-surgical nursing: Foundations for clinical practice* (2nd ed.). Philadelphia: W. B. Saunders, p. 559.

269. The client with a cuffed tracheostomy has a nursing diagnosis of Altered Nutrition: Less Than Body Requirements. The client is able to take a diet orally. The nurse would do which of the following during meals for this client?

1 Provide frequent mouth care
2 Hyperoxygenate the client
3 Inflate the tracheostomy cuff
4 Place a T-piece on the tracheostomy

Answer: 3

Rationale: For safety during meals, the client with a tracheostomy who is able to tolerate a diet should have the cuff inflated. This minimizes the risk of aspiration. Frequent mouth care is a general measure that is beneficial to the client with an altered airway. Hyperoxygenation is done before and after suctioning. A T-piece is used for some clients during weaning from a ventilator and has nothing to do with meals.

Test-Taking Strategy: Note the key phrases in this question, which are "cuffed tracheostomy" and "during meals." This guides you to look for a response that addresses prevention of aspiration. Note that option 3 addresses the issue "tracheostomy cuff." Using this as your frame of reference, you will easily eliminate each of the incorrect responses.

Level of Cognitive Ability: Application
Phase of Nursing Process: Implementation
Client Needs: Physiological Integrity
Content Area: Adult Health/Respiratory

Reference

Monahan, F., & Neighbors, M. (1998). *Medical-surgical nursing: Foundations for clinical practice* (2nd ed.). Philadelphia: W. B. Saunders, p. 563.

---

270. The client is receiving mechanical ventilation. The nurse takes which of the following most important actions in the management of this client?

1 Avoids shutting off ventilator alarms
2 Suctions the client every 2 hours
3 Listens to breath sounds every shift
4 Gives medication hourly so the client doesn't "buck" the ventilator

Answer: 1

Rationale: It is critically important that ventilator alarms should never be shut off. The alarm indicates whether the system pressure has risen, whether other problems are occurring, or whether the client has become disconnected from the ventilator. The client is suctioned as needed. Breath sounds are auscultated at least every 2 hours. The client is sedated on a PRN basis to be able to tolerate the ventilator.

Test-Taking Strategy: The key phrases in this question are "mechanical ventilation" and "most important." Eliminate each of the incorrect responses because the frequencies listed are incorrect, although the actions themselves are proper. Remember that in questions that are worded like this one, the incorrect options may be partially correct. Review care of a client on a ventilator now if you had difficulty with this question!

Level of Cognitive Ability: Application
Phase of Nursing Process: Implementation
Client Needs: Safe, Effective Care Environment
Content Area: Adult Health/Respiratory

Reference

Monahan, F., & Neighbors, M. (1998). *Medical-surgical nursing: Foundations for clinical practice* (2nd ed.). Philadelphia: W. B. Saunders, p. 570.

271. A client hospitalized with a paranoid disorder refuses to turn off the lights in the room at night because the roommates will "steal me blind." The nurse questions the client's refusal to allow the lights to be turned off and, upon hearing the client's reason, initially states

1 "Tell me more about the details of your belief."
2 "Why do you believe this?"
3 "If you want a pass for tomorrow evening's movie, you'd better turn that light off this minute."
4 "I hear what you are saying, but I don't share your belief."

Answer: 4

Rationale: Paranoid beliefs are coping mechanisms and thus are not easily relinquished. They can be reinforced by challenging behaviors such as that in option 3. It is important that the nurse not support the belief and yet not ridicule, argue, or criticize it either. Therefore, option 4 is the appropriate answer. Option 1 encourages the client to expound on the belief when discussion should instead be limited. Option 2 places the client in a defensive position by asking "why." Option 3 threatens the client.

Test-Taking Strategy: You will need to know the dynamics of the paranoid thought process to answer the question. Although option 1 meets criteria for encouraging communication, it is incorrect because it encourages the client to fixate on the paranoid belief. Thus you would be focusing on inappropriate issues, making option 1 incorrect. Option 2 is requesting an explanation, and option 3 shows disapproval and is challenging. Both options may cause the client to become defensive. Option 4 does not devalue the client's belief but does reinforce reality.

Level of Cognitive Ability: Application
Phase of Nursing Process: Implementation
Client Needs: Psychosocial Integrity
Content Area: Mental Health

Reference
Wilson, H., & Kneisl, C. (1996). *Psychiatric nursing* (5th ed.). Menlo Park, CA: Addison-Wesley, p. 478.

---

272. The West Virginian (Appalachian American) client says to the nurse, "I've had the blind staggers, been deader than four o'clock ever since the running off stopped 2 days ago." Which of the following is the most culturally congruent therapeutic response by the nurse?

1 "So, you're saying you've suffered from dizziness, lightheadedness, and syncope ever since the diarrhea stopped 2 days ago?"
2 "Some of the things you're saying make no sense to me. I'll have to get an interpreter from the college language department."
3 "Do you have someone who speaks the English language who can come here and explain what you're telling me?"
4 "So, you're saying that you've been 'staggering like a blind man' and 'felt dead since 4 P.M.' ever since the 'running off' occurred 2 days ago?"

Answer: 1

Rationale: The therapeutic communication technique employed by the nurse is restating, which affords an opportunity for the nurse to validate the nurse's interpretation of the client's stated problem. Transcultural nursing is evident in the nurse's ability to identify the culturally congruent terms that assist in understanding the client's complaints.

Test-Taking Strategy: This question tests your knowledge of the appropriate therapeutic communication technique and the most culturally congruent interpretations of the client's language. Options 2 and 3 are critical and demeaning because they imply that the nurse's lack of understanding stems from the client's language. Option 4 is a fine attempt, but the use of restating exactly does not clarify the client's meaning for the nurse's understanding.

Level of Cognitive Ability: Application
Phase of Nursing Process: Implementation
Client Needs: Psychosocial Integrity
Content Area: Fundamental Skills

Reference
Antai-Otong, D. (1995). *Psychiatric nursing: Biological and behavioral concepts.* Philadelphia: W. B. Saunders, pp. 543–576.

273. The client taking a daily dose of an anticoagulant says to the nurse, "I'm having my teeth cleaned tomorrow, so I'm sure the gum bleeding I get when I brush my teeth will disappear." Which of the following would be the most appropriate response by the nurse?

1. "You may need to use a softer bristle brush and avoid flossing. Your dentist and other health care providers need to know about the anticoagulant you're taking."
2. "If you experience any prolonged bleeding, you need to report it to the physician."
3. "Your dentist will need to take extra care when cleaning your teeth."
4. "Cleaning your teeth is forbidden. Please cancel your appointment and tell me more about your bleeding gums."

Answer: 1

Rationale: All health care providers are to be informed when a client is placed on anticoagulants. Clients should discuss with the physician whether procedures such as cleaning teeth and flossing are allowed. They are often avoided until the anticoagulant therapy can be discontinued.

Test-Taking Strategy: Note the key phrase "most appropriate" in the stem of the question. Eliminate option 2 because of the word "prolonged." Any evidence of bleeding should be reported to the physician immediately. In option 3, although the advice is probably wise, there is nothing to indicate that permission for cleaning teeth has been given or that the dentist is aware that the client is taking anticoagulants. Eliminate option 4, because of the word "forbidden." In addition, the dogmatic or "bossy" communication style probably alerted you that this is an incorrect answer.

Level of Cognitive Ability: Application
Phase of Nursing Process: Implementation
Client Needs: Physiological Integrity
Content Area: Pharmacology

Reference

Clark, J., Queener, S., & Karb, V. (1997). *Pharmacologic basis of nursing practice* (5th ed.). St. Louis: Mosby–Year Book, pp. 263–265.

---

274. The nurse is caring for a client who is on warfarin sodium (Coumadin). The client asks for assistance in selecting meals. Which of the following would be the most appropriate selections for this client?

1. Bran cereal, milk, cooked spinach, margarine, and salad with iceberg lettuce and tomatoes
2. Peanut butter, mixed nuts, cashews, and Waldorf salad with dressing
3. Bran cereal, milk, raw cabbage, cooked Brussels sprouts, and canned green peas
4. Toast with jelly; cereal; boiled egg; salad with romaine lettuce, onions, and mushrooms; turkey; banana; and orange

Answer: 4

Rationale: Clients receiving Coumadin can develop serious hemorrhaging problems if they consume high amounts of vitamin E. Large amounts of foods that are high in vitamin K, the antidote for warfarin overdose, are also contraindicated. It is important to remember that cooked foods do not alter the amounts of vitamin K because it is stable in heat, as is vitamin E (although freezing may cause some loss of E). Sources of vitamin E include vegetable oils, vegetable oil–based margarine, whole-grain or fortified cereals, wheat germ, nuts, green leafy vegetables, apples, peaches, and apricots. Sources rich in vitamin K include green leafy vegetables, tomatoes, cauliflower, fish, liver, egg yolks, fats from red meats, raw cabbage, cooked spinach, and Brussels sprouts.

Test-Taking Strategy: This question test your knowledge of nutrition and diet therapy for clients who take Coumadin. Options 1, 2, and 3 all list foods that are rich in either vitamin E or vitamin K. Review this medication and foods high in vitamins E and K if you had difficulty with this question!

Level of Cognitive Ability: Application
Phase of Nursing Process: Implementation
Client Needs: Physiological Integrity
Content Area: Pharmacology

Reference

Kee, J., & Hayes, E. (1997). *Pharmacology: A nursing process approach* (2nd ed.). Philadelphia: W. B. Saunders, p. 521.

275. The nurse is caring for a male client who is to be treated with an antiplatelet agent for prophylaxis after a transient ischemic attack (TIA). The nurse would anticipate that the most likely medication to be administered would be

1 Aspirin.
2 Dextran 70.
3 Sulfinpyrazone (Anturane).
4 Dipyridamole (Persantine).

Answer: 1

Rationale: Aspirin has been found to prevent venous thrombus formation by inhibiting platelet aggregation. Aspirin, an antiplatelet agent, has been determined to be an effective prophylaxis treatment for male clients who have experienced a TIA. Dextran 70, a medication that alters the platelet surface membrane and inhibits the von Willebrand factor, is used before and after the placement of intracoronary stents. Sulfinpyrazone (Anturane), a medication that inhibits platelet adhesion, is used for prosthetic heart valves. Dipyridamole (Persantine), a medication that increases platelet cyclic adenosine monophosphate (AMP) levels, is used for prosthetic heart valves and in peripheral vascular disease.

Test-Taking Strategy: This question tests your knowledge of aspirin and its uses for prophylaxis related to stroke or heart attack. Options 2, 3, and 4 are incorrect, although they too are antiplatelet agents. Review the uses of aspirin now if you had difficulty with question!

Level of Cognitive Ability: Application
Phase of Nursing Process: Implementation
Client Needs: Physiological Integrity
Content Area: Pharmacology

Reference
Clark, J., Queener, S., & Karb, V. (1997). *Pharmacologic basis of nursing practice* (5th ed.). St. Louis: Mosby–Year Book, pp. 257–259.

276. The nurse is caring for the hyperthermic client. Which of the following actions is the least helpful in the care of this client?

1 Cooling the room to 62°
2 Encouraging fluids up to 3000 mL in 24 hours
3 Providing mouth care every 4 hours
4 Changing bed linens and pajamas when damp

Answer: 1

Rationale: The room temperature should be cooled only as low as 70 degrees, to prevent overcooling and chilling. Pushing fluids to 3000 mL helps maintain fluid balance. Providing mouth care every 4 hours maintains moist mucous membranes, which become dry from mouth breathing with fever. Keeping pajamas and bed linens dry helps prevent the client from shivering.

Test-Taking Strategy: The question asks for the "least helpful" action, which would be one that is either contraindicated or excessive. Options 3 and 4 are good actions for basic nursing care and are eliminated first. The stem does not mention that the client cannot drink, so option 2 is acceptable also. Excessive cooling is the least helpful item.

Level of Cognitive Ability: Application
Phase of Nursing Process: Implementation
Client Needs: Physiological Integrity
Content Area: Fundamental Skills

Reference
Cox, H., Hinz, M., Lubno, M., et al. (1997). *Clinical applications of nursing diagnosis: Adult, child, women's, psychiatric, gerontic, and home health considerations* (3rd ed.). Philadelphia: F. A. Davis, p. 146.

277. The nurse is performing a bladder catheterization with an indwelling catheter. Which of the following represents an incorrect action of the nurse while completing this procedure?

1. Inflating the balloon to test patency before catheter insertion
2. Advancing the catheter just until urine appears in the catheter tubing
3. Inflating the balloon with 4–5 mL more than the stated balloon capacity
4. Placing the bag lower than bladder level, with no kinks in the tubing

Answer: 2

Rationale: The catheter should be advanced for 1–2 more inches beyond the point where the flow of urine is first noted. This ensures that the balloon is fully in the bladder before it is inflated. Each of the other statements represents correct procedure.

Test-Taking Strategy: Options 1 and 4 are most obviously correct actions and are therefore eliminated as possible answers to the question as stated. To discriminate among the last two options, you need to know either that the catheter is advanced 1–2 more inches or that extra fluid is needed to fill the lumen that runs between the external port and the balloon at the tip of the catheter.

Level of Cognitive Ability: Application
Phase of Nursing Process: Implementation
Client Needs: Physiological Integrity
Content Area: Fundamental Skills

Reference

Taylor, C., Lillis, C., & LeMone, P. (1997). *Fundamentals of nursing: The art and science of nursing care* (3rd ed.). Philadelphia: Lippincott-Raven, p. 1237.

278. The nurse has an order from the surgeon to irrigate the nephrostomy tube of a client. The nurse correctly implements this order by irrigating with

1. 30 mL of sterile saline.
2. 30 mL of sterile water.
3. 10 mL of sterile saline.
4. 10 mL of sterile water.

Answer: 3

Rationale: Sterile normal saline is used to irrigate a nephrostomy tube because it is an isotonic solution. The volume is limited to 10 mL because the renal pelvis is small and could be damaged by excessive volume and pressure. The nurse never irrigates a nephrostomy tube without a specific order. Some surgeons prefer to irrigate these catheters themselves.

Test-Taking Strategy: Begin to answer this question by eliminating the options with sterile water, because this is not a physiological solution. To discriminate between the last two, it is necessary to understand that the kidney cannot tolerate undue stress and distention; thus option 3 is correct.

Level of Cognitive Ability: Application
Phase of Nursing Process: Implementation
Client Needs: Physiological Integrity
Content Area: Adult Health/Renal

Reference

Smeltzer, S., & Bare, B. (1996). *Brunner and Suddarth's Textbook of medical-surgical nursing* (8th ed.). Philadelphia: Lippincott-Raven, p. 1169.

279. The nurse is caring for the client who has had a renal biopsy. Which of the following interventions would the nurse avoid in the care of the client after this procedure?

1. Forcing fluids to at least 3 liters in the first 24 hours
2. Administering PRN narcotics
3. Testing serial urine samples with dipsticks for occult blood
4. Ambulating the client in the room and hall for short distances

Answer: 4

Rationale: After renal biopsy, the nurse ensures that the client remains in bed for at least 24 hours. Vital signs and puncture site assessments are done frequently during this time. Forcing fluids is done to reduce possible clot formation at the biopsy site. Serial urine samples are evaluated for occult blood with urine dipsticks to evaluate bleeding. Narcotic analgesics are often needed to manage the renal colic pain that some clients feel after this procedure.

Test-Taking Strategy: Begin to answer this question by recalling that pain and bleeding are potential concerns after this procedure. This would allow you to eliminate options 2 and 3 as possible responses. To discriminate between the other two options, you would need to recall that forcing fluids will reduce clotting at the site, whereas ambulation could initiate or enhance bleeding at the biopsy site.

Level of Cognitive Ability: Application
Phase of Nursing Process: Implementation
Client Needs: Physiological Integrity
Content Area: Adult Health/Renal

Reference

Black, J., & Matassarin-Jacobs, E. (1997). *Medical-surgical nursing: Clinical management for continuity of care* (5th ed.). Philadelphia: W. B. Saunders, p. 1569.

---

280. The client has been hospitalized with a diagnosis of acute glomerulonephritis. The nurse would avoid which of the following activities in the care of this client?

1 Offering hard candies or ice chips
2 Monitoring daily weight
3 Performing serial measurements of edematous areas
4 Encouraging intake of high-protein milk shakes

Answer: 4

Rationale: The client with glomerulonephritis has fluids restricted and is encouraged to limit protein intake. The client's thirst with limited fluids may be alleviated with hard candies or ice chips instead of glasses of fluids to drink. Fluid status is tracked by measuring intake and output, daily weight, and edema.

Test-Taking Strategy: This question is testing knowledge of protein and fluid restriction in the client with glomerulonephritis. Because the question asks for an item to avoid, you are looking for an incorrect nursing action. Knowing that this disorder causes problems with edema and fluid balance, you would eliminate options 2 and 3 because they are obviously helpful. To choose correctly between options 1 and 4, it is necessary to know either that the client is placed on a fluid restriction (and therefore should not have water available at the bedside), or that protein intake in the diet is limited. Knowledge of either of these concepts would allow you to choose option 4 as the action to avoid.

Level of Cognitive Ability: Application
Phase of Nursing Process: Implementation
Client Needs: Physiological Integrity
Content Area: Adult Health/Renal

Reference

Black, J., & Matassarin-Jacobs, E. (1997). *Medical-surgical nursing: Clinical management for continuity of care* (5th ed.). Philadelphia: W. B. Saunders, p. 1632.

---

281. The nurse is giving the client with polycystic kidney disease instructions in replacing elements lost in the urine as a result of impaired kidney function. The nurse instructs the client to increase intake of which of the following in the diet?

1 Sodium and potassium
2 Sodium and water
3 Water and phosphorus
4 Calcium and phosphorus

Answer: 2

Rationale: Clients with polycystic kidney disease waste sodium rather than retain it and therefore need an increase in sodium and water in the diet. Potassium, calcium, and phosphorus levels need no special attention.

Test-Taking Strategy: In reviewing the possible answers to this question, notice that either sodium or phosphorus appears in each of the options. Remember also that when an answer has two parts to it, both of the parts must be correct for the option to be correct. Knowing this, begin to answer this question by eliminating options 3 and 4 first because the disorder causes sodium, not phosphorus, to be wasted. To discriminate between options 1 and 2, you should recall that when the kidney excretes sodium, water is carried with it. This would allow you to choose option 2 over option 1 as the correct answer.

Level of Cognitive Ability: Application
Phase of Nursing Process: Implementation
Client Needs: Health Promotion and Maintenance
Content Area: Adult Health/Renal

Reference

Black, J., & Matassarin-Jacobs, E. (1997). *Medical-surgical nursing: Clinical management for continuity of care* (5th ed.). Philadelphia: W. B. Saunders, pp. 2070–2071.

282. The client with urolithiasis who is scheduled for lithotripsy has a sudden decrease in urine output. The nurse would take which of the following priority actions?

1 Call the physician
2 Replace the Foley catheter with a new one
3 Assess the client for increased pain
4 Measure urine specific gravity

Answer: 1

Rationale: A sudden drop in urine output, as a result of either oliguria or anuria, represents obstruction of the urinary tract, usually at the bladder neck or urethra. This represents a medical emergency, necessitating prompt treatment to preserve kidney function. In this instance, the nurse would call the physician to report the findings immediately.

Test-Taking Strategy: Begin to answer this question by eliminating options 2 and 4 as the least plausible of all options. You would choose option 1 over option 3, knowing that the condition constitutes a medical emergency and that the client may not experience pain from obstruction immediately.

Level of Cognitive Ability: Analysis
Phase of Nursing Process: Implementation
Client Needs: Physiological Integrity
Content Area: Adult Health/Renal

Reference

Ignatavicius, D. D., Workman, M. L., & Mishler, M. A. (1995). *Medical-surgical nursing: A nursing process approach* (2nd ed.). Philadelphia: W. B. Saunders, p. 2068.

---

283. The nurse is caring for the client who is undergoing extracorporeal shock wave lithotripsy. The nurse ensures that which of the following most essential items is in place before the start of the procedure?

1 Foley catheter
2 Oxygen saturation monitor
3 Blood pressure cuff
4 Cardiac monitor

Answer: 4

Rationale: It is essential that the client undergoing extracorporeal shock wave lithotripsy is placed on a cardiac monitor for this procedure. This is because the shock waves are administered in synchrony of the R wave on the electrocardiogram (ECG). General or epidural anesthesia is used if performed with a water bath. The other items listed are also helpful in the care of this client; however, the ECG monitor is most critical because of the timing of the sound waves in conjunction with the R wave of the ECG.

Test-Taking Strategy: The question asks for the most essential item, which implies that more than one or all of the options may be used in the care of this client. Begin to answer this question by eliminating options 1 and 3 because they are not used for ongoing monitoring of the client during this procedure. To choose between options 2 and 4, it is necessary to know that the cardiac monitor is used to time the delivery of the shock waves.

Level of Cognitive Ability: Application
Phase of Nursing Process: Implementation
Client Needs: Physiological Integrity
Content Area: Adult Health/Renal

Reference

Ignatavicius, D. D., Workman, M. L., & Mishler, M. A. (1995). *Medical-surgical nursing: A nursing process approach* (2nd ed.). Philadelphia: W. B. Saunders, pp. 2070–2071.

284. The client is having difficulty coughing and deep breathing as a result of pain after nephrectomy. Which of the following actions by the nurse would be least helpful in promoting optimal respiratory function?

1. Administering pain medication only before ambulation
2. Encouraging use of incentive spirometer hourly
3. Assisting the client to splint the incision during respiratory exercise
4. Offering PRN pain medication every 4 hours when due

Answer: 1

Rationale: The client who has had a nephrectomy may have pain with coughing and deep breathing and other respiratory exercise because the incision is very close to the diaphragm. The nurse assists the client by administering narcotic analgesics liberally, encouraging incentive spirometer use, and assisting the client to splint the incision during coughing. If the client takes pain medication only before ambulation, this may be insufficient and may not promote optimal respiratory function.

Test-Taking Strategy: By asking for the "least helpful" action in promoting respiratory function, the question is seeking the response that is the most incorrect. Options 2 and 3 are obviously helpful and are eliminated first. Because option 4 is more helpful than option 1, you would choose option 1 as the answer to the question as stated.

Level of Cognitive Ability: Application
Phase of Nursing Process: Implementation
Client Needs: Physiological Integrity
Content Area: Adult Health/Renal

Reference

Black, J., & Matassarin-Jacobs, E. (1997). *Medical-surgical nursing: Clinical management for continuity of care* (5th ed.). Philadelphia: W. B. Saunders, p. 1673.

285. The nurse is doing a physical assessment of the musculoskeletal system. The nurse would document the presence of which of the following as a normal finding?

1. Presence of fasciculations
2. Muscle strength graded 3/5
3. Hypertrophy on the client's dominant side
4. Atrophy on the client's nondominant side

Answer: 3

Rationale: Hypertrophy, or increased muscle size, on the client's dominant side of up to 1 cm is considered normal. Atrophy on either side is considered an abnormal finding. Muscle strength is graded from 0/5 (paralysis) to 5/5 (normal power). Fasciculations are fine muscle twitches that are not normally present.

Test-Taking Strategy: Options 2 and 4 should be ruled out first; atrophy is not a normal finding, and muscle strength of 3/5 is less than the maximum of 5/5, which is normal power. Knowing that fasciculations are not normal helps you to select option 3 over option 1.

Level of Cognitive Ability: Application
Phase of Nursing Process: Implementation
Client Needs: Health Promotion and Maintenance
Content Area: Adult Health/Musculoskeletal

Reference

Black, J., & Matassarin-Jacobs, E. (1997). *Medical-surgical nursing: Clinical management for continuity of care* (5th ed.). Philadelphia: W. B. Saunders, p. 2086.

286. The nurse is teaching the client who is to have a gallium scan about the procedure. The nurse would include which of the following items as part of the instructions?

1. The gallium will be injected intravenously 2–3 hours before the procedure
2. The procedure takes about 15 minutes to perform
3. The client must stand erect during the filming
4. The client should remain on bed rest for the remainder of the day after the scan

Answer: 1

Rationale: A gallium scan is similar to a bone scan but with injection of gallium isotope instead of technetium Tc 99m. Gallium is injected 2–3 hours before the procedure. The procedure takes 30–60 minutes to perform. The client must lie still during the procedure. There is no special aftercare.

Test-Taking Strategy: If you know that a gallium scan is similar to a bone scan, you can begin by eliminating options 3 and 4. The time frame in option 2 is too brief, which allows you to choose option 1 as the correct answer.

Level of Cognitive Ability: Application
Phase of Nursing Process: Implementation
Client Needs: Physiological Integrity
Content Area: Fundamental Skills

Reference

Black, J., & Matassarin-Jacobs, E. (1997). *Medical-surgical nursing: Clinical management for continuity of care* (5th ed.). Philadelphia: W. B. Saunders, p. 2094.

287. The client has a fiberglass (nonplaster) cast applied to the lower leg. The client asks the nurse when he or she will be able to walk on the cast. The nurse replies that the client will be able to bear weight on the cast

1. Within 20–30 minutes of application.
2. In approximately 8 hours.
3. In 24 hours.
4. In 48 hours.

Answer: 1

Rationale: A fiberglass cast is made of water-activated polyurethane materials that are dry to the touch within minutes and reach full rigid strength in about 20 minutes. Because of this, the client can bear weight on the cast within 20–30 minutes.

Test-Taking Strategy: Familiarity with nonplaster casts is needed to answer this question precisely. Options 3 and 4 should be eliminated first, because these time frames are similar to the drying times for plaster casts. Knowing that the nonplaster type of cast is lighter and dries extremely quickly may help you to choose the 20- to 30-minute time frame as correct.

Level of Cognitive Ability: Application
Phase of Nursing Process: Implementation
Client Needs: Health Promotion and Maintenance
Content Area: Adult Health/Musculoskeletal

Reference

Black, J., & Matassarin-Jacobs, E. (1997). *Medical-surgical nursing: Clinical management for continuity of care* (5th ed.). Philadelphia: W. B. Saunders, p. 2147.

288. The client in skeletal leg traction with an overbed frame is not allowed to turn from side to side. Which of the following actions by the nurse would be most useful in trying to provide good skin care to the client?

1. Asking the client to lift up by digging into the mattress with the unaffected leg
2. Pushing down on the mattress of the bed while administering care
3. Having another nurse turn the client anyway
4. Asking the client to pull up on a trapeze to lift the hips off the bed

Answer: 4

Rationale: If the client in skeletal traction may not turn from side to side, the nurse should have the client pull up on a trapeze and try to lift the hips off the bed for skin care, bed pan use, and linen changes. If the client is unable to pull up on a trapeze, the nurse can push down on the mattress with one hand while administering care with the other.

Test-Taking Strategy: Option 3 is contraindicated because it ignores a medical order. Option 1 is not feasible as stated; the client cannot lift up from the bed by using only one foot. Both options 2 and 4 are acceptable alternatives. Because the question asks which would be "most useful," the answer is option 4. Providing care to the client who can lift the hips off the bed using a trapeze is easier and more efficient than providing care to one who cannot.

Level of Cognitive Ability: Application
Phase of Nursing Process: Implementation
Client Needs: Physiological Integrity
Content Area: Adult Health/Musculoskeletal

Reference

Smeltzer, S., & Bare, B. (1996). *Brunner and Suddarth's Textbook of medical-surgical nursing* (8th ed.). Philadelphia: Lippincott-Raven, p. 1862.

---

289. The nurse is caring for the client who had skeletal traction applied to the left leg. The client is complaining of severe left leg pain. Which of the following actions should the nurse take first?

1. Medicate the client with an analgesic
2. Provide pin care
3. Call the physician
4. Check the client's alignment in bed

Answer: 4

Rationale: A client who complains of severe pain may need realignment or may have traction weights ordered that are too heavy. The nurse realigns the client and, if that is ineffective, then calls the physician. Severe leg pain, once traction has been established, indicates a problem. Medicating the client should be done after the nurse tries to determine and treat the cause. Providing pin care is unrelated to the problem as described.

Test-Taking Strategy: On first reading, the only option that can be readily eliminated is option 2, providing pin care. The question asks you which should be done "first," which tells you that more than one answer is correct. Because it would be unwise to medicate a client without determining the true cause of the pain, option 1 is also eliminated. Of the remaining choices, checking the client's alignment is a prudent choice before calling the physician. At the very least, it would provide one more piece of data for the physician to work with.

Level of Cognitive Ability: Application
Phase of Nursing Process: Implementation
Client Needs: Physiological Integrity
Content Area: Adult Health/Musculoskeletal

Reference

Ignatavicius, D. D., Workman, M. L., & Mishler, M. A. (1995). *Medical-surgical nursing: A nursing process approach* (2nd ed.). Philadelphia: W. B. Saunders, p. 1463.

---

290. The client is complaining of skin irritation from the edges of a cast applied the previous day. The nurse should take which of the following actions?

1. Massage the skin at the rim of the cast
2. Apply lotion to the skin at the rim of the cast
3. Use a rough file to smooth the cast edges
4. Petal the cast edges with adhesive tape

Answer: 4

Rationale: The nurse petals the edges of the cast with tape to minimize skin irritation. If a client has a cast applied and returns home, the client can be taught to do the same.

Test-Taking Strategy: Options 1 and 2 are similar, and neither helps to get rid of the cause of the irritation, so they are eliminated first. Imagine the use of a "rough file"; it would create plaster chips and dust, which could go underneath the cast, and so it is not practical. By the process of elimination, you would choose to petal the cast to cushion the skin from the irritating cast material.

Level of Cognitive Ability: Application
Phase of Nursing Process: Implementation
Client Needs: Physiological Integrity
Content Area: Adult Health/Musculoskeletal

Reference

Smeltzer, S., & Bare, B. (1996). *Brunner and Suddarth's Textbook of medical-surgical nursing* (8th ed.). Philadelphia: Lippincott-Raven, pp. 1851, 1853.

291. The client who is learning to use a cane is afraid it will slip with ambulation, causing a fall. The nurse provides the client with the greatest reassurance by telling the client that

1. Canes prevent falls, not cause them.
2. The cane has a flared tip with concentric rings to give stability.
3. The physical therapist will determine whether the cane is inadequate.
4. The cane would help to break a fall, even if the client does slip.

Answer: 2

Rationale: A cane should have a slightly flared tip with flexible concentric rings. This tip acts as a shock absorber and provides optimal stability. Other advantages include greater speed with ambulation and less fatigue.

Test-Taking Strategy: Options 1 and 4 are the least plausible of all the choices and may be eliminated first. Neither of these statements provides any reassurance for the client. Option 3 also provides no information to relieve the client's anxiety. Option 2 is the best answer. It is a true statement and addresses the client's concerns about safety in a factual way.

Level of Cognitive Ability: Application
Phase of Nursing Process: Implementation
Client Needs: Psychosocial Integrity
Content Area: Adult Health/Musculoskeletal

Reference

Smeltzer, S., & Bare, B. (1996). *Brunner and Suddarth's Textbook of medical-surgical nursing* (8th ed.). Philadelphia: Lippincott-Raven, p. 341.

---

292. The nurse is caring for a child with a hernia. Which nursing action would be most appropriate to assist in reducing the hernia?

1. A saline water enema
2. Increasing client's physical activity
3. A warm bath
4. Instructing the client to cough

Answer: 3

Rationale: A warm bath, avoidance of upright positioning, and comfort measures to reduce crying all are simple measures to reduce a hernia. Coughing and crying increase the strain on the hernia. Enemas of any type would increase the strain on the hernia.

Test-Taking Strategy: Use the process of elimination. The issue of the question is an appropriate nursing action to reduce a hernia. Options 1, 2, and 4 all increase pressure and strain on the hernia site. Review nursing measures for a hernia now if you had difficulty with this question!

Level of Cognitive Ability: Application
Phase of Nursing Process: Implementation
Client Needs: Physiological Integrity
Content Area: Child Health

Reference

Wong, D. (1995). *Whaley and Wong's Nursing care of infants and children* (5th ed.). St. Louis: Mosby–Year Book, pp. 493–494.

---

293. The nurse is caring for a newborn with spina bifida (meningomyelocele type). The newborn is scheduled for the removal of the gibbus (sac on the back filled with cerebrospinal fluid, meninges, and some of the spinal cord). In the preoperative period, the priority nursing action would be to monitor

1. Blood pressure.
2. Moisture of the normal saline dressing on the gibbus area.
3. Specific gravity.
4. Anterior fontanel for depression.

Answer: 2

Rationale: The newborn is at risk for infection before closure of the gibbus. A sterile normal saline dressing is placed over the gibbus to maintain moisture of the gibbus and its contents. This prevents tearing or breakdown of the skin integrity at the site. Blood pressure is difficult to assess during the newborn period and is not the best indicator of infection. Urine concentration is not well developed in the newborn stage of development. Depression of the anterior fontanel is a sign of dehydration. With spina bifida, an increase in intracranial pressure is more of a priority. A bulging or taut anterior fontanel would signal a complication of spina bifida.

Test-Taking Strategy: Knowledge of the characteristics of spina bifida and the potential complications is needed to correctly answer this question. Read the question carefully. The question asks for a preoperative priority nursing action. Blood pressure and specific gravity are common preoperative assessments but are not as reliable as indicators of changes in newborn status as they would be for an older child. Knowledge of the newborn development of organ maturity and body functioning is also needed to make the correct selection. Option 2 is the only correct choice. Review preoperative care now if you had difficulty with this question!

Level of Cognitive Ability: Application
Phase of Nursing Process: Implementation
Client Needs: Physiological Integrity
Content Area: Child Health

Reference

Ashwill, J., & Droske, S. (1997). *Nursing care of children: Principles and practice.* Philadelphia: W. B. Saunders, p. 1234.

---

294. Exercise stress testing is ordered for a client with coronary artery disease. The nurse teaches the client to

1 Eat a light snack just before the procedure.
2 Wear loose clothing with a shirt that buttons in front.
3 Wear firm, rigid shoes such as work boots.
4 Avoid cigarettes for 30 minutes before the procedure.

Answer: 2

Rationale: The client wears loose, comfortable clothing for the procedure. A shirt that buttons in front is helpful for electrocardiogram (ECG) lead placement. The client is advised to wear rubber-soled, supportive shoes, such as sneakers. The client should be on NPO status after bedtime or for a minimum of 2 hours before the test and should avoid smoking, alcohol, and caffeine on the day of the test.

Test-Taking Strategy: Inadequate or incorrect preparation can interfere with the test, yielding false-positive findings. Thus the nurse would teach the client to avoid negative influences, such as eating, alcohol, caffeine, smoking, and restrictive or uncomfortable clothing. The question is worded to elicit an appropriate response by the nurse. Review test preparation for this procedure now if you had difficulty with this question!

Level of Cognitive Ability: Application
Phase of Nursing Process: Implementation
Client Needs: Physiological Integrity
Content Area: Adult Health/Cardiovascular

Reference

Ignatavicius, D. D., Workman, M. L., & Mishler, M. A. (1995). *Medical-surgical nursing: A nursing process approach* (2nd ed.). Philadelphia: W. B. Saunders, p. 806.

---

295. A client with coronary artery disease has an order to wear a Holter monitor for the next 24 hours. The nurse implements this order by

1 Shaving the anterior chest.
2 Providing a sling or holder for the monitor.
3 Encouraging the client to do very little activity for the next 24 hours.
4 Instructing the client to put the monitor in a plastic bag before showering.

Answer: 2

Rationale: Clients undergoing Holter monitoring are instructed to maintain a normal schedule and to keep a diary of all activity and symptoms. The client is told to avoid activities that could interfere with the ECG recorder, such as using heavy machinery, using electric shavers, using hair dryers, bathing, or showering. The nurse applies the leads to the chest and provides a sling to hold the transistor-sized monitor, which is worn around the chest or waist.

Test-Taking Strategy: The question is eliciting information about usual procedures for ambulatory cardiac monitoring. Options 1 and 4 are immediately eliminated because they are not standard practice. Option 3 is eliminated next because it could prevent the diagnostic procedure from picking up dysrhythmias that might have occurred with normal activity.

Level of Cognitive Ability: Application
Phase of Nursing Process: Implementation
Client Needs: Physiological Integrity
Content Area: Adult Health/Cardiovascular

Reference

Ignatavicius, D. D., Workman, M. L., & Mishler, M. A. (1995). *Medical-surgical nursing: A nursing process approach* (2nd ed.). Philadelphia: W. B. Saunders, p. 806.

296. The hospitalized client with a history of angina pectoris begins to complain of severe substernal chest pain. The nurse would take which of the following actions first?

1 Administer sublingual nitroglycerin
2 Assist the client to sit or lie down
3 Apply nasal oxygen at a rate of 2 liters/minute
4 Measure the client's vital signs

Answer: 2

Rationale: Chest pain is caused by an imbalance between myocardial oxygen supply and demand. During episodes of pain, the nurse limits the client's activity, assists the client to a position of comfort, obtains vital signs and a 12-lead ECG, and administers medication and oxygen according to protocol.

Test-Taking Strategy: The word "first" implies that more than one option is correct, as well as a proper time sequence. In this case, all answers are correct. The client needs to stop activity and assume a position of comfort to reduce myocardial oxygen demand. The other options cannot be performed while the client is engaged in activity.

Level of Cognitive Ability: Application
Phase of Nursing Process: Implementation
Client Needs: Physiological Integrity
Content Area: Adult Health/Cardiovascular

Reference

Luckmann, J. (1997). *Saunders manual of nursing care.* Philadelphia: W. B. Saunders, p. 1040.

---

297. The nurse is teaching a client with left-sided heart failure how to recognize early signs of exacerbation. The nurse includes which of the following in the list of signs and symptoms?

1 Difficulty breathing
2 Distended neck veins
3 Nausea and vomiting
4 Enlarged abdomen

Answer: 1

Rationale: Dyspnea, cough, fatigue, tachycardia, S_3 heart sound, anxiety, and restlessness are typical signs and symptoms of left-sided heart failure. The others listed in options 2, 3, and 4 are indicators of right-sided heart failure.

Test-Taking Strategy: Remember that blood pools in the area behind the failing chamber. In the case of left-sided heart failure, that area is the lungs. This will help eliminate the other options successfully. Remember "left" and "lungs." Left-sided heart failure results in respiratory symptoms.

Level of Cognitive Ability: Application
Phase of Nursing Process: Implementation
Client Needs: Physiological Integrity
Content Area: Adult Health/Cardiovascular

Reference

Smeltzer, S., & Bare, B. (1996). *Brunner and Suddarth's Textbook of medical-surgical nursing* (8th ed.). Philadelphia: Lippincott-Raven, p. 664.

---

298. The nurse is discussing dietary sodium restrictions with the client experiencing heart failure. The nurse gives the client a list that includes which of the following foods that can be used?

1 Tuna packed in water
2 Pasteurized processed cheese
3 Commercial salad dressings
4 Tomato juice

Answer: 1

Rationale: Sodium-restricted diets generally require avoiding the use of commercially prepared and highly processed foods. Fruits (and fresh fruit juices) and vegetables are acceptable, with the exception of tomato juice and V8 juice. Cheese and commercial salad dressings contain sodium. Tuna packed in water is acceptable.

Test-Taking Strategy: Most commercial products contain preservatives and therefore contain sodium, unless they are labeled otherwise. Evaluate any questions of this nature by using this concept. Review foods that are high in sodium now if you had difficulty with this question!

Level of Cognitive Ability: Application
Phase of Nursing Process: Implementation
Client Needs: Health Promotion and Maintenance
Content Area: Adult Health/Cardiovascular

Reference

Black, J., & Matassarin-Jacobs, E. (1997). *Medical-surgical nursing: Clinical management for continuity of care* (5th ed.). Philadelphia: W. B. Saunders, p. 1286.

299. The client with pulmonary edema has a multilumen pulmonary artery catheter inserted for hemodynamic monitoring. After the nurse obtains a pulmonary capillary wedge pressure reading, it is critical for the nurse to

1 Purge the system of air.
2 Pull the catheter back slightly.
3 Deflate the balloon.
4 Flush the system with heparin.

Answer: 3

Rationale: Pulmonary capillary wedge pressure readings are obtained by inflating the tiny distal balloon so that the catheter migrates (wedges) into a smaller branch of the pulmonary artery and detects the pressure proximal to the catheter in the pulmonary capillaries. It is vital after this measurement to deflate the balloon in order to avoid segmental lung infarction from mechanical vessel occlusion by the balloon.

Test-Taking Strategy: This is a difficult question, and a basic understanding of the function of this catheter is needed to answer the question correctly. The word "critical" in the stem may help you eliminate options 2 and 4. It is not usual nursing practice to withdraw hemodynamic catheters in any manner. Heparin flush may not be plausible because no blood was withdrawn from the catheter. No fluid system going into a client's blood vessel should have air in it after the tubing is originally primed. Review this procedure now if you had difficulty with this question!

Level of Cognitive Ability: Application
Phase of Nursing Process: Implementation
Client Needs: Physiological Integrity
Content Area: Adult Health/Cardiovascular

Reference

Smeltzer, S., & Bare, B. (1996). *Brunner and Suddarth's Textbook of medical-surgical nursing* (8th ed.). Philadelphia: Lippincott-Raven, p. 667.

---

300. The client who underwent cardiac surgery 6 weeks ago has a pleural effusion detected on follow-up office visit. The physician schedules the client for thoracentesis. In preparing the client for the procedure, the nurse positions the client

1 In the dorsal recumbent position.
2 In the left lateral position with right arm supported by a pillow.
3 Sitting upright and forward with arms resting on an over-the-bed table.
4 Lying on the right side, curled into a fetal position.

Answer: 3

Rationale: The client undergoing thoracentesis usually sits in an upright position, with the anterior thorax supported by pillows, or leaning over an over-the-bed table.

Test-Taking Strategy: If you have any difficulty with this question, think about the procedure and the effects of gravity on fluid in the lungs. The correct option is the only one that uses gravity to consolidate the fluid in an easily accessible area to be aspirated. Any form of side-lying position will cause fluid to accumulate under that side, which is inaccessible to the physician.

Level of Cognitive Ability: Application
Phase of Nursing Process: Implementation
Client Needs: Physiological Integrity
Content Area: Adult Health/Cardiovascular

Reference

Potter, P., & Perry, A. (1997). *Fundamentals of nursing: Concepts, process, and practice* (4th ed.). St. Louis: Mosby–Year Book, p. 1215.

REFERENCES

Antai-Otong, D. (1995). *Psychiatric nursing: Biological and behavioral concepts.* Philadelphia: W. B. Saunders.

Ashwill, J., & Droske, S. (1997). *Nursing care of children: Principles and practices.* Philadelphia: W. B. Saunders.

Ball, J., & Bindler, R. (1995). *Pediatric nursing: Caring for children.* Stamford, CT: Appleton & Lange.

Black, J., & Matassarin-Jacobs, E. (1997). *Medical-surgical nursing: Clinical management for continuity of care* (5th ed.). Philadelphia: W. B. Saunders.

Bolander, V. (1994). *Sorenson and Luckmann's Basic nursing: A psychophysiologic approach* (3rd ed.). Philadelphia: W. B. Saunders.

Burrell, P., Gerlach, M., & Pless, B. (1997). *Adult nursing: Acute and community care* (2nd ed.). Stamford, CT: Appleton & Lange.

Carson, V., & Arnold, E. (1996). *Mental health nursing: The nurse-patient journey.* Philadelphia: W. B. Saunders.

Chernecky, C., & Berger, B. J. (1997). *Laboratory tests and diagnostic procedures* (2nd ed.). Philadelphia: W. B. Saunders.

Clark, J., Queener, S., & Karb, V. (1997). *Pharmacologic basis of nursing practice* (5th ed.). St. Louis: Mosby–Year Book.

Clark, M. (1996). *Nursing in the community* (2nd ed.). Stamford, CT: Appleton & Lange.

Cox, H., Hinz, M., Lubno, M., et al. (1997). *Clinical applications of nursing diagnosis: Adult, child, women's, psychiatric, gerontic, and home health considerations* (3rd ed.). Philadelphia: F. A. Davis.

Deglin, J., & Vallerand, A. (1997). *Davis's drug guide for nurses* (5th ed.). Philadelphia: F. A. Davis.

Ellis, J., & Hartley, C. (1995). *Nursing in today's world: Challenges, issues, and trends* (5th ed.). Philadelphia: Lippincott-Raven.

Gorrie, T. M., McKinney, E. S., & Murray, S. S. (1998). *Foundations of maternal newborn nursing* (2nd ed.). Philadelphia: W. B. Saunders.

Haber, J. (1997). *Comprehensive psychiatric nursing* (5th ed.). St. Louis: Mosby–Year Book.

Hartshorn, J., Sole, M., & Lamborn, M. (1997). *Introduction to critical care nursing* (2nd ed.). Philadelphia: W. B. Saunders.

Hodgson, B., & Kizior, R. (1998). *Saunders nursing drug handbook 1998.* Philadelphia: W. B. Saunders.

Ignatavicius, D. D., Workman, M. L., & Mishler, M. A. (1995). *Medical-surgical nursing: A nursing process approach* (2nd ed.). Philadelphia: W. B. Saunders.

Johnson, B. (1997). *Psychiatric-mental health nursing: Adaptation and growth* (4th ed.). Philadelphia: Lippincott-Raven.

Kee, J., & Hayes, E. (1997). *Pharmacology: A nursing process approach* (2nd ed.). Philadelphia: W. B. Saunders.

Kee, J., & Marshall, S. (1996). *Clinical calculation with applications to general and specialty areas* (3rd ed.). Philadelphia: W. B. Saunders.

Kozier, B., Glenora, E., & Blais, K. (1995). *Fundamentals of nursing* (5th ed.). Menlo Park, CA: Addison-Wesley.

Lammon, C. B., Foote, A. W., Leli, P. G., et al. (1995). *Clinical nursing skills.* Philadelphia: W. B. Saunders.

Lehne, R. A. (1998). *Pharmacology for nursing care* (3rd ed.). Philadelphia: W. B. Saunders.

LeMone, P., & Burke, K. (1996). *Medical-surgical nursing: Critical thinking in client care.* Menlo Park, CA: Addison-Wesley.

Lewis, S., Collier, I., & Heitkemper, M. (1996). *Medical-surgical nursing: Assessment and management of clinical problems* (4th ed.). St. Louis: Mosby–Year Book.

Lowdermilk, D., Perry, S., & Bobak, I. (1997). *Maternity and women's health care* (6th ed.). St. Louis: Mosby–Year Book.

Luckmann, J. (1997). *Saunders manual of nursing care.* Philadelphia: W. B. Saunders.

Monahan, F., & Neighbors, M. (1998). *Medical-surgical nursing: Foundations for clinical practice* (2nd ed.). Philadelphia: W. B. Saunders.

Nichols, F., & Zwelling, E. (1997). *Maternal-newborn nursing: Theory and practice.* Philadelphia: W. B. Saunders.

Olds, S., London, M., & Ladewig, P. (1996). *Clinical handbook for maternal-newborn nursing: A family-centered approach* (5th ed.). Menlo Park, CA: Addison-Wesley.

Phipps, W., Cassmeyer, V., Sands, J., et al. (1995). *Medical-surgical nursing: Concepts and clinical practice* (5th ed.). St. Louis: Mosby–Year Book.

Pillitteri, A. (1995). *Maternal and child health nursing: Care of the childbearing and childrearing family* (2nd ed.). Philadelphia: Lippincott-Raven.

Pinnell, N. L. (1996). *Nursing pharmacology.* Philadelphia: W. B. Saunders.

Polaski, A., & Tatro, S. (1996). *Luckmann's Core principles and practice of medical-surgical nursing.* Philadelphia: W. B. Saunders.

Potter, P., & Perry, A. (1997). *Fundamentals of nursing: Concepts, process, and practice* (4th ed.). St. Louis: Mosby–Year Book.

Reeder, S., Martin, L., & Koniak-Griffin, D. (1997). *Maternity nursing: Family, newborn, and women's health care* (18th ed.). Philadelphia: Lippincott-Raven.

Rice, R. (1996). *Home health nursing practice: Concepts and application* (2nd ed.). St. Louis: Mosby–Year Book.

Sieh, A., & Brentin, L. (1997). *The nurse communicates.* Philadelphia: W. B. Saunders.

Smeltzer, S., & Bare, B. (1996). *Brunner and Suddarth's Textbook of medical-surgical nursing* (8th ed.). Philadelphia: Lippincott-Raven.

Stuart, G., & Sundeen, S. (1995). *Principles and practice of psychiatric nursing.* St. Louis: Mosby–Year Book.

Taylor, C., Lillis, C., & LeMone, P. (1997). *Fundamentals of nursing: The art and science of nursing care* (3rd ed.). Philadelphia: Lippincott-Raven.

Tierney, L., McPhee, S., & Papadakis, M. (1997). *Current medical diagnosis and treatment* (36th ed.). Stamford, CT: Appleton & Lange.

Townsend, M. (1996). *Psychiatric-mental health nursing: Concepts of care* (2nd ed.). Philadelphia: F. A. Davis.

VanRiper, S., & VanRiper, J. (1997). *Cardiac diagnostic tests: A guide for nurses.* Philadelphia: W. B. Saunders.

Wilson, B., Shannon, M., & Stang, C. (1997). *Nurses drug guide.* Stamford, CT: Appleton & Lange.

Wilson, H., & Kneisl, C. (1996). *Psychiatric nursing* (5th ed.). Menlo Park, CA: Addison-Wesley.

Wong, D. (1995). *Whaley and Wong's Nursing care of infants and children* (5th ed.). St. Louis: Mosby–Year Book.

Wong, D. (1997). *Whaley and Wong's Essentials of pediatric nursing* (5th ed.). St. Louis: Mosby–Year Book.

Wong, D., & Perry, S. (1998). *Maternal-child nursing care.* St. Louis: Mosby–Year Book.

Zang, S., & Bailey, N. (1997). *Home care manual: Making the transition.* Philadelphia: Lippincott-Raven.

CHAPTER 9

The Process of Evaluation

Evaluation is the fifth and final step of the nursing process. The process of evaluation identifies the degree to which the nursing diagnoses, plans for care, and interventions have been successful.

Although evaluation is the final step of the nursing process, it is an ongoing and integral component of each step. The process of data collection and assessment is reviewed to determine whether sufficient information was obtained and whether the information obtained was specific and appropriate. The nursing diagnoses are evaluated for accuracy and completeness on the basis of the specific needs of the client. The plan and expected outcomes are examined to determine whether they are realistic, achievable, measurable, and effective. Interventions are examined to determine their effectiveness in achieving the expected outcomes.

Because evaluation is an ongoing process, it is vital to all steps of the nursing process. It is the continuous process of comparing actual outcomes with expected outcomes of care, and it provides the means for determining the need to modify the plan of care. Inherent in this step of the nursing process is the communication of evaluation findings and the process of documenting the client's response to treatment, care, and/or teaching.

PRACTICE TEST

1. A client with angina pectoris expresses concerns to the nurse about not being able to return to a normal lifestyle in view of the newly diagnosed cardiac condition. Which response by the client demonstrates effective coping?

1 "If I die, I die. There's nothing left to say."
2 "Can we talk about my heart now?"
3 "I don't want to talk about this now."
4 "I guess I'll just retire from my job."

Answer: 2

Rationale: The client expresses a desire to verbalize concerns and anxieties. Expressing emotions can decrease the perceived intensity of the stressor, indicating effective coping. Option 1 indicates an inability to solve problems effectively. Option 3 indicates denial of the problem. Although option 4 may be a decision the client will face, it is premature at this time and does not reflect effective coping.

Test-Taking Strategy: Use the process of elimination in answering the question. The stem seeks a client response that indicates effective coping. Option 1 indicates an inability to effectively problem solve. Option 3 indicates denial. Option 4 indicates a premature decision. Option 2 reflects effective coping.

Level of Cognitive Ability: Analysis
Phase of Nursing Process: Evaluation
Client Needs: Psychosocial Integrity
Content Area: Adult Health/Cardiovascular

Reference
Kozier, B., Glenora, E., & Blais, K. (1995). *Fundamentals of nursing: Concepts, process, and practice* (5th ed.). Menlo Park, CA: Addison-Wesley, p. 844.

2. An infant with a diagnosis of pyloric stenosis undergoes a pyloromyotomy. Postoperatively, the nurse provides the mother with instructions regarding care of the infant. Which of the following statements, if made by this mother, indicates a need for additional instruction?

1 "Last night, the nurse told me that my baby would gain weight now that the pyloric stenosis has been corrected."
2 "My pediatrician told me that babies come in all sizes and the important thing is to follow my baby's growth pattern."
3 "Since my baby has been so sick, I will wait to begin the 'baby shots' until the baby is 6 months old."
4 "I can't wait to see my baby smile again. My baby has been so sick."

Answer: 3

Rationale: The convalescent phase of illnesses is not a contraindication for immunizations. The general contraindication for all immunizations is a severe febrile illness or immunocompromise. The normal schedule for immunizations is recommended for this infant to provide protection from life-threatening diseases. Options 1, 2, and 4 indicate an appropriate understanding of growth and development.

Test-Taking Strategy: Read the stem of the question carefully. Evaluation questions frequently use false response stems. The question asks for the client's statement that indicates a need for further teaching. Use the process of elimination to select the option that indicates the need for further instructions. If you had difficulty with this question, take time now to review the contraindications associated with immunizations and the postoperative care associated with pyloromyotomy!

Level of Cognitive Ability: Analysis
Phase of Nursing Process: Evaluation
Client Needs: Health Promotion and Maintenance
Content Area: Child Health

Reference

Wong, D., & Perry, S. (1998). *Maternal-child nursing care.* St. Louis: Mosby–Year Book, p. 1429.

---

3. The nurse has been conducting a community support group for grief education and resolution issues. In the termination stage, the nurse would best evaluate the group experience by inviting clients to engage in which of the following?

1 Idea review of what the clients had learned about handling their grief on a day-to-day basis and how they were now handling "saying good-by" to other clients
2 Ideas about how the clients could help themselves and others when they leave the group
3 Ideas of how clients would handle loss and grieving in the future
4 Ideas pertaining to handling conflict and decision making in the group

Answer: 1

Rationale: During the termination phase of a support group, the nurse addresses evaluation by exploring clients' thoughts and feelings about the group experience and separating from the group. Loss and grieving as part of the human experience are addressed. Options 2 and 3 are premature evaluative techniques and do not specifically evaluate group experience as the question asks. Option 4 relates to tasks in the working stage of group process.

Test-Taking Strategy: Knowledge of the tasks during the evaluative stage of group process is essential for responding to the question correctly. Options 2 and 3 are similar; therefore, neither one is likely to be the correct answer. Option 4 is related to the working stage of group process. If you had difficulty with this question, take time now to review the stages of group process!

Level of Cognitive Ability: Analysis
Phase of Nursing Process: Evaluation
Client Needs: Psychosocial Integrity
Content Area: Mental Health

Reference

Johnson, B. (1997). *Psychiatric mental health nursing: Adaptation and growth* (4th ed.). Philadelphia: Lippincott-Raven, p. 270.

4. The nurse evaluates a client in a hip spica cast. The client complains of abdominal pain, nausea, and shortness of breath. On the basis of the evaluation of the client's symptoms, the nurse determines that the appropriate action requires
   1 Repositioning the client in a side-lying position.
   2 Preparing the client for immediate fasciotomy.
   3 Bivalving the cast to relieve pressure.
   4 Cutting the cast down the center over the chest.

Answer: 3

Rationale: Repositioning the client will not alleviate the symptoms. A fasciotomy is a treatment for compartment syndrome. Cutting the cast over the chest is an appropriate measure for performing cardiac compression. Because this is an emergency situation indicating compression, bivalving the cast is the appropriate action.

Test-Taking Strategy: Identify the client's symptoms and determine the cause of the symptoms. Read each option carefully, considering what the particular action would accomplish. Consider the ABCs: airway, breathing, and circulation; option 3 addresses circulation. If you had difficulty with this question, take time now to review cast therapy and its complications!

Level of Cognitive Ability: Analysis
Phase of Nursing Process: Evaluation
Client Needs: Physiological Integrity
Content Area: Adult Health/Musculoskeletal

Reference
Burrell, P., Gerlach, M., & Pless, S. (1997). *Adult nursing: Acute and community care* (2nd ed.). Stamford, CT: Appleton & Lange, pp. 1588, 1590–1593.

5. The community health nurse is caring for a client who has had a parathyroidectomy with autotransplantation of some parathyroid tissue into the forearm. The client has been taking oral calcium and vitamin D supplements since discharge 2 weeks ago. Which statement by the client indicates a good understanding of the medical management after this type of surgical procedure?
   1 "Well, I guess the transplant isn't working because my calcium levels are still low."
   2 "The thought of taking these pills for the rest of my life makes me shudder!"
   3 "I can't wait for the transplant to start working, I'm tired of taking all these pills!"
   4 "Do you think I'll always have to take these pills?"

Answer: 3

Rationale: In autotransplantation of parathyroid tissue, the transplant takes some time to mature. Oral calcium and vitamin D supplements must be taken to prevent hypoparathyroidism until the transplant matures and becomes an active endocrine gland.

Test-Taking Strategy: Knowledge regarding parathyroid transplant surgery is helpful for answering this question. Use the process of elimination to answer the question. Options 2 and 4 can be eliminated because they are similar and both seem to negate the purpose of transplants, that of gaining function of the organ. Eliminate option 1 because the question does not address low calcium levels. If you had difficulty with this question, take time now to review parathyroid transplant surgery!

Level of Cognitive Ability: Analysis
Phase of Nursing Process: Evaluation
Client Needs: Health Promotion and Maintenance
Content Area: Adult Health/Endocrine

Reference
Black, J., & Matassarin-Jacobs, E. (1997). *Medical-surgical nursing: Clinical management for continuity of care* (5th ed.). Philadelphia: W. B. Saunders, p. 2035.

6. A child with Hirschsprung's disease is scheduled for surgery. A temporary colostomy is performed on the child. Postoperatively, the nurse teaches the child and parents about colostomy care at home. Which of these actions by the parents indicates the teaching was effective?

1 Reporting early evidence of skin breakdown
2 Application of a heat lamp to moist red tissue around the stoma
3 Administration of antidiarrheal medications
4 Administration of saline water enema because of absent stools

Answer: 1

Rationale: Option 1 is the only correct action. The family is instructed to report early evidence of skin breakdown or stomal complications, such as ribbon-like stools or excessive failure to pass flatus or stools, to the physician or the nurse. Moist, red granulation tissue may grow around an ostomy site and does not require special treatment. Options 3 and 4 would be incorrect actions and are contraindicated.

Test-Taking Strategy: The stem of the question asks you to select an option that indicates that the parents understand their responsibilities in the child's colostomy care. Look for the one option that is the correct action for the parents to take. Use the process of elimination to eliminate the incorrect options. If you had difficulty with this question, take time now to review parent teaching and colostomy care!

Level of Cognitive Ability: Analysis
Phase of Nursing Process: Evaluation
Client Needs: Health Promotion and Health Maintenance
Content Area: Child Health

Reference

Wong, D. (1995). *Whaley and Wong's Nursing care of infants and children* (5th ed.). St. Louis: Mosby–Year Book, pp. 1158–1160, 1195–1197.

---

7. The nurse is engaged in preparing a client for electroconvulsive therapy (ECT). The client's family is present during the discussion. The nurse has discussed the treatment process, preparation for treatment, treatment procedure, and aftereffects of treatment with the client and family. The client has signed the informed consent form. Upon departure from the session, a family member states, "I don't know. . . . I don't think that this ECT will be helpful if it is going to make people's memory worse. People who are depressed are bad enough off . . . without making them any worse." The nurse would then

1 Involve the family member in a dialogue to ascertain how the family member arrived at this conclusive statement.
2 Inquire with other family members and the client if they thought the same way about ECT making people worse.
3 Immediately reassure the client that the ECT will help and that memory loss or confusion is minimal and temporary.
4 Reinforce with the family member that depression causes more memory impairment than ECT.

Answer: 1

Rationale: In option 1, the nurse is exploring for data to assist in clarification of a faulty judgment. If the nurse gathers additional data from the family member, the nurse may use the data to explore the family member's questions. While inviting the client's and family's feedback to the ECT process, the nurse is supporting the family's presence and encouraging the client's self-care and family support system. Option 2 may place family members on the defensive and promote conflict among family members. Option 3 would not acknowledge the family member's statement and concern. Option 4 addresses content clarification but not the evaluative process and feedback from clients.

Test-Taking Strategy: Remember that assessment is the first step in the nursing process. Identify the client of the question, which in this question, is the family member. This evaluation question addresses the family member's response to an educationally oriented session presented by the nurse. In option 1, the nurse gathers more data and addresses the family member's thoughts and feelings first. The nurse has given out information but now is involved in further clarification with the family member.

Level of Cognitive Ability: Analysis
Phase of Nursing Process: Evaluation
Client Needs: Psychosocial Integrity
Content Area: Mental Health

Reference

Carson, V., & Arnold, E. (1996). *Mental health nursing: The nurse-patient journey.* Philadelphia: W. B. Saunders, p. 785.

8. A client has had a cerebrovascular accident (CVA) with damage to the nondominant cerebral hemisphere and has unilateral neglect. Before discharge from the hospital, the nurse determines that the client has compensated for the neglect when it is observed that the client

1 Allows the affected lower extremity to be abducted and externally rotated in bed.
2 Scans the environment before beginning to bathe the affected side first.
3 Focuses attention only on visitors who stand or sit on the client's unaffected side.
4 Misplaces objects and then finds them later on the affected side.

Answer: 2

Rationale: The client with unilateral neglect must learn to scan the environment and gradually come to a realization of the affected side. Options 1, 3, and 4 present examples of the client neglecting the affected side through loss of position sense, focus of attention, and forgetting to scan.

Test-Taking Strategy: Read the question carefully to be sure that you understand that the client has met the goal, has compensated for the neglect, and can care for the affected side. In option 1, the extremity is positioned unsafely. In option 3, the absolute term "only" appears, most likely making it an incorrect option. In option 4, the client neglects the affected side.

Level of Cognitive Ability: Analysis
Phase of Nursing Process: Evaluation
Client Needs: Health Promotion and Maintenance
Content Area: Adult Health/Neurological

References
Black, J., & Matassarin-Jacobs, E. (1997). *Medical-surgical nursing: Clinical management for continuity of care* (5th ed.). Philadelphia: W. B. Saunders, p. 806.

---

9. The clinic nurse is teaching the parents of a 5-year-old child about safety issues. Which statement, if made by the parents, indicates a need for further teaching?

1 "All medications and dangerous fluids are stored in areas inaccessible to a child."
2 "We always watch our child in the bathtub."
3 "Bicycle helmets are necessary only when riding in the street."
4 "The safest way for a child to ride in a car is in the center back seat with a seatbelt on."

Answer: 3

Rationale: Bicycle safety requires always wearing a helmet when riding. Most injuries occur near home, and there is potential for falls on bike paths and off roads. Five is also a young age to be riding in the street. All other answers are age-appropriate safety measures.

Test-Taking Strategy: The key phrase, "need for further teaching," alerts you to a false response stem often used in evaluation questions. Note the child's age, and use the process of elimination in answering the question. Look for the option that identifies an incorrect statement, if made by the parents. The absolute terminology "only" in option 3 tends to make a statement false and would also help to direct you to the correct option for this question as stated. If you had difficulty with this question, take time now to review safety issues related to a 5-year-old!

Level of Cognitive Ability: Analysis
Phase of Nursing Process: Evaluation
Client Needs: Health Promotion and Maintenance
Content Area: Child Health

Reference
Wong, D. (1997). *Whaley and Wong's Essentials of pediatric nursing* (5th ed.). St. Louis: Mosby–Year Book, p. 459.

10. The nurse has cared for a client who died a few minutes ago. The nurse reflects on the care given to the client. Which of the following statement supports the nurse's belief that the client died with dignity?

1 The family thanks the nurse and states that the client was not in pain and was peaceful at the end.
2 The physician recognizes that all the orders were carried out and there were no questions.
3 A new nurse states it would be very difficult to give that kind of care to a dying client.
4 The nurse gave increasing doses of pain medication to keep the client well sedated.

Answer: 1

Rationale: The family response is an external perception, which is extremely important. Families derive a great deal of comfort knowing their loved one received the best care possible. The nurse needs to keep the family aware of what is happening and allow them to participate as much as possible. The family's perception is what remains after the death of the client.

Test-Taking Strategy: Use the process of elimination to answer the question. Option 1 provides external validation that the client received comprehensive, quality care. Option 2 focuses on physician orders rather than client care. Option 3 focuses on the feelings of a new nurse who may be expressing his or her own anxiety. Option 4 reflects only one aspect of caring for a dying client.

Level of Cognitive Ability: Analysis
Phase of Nursing Process: Evaluation
Client Needs: Psychosocial Integrity
Content Area: Fundamental Skills

Reference

Bandman, E., & Bandman, B. (1995). *Nursing ethics through the life span.* Stamford, CT: Appleton & Lange, pp. 297–302.

---

11. After identifying a possible occult prolapsed umbilical cord in a client in early second-stage labor, the nurse turns the client to a modified Sim's position. The nurse then starts oxygen at 10 liters per minute by mask, increases the rate of intravenous fluids, alerts the physician and other staff, and explains the situation to the client. Which of the following criteria would the nurse use to determine whether this plan of care is effective?

1 Arrival time of the physician
2 Vital signs of the woman and her emotional state
3 Client anxiously cooperates with instructions to stay on her side
4 Fetal monitor indicating a normal baseline rate and variability of the fetal heart

Answer: 4

Rationale: The fetus is at risk in this situation. The greatest danger of a prolapsed cord is fetal cord compression, which is indicated by changes in the fetal monitor pattern. Fetal heart rate and variability are the cardinal measures of fetal well-being and are thus the most vital indicators of the success of the nursing care measures. If the plan is unsuccessful, the fetal heart monitor will show a pattern of increasing early decelerations and a decreasing baseline as the situation deteriorates.

Test-Taking Strategy: To determine the focus of your evaluation, determine which of the obstetrical couplet (woman and fetus) is primarily at risk. Look at the stem of the question carefully and determine which step of the nursing process is to be addressed. Because this is an evaluation question, determine which option evaluates the nursing plan or action. Use the ABCs—airway, breathing, and circulation—to assist in answering the question!

Level of Cognitive Ability: Analysis
Phase of Nursing Process: Evaluation
Client Needs: Physiological Integrity
Content Area: Maternity

Reference

Lowdermilk, D., Perry, S., & Bobak, I. (1997). *Maternity and women's health care* (6th ed.). St. Louis: Mosby–Year Book, pp. 328, 952, 973.

12. A client is admitted with a bowel obstruction secondary to a recurrent malignancy. The physician plans to insert a Miller-Abbott tube. When the nurse tries to explain the procedure, the client interrupts the nurse and states, "I don't want to hear about that. Just let the doctor do it." On the basis of the client's statement, the nurse evaluates that the best action is to

1 Leave the room.
2 Ask the client whether he or she would like another nurse to care for him or her.
3 Explain to the client that all clients have the right to know about medical procedures.
4 Remain with the client and be silent.

Answer: 4

Rationale: The nurse evaluates a situation and attempts to educate the client. In this particular situation, the client has a greater need for security and acceptance than education. The nurse needs to recognize the client's need. In option 4, the nurse conveys acceptance of the client and uses the therapeutic tool of silence. Options 1, 2, and 3 block communication and do not address the client's need.

Test-Taking Strategy: Using teaching-learning theory, the nurse should assess for client motivation and readiness. Use the process of elimination and eliminate the nontherapeutic actions. The nursing actions in options 1, 2, and 3 could be blocks to communication. Remaining with the client demonstrates acceptance.

Level of Cognitive Ability: Application
Phase of Nursing Process: Evaluation
Client Needs: Psychosocial Integrity
Content Area: Adult Health/Gastrointestinal

Reference
Potter, P., & Perry, A. (1997). *Fundamentals of nursing: Concepts, process, and practice* (4th ed.). St. Louis: Mosby–Year Book, pp. 233–235.

---

13. The community health nurse visits a client who is receiving continuous total parenteral nutrition (TPN) through a central venous catheter in the home. The nurse visits the client twice per week. The client's spouse manages the administration of the solution. Which of the following statements, if made by the client, indicates the need for further teaching?

1 "My spouse checks my temperature each evening."
2 "My blood sugars have been running around 110."
3 "I have had my blood work drawn every week like the physician ordered."
4 "I told my spouse to slow the IV down yesterday because I was feeling full."

Answer: 4

Rationale: Clients receiving TPN at home require education and nurse supervision. Clients and caregivers need to follow prescribed protocols for management of TPN. Measures for managing the administration and prevention of complications are modified for in the home. Clients should report concerns to the nurse before changing management methods. TPN infusions should be maintained at a constant flow rate. Too rapid a flow of solution could result in hyperglycemia. Too slow of a flow solution will not deliver the prescribed nutrients and fluids.

Test-Taking Strategy: Read the stem carefully and identify the key phrase "need for further education." Use the process of elimination. Options 1, 2, and 3 are examples of measures necessary for correct TPN management. Option 4 should not be performed independently by the client. If you had difficulty with this question, take time now to review home care management of TPN!

Level of Cognitive Ability: Analysis
Phase of Nursing Process: Evaluation
Client Needs: Health Promotion and Maintenance
Content Area: Adult Health/Gastrointestinal

Reference
Black, J., & Matassarin-Jacobs, E. (1997). *Medical-surgical nursing: Clinical management for continuity of care* (5th ed.). Philadelphia: W. B. Saunders, pp. 1754–1756.

---

14. A client is being taught to eliminate factors that might cause a future attack of acute pancreatitis. The nurse's teaching is effective when the client states which of the following?

1 "A glass of wine before dinner will be good for my appetite."
2 "It's okay to drink my favorite brands of coffee."
3 "Starchy foods are strictly taboo."
4 "I'm going to try using a nicotine patch."

Answer: 4

Rationale: Alcohol can precipitate an attack of pancreatitis. Coffee and soft drinks, which contain caffeine, stimulate the pancreas. Carbohydrates actually should be encouraged because they are less stimulating to the pancreas. Because smoking can overstimulate the pancreas, the nurse's teaching is effective when the client will try to stop smoking.

Test-Taking Strategy: Knowledge of what stimulates the pancreas is helpful in answering this question. Eliminate options 1 and 2 because both these options can stimulate the pancreas. Note the absolute term "strictly" in option 3; such an absolute term would tend to make the option incorrect. This leaves option 4 as the correct option. If you had difficulty with this question, take time now to review the factors that can precipitate an attack of pancreatitis!

Level of Cognitive Ability: Analysis
Phase of Nursing Process: Evaluation
Client Needs: Health Promotion and Maintenance
Content Area: Adult Health/Gastrointestinal

Reference

Lewis, S., Collier, I., & Heitkemper, M. (1996). *Medical-surgical nursing: Assessment and management of clinical problems* (4th ed.). St. Louis: Mosby–Year Book, p. 1293.

---

15. The home health nurse is caring for a client with tuberculosis. In evaluating the client's knowledge regarding respiratory precautions at home, the home health nurse would examine compliance with which of the following respiratory precautions?

1 Keeping an oxygen mask on at all times
2 Keeping the client secluded in the bedroom
3 Keeping the house closed up to minimize spread of disease
4 Disposing of contaminated tissues in container-lined receptacles

Answer: 4

Rationale: Keeping an oxygen mask on at all times is not a respiratory precaution. Clients do not need to be in seclusion. The client would not be at home if he or she were infectious; however, proper respiratory precautions are needed. The house should be properly ventilated, and opening the windows as much as possible is preferred. Contaminated tissues should be discarded in container-lined receptacles and then put in the outdoor trash as frequently as possible. Tissues should not be lying around on the floor, tables, or other furniture.

Test-Taking Strategy: Use the process of elimination to answer this question. Knowledge regarding the transmission and home care of a client with tuberculosis is necessary to answer this question correctly. If you had difficulty answering this question, take the time now to review this important content area. You are likely to find questions related to tuberculosis on NCLEX-RN!

Level of Cognitive Ability: Analysis
Phase of Nursing Process: Evaluation
Client Needs: Health Promotion and Maintenance
Content Area: Adult Health/Respiratory

Reference

Zang, S., & Bailey, N. (1997). *Home care manual: Making the transition.* Philadelphia: Lippincott-Raven, p. 281.

---

16. After instructing a mother on how to feed an infant who has a cleft palate, the nurse observes the mother feeding the child. Which of these observations would indicate a need for further teaching?

1 The mother uses a bottle with a lamb's nipple to administer formula
2 The mother places the nipple between the existing palate and tongue
3 The mother follows the formula feeding with a small amount of water
4 The mother frequently interrupts the feeding to check for choking

Answer: 4

Rationale: The mother should be taught to maintain constant pressure to the bottom of the bottle to decrease the risk of choking. The mother should also be taught to expect noise from the baby while feeding and to watch facial expressions as a cue to stop the feeding. Options 1, 2, and 3 are appropriate feeding techniques. Frequently interrupting the feeding to check for choking is not an appropriate feeding technique.

Test-Taking Strategy: The key phrase in the stem is "a need for further teaching." This phrase should direct you to look for the option that is inappropriate. Use the process of elimination and knowledge regarding the feeding techniques appropriate for a child with cleft palate. If you had difficulty with this question, take time now to review feeding techniques associated with cleft palate!

Level of Cognitive Ability: Analysis
Phase of Nursing Process: Evaluation
Client Needs: Physiological Integrity
Content Area: Child Health

Reference

Wong, D. L. (1995). *Whaley and Wong's Nursing care of infants and children* (5th ed.). St. Louis: Mosby–Year Book, pp. 475–476.

17. After three defibrillation attempts, the client continues to be in a pulseless, ventricular tachycardia. A lidocaine bolus of 100 mg IV is administered. The nurse would expect that a therapeutic response would result in

1 The client's converting from a ventricular tachycardia to a ventricular fibrillation.
2 The client's heart rate slowing to 80 beats per minute.
3 A decrease in ventricular irritability.
4 An increase in the level of consciousness.

Answer: 3

Rationale: Lidocaine is the primary medication used to treat ventricular dysrhythmias. Lidocaine exerts a local anesthetic effect on the heart, thus decreasing myocardial irritability.

Test-Taking Strategy: The question asks for an evaluation of the effects of a medication. Even without a familiarity of lidocaine, the similarities in the words "ventricular" in the question and in options 1 and 3 should guide the nurse to these options. From this point, in evaluating the effectiveness of a medication used for a life-threatening dysrhythmia, it is not logical to expect a ventricular tachycardia to convert to a ventricular fibrillation, which is more dangerous; thus option 1 is eliminated. Option 3 is the desired effect of a medication administered for ventricular tachycardia. If you had difficulty with this question, take time now to review the therapeutic effects of this medication!

Level of Cognitive Ability: Analysis
Phase of Nursing Process: Evaluation
Client Needs: Physiological Integrity
Content Area: Pharmacology

Reference

Kee, J., & Hayes, E. (1997). *Pharmacology: A nursing process approach* (2nd ed.). Philadelphia: W. B. Saunders, p. 754.

18. The client with congestive heart failure is being discharged home and will be taking furosemide (Lasix). The nurse evaluates that teaching has been effective if the client states which of the following?

1 "I will check my ankles every day for swelling."
2 "I will take my pulse every day."
3 "I will measure my urine output."
4 "I will weigh myself every day."

Answer: 4

Rationale: A client taking furosemide (Lasix) must be able to monitor fluid status throughout therapy. Monitoring weight daily is the easiest and most accurate way to accomplish this. Options 1 and 3 are incorrect because of the difficulty of assessing fluid status accurately in this way. In addition, in order for option 3 to be correct, fluid intake would need to be measured. Option 2 is incorrect and unrelated to the administration of furosemide (Lasix).

Test-Taking Strategy: Use the process of elimination. In client teaching questions, try to select the response that would be the easiest and most effective for a nurse to teach and for the client to understand. Remember, if you instruct a client to do something that is too complicated, there will be no compliance. Option 4 provides the easiest and most accurate way to measure fluid status. If you had difficulty with this question, take time now to review the measures that will effectively determine a therapeutic response to furosemide!

Level of Cognitive Ability: Analysis
Phase of Nursing Process: Evaluation
Client Needs: Health Promotion and Maintenance
Content Area: Pharmacology

Reference

Hodgson, B., & Kizior, R. (1998). *Saunders nursing drug handbook 1998.* Philadelphia: W. B. Saunders, pp. 452–454.

19. A client is being treated for acute congestive heart failure (CHF). The client is receiving digoxin (Lanoxin). The client's vital signs are as follows: blood pressure, 85/50; pulse, 96; respiration, 26. To evaluate a therapeutic effectiveness of this medication, the nurse would expect which of the following changes in the client's vital signs?

1 Blood pressure 85/50, pulse 60, respirations 26
2 Blood pressure 98/60, pulse 80, respirations 24
3 Blood pressure 130/70, pulse 104, respirations 20
4 Blood pressure 110/40, pulse 110, respirations 20

Answer: 2

Rationale: The main function of digoxin is inotropic. The increased myocardial contractility is associated with increased cardiac output, causing a rise in blood pressure in a client with CHF. Digoxin has a negative chronotropic effect (decreases heart rate) and will therefore cause a slowing of heart rate. As cardiac output improves, there should be an improvement in respiration as well.

Test-Taking Strategy: This question requires knowledge of the action of digoxin. Evaluation questions require that you compare actual outcomes with expected outcomes. Knowing that digoxin slows the heart rate will allow you to eliminate options 3 and 4. Knowing that digoxin improves cardiac output will assist you in eliminating option 1. This leaves option 2 as the correct option. If you had difficulty with this question, take time now to review the therapeutic effects of digoxin (Lanoxin)!

Level of Cognitive Ability: Analysis
Phase of Nursing Process: Evaluation
Client Needs: Physiological Integrity
Content Area: Pharmacology

Reference

Hodgson, B., & Kizior, R. (1998). *Saunders nursing drug handbook 1998.* Philadelphia: W. B. Saunders, pp. 324–326.

---

20. A client with a partial right adrenalectomy is placed on corticosteroid replacement therapy. Which of the following signs/symptoms would indicate that the client is experiencing an adverse effect related to the pharmacological treatment?

1 Hypoglycemia
2 Hypotension
3 Dry mouth
4 Tarry stools

Answer: 4

Rationale: Glucocorticoids increase gastric secretion, and this can result in peptic ulcers and gastrointestinal bleeding. Corticosteroids increase blood glucose levels. Hypotension and a dry mouth are not side effects of corticosteroid therapy.

Test-Taking Strategy: Knowledge regarding the adverse effects associated with corticosteroid therapy is necessary to answer this question. Take time to review the adverse effects associated with corticosteroids now if you had difficulty with this question. You are likely to see a question related to corticosteroids on NCLEX-RN!

Level of Cognitive Ability: Analysis
Phase of Nursing Process: Evaluation
Client Needs: Physiological Integrity
Content Area: Pharmacology

Reference

Pinnell, N. (1996). *Nursing pharmacology.* Philadelphia: W. B. Saunders, pp. 564–565.

---

21. The client with valvular heart disease develops congestive heart failure (CHF). Which of the following assessments most accurately evaluates the onset of CHF?

1 Heart rate
2 Blood pressure
3 Breath sounds
4 Activity tolerance

Answer: 3

Rationale: Breath sounds are the best way to evaluate the onset of CHF. The presence of crackles or rales or an increase in crackles is an indicator of fluid in the lungs caused by CHF. Options 1, 2, and 4, although components of the assessment, are less reliable indicators.

Test-Taking Strategy: Understanding that the best indicator of CHF available to the nurse is listening to the lungs provides the key to this question. The word "congestive" should direct you to the correct option. If you had difficulty with this question, take time now to review assessment of CHF!

Level of Cognitive Ability: Analysis
Phase of Nursing Process: Evaluation
Client Needs: Physiological Integrity
Content Area: Adult Health/Cardiovascular

Reference
Black, J., & Matassarin-Jacobs, E. (1997). *Medical-surgical nursing: Clinical management for continuity of care* (5th ed.). Philadelphia: W. B. Saunders, p. 1349.

---

22. To protect the newborn from hypothermia during a bath, the nurse exposes only the body part being washed. Which of the following signs would indicate hypothermia?

1. Pallor or mottling, flexed position, increased activity
2. Pallor or mottling, decreased activity, open position
3. Poor eating, decreased activity, sleepiness
4. Cool hands and feet, acrocyanosis, flexed position

Answer: 1

Rationale: Signs of cold stress include drop in skin temperature; increased activity; poor eating; pallor or mottling; cool skin, hands, and feet; and a flexed position. The newborn attempts to maintain temperature by vasoconstriction, increasing muscle activity, metabolizing brown fat, and increasing metabolism. A flexed position decreases body surface through which heat can be lost. Cooling leads to peripheral vasoconstriction and to pallor and mottling.

Test-Taking Strategy: Use the process of elimination. Option 2 is incorrect; the open posture would increase heat loss. Option 3 is incorrect because of the decreased activity. Option 4 is incorrect because acrocyanosis is a normal finding in a newborn that results from decreased peripheral blood flow. Review the principles related to hypothermia in a newborn now if you had difficulty with this question!

Level of Cognitive Ability: Analysis
Phase of Nursing Process: Evaluation
Client Needs: Physiological Integrity
Content Area: Maternity

Reference
Nichols, F., & Zwelling, E. (1997). *Maternal-newborn nursing: Theory and practice.* Philadelphia: W. B. Saunders, pp. 1072–1073.

---

23. A client is being discharged after treatment for left-sided heart failure. The nurse is teaching the client the purpose, actions, adverse effects, and use of digoxin (Lanoxin), 0.25 mg daily, and hydrochlorothiazide (HydroDIURIL), 50 mg daily. Which statement, if made by the client, indicates that further discharge teaching is needed?

1. "I should decrease my intake of foods high in potassium, such as bananas."
2. "I should take my radial pulse before taking these medications."
3. "These medications will cause an increase in urine output."
4. "These medications should be taken at the same time in the morning rather than in the evening."

Answer: 1

Rationale: The diet should be high in potassium. Clients taking digitalis have an increased risk of digitalis toxicity from the potassium-depleting effect of hydrochlorothiazide. The client should take his or her pulse before taking cardiac glycosides. For the best therapeutic effects, these medications should be taken at the same time in the morning. A combined therapeutic effect of these medications is to increase urine output. The increased blood flow to the kidneys from enhanced cardiac contractility from the digitalis will promote urinary output. Hydrochlorothiazide increases urine excretion of sodium and water by inhibiting sodium reabsorption in the nephron.

Test-Taking Strategy: The question asks for the client's statement that indicates the need for further teaching, Look for the response with inaccurate information. Knowledge of the actions of these medications will assist in eliminating the incorrect options. If you had difficulty with this question, take time now to review these medications!

Level of Cognitive Ability: Analysis
Phase of Nursing Process: Evaluation
Client Needs: Health Promotion and Maintenance
Content Area: Pharmacology

Reference
Black, J., & Matassarin-Jacobs, E. (1997). *Medical-surgical nursing: Clinical management for continuity of care* (5th ed.). Philadelphia: W. B. Saunders, p. 1284.

24. The nurse is performing discharge teaching with a client with multiple myeloma. Which of the following activities will the nurse encourage to prevent the risk of pathological fractures associated with the disease?

1. Use of splints on extremities
2. Daily regimen of ambulation
3. Daily vital sign measurement
4. Aerobic exercise three times weekly

Answer: 2

Rationale: Hypercalcemia is a phenomenon associated with multiple myeloma. Because of hypercalcemia, pathological fractures are possible. Ambulation is important because bed rest only increases the likelihood of hypercalcemia. Most clients with multiple myeloma will not tolerate aerobic exercise because of anemia. Splints on the extremities will not prevent pathological fractures to other body areas such as the vertebrae. Vital signs are unrelated to the issue of the question.

Test-Taking Strategy: Use the process of elimination, the principles of hypercalcemia, and the pathophysiology associated with multiple myeloma to answer the question. Identifying the issue of the question will assist in eliminating options 3 and 4. Of the remaining options, option 2 is the one most likely to prevent pathological fractures. If you had difficulty with this question, take time now to review the nursing care associated with the prevention of pathological fractures in a client with multiple myeloma!

Level of Cognitive Ability: Application
Phase of Nursing Process: Evaluation
Client Needs: Health Promotion and Maintenance
Content Area: Adult Health/Oncology

Reference

Smeltzer, S., & Bare, B. (1996). *Brunner and Suddarth's Textbook of medical-surgical nursing* (8th ed.). Philadelphia: Lippincott-Raven, p. 798.

---

25. Which of the following nursing diagnoses is most appropriate for a client with newly diagnosed testicular cancer?

1. High Risk for Infection related to surgical incision
2. Alteration in Skin Integrity related to radiation
3. Ineffective Coping related to poor support systems
4. Body Image Disturbance related to diagnosis of cancer

Answer: 4

Rationale: Even if testicular cancer is detected in an early stage, the young adult may be afraid that he will be sexually handicapped, and feelings of sexual inadequacy may occur. An appropriate nursing diagnosis would be Body Image Disturbance. Altered Role Performance is an additional appropriate nursing diagnosis.

Test-Taking Strategy: Use the process of elimination. Do not read into the question. The question does not mention support systems, so eliminate option 3. The question states "newly diagnosed," so eliminate options 1 and 2 because treatment has not begun yet.

Level of Cognitive Ability: Analysis
Phase of Nursing Process: Evaluation
Client Needs: Psychosocial Integrity
Content Area: Adult Health/Oncology

Reference

Ignatavicius, D. D., Workman, M. L., & Mishler, M. A. (1995). *Medical-surgical nursing: A nursing process approach* (2nd ed.). Philadelphia: W. B. Saunders, pp. 1069–1070.

---

26. The nurse obtains a reading of 6 mm induration from a Mantoux tuberculin skin test in an HIV-positive client. The nurse would evaluate this finding as indicating the client

1. Definitely has active tuberculosis.
2. May have tuberculosis.
3. Is indeed HIV-positive.
4. Does not have active tuberculosis.

Answer: 2

Rationale: Purified protein derivative (PPD) of tuberculin is used primarily to detect the delayed hypersensitivity response. Once acquired, sensitivity to tuberculin tends to persist throughout life. A positive reaction indicates the presence of a tuberculosis infection, but it does not show whether the infection is dormant or active (causing a clinical illness). Because the response to tuberculosis skin testing may be decreased in the immunosuppressed client, an induration of 5 mm or greater may be considered positive.

Test-Taking Strategy: This question asks for evaluation of the assessment data. Note that the client is HIV-positive and has a 6-mm induration reaction to the Mantoux tuberculin skin test. Draw upon the knowledge that the immune system is compromised in the HIV-positive person and that the full expected 10-mm induration reaction may not occur in this client. Note the word "definitely" in option 1 and "does not" in option 4. Use of these words will more than likely make an option incorrect. Eliminate option 3 because the tuberculin test is not related to diagnosis in an HIV-positive client.

Level of Cognitive Ability: Analysis
Phase of Nursing Process: Evaluation
Client Needs: Physiological Integrity
Content Area: Adult Health/Respiratory

Reference

Lewis, S., Collier, I., & Heitkemper, M. (1996). *Medical-surgical nursing: Assessment and management of clinical problems* (4th ed.). St. Louis: Mosby–Year Book, pp. 583, 638.

---

27. The home health nurse visits a 4-day-old full-term small-for-gestational-age (SGA) infant at home. The nurse observes that the infant is jaundiced and dehydrated. Which of the following statements, if made by the infant's mother, indicates that she understood the discharge teaching for the infant?

1 "My baby is so good. She is already sleeping through the night."
2 "My baby looks so yellow. I am going to call the doctor."
3 "My baby has been drinking one-half ounce of formula every 6 hours."
4 "My baby is wetting her diaper about three times per day."

Answer: 2

Rationale: Jaundice is a complication of the full-term SGA infant that results from increased hematocrit. Jaundice in the 4-day-old infant should be reported to the physician, as a bilirubin level may need to be measured. Four-day-old SGA infants should be fed at least every 3 hours because they require more calories per kilogram as a result of increased metabolical activity and oxygen consumption. The newborn should be fed with small feedings of high-calorie formula or breast milk because of decreased stomach capacity. Feedings should be done even through the night. Newborns usually wet at least 6 to 8 diapers per day; urine output less than this amount indicates dehydration.

Test-Taking Strategy: Knowledge of discharge teaching is necessary to answer this question. Use the process of elimination to answer the question. Read each option carefully, noting the time frames specified in the options. If you had difficulty with this question, take time now to review the appropriate discharge instructions for an infant with SGA!

Level of Cognitive Ability: Analysis
Phase of Nursing Process: Evaluation
Client Needs: Health Promotion and Maintenance
Content Area: Child Health

Reference

Olds, S., London, M., & Ladewig, P. (1996). *Maternal-newborn nursing: A family-centered approach* (5th ed.). Menlo Park, CA: Addison-Wesley, p. 927.

---

28. A registered nurse is mentoring a new nurse hired to work in the nursing unit. The registered nurse evaluates that the new nurse is competent in providing care to a client on a ventilator, when the registered nurse notes that the new nurse

1 Has the ventilator routinely assessed by the respiratory therapist.
2 Realizes the ventilator readings provide information without human error.
3 Teaches family members how to reset controls during their visits if necessary.
4 Establishes a rest pattern before morning care.

Answer: 1

Rationale: Ventilators need to be routinely assessed by the respiratory specialist. Ventilators are machines, and machines can fail; therefore option 2 is not a reasonable option. Family members should not reset ventilator controls. Although option 4 is considered good nursing practice for the comfort of client, it is not the priority option.

Test-Taking Strategy: Note the key word "competent." Use the ABCs to answer the question. Option 1 is the only option that addresses the airway. If you had difficulty with this question, take time now to review nursing care to a client on a ventilator!

Level of Cognitive Ability: Analysis
Phase of Nursing Process: Evaluation
Client Needs: Safe, Effective Care Environment
Content Area: Adult Health/Respiratory

Reference

Potter, P., & Perry, A. (1997). *Fundamentals of nursing: Concepts, process, and practice* (4th ed.). St. Louis: Mosby–Year Book, p. 303.

29. The community health nurse visits a diabetic client at home. The client has cut the blood glucose monitoring strips in half lengthwise to save money. After evaluation of this client action, the most appropriate statement by the nurse would be

1 "What a great idea, I'll tell all my clients about this."
2 "You must find the money for your supplies or you'll end up in the hospital."
3 "Why did you do this?"
4 "You need to be careful doing this. A lot of times the blood glucose value is underestimated with such a small area to read."

Answer: 4

Rationale: Visual interpretation of blood glucose monitoring strips by clients can be difficult because of decreased visual acuity levels. Tearing the strips in half may affect the accuracy in reading. Option 1 is inappropriate, according to this rationale. Option 2 places a demand on the client. Asking a client "Why" needs to be avoided because it requires an explanation from the client and may cause the client to become defensive.

Test-Taking Strategy: Use the process of elimination. Option 1 is an inappropriate nursing response. Options 2 and 3 are blocks to communication. If you had difficulty with this question, take time now to review therapeutic communication techniques!

Level of Cognitive Ability: Application
Phase of Nursing Process: Evaluation
Client Needs: Health Promotion and Maintenance
Content Area: Adult Health/Endocrine

Reference

Lammon, C. B., Foote, A. W., Leli, P. G., et al. (1995). *Clinical nursing skills.* Philadelphia: W. B. Saunders, pp. 177–178.

30. A client describes a rash that is red, raised, and itchy. The client used an over-the-counter hydrocortisone cream for 1 week, and the rash seems to be worse. After evaluation of the situation, which of the following statements, if made by the nurse, would be most appropriate at this time?

1 "Give the hydrocortisone another week."
2 "You should call your primary care provider for an appointment and have that looked at."
3 "Ask your pharmacist what to use."
4 "Take diphenhydramine hydrochloride (Benadryl), because you must be allergic to the cream."

Answer: 2

Rationale: Hydrocortisone is the topical treatment of choice for cutaneous inflammation and pruritus associated with contact dermatitis. If the rash hasn't responded to this over-the-counter medication, it needs to be evaluated by a health care provider.

Test-Taking Strategy: Read the question carefully, noting that the client has been using the hydrocortisone cream for 1 week. This information should direct you to the correct option. If you had difficulty with this question, take time now to review client instruction regarding dermatitis!

Level of Cognitive Ability: Analysis
Phase of Nursing Process: Evaluation
Client Needs: Physiological Integrity
Content Area: Adult Health/Integumentary

Reference

Hodgson, B., & Kizior, R. (1998). *Saunders nursing drug handbook 1998.* Philadelphia: W. B. Saunders, pp. 498–500.

31. The nurse administers medications to the wrong client. During the investigation of the incident, it was determined that the nurse failed to check the client's identification bracelet before administering the medications. The nursing supervisor evaluates the situation and determines that the nurse can be guilty of negligence because

1 Negligence is defined as the failure to meet established standards of care.
2 Negligence is defined as a crime that results in the injury of a client.
3 Negligence is strictly prohibited by the State's Nurse Practice Act.
4 Negligence is strictly prohibited by the institution's own policies.

Answer: 1

Rationale: The legal definition of negligence is the failure to meet accepted standards of care. Option 2 is an incorrect definition of negligence, although injury may have indeed come to the client as a result of negligence. Both the institution and the Nurse Practice Act have provisions that identify and discourage acts of negligence.

Test-Taking Strategy: In order to answer this question correctly, you must know the definition of negligence as applied to the profession of nursing. Options 3 and 4 are true in that the purpose of the Nurse Practice Act and institutional policies and procedures is to protect the public from harm, but they identify and discourage acts of negligence rather than "strictly prohibit" negligence. Of the remaining two responses, option 1 is more global. If you had difficulty with this question, take time now to review the concepts related to negligence!

Level of Cognitive Ability: Analysis
Phase of Nursing Process: Evaluation
Client Needs: Safe, Effective Care Environment
Content Area: Fundamental Skills

Reference

Potter, P., & Perry, A. (1997). *Fundamentals of nursing: Concepts, process, and practice.* (4th ed.). St. Louis: Mosby–Year Book, pp. 335–336.

---

32. The nurse has been working with a morbidly obese man to implement a plan for weight reduction. Which of the following statements, if made by the client, indicates the need for additional teaching?

1 "I wish my mother could have seen me lose the 60 pounds in the last 9 months."
2 "It is so difficult to find food exchanges that taste good and fill me up."
3 "My wife was kidding me the other night about my being a whole new husband."
4 "This diet doesn't let me go to out for lunch with my friends at work anymore."

Answer: 4

Rationale: Both options 1 and 3 are responses indicating a positive perception of self: that another person has recognized these changes, and that the client wishes to have been able to share these changes with his mother. In the absence of any other data, option 2, although apparently a negative response, is likely a normal response to the changes in eating habits. Option 4 indicates either that the client may be having difficulty in making appropriate dietary choices when going out for lunch or that he may perceive his coworkers as being uncomfortable with his need to eat differently. A sense of not fitting in can leave the obese individual isolated and therefore make it more difficult to maintain the diet at work.

Test-Taking Strategy: This question asks you to determine which of the four statements is a negative indicator of potential success. Read each carefully and determine whether it is a positive indicator or a negative one. Eliminate options 1 and 3 first. Option 2 is a common response by persons who have had to make dietary changes. Option 4 clearly states that the client perceives a definite barrier to pursuing his accustomed lifestyle.

Level of Cognitive Ability: Analysis
Phase of Nursing Process: Evaluation
Client Needs: Health Promotion and Maintenance
Content Area: Fundamental Skills

Reference

Barry, P. (1997). *Psychosocial nursing: Care of physically ill patients and their families* (3rd ed.). Philadelphia: Lippincott-Raven, p. 355.

---

33. A community health nurse is evaluating the effectiveness of a class for adolescent girls about fetal alcohol syndrome. Which of the following statements, if made by one student, suggests the need for further teaching?

1 "Fetal alcohol syndrome is a preventable cause of mental retardation."
2 "Symptoms include retarded growth of the baby and abnormalities of the central nervous system."
3 "Diagnosis of fetal alcohol syndrome is based on symptoms manifested by the infant and the mother's history of alcohol use."
4 "Only heavy use of alcohol by the pregnant woman is a problem; moderate alcohol ingestion is acceptable during pregnancy."

Answer: 4

Rationale: Both low amounts and excessive amounts of alcohol ingestion during pregnancy place the fetus at risk. Options 1, 2, and 3 demonstrate a good understanding of fetal alcohol syndrome.

Test-Taking Strategy: This question focuses on analyzing the knowledge of the client with regard to evaluating the nursing intervention of teaching. Remembering that alcohol needs to be avoided during pregnancy will assist in answering the question. If you had difficulty with this question, take time now to review FAS!

Level of Cognitive Ability: Analysis
Phase of Nursing Process: Evaluation
Client Needs: Health Promotion and Maintenance
Content Area: Maternity

Reference

Nichols, F., & Zwelling, E. (1997). *Maternal-newborn nursing: Theory and practice.* Philadelphia: W. B. Saunders, pp. 124–125.

34. The school nurse is evaluating the effectiveness of providing mass influenza virus vaccine to all students and teachers in the school last year. What information would indicate that the expected outcome was achieved?

1. There was a 60% reduction in absences caused by influenza-like symptoms
2. No students or teachers were diagnosed with pneumonia
3. There was a 10% reduction in absences caused by influenza-like symptoms
4. No *Haemophilus influenzae* type B (HIB) infections were reported by students or teachers

Answer: 1

Rationale: The strains of the A and B influenza viruses are reformulated annually to provide the anticipated best protection for 60%–75% of the population during one high-risk season. The 60% figure is in the anticipated range; 10% is not. Option 4 is expected without any vaccine, because this is not a population at high risk for HIB.

Test-Taking Strategy: Don't confuse HIB and influenza vaccine. The strains and the target populations are different. Options 1 and 3 used the word "influenza" as in the stem. When unsure of measurements for expected outcomes, the higher percentage is more effective and therefore is a better choice.

Level of Cognitive Ability: Analysis
Phase of Nursing Process: Evaluation
Client Needs: Health Promotion and Maintenance
Content Area: Adult Health/Respiratory

Reference

Wong, D. (1997). *Whaley and Wong's Essentials of pediatric nursing* (5th ed.). St. Louis: Mosby–Year Book, p. 319.

---

35. The client is being discharged after cesarean section. The nurse would be alerted to the need for more education about postdischarge complications if the client states that she will report

1. Fever over 102°F.
2. Painful urination.
3. Flow heavier than a normal period.
4. Redness at the incision site.

Answer: 1

Rationale: By definition, a postpartum infection is defined as a temperature of greater than 100.4°F or more on 2 successive days, not counting the first 24 hours after birth. Temperatures of this magnitude must be considered a sign of a postpartum infection unless proven otherwise. The client needs to notify the physician under these conditions and not wait until the temperature rises to 102°F.

Test-Taking Strategy: Read the stem of the question carefully. Eliminate options 2, 3, and 4 systematically. These options indicate that the client would correctly be alerted to call the physician. The client should notify the physician before the temperature rises to 102°F.

Level of Cognitive Ability: Analysis
Phase of Nursing Process: Evaluation
Client Needs: Health Promotion and Maintenance
Content Area: Maternity

Reference

Lowdermilk, D., Perry, S., & Bobak, I. (1997). *Maternity and women's health care* (6th ed.). St. Louis: Mosby–Year Book, pp. 750–751.

---

36. The nurse has given the client instructions regarding crutch safety. The nurse evaluates that the client needs reinforcement of information if the client states

1. The need to have spare crutches and tips available.
2. That the crutch tips will not slip even when wet.
3. Not to use someone else's crutches.
4. That crutch tips should be inspected periodically for wear.

Answer: 2

Rationale: Crutch tips should remain dry. Water could cause slipping by decreasing the surface friction of the rubber tip on the floor. If crutch tips get wet, the client should dry them with a cloth or paper towel. The client should use only crutches measured for the client. The tips should be inspected for wear, and spare crutches and tips should be available if needed.

Test-Taking Strategy: The wording of the question directs you to look for a statement that is incorrect. Options 1, 3, and 4 are certainly correct statements and are therefore eliminated. This leaves option 2 as the correct answer. Crutch tips can slip when they get wet, posing a possible threat to the unsuspecting client.

Level of Cognitive Ability: Analysis
Phase of Nursing Process: Evaluation
Client Needs: Health Promotion and Maintenance
Content Area: Adult Health/Musculoskeletal

Reference

Potter, P., & Perry, A. (1997). *Fundamentals of nursing: Concepts, process, and practice* (4th ed.). St. Louis: Mosby–Year Book, p. 936.

---

37. The client with AIDS has been receiving amphotericin B for a fungal respiratory infection. Which of the following would the nurse evaluate as indicating an adverse reaction?

1 Hypocalcemia
2 Hypokalemia
3 Hypercalcemia
4 Hyperkalemia

Answer: 2

Rationale: Clients receiving amphotericin B may develop hypokalemia, which can be severe and lead to extreme muscle weakness and electrocardiogram (ECG) changes. Distal renal tubular acidosis commonly occurs, contributing to the development of hypokalemia. High potassium levels do not occur. The medication does not cause calcium levels to fluctuate.

Test-Taking Strategy: Knowledge that an adverse reaction to amphotericin B is hypokalemia is necessary to answer the question. Review this medication now if you had difficulty with this question!

Level of Cognitive Ability: Analysis
Phase of Nursing Process: Evaluation
Client Needs: Physiological Integrity
Content Area: Pharmacology

Reference

Baer, C., & Williams, B. (1996). *Clinical pharmacology and nursing* (3rd ed.). Springhouse, PA: Springhouse, p. 1082.

---

38. The community health nurse visits a diabetic client at home. The nurse consults with the physician, who mentions considering ordering valproic acid (Depakene) to treat the client's absence epilepsy. Which of the following statements, if made by the nurse, would indicate knowledge of the medication?

1 "I will teach the client to take daily weights each morning to monitor for edema."
2 "I will need to have an order for the client to take insulin for 4 weeks until the medicine reaches its therapeutic level."
3 "I will teach the client to monitor the urine for glucose three times a day to observe for increased glycosuria."
4 "I will teach the client to monitor blood glucose because this drug alters the urine ketone and gives false-positive results."

Answer: 4

Rationale: Clients who are placed on valproic acid are instructed that this medication may alter urine tests for ketones by providing a false-positive result. Options 1, 2, and 3 are statements unrelated to this medication.

Test-Taking Strategy: This question is straightforward and depends on your knowledge of the specific interactions caused by valproic acid. Remembering that it specifically affects ketones will assist in answering the question. If you had difficulty with the question, take time now to review this medication!

Level of Cognitive Ability: Application
Phase of Nursing Process: Evaluation
Client Needs: Health Promotion and Maintenance
Content Area: Pharmacology

Reference

Clark, J., Queener, S., & Karb, V. (1997). *Pharmacologic basis of nursing practice* (5th ed.). St. Louis: Mosby–Year Book, pp. 693–695.

39. Which client statement indicates that the nurse's teaching, to a human immunodeficiency virus (HIV)–infected pregnant client, about the prevention of an opportunistic infection has been successful?

1. "My husband is taking care of the cat's litter box."
2. "I plan to have a natural childbirth experience."
3. "I know I must have a cesarean section to avoid infecting my baby."
4. "I am trying to lead a normal life. Tomorrow I will go to my niece's sixth birthday party."

Answer: 1

Rationale: Clients should be taught proper handwashing techniques, to avoid persons who are ill, not to care for fish tanks or litter, and to avoid undercooked meat, raw eggs, and unpasteurized dairy products. An HIV-infected mother may have a normal, spontaneous vaginal delivery; however, this is not related to methods of preventing infection. It is critical to limit trauma during delivery to avoid the risk of HIV transmission to the neonate. Attending a party with a number of preschool children may increase exposure to colds and opportunistic infections.

Test-Taking Strategy: Read the stem of the question carefully. Option 2 is unrelated to infection. Option 3 will increase the risk of transmission of HIV to the neonate. Option 4 exposes the client to the risk of infection. If you had difficulty with this question, take time to now to review content related to the development of opportunistic infections!

Level of Cognitive Ability: Analysis
Phase of Nursing Process: Evaluation
Client Needs: Health Promotion and Maintenance
Content Area: Maternity

Reference

Nichols, F., & Zwelling, E. (1997). *Maternal-newborn nursing: Theory and practice.* Philadelphia: W. B. Saunders, p. 1500.

---

40. A client is being discharged after recovery from an acute anterior myocardial infarction with recurrent angina. The nurse is teaching the client the purpose, actions, adverse effects, and use of the following medications: diltiazem (Cardizem SR), 90 mg orally two times daily; isosorbide dinitrate (Isordil), 10 mg orally three times daily; and nitroglycerin (Nitrostat), 0.4 mg sublingually as needed. Which statement, if made by the client, indicates that further discharge teaching is needed?

1. "I should notify my doctor if I experience headaches with any of these medications."
2. "All three of these medications will increase blood flow to my heart."
3. "All three of these medications will help to decrease the intensity of my chest pain."
4. "I will store these medications in a cool place, away from light."

Answer: 1

Rationale: Because of the vasodilating effects of nitrates, headache is a common side effect. Medical attention is not needed unless the headaches increase in severity or frequency. All three medications are nitrates, which improve myocardial circulation by dilating coronary arteries and collateral vessels, thus increasing blood flow to the heart. These medications are used to help prevent the frequency, intensity, and duration of anginal attacks. Nitrates should be stored in a cool place and in dark containers; heat and light cause these medications to break down and lose their potency.

Test-Taking Strategy: Knowledge of nitrate medications is necessary to assist you in answering this question. Be careful with questions that ask you to select the response that indicates that the client needs further teaching. Look for the response that is an inaccurate statement, because this would reflect the need for further teaching. If you had difficulty with this question, take time to review these important cardiac medications!

Level of Cognitive Ability: Analysis
Phase of Nursing Process: Evaluation
Client Needs: Health Promotion and Maintenance
Content Area: Pharmacology

Reference

Black, J., & Matassarin-Jacobs, E. (1997). *Medical-surgical nursing: Clinical management for continuity of care* (5th ed.). Philadelphia: W. B. Saunders, p. 1254.

41. The nurse instructs a client with mild preeclampsia on home care. The nurse evaluates that the teaching has been effective concerning assessment of complications when the client states

1 "As long as the health nurse is visiting me daily, I do not have to keep my next physician's appointment."
2 "I need to take my blood pressure each morning and alternate arms each time."
3 "I need to check my weight every day at different times during the day."
4 "I need to check my urine with a dipstick every day for protein and call the physician if it is 2+ or more."

Answer: 4

Rationale: It is still important to keep physician appointments to assess for any other physical changes in the mother or baby. Blood pressure measurements need to be taken in the same arm, in a sitting position, every day in order to obtain a consistent and accurate reading. The weight needs to be checked at the same time each day, with the client wearing the same clothes, before breakfast and after voiding in order to obtain reliable weights. Option 4 is a true statement as written.

Test-Taking Strategy: All of the options are procedures that the client must perform at home. You must then look at the correctness of each procedure. Knowledge of the principles related to blood pressure measurement and weight will assist in eliminating options 2 and 3. Remembering that follow-up care is necessary will assist in eliminating option 1.

Level of Cognitive Ability: Analysis
Phase of Nursing Process: Evaluation
Client Needs: Health Promotion and Maintenance
Content Area: Maternity

Reference
Lowdermilk, D., Perry, S., & Bobak, I. (1997). *Maternity and women's health care* (6th ed.). St. Louis: Mosby–Year Book, p. 710.

42. The client undergoing peritoneal dialysis who is also diabetic has had insulin added to the dialysate before instillation. The nurse would evaluate that the dose is optimal if the client has a random blood glucose level of

1 75 mg/dL.
2 115 mg/dL.
3 140 mg/dL.
4 200 mg/dL.

Answer: 2

Rationale: The normal random blood glucose level is 70–115 mg/dL but may vary, depending on the time of the last meal. In the diabetic client, the glucose level is usually elevated. Options 3 and 4 are incorrect because they exceed the normal range. Option 2 is better than option 1 because it does not put the client at the lower end of the normal range, at which point hypoglycemia could more easily result.

Test-Taking Strategy: Note that the key word "optimal" in the stem. This implies that more than one of the options may be partially or totally correct. You may eliminate options 3 and 4 first by knowing that these values are elevated. You would choose correctly between the two remaining options by knowing that the client who is insulin dependent can also experience hypoglycemia, which makes option 1 less than "optimal."

Level of Cognitive Ability: Analysis
Phase of Nursing Process: Evaluation
Client Needs: Physiological Integrity
Content Area: Adult Health/Endocrine

Reference
Black, J., & Matassarin-Jacobs, E. (1997). *Medical-surgical nursing: Clinical management for continuity of care* (5th ed.). Philadelphia: W. B. Saunders, p. 1650.

43. The client had thoracic surgery earlier in the week and has had chest tubes removed in preparation for discharge. The nurse evaluates that the client needs further instruction in acceptable discharge instructions if the client states that he or she will

1 Avoid heavy lifting for the first 4–6 weeks.
2 Monitor temperature as an indication of possible infection.
3 Remove the chest tube site dressing as soon as the client gets home.
4 Report signs of respiratory difficulty to the physician.

Answer: 3

Rationale: Upon removal of a chest tube, an occlusive dressing consisting of petrolatum gauze covered by a dry sterile dressing (DSD) is placed over the chest tube site dressing. This is maintained in place until the physician states that it may be removed. Monitoring and reporting respiratory difficulty and increased temperature are appropriate client activities upon discharge. The client should avoid heavy lifting for the first 4–6 weeks after discharge to facilitate continued wound healing.

Test-Taking Strategy: The wording of the question guides you to seek an incorrect statement on the part of the client. Knowing that signs of infection and respiratory difficulty should be monitored and reported helps you eliminate options 2 and 4 first. You would choose option 3 over option 1 as the answer because avoiding heavy lifting is also a routine instruction after surgery, whereas removal of the dressing disturbs the occlusive seal provided over the chest tube insertion site.

Level of Cognitive Ability: Analysis
Phase of Nursing Process: Evaluation
Client Needs: Health Promotion and Maintenance
Content Area: Adult Health/Respiratory

Reference

Black, J., & Matassarin-Jacobs, E. (1997). *Medical-surgical nursing: Clinical management for continuity of care* (5th ed.). Philadelphia: W. B. Saunders, p. 1162.

44. Which of the following statements, if made by a client with Parkinson's disease who is taking L-dopa, indicates the need for further instruction?

1 "I will take the medication just before meals to avoid nausea."
2 "I will eat lots of foods high in vitamin B_6."
3 "I will get up slowly to prevent dizziness."
4 "I may need to take this medication for the rest of my life."

Answer: 2

Rationale: Foods high in vitamin B_6 can counteract the effects of L-dopa. Options 1, 3, and 4 are accurate statements regarding this medication.

Test-Taking Strategy: This is a false response stem, which requires you to select an answer that is not true. If you had difficulty with this question, take time now to review this medication!

Level of Cognitive Ability: Analysis
Phase of Nursing Process: Evaluation
Client Needs: Health Promotion and Maintenance
Content Area: Pharmacology

Reference

Deglin, J. H., & Vallerand, A. H. (1997). *Davis's drug guide for nurses* (5th ed.). Philadelphia: F. A. Davis, pp. 692–694.

45. The client has received teaching about postoperative care after a parathyroidectomy. Which of the following actions, if performed by the client, would indicate to the nurse that the client understood the instructions?

1 The client places hands at the back of the head when moving the neck
2 The client speaks frequently to exercise the vocal cords
3 The client splints chest when deep breathing and coughing
4 The client drinks nothing by mouth (NPO) for 24–48 hours

Answer: 1

Rationale: The weight of the client's head must be supported when the client flexes the neck or moves the head. This decreases the stress on the suture line, which prevents bleeding. Options 2 and 4 are inaccurate information and actually could be harmful to the client. Option 3 is really not necessary because the incision is on the neck, not the chest.

Test-Taking Strategy: In order to answer this question, you must have knowledge of what is necessary for the client to know after a parathyroidectomy. Eliminate options 2 and 3 by considering the anatomical location of the parathyroids. Eliminate option 4 because NPO status is indicated preoperatively. Review postoperative care after a parathyroidectomy if you had difficulty with this question!

Level of Cognitive Ability: Analysis
Phase of Nursing Process: Evaluation
Client Needs: Health Promotion and Maintenance
Content Area: Adult Health/Endocrine

Reference

Luckmann, J. (1997). *Saunders manual of nursing care.* Philadelphia: W. B. Saunders, p. 1043.

---

46. The client recovering from acute renal failure (ARF) has been given dietary instructions that include restriction of potassium in the diet. The nurse evaluates that the client understands the information if the client indicates that meal preparation should include

1 Using salt substitutes instead of salt.
2 Boiling vegetables and discarding the water.
3 Increased servings of bananas and oranges.
4 At least 10 oz of meats per day.

Answer: 2

Rationale: The potassium content of vegetables can be decreased by boiling the vegetables and discarding the water. Bananas and oranges are high in potassium and should be avoided. Meats should be limited to 6 oz. per day. Salt substitutes are often high in potassium and are also avoided.

Test-Taking Strategy: Specific knowledge of dietary items high in potassium helps you to eliminate options 1 and 3. Option 4 is unrelated to potassium but contains an amount of protein that is too high for this client, and so that option may also be eliminated. This leaves option 2 as the correct answer. Boiling vegetables does decrease the potassium content, especially when the fluid is then discarded. Review foods high in potassium now if you had difficulty with this question!

Level of Cognitive Ability: Analysis
Phase of Nursing Process: Evaluation
Client Needs: Health Promotion and Maintenance
Content Area: Adult Health/Renal

Reference

Lutz, C., & Przytulski, K. (1997). *Nutrition and diet therapy* (2nd ed.). Philadelphia: F. A. Davis, pp. 390–391.

---

47. The client has refractory myasthenia gravis and undergoes plasmapheresis therapy. The nurse would evaluate that the client obtained the intended effects of therapy if the client demonstrates improvement in

1 Vital capacity.
2 Leg strength.
3 Ptosis.
4 Diplopia.

Answer: 1

Rationale: Plasmapheresis is a process which separates the plasma from the blood elements, so that plasma proteins that contain antibodies can be removed. It is used as an adjunct therapy in myasthenia gravis and may give temporary relief to clients with actual or impending respiratory failure. Usually three to five treatments are required.

Test-Taking Strategy: Begin to answer this question by looking at the severity of the symptoms. Options 3 and 4 are similar and probably not as potentially distressing as options 1 and 2. Of the two remaining choices, respiratory problems would be a more acute problem for the client than would decreased leg strength. Thus, this is the answer to the question as it addresses respiratory capacity. Review the purpose of plasmapheresis now if you had difficulty with this question!

Level of Cognitive Ability: Analysis
Phase of Nursing Process: Evaluation
Client Needs: Physiological Integrity
Content Area: Adult Health/Neurological

Reference

Black, J., & Matassarin-Jacobs, E. (1997). *Medical-surgical nursing: Clinical management for continuity of care* (5th ed.). Philadelphia: W. B. Saunders, p. 885.

48. The client with adult respiratory distress syndrome (ARDS) being mechanically ventilated has received a dose of vecuronium (Norcuron). The nurse would evaluate that the medication had the intended effect if the client

1. Fell asleep.
2. Gave weak but equal hand grasps on command.
3. Stopped fighting (bucking) the ventilator.
4. Produced thinner respiratory secretions.

Answer: 3

Rationale: The client with ARDS often requires mechanical ventilation to manage the respiratory status. The client may develop tachypnea or restlessness or may begin to fight (buck) the ventilator. Intravenous sedation is usually tried first, and if unsuccessful, a neuromuscular blocking agent such as vecuronium may be given to paralyze the client.

Test-Taking Strategy: To answer this question accurately, it is necessary to know that this medication has a paralyzing effect on the muscles and prevents any type of client movement. Knowing this you would first eliminate option 2. Options 1 and 4 would be eliminated next because the medication does not have either a sedative or mucolytic effect.

Level of Cognitive Ability: Analysis
Phase of Nursing Process: Evaluation
Client Needs: Physiological Integrity
Content Area: Adult Health/Respiratory

References

Black, J., & Matassarin-Jacobs, E. (1997). *Medical-surgical nursing: Clinical management for continuity of care* (5th ed.). Philadelphia: W. B. Saunders, p. 1172.

Deglin, J. H., & Vallerand, A. H. (1997). *Davis's drug guide for nurses* (5th ed.). Philadelphia: F. A. Davis, p. 852.

---

49. The nurse has conducted discharge teaching with the client with chronic airflow limitation (CAL) about energy conservation techniques. The nurse evaluates that the client needs further instruction if the client says that he or she will

1. Sit for as many activities as possible.
2. Hold the breath while performing activities.
3. Keep objects near or below shoulder level.
4. Rest in between activities during the day.

Answer: 2

Rationale: The client with CAL should use energy conservation techniques to conserve oxygen. These include sitting to perform many household chores or activities and alternating activity with rest periods. The client should avoid raising the arms above the head because use of the arms could increase dyspnea. The client should never hold the breath during an activity.

Test-Taking Strategy: The wording of the question guides you to look for a response that is an incorrect item. Options 1 and 4 are obviously correct and are eliminated as possible answers to this question. Keeping objects below shoulder level will help conserve energy because the client will not have to reach overhead, which is taxing. Holding the breath is not helpful for energy conservation and could make the client become short of breath. Thus you would choose option 2 over option 3 as the answer to the question as it is stated.

Level of Cognitive Ability: Analysis
Phase of Nursing Process: Evaluation
Client Needs: Health Promotion and Maintenance
Content Area: Adult Health/Respiratory

Reference

Ignatavicius, D. D., Workman, M. L., & Mishler, M. A. (1995). *Medical-surgical nursing: A nursing process approach* (2nd ed.). Philadelphia: W. B. Saunders, p. 688.

50. A diabetic mother delivered her infant an hour ago. The nurse interprets that which of the following statements of the parents indicates a lack of understanding of the needs of their infant?

1. "I don't think the baby needs to eat right now. It's only an hour old and is very sleepy."
2. "I need to keep the baby's temperature just right, so that it will not use up any extra glucose, causing hypoglycemia."
3. "The baby is jittery. I need to feed the baby right away."
4. "My baby is having some problems breathing. My diabetes must have caused a delay in lung maturity."

Answer: 1

Rationale: Parents need to be taught to feed their newborn early, and often, as a prophylactic measure to decrease the possibility of hypoglycemia. These newborns may become hypoglycemic within 15 minutes of delivery as exhibited by lethargy and poor feeding in the first hour after delivery. Hypoglycemia is a result of hyperinsulinism and loss of maternal glucose. Cold stress increases the metabolism of glucose. Jitteriness is one of the classical symptoms of hypoglycemia. A risk faced by a newborn of a diabetic mother is immature lungs.

Test-Taking Strategy: Use the process of elimination considering the issue of the question: a newborn of a diabetic mother. If you had difficulty with this question, take time now to review concepts related to diabetes in pregnancy and its effect on the newborn!

Level of Cognitive Ability: Analysis
Phase of Nursing Process: Evaluation
Client Needs: Physiological Integrity
Content Area: Maternity

Reference

Nichols, F. H., & Zwelling, E. (1997). *Maternal-newborn nursing: Theory and practice.* Philadelphia: W. B. Saunders, pp. 1357–1359.

51. The nurse is caring for a client in pelvic traction. Which of the following physician's orders would the nurse evaluate as requiring clarification?

1. "Apply girdle snugly over the client's pelvis and iliac crest."
2. "Raise the head of the bed 30 degrees."
3. "Observe for pressure points over the iliac crest."
4. "Keep the client in good alignment."

Answer: 2

Rationale: The foot end of the bed is raised to prevent the client from being pulled down in bed by the traction. The head of the bed is usually kept flat. The girdle should be applied snugly so it does not slip off of the client, and therefore skin should be checked for pressure sores.

Test-Taking Strategy: Use the process of elimination. Options 3 and 4 are basic fundamental principles. Pelvic traction is accomplished by applying a belt just above and encircling the iliac crest. Visualizing the procedure in your mind will assist in directing you to the correct option for this question. If you had difficulty with this question, take time now to review the procedure for pelvic traction!

Level of Cognitive Ability: Analysis
Phase of Nursing Process: Evaluation
Client Needs: Physiological Integrity
Content Area: Adult Health/Musculoskeletal

Reference

Black, J., & Matassarin-Jacobs, E. (1997). *Medical-surgical nursing: Clinical management for continuity of care* (5th ed.). Philadelphia, W. B. Saunders, p. 2139.

52. Which of the following statements by the client indicates adequate understanding of the antidepressant fluoxetine (Prozac)?

1. "I know that there are no side effects with this medication."
2. "The sexual dysfunction should be a passing symptom."
3. "I have been on this medication for 3 days and already feel cured."
4. "I know that it will take some time before I feel normal again."

Answer: 4

Rationale: Prozac tends to improve energy level of clients, and if it is taken late in the day, insomnia may occur. Many clients suffer from sexual dysfunction throughout treatment, such as anorgasmia or decreased libido. Side effects can be expected to some degree with any medication. The lag time between when the medication is started to when therapeutic effects are achieved is 2–4 weeks or longer. This is true with any antidepressant.

Test-Taking Strategy: Look for the inaccurate statements that you can easily identify. Remember that sexual dysfunction is a common side effect of most antidepressants. The word "cure" is an indicator that option 3 is incorrect. Remembering that the lag time between when the medication is started and when therapeutic effects are achieved is

2–4 weeks or longer with any antidepressant will assist in directing you to the correct option!

Level of Cognitive Ability: Analysis
Phase of Nursing Process: Evaluation
Client Needs: Health Promotion and Maintenance
Content Area: Pharmacology

Reference

Wilson, B., Shannon, M., & Stang, C. (1996). *Nurse's drug guide.* Stamford, CT: Appleton & Lange, pp. 589–591.

---

53. The community health nurse visits the client at home 4 days after a cast has been applied. Which of the following statements, if made by the client, would indicate a need for further instruction?

1 "I am to look for any musty, unpleasant odor coming from the cast or at the end of the cast."
2 "I am to inspect the cast for any drainage through the cast or cast opening."
3 "I am to keep my cast away from any hard surfaces or counters."
4 "I am to check for any hot spots on the cast."

Answer: 3

Rationale: Option 3 would indicate the need for further instruction. This is to be done only when the cast is drying. Synthetic casts take approximately 20 minutes to set completely. Plaster casts set rapidly but may take several hours to dry completely. Options 1, 2, and 4 are all potential signs of tissue necrosis and infection for which the client should be observing.

Test-Taking Strategy: Knowledge regarding the signs of infection will assist you in answering this question correctly. Options 1, 2, and 4 can be eliminated because they are correct findings of infection. Option 3 is an inaccurate statement about cast drying. If you had difficulty with this question, take time now to review cast care after application!

Level of Cognitive Ability: Application
Phase of Nursing Process: Evaluation
Client Needs: Health Promotion and Maintenance
Content Area: Adult Health/Musculoskeletal

Reference

Black, J., & Matassarin-Jacobs, E. (1997). *Medical-surgical nursing: Clinical management for continuity of care* (5th ed.). Philadelphia: W. B. Saunders, p. 2147.

---

54. The client's priority nursing diagnosis has been Risk for Injury related to High Risk for Suicide. The client has been gradually exhibiting a lifting of mood, has been having no suicidal thoughts for the past 3 days, and is making plans for a return to the vocational school upon discharge from the hospital. The nurse evaluates these findings and documents that this nursing diagnosis

1 Is still a concern to the nursing staff.
2 Requires further assessment.
3 Seems to have been resolved.
4 Suggests need for close monitoring.

Answer: 3

Rationale: Option 3 is the best answer according to the documenting data in the stem. The client's mood is improving, and future goals are being made. The client has not experienced suicidal thoughts recently, so the nurse and the staff can probably safely conclude that the client has passed the danger point. With the documenting data, further assessment does not seem warranted; therefore, option 2 can be eliminated. The documenting data in the stem also do not suggest a need for close supervision at this time.

Test-Taking Strategy: Use the process of elimination. Options 1, 3, and 4 are similar and are basically saying the same thing. If you had difficulty with this question, take time now to review the critical assessment process required in a suicidal client!

Level of Cognitive Ability: Analysis
Phase of Nursing Process: Evaluation
Client Needs: Physiological Integrity
Content Area: Mental Health

Reference

Johnson, B. (1997). *Psychiatric mental health nursing: Adaptation and growth* (4th ed.). Philadelphia: Lippincott-Raven, p. 872.

55. After instructing a mother about measures to take to reduce the incidence of gastroesophageal reflux (GER) in her child, which statement by the mother indicates a need for further teaching?

1. "I give my child small feedings often throughout the day."
2. "I buy bottle nipples that have smaller holes for my child."
3. "I add a small amount of cereal to my child's formula."
4. "I give my child a pacifier and maintain an upright position after meals."

Answer: 2

Rationale: This child's formula will most likely be thickened with cereal. The nipple holes will need to be larger to allow for easy flow of thicker formula. The child should receive smaller feedings throughout the day. Cereal is added to the formula to increase the consistency and decrease the incidence of regurgitation. Sucking on a pacifier in an upright position facilitates the flow of food through the esophagus.

Test-Taking Strategy: Use the process of elimination to answer the question. Note the key phrases in the options: "small feedings," "add a small amount of cereal," "maintain an upright position." This should direct you to the correct option for this question as it is stated. If you had difficulty with this question, take time now to review the feeding procedures for a child with GER!

Level of Cognitive Ability: Analysis
Phase of Nursing Process: Evaluation
Client Needs: Physiological Integrity
Content Area: Child Health

Reference

Wong, D. L. (1995). *Whaley and Wong's Nursing care of infants and children* (5th ed.). St. Louis: Mosby–Year Book, p. 1462.

---

56. In evaluating a client's understanding of health measures to prevent coronary artery disease (CAD), the nurse evaluates which of the following client statements as a need for more teaching?

1. "I should restrict the amount of fried foods I eat."
2. "If I exercise, I could bring on a heart attack."
3. "I should take my medicines at the same times each day."
4. "If I quit smoking, I will eventually lose my risk for heart disease caused by smoking."

Answer: 2

Rationale: A sedentary lifestyle is a major risk factor for development of CAD. Exercise may reduce the risk of CAD by decreasing weight, reducing blood pressure, and elevating high-density lipoprotein (HDL). All of the other options are health measures to prevent CAD.

Test-Taking Strategy: Understanding the risk factors associated with CAD will assist in answering the question. Remember that exercise is a key component of preventing this disease. If you had difficulty with this question, take time now to review prevention measures for CAD!

Level of Cognitive Ability: Analysis
Phase of Nursing Process: Evaluation
Client Needs: Health Promotion and Maintenance
Content Area: Adult Health/Cardiovascular

Reference

Black, J., & Matassarin-Jacobs, E. (1997). *Medical-surgical nursing: Clinical management for continuity of care* (5th ed.). Philadelphia: W. B. Saunders, p. 1239.

57. A client with polycystic kidney disease has developed a urinary tract infection (UTI). The nurse has been discussing discharge instructions with the client. Which statement by the client indicates a need for further teaching?

1 "I continue to take my antibiotics until I finish the prescription as prescribed."
2 "Once the symptoms of my infection go away, I can stop taking my antibiotics."
3 "I should clean my perineal area from front to back after every voiding."
4 "I should drink at least 8 glasses of fluid a day."

Answer: 2

Rationale: Traditional treatment of a urinary tract infection involves 7–10 days of administration of oral antimicrobial therapy. It is important to take antibiotics even if the client is feeling better. While taking these medications, the client should drink at least 8 glasses of water of fluid per day to keep urine dilute. Voiding regularly will flush bacteria out of the bladder and urethra. Teaching the client to cleanse the perineal area from front to back helps to prevent urinary tract infection.

Test-Taking Strategy: Use the process of elimination to answer the question. The key is to remember that the entire prescription of antibiotics needs to be taken even if symptoms resolve. If you had difficulty with this question, take time now to review treatment measures for UTI!

Level of Cognitive Ability: Analysis
Phase of Nursing Process: Evaluation
Client Needs: Health Promotion and Maintenance
Content Area: Adult Health/Renal

Reference

LeMone, P., & Burke, K. M. (1996). *Medical-surgical nursing: Critical thinking in client care.* Menlo Park, CA: Addison-Wesley, pp. 888–891.

58. The client is taking phenytoin (Dilantin). The blood level is within therapeutic range and seizures are controlled. Which of the following, however, if observed by the nurse, would require physician notification and possible discontinuation of the medication?

1 Stevens-Johnson syndrome
2 Bleeding gums
3 Mental impairment
4 Diplopia

Answer: 1

Rationale: Stevens-Johnson syndrome is a rash indicating an allergy; therefore, the physician needs to be notified for consideration of medication discontinuation. Options 2, 3, and 4 are also side effects of the medication but may be reversed with medication dose alteration rather that medication discontinuation.

Test-Taking Strategy: The stem of the question asks you to identify the option that requires physician notification. The key phrase is "possible discontinuation." Options 2, 3, and 4 require attention, but a rash indicates an allergic response, and an allergy can be life-threatening. If you are unfamiliar with this medication, review it now. You will surely note questions related to this medication on NCLEX-RN!

Level of Cognitive Ability: Analysis
Phase of Nursing Process: Evaluation
Client Needs: Physiological Integrity
Content Area: Pharmacology

Reference

Lehne, R. A. (1998). *Pharmacology for nursing care* (3rd ed.). W. B. Saunders, p. 208.

59. A nurse instructs a mother caring for an infant with acute infectious diarrhea about measures to prevent the spread of pathogens. Which action by the mother indicates a need for further teaching?

1 Washes the child's hands after changing the diaper
2 Applies a cloth diaper snugly after cleaning perineum
3 Restrains the child's hands when changing the diaper
4 Places the soiled diaper in a sealed, double plastic bag

Answer: 2

Rationale: Cloth diapers do not have elastic in the legs. This could allow for seepage of the infectious stool and cause spread of pathogens. Second, the liquid stool makes the diaper wet, which also promotes the spread of disease. Disposable, plastic diapers have elastic in the legs, high absorbency, and plastic on the outside. These features decrease transmission of pathogens. Option 1 prevents the spread of pathogens through handwashing. Option 3 prevents the child from coming into contact with the infectious material. Option 4 is appropriate disposal of infectious waste.

Test-Taking Strategy: Use the principles of universal precautions—which include handwashing, proper disposal of body fluid and waste, and avoiding contact with body fluids—when answering the question.

The only option that does not accurately reflect universal precautions is option 2.

Level of Cognitive Ability: Analysis
Phase of Nursing Process: Evaluation
Client Needs: Safe, Effective Care Environment
Content Area: Child Health

Reference

Wong, D. L. (1995). *Whaley and Wong's Nursing care of infants and children* (5th ed.). St. Louis: Mosby–Year Book, pp. 1164–1166, 1241.

---

60. The nurse is evaluating the client's use of a cane for left-sided weakness. The nurse would intervene and correct the client if the nurse observed that the client

1 Holds the cane on the right side.
2 Keeps the cane 6 inches out to the side of the right foot.
3 Moves the cane when the right leg is moved.
4 Leans on the cane when the right leg swings through.

Answer: 3

Rationale: The cane is held on the stronger side to minimize stress on the affected extremity and provide a wide base of support. The cane is held 6 inches lateral to the fifth toe. The cane is moved forward with the affected leg. The client leans on the cane for added support while the stronger side swings through.

Test-Taking Strategy: The wording of this question guides you to look for an incorrect action. Knowing that the cane is held on the stronger side helps you eliminate options 1 and 2 first; both are correct. To discriminate between the two remaining choices, recall that the client moves the cane with the weaker leg and leans on it for support when the stronger leg swings through. This will help you to choose option 3 as the answer to this question. Review the use of a cane now if you had difficulty with this question!

Level of Cognitive Ability: Analysis
Phase of Nursing Process: Evaluation
Client Needs: Safe, Effective Care Environment
Content Area: Adult Health/Musculoskeletal

Reference

Smeltzer, S., & Bare, B. (1996). *Brunner and Suddarth's Textbook of medical-surgical nursing* (8th ed.). Philadelphia: Lippincott-Raven, p. 341.

---

61. The nurse is caring for a client being treated for fat embolus after multiple fractures. Which of the following data would the nurse evaluate as the most favorable indication of resolution of the fat embolus?

1 Arterial oxygen level: 78 mmHg
2 Minimal dyspnea
3 Clear chest x-ray
4 Oxygen saturation: 85%

Answer: 3

Rationale: A clear chest x-ray is a good indicator that fat embolus is resolving. When fat embolism occurs, there is a "snowstorm" appearance to chest x-ray. Eupnea, not minimal dyspnea, is a normal sign. Arterial oxygen levels should be 80–100 mmHg. Oxygen saturation should be greater than 95%.

Test-Taking Strategy: Knowledge of normal baseline respiratory values is helpful in answering this question. Knowing that the arterial oxygen and oxygen saturation levels are below normal helps you to eliminate these as possible correct answers. Dyspnea, even at a minimal level, is not normal, and option 2 can be eliminated quickly. A clear chest x-ray is a normal finding and is the answer to the question as stated.

Level of Cognitive Ability: Analysis
Phase of Nursing Process: Evaluation
Client Needs: Physiological Integrity
Content Area: Adult Health/Musculoskeletal

Reference

Smeltzer, S., & Bare, B. (1996). *Brunner and Suddarth's Textbook of medical-surgical nursing* (8th ed.). Philadelphia: Lippincott-Raven, p. 1917.

62. Adenosine (Adenocard) is to be administered to a client in the emergency room. Before the preparation of the medication, the nurse evaluates the client's room to ensure the presence of

1 A pulse oximetry machine.
2 An IV pole.
3 A cardiac monitor.
4 An endotracheal tube.

Answer: 3

Rationale: Adenosine (Adenocard) is an antidysrhythmic used in the treatment of paroxysmal supraventricular tachycardia. Cardiac performance must be assessed before and throughout treatment by cardiac monitor. An endotracheal tube may be used if an emergency arose necessitating mechanical ventilation, but the tube itself is a rather isolated item. An IV pole may be needed but is not the priority. A pulse oximetry machine may be helpful in assessing oxygenation but is not the priority item.

Test-Taking Strategy: Knowledge that the medication is an antidysrhythmic and use of the ABCs will assist in directing you to the correct option. Review this medication now if you had difficulty with this question!

Level of Cognitive Ability: Analysis
Phase of Nursing Process: Evaluation
Client Needs: Physiological Integrity
Content Area: Pharmacology

Reference
Hodgson, B., & Kizior, R. (1998). *Saunders nursing drug handbook 1998.* Philadelphia: W. B. Saunders, pp. 13–14.

---

63. A client who was treated successfully with streptokinase for an occluded arterial graft is being prepared for discharge. The nurse would evaluate that the client is best prepared for self-management at home if the client made which of the following statements?

1 "I'll have to check the circulation to my leg at least once a week."
2 "As long as I take one baby aspirin a day, I should do well."
3 "I'll try not to walk around too much on that leg."
4 "I'll be sure to check the condition of my leg and foot every day."

Answer: 4

Rationale: After restoring circulation to the affected limb, the nurse reinforces teaching that was done after original surgery. This includes exercise and dietary recommendations, as well as instructions on foot care and prevention of injury to the limb.

Test-Taking Strategy: The wording of the question guides you to look for a correct statement. Because streptokinase therapy cannot ensure that no future thrombosis will occur, the client must continue to monitor circulation. Thus you would choose option 4. If you had difficulty with this question, take time now to review the effects of this medication!

Level of Cognitive Ability: Analysis
Phase of Nursing Process: Evaluation
Client Needs: Health Promotion and Maintenance
Content Area: Adult Health/Cardiovascular

Reference
Ignatavicius, D. D., Workman, M. L., & Mishler, M. A. (1995). *Medical-surgical nursing: A nursing process approach* (2nd ed.). Philadelphia: W. B. Saunders, p. 946.

---

64. The nurse has given instructions to the client with aortoiliac bypass grafting about measures to improve circulation while in the hospital. The nurse would evaluate the teaching as successful if the nurse observed the client doing which of the following?

1 Using the knee gatch
2 Keeping knees and ankles uncrossed
3 Flexing the knee and hip
4 Placing pillows under the knees

Answer: 2

Rationale: Clot formation in the graft can result from any form of pressure that impairs blood flow through the graft, including bending at the hip or knee, crossing knees or ankles, or using the knee gatch or pillows. All of these are to be avoided in the postoperative period.

Test-Taking Strategy: This question is fairly straightforward. Think about concepts related to blood flow and obstruction to flow while answering this question. Doing so will help you eliminate each of the incorrect options. Option 2 is the only option that will prevent obstruction to blood flow. These are important points to know, so review them now if needed.

Level of Cognitive Ability: Analysis
Phase of Nursing Process: Evaluation
Client Needs: Health Promotion and Maintenance
Content Area: Adult Health/Cardiovascular

References

Black, J., & Matassarin-Jacobs, E. (1997). *Medical-surgical nursing: Clinical management for continuity of care* (5th ed.). Philadelphia: W. B. Saunders, p. 1416.

Ignatavicius, D. D., Workman, M. L., & Mishler, M. A. (1995). *Medical-surgical nursing: A nursing process approach* (2nd ed.). Philadelphia: W. B. Saunders, p. 944.

---

65. The nurse has conducted teaching with a client in an arm cast about signs and symptoms of compartment syndrome. The nurse would evaluate that the client understands the information if the client stated which of the following early symptoms of compartment syndrome?

1 Pain that is relieved only by oxycodone and aspirin (Percodan)
2 Pain that increases when the arm is dependent
3 Cold, bluish fingers
4 Numbness and tingling in the fingers

Answer: 4

Rationale: The earliest symptom of compartment syndrome is paresthesias (numbness and tingling in the fingers). Other symptoms include pain unrelieved by narcotics, pain that increases with limb elevation, and pallor and coolness to the distal limb. Cyanosis is a late sign.

Test-Taking Strategy: This question asks for an "early" symptom of compartment syndrome. Because cyanosis is a late sign, eliminate option 3 first. Knowing that compartment syndrome is characterized by insufficient circulation and ischemia secondary to pressure, you would look for symptoms that are consistent with this process. Pain would be increased with elevation rather than dependency, so eliminate option 2 also. Because the pain of ischemia is generally not relieved with analgesics, this cannot be an early symptom either. This leaves numbness and tingling as the answer.

Level of Cognitive Ability: Analysis
Phase of Nursing Process: Evaluation
Client Needs: Health Promotion and Maintenance
Content Area: Adult Health/Musculoskeletal

Reference

Black, J., & Matassarin-Jacobs, E. (1997). *Medical-surgical nursing: Clinical management for continuity of care* (5th ed.). Philadelphia: W. B. Saunders, p. 2139.

---

66. A client with a thoracic cord injury is receiving dantrolene sodium (Dantrium). Which statement by the client indicates to the nurse that the client is having an undesired medication effect?

1 "I'm feeling drowsy."
2 "My legs are very relaxed."
3 "I can't seems to get enough to eat."
4 "My urine has a bluish color."

Answer: 1

Rationale: Drowsiness, diarrhea, and hepatotoxicity are the major adverse effects of this muscle relaxant, which is used to treat the chronic spasticity seen in spinal cord injury. The drowsiness may interfere with the client's rehabilitation. Some clients have anorexia and hematuria.

Test-Taking Strategy: The stem is a false response question that required identification of an undesired medication effect. Option 2 is a desired effect. Options 3 and 4 are unrelated to this medication. If you have to guess, remember that many medications cause nausea or gastric irritation, so option 3 could be eliminated. Very few drugs cause blue urine, making option 4 a poor choice. If you had difficulty with this question, take time now to review the undesired effects of this medication!

Level of Cognitive Ability: Analysis
Phase of Nursing Process: Evaluation
Client Needs: Physiological Integrity
Content Area: Pharmacology

Reference

Smeltzer, S., & Bare, B. (1996). *Brunner and Suddarth's Textbook of medical-surgical nursing* (8th ed.). Philadelphia: Lippincott-Raven, p. 1808.

67. The nurse administers hydralazine hydrochloride (Apresoline) to a client with autonomic dysreflexia. Which evaluation finding most accurately indicates that the medication is effective?

1 Muscle spasms subside
2 Blood pressure declines
3 Intensity of seizure activity declines
4 Client states that he or she feels better

Answer: 2

Rationale: Apresoline is a potent ganglionic blocking agent that decreases the blood pressure by vasodilation. It may be given by slow IV push during an episode of extreme hypertension. A variety of beta-adrenergic blocking agents may be used to prevent dysreflexic episodes.

Test-Taking Strategy: The question requires knowledge about the drug involved: an antihypertensive agent. If you are unfamiliar with a medication, try to make a relationship between the name of the medication and the action: in this case, A*pres*oline and *pres*sure. If you had difficulty with this question, take time now to review the action of this medication!

Level of Cognitive Ability: Analysis
Phase of Nursing Process: Evaluation
Client Needs: Physiological Integrity
Content Area: Pharmacology

Reference
Kee, J., & Hayes, E. (1997). *Pharmacology: A nursing process approach* (2nd ed.). Philadelphia: W. B. Saunders, pp. 510–511.

---

68. Which evaluation finding indicates successful outcomes of the treatment plan for the altered urinary elimination encountered by a client who had a T2 spinal cord injury 2 weeks ago?

1 The client's urine is clear and yellow
2 The urinary output matches the intake
3 The client promptly reports the voiding sensation
4 The client knows to take an anticholinergic before attempting to void

Answer: 1

Rationale: Spinal shock lasts 3–6 weeks after spinal cord injury and is characterized by a flaccid neurogenic bladder with urinary retention. Intermittent catheterization used to empty the bladder should be carried out in a manner that prevents urinary tract infection. Cloudy or blood-tinged urine may indicate the onset of infection. Because fluid is lost through skin, lungs, and bowel, intake does not normally equal output. Sensations of the need to void require an intact cord. Cholinergic action stimulates bladder emptying, so anticholinergics would produce the undesirable effect of relaxation of the bladder for this client.

Test-Taking Strategy: The question requires knowledge of urinary function and management and physiology related to spinal cord injury. Use the process of elimination. Read the option carefully, and consider the client's condition in determining whether the option is realistic. If you had difficulty with this question, take time now to review spinal cord injury!

Level of Cognitive Ability: Analysis
Phase of Nursing Process: Evaluation
Client Needs: Physiological Integrity
Content Area: Adult Health/Neurological

Reference
Smeltzer, S., & Bare, B. (1996). *Brunner and Suddarth's Textbook of medical-surgical nursing* (8th ed.). Philadelphia: Lippincott-Raven, pp. 1150, 1153–1154, 1800.

69. A community health nurse is assigned to teach unwed teenaged mothers sexually transmitted disease–prevention measures. The nurse determines that appropriate learning has occurred when the participants

1 Report a weight gain of 10 pounds per month.
2 Demonstrate proper method for bathing a baby.
3 State that the father of the baby will attend birthing classes.
4 Understand the concept of using condoms.

Answer: 4

Rationale: Use of condoms is the best way to prevent sexually transmitted disease. Options 1, 2, and 3 do not directly relate to sexually transmitted disease–prevention measures.

Test-Taking Strategy: Use the process of elimination. The key words are "sexual disease prevention." Option 1 is subjective assessment. Demonstration of skill for bathing is implementation of a goal. The father may or may not be identified; the stem does not address psychosocial interactions of significant others. Research is ongoing; however, it is shown that use of condoms is the best way to prevent sexually transmitted diseases.

Level of Cognitive Ability: Analysis
Phase of Nursing Process: Evaluation
Client Needs: Health Promotion and Maintenance
Content Area: Maternity

Reference

Nichols, F., & Zwelling, E. (1997). *Maternal-newborn nursing: Theory and practice.* Philadelphia: W. B. Saunders, pp. 247–252.

---

70. A nurse is performing an assessment on a client admitted with chest pain. Upon evaluating the rhythm strip, the nurse discovers the client is in first-degree heart block. Which of the following statements, if made by the client, would indicate an understanding of this rhythm?

1 "I understand there is slowed conduction from one point to another point in the heart."
2 "If I lie very still, this problem will go away."
3 "I understand this is a serious problem, and I will need a pacemaker."
4 "I will need to take a special medication for this heart problem."

Answer: 1

Rationale: First-degree heart block indicates a delayed conduction somewhere between the junctional tissue and the Purkinje network, prolonging the PR interval. Lying still will not relieve the problem. A pacemaker is not necessary for first-degree heart block. Medication may be prescribed, but the issue of the question is an "understanding of this rhythm."

Test-Taking Strategy: To respond correctly to this question, basic knowledge of ECGs is required. Eliminate option 2 because this is unlikely. Eliminate option 4 because it is not directly related to the issue of the question. Knowing that there are more than one type of heart block and that first-degree is the least serious should assist you in eliminating option 3. Review basic ECG concepts now if you had difficulty with this question!

Level of Cognitive Ability: Analysis
Phase of Nursing Process: Evaluation
Client Needs: Physiological Integrity
Content Area: Adult Health/Cardiovascular

Reference

Smeltzer, S., & Bare, B. (1996). *Brunner and Suddarth's Textbook of medical-surgical nursing* (8th ed.). Philadelphia: Lippincott-Raven, p. 625.

---

71. A client has been taught to use a walker to aid in mobility after internal fixation of a hip fracture. The nurse evaluates that the client is using the walker incorrectly if the client

1 Holds the walker by using the hand grips.
2 Leans forward slightly when advancing the walker.
3 Advances the walker with reciprocal motion.
4 Supports body weight on the hands while advancing the weaker leg.

Answer: 3

Rationale: The client should use the walker by placing the hands on the hand grips for stability. The client lifts the walker to advance it and leans forward slightly while moving it. The client walks into the walker, supporting the body weight on the hands while moving the weaker leg. A disadvantage of the walker is that it does not allow for reciprocal walking motion. If the client were to try to use reciprocal motion with a walker, the walker would advance forward one side at a time as the client walks; thus the client would not be supporting the weaker leg with the walker during ambulation.

Test-Taking Strategy: The question asks for an incorrect movement on the part of the client. Holding the walker by using the hand grips is obviously a correct action and is eliminated first. The client must lean forward slightly in order to move the walker forward, so this option is eliminated as well. Reciprocal motion is moving one leg and the opposite arm at the same time. If the client were trying to do this with a walker, the client would be twisting the walker from side to side as it advances. This would be incorrect and is therefore the answer to the question as stated.

Level of Cognitive Ability: Analysis
Phase of Nursing Process: Evaluation
Client Needs: Safe, Effective Care Environment
Content Area: Adult Health/Musculoskeletal

Reference

Smeltzer, S., & Bare, B. (1996). *Brunner and Suddarth's Textbook of medical-surgical nursing* (8th ed.). Philadelphia: Lippincott-Raven, p. 341.

---

72. The client with AIDS has an opportunistic respiratory fungal infection and is receiving IV amphotericin B treatment. Which of the following statements, if made by the client, indicates an accurate understanding of the points taught about amphotericin B?

1 "I will notify the nurse if I notice cloudy urine, blood in my urine, or little or no urine output."
2 "Amphotericin will color my urine orange."
3 "I will notify the nurse if I notice dark, amber urine or pale stools."
4 "I may notice some pain or burning when I urinate, which is normal."

Answer: 1

Rationale: Some clients receiving amphotericin B develop nephrotoxicity. Clients should be taught to report oliguria, hematuria, cloudy urine, and lack of urine output. Rifampin stains urine and other secretions red or orange, but amphotericin does not. Dark, amber urine or pale stools are symptoms of jaundice. Because amphotericin is cleared by the kidneys, not the liver, jaundice would not be an expected adverse effect. Pain or burning upon urination is not an expected or normal side effect and is also an inaccurate statement.

Test-Taking Strategy: This question requires you to know that nephrotoxicity is a common adverse effect of amphotericin B. You could eliminate option 4 because pain and burning on urination are not normal symptoms. From this point, knowledge that this medication is nephrotoxic will direct you to the correct option.

Level of Cognitive Ability: Analysis
Phase of Nursing Process: Evaluation
Client Needs: Physiological Integrity
Content Area: Pharmacology

Reference

Baer, C., & Williams, B. (1996). *Clinical pharmacology and nursing* (3rd ed.). Springhouse, PA: Springhouse, pp. 1053, 1080–1083.

---

73. The nurse is evaluating the status of a 4-day postoperative client with a chest tube and Pleur-Evac drainage system in place. There is no fluctuation or bubbling in the water seal chamber. The fluid level in the drainage collection chamber has not increased. The nurse evaluates that

1 There is an air leak in the system.
2 The level of suction needs to be increased.
3 The tube is probably occluded by a clot.
4 The lung is probably fully reexpanded.

Answer: 4

Rationale: Within 2 or 3 days of surgery, a lung is generally fully reexpanded. The nurse notes an absence of fluctuation, bubbling, or drainage from the chest tube. At this time, the client's status is confirmed by chest x-ray. If the lung is fully reexpanded, the physician may remove the chest tube.

Test-Taking Strategy: To answer this question correctly, it is necessary to know that a chest tube stops functioning either if the lung is fully reexpanded or if the system becomes occluded. This helps you eliminate options 1 and 2. Because the client has had the chest tube in place for 4 days, the lung is probably reexpanded, which would help you choose option 4 over option 3.

Level of Cognitive Ability: Analysis
Phase of Nursing Process: Evaluation
Client Needs: Physiological Integrity
Content Area: Adult Health/Respiratory

Reference

Black, J., & Matassarin-Jacobs, E. (1997). *Medical-surgical nursing: Clinical management for continuity of care* (5th ed.). Philadelphia: W. B. Saunders, p. 1165.

74. The client experiencing irreversible cardiogenic shock reaches for the nurse's hand. Which statement by the client reflects an understanding of his/her condition?

1. "Please help my family now. I have had a good life."
2. "I will soon be playing golf again."
3. "I know I won't be able to do much activity from now on."
4. "This is hard on my family, please teach them how to take care of me when I go home."

Answer: 1

Rationale: Irreversible stage of cardiogenic shock represents the point along the shock continuum at which organ damage is so severe that the client does not respond to treatment and is unable to survive. Multiple organ failure has occurred, and death is imminent. As it becomes obvious that the client is unlikely to survive, the client's family needs to be informed about prognosis and outcome. Support to the grieving family members becomes an integral part of the nursing care plan.

Test-Taking Strategy: Use the process of elimination. In option 1, the client has resolved that the condition is terminal and requests support to those remaining upon his or her demise. Options 2, 3, and 4 do not acknowledge the client's condition as terminal or that death is imminent; the client instead expresses unrealistic hopes of survival. If you had difficulty with this question, take time to review the outcome associated with cardiogenic shock!

Level of Cognitive Ability: Analysis
Phase of Nursing Process: Evaluation
Client Needs: Psychosocial Integrity
Content Area: Adult Health/Cardiovascular

Reference

Smeltzer, S., & Bare, B. (1996). *Brunner and Suddarth's Textbook of medical-surgical nursing* (8th ed.). Philadelphia: Lippincott-Raven, p. 259.

75. The nurse evaluates the client for the presence of extrapyramidal side effects (EPS) from the use of antipsychotic medications. These side effects include

1. Akathisia (spasms of the tongue, face, neck, and back).
2. Agraphia (inability to recognize familiar sounds).
3. Tardive dyskinesia (involuntary movements of the tongue, jaw, lips, and facial muscles).
4. Dystonia (motor restlessness, jitteriness).

Answer: 3

Rationale: Options 1, 3, and 4 are manifestations of EPS; however, akathisia is characterized by motor restlessness, tapping feet, and rocking backwards and forwards. Dystonia is characterized by acute spasms of the tongue, neck, face, and back, laryngospasms, torticollis, and eyes locked upwards. Agraphia, the inability to read or write, is not a characteristic of EPS.

Test-Taking Strategy: Remember that for the option to be correct, the entire option needs to contain correct information. Options 1 and 4 contain distracters with correct terms but with incorrect descriptions. Option 2 is not a characteristic of EPS. If you had difficulty with this question, take time now to review these terms and the characteristics of EPS!

Level of Cognitive Ability: Analysis
Phase of Nursing Process: Evaluation
Client Needs: Physiological Integrity
Content Area: Mental Health

Reference

Carson, V., & Arnold, E. (1996). *Mental health nursing: The nurse-patient journey.* Philadelphia: W. B. Saunders, p. 529.

76. A nurse manager on a telemetry unit is assessing the knowledge level of a new nurse regarding ECG monitoring. Which statement by the nurse would indicate a need for further instruction?

1 "The ECG yields valuable information on the heart during resting and recovery phases."
2 "Telemetry monitoring allows the client more freedom than the hardwire monitoring system."
3 "In preparing for electrode placement, sites should be shaved of hair that could interfere with good contact between electrode pads and the skin."
4 "Modern ECG monitoring systems are so well grounded that electrical interference is seldom a problem."

Answer: 4

Rationale: The purpose of ECG monitoring is to record cardiac electrical activity during the depolarization and repolarization phases. The two types of single-lead monitoring are hardwire and telemetry. With a wireless battery-operated telemetry system, the client is afforded more freedom and mobility than with the hardwire system. The most common problems with ECG monitoring are related to client movement, electrical interference from equipment in the room, poor choice of monitoring leads, and poor contact between skin and electrode.

Test-Taking Strategy: The question is asking the nurse to identify the statement that indicates the need for more teaching; thus the correct options are the ones eliminated. Basic knowledge of ECG monitoring is needed to answer this question. If you had difficulty with this question, take time now to review these basics!

Level of Cognitive Ability: Analysis
Phase of Nursing Process: Evaluation
Client Needs: Safe, Effective Care Environment
Content Area: Adult Health/Cardiovascular

Reference

Huff, J. (1997). *ECG workout: Exercises in arrhythmia interpretation* (3rd ed.). Philadelphia: Lippincott-Raven, pp. 28–35.

---

77. The nurse is caring for an infant with ABO incompatibility who is receiving phototherapy. The infant's blood type is A positive. The laboratory reports that the mother's blood type is O positive, and the direct Coombs' test yields a positive result. Which of the following outcome criteria indicates that the infant's condition is improving?

1 The infant's reticulocyte count increases to 5.5%
2 The infant's stools become loose and green in color
3 An increase in the total bilirubin of 2 mg/dL after 6 hours of phototherapy
4 The infant's urine becomes pale yellow

Answer: 2

Rationale: The infant's stools often become loose and bright green because of the excretion of excessive bilirubin as a result of the phototherapy. The infant's urine may become a dark color from urobilinogen formation. In option 1, normal reticulocyte count in an infant 1 to 3 days of age is 1.8%–4.6%. An increasing reticulocyte count indicates continued destruction of the infant's red blood cells by the maternal acquired anti-A antibodies. Phototherapy works by a process of photoisomerization and photo-oxidation, which results in more water-soluble bilirubin end products, which can then be more rapidly excreted in the urine and stool.

Test-Taking Strategy: This question asks you to identify an outcome criterion that indicates improvement in the infant with ABO incompatibility. You must know the pathophysiological process of ABO incompatibility to answer the question correctly. If you had difficulty with this question, take time now to review this content area!

Level of Cognitive Ability: Analysis
Phase of Nursing Process: Evaluation
Client Needs: Physiological Integrity
Content Area: Child Health

Reference

Pillitteri, A. (1995). *Maternal and child health nursing: Care of the childbearing and childrearing family* (2nd ed.). Philadelphia: Lippincott-Raven, pp. 766–768, 1813.

78. The nurse is preparing the client for discharge to home. Cold therapy daily has been prescribed for the client. Which of the following statements, if made by the client, indicates adequate understanding of cold therapy techniques?

1 "I need to apply the cold pack for at least 60 minutes."
2 "I can lie on the ice by placing it between the bed and my body."
3 "I should wrap the frozen ice pack in a warm towel to help adjust the cold."
4 "I should check my pulse before using the ice on my joints."

Answer: 3

Rationale: Cold therapy should be used for only 15–20 minutes two or three times a day. The client needs to be instructed not to place ice cubes directly between the skin and a firm surface. The weight of the body and the lowered temperature may produce ischemia. The skin should be checked for signs of injury. The slush pack is taken from the freezer and should be wrapped in a warm towel to adjust the cold.

Test-Taking Strategy: Use the process of elimination, trying to visualize the procedure in your mind. This should help you eliminate options 1 and 2. Option 4 is not relevant to the issue of the question. If you had difficulty with this question, take time now to review the procedure for cold pack therapy!

Level of Cognitive Ability: Analysis
Phase of Nursing Process: Evaluation
Client Needs: Health Promotion and Maintenance
Content Area: Fundamental Skills

Reference

Burrell, P., Gerlach, M., & Pless, S. (1997). *Adult nursing: Acute and community care* (2nd ed.). Stamford, CT: Appleton & Lange, pp. 1608–1609.

---

79. The client with AIDS has a T_4 count below 200. The nurse initiates prophylactic treatment as prescribed with aerosolized pentamidine isethionate (Nebupent). Which of the following is an expected outcome?

1 The client has a respiratory rate and depth within normal limits for activity level
2 Strict universal precautions will be maintained until the T_4 count is above 200
3 The client shows no weight loss
4 The client maintains serum sodium, potassium, calcium, and chloride values within normal ranges

Answer: 1

Rationale: Aerosolized pentamidine is given prophylactically in clients with a T_4 count below 200 to prevent *Pneumocystis carinii* pneumonia (PCP). PCP is the most common opportunistic infection and occurs in 75%–80% of persons with HIV. A respiratory rate and depth within normal limits for activity level would indicate that the client was not experiencing respiratory difficulty (i.e., PCP pneumonia). Universal precautions are always maintained on all clients, so eliminate option 2. This question is referring to the client's respiratory status, not to nutritional status or fluid and electrolyte balance; therefore, eliminate options 3 and 4 also.

Test-Taking Strategy: Use the principles associated with prioritizing when answering the question. Remember the ABCs: airway, breathing, and circulation. A method for preventing breathing difficulty caused by *P. carinii* pneumonia is to give prophylactic aerosolized pentamidine isethionate. If you had difficulty with this question, take time now to review this medication!

Level of Cognitive Ability: Analysis
Phase of Nursing Process: Evaluation
Client Needs: Physiological Integrity
Content Area: Adult Health/Respiratory

Reference

Ignatavicius, D. D., Workman, M. L., & Mishler, M. A. (1995). *Medical-surgical nursing: A nursing process approach* (2nd ed.). Philadelphia: W. B. Saunders, pp. 505, 510–511.

80. The community health nurse visits the client with tuberculosis at home 2 weeks after diagnosis. Which of the following statements, if made by the client, indicates that further teaching is needed?

1. "I know I am no longer able to infect others after 2–3 weeks."
2. "I am gradually resuming my activities."
3. "When the fatigue is gone, I can stop my medication."
4. "I know that eating well will help prevent the infection from coming back."

Answer: 3

Rationale: The client must continue the prescribed medication for 6 months or longer as prescribed and cannot discontinue the medication on his or her own. Options 1, 2, and 4 are correct statements.

Test-Taking Strategy: By the process of elimination, you should be directed toward the correct option. Remember that clients should not discontinue medication. If you had difficulty with this question, take time now to review medication therapy and tuberculosis!

Level of Cognitive Ability: Analysis
Phase of Nursing Process: Evaluation
Client Needs: Health Promotion and Maintenance
Content Area: Adult Health/Respiratory

Reference

Ignatavicius, D. D., Workman, M. L., & Mishler, M. A. (1995). *Medical-surgical nursing: A nursing process approach* (2nd ed.). Philadelphia: W. B. Saunders, p. 722.

---

81. A client with a high risk for coronary artery closure is being prepared for percutaneous transluminal coronary angioplasty (PTCA). Abciximab (ReoPro) is being administered by infusion. The nurse evaluates the assessment data and determines that a potential adverse effect of the medication may be occurring when the nurse notes

1. A widened pulse pressure.
2. A hemoglobin of 12 g/dL.
3. An apical rate of 88.
4. A blood pressure of 112/60.

Answer: 1

Rationale: Abciximab (ReoPro) is an antiplatelet, antithrombotic agent that is used as an adjunct to aspirin and heparin to prevent acute cardiac ischemic complications in clients at high risk for abrupt closure of treated coronary blood vessel undergoing PTCA. Bleeding is a concern when this medication is administered. A widened pulse pressure is a sign of increased intracranial pressure, which could indicate intracranial bleeding. A hemoglobin of 12 g/dL, an apical rate of 88, and a blood pressure reading of 112/60 are not abnormal findings.

Test-Taking Strategy: Use knowledge of normal assessment findings and the process of elimination to answer the question. Eliminate options 2, 3, and 4 because these are normal findings. Take time now to review this medication if you had difficulty with this question!

Level of Cognitive Ability: Analysis
Phase of Nursing Process: Evaluation
Client Needs: Physiological Integrity
Content Area: Pharmacology

Reference

Hodgson, B., & Kizior, R. (1998). *Saunders nursing drug handbook 1998.* Philadelphia: W. B. Saunders, pp. 1–2.

---

82. The client informs the clinic nurse that he or she has been taking acarbose (Precose) as prescribed. The clinic nurse evaluates that a therapeutic effect of the medication has occurred when the nurse notes

1. A serum lipase level of 100 U/liter.
2. A 2-hour postprandial serum glucose level of 120 mg/dL.
3. A sodium level of 140 mEq/liter.
4. A blood urea nitrogen (BUN) level of 15 mg/dL.

Answer: 2

Rationale: Acarbose (Precose) is an oral antidiabetic medication used as an adjunct to diet in order to lower blood glucose in clients with non–insulin-dependent diabetes mellitus whose hyperglycemia cannot be managed by diet alone. All laboratory values presented in the options are within normal ranges. Lipase level is used to determine the presence of pancreatitis. Sodium is an electrolyte. BUN is a measure of renal function. A 2-hour postprandial serum glucose of 120 mg/dL would identify a therapeutic effect of the medication.

Test-Taking Strategy: Knowledge of the action and classification of this medication is necessary to answer the question. If you were unfamiliar with this medication, a key is the medication name *Pre*cose. This can provide you with a clue that the medication is administered before something. Knowing that antidiabetics are administered before the meal may assist with directing you to the correct option. Review the purpose of this medication now if you had difficulty with this question!

Level of Cognitive Ability: Analysis
Phase of Nursing Process: Evaluation
Client Needs: Physiological Integrity
Content Area: Pharmacology

Reference
Hodgson, B., & Kizior, R. (1998). *Saunders nursing drug handbook 1998.* Philadelphia: W. B. Saunders, p. 3.

---

83. The client is breathing independently with a Shiley tracheostomy. The client coughs up large amounts of secretions onto the tracheostomy dressing. The nurse evaluates that which of the following modifications needs to be made in the care plan?

1 Change the oxygen collar every 8 hours instead of every 24 hours
2 Continue to do tracheostomy care every 8 hours, and add PRN dressing changes
3 Cleanse the inner cannula every 4 hours instead of every 8 hours
4 Decrease fluid intake to decrease production of secretions

Answer: 2

Rationale: Tracheostomy dressings should be changed whenever they get wet or damp. A soiled dressing promotes microorganism growth and enhances tissue irritation and breakdown. The oxygen collar may be cleaned if it becomes soiled between collar and tubing changes, which is done every 24 hours. Tracheostomy care should be done every 8 hours. It would not be beneficial to the client to limit fluids, because thicker secretions pose added problems with airway management.

Test-Taking Strategy: The question focuses on secretions that accumulate on the tracheostomy dressing. This could lead to bacterial growth and skin breakdown when the dressing becomes saturated. According to this line of reasoning, the intervention of choice would be to do more frequent dressing changes. This leads you to select option 2 as the correct answer.

Level of Cognitive Ability: Application
Phase of Nursing Process: Evaluation
Client Needs: Physiological Integrity
Content Area: Adult Health/Respiratory

Reference
Black, J., & Matassarin-Jacobs, E. (1997). *Medical-surgical nursing: Clinical management for continuity of care* (5th ed.). Philadelphia: W. B. Saunders, p. 1074.

---

84. The emergency room receives a telephone call from the emergency alert system informing the department that a child who ingested a bottle of acetaminophen (Tylenol) is en route to the emergency room. The nurse prepares the room for the arrival of the child and evaluates the medication supply to determine that which medication is available?

1 Phytonadione (vitamin K)
2 Protamine sulfate
3 Acetylcysteine (Mucomyst)
4 Pancreatin

Answer: 3

Rationale: Acetylcysteine (Mucomyst) is the antidote for acetaminophen (Tylenol). Protamine sulfate is the antidote for heparin. Phytonadione (vitamin K) is the antidote for warfarin (Coumadin). Pancreatin is a pancreatic enzyme replacement or supplement.

Test-Taking Strategy: Knowledge regarding the appropriate antidote for acetaminophen (Tylenol) is necessary to answer the question. Review the various medication antidotes now if you had difficulty with this question!

Level of Cognitive Ability: Application
Phase of Nursing Process: Evaluation
Client Needs: Safe, Effective Care Environment
Content Area: Pharmacology

Reference
Hodgson, B., & Kizior, R. (1998). *Saunders nursing drug handbook 1998.* Philadelphia: W. B. Saunders, pp. 8, 786, 1064, 1098.

85. The nurse is caring for a client who has been taking acetazolamide (Diamox) for glaucoma. The nurse evaluates the assessment data and determines that a potential adverse effect of the medication may be occurring when the nurse notes

1. No change in the level of peripheral vision.
2. Jaundice.
3. Pupillary constriction in response to light.
4. Tinnitus.

Answer: 2

Rationale: Acetazolamide (Diamox) is a carbonic anhydrase inhibitor used in the treatment of open-angle, secondary, or angle-closure glaucoma to reduce the rate of aqueous humor formation and to lower intraocular pressure. Adverse effects are related to nephrotoxicity, hepatotoxicity, and bone marrow depression. Jaundice is a sign of hepatotoxicity. A decrease in the level of peripheral vision would indicate a complication of glaucoma. Pupillary constriction in response to light is a normal response. Tinnitus is unrelated to this medication.

Test-Taking Strategy: Read the options carefully. Eliminate options 1 and 3 because these are normal responses. With the remaining two options, remembering that nephrotoxicity, hepatotoxicity, and bone marrow depression indicate adverse effects will direct you to the correct option!

Level of Cognitive Ability: Analysis
Phase of Nursing Process: Evaluation
Client Needs: Physiological Integrity
Content Area: Pharmacology

Reference

Hodgson, B., & Kizior, R. (1998). *Saunders nursing drug handbook 1998.* Philadelphia: W. B. Saunders, p. 10.

86. The client with a tracheostomy is being considered for long-term home ventilator therapy. The nurse evaluates that the client is not yet ready for discharge if which of the following items is noted?

1. A ventilator is available with a mechanism for converting from electricity to an internal battery source
2. The electrical service to the home is sufficient to handle the equipment
3. The family is cardiopulmonary resuscitation (CPR)–certified through a course designed for lay people in the community
4. The home environment is free of drafts and has adequate ventilation

Answer: 3

Rationale: Before discharging a ventilator-dependent client to home, the nurse determines that the family is able to perform CPR, including mouth-to-tracheostomy ventilation. The CPR course designed for the general community does not include this element of care. The electrical service to the home must be sufficient for the equipment that will be used. The ventilator should have a built-in converter to battery power if the electrical power should fail; otherwise, a generator must be installed. The home itself should be free of drafts and provide adequate air circulation.

Test-Taking Strategy: On first reading, each of the options seems like a plausible answer. On closer scrutiny, however, notice that the stem discusses a client who will be managed on a ventilator and who has a tracheostomy. Knowing that resuscitation as taught in a community-level CPR course does not include ventilation with artificial airways, you would then select option 3 as the only plausible option.

Level of Cognitive Ability: Analysis
Phase of Nursing Process: Evaluation
Client Needs: Health Promotion and Maintenance
Content Area: Adult Health/Respiratory

Reference

Smeltzer, S., & Bare, B. (1996). *Brunner and Suddarth's Textbook of medical-surgical nursing* (8th ed.). Philadelphia: Lippincott-Raven, p. 566.

87. During a prenatal visit, the nurse is explaining dietary management to a client with diabetes. The nurse evaluates that the teaching has been effective when the client states

1 "I can eat more sweets now because I need more calories."
2 "I need more fat in my diet so the baby can gain enough weight."
3 "I need to eat a high-protein, low-carbohydrate diet now in order to control my blood sugar."
4 "I need to increase the fiber in my diet to control my blood glucose and prevent constipation."

Answer: 4

Rationale: An increase in calories is needed with pregnancy, but concentrated sugars should be avoided because they may cause hyperglycemia. The fat intake should remain at 30% of the total calories. The fetus of a diabetic mother is prone to macrosomia. The diabetic client needs about 40%–50% of the diet from carbohydrates and about 20%–25% of the diet from protein. High-fiber foods will cause blood glucose levels to rise more slowly by delaying gastrointestinal absorption.

Test-Taking Strategy: Use the process of elimination. You can easily eliminate options 1 and 2. Of the remaining options, option 4 is the correct statement because a low carbohydrate diet will not maintain or control an adequate blood glucose level. If you had difficulty with this question, take time now to review dietary management with diabetes in pregnancy!

Level of Cognitive Ability: Analysis
Phase of Nursing Process: Evaluation
Client Needs: Health Promotion and Maintenance
Content Area: Maternity

Reference
Lowdermilk, D., Perry, S., & Bobak, I. (1997). *Maternity and women's health care* (6th ed.). St. Louis: Mosby–Year Book, p. 816.

---

88. The client reports to the clinic for follow-up after a 1-month treatment with acebutolol (Sectral). The clinic nurse evaluates that a therapeutic effect of the medication has occurred when the nurse notes

1 A blood pressure of 130/84.
2 An apical rate of 88.
3 Palpable peripheral pulses.
4 Maintenance of desired weight.

Answer: 1

Rationale: Acebutolol (Sectral) is a beta-adrenergic blocker used primarily to manage mild to moderate hypertension or cardiac dysrhythmias. The expected therapeutic response is a controlled blood pressure within normal limits. Although a pulse rate of 88 is also normal, no reference is made regarding the quality or regularity of the pulse. Options 3 and 4 are unrelated to the action of the medication.

Test-Taking Strategy: Remember that medication names that end in "lol" are beta-blockers and that beta-blockers lower blood pressure. This should assist you in determining the correct option. Review this medication now if you had difficulty with the question!

Level of Cognitive Ability: Analysis
Phase of Nursing Process: Evaluation
Client Needs: Physiological Integrity
Content Area: Pharmacology

Reference
Hodgson, B., & Kizior, R. (1998). *Saunders nursing drug handbook 1998.* Philadelphia: W. B. Saunders, p. 5.

---

89. The nurse is administering, as prescribed, a high but acceptable dose of acyclovir (Zovirax) to a client with severe herpes genitalis. During administration of the medication, the nurse evaluates assessment data for adverse effects. Which of the following would be indicative of an adverse reaction?

1 Lightheadedness
2 Decreased urinary output
3 Headache
4 Tremors

Answer: 2

Rationale: Acyclovir (Zovirax) is an antiviral medication used to treat the herpesvirus. Rapid parenteral administration, excessively high doses, or fluid and electrolyte imbalances may produce renal failure, and signs and symptoms that include abdominal pain, decreased urination, decreased appetite, increased thirst, nausea, and vomiting. Lightheadedness and headache are occasional side effects of oral use. Tremors are a rare side effect of parenteral use.

Test-Taking Strategy: Note that options 1, 3, and 4 are all neurologically related symptoms. The option that is different is option 2. Review this important medication now if you had difficulty with this question!

Level of Cognitive Ability: Analysis
Phase of Nursing Process: Evaluation
Client Needs: Physiological Integrity
Content Area: Pharmacology

Reference

Hodgson, B., & Kizior, R. (1998). *Saunders nursing drug handbook 1998.* Philadelphia: W. B. Saunders, pp. 13–14.

---

90. The client who has undergone abdominal aortic aneurysm (AAA) repair complains of back pain. The nurse evaluates this client complaint as indicating the need to

1 Massage the back.
2 Auscultate breath sounds.
3 Auscultate bowel sounds.
4 Report this to the physician immediately.

Answer: 4

Rationale: Back pain after AAA repair may indicate a problem with the repair. It should be reported immediately. Options 1, 2, and 3 are not helpful.

Test-Taking Strategy: Recognizing the symptom of back pain as being indicative of hemorrhage in a client after AAA repair will assist in directing you to the correct option. If you had difficulty with this question, take time now to review signs of complications after AAA repair!

Level of Cognitive Ability: Analysis
Phase of Nursing Process: Evaluation
Client Needs: Physiological Integrity
Content Area: Adult Health/Cardiovascular

Reference

Black, J., & Matassarin-Jacobs, E. (1997). *Medical-surgical nursing: Clinical management for continuity of care* (5th ed.). Philadelphia: W. B. Saunders, p. 1472.

---

91. The nurse has a teaching session with a malnourished client regarding iron supplementation to prevent anemia during pregnancy. Which of the following statements, if made by the client, would indicate successful learning?

1 "The iron is needed to make red blood cells to supply my baby with food."
2 "Meat does not provide iron and should be avoided."
3 "Iron supplements will give me diarrhea."
4 "My body has all the iron it needs and I don't need to take supplements."

Answer: 1

Rationale: The nutritional supplement most commonly needed during pregnancy is iron. Anemia of pregnancy is primarily caused by iron deficiency. Iron supplements usually cause constipation. Meat is an excellent source of iron. Iron for the fetus comes from the maternal serum.

Test-Taking Strategy: Options 2 and 4 have absolute terminology such as "not" and "all," therefore eliminate these options. Note the key word "malnourished" in the question. This would eliminate option 4 as a possibility. Knowledge regarding the effects of iron supplements would assist in eliminating option 3. If you had difficulty with this question, take time now to review the effects of iron medications!

Level of Cognitive Ability: Analysis
Phase of Nursing Process: Evaluation
Client Needs: Physiological Integrity
Content Area: Maternity

Reference

Lowdermilk, D., Perry, S., & Bobak, I. (1997). *Maternity and women's health care* (6th ed.). St. Louis: Mosby–Year Book, pp. 168, 183, 846.

92. The nurse instructs the client with myxedema about the dosage, method of administration, and side effects of levothyroxine sodium (Synthroid). Which of the following responses by the client would indicate an understanding of the nurse's instructions?

1 "I can expect to have diarrhea, insomnia, and excessive sweating."
2 "If I feel nervous or have tremors, I should only take half the dose."
3 "I should apply the topical patch to a nonhairy area."
4 "I will report any episodes of palpitations, chest pain, or dyspnea."

Answer: 4

Rationale: A major concern when initiating thyroid hormone replacement therapy is that the dose may be too high, which can lead to cardiovascular problems. As a result, clients need to be aware of the early signs and symptoms of toxicity and that they must report these immediately to their physician. Diarrhea, insomnia, and excessive sweating are signs and symptoms of hyperthyroidism, and although they can occur with thyroid replacement therapy, they are not expected and should be reported. Tremors and nervousness are also signs of toxicity, which need to be reported. Clients should never take it upon themselves to adjust hormone dosage. Synthroid is not administered topically.

Test-Taking Strategy: Knowledge of the major side effects and method of administration, as well as signs of toxicity related to hormone replacement therapy with Synthroid, is necessary to assist you in answering the question. It is important to remember that clients should always report adverse side effects to the physician, who will then determine whether adjusting the medication dosage is warranted. Use the ABCs—airway, breathing, and circulation—to direct you toward the correct option. If you had difficulty with this question, take time now to review this medication!

Level of Cognitive Ability: Analysis
Phase of Nursing Process: Evaluation
Client Needs: Health Promotion and Maintenance
Content Area: Pharmacology

Reference

Ignatavicius, D. D., Workman, M. L., & Mishler, M. A. (1995). *Medical-surgical nursing: A nursing process approach* (2nd ed.). Philadelphia: W. B. Saunders, p. 1847.

93. The nurse is discharging a client who had been treated with a Sengstaken-Blakemore tube for bleeding esophageal varices. The client asks the nurse why the bleeding occurs from the esophagus when the problem is with the liver. The nurse explains to the client that

1 Because of the hardening of the liver, the blood that circulates through the liver backs up and causes dilated esophageal veins, which can bleed.
2 Because of poor nutrition, the blood vessels in the esophagus weaken and bleed.
3 Because of poor liver function, the blood does not clot correctly, and bleeding occurs in the esophagus.
4 Alcohol weakens the veins in the esophagus, and then coughing causes the veins to rupture.

Answer: 1

Rationale: Disease processes such as cirrhosis damage the blood flow through the liver, resulting in hypertension in the portal venous system. The increased portal pressure causes esophageal varices, which are swollen and distended veins. Factors such as increased intrathoracic pressure or irritations can cause these varices to rupture with subsequent hemorrhage.

Test-Taking Strategy: The issue of this question is specific content relating to how liver disease, such as cirrhosis, leads to the development of esophageal varices. Option 1 correctly describes the development of esophageal varices. All other options are incorrect. Review the pathophysiology of cirrhosis now if you had difficulty with this question!

Level of Cognitive Ability: Analysis
Phase of Nursing Process: Evaluation
Client Needs: Physiological Integrity
Content Area: Adult Health/Gastrointestinal

Reference

Black, J., & Matassarin-Jacobs, E. (1997). *Medical-surgical nursing: Clinical management for continuity of care* (5th ed.). Philadelphia: W. B. Saunders, p. 1885.

94. Which of the following statements, if made by the client, indicates a need for more client teaching regarding cryosurgery?

1 "I may experience some cramping during the procedure."
2 "I may feel faint during cryosurgery."
3 "I will be under general anesthesia."
4 "I may have watery cervical discharge after the procedure."

Answer: 3

Rationale: Cryosurgery entails freezing cervical tissue with nitrous oxide. It is performed in the outpatient setting. Cryotherapy may result in cramping and in a vasovagal response, which may cause faintness. A watery discharge is normal for a few weeks after the procedure.

Test-Taking Strategy: Options 1, 2, and 4 contain the word "may," which tends to make a statement correct. Option 3 contains the word "will," which is an absolute term and often makes the statement incorrect. If you had difficulty with this question, take time now to review cryosurgery!

Level of Cognitive Ability: Analysis
Phase of Nursing Process: Evaluation
Client Needs: Physiological Integrity
Content Area: Adult Health/Oncology

Reference

Smeltzer, S., & Bare, B. (1996). *Brunner and Suddarth's Textbook of medical-surgical nursing* (8th ed.). Philadelphia: Lippincott-Raven, pp. 1239–1240.

---

95. The nurse evaluates the effectiveness of preventive teaching done with parents of an infant with recurring acute otitis media. Which statement indicates more teaching is needed?

1 "No one is permitted to smoke around the baby."
2 "The baby continues to be breast-fed."
3 "We stopped giving the antibiotics to the baby when the fever subsided."
4 "The baby received *Haemophilus influenzae* (HIB) vaccine."

Answer: 3

Rationale: All antibiotics should be given for the prescribed time even if symptoms disappear, because the infection may not be completely eradicated, in which case it recurs. HIB is a common cause of acute otitis media, so the vaccine should reduce this source. Breast feeding can continue. Some infection and allergy protection also comes from breast milk. Passive smoking can cause upper respiratory irritation.

Test-Taking Strategy: Read the question carefully. Option 3 is the only option that is not preventive. In addition, all antibiotics should be given for the prescribed time even if symptoms disappear. If you had difficulty with this question, take time now to review preventative measures and otitis media!

Level of Cognitive Ability: Analysis
Phase of Nursing Process: Evaluation
Client Needs: Health Promotion and Maintenance
Content Area: Child Health

Reference

Wong, D. (1997). *Whaley and Wong's Essentials of pediatric nursing* (5th ed.). St. Louis: Mosby–Year Book, pp. 760–762.

---

96. The clinic nurse evaluates the effectiveness of a client's involvement in a Reach to Recovery group after undergoing a mastectomy. What is the most crucial indicator of successful involvement in the group?

1 The client states that she attends the group every month
2 The client states that she is thrilled with her involvement in the group
3 The client attributes her positive attitude about her recovery to her group involvement
4 The client states that she looks forward to group meetings

Answer: 3

Rationale: Option 1 indicates that the client attends the meetings but gives no indication about participation in the group. Option 2 shows enthusiasm but gives no reason for her elation; perhaps she merely uses the group as an opportunity for socialization, not a place to work on problems. Option 3 indicates a deeper comprehension of the supportive and educational components of the group work. Option 4 states that she enjoys attendance but does not give information as to the reason, which could be purely social.

Test-Taking Strategy: Seek the option that identifies the most active involvement in the group. Option 3 is the most accurate indicator of successful involvement in the group.

Level of Cognitive Ability: Analysis
Phase of Nursing Process: Evaluation
Client Needs: Health Promotion and Maintenance
Content Area: Adult Health/Oncology

Reference

Varcarolis, E. M. (1998). *Foundations of psychiatric mental health nursing* (3rd ed.). Philadelphia: W. B. Saunders, pp. 258–260.

---

97. The client has epididymitis as a complication of urinary tract infection (UTI). The nurse is giving the client instructions to prevent a recurrence. The nurse would evaluate that the client needs further instruction if the client states that he will

1 Drink increased amounts of fluids.
2 Discontinue antibiotics once all symptoms are gone.
3 Limit the force of the stream during voiding.
4 Use condoms to eliminate risk from chlamydia and gonorrhea.

Answer: 2

Rationale: The client who experiences epididymitis from urinary tract infection should increase intake of fluids to flush the urinary system. Because organisms can be forced into the vas deferens and epididymis from strain or pressure during voiding, the client may limit the force of the stream. Condom use can help to prevent urethritis and epididymitis from sexually transmitted diseases (STDs). Antibiotics are always taken until the full course of therapy is completed.

Test-Taking Strategy: The wording of the question guides you to look for an incorrect response. Because option 1 is consistent with good practices in the prevention of UTI, this option 1 may be eliminated first. It is necessary to know that the force of stream should be limited to prevent backflow into the epididymis and that condoms are helpful in preventing this disorder from occurring as a complication of an STD. Review treatment of epididymitis now, if you had difficulty with this question.

Level of Cognitive Ability: Analysis
Phase of Nursing Process: Evaluation
Client Needs: Health Promotion and Maintenance
Content Area: Adult Health/Renal

Reference

Black, J., & Matassarin-Jacobs, E. (1997). *Medical-surgical nursing: Clinical management for continuity of care* (5th ed.). Philadelphia: W. B. Saunders, p. 2381.

---

98. The client with prostatitis secondary to kidney infection has received instructions on management of the condition at home and prevention of recurrence. The nurse evaluates that the client understood the instructions if the client committed to

1 Keep fluid intake to a minimum to decrease the need to void.
2 Exercise as much as possible to stimulate circulation.
3 Stop antibiotic therapy when pain subsides.
4 Use warm sitz baths and analgesics to increase comfort.

Answer: 4

Rationale: Treatment of prostatitis includes medication with antibiotics, analgesics, and stool softeners. The client is also taught to rest, increase fluid intake, and use sitz baths for comfort. Antimicrobial therapy is always continued until the prescription is completely finished.

Test-Taking Strategy: Eliminate option 3 because stopping medication therapy before the end of the course is contraindicated. Option 1 is also eliminated, because fluid intake should be increased. To discriminate between the last two options correctly, it is necessary to understand that sitz baths provide comfort or that rest is helpful in the healing process. Knowledge of either of these concepts would help you to choose option 4 as the correct answer.

Level of Cognitive Ability: Analysis
Phase of Nursing Process: Evaluation
Client Needs: Health Promotion and Maintenance
Content Area: Adult Health/Renal

Reference

Black, J., & Matassarin-Jacobs, E. (1997). *Medical-surgical nursing: Clinical management for continuity of care* (5th ed.). Philadelphia: W. B. Saunders, p. 2372.

99. The client has a prescription for niacin (Nicobid, Niacor). The nurse would evaluate that the client understands the importance of this therapy if the client verbalized the importance of periodic monitoring of

1 Serum cholesterol and chylomicrons.
2 Serum cholesterol and triglycerides.
3 Triglycerides and chylomicrons.
4 Triglycerides and low-density lipoproteins.

Answer: 2

Rationale: Niacin is used as adjunctive therapy in the management of hyperlipidemia. This is used in conjunction with a low-fat and low-cholesterol diet, exercise, and smoking cessation. Serum cholesterol and triglyceride levels are monitored periodically to assess the effectiveness of therapy.

Test-Taking Strategy: To answer this question, you need to know that niacin is used to lower blood cholesterol levels. This would help you eliminate options 3 and 4. Of the remaining two options, the most likely choice is option 2, because chylomicron levels are not monitored. Review this medication now if you had difficulty with this question!

Level of Cognitive Ability: Analysis
Phase of Nursing Process: Evaluation
Client Needs: Health Promotion and Maintenance
Content Area: Pharmacology

Reference

Deglin, J. H., & Vallerand, A. H. (1997). *Davis's drug guide for nurses* (5th ed.). Philadelphia: F. A. Davis, pp. 858, 861.

---

100. The nurse is evaluating the effectiveness of electroconvulsive therapy (ECT). An expected outcome includes which of the following?

1 No seizure activity accompanies the treatment
2 Minor memory deficits are present after 3 months
3 No long-term or short-term memory deficits occur
4 All symptoms of depression are absent

Answer: 2

Rationale: Sensitive testing of memory has revealed minor memory deficits after 3 months, but these resolve within 6 months. Option 1 is incorrect; ECT induces a seizure by applying electrical current. Option 3 is not true. Option 4 is not true; in fact, many clients require the addition of antidepressants after ECT treatments are complete.

Test-Taking Strategy: Use the process of elimination and knowledge regarding ECT therapy. Review the expected effects of ECT now if you had difficulty with this question!

Level of Cognitive Ability: Analysis
Phase of Nursing Process: Evaluation
Client Needs: Physiological Integrity
Content Area: Mental Health

Reference

Carson, V., & Arnold, E. (1996). *Mental health nursing: The nurse-patient journey.* Philadelphia: W. B. Saunders, p. 785.

---

101. Which statement by a client with a new ileostomy demonstrates a positive outcome for the nursing diagnosis of body image disturbance?

1 "As long as none of my friends find out, I will be fine."
2 "This really won't change my life that much; it is just a different exit for my bowel."
3 "I will go to the ostomy support group to learn how to make things easier."
4 "I can work hard to regulate ostomy movements so I can get rid of this bag."

Answer: 3

Rationale: The client's statement reflects acceptance of a changed body image by participation in the support group. The other options reflect denial to some extent, embarrassment, and the desire to hide the change in body image.

Test-Taking Strategy: The desired outcome for altered body image is acceptance; therefore, look for the option that most closely reflects acceptance. Option 3 is the only option that reflects acceptance!

Level of Cognitive Ability: Analysis
Phase of Nursing Process: Evaluation
Client Needs: Psychosocial Integrity
Content Area: Adult Health/Gastrointestinal

Reference

Wong, D. (1997). *Whaley and Wong's Essentials of pediatric nursing* (5th ed.). St. Louis: Mosby–Year Book, pp. 616, 1214.

102. A client with borderline disorder tells the nurse that he or she is going to "put an end to my misery." Which of the following would be the most effective response by the nurse evaluating the seriousness of the client's statement?

1 "We all feel like that at times."
2 "Why do you feel like you need to say that?"
3 "Can you tell me more about what you plan to do?"
4 "You feel like that now, but soon you'll regain your will to live."

Answer: 3

Rationale: All suicidal threats must be taken seriously, and their meaning must be thoroughly explored. Options 1 and 4 devalue the client. Option 2 is incorrect because "why" questions are demeaning and make the client feel belittled and filled with guilt.

Test-Taking Strategy: Identify the communication blocks. Devaluing the client should be avoided, as should making him or her feel guilty. Always reflect and focus on client's feeling. If you had difficulty with this question, take time now to review therapeutic communication techniques!

Level of Cognitive Ability: Application
Phase of Nursing Process: Evaluation
Client Needs: Psychosocial Integrity
Content Area: Mental Health

Reference

Antai-Otong, D. (1995). *Psychiatric nursing: Biological and behavioral concepts.* Philadelphia: W. B. Saunders, p. 343.

103. The home health nurse has instructed the client in safety measures for using oxygen in the home. The nurse would evaluate that the client has not fully understood the directions if the client verbalized that he or she will

1 Keep the oxygen concentrator slightly away from the walls or corners of the room.
2 Use an electric razor while wearing the oxygen.
3 Follow the oxygen prescription exactly.
4 Forbid smoking or open flames within 10 feet of the oxygen source.

Answer: 2

Rationale: The use of electric razors or other equipment that could emit sparks should be avoided while oxygen is in use. This could result in fire and injury to the client. The oxygen concentrator is kept slightly away from the walls and corners to permit adequate air flow. The client should follow the oxygen prescription exactly. The client should not allow smoking or any type of flame within 10 feet of the oxygen source.

Test-Taking Strategy: The major hazard associated with oxygen is ignition, which could result from heat in the form of flame, or spark. From this perspective, option 3 is safe and is eliminated first. Options 1 and 4 also control heat and flame, respectively, and are also eliminated. This leaves option 2 as the answer, because an electric razor could emit a spark, which could ignite the oxygen.

Level of Cognitive Ability: Analysis
Phase of Nursing Process: Evaluation
Client Needs: Safe, Effective Care Environment
Content Area: Fundamental Skills

Reference

Taylor, C., Lillis, C., & LeMone, P. (1997). *Fundamentals of nursing: The art and science of nursing care* (3rd ed.). Philadelphia: Lippincott-Raven, p. 1344.

104. The most appropriate outcome for effective pain management in a 6-year-old child is

1 The child will be free of restlessness, irritability, and disturbed sleep.
2 The child will request pain medication only when needed.
3 The child will use imagery and relaxation when perceiving pain.
4 The child will state that it only hurts a little or not at all.

Answer: 4

Rationale: Children of early school age can accurately describe pain in simple terms. Pain is subjective, so a statement from the client is the best indication of relief. Options with only objective data or inappropriate expectations for this age are incorrect.

Test-Taking Strategy: Use your knowledge of the nursing process to eliminate option 3 because it is not such a measurable outcome. Your nursing experience with pain can eliminate option 1 because these are objective signs, and pain is subjective. Option 2 is not appropriate because of the client's age. This leaves option 4, which is age-appropriate and a specific, observable outcome.

Level of Cognitive Ability: Analysis
Phase of Nursing Process: Evaluation
Client Needs: Physiological Integrity
Content Area: Child Health

Reference

Ball, J., & Bindler, R. (1995). *Pediatric nursing: Caring for children.* Stamford, CT: Appleton & Lange, pp. 184–186.

---

105. The client has a nursing diagnosis of Ineffective Individual Coping related to decreased activity tolerance and secondary to respiratory disease. The home care nurse would evaluate that the client is showing an adaptive response if which of the following behaviors was observed?

1. Tries to increase ambulation and completion of small tasks each day
2. Secludes self in one room of the home to decrease fatigue
3. States that appetite is decreased.
4. Has increased use of medication to aid in sleep

Answer: 1

Rationale: The client with pulmonary disease may have Ineffective Individual Coping related to inability to tolerate activity and work and to social isolation. The client demonstrates adaptive responses by increasing the activity to the highest level possible before symptoms are triggered, using relaxation or other learned coping skills, or enrolling in a pulmonary rehabilitation program. Enhancing one's own seclusion, anorexia, and insomnia are not adaptive responses.

Test-Taking Strategy: This question asks you to select a healthy coping response. Anorexia and insomnia are therefore eliminated first because they are maladaptive responses. Although seclusion in a single room (option 2) may minimize fatigue, it is likely to have a negative effect on morale and coping skills over time. On the other hand, active participation in ambulation and activities of daily living will have the two-fold benefit of increasing endurance and helping the client feel more in control of his or her own health. This makes option 1 preferable to option 2.

Level of Cognitive Ability: Analysis
Phase of Nursing Process: Evaluation
Client Needs: Health Promotion and Maintenance
Content Area: Adult Health/Respiratory

Reference

Smeltzer, S., & Bare, B. (1996). *Brunner and Suddarth's Textbook of medical-surgical nursing* (8th ed.). Philadelphia: Lippincott-Raven, p. 515.

---

106. Which statement of first-time parents demonstrates adequate knowledge of an infant's nutritional needs?

1. "Whole milk can be given by bottle at 6 months or in a cup at 9 months."
2. "Rice cereal should be introduced in the second month and add a new grain weekly."
3. "Breast milk or infant formula is all that is needed for the first 6 months."
4. "Babies need feedings every 2 to 3 hours for 8 to 10 months."

Answer: 3

Rationale: Human milk or formula provides all the nutrients required for growth for the first 6 months. Whole milk is not recommended for the first year. Cereals and baby food are not recommended before 4 to 6 months because they are difficult to digest and may lead to allergies. Frequency of feeding is individual, the average being every 4 to 6 hours by the age of 6 months.

Test-Taking Strategy: Notice the key word "adequate" in the stem. Even if you were unfamiliar with the information on infant nutrition, the information in option 3 is the only response inclusive enough to be considered adequate and is therefore the best choice. If you had difficulty with this question, take time now to review infant nutrition!

Level of Cognitive Ability: Analysis
Phase of Nursing Process: Evaluation
Client Needs: Health Promotion and Maintenance
Content Area: Child Health

Reference

Ashwill, J., & Droske, S. (1997). *Nursing care of children: Principles and practice.* Philadelphia: W. B. Saunders, pp. 272–273, 276.

107. The nurse is caring for a client receiving tranylcypromine (Parnate), 30 mg PO BID. Which of the following statements, if made by the client, indicates that health teaching has been successful?

1 "I need sunscreen when I go in the sun."
2 "I must avoid mouthwashes and gargles."
3 "I can no longer eat cheese pizza."
4 "I need to increase my salt intake."

Answer: 3

Rationale: Clients who are taking monoamine oxidase inhibitors (MAOIs) must maintain a low-tyramine diet and receive health teaching regarding the food, beverage, and medication restrictions that must be avoided. Foods with aged cheese are responsible for 80% of all hypertensive crises associated with MAOIs.

Test-Taking Strategy: Knowledge of medications and side effects is necessary to assist you in answering this question. If you know that Parnate is an MAOI, you would select this option. If you are unfamiliar with the medication addressed in this question and this classification of antidepressants, it is important to review them now!

Level of Cognitive Ability: Application
Phase of Nursing Process: Evaluation
Client Needs: Health Promotion and Maintenance
Content Area: Pharmacology

Reference

Varcarolis, E. M. (1998). *Foundations of psychiatric mental health nursing* (3rd ed.). Philadelphia: W. B. Saunders, pp. 573, 576.

108. One week after teaching the client about the relationship of the intake of large amounts of alcohol to liver cancer, the nurse visits the home health client. The nurse evaluates whether the teaching from the last visit was effective by asking what the client remembers from the last nursing visit. The client responds, "You said I can never have another drink." The nurse evaluates that

1 The client understood what was taught.
2 The client understood but reinforcement is necessary.
3 The client needs clarification and reinforcement.
4 The client should never drink again.

Answer: 3

Rationale: Large quantities of alcohol have been associated with increased risk of liver cancer. However, the client understood that no alcohol may be consumed. Thus the client requires reinforcement that alcohol is the substance associated with liver cancer; however, clarification is needed that it is excessive intake that is associated with liver cancer.

Test-Taking Strategy: The issue of the question is large amounts of alcohol. This should assist in eliminating option 4. Focus on the client's statement. The statement indicates the need for additional teaching. Option 3 is the correct choice.

Level of Cognitive Ability: Analysis
Phase of Nursing Process: Evaluation
Client Needs: Health Promotion and Maintenance
Content Area: Adult Health/Gastrointestinal

Reference

Smeltzer, S., & Bare, B. (1996). *Brunner and Suddarth's Textbook of medical-surgical nursing* (8th ed.). Philadelphia: Lippincott-Raven, p. 273.

109. A client with Addison's disease has been instructed on follow-up care to avoid complications. The nurse evaluates that teaching was effective when the client verbalizes that he or she will avoid

1 Salty food.
2 Snacks between meals.
3 Taking corticosteroids.
4 Becoming dehydrated.

Answer: 4

Rationale: Decreased aldosterone secretion results in fluid volume deficit. Clients are encouraged to maintain an oral intake of 3000 mL per day to avoid dehydration. Clients require a high-sodium diet to replace losses. Snacks between meals are encouraged, to prevent hypoglycemia. Clients with Addison's disease require hormone replacement therapy with corticosteroids.

Test-Taking Strategy: Beware of the key word "avoid" in the stem. Use knowledge related to Addison's disease to eliminate options and answer the question. If you had difficulty with this question, take time now to review Addison's disease. You will surely find questions related to this content in NCLEX-RN!

Level of Cognitive Ability: Analysis
Phase of Nursing Process: Evaluation
Client Needs: Health Promotion and Maintenance
Content Area: Adult Health/Endocrine

Reference

LeMone, P., & Burke, K. M. (1996). *Medical-surgical nursing: Critical thinking in client care.* Menlo Park, CA: Addison-Wesley, p. 699.

---

110. A client with aldosteronism has been instructed on spironolactone (Aldactone) treatment. Which of the following evaluative statements indicates that the client needs further teaching?

1 "This medication will make me void frequently."
2 "This medication will decrease my blood sugar."
3 "My blood pressure should get back to normal."
4 "My plasma potassium should increase."

Answer: 2

Rationale: Aldactone does not lower blood glucose. Aldactone counteracts the effect of aldosterone and promotes sodium and water excretion, decreases circulating volume, and therefore decreases blood pressure and inhibits the excretion of potassium.

Test-Taking Strategy: A key word in the stem is "needs further instruction." Knowledge that this medication is a potassium-sparing diuretic will assist in eliminating option 4. Knowledge that the medication also is prescribed for blood pressure control will assist in eliminating options 1 and 3. If you had difficulty with this question, take time now to review this important diuretic!

Level of Cognitive Ability: Analysis
Phase of Nursing Process: Evaluation
Client Needs: Physiological Integrity
Content Area: Pharmacology

Reference

Hodgson, B., & Kizior, R. (1998). *Saunders nursing drug handbook 1998.* Philadelphia: W. B. Saunders, pp. 942–944.

---

111. The nurse has completed discharge teaching with the family of a client who is to have enteral feedings at home. Which method of evaluation should the nurse use to best determine the family's competence in performing the feeding procedure?

1 Return demonstration of the feeding procedure
2 Selection of appropriate equipment for the feeding procedure
3 Written testing on the steps of the feeding procedure
4 Verbal description of the feeding procedure by each member of the family

Answer: 1

Rationale: Return demonstration is the most reliable evaluation of procedure performance. Selection of equipment is included in a return demonstration. Written testing is not useful for performance testing of procedures. Verbal description does not allow the nurse to observe the psychomotor skill needed to perform the procedure.

Test-Taking Strategy: Similar words are found in the question and option. "Performing" in the question and "demonstration" in the option indicate action. Option 2 is contained within option 1. Options 3 and 4 do not involve procedure performance.

Level of Cognitive Ability: Analysis
Phase of Nursing Process: Evaluation
Client Needs: Health Promotion and Maintenance
Content Area: Fundamental Skills

Reference

Burrell, P., Gerlach, M., & Pless, S. (1997). *Adult nursing: Acute and community care* (2nd ed.). Stamford, CT: Appleton & Lange, p. 1349.

---

112. The nurse has completed diet teaching for a client on a low-sodium diet for hypertension. The nurse evaluates that further teaching is necessary when the client makes which of these statements?

1 "This diet will help to lower my blood pressure."
2 "The reason I need lower salt intake is to reduce fluid retention."
3 "This diet is not a replacement for my antihypertensive medications."
4 "Frozen dinners are an important part of a low-sodium diet."

Answer: 4

Rationale: A low-sodium diet is used as an adjunct to antihypertensive medications for the treatment of hypertension. High sodium levels cause fluid retention, which leads to hypertension secondary to increased fluid volume. Frozen dinners contain salt as a preservative and should not be encouraged as part of a low-sodium diet.

Test-Taking Strategy: The direction of the question stem, "further teaching is necessary," is to seek the incorrect answer. Option 1 presents a term ("blood pressure") similar to that found in the case situation ("hypertension"). Option 2 addresses the relationship of low salt and reducing fluid retention. With option 3, remember that lifelong medication is necessary in the treatment of hypertension. Options 1, 2, and 3 are correct. Only option 4 is incorrect. Review low-sodium diets now if you had difficulty with this question!

Level of Cognitive Ability: Analysis
Phase of Nursing Process: Evaluation
Client Needs: Health Promotion and Maintenance
Content Area: Fundamental Skills

Reference

Mahan, L., & Escott-Stump, S. (1996). *Krause's Food, nutrition, and diet therapy* (9th ed.). Philadelphia: W. B. Saunders, p. 561.

---

113. The nurse teaches a client with Addison's disease about the signs of Addisonian crisis. The nurse evaluates that teaching was effective when the client states that which of the following is a sign of this crisis?

1 Profuse diaphoresis
2 Severe agitation
3 Malignant hypertension
4 Sudden, profound weakness

Answer: 4

Rationale: Addison's crisis is a serious, life-threatening response to acute adrenal insufficiency that is most commonly precipitated by a major stressor. The client with Addisonian crisis may have any of the symptoms of Addison's disease, but the primary problems are sudden, profound weakness; severe abdominal, back, and leg pain; hyperpyrexia followed by hypothermia; peripheral vascular collapse; coma; and renal shutdown.

Test-Taking Strategy: Knowledge of adrenal gland function can be used to select the correct answer. Because adrenal hormones are used to fight stress and maintain fluid volume balance, an acute loss of these hormones will produce severe weakness. If you had difficulty with this question, take time to now to review the signs of Addisonian crisis!

Level of Cognitive Ability: Application
Phase of Nursing Process: Evaluation
Client Needs: Psychosocial Integrity
Content Area: Adult Health/Endocrine

Reference

Polaski, A., & Tatro, S. (1996). *Luckmann's Core principles and practice of medical-surgical nursing.* Philadelphia: W. B. Saunders, p. 1235.

---

114. The nurse is conducting a home visit to a mother and infant 1 week post partum. The home health nurse concludes that the infant should be evaluated for congenital neonatal syphilis if which of the following neonatal symptoms is observed at this time?

1 Irregular heart rate with no episodes of apnea
2 Hypothermia and loose stools
3 High-pitched cry and rigorous feeding habits
4 A copper-colored maculopapular dermal rash on the palms of the hands, soles of the feet, mouth, and anal areas

Answer: 4

Rationale: Signs of congenital neonatal syphilis may be nonspecific at first and include poor feedings, slight hyperthermia, and "snuffles." *Snuffles* refers to copious, clear serosanguineous mucus discharge from the nose. By the end of the first week, a copper-colored maculopapular dermal rash is characteristically observed on the palms of the hands, soles of the feet, and around the mouth and anus.

Test-Taking Strategy: The correct response demonstrates the home care nurse's ability to analyze the symptoms presented by the newborn and evaluate findings on the basis of appropriate knowledge of the manifestations of congenital neonatal syphilis. Knowledge of these signs guides you to eliminate each of the incorrect options in turn. If you had difficulty with this question, take time now to review the signs of congenital neonatal syphilis.

Level of Cognitive Ability: Analysis
Phase of Nursing Process: Evaluation
Clients Needs: Physiological Integrity
Content Area: Child Health

Reference

Lowdermilk, D., Perry, S., & Bobak, I. (1997). *Maternity and women's health care* (6th ed.). St. Louis: Mosby–Year Book, p. 1087.

115. The client with chronic atrial fibrillation is being started on quinidine sulfate (Quinidex Extentabs) as maintenance therapy for dysrhythmia suppression. The nurse would evaluate that the client needs further instruction about this medication if the client stated that he or she would

1. Take the dose at the same times each day.
2. Avoid chewing the sustained-release tablets.
3. Take the medication with food if gastrointestinal (GI) upset occurred.
4. Stop taking the prescribed digoxin (Lanoxin) after starting this new medication.

Answer: 4

Rationale: Medication-specific teaching points for quinidine include taking the medication exactly as prescribed; not chewing the sustained-release tablets; taking with food if GI upset occurs; carrying identification describing medication regimen; and receiving periodic checks of heart rhythm and blood counts. This medication is started for atrial flutter or fibrillation only after the client is digitalized.

Test-Taking Strategy: Options 1 and 2 are good general instructions for medication use and are therefore eliminated first. If you can't choose between options 3 and 4, look at the wording of the latter. It is not usual practice to "stop taking" a "prescribed" medication. This would lead you to choose option 4 as the answer.

Level of Cognitive Ability: Analysis
Phase of Nursing Process: Evaluation
Client Needs: Health Promotion and Maintenance
Content Area: Pharmacology

Reference

Karch, A. (1997). *1997 Lippincott's nursing drug guide.* Philadelphia: Lippincott-Raven, p. 943.

---

116. The client with insertion of an automatic internal cardioverter-defibrillator (AICD) has received directions about managing the circumstances surrounding device activation. The nurse would evaluate that the client needs further instruction if the client made which of the following statements?

1. "I should sit or lie down if I feel dizzy or faint, so I won't fall if the AICD fires."
2. "I should take an extra dose of antidysrhythmic medication the day after the AICD is activated."
3. "I should contact my doctor before going out of town so I can plan access to health care if I need it."
4. "I should tell the emergency medical technicians at the fire department about the device, so they will know what to do if they are called."

Answer: 2

Rationale: Typical discharge instructions after AICD implantation include reporting to the physician symptoms indicating dysrhythmias, such as fainting, blackouts, rapid pulse, weakness, or nausea. The physician may want to be called each time the device discharges. At a minimum, the client should keep a log, recording date, time, symptoms, and activity before the shock; number of shocks delivered; and how the client felt afterward. The physician will use this information in managing the ongoing medication regimen. The community emergency medical system (EMS) should be notified about the device, so they are prepared if they are called to the home. Contingency plans for health care should be made before travel. The family should also become trained in cardiopulmonary resuscitation (CPR).

Test-Taking Strategy: If you are unfamiliar with this content, you can nonetheless answer this question by looking at the plausibility of each answer. Each of them makes sense, with the exception of option 2. Clients are not generally advised to independently change their medication dosages or timing on the basis of symptoms, especially with medications that are so vital to the client's health.

Level of Cognitive Ability: Analysis
Phase of Nursing Process: Evaluation
Client Needs: Physiological Integrity
Content Area: Adult Health/Cardiovascular

Reference

Ignatavicius, D. D., Workman, M. L., & Mishler, M. A. (1995). *Medical-surgical nursing: A nursing process approach* (2nd ed.). Philadelphia: W. B. Saunders, p. 886.

117. Which of the following statements, if made by the parents of a child with congenital hypothyroidism, indicates the need for further instructions?

1 "Giving my child levothyroxine (Synthroid) for this disorder may help prevent further damage."
2 "If my child is not getting enough medicine, he or she will probably be more tired and sleepy."
3 "I will check my child's pulse on a daily basis to observe for signs of medication overdose."
4 "The only reason this could have happened to my child is that I took asthma medicine while I was pregnant."

Answer: 4

Rationale: Congenital hypothyroidism may have a number of etiologies and can be either permanent or transient. Congenital hypothyroidism may be caused by an embryonic defect in the development or placement of the thyroid gland or by inborn errors of thyroid hormone synthesis, secretion, or use. Genetic counseling may be needed because an inborn error of thyroid hormone synthesis is an autosomal recessive trait. Transient primary hypothyroidism is often caused by a maternal ingestion of medication during pregnancy such as iodides for asthma, antithyroid drugs, or maternal antibodies.

Test-Taking Strategy: The word "only" in option 4 is an absolute term that should warn you that it is an incorrect statement. Be careful with this type of question and read it carefully; otherwise, it can easily confuse you. Read each statement and eliminate the answers that are accurate statements made by the client. If you had difficulty with this question, take time now to review the causes of congenital hypothyroidism!

Level of Cognitive Ability: Analysis
Phase of Nursing Process: Evaluation
Client Needs: Physiological Integrity
Content Area: Child Health

Reference

Wong, D. (1997). *Whaley and Wong's Essentials of pediatric nursing* (5th ed.). St. Louis: Mosby–Year Book, p. 277.

118. The nurse uses the proverb "While the cat's away, the mice will play!" to evaluate for abstract thinking ability in a schizophrenic client. Which of the following client responses demonstrates appropriate abstract thinking?

1 "Cats and mice don't play. They fight."
2 "I don't have a cat."
3 "When the boss is gone, everyone relaxes in the office."
4 "When the cat is gone, then the mice can get the cheese."

Answer: 3

Rationale: Often seen in response to simple proverbs, symbolism is the ability to abstract meaning from a situation. Responses may be inappropriate because words are interpreted literally (concretely) rather than abstractly. The schizophrenic has difficulty with concreteness and symbolism. Thinking is characterized by being overly symbolic as well as overly concrete.

Test-Taking Strategy: The question asks you to select the response that indicates that the client is perceiving reality and relationships accurately. Look for the response that is an accurate statement of what people do and how they act in the real world: for example, ability to make accurate progression from the concrete images of "cat" and "mice playing" to the concepts of authority and relationships. Also note that option 3 is different from the others.

Level of Cognitive Ability: Analysis
Phase of Nursing Process: Evaluation
Client Needs: Psychosocial Integrity
Content Area: Mental Health

Reference

Carson, V., & Arnold, E. (1996). *Mental health nursing: The nurse-patient journey.* Philadelphia: W. B. Saunders, p. 739.

119. A drug-addicted male newborn is ready for discharge. The infant has been in the hospital for 2 weeks in withdrawal. The nurse observes the infant to evaluate the outcomes of the plan of care. Which of the following observations indicates that the infant is adjusting to life without drugs?

1. Face is calm, eyes are open, and infant is looking into caregiver's face
2. Color changes when infant is exposed to noise
3. Spits up, hiccups, and frequently sneezes when exposed to bright light
4. Weight loss every other day

Answer: 1

Rationale: An infant who is adjusting to drug withdrawal is calm and quiet and interacts with caregivers and parents. If the infant remains distressed by light or noise, or if the infant is not exhibiting weight gain appropriate for healthy infants, the problem of drug addiction is not resolved.

Test-Taking Strategy: This question asks you to evaluate the infant's outcome on the basis of the problem of drug addiction. In order to make a judgment, review the needs and problems of a drug-addicted infant. Eliminate the options that show signs of failure or the client's inability to control him- or herself or the environment. If you had difficulty with this question, take time to review resolved drug addiction in a newborn!

Level of Cognitive Ability: Analysis
Phase of Nursing Process: Evaluation
Client Needs: Physiological Integrity
Content Area: Child Health

Reference

Ashwill, J., & Droske, S. (1997). *Nursing care of children: Principles and practice.* Philadelphia: W. B. Saunders, pp. 575–576.

---

120. Which of the following statements indicates that a client with Addison's disease knows how to safely manage a medication regimen that consists of daily doses of glucocorticoids?

1. "I will need to call my doctor for an increase in medication dose when I'm experiencing a lot of stress."
2. "I should stop my medication if I begin to experience any unpleasant side effects."
3. "The medication I am taking is very safe and causes only a few minor side effects."
4. "If I'm nauseated and can't take my medicine for a few days, I can do without it."

Answer: 1

Rationale: The client with Addison's disease will require lifelong replacement of adrenal hormones. The medications must be taken daily, and an alternative route of administration must be used if the client cannot take oral medications for any reason, such as nausea and vomiting. Additional doses of glucocorticoids will be needed during times of acute stress. The nurse must emphasize to the client that the client must call the physician to get a dosage increase when experiencing stressful situations. Abrupt withdrawal of this medication can result in Addisonian crisis. Although side effects are not severe at lower doses, side effects may be experienced with glucocorticoid administration. It is very unsafe to stop taking the medication without first consulting the physician.

Test-Taking Strategy: To answer this question correctly, you must recall and apply information about glucocorticoids and the stress response. The correct option makes the correlation between stress and the increased need of corticosteroids. If you had difficulty with this question, take time now to review glucocorticoids.

Level of Cognitive Ability: Analysis
Phase of Nursing Process: Evaluation
Client Needs: Physiological Integrity
Content Area: Pharmacology

Reference

Polaski, A., & Tatro, S. (1996). *Luckmann's Core principles and practice of medical-surgical nursing.* Philadelphia: W. B. Saunders, p. 1235.

121. A perinatal client with a history of heart disease has been instructed on care at home. Which of the following statements, if made by the client, would indicate that the client understands her needs?

1 "There is no restriction on people who visit me."
2 "I should avoid stressful situations."
3 "My weight gain is not important."
4 "I should rest on my right side."

Answer: 2

Rationale: To avoid infections, visitors with active infections should not be allowed to visit the client. Stress causes increased heart workload. Too much weight gain causes an increase in body requirements and in stress on the heart. Resting should be on the left side to promote blood return.

Test-Taking Strategy: Avoid absolute terminology such as in options 1 and 3, in which "no" and "not" are used. Knowledge regarding blood return during pregnancy would assist in eliminating option 4. If you had difficulty with this question, take time now to review the perinatal client with heart disease!

Level of Cognitive Ability: Analysis
Phase of Nursing Process: Evaluation
Client Needs: Health Promotion and Maintenance
Content Area: Maternity

Reference

Pillitteri, A. (1995). *Maternal and child health nursing: Care of the childbearing and childrearing family* (2nd ed.). Philadelphia: Lippincott-Raven, pp. 353–355.

122. The client began taking amantadine (Symmetrel) approximately 2 weeks ago. The nurse would evaluate that the medication was having a therapeutic effect if the client exhibited decreased

1 White blood cell count.
2 Voiding.
3 Rigidity and akinesia.
4 Blood pressure.

Answer: 3

Rationale: Amantadine is an antiparkinson agent that potentiates the action of dopamine in the central nervous system (CNS). The expected effect of therapy is a decrease in akinesia and in rigidity. Leukopenia, urinary retention, and hypotension are all adverse effects of the medication.

Test-Taking Strategy: Begin to answer this question by recalling that this medication is used to treat Parkinson's disease. This would lead you to choose option 3 as the expected effects of the medication. Thorough knowledge of the medication reinforces that the other options are incorrect, because they are all side effects of the medication. Review this medication now if you had difficulty with this question!

Level of Cognitive Ability: Analysis
Phase of Nursing Process: Evaluation
Client Needs: Physiological Integrity
Content Area: Pharmacology

Reference

Hodgson, B., & Kizior, R. (1998). *Saunders nursing drug handbook 1998.* Philadelphia: W. B. Saunders, pp. 35–37.

123. The client suspected of bone metastasis is scheduled for a bone scan. The nurse would evaluate that the client understands the elements of follow-up care if the client states that he or she will

1 Report any feelings of nausea or flushing.
2 Ambulate at least three times before the end of the day.
3 Eat only small meals for the remainder of the day.
4 Drink plenty of water for a day or two after the procedure.

Answer: 4

Rationale: There are no special restrictions after a bone scan. The client is encouraged to drink large amounts of water for 24–48 hours to flush the radioisotope from the system. There are no hazards to the client or staff from the minimal amount of radioactivity of the isotope.

Test-Taking Strategy: There is no therapeutic purpose for options 2 or 3, which allows you to eliminate them first. Nausea and flushing could accompany dye injection during a procedure, but this procedure uses radioisotopes and the question relates to care after the procedure; thus this option is also eliminated. The only option left is pushing fluids, which will hasten elimination of the isotope from the client's system.

Level of Cognitive Ability: Analysis
Phase of Nursing Process: Evaluation
Client Needs: Physiological Integrity
Content Area: Adult Health/Oncology

Reference

Black, J., & Matassarin-Jacobs, E. (1997). *Medical-surgical nursing: Clinical management for continuity of care* (5th ed.). Philadelphia: W. B. Saunders, p. 2094.

---

124. The nurse is evaluating the pin sites of a client in skeletal traction. The nurse would be least concerned with which of the following findings?

1 Purulent drainage
2 Serous drainage
3 Pain at a pin site
4 Inflammation

Answer: 2

Rationale: A small amount of serous oozing is expected at pin insertion sites. Signs of infection such as inflammation, purulent drainage, and pain at the pin site are not expected findings and should be reported to the physician.

Test-Taking Strategy: Options 1 and 4 indicate an infectious problem and are eliminated as answers to be "least concerned with." To discriminate between options 2 and 3, look at them carefully. The complaint of pain is at "a pin site" only. It gives no indication that the pain is related to the fracture or muscle spasm. Because serous drainage is an expected finding, you would choose this over the complaint of pain as the answer to the question.

Level of Cognitive Ability: Analysis
Phase of Nursing Process: Evaluation
Client Needs: Physiological Integrity
Content Area: Adult Health/Musculoskeletal

Reference

Smeltzer, S., & Bare, B. (1996). *Brunner and Suddarth's Textbook of medical-surgical nursing* (8th ed.). Philadelphia: Lippincott-Raven, p. 1863.

---

125. The nurse has suggested specific leg exercises for the client immobilized in right skeletal lower leg traction. The nurse evaluates that the client needs further instruction if the nurse observes the client

1 Pulling up on the trapeze.
2 Flexing and extending the feet.
3 Performing active range-of-motion (ROM) exercises with the right ankle and knee.
4 Doing quadriceps-setting and gluteal-setting exercises.

Answer: 3

Rationale: Exercise within therapeutic limits is indicated for the client in skeletal traction to maintain muscle strength and range of motion. The client may pull up on the trapeze, perform active ROM exercises with uninvolved joints, and do isometric muscle-setting exercises (such as quadriceps- and gluteal-setting exercises). The client may also flex and extend the feet.

Test-Taking Strategy: Options 1 and 4 are most easily identified as correct actions and are therefore eliminated as possible answers to this question. To discriminate between options 2 and 3, imagine the lines of pull on the fracture site with the movements described. Whereas flexing and extending the feet do not disrupt the line of pull from the traction, performing active ROM exercises with the affected knee and ankle does. Thus, active ROM exercises are the answer to the question, which is seeking an item that is an incorrect action.

Level of Cognitive Ability: Analysis
Phase of Nursing Process: Evaluation
Client Needs: Physiological Integrity
Content Area: Adult Health/Musculoskeletal

Reference

Smeltzer, S., & Bare, B. (1996). *Brunner and Suddarth's Textbook of medical-surgical nursing* (8th ed.). Philadelphia: Lippincott-Raven, p. 1863.

126. An insulin-dependent client is visited at home by the community health nurse. The client takes NPH insulin every morning and checks the blood glucose level four times per day. The client tells the nurse that yesterday, the late afternoon blood glucose level was 60 mg/dL and that he or she felt funny. Which statement by the client would indicate an understanding of this occurrence?

1 "My blood sugars are running low because I'm tired."
2 "I forgot to take my usual afternoon snack yesterday."
3 "I took less insulin this morning so I won't feel funny today."
4 "I don't know why I have to check my blood sugar four times a day. That seems too much."

Answer: 2

Rationale: Hypoglycemia is a blood glucose level of 60 mg/dL or less. The causes are multiple, but in this case, omitting the afternoon snack is the only appropriate conclusion drawn from the case. Fatigue and self-adjustment of dose are incorrect options. Recommended frequency of blood glucose testing for insulin-dependent diabetics is four times a day.

Test-Taking Strategy: The stem of the question seeks for a cause of this occurrence. Option 4 does not identify a cause but rather questions an action. Option 3 is a treatment, not a cause, and option 1 is an illogical conclusion; fatigue does not cause hypoglycemia. If you had difficulty with this question, take time now to review the causes of hypoglycemia!

Level of Cognitive Ability: Analysis
Phase of Nursing Process: Evaluation
Client Needs: Physiological Integrity
Content Area: Adult Health/Endocrine

Reference

Black, J., & Matassarin-Jacobs, E. (1997). *Medical-surgical nursing: Clinical management for continuity of care* (5th ed.). Philadelphia: W. B. Saunders, p. 1988.

---

127. The community health nurse visits the client at home with a diagnosis of primary hyperparathyroidism. Which of the following statements, if made by the client, indicates that the client has a knowledge deficit regarding the treatment of this condition?

1 "I take the diuretic every day because it helps get rid of the extra calcium in my blood."
2 "I'm not feeling so sad now as I used to before I started the medication."
3 "I urinate frequently, so I only take half of my fluid pill."
4 "I love milk shakes with ice cream, but I guess I can't have that as much now."

Answer: 3

Rationale: Medical management of hyperparathyroidism includes increasing urinary calcium excretion with diuretics. Option 1 reflects the client's knowledge of this, whereas option 3 does not. Option 4 identifies high-calcium foods, which would need to be limited, and option 2 identifies psychosocial manifestations of hyperparathyroidism, which diminish as serum calcium levels are lowered with treatment.

Test-Taking Strategy: Knowledge of diuretic and diet therapy as well as of clinical manifestations of hyperparathyroidism is necessary to assist you in answering the question. However, the correct answer reflects a client-generated change in the medication regimen. This should never be done without first consulting the physician. Thus this would be a good selection if you were unsure.

Level of Cognitive Ability: Analysis
Phase of Nursing Process: Evaluation
Client Needs: Health Promotion and Maintenance
Content Area: Adult Health/Endocrine

Reference

Black, J., & Matassarin-Jacobs, E. (1997). *Medical-surgical nursing: Clinical management for continuity of care* (5th ed.). Philadelphia: W. B. Saunders, pp. 2031, 2033.

128. The nurse caring for a client with hypoparathyroidism evaluates achievement of the expected outcomes. Which of the following would be an appropriate expected outcome of nursing care for this client?

1 The client verbalizes that therapy for hypocalcemia is lifelong
2 The client describes the signs and symptoms of thrombocytopenia
3 The client maintains an ideal body weight
4 The client experiences less protrusion exophthalmos

Answer: 1

Rationale: Clients with hypoparathyroidism experience symptoms related to hypocalcemia ranging from mild paresthesias to tetany. Options 2, 3, and 4 do not relate to the problem. Treatment for the disorder involves correction of the hypocalcemia and vitamin D deficiency with pharmacological intervention such as calcium chloride and calcitriol. Nurses need to encourage compliance with the prescription regimen as well as teaching the client that treatment for this disorder is lifelong. In addition to pharmacological compliance, they will need to abide by certain dietary guidelines (high calcium, low phosphorus) if the disease is to be controlled.

Test-Taking Strategy: Use the process of elimination. Options 2, 3, and 4 are false and have nothing to do with hypoparathyroidism. On the other hand, option 1 is true because it focuses on the fact that with this disorder, the client must observe certain guidelines such as lifelong dietary management with foods high in calcium and low in phosphate. If you had difficulty with this question, take time now to review the treatment for hypoparathyroidism.

Level of Cognitive Ability: Analysis
Phase of Nursing Process: Evaluation
Client Needs: Physiological Integrity
Content Area: Adult Health/Endocrine

Reference

Ignatavicius, D. D., Workman, M. L., & Mishler, M. A. (1995). *Medical-surgical nursing: A nursing process approach* (2nd ed.). Philadelphia: W. B. Saunders, p. 1854.

---

129. The nurse is caring for a mother receiving betamethasone (Celestone) to prevent neonatal respiratory distress syndrome during premature labor. The nurse evaluates the impact of the medication on the newborn. What evidence in the infant would demonstrate side effects secondary to betamethasone administration?

1 Frequent meconium stools
2 Jaundiced skin
3 Hypoglycemia
4 Irregular sleep patterns

Answer: 3

Rationale: Hypoglycemia in the newborn may suggest hypoadrenalism secondary to betamethasone administration. Betamethasone is a synthetic glucocorticoid. Frequent meconium stools, jaundice, or irregular sleep patterns in an infant would not be related to betamethasone (Celestone) administration, but they could be important symptoms of other difficulties in a newborn.

Test-Taking Strategy: Knowledge of the side effects related to betamethasone is necessary to answer this question. Take time now to review this important medication, if you had difficulty with this question!

Level of Cognitive Ability: Analysis
Phase of Nursing Process: Evaluation
Client Needs: Physiological Integrity
Content Area: Pharmacology

Reference

Hodgson, B., & Kizior, R. (1998). *Saunders nursing drug handbook 1998.* Philadelphia: W. B. Saunders, pp. 107–111.

130. The nurse is evaluating the effectiveness of meperidine hydrochloride (Demerol) for pain management for a laboring client at term. The effectiveness of this medication therapy can be demonstrated by

1. Complete pain relief and a period of rest from labor contractions.
2. Moderate pain relief while a progressive labor pattern continues.
3. Moderate pain relief with increased amounts of bloody show.
4. Contractions that are longer, stronger, and closer together.

Answer: 2

Rationale: Effective pain management during labor does not interrupt the labor process but does provide relaxation and moderate pain relief to the mother. The increased bloody show and the intensity of the contractions are not measures of effective pain management.

Test-Taking Strategy: Use the process of elimination to answer the question. Eliminate options 3 and 4 first because the increased bloody show and intensity of the contractions are not measures of effective pain management. For the remaining two options, the key phrase is "progressive labor pattern continues." This should direct you to the correct option!

Level of Cognitive Ability: Analysis
Phase of Nursing Process: Evaluation
Client Needs: Health Promotion and Maintenance
Content Area: Maternity

Reference

Hodgson, B., & Kizior, R. (1998). *Saunders nursing drug handbook 1998.* Philadelphia: W. B. Saunders, pp. 638–640.

---

131. A nursing priority with a client with a diagnosis of placental abruption is to minimize alterations in fetal tissue perfusion. The nurse recognizes the goal has been met when which of the following is assessed?

1. Decreased fetal heart rate variability
2. Presence of late decelerations
3. Presence of accelerations
4. Evidence of fetal bradycardia

Answer: 3

Rationale: Accelerations are an indication of fetal well-being and an oxygenated central nervous system. Bradycardia, late decelerations, and decreased variability are representative of decreased oxygenation of the fetus. An understanding of the effects of hypoxia on the fetus is necessary.

Test-Taking Strategy: Eliminate options 1, 2, and 4 by knowing that accelerations are an indication of fetal well-being. If you had difficulty with this question, take time now to review bradycardia, late decelerations, and decreased variability!

Level of Cognitive Ability: Analysis
Phase of Nursing Process: Evaluation
Client Needs: Physiological Integrity
Content Area: Maternity

Reference

Gorrie, T. M., McKinney, E. S., & Murray, S. S. (1994). *Foundations of maternal-newborn nursing.* Philadelphia: W. B. Saunders, p. 677.

---

132. The community health nurse visits the family of a 2-year-old boy recently discharged from the hospital after treatment for nephrotic syndrome. Which of the following statements, if made by the parents, indicates that further teaching is needed?

1. "We're preparing his diet the same as before, except being careful not to add salt."
2. "We're monitoring his urine every day for protein and keeping the results in a diary."
3. "We're giving him his prednisone whenever he gains more than a pound a day."
4. "We're keeping him with private babysitters instead of at the day-care center."

Answer: 3

Rationale: Prednisone dosage needs to be maintained at ordered levels and dosage adjustments must be made only by physician. To prevent withdrawal syndrome, doses are gradually reduced, never stopped or started at will.

Test-Taking Strategy: Use the process of elimination. Options 1 and 2 are part of treatment regimen for nephrotic syndrome. Option 4 will reduce the chance of exposure to infection. Option 3 reflects medication dosage adjustment, which should be done only by the physician!

Level of Cognitive Ability: Analysis
Phase of Nursing Process: Evaluation
Client Needs: Health Promotion and Maintenance
Content Area: Child Health

Reference

Ball, J., & Bindler, R. (1995). *Pediatric nursing: Caring for children.* Norwalk, CT: Appleton & Lange, pp. 633–634.

133. Which of the following would not be a component of the plan of care for a child with a head injury?

1. Keep the child in a sitting-up position
2. Force fluids
3. Keep the child awake as much as possible
4. Perform neurological assessment

Answer: 2

Rationale: A child with a head injury is at risk for increased intracranial pressure (ICP). Sitting up will decrease fluid retention in cerebral tissue and promote drainage. Keeping the child awake will assist in accurate evaluation of cerebral edema present and will detect early coma. Increased fluids may cause fluid overload and increased ICP. Neurological assessments need to be performed to monitor for increased ICP.

Test-Taking Strategy: To answer this question correctly, use the process of elimination and knowledge regarding intracranial pressure. Eliminate options 1, 3, and 4 because they are correct in terms of monitoring for and preventing intracranial pressure. Take time now to review measures to prevent intracranial pressure, if you had difficulty with this question!

Level of Cognitive Ability: Analysis
Phase of Nursing Process: Evaluation
Client Needs: Physiological Integrity
Content Area: Child Health

Reference

Ashwill, J. W., & Droske, S. C. (1997). *Nursing care of children: Principles and practice.* Philadelphia: W. B. Saunders, pp. 1261–1262.

---

134. Which of the following diagnostic tests would best indicate that there is a reduction in thyroid hormone secretion and synthesis in the client who is in thyroid storm and is being treated with propylthiouracil (PTU)?

1. Serum thyroid antibodies (TA test)
2. Thyroid scan
3. Serum T_3 and T_4
4. Thyroid stimulation test (TSH stimulation)

Answer: 3

Rationale: PTU is administered to clients in thyroid storm in order to block thyroid hormone synthesis of T_3 and T_4. Thyroid antibodies indicate whether there is an autoimmune disease causing the client's symptoms. A thyroid scan provides information about whether there is excessive or diminished activity present in the gland but does not provide information about the degree of hormone synthesis. The TSH stimulation test differentiates primary from secondary hypothyroidism.

Test-Taking Strategy: Knowledge of the actions of PTU as well as the diagnostic test used to evaluate the effectiveness of the medication will assist you in answering this question. By the process of elimination, you can select the correct response. Options 1, 2, and 4 will not provide information regarding thyroid hormone secretion or synthesis (T_3 and T_4). If you had difficulty with this question, take time now to review these tests!

Level of Cognitive Ability: Analysis
Phase of Nursing Process: Evaluation
Client Needs: Physiological Integrity
Content Area: Adult Health/Endocrine

Reference

Ignatavicius, D. D., Workman, M. L., & Mishler, M. A. (1995). *Medical-surgical nursing: A nursing process approach* (2nd ed.). Philadelphia: W. B. Saunders, pp. 1838–1839.

135. The client has had creation of a neobladder after cystectomy. The nurse evaluates that the client understands how to initiate voiding when the client states that it is necessary to

1 Tighten the external sphincter and relax the abdominal muscles.
2 Tighten the external sphincter and the abdominal muscles.
3 Relax the external sphincter while performing the Valsalva maneuver.
4 Relax the external sphincter and the abdominal muscles.

Answer: 3

Rationale: The client learns to void after creation of a neobladder by relaxing the external sphincter while increasing the intra-abdominal pressure (Valsalva maneuver). If this procedure cannot be accomplished by the client, then the client must learn to do intermittent catheterization of the neobladder.

Test-Taking Strategy: Begin to answer this question by eliminating options 1 and 2 first. A client cannot void effectively by tightening an external sphincter. The external sphincter is normally tight and must be relaxed for urine to pass. You would choose option 3 over option 4 by realizing that force from the Valsalva maneuver is needed to push the urine out of the neobladder.

Level of Cognitive Ability: Analysis
Phase of Nursing Process: Evaluation
Client Needs: Physiological Integrity
Content Area: Adult Health/Renal

Reference

Black, J., & Matassarin-Jacobs, E. (1997). *Medical-surgical nursing: Clinical management for continuity of care* (5th ed.). Philadelphia: W. B. Saunders, pp. 1586–1587.

---

136. The nurse has planned and conducted a stress management seminar for clients in an ambulatory care setting. Which of the following responses, if made by an attendee, would indicate that further instruction is needed?

1 "Biofeedback might be nice, but I don't like the idea of having to use equipment."
2 "I can use guided imagery anywhere and anytime."
3 "The progressive muscle relaxation technique should ease my tension headaches."
4 "Using confrontation with coworkers should solve my problems at work quickly."

Answer: 4

Rationale: Biofeedback, progressive muscle relaxation, meditation, and guided imagery are techniques that the nurse can teach the client to reduce the physical impact of stress on the body and promote a feeling of self-control for the client. Biofeedback entails electronic equipment, whereas the others require no adjuncts, such as tapes, once the technique is learned. Confrontation is a communication technique, not a stress-management technique. It may also exacerbate stress, at least in the short term, rather than alleviate it.

Test-Taking Strategy: The wording of the question guides you to look for an incorrect statement. Read each option carefully. Knowledge of stress management techniques guides you to option 4, which is a communication technique.

Level of Cognitive Ability: Analysis
Phase of Nursing Process: Evaluation
Client Needs: Psychosocial Integrity
Content Area: Mental Health

Reference

Ignatavicius, D. D., Workman, M. L., & Mishler, M. A. (1995). *Medical-surgical nursing: A nursing process approach* (2nd ed.). Philadelphia: W. B. Saunders, p. 114.

137. A client is trying to modify potential risk factors for coronary artery disease. Laboratory screening shows that the total cholesterol level is 183 mg/dL, the low-density lipoprotein (LDL) level is 110 mg/dL, and the high-density lipoprotein (HDL) level is 65 mg/dL. The nurse evaluates that these results

1 Put the client at very high risk for heart disease.
2 Put the client at slight to moderately high risk for heart disease.
3 Put the client at low risk for heart disease.
4 Are inconclusive unless triglyceride level is also screened.

Answer: 3

Rationale: In the absence of documented heart disease, the desired goal is to have total cholesterol level less than 200 mg/dL, LDL values less than 130 mg/dL, and HDL levels higher than 50 mg/dL. In the absence of documented heart disease or significant risk factors, the values listed in the question place the client at low risk for heart disease.

Test-Taking Strategy: The word "potential" before risk factors indicates that the client does not have documented heart disease, so the standard recommended values apply. Knowing that the total cholesterol should be less than 200 mg/dL helps you choose your answer correctly.

Level of Cognitive Ability: Analysis
Phase of Nursing Process: Evaluation
Client Needs: Health Promotion and Maintenance
Content Area: Adult Health/Cardiovascular

Reference
Smeltzer, S., & Bare, B. (1996). *Brunner and Suddarth's Textbook of medical-surgical nursing* (8th ed.). Philadelphia: Lippincott-Raven, p. 640.

---

138. Upon reviewing the health promotion activities of an HIV-infected pregnant mother, the nurse evaluates which factor as problematic for the client?

1 The client has been avoiding contact with friends who have fevers or coughs
2 The client continues to clean the cat litter box once a week only
3 The client states she has avoided eating fish or meats that are uncooked
4 The client has taken prescribed antiviral drugs and prenatal vitamins routinely

Answer: 2

Rationale: Prevention of maternal opportunistic infections during pregnancy for the HIV infected client involves both education and pharmacological prophylaxis, when indicated. Client education includes the need to avoid contact with fish tanks and cat feces or litter, to avoid coming into contact with persons who are ill, and to avoid eating uncooked meats, fish, and unpasteurized dairy products.

Test-Taking Strategy: The correct response involves applying the knowledge of antenatal health promotion to the pregnant woman and evaluating stated behaviors. Options 1, 3, and 4 minimize risks of opportunistic infections for the HIV-positive mother and promote physiological integrity during pregnancy. If you had difficulty with this question, take time now to review these preventive measures!

Level of Cognitive Ability: Application
Phase of Nursing Process: Evaluation
Clients Needs: Health Promotion and Maintenance
Content Area: Maternity

Reference
Nichols, F., & Zwelling, E. (1997). *Maternal-newborn nursing: Theory and practice.* Philadelphia: W. B. Saunders, p. 1500.

139. A client with adult respiratory distress syndrome (ARDS) will be discharged to home with a tracheostomy, which will require suctioning by a family member. Which statement, if made by a family member, would alert the nurse that further teaching about tracheostomy suctioning is needed?

1 "When I am done suctioning the trachea, I can suction the mouth."
2 "I will wait 30 seconds to 1 minute between times that I insert the suction catheter."
3 "I will not apply negative suction over 120 mmHg."
4 "I will leave the suction catheter in place until all the mucus is removed.'

Answer: 4

Rationale: The oropharynx should be suctioned last to prevent introducing oral bacteria into the lung field. Allowing at least 30-second intervals between suctioning times will allow the client to equilibrate. Negative pressure beyond 120 mmHg will damage the mucous membranes. The suction catheter should not be left in the trachea for more than 15 seconds or the client will experience hypoxia.

Test-Taking Strategy: Remember the ABCs: airway, breathing, and circulation. Option 4 suggests that the airway will be blocked and that removal of oxygen will occur at the same time for an extended period. If, however, you had difficulty with this question, be sure to stop and review the principles related to suctioning now. You will surely note questions related to suctioning on NCLEX-RN!

Level of Cognitive Ability: Analysis
Phase of Nursing Process: Evaluation
Client Needs: Physiological Integrity
Content Area: Adult Health/Respiratory

Reference

Lammon, C. B., Foote, A. W., Leli, P. G., et al. (1995). *Clinical nursing skills.* Philadelphia: W. B. Saunders, p. 504.

140. A client is admitted to the labor and delivery suite with intrauterine fetal demise. The nurse evaluates that the discussion with the parents was most effective in preparing them for the delivery when the parents

1 State that they have no questions.
2 Request to hold the infant.
3 Are surprised by the appearance of the infant.
4 Refuse a footprint and picture of the infant to take home.

Answer: 2

Rationale: Holding and viewing the dead infant can help put to rest any negative images the mother or her partner may have fantasized. Providing a picture or other mementos at the time of discharge will help preserve the memory. If the parent refuses a picture, most hospitals will keep a picture and copy of the footprints on file for access by parents later. Parents should be encouraged to verbalize their feelings, ask questions about the process, and make their own decisions about care as much as possible.

Test-Taking Strategy: Use the process of elimination to seek an option that identifies preparedness of the parents for delivery. Option 2 is the option that most clearly identifies this preparedness.

Level of Cognitive Ability: Analysis
Phase of Nursing Process: Evaluation
Client Needs: Psychosocial Integrity
Content Area: Maternity

Reference

Nichols, F., & Zwelling, E. (1997). *Maternal-newborn nursing: Theory and practice.* Philadelphia: W. B. Saunders, p. 903.

141. A client with a pacemaker is being scheduled for a series of tests to determine the presence of an intestinal tumor. The nurse evaluates that preprocedure teaching was effective when the client says

1 "My heartbeat may act up during the x-ray exams."
2 "We will deactivate the pacemaker during the barium enema test."
3 "I will take a nitroglycerin tablet before each test."
4 "I must inform my physician that I have a pacemaker in case an MRI is planned."

Answer: 4

Rationale: Magnetic resonance imaging (MRI) is a test that involves an external magnetic field to visualize soft tissues. Because of the magnetic field, this test is contraindicated in clients with pacemakers because it can reprogram the pacemaker. This information should be given to all clients with pacemakers. Options 1, 2, and 3 are inaccurate.

Test-Taking Strategy: Note the key words "teaching was effective." Option 1 is incorrect because the pacemaker should not cause a problem with heart rate for any GI diagnostic tests except the MRI. Option 2 is incorrect because the barium enema should not affect the pacemaker and a pacemaker would not be deactivated. Option 3 is incorrect because nitroglycerin should not be required before these tests unless chest pain occurs.

Level of Cognitive Ability: Analysis
Phase of Nursing Process: Evaluation
Client Needs: Physiological Integrity
Content Area: Adult Health/Cardiovascular

Reference
Black, J., & Matassarin-Jacobs, E. (1997). *Medical-surgical nursing: Clinical management for continuity of care* (5th ed.). Philadelphia: W. B. Saunders, p. 1713.

---

142. A client who was recently hospitalized for bleeding esophageal varices returns to the clinic for a follow-up visit. The nurse evaluates that more teaching needs to be done when the client says

1 "I no longer eat Mexican foods."
2 "I have not had any alcohol since I was in the hospital."
3 "I've put all my emergency numbers on my speed dial phone."
4 "I've started working out in a gym lifting weights."

Answer: 4

Rationale: Although esophageal varices are caused by portal pressure, rupture of varices may be caused by increased intrathoracic pressure such as coughing and straining. This pressure may occur during heavy weight lifting. Options 1, 2, and 3 indicate understanding of the self-care measures necessary after treatment for bleeding esophageal varices.

Test-Taking Strategy: This question is asking for the inappropriate response. Options 1, 2, and 3 are all important and accurate care issues that the client apparently learned from teaching. Option 4 is the inaccurate statement.

Level of Cognitive Ability: Analysis
Phase of Nursing Process: Evaluation
Client Needs: Health Promotion and Maintenance
Content Area: Adult Health/Gastrointestinal

Reference
Black, J., & Matassarin-Jacobs, E. (1997). *Medical-surgical nursing: Clinical management for continuity of care* (5th ed.). Philadelphia: W. B. Saunders, p. 1884.

---

143. The nurse evaluates that client teaching is effective for a client with a hiatal hernia when the client says

1 "I will lie down to rest right after eating."
2 "I will eat four to six small meals per day."
3 "I will avoid fluids at mealtime."
4 "I have no dietary restrictions."

Answer: 2

Rationale: A major goal of care for the client with a hiatal hernia is to prevent regurgitation and aspiration. The client who is taught to eat four to six small meals a day and practices this will have less food in the stomach and thereby decrease the chances of regurgitation. Lying down to rest right after eating will increase the risk for regurgitation. Fluids should be encouraged to assist food passage. There are dietary restrictions for this disorder.

Test-Taking Strategy: Read the question and options carefully. Use the process of elimination. A recumbent position allows reflux to occur more easily in the client with a hiatal hernia, so option 1 is incorrect. Fluids should be encouraged to assist food passage, so option 3 is incorrect. Although there may be no specific foods to avoid, large meals and alcohol should be avoided. Review teaching points for the client with hiatal hernia now if you had difficulty with this question!

Level of Cognitive Ability: Analysis
Phase of Nursing Process: Evaluation
Client Needs: Health Promotion and Maintenance
Content Area: Adult Health/Gastrointestinal

Reference

Black, J., & Matassarin-Jacobs, E. (1997). *Medical-surgical nursing: Clinical management for continuity of care* (5th ed.). Philadelphia: W. B. Saunders, pp. 1738, 1741.

---

144. The nurse is caring for a client with a peptic ulcer. In assessing the client for gastrointestinal perforation (GI), the nurse will monitor for

1. Increase in bowel sounds.
2. Sudden, severe abdominal pain.
3. Positive guaiac test results.
4. Slow, strong pulses.

Answer: 2

Rationale: Sudden, severe abdominal pain is the most indicative sign of perforation of the intestine. When perforation of an ulcer occurs, the nurse may be unable to auscultate bowel sounds at all. When perforation occurs, the pulse will most likely be weak and rapid. Positive guaiac test results may be obtained from clients with perforation but are also obtained from clients with other disorders.

Test-Taking Strategy: Use the process of elimination and knowledge regarding the signs of perforation. Correlate perforation with sudden, severe abdominal pain. Remember that the nurse may be unable to auscultate bowel sounds and that the pulse will most likely be weak and rapid. Positive guaiac test results are not specific to perforation. If you had difficulty with this question, take time now to review signs of perforation!

Level of Cognitive Ability: Analysis
Phase of Nursing Process: Evaluation
Client Needs: Physiological Integrity
Content Area: Adult Health/Gastrointestinal

Reference

Lewis, S., Collier, I., & Heitkemper, M. (1996). *Medical-surgical nursing: Assessment and management of clinical problems* (4th ed.). St. Louis: Mosby–Year Book, p. 1193.

---

145. A manic client has been hospitalized for 4 weeks and is ready to be discharged. Lithium carbonate (Eskalith) was administered until a therapeutic level was attained, and then it was decreased gradually until a maintenance level of 1.0 mEq/liter was reached. Which of the following client statements indicates that additional teaching about lithium carbonate is needed?

1. "My diet must include adequate salt and liquids."
2. "I need to have blood tests to monitor blood levels of the medication."
3. "I will vary my dose, depending upon how I feel."
4. "I will call my doctor if I vomit or have diarrhea."

Answer: 3

Rationale: The dosage of lithium carbonate needs to remain constant to maintain blood levels between 0.6 and 1.2 mEq/liter. There is a narrow margin between therapeutic and toxic levels. It is necessary to assess blood levels for this narrow range. Adequate salt and fluids are necessary to prevent toxicity. Vomiting and diarrhea could be signs of toxicity and need to be reported. Dosages should never be adjusted.

Test-Taking Strategy: This question should be relatively easy if you read the stem carefully. Clients should never adjust medication dosages. This should direct you toward the correct option. This is an extremely important medication. You are likely to find questions regarding this medication on NCLEX-RN!

Level of Cognitive Ability: Analysis
Phase of Nursing Process: Evaluation
Client Needs: Physiological Integrity
Content Area: Mental Health

Reference

Hodgson, B., & Kizior, R. (1998). *Saunders nursing drug handbook 1998.* Philadelphia: W. B. Saunders, pp. 598–600.

146. The community health nurse visits a client newly discharged after hospitalization for depression. The nurse reviews the client's medication and notes that the client is taking amitriptyline (Elavil). Which of the following statements, if made by the client, indicates the need for further teaching?

1. "I only have to take my medicine once a day."
2. "I chew sugarless gum all the time."
3. "I tend to nod off in the morning after I take my amitriptyline (Elavil)."
4. "I have prunes every other day at breakfast."

Answer: 3

Rationale: Amitriptyline (Elavil) has a sedative effect and a single maintenance dose should be taken at bedtime. This also precludes the need for insomnia medication. All of the other options are clinically appropriate for a client taking Elavil.

Test-Taking Strategy: Read the stem carefully. The question is asking you to analyze which client statement is inappropriate, necessitating the need for further teaching. Knowledge that this medication should be taken at bedtime is necessary to answer the question. If you are unfamiliar with this medication, take time now to review!

Level of Cognitive Ability: Analysis
Phase of Nursing Process: Evaluation
Client Needs: Physiological Integrity
Content Area: Mental Health

Reference

Hodgson, B., & Kizior, R. (1998). *Saunders nursing drug handbook 1998.* Philadelphia: W. B. Saunders, pp. 49–51.

---

147. The community health nurse visits a client newly discharged after a hospitalization for depression. The client is taking 20 mg of tranylcypromine (Parnate) daily. Which of the following statements, if made by the client, indicates the need for further teaching?

1. "I chew sugarless gum all the time."
2. "I take aspirin for headaches."
3. "I eat a low-tyramine diet."
4. "I eat dry crackers if I get nauseated."

Answer: 2

Rationale: Tranylcypromine (Parnate) is a monoamine oxidase inhibitor (MAOI). Clients taking MAOIs should report any headache to the physician because it may signal an impending hypertensive crisis. A low-tyramine diet needs to be consumed. Dry crackers can be eaten if the client becomes nauseated. Chewing sugarless gum is appropriate.

Test-Taking Strategy: Read the stem carefully. This question is asking you to analyze which client statement is inappropriate. Knowledge regarding MAOIs is necessary to answer the question. Review the pharmacology of MAOIs now if you had difficulty with this question. You are likely to find questions related to these medications on NCLEX-RN!

Level of Cognitive Ability: Analysis
Phase of Nursing Process: Evaluation
Client Needs: Health Promotion and Maintenance
Content Area: Mental Health

Reference

Hodgson, B., & Kizior, R. (1998). *Saunders nursing drug handbook 1998.* Philadelphia: W. B. Saunders, pp. 1012–1014.

---

148. Which of the following describes the most positive outcome for a client discharged after an episode of severe depression?

1. The client is able to meet self-care needs and interact socially
2. The client is able to attend outpatient group therapy
3. The client is able to start a new hobby
4. The client is able to comply with medication regimen

Answer: 1

Rationale: All of the items are positive outcomes for a depressed client. Option 1 is the broadest and most specifically related to the abatement of the signs and symptoms of depression. Meeting self-care needs and interacting socially will promote self-esteem.

Test-Taking Strategy: Note that the question asks for the "most" positive outcome. This could indicate that more than one option is correct. Option 1 is the most global response and encompasses the other responses.

Level of Cognitive Ability: Application
Phase of Nursing Process: Evaluation
Client Needs: Psychosocial Integrity
Content Area: Mental Health

Reference

Wilson, H., & Kneisl, C. (1996). *Psychiatric nursing* (5th ed.). Menlo Park, CA: Addison-Wesley, p. 341.

149. The home care nurse is assessing a client who was discharged with mild preeclampsia. Which of the following data indicates that the preeclampsia is not resolving?

1 Blood pressure reading has returned to the prenatal baseline
2 Urinary output has increased
3 The client complains of a daily headache and developed blurred vision this morning
4 There is no evidence of dependent edema

Answer: 3

Rationale: Options 1, 2, and 4 are all signs that the preeclampsia is resolving. Option 3 is a symptom of worsening of the preeclampsia.

Test-Taking Strategy: It is important to note in this question what the question is specifically asking. The stem asks which data does "not" show resolution. From this point, use the process of elimination, identifying the sign that would indicate a concern. If you had difficulty with this question, take time now to review signs of preeclampsia!

Level of Cognitive Ability: Analysis
Phase of Nursing Process: Evaluation
Client Needs: Physiological Integrity
Content Area: Maternity

Reference

Lowdermilk, D., Perry, S., & Bobak, I. (1997). *Maternity and women's health care* (6th ed.). St. Louis: Mosby–Year Book, p. 719.

---

150. In evaluating the client at risk for disseminated intravascular coagulation (DIC), which of the following factors would the nurse consider to be the most significant?

1 A gravida six who delivered 10 hours ago and has lost 450 mL of blood
2 A gravida two in whom dead fetus syndrome has just been diagnosed and fetal demise occurred 2 months ago
3 A primigravida with mild preeclampsia
4 A primigravida who delivered a 10-pound baby 3 hours ago

Answer: 2

Rationale: Hemorrhage is a risk factor with DIC; however, a loss of 450 mL is not considered hemorrhage. Dead fetus syndrome is considered a risk factor for DIC. Severe preeclampsia is considered a risk factor for DIC; a mild case is not. Delivering a large baby is not considered a risk factor for DIC.

Test-Taking Strategy: In answering this question, understanding risk factors of DIC is important. Use the process of elimination and prioritize by focusing on which option is most serious. Eliminate options 1 and 4 first as the least likely risk factors. Eliminate option 3, noting "mild" preeclampsia. If you had difficulty with this question, take time now to review risk factors associated with DIC!

Level of Cognitive Ability: Analysis
Phase of Nursing Process: Evaluation
Client Needs: Physiological Integrity
Content Area: Maternity

Reference

Lowdermilk, D., Perry, S., & Bobak, I. (1997). *Maternity and women's health care* (6th ed.). St. Louis: Mosby–Year Book, p. 792.

---

151. The nurse receives an initial report of a urine culture that identifies the presence of several different organisms. The nurse evaluates that this most likely means

1 The client has a bladder infection.
2 The client has a kidney infection.
3 The specimen was contaminated.
4 The specimen was mishandled in the laboratory.

Answer: 3

Rationale: The presence of multiple organisms in a urine culture usually indicates that contamination has occurred. The urinary tract is normally sterile, and infection, if it occurs, is usually with one organism. A repeat of the urine culture is indicated.

Test-Taking Strategy: The question asks for the "most likely" cause of the culture result. There is no logical reason to assume that the laboratory personnel mishandled the specimen, so this is eliminated as the "most likely" cause. The urine culture will not discriminate between bladder or kidney infection; the clinical picture would help differentiate this. On this basis, select option 3 as the most likely cause of the result. Remember that specimen contamination is the most frequent reason why multiple organisms would be cultured; most urinary tract infections are caused by a single organism, such as *Escherichia coli*.

Level of Cognitive Ability: Analysis
Phase of Nursing Process: Evaluation
Client Needs: Safe, Effective Care Environment
Content Area: Adult Health/Renal

Reference

Black, J., & Matassarin-Jacobs, E. (1997). *Medical-surgical nursing: Clinical management for continuity of care* (5th ed.). Philadelphia: W. B. Saunders, p. 1559.

---

152. The nurse is caring for the client who has undergone renal angiography, with the left femoral artery used for access. The nurse evaluates that the client is experiencing a complication of the procedure if which of the following observations is made?

1 Urine output is 50 mL/hour
2 Absence of hematoma in the left groin
3 Blood pressure is 110/74
4 Pallor and coolness of the left leg

Answer: 4

Rationale: Potential complications after renal angiography include allergic reaction to the dye, renal damage from the dye, and a number of vascular complications, which include hemorrhage, thrombosis, and embolism. The nurse detects these complications by noting signs and symptoms of allergic reaction, decreased urine output, hematoma or hemorrhage at the insertion site, or signs of decreased circulation to the affected leg.

Test-Taking Strategy: Begin to answer this question by eliminating options 1 and 3, because they are normal findings; thus they cannot be complications of this procedure. Because a hematoma is abnormal, "absence of hematoma" is a normal finding, which eliminates option 2 also. Thus option 4 is the answer to the question as stated. This is the only option that has any abnormal clinical findings.

Level of Cognitive Ability: Analysis
Phase of Nursing Process: Evaluation
Client Needs: Physiological Integrity
Content Area: Adult Health/Renal

Reference

Black, J., & Matassarin-Jacobs, E. (1997). *Medical-surgical nursing: Clinical management for continuity of care* (5th ed.). Philadelphia: W. B. Saunders, pp. 1564–1565.

---

153. The nurse is caring for the client who has had a cystoscopy. The nurse evaluates that the client does not understand postdischarge instructions if the client verbalizes that he or she will

1 Take warm tub baths.
2 Expect small amounts of bright red bleeding.
3 Drink more fluids.
4 Take acetaminophen (Tylenol) to increase comfort.

Answer: 2

Rationale: Pink-tinged urine is common after cystoscopy, but not bright red bleeding. Increased intake of fluids helps prevent this from occurring. Clients often experience bladder spasm and bladder pain, feelings of bladder fullness and burning, and burning sensation on urination after this procedure. Mild analgesics and warm tub baths are recommended to relieve these discomforts. Bladder spasms may be relieved with antispasmodics or belladonna and opium (B&O) suppositories. Because clients may be discharged within a few hours of this procedure, it is imperative that clients understand the elements of self-care after discharge.

Test-Taking Strategy: To answer this question correctly, it is necessary to know that bright red bleeding is abnormal after this procedure; thus eliminate option 3, because flushing the kidneys is a helpful action. Because options 1 and 4 represent reasonable comfort measures, both should be eliminated next. This leaves the bright red bleeding as the answer to the question. This is not expected and should be reported to the physician.

Level of Cognitive Ability: Analysis
Phase of Nursing Process: Evaluation
Client Needs: Physiological Integrity
Content Area: Adult Health/Renal

Reference

Black, J., & Matassarin-Jacobs, E. (1997). *Medical-surgical nursing: Clinical management for continuity of care* (5th ed.). Philadelphia: W. B. Saunders, p. 1568.

154. The nurse has conducted dietary teaching for the client with acute glomerulonephritis. The nurse evaluates the session as successful if the client states that he or she will limit intake of which of the following foods?

1 Summer squash
2 Pineapple
3 Baked chicken
4 Toasted bagel

Answer: 3

Rationale: The diet in glomerulonephritis should be high in calories but low in protein. This diet allows the kidneys to rest by handling fewer protein molecules and metabolites. In addition, the high-calorie diet will prevent protein catabolism and negative nitrogen balance. Because meat and milk products are good sources of protein, these foods are restricted or limited for the client with glomerulonephritis.

Test-Taking Strategy: Knowledge that a low-protein diet is best will assist in the process of elimination and in answering the question. Knowing that fruits and vegetables are normally not high in protein eliminates options 1 and 2 as foods to limit in the diet. To discriminate between options 3 and 4, it is necessary to know that animal sources are highest in protein.

Level of Cognitive Ability: Analysis
Phase of Nursing Process: Evaluation
Client Needs: Health Promotion and Maintenance
Content Area: Adult Health/Renal

References

Black, J., & Matassarin-Jacobs, E. (1997). *Medical-surgical nursing: Clinical management for continuity of care* (5th ed.). Philadelphia: W. B. Saunders, p. 1632.

Lutz, C., & Przytulski, K. (1997). *Nutrition and diet therapy* (2nd ed.). Philadelphia: F. A. Davis, p. 75.

---

155. The nurse has conducted client teaching to prevent return of calcium oxalate stones. The nurse evaluates that the client has understood the instructions if the client selects which of the following vegetables on the dietary menu?

1 Beets
2 Green beans
3 Peas
4 Spinach

Answer: 3

Rationale: Vegetables that are high in oxalic acid include beets, carrots, green beans, rhubarb, and spinach. Fruits high in oxalic acid include blackberries, gooseberries, and plums. Dry cocoa, Ovaltine powder, instant dry coffee, and brewed tea are also high in oxalic acid.

Test-Taking Strategy: This question is difficult to answer without specific knowledge of which foods are high in oxalates. If you had difficulty with this question, take time now to review food sources of oxalates!

Level of Cognitive Ability: Analysis
Phase of Nursing Process: Evaluation
Client Needs: Health Promotion and Maintenance
Content Area: Adult Health/Renal

Reference

Black, J., & Matassarin-Jacobs, E. (1997). *Medical-surgical nursing: Clinical management for continuity of care* (5th ed.). Philadelphia: W. B. Saunders, pp. 1670–1671.

---

156. The nurse is caring for a child with leukemia. The nurse determines that the child is most susceptible to overwhelming infection

1 During the blood transfusion.
2 Before immunosuppressive therapy.
3 After prolonged antibiotic therapy.
4 During remission.

Answer: 3

Rationale: Prolonged antibiotic therapy predisposes the client to growth of resistant organisms. Overwhelming infection is more likely to occur during or after immunosuppressive therapy, not before. During remission, the amount of cancer cells is minimal and the body is more resistive to infection. Blood transfusions restore blood components.

Test-Taking Strategy: Read the stem carefully. "Most" susceptible could mean that there may be more than one correct answer. Use the process of elimination, remembering that antibiotics affect normal flora. This may assist in directing you to the correct option!

Level of Cognitive Ability: Analysis
Phase of Nursing Process: Evaluation
Client Needs: Physiological Integrity
Content Area: Child Health

Reference

Wong, D. (1997). *Whaley and Wong's Essentials of pediatric nursing* (5th ed.). St. Louis: Mosby–Year Book, p. 925.

---

157. Human albumin (Albuminar) IV is prescribed for the client with second- and third-degree burns of the anterior chest and both legs. Before administering the albumin, the nurse evaluates the documented client history to identify the presence of any existing conditions that would be a contraindication to its use. Which of the following, if noted on the chart, would be a contraindication?

1 Lymphocytic leukemia
2 Multiple myeloma
3 Diabetes mellitus
4 Renal insufficiency

Answer: 4

Rationale: Human albumin (Albuminar) is classified as a blood derivative and is contraindicated in clients with severe anemia, cardiac failure, history of allergic reaction, or renal insufficiency and when no albumin deficiency is present. It is used with caution in clients with low cardiac reserve, pulmonary disease, or hepatic or renal failure.

Test-Taking Strategy: Use the process of elimination and eliminate options 1 and 2 first because they are similar in that they are both oncological disorders. Because albumin restores intravascular volume, you should be directed to option 4. Review this blood derivative now if you had difficulty with this question!

Level of Cognitive Ability: Analysis
Phase of Nursing Process: Evaluation
Client Needs: Physiological Integrity
Content Area: Pharmacology

Reference

Hodgson, B., & Kizior, R. (1998). *Saunders nursing drug handbook 1998.* Philadelphia: W. B. Saunders, pp. 16–17.

---

158. The client being discharged to home after renal transplantation has a nursing diagnosis of Risk for Infection related to immunosuppressive therapy. The nurse evaluates that the client needs further instruction on measures to prevent and control infection if the client states that he or she will

1 Take oral temperature daily.
2 Use good handwashing technique.
3 Take all scheduled medications exactly as prescribed.
4 Monitor urine character and output at least 1 day each week.

Answer: 4

Rationale: The client receiving immunosuppressive medication therapy must learn and use infection control methods for use at home. The client must learn proper handwashing technique and should take the temperature daily to detect early infection. This is especially important because this client also takes corticosteroids, which mask signs and symptoms of infection. The client monitors own urine output and its characteristics on a daily basis. All medications should be taken exactly as ordered.

Test-Taking Strategy: Options 1 and 2 are the most obviously correct and are therefore eliminated as possible choices. Because the client may be taking a combination of anti-infectives on a routine basis, along with immunosuppressive medication, it would be important to take scheduled medications on time. Thus option 3 is correct and cannot be the answer to the question. This leaves option 4 as the answer. Knowing that the "once a week" frequency is insufficient makes this the answer to the question as stated.

Level of Cognitive Ability: Analysis
Phase of Nursing Process: Evaluation
Client Needs: Health Promotion and Maintenance
Content Area: Adult Health/Renal

Reference

Black, J., & Matassarin-Jacobs, E. (1997). *Medical-surgical nursing: Clinical management for continuity of care* (5th ed.). Philadelphia: W. B. Saunders, p. 1664.

159. A male newborn is in the intensive care for respiratory distress syndrome (RDS) and needs mechanical ventilation for support. Surfactant replacement therapy has been given. The nurse evaluates the infant 1 hour after the surfactant therapy and determines that the infant's condition has somewhat improved. Which of the following, if observed by the nurse, would indicate improvement?

1. Decreased need for supplemental oxygen
2. Increased work of breathing
3. Unequal breath sounds
4. Increased level of CO_2 in blood gas

Answer: 1

Rationale: A decreased need for supplemental oxygen indicates an improvement in the infant's ability to use oxygen. The increased work of breathing shows air hunger and need for further support. Unequal breath sounds may indicate atelectasis or blocked airways. Increased levels of CO_2 would indicate increasing respiratory acidosis, not improvement of oxygenation.

Test-Taking Strategy: The issue of this question focuses on "improvement." The fact that two of the options use the same idea or thought, such as "increased" work of breathing and "increased" CO_2, may indicate that neither of these options can be the answer. From the remaining options, "unequal" does not indicate improvement. In this case, the correct choice is option 1.

Level of Cognitive Ability: Analysis
Phase of Nursing Process: Evaluation
Client Needs: Physiological Integrity
Content Area: Child Health

References

Ashwill, J., & Droske, S. (1997). *Nursing care of children: Principles and practice.* Philadelphia: W. B. Saunders, pp. 550–556.

Nichols, F., & Zwelling, E. (1997). *Maternal-newborn nursing: Theory and practice.* Philadelphia: W. B. Saunders, pp. 1340–1345.

160. A newborn infant is suspected to be HIV-positive. The nurse is preparing the parents for the discharge of their infant. Which of the following outcomes indicates to the nurse that the parents need further reinforcement in the care of an HIV-positive infant?

1. Parents state that they will not allow anyone with a cold to hold and kiss the baby
2. Parents are able to verbalize signs and symptoms of failure to thrive
3. Parents ask for a prescription for an antiretroviral medication
4. Parents plan to use rice cereal to help with watery stools when they occur

Answer: 4

Rationale: If an infant is having diarrhea, the parents need to seek medical attention because this could be the beginning of an opportunistic infection. Asking for antiretroviral therapy, understanding signs and symptoms of progressive disease, and being protective of an immunocompromised infant are evidence of understanding the needs of the infant.

Test-Taking Strategy: Knowledge of how the HIV infection affects the newborn and education required by the parents is needed to use the process of elimination in selecting the correct response. If you had difficulty with this question, take time now to review parent education points for the newborn with HIV!

Level of Cognitive Ability: Analysis
Phase of Nursing Process: Evaluation
Client Needs: Physiological Integrity
Content Area: Maternity

Reference

Nichols, F., & Zwelling, E. (1997). *Maternal-newborn nursing: Theory and practice.* Philadelphia: W. B. Saunders, pp. 1187–1188.

161. Three days after a suicide attempt by a 26-year-old male client, the family states, "We are so glad that this has happened and now is out of his system." This nurse evaluates this comment as indicating which of the following?

1. The need to provide the family additional education on suicide
2. Follow-up counseling will not be needed by this client
3. The family will not be able to contribute to the client's recovery
4. Repeat self-harm acts are unlikely

Answer: 1

Rationale: The family's comment reflects an inaccurate perception regarding the seriousness related to the suicide attempt. The family needs education on suicidal actions and indications. Options 2 and 4 focus on the client and not the family. Option 3 lacks supporting data. Remember that family support is always helpful in client recovery.

Test-Taking Strategy: If you are unsure of the answer, note the similarities in options 2, 3, and 4. Note the terms "will not" in options 2 and 3 and "unlikely" in option 4. Select option 1, the option that is different!

Level of Cognitive Ability: Analysis
Phase of Nursing Process: Evaluation
Client Needs: Psychosocial Integrity
Content Area: Mental Health

Reference

Fortinash, K. M., & Holoday-Worret, P. A. (1996). *Psychiatric–mental health nursing.* St. Louis: Mosby–Year Book, p. 623.

---

162. An 83-year-old client with dementia and dysphagia is frequently agitated and hyperactive as a result of insomnia. Amitriptyline hydrochloride (Elavil), 50 mg by mouth, will be administered at home each evening. Elavil is supplied in 25-mg and 50-mg tablets. Which of the following does the nurse evaluate as the most appropriate method of administering the medication?

1. Administer two 25-mg tablets each evening
2. Administer five tiny 10-mg tablets each evening
3. Administer the medication sprinkled evenly over the evening meal
4. Administer the medication crushed in 1 tablespoon of apple sauce

Answer: 4

Rationale: The client has dysphagia, and choking is a concern. If swallowing is difficult, avoid tablets and capsules when possible. Sprinkling the medication over the evening meal cannot ensure that the whole dose will be consumed. Crushed medication placed in a small quantity of sweet, soft food facilitates ease in swallowing and provides a pleasant taste.

Test-Taking Strategy: Dementia and dysphagia are important issues in this question. Remembering that tablets and capsules should be avoided by the client with dysphagia will assist in eliminating options 1 and 2. When choosing from the remaining two options, think about the process of measuring or evaluating accurate dosage. Option 4 provides the most accurate measurement!

Level of Cognitive Ability: Analysis
Phase of Nursing Process: Evaluation
Client Needs: Physiological Integrity
Content Area: Pharmacology

Reference

Fortinash, K. M., & Holoday-Worret, P. A. (1996). *Psychiatric–mental health nursing.* St. Louis: Mosby–Year Book, p. 387.

---

163. The client undergoing peritoneal dialysis has experienced peritonitis. The nurse would evaluate that the client is recovering most adequately from the infection if which of the following outcomes were noted?

1. Oral temperature decreased to 99.8°F
2. Reduction of rebound tenderness from moderate to mild
3. Dialysate drainage is only slightly hazy in appearance
4. White blood cell (WBC) count is 8000/μL

Answer: 4

Rationale: Outcomes indicating that peritonitis has resolved include absence of fever, absence of rebound tenderness, clear appearance of dialysate, absence of bacteria in dialysate, normal WBC count (4500–11,000/μL), and no redness or swelling at the catheter site.

Test-Taking Strategy: Note that the question asks for the indicator that the client is recovering "most adequately" from the infection. All of the options except the correct one show a reduction, not an absence, of a sign of infection. This makes option 4 the only correct choice.

Level of Cognitive Ability: Analysis
Phase of Nursing Process: Evaluation
Client Needs: Physiological Integrity
Content Area: Adult Health/Renal

Reference

Black, J., & Matassarin-Jacobs, E. (1997). *Medical-surgical nursing: Clinical management for continuity of care* (5th ed.). Philadelphia: W. B. Saunders, p. 1658.

---

164. The client has been receiving nitrofurantoin (Macrodantin). The nurse evaluates that the therapy is effective if which of the following outcomes is noted?

1 Cessation of cough
2 Absence of dysuria
3 Relief of chest pain
4 Decreased urge for cigarettes

Answer: 2

Rationale: Nitrofurantoin (Macrodantin) is used to treat acute urinary tract infection or for the chronic suppressive treatment of urinary tract infection. It is not effective with systemic bacterial infections. Because dysuria is a sign of urinary tract infection, this is the only correct answer.

Test-Taking Strategy: Familiarity with the classification of this medication is needed to answer this question correctly. Take time now to review this medication, if you had difficulty with this question!

Level of Cognitive Ability: Analysis
Phase of Nursing Process: Evaluation
Client Needs: Physiological Integrity
Content Area: Pharmacology

Reference

Deglin, J. H., & Vallerand, A. H. (1997). *Davis's drug guide for nurses* (5th ed.). Philadelphia: F. A. Davis, p. 864.

---

165. The nurse is monitoring the fluid balance of an assigned client. The nurse evaluates that the client has proper fluid balance if which of the following 24-hour intake and output totals is noted?

1 Intake, 1500 mL; output, 800 mL
2 Intake, 3000 mL; output, 2400 mL
3 Intake, 2400 mL; output, 2900 mL
4 Intake, 1800 mL; output, 1750 mL

Answer: 4

Rationale: For the client taking a normal diet, the normal fluid intake is approximately 1200–1800 mL of measurable fluids per day. The client's output in the same period should be about the same and should not include insensible losses, which are extra. This is offset by the fluid in solid foods, which is also not measured.

Test-Taking Strategy: This question tests a fundamental concept and is straightforward in wording. Knowing that intake should approximately equal output helps you eliminate each of the incorrect choices. If this question was difficult, take a few moments to review this core principle.

Level of Cognitive Ability: Analysis
Phase of Nursing Process: Evaluation
Client Needs: Physiological Integrity
Content Area: Fundamental Skills

Reference

Black, J., & Matassarin-Jacobs, E. (1997). *Medical-surgical nursing: Clinical management for continuity of care* (5th ed.). Philadelphia: W. B. Saunders, p. 1554.

---

166. The nurse is evaluating the effectiveness of antimicrobial therapy for the client with infective endocarditis. The nurse knows that which of the following assessments about the client is the least reliable indicator of success?

1 Clear breath sounds
2 Systolic heart murmur
3 Oral temperature, 98.8°F
4 Negative blood cultures

Answer: 2

Rationale: A systolic heart murmur, once present, will not resolve spontaneously and is therefore the least reliable indicator. Negative blood cultures and normothermia indicate resolution of infection. Clear breath sounds are a normal finding, and in this instance could mean resolution of heart failure if that was accompanying the endocarditis.

Test-Taking Strategy: The question is worded so that you will look for something that will not respond to antimicrobial therapy and that is an abnormal evaluative finding. The only option that meets these criteria is option 2, which does not resolve once it has developed.

Level of Cognitive Ability: Application
Phase of Nursing Process: Evaluation
Client Needs: Physiological Integrity
Content Area: Adult Health/Cardiovascular

Reference

Ignatavicius, D. D., Workman, M. L., & Mishler, M. A. (1995). *Medical-surgical nursing: A nursing process approach* (2nd ed.). Philadelphia: W. B. Saunders, p. 913.

---

167. The nurse has conducted health teaching for the client with a cardiac valvular disorder. The nurse would evaluate the session as successful if the client stated the need to use which of the following measures for oral hygiene?

1 Brush with a soft manual toothbrush, followed by an oral rinse
2 Use an electric toothbrush, followed by an oral rinse
3 Use an irrigating device for oral care
4 Floss at least two times every day

Answer: 1

Rationale: To reduce the risk of infective endocarditis, the nurse teaches the client to brush teeth at least twice daily with a soft, manual toothbrush and then do an oral rinse. Irrigation devices, electric toothbrushes, and use of dental floss are to be avoided. Their use is prohibited because they could cause gums to bleed, allowing bacteria to enter mucous membranes and then the blood stream. The client should have regular dental care by a dentist who is aware of the client's valve disorder.

Test-Taking Strategy: The principles of oral hygiene are the same as for the client with infectious endocarditis. If you are still uncertain of the answer, evaluate the question from the perspective of gum trauma. This will lead you to the correct option, which is brushing with a soft, manual toothbrush and oral rinses.

Level of Cognitive Ability: Analysis
Phase of Nursing Process: Evaluation
Client Needs: Health Promotion and Maintenance
Content Area: Adult Health/Cardiovascular

Reference

Ignatavicius, D. D., Workman, M. L., & Mishler, M. A. (1995). *Medical-surgical nursing: A nursing process approach* (2nd ed.). Philadelphia: W. B. Saunders, p. 909.

---

168. The home care nurse has discussed measures to prevent recurrence of venous stasis ulcers with a client. The client demonstrates that there is a need for further instruction if the client makes which of the following statements?

1 "I should elevate my legs for about 20 minutes whenever I am able during the day."
2 "I'll buy some lotion with lanolin for my legs and use it every day."
3 "I can cross my knees as long as they don't ache and swell up."
4 "It's important for the top of the elastic stockings not to get twisted."

Answer: 3

Rationale: Antigravity measures, such as intermittent leg elevation during the day and elevation during sleep, are used. Factors that interfere with the return of blood to the heart are also counteracted. The client is advised to avoid crossing the legs, avoid putting pressure on the popliteal space, and avoid any ill-fitting garments that bind or twist. Lanolin-based lotion is applied to the legs daily to prevent cracking of dry, scaly skin.

Test-Taking Strategy: Use concepts of gravity and common sense to answer this question. The wording of the question makes you look for an incorrect statement. Eliminate options 1 and 4 first, followed by option 2. The client should always avoid crossing the legs at the knees.

Level of Cognitive Ability: Analysis
Phase of Nursing Process: Evaluation
Client Needs: Health Promotion and Maintenance
Content Area: Adult Health/Cardiovascular

Reference

Black, J., & Matassarin-Jacobs, E. (1997). *Medical-surgical nursing: Clinical management for continuity of care* (5th ed.). Philadelphia: W. B. Saunders, p. 1438.

169. The nurse is caring for a client with continuous electrocardiogram (ECG) monitoring. The nurse notes that the electrocardiogram complexes are very small and hard to evaluate. The nurse checks which setting on the ECG monitor console?

1 Power button
2 Low rate alarm
3 Amplitude or "gain"
4 High rate alarm

Answer: 3

Rationale: The power button turns the machine on and off. The high and low alarm settings indicate the heart rate limits beyond which an alarm will sound. The amplitude, commonly called "gain," regulates the size of the complex and can be adjusted up and down to some degree.

Test-Taking Strategy: This question is fairly easy to decipher, without sophisticated ECG knowledge, using general principles and experience with electrical equipment. Option 1 is eliminated first. The word "rate" in options 2 and 4 is a clue that they are incorrect. This leaves you with the amplitude (meaning size or strength) as the correct choice.

Level of Cognitive Ability: Analysis
Phase of Nursing Process: Evaluation
Client Needs: Physiological Integrity
Content Area: Adult Health/Cardiovascular

Reference

Black, J., & Matassarin-Jacobs, E. (1997). *Medical-surgical nursing: Clinical management for continuity of care* (5th ed.). Philadelphia: W. B. Saunders, pp. 1221–1222.

---

170. The client has received antidysrhythmic therapy for treatment of premature ventricular contractions (PVCs). The nurse would evaluate this therapy as being less than optimal if the client's PVCs continued to

1 Be fewer than six per minute.
2 Be unifocal in appearance.
3 Fall after the end of the T wave.
4 Occurred in pairs.

Answer: 4

Rationale: PVCs are considered dangerous when they are frequent (more than six per minute), occur in pairs or couplets, are multifocal (multiform), or fall on the T wave.

Test-Taking Strategy: Any questions you may find on NCLEX-RN regarding PVCs will probably relate to these cardinal rules of when PVCs are dangerous. Review these now, if needed.

Level of Cognitive Ability: Analysis
Phase of Nursing Process: Evaluation
Client Needs: Physiological Integrity
Content Area: Adult Health/Cardiovascular

Reference

Black, J., & Matassarin-Jacobs, E. (1997). *Medical-surgical nursing: Clinical management for continuity of care* (5th ed.). Philadelphia: W. B. Saunders, p. 1305.

---

171. The nurse is evaluating the effects of care for the client with deep vein thrombosis. Which of the following limb observations would the nurse note as indicating success in meeting the outcome criteria for this problem?

1 Pedal edema that is graded 1+
2 Slight residual calf tenderness
3 Warm skin, equal temperature in both legs
4 Calf girth 1/2 inch larger than unaffected limb

Answer: 3

Rationale: Successful resolution of the deep vein thrombosis is marked by the absence of original symptoms used to diagnose the problem (leg warmth, redness, edema, tenderness, enlarged calf).

Test-Taking Strategy: By the wording of the question, you are looking for return of indicators of normal circulation. Use the process of elimination and eliminate the options that are abnormal. Options 1, 2, and 4 show slight residual alterations from normal.

Level of Cognitive Ability: Analysis
Phase of Nursing Process: Evaluation
Client Needs: Physiological Integrity
Content Area: Adult Health/Cardiovascular

Reference

Ignatavicius, D. D., Workman, M. L., & Mishler, M. A. (1995). *Medical-surgical nursing: A nursing process approach* (2nd ed.). Philadelphia: W. B. Saunders, pp. 953, 957.

172. The client with chronic airway limitation (CAL) has received instructions to limit the carbohydrate in the diet to reduce the metabolical demands on the body. This measure has been effective if the client has which of these findings?

1 Oxygen partial pressure (PO_2) within normal limits
2 Carbon dioxide partial pressure (PCO_2) lowered
3 Total carbon dioxide (TCO_2) elevated
4 Oxygen saturation (SaO_2) returning to the normal range

Answer: 2

Rationale: Carbohydrate (glucose) metabolism results in increased CO_2 levels in the body. The more the carbohydrate intake is reduced, the less CO_2 will be produced.

Test-Taking Strategy: Remembering that decreased carbohydrates leads to decreased CO_2 will assist in answering the question. If you had difficulty with this question, take time now to review the relationship of CO_2 and carbohydrates!

Level of Cognitive Ability: Analysis
Phase of Nursing Process: Evaluation
Client Needs: Physiological Integrity
Content Area: Adult Health/Respiratory

Reference

Luckmann, J. (1997). *Saunders manual of nursing care.* Philadelphia: W.B. Saunders, p. 927.

---

173. The nurse checks the client's arterial blood gases (ABGs). Which of these findings would indicate respiratory acidosis?

1 pH 7.5, PCO_2 30
2 pH 7.3, PCO_2 50
3 pH 7.3, HCO_3 19
4 pH 7.5, HCO_3 30

Answer: 2

Rationale: In respiratory acidosis, the pH is decreased and an opposite effect is seen in the PCO_2 (pH decreased, PCO_2 elevated). Option 1 indicates respiratory alkalosis. Option 3 indicates metabolic acidosis, and option 4 indicates metabolic alkalosis.

Test-Taking Strategy: Recalling that the pH is decreased in a respiratory problem will assist in eliminating options 1 and 4. In respiratory acidosis, the PCO_2 has an opposite effect from the pH. This will easily direct you to option 2.

Level of Cognitive Ability: Analysis
Phase of Nursing Process: Evaluation
Client Needs: Physiological Integrity
Content Area: Adult Health/Respiratory

Reference

Luckmann, J. (1997). *Saunders manual of nursing care.* Philadelphia: W.B. Saunders, p. 918.

---

174. A person with post-traumatic stress disorder (PTSD) who has succeeded in focusing the trauma in a healthy perspective might make which of the following statements?

1 "I don't know why I was sitting out there at night."
2 "I guess this was payback for all the things I have done wrong."
3 "I guess I am a poor judge of character."
4 "It was bad luck. I was in the wrong place at the wrong time."

Answer: 4

Rationale: Clients need to be able to put the trauma into a new context in which the client is not to blame. The client needs to realize that the trauma did not occur because they did something wrong, used poor judgment, or somehow deserved it.

Test-Taking Strategy: Clients will often express feelings of guilt, but the goal is to assist in putting the traumatic incident in perspective and eventually to be able to work through their feelings of guilt. Options 1, 2, and 3 are allowing the client to accept some guilt and responsibility when none is warranted. If you had difficulty with this question, take time now to review PTSD!

Level of Cognitive Ability: Analysis
Phase of Nursing Process: Evaluation
Client Needs: Psychosocial Integrity
Content Area: Mental Health

Reference

Carson, V., & Arnold, E. (1996). *Mental health nursing: The nurse-patient journey.* Philadelphia: W. B. Saunders, pp. 702–707.

175. The client is taking the benzodiazepine diazepam (Valium), 5 mg PO TID. During the client visit the nurse evaluates the client's understanding of this medication. Which statement by the client indicates the need for additional medication instruction?

1 "A glass of wine every day with dinner helps me to relax."
2 "I was very drowsy when I began to take this medication, but now I feel all right."
3 "When do you think I'll be able to start tapering off the Valium?"
4 "I think I am coming down with the flu. What can I take that will not interfere with the Valium?"

Answer: 1

Rationale: If taken with benzodiazepines, CNS depressants such as alcohol will produce additive effects, which can be lethal, and they may also cause respiratory depression. The other responses are appropriate concerns that the client should have. Valium may cause initial drowsiness. Valium should not be discontinued abruptly, because the client may develop withdrawal symptoms. Many of the over-the-counter medications used to treat the flu contain medication that should not be taken with Valium.

Level of Cognitive Ability: Application
Phase of Nursing Process: Evaluation
Client Needs: Health Promotion and Maintenance
Content Area: Pharmacology

Reference
Hodgson, B., & Kizior, R. (1998). *Saunders nursing drug handbook 1998.* Philadelphia: W. B. Saunders, pp. 307–308.

---

176. The nurse is caring for a client with a chest tube attached to closed chest drainage. The nurse would evaluate that the client's lung has completely expanded if

1 Oxygen saturation is greater than 92%.
2 Bubbling in the water seal chamber has ceased.
3 Pleuritic chest pain has resolved.
4 Suction in the chest drainage system is no longer needed.

Answer: 2

Rationale: When the lung has completely expanded, there is no longer air or fluid in the pleural space to be drained into the bottle/chamber or the water seal chamber. Thus an indication that a chest tube is ready for removal is when bubbling in the water seal chamber ceases and drainage of fluid into the collection bottle/chamber ceases. Adequate oxygen saturation does not imply that the lung has fully reexpanded. Although air is known to be an irritant to pleural tissue, cessation of pleuritic pain may not occur when the lung is expanded. The chest tube acts as an irritant and therefore contributes to pain. Use or nonuse of suction in the chest drainage system is not necessarily governed by the degree of lung expansion. Suction is indicated when gravity is not sufficient to drain air and pleural fluid or if the client has a poor respiratory effort and cough. Suction increases the speed at which air and fluid is removed from the pleural space.

Test-Taking Strategy: The key phrase is "completely expanded." This phrase and knowledge of the functioning of chest tubes should direct you to the correct option. Review chest tube drainage systems now if you had difficulty with this question. You are very likely to find questions related to this content on NCLEX-RN!

Level of Cognitive Ability: Analysis
Phase of Nursing Process: Evaluation
Client Needs: Physiological Integrity
Content Area: Adult Health/Respiratory

Reference
Ignatavicius, D. D., Workman, M. L., & Mishler, M. A. (1995). *Medical-surgical nursing: A nursing process approach* (2nd ed.). Philadelphia: W. B. Saunders, p. 745.

177. The nurse is providing teaching regarding prevention of hepatitis A to a client who will be traveling overseas. The nurse realizes continued health teaching is needed when the client states

1. "I should boil all of the water that I drink and avoid ice cubes."
2. "I should be cautious of animals because they can carry hepatitis A."
3. "Handwashing is one of the best methods of preventing infection."
4. "There is no type of immunization against hepatitis A."

Answer: 4

Rationale: In 1995, a hepatitis A vaccine was approved by the U.S. Food and Drug Administration (FDA). In addition, there is a standard immunoglobulin for passive immunization that can be given prophylactically or after exposure. The immunoglobulin for passive immunization provides protection from infection for approximately 2 months. Hepatitis A is transmitted via the fecal-oral route; thus precautions in options 1, 2, and 3 are appropriate.

Test-Taking Strategy: Look for similar distracters. Options 1, 2, and 3 all relate to prevention of transmission of hepatitis A. Option 4 is different because it addresses immunization. If you had difficulty with this question, take time now to review preventive measures associated with hepatitis A!

Level of Cognitive Ability: Analysis
Phase of Nursing Process: Evaluation
Client Needs: Health Promotion and Maintenance
Content Area: Adult Health/Gastrointestinal

Reference

Polaski, A., & Tatro, A. (1996). *Luckmann's Core principles and practice of medical-surgical nursing.* Philadelphia: W. B. Saunders, p. 1114.

178. The nurse has just administered the tuberculin skin test to an elderly client as part of a routine health physical. The nurse realizes further education is necessary when the client states

1. "If this is positive, I will need to have a chest x-ray done."
2. "I should come back in 2–3 days to have you check the reaction on my arm."
3. "If there is no reaction, then I do not have tuberculosis."
4. "Redness on my arm does not mean I have tuberculosis."

Answer: 3

Rationale: Elderly and immunocompromised clients may not have a positive reaction to the initial tuberculin skin test, even if they have had prior exposure to the tubercle bacillus. These clients may have a delayed reaction and should have a repeat tuberculin skin test in 1–2 weeks. The second test should reveal positive results if the client has had prior exposure. Options 1, 2, and 4 are correct. The tuberculin skin test is read in 48–72 hours. Erythema or redness alone is not considered significant. The size of induration, if any, is what determines the significance of the test. A positive test result does not, however, indicate active disease. Persons with a positive reaction receive follow-up monitoring with a chest radiograph.

Test-Taking Strategy: Knowledge of screening tests for tuberculosis is essential to answer this question accurately. From this point, use the process of elimination. If you had difficulty with this question, take time now to review interpretation of the tuberculin test!

Level of Cognitive Ability: Analysis
Phase of Nursing Process: Evaluation
Client Needs: Health Promotion and Maintenance
Content Area: Adult Health/Respiratory

Reference

Polaski, A., & Tatro, A. (1996). *Luckmann's Core principles and practice of medical-surgical nursing.* Philadelphia: W. B. Saunders, pp. 590–591.

179. Which of the following statements about a hospitalized client diagnosed with chronic schizophrenia who is taking fluphenazine decanoate (Prolixin) identifies an effective client response to the medication?

1. "This one's a lost cause and will never be well."
2. "The client is able to dress, bathe, and eat without reminders."
3. "It's hard to determine the client's needs."
4. "It would be nice if the client was always this good."

Answer: 2

Rationale: Option 2 recognizes client change as an observation. Option 1 is judgmental about prognosis and ignores the effect of medication while labeling the client. Options 3 and 4 may be true but focus on the nurse and not on responses to medication and/or physiological change.

Test-Taking Strategy: The issue of the question is the effectiveness of the medication. Focusing on the issue should assist in eliminating the incorrect options. In addition, use therapeutic communication techniques. These strategies should direct you to the correct option!

Level of Cognitive Ability: Analysis
Phase of Nursing Process: Evaluation
Client Needs: Psychosocial Integrity
Content Area: Mental Health

Reference

Hodgson, B., & Kizior, R. (1998). *Saunders nursing drug handbook 1998.* Philadelphia: W. B. Saunders, pp. 434–436.

---

180. The client who has received a diagnosis of being in the manic phase of bipolar disorder is quietly attending to the group session, and the client is offering appropriate suggestions to other newly admitted clients about complying with medications. How should the nurse evaluate this behavior?

1. The client has achieved the goals of the treatment plan
2. The client may be manipulating the group process
3. The client may need a longer stay at the hospital
4. The client may need some change in the current medication regimen

Answer: 1

Rationale: The behavior described in the stem of the question is what the physician and nursing staff hope the client will achieve before discharge. The behavior shows adequate attention span, an "other-centered" approach, and adequate knowledge of medication as a method of treatment of illness. The participation with others is an expected outcome of any group session in which clients support and teach each other.

Test-Taking Strategy: All items except option 1 are negative responses. The behavior described is very appropriate, so the answer must be the positive response. Note the key words "manic" and "quietly." This should assist in directing you to the option that reflects a positive response!

Level of Cognitive Ability: Analysis
Phase of Nursing Process: Evaluation
Client Needs: Psychosocial Integrity
Content Area: Mental Health

Reference

Johnson, B. (1997). *Psychiatric mental health nursing: Adaptation and Growth* (4th ed.). Philadelphia: Lippincott-Raven, p. 552.

181. A 16-year-old with a history of type I diabetes for 10 years comes into the physician's office for a sports physical. In looking at the record, the nurse determines that the client had four hyperglycemic reactions in the past year. In evaluating the causes of these reactions, the most appropriate nursing action would be to

1 Ask the mother what time of day the hyperglycemic reactions occur.
2 Complete the basic preparation for a physical before the physician arrives.
3 Ask the mother to step outside so that the nurse can discuss the hyperglycemic reactions with the client.
4 Complete the basic preparation for a physical and discuss sports with the client.

Answer: 3

Rationale: Consider the developmental level (16-year-old) of the client. Self-management is key to close control of diabetes. On the basis of the age and developmental level of the client, the best action to evaluate these reactions is to discuss their occurrences with the 16-year-old in private.

Test-Taking Strategy: Use the process of elimination, considering the developmental level of the client and the issue of the question: hyperglycemic reactions. Eliminate options 2 and 4 because they are similar. Of the remaining two options, option 3 is most thorough and is directly focused toward the client. If you had difficulty with this question, take time now to review the developmental stage of a 16-year-old!

Level of Cognitive Ability: Analysis
Phase of Nursing Process: Evaluation
Client Needs: Psychosocial Integrity
Content Area: Child Health

Reference
Wong, D. (1997). *Whaley and Wong's Essentials of pediatric nursing* (5th ed.). St. Louis: Mosby–Year Book, pp. 479–480, 1058.

---

182. The mother and grandmother of a 2-month-old infant are speaking to the physician about the baby's immunization schedule. The physician is told that the grandmother is visiting with her daughter for the next 6 months while receiving chemotherapy at a local hospital. Which of the following statements, if made by the mother, indicates that she understands which immunizations can be administered this visit?

1 "The baby will receive the first oral poliovirus vaccine [OPV] today."
2 "The baby takes oral medication very well for an infant."
3 "The baby will receive a shot of inactivated poliovirus vaccine [IPV] today."
4 "The baby won't get any immunizations this visit."

Answer: 3

Rationale: OPV is a live attenuated poliovirus and is shed in the stool. It should never be administered to any child who is in contact with an immunosuppressed person (the visiting grandmother). IPV is an inactivated poliovirus vaccine and is the recommended immunization for infants in contact with an immunosuppressed person.

Test-Taking Strategy: The key words are "immunization" and "chemotherapy." The grandmother is immunosuppressed from the chemotherapy. Option 1 refers to administering OPV and option 2 also refers to oral medication to an infant. Option 4 refers to not being immunized. If you had difficulty with this question, take time now to review the contraindications associated with immunizations!

Level of Cognitive Ability: Application
Phase of Nursing Process: Evaluation
Client Needs: Health Promotion and Maintenance
Content Area: Child Health

Reference
Ashwill, J. & Droske, S. (1997). *Nursing Care of Children: Principles and Practice.* Philadelphia: W.B. Saunders, p. 1005.

---

183. The nurse is evaluating for the presence of bleeding tendencies in a child with leukemia. Which of the following will assist in confirming the presence of bleeding?

1 Decreased erythrocyte count
2 Decreased platelet production
3 Decreased white blood cell count
4 Decreased eosinophil count

Answer: 2

Rationale: Platelets are necessary for the clotting of blood. Therefore, a decreased number would promote bleeding tendencies. Decreased erythrocyte count may indicate that the bone marrow function is decreased but not necessarily causing a decreased platelet count. A decreased white blood cell count is not necessarily related to bleeding. Decreased eosinophil count indicates a decreased allergic reaction.

Test-Taking Strategy: The issue of the question is bleeding tendencies. Use the process of elimination to identify the laboratory test that reflects bleeding. This should direct you to the correct option. If you are unsure of the meaning of the laboratory tests presented in the options, review them now!

Level of Cognitive Ability: Analysis
Phase of Nursing Process: Evaluation
Client Needs: Physiological Integrity
Content Area: Child Health

Reference

Wong, D., & Perry, S. (1998). *Maternal-child nursing care.* St. Louis: Mosby–Year Book, pp. 1500, 1518.

---

184. The nurse is caring for a child with leukemia. The nurse notes that the platelet count is 20,000/mm³. Which of the following would not be a component of the plan of care?

1. Assess stools for blood
2. Clean oral cavity with a toothette
3. Administer acetaminophen (Tylenol) suppositories for fever
4. Provide quiet play activities

Answer: 3

Rationale: A platelet count of 20,000/mm³ places the child at risk for bleeding. Options 1, 2, and 4 are accurate interventions. The use of suppositories is avoided because of the risk of rectal bleeding.

Test-Taking Strategy: Note the key word "not" in the stem of the question. Noting the issue of the question—bleeding—and using the process of elimination will easily direct you to option 3.

Level of Cognitive Ability: Analysis
Phase of Nursing Process: Evaluation
Client Needs: Physiological Integrity
Content Area: Child Health

Reference

Ashwill, J., & Droske, S. (1997). *Nursing care of children: Principles and practice.* Philadelphia: W. B. Saunders, p. 1005.

---

185. The nurse provides teaching for a client with Buerger's disease. Which of the following data would indicate the need for further teaching?

1. The client is performing Buerger-Allen exercises three times a day.
2. The client states, "I'm using gloves when I go out in the cold."
3. The client states, "I'm still smoking but I gave up coffee."
4. The client is following the guidelines for foot care.

Answer: 3

Rationale: Smoking is a risk factor for Buerger's disease. The client should be counseled with regard to how important it is to stop smoking immediately. Options 1, 2, and 4 are appropriate measures.

Test-Taking Strategy: Options 1, 2, and 4 describe the appropriate and correct lifestyle measures to be taken by the client with Buerger's disease. Buerger-Allen exercises promote circulation. Using gloves to protect the upper extremities from extremes in temperature is often recommended. Daily foot care is another health promotion measure to prevent skin breakdown. If you had difficulty with this question, take time now to review teaching measures for the client with Buerger's disease!

Level of Cognitive Ability: Analysis
Phase of Nursing Process: Evaluation
Client Needs: Physiological Integrity
Content Area: Adult Health/Cardiovascular

Reference

Luckmann, J. (1997). *Saunders manual of nursing care.* Philadelphia: W. B. Saunders, pp. 1102–1115.

186. The community health nurse visits the client with Raynaud's disease at home. Nifedipine (Procardia) has been prescribed, and the nurse teaches the client about the medication. Which of the following statements, if made by the client, indicates that the client does not know the side effects of the medication?

1 "I need to get up slowly when I change positions because the medicine causes hypotension."
2 "I will contact my doctor if I get any swelling in my feet or fingers."
3 "I will call my doctor if I begin to get an increase in headaches or facial flushing."
4 "I will use a magnifying glass until my blurred vision from the medication goes away."

Answer: 4

Rationale: Nifedipine is a calcium antagonist that reduces smooth muscle contractility by inhibiting the movement of calcium ions in slow channels. Its side effects include headache, flushing, peripheral edema, and postural hypotension.

Test-Taking Strategy: This question assesses your knowledge of medication used to treat Raynaud's disease. Options 1, 2, and 3 are all correct client responses and indicate understanding of the side effects of the medication. Option 4 is incorrect and refers to a side effect of psychotropic medication. Use the process of elimination. From basic knowledge regarding medications, you should be able to eliminate options 1, 2, and 3. If you had difficulty with this question, take time now to review the side effects of this medication!

Level of Cognitive Ability: Analysis
Phase of Nursing Process: Evaluation
Client Needs: Physiological Integrity
Content Area: Pharmacology

Reference
Hodgson, B., & Kizior, R. (1998). *Saunders nursing drug handbook 1998.* Philadelphia: W. B. Saunders, pp. 744–745.

---

187. The community health nurse visits a client who has just received a permanent pacemaker at home. The nurse instructs the client about pulse checks. Which of the following statements, if made by the client, indicates that the nurse's teaching was effective?

1 "I will take my pulse the same time every day, and if I notice it slowing, I'll call the doctor."
2 "I will take my pulse the same time every day, and if I notice any change in the rate or rhythm, I'll call the doctor immediately."
3 "It's important that I take my pulse at the same time every day and that I count for 15 full seconds, using a watch with the second hand."
4 "It's important that I take my pulse at the same time every day, preferably after I've been physically active, to determine my progress."

Answer: 2

Rationale: The client should be taught to take the pulse in the wrist or neck every day at the same time, preferably in the morning, and to rest a full 5 minutes before taking the pulse. The pulse should be counted for 1 full minute by a watch or clock that has an accurate second hand, and the pulse should be recorded every day in a log containing a description of the rate, rhythm, date, and time of day.

Test-Taking Strategy: In option 1, the client's response seems to be correct, but the client's answer is actually vague in terms of what is being assessed. A mere slowing of the rate is not sufficient measurement. In option 3, the time frame used when teaching accurate pulse taking is 1 full minute, not 15 seconds. In option 4, it is important to take the pulse when the client is relaxed or has been at rest. If the client has been physically active, resting for 5 full minutes before pulse assessment is necessary to obtain an accurate reading. If you had difficulty with this question, take time now to review the appropriate method to assess a pulse!

Level of Cognitive Ability: Analysis
Phase of Nursing Process: Evaluation
Client Needs: Health Promotion and Maintenance
Content Area: Adult Health/Cardiovascular

Reference
Luckmann, J. (1997). *Saunders manual of nursing care.* Philadelphia: W. B. Saunders, pp. 1019–1020.

188. The nurse visits a client with deep vein thrombosis who is on bed rest at home. Which of the following statements, if made by the client, indicates that the client identifies the clinical manifestations for pulmonary embolism?

1 "I will notify the doctor immediately if I develop coughing, profuse sweating, difficulty breathing, and/or chest pain."
2 "I will notify you if anything unusual occurs."
3 "I will notify the doctor immediately if I develop tingling in my legs, become nauseated, start vomiting, and have diarrhea."
4 "I will call you if I begin to develop ataxia, intentional tremor, and coughing."

Answer: 1

Rationale: Of the clinical manifestations of a pulmonary embolism, chest pain is the most common. Coughing, diaphoresis, dyspnea, and apprehension are the other clinical manifestations. Pleuritic chest pain (sudden onset and aggravated by breathing) is caused by an inflammatory reaction of the lung parenchyma or occurs when there is a pulmonary infarction or ischemia caused by an obstruction of small pulmonary arterial branches.

Test-Taking Strategy: This question tests your knowledge of the symptoms of pulmonary embolism, an acute lethal complication of deep vein thrombosis. Focus on the issue of the question. Options 2, 3, and 4 all provide inaccurate clinical descriptions of pulmonary embolism. If you had difficulty with this question, take time now to review the clinical manifestations of pulmonary embolism!

Level of Cognitive Ability: Analysis
Phase of Nursing Process: Evaluation
Client Needs: Health Promotion and Maintenance
Content Area: Adult Health/Cardiovascular

Reference

Luckmann, J. (1997). *Saunders manual of nursing care.* Philadelphia: W. B. Saunders, p. 1019.

189. The community health nurse visits a client with varicose veins at home. A venogram has been prescribed for the client. The nurse teaches the client about the venogram. Which of the following statements, if made by the client, indicates that the client understands the procedure?

1 "I expect that the test dye the physician injects will be painless."
2 "I imagine that the procedure will eliminate my leg problems."
3 "I know that the dye the physician injects can irritate my veins and be somewhat painful afterwards."
4 "I'm being tested to determine whether I can discontinue using my support stockings."

Answer: 3

Rationale: The purpose of a venogram is to assess the severity of venous obstruction and to locate the obstructions and/or thrombi by x-ray films after a radiopaque dye is injected into a vein. This test is a diagnostic procedure and will not eliminate leg problems or determine whether the support stockings can be discontinued. Injections can cause pain.

Test-Taking Strategy: This question assesses your knowledge of an invasive procedure: the venogram for clients who may have venous disease. You can easily eliminate options 2 and 4 because this is a diagnostic procedure, not a treatment procedure. Of the remaining two options, it is more realistic that some pain would be expected after the injection. If you had difficulty with this question, take time now to review this diagnostic procedure!

Level of Cognitive Ability: Analysis
Phase of Nursing Process: Evaluation
Client Needs: Physiological Integrity
Content Area: Adult Health/Cardiovascular

Reference

Luckmann, J. (1997). *Saunders manual of nursing care.* Philadelphia: W. B. Saunders, p. 1019.

190. Which of the following would indicate that the lung has reexpanded after a spontaneous pneumothorax that was treated with insertion of a chest tube?

1 The client's respiratory rate is low
2 Bubbling is noted in the suction control chamber
3 There is no bubbling in the water seal chamber
4 The PCO_2 is 40

Answer: 3

Rationale: A lack of bubbling in the water seal chamber can indicate that the lung has reexpanded. Bubbling in the suction control chamber is expected and does not indicate reexpansion of the lung. Options 1 and 4 do not determine lung reexpansion.

Test-Taking Strategy: The issue of the question is reexpansion of the lung. Eliminate options 1 and 2 because they do not relate to the issue of evaluating whether lung reexpansion has occurred. Although the PCO_2 in option 4 is normal, it also does not determine whether lung reexpansion has occurred. If you had difficulty with this question, take time now to review chest tubes!

Level of Cognitive Ability: Analysis
Phase of Nursing Process: Evaluation
Client Needs: Physiological Integrity
Content Area: Adult Health/Respiratory

Reference

Black, J., & Matassarin-Jacobs, E. (1997). *Medical-surgical nursing: Clinical management for continuity of care* (5th ed.). Philadelphia: W. B. Saunders, pp. 1165–1166.

---

191. The client with chronic airway limitation (CAL, chronic obstructive pulmonary disease [COPD]) has received dietary instructions to reduce the metabolical demands on the body. This teaching has been effective if the client selects which of the following?

1 Cabbage
2 Grapes
3 Broccoli
4 Milkshake

Answer: 2

Rationale: High bulk and fiber foods may produce intestinal bloating that reduces lung expansion. Milk products can thicken secretions.

Test-Taking Strategy: Eliminate options 1 and 3 because they are similar food items. Recalling that milk products thicken secretions will easily direct you to option 2. If you had difficulty with this question, take time now to review the diet recommended for the client with CAL. You are likely to find a question related to this concept in NCLEX-RN!

Level of Cognitive Ability: Analysis
Phase of Nursing Process: Evaluation
Client Needs: Physiological Integrity
Content Area: Adult Health/Respiratory

Reference

Luckmann, J. (1997). *Saunders manual of nursing care.* Philadelphia: W. B. Saunders, p. 927.

---

192. The nurse evaluates the client's ABGs. Which of these findings would indicate that the FIO_2 was sufficient?

1 A PCO_2 of 58 mmHg
2 A PO_2 of 60 mmHg
3 An SaO_2 of 88
4 A TCO_2 of 32

Answer: 2

Rationale: Keeping the PO_2 at 60 mmHg will indicate that the hemoglobin is 90% saturated (unless the pH varies).

Test-Taking Strategy: In order to answer the question, you must know which parameter to look at before you can apply this information to evaluate the results of the oxygen therapy. Note that options 1, 3, and 4 are abnormal values. This is a difficult question, and if you had difficulty with it, take time now to review normal blood gas values and the effect of the FIO_2!

Level of Cognitive Ability: Analysis
Phase of Nursing Process: Evaluation
Client Needs: Physiological Integrity
Content Area: Adult Health/Respiratory

Reference

Black, J., & Matassarin-Jacobs, E. (1997). *Medical-surgical nursing: Clinical management for continuity of care* (5th ed.). Philadelphia: W. B. Saunders, p. 1055.

193. The nurse evaluates the client admitted with rib fractures in order to identify the risk for potential complications. The client has a history of chronic bronchitis. All of the following actions were in the care plan. Which one indicates that the nurse has most appropriately evaluated the assessment information?

1 Have the client cough and breathe deeply 20 minutes after pain medication is given
2 Administer low-flow oxygen at 3 liters/minute
3 Assist the client to a position of comfort
4 Administer small, frequent meals with plenty of fluids

Answer: 2

Rationale: Giving the client with chronic bronchitis a high flow of oxygen would stop the hypoxic drive and cause apnea. Although options 1, 3, and 4 may be appropriate nursing interventions, option 2 specifically addresses the issue of the question.

Test-Taking Strategy: Use only the data presented in the question to answer the question. Note the key phrase "most appropriately" and the issues "chronic bronchitis" and "potential complications." Focusing on these points should direct you to the correct option. In addition, using the ABCs—airway, breathing, and circulation—will direct you to the correct option!

Level of Cognitive Ability: Analysis
Phase of Nursing Process: Evaluation
Client Needs: Physiological Integrity
Content Area: Adult Health/Respiratory

Reference

Black, J., & Matassarin-Jacobs, E. (1997). *Medical-surgical nursing: Clinical management for continuity of care* (5th ed.). Philadelphia: W. B. Saunders, p. 2526.

194. The community health nurse visits a client at home. Azidothymidine (AZT) has recently been prescribed for the client. The client states, "I've been getting a little nauseated, and I've had a couple of headaches since I started the AZT. Does this mean I can't take the medicine?" The nurse evaluates the client's concerns. On the basis of the nurse's evaluation, which of the following would be the most appropriate response?

1 "These symptoms may become more tolerable as you adjust to ongoing therapy."
2 "Don't worry. There are so many other medications these days that the doctor can give you."
3 "I know you're worried you won't be able to take AZT, but you only have a slight neutropenia."
4 "I do not see the need for you to worry because your neutrophil counts are normal."

Answer: 1

Rationale: The initial adverse effects of AZT include headache, malaise, insomnia, rash, diarrhea, and fever. As AZT therapy proceeds, these symptoms become more tolerable. Side effects of anemia and neutropenia (count below 500) are the side effects that would cause the medication to be discontinued or therapy to be interrupted.

Test-Taking Strategy: This test assesses your knowledge of antiviral therapy such as AZT. Use the process of elimination. In options 2, 3, and 4, telling the client, "Don't worry" is false reassurance; furthermore, it is inappropriate to assume that you know what the client is thinking. If you had difficulty with this question, take time now to review the side effects of AZT!

Level of Cognitive Ability: Application
Phase of Nursing Process: Evaluation
Client Needs: Physiological Integrity
Content Area: Pharmacology

Reference

Black, J., & Matassarin-Jacobs, E. (1997). *Medical-surgical nursing: Clinical management for continuity of care* (5th ed.). Philadelphia: W. B. Saunders, pp. 614–651.

195. The nurse prepares a report for the case management group on a client with HIV/AIDs. Which of the following criteria may be used as outcomes for evaluation by the nurse?

1. The client does not experience respiratory distress
2. The client has no increased platelet aggregation
3. The client has no evidence of dissecting aortic aneurysm
4. The client has a urinary output of 50 mL per hour

Answer: 1

Rationale: The absence of respiratory distress is one of the goals that the nurse sets as a priority. The most common, life-threatening opportunistic infection that attacks clients with HIV/AIDS is *Pneumocystis carinii* pneumonia. Its symptoms include fever, exertional dyspnea, and nonproductive cough. Options 2, 3, and 4 are not specifically related to the issue of the question.

Test-Taking Strategy: Note the issue of the question. Option 1 is the only option that is directly related. In addition, use the ABCs—airway, breathing, and circulation—to answer the question. If you had difficulty with this question, take time now to review the expected outcomes with the client with HIV/AIDS!

Level of Cognitive Ability: Analysis
Phase of Nursing Process: Evaluation
Client Needs: Physiological Integrity
Content Area: Adult Health/Respiratory

Reference

Black, J., & Matassarin-Jacobs, E. (1997). *Medical-surgical nursing: Clinical management for continuity of care* (5th ed.). Philadelphia: W. B. Saunders, pp. 614–651.

---

196. The nurse is caring for a preoperative client who has a diagnosis of pedophilia and says, "I thought I wanted to be 'neutered,' but now I don't know if it is the best way to treat my problem." After evaluation of the client's statement, the most therapeutic response by the nurse would be

1. "Let's talk about the vasectomy that you have requested the surgeon to perform, its purpose, and the realistic expectations."
2. "I'll rip up the informed consent you've signed and notify the surgeon if you want."
3. "This surgery is mandatory if you wish to remain out of prison."
4. "Think what this will mean if you have a relapse. You need to remake your life and this is a safeguard as much for you as for your victims if your treatment relapses."

Answer: 1

Rationale: Because the diagnosis of pedophilia does not bring with it mandatory vasectomy, the procedure must be elective. The client ought to understand what an elective vasectomy will ensure and what it will not ensure. For example, it will not treat pedophilia, which is implied by the client's comments. The nurse has a responsibility to explain and to assess that the surgical procedure is understood for the purposes of informed consent. A vasectomy is an elected surgical procedure performed as a permanent method of contraception (although occasionally a vasectomy can be surgically reversed). The procedure can also frequently be performed after a prostatectomy to prevent retrograde epididymitis.

Test-Taking Strategy: Use therapeutic communication techniques to answer the question. In option 2, the nurse's offer is an incorrect nursing action because it does not allow the client to control and determine the process. In option 3, the nurse's response contains incorrect information; legal punishment does not include punitive surgeries. Even if you were uncertain about this fact, the threat that the nurse presents in option 3 is a nontherapeutic communication. In option 4, the nurse's response is cajoling and holds an implied threat.

Level of Cognitive Ability: Application
Phase of Nursing Process: Evaluation
Client Needs: Psychosocial Integrity
Content Area: Mental Health

Reference

Antai-Otong, D. (1995). *Psychiatric nursing: Biological and behavioral concepts.* Philadelphia: W. B. Saunders, pp. 407–426.

197. The community health nurse is visiting a male with trigeminal neuralgia at home. As part of the nursing care plan, the nurse teaches the client to avoid factors that trigger pain. Which of the following statements, if made by the client, indicates that further teaching is necessary?

1. "Don't worry, I'm taking an early retirement and I won't be going out much to start the pain again."
2. "I'm going to begin biofeedback this week."
3. "I'm going to grow a beard so I won't have to shave."
4. "I've bought a water jet to use to clean my teeth instead of a toothbrush."

Answer: 1

Rationale: It is important for the client to learn to avoid which factors can trigger trigeminal pain, but it is also important to ensure that these behaviors do not become avoidance behaviors that are maladaptive, such as failure to eat, poor dental hygiene, and withdrawal and isolation.

Test-Taking Strategy: This question assesses your critical thinking in educating clients with trigeminal neuralgia. In option 1, the client is withdrawing and isolating himself, which is an unnecessary and potentially maladaptive behavior. Options 2, 3, and 4 are adaptive and appropriate behaviors. If you had difficulty with this question, take time now to review teaching points for the client with trigeminal neuralgia!

Level of Cognitive Ability: Analysis
Phase of Nursing Process: Evaluation
Client Needs: Health Promotion and Maintenance
Content Area: Adult Health/Neurological

Reference

Black, J., & Matassarin-Jacobs, E. (1997). *Medical-surgical nursing: Clinical management for continuity of care* (5th ed.). Philadelphia: W. B. Saunders, pp. 915–932.

---

198. The nurse is caring for a newly admitted client who has a history of depressive illness for over 20 years with three suicide attempts. Which of the following indicates that the treatment for this depressive disorder has been successful?

1. "I am going to therapy and I have decided that suicide is not the answer to my problems."
2. "While I'm on this antidepressant, I can finally have a baby!"
3. "I can discontinue my antidepressant gradually after 3 months without any depressive illness."
4. "I still believe suicide will probably be my best bet, but I have agreed not to do anything without first talking to my psychiatrist."

Answer: 1

Rationale: Desired outcomes of a suicidal client include verbalization of suicidal feelings and thoughts and their precipitants, rather than acting on them. Actively attending therapy and giving up suicidal ideation are positive outcomes in the evaluation. Antidepressants are administered for at least 1 year after the termination of depressive symptoms, and many clients are on low maintenance doses for life.

Test-Taking Strategy: Remember that when answers do not seem logical, they are usually wrong answers. For example, taking an antidepressant does not provide an opportunity to have babies; it frees the client from depressive illness. The retention of suicidal ideation is a negative outcome, even if the client has agreed to a "no-suicide" contract. Option 1 presents the positive outcome!

Level of Cognitive Ability: Analysis
Phase of Nursing Process: Evaluation
Client Needs: Psychosocial Integrity
Content Area: Mental Health

Reference

Antai-Otong, D. (1995). *Psychiatric nursing: Biological and behavioral concepts.* Philadelphia: W. B. Saunders, pp. 554–556.

199. Which of the following questions would the nurse ask in order to evaluate the goals of care for a client admitted for a manic episode of a bipolar disorder?

1. "Is the client decreasing psychomotor activity and speech and becoming less distractible?"
2. "Is the client able to recognize me and address me by name?"
3. "Is the client's family willing to commit to 1 month of careful observation and support?"
4. "Is the client returning from the waxy flexibility of the manic episode?"

Answer: 1

Rationale: The outcomes that the nursing care plan would set include increased ability to control behavior and motivation to participate in activities of daily living (ADLs). Evaluation would search for evidence of decreased psychomotor activity and speech; increased concentration span with decreased distractibility; increased recognition of realistic self-perception of influence and abilities; increased introspection; increased appropriateness of dress and makeup; and increased sleep and ability to monitor own physical needs.

Test-Taking Strategy: This question asks you to apply your knowledge of the nursing care for a client who had experienced a manic episode. Use the process of elimination. Option 2 is a question that might be asked of any client in the mental status examination. Option 3 is family focused and is a question that seeks to ascertain support systems for any clients. In option 4, waxy flexibility, a condition in which a client remains in any body position in which they are placed, was frequently seen before the advent of psychotropic medication.

Level of Cognitive Ability: Application
Phase of Nursing Process: Evaluation
Client Needs: Physiological Integrity
Content Area: Mental Health

Reference

Antai-Otong, D. (1995). *Psychiatric nursing: Biological and behavioral concepts.* Philadelphia: W. B. Saunders, pp. 172–173.

---

200. A pregnant woman has tested positive for HIV (human immunodeficiency virus). The nurse counsels the client and determines that more teaching is necessary when the client states

1. "Breast-feeding after delivery is best for my baby."
2. "I can continue to hug and hold my other children."
3. "It may be 2 years before I know if the baby has HIV."
4. "My husband and I can still sleep together in the same bed."

Answer: 1

Rationale: Breast-feeding is contraindicated because current data indicate that the virus may be transmitted through the breast milk. HIV is not spread through casual contact, so holding, hugging, and sleeping with other family members is not prohibited. A newborn may test positive for HIV for up to 2 years after birth because of placental transfer of maternal antibodies. It is vital that the nurse ascertains that the client has correct knowledge regarding the transmission of the disease and precautions necessary to prevent the transmission and spread of HIV.

Test-Taking Strategy: Knowing that HIV is transmitted by direct contact with infected bodily fluids should help make the correct answer apparent. A similarity exists between options 2 and 4 in that both describe relational behaviors. If you had difficulty with this question, take time now to review transmission of the AIDS virus!

Level of Cognitive Ability: Analysis
Phase of Nursing Process: Evaluation
Client Needs: Health Promotion and Maintenance
Content Area: Maternity

Reference

Nichols, F., & Zwelling, E. (1997). *Maternal-newborn nursing: Theory and practice.* Philadelphia: W. B. Saunders, pp. 1497–1498.

201. The nurse evaluates that further education is necessary when a client with gestational diabetes states

1. "I'm aware that the possibility of a cesarean birth is greater for me."
2. "I know that I might need to take insulin at some point in my pregnancy."
3. "I'm disappointed that I will be unable to breast-feed my baby."
4. "I intend to continue walking every day."

Answer: 3

Rationale: Breast-feeding is not contraindicated for a diabetic woman. Women with gestational diabetes may need insulin in order to maintain good glycemic control during pregnancy. Exercise is an important aspect of care, and clients should be encouraged to continue their usual exercise program. Cesarean births are often necessary for diabetic clients because of early placental degeneration.

Test-Taking Strategy: This question is asking you to identify the response that indicates that the client needs further teaching. Knowledge of the concepts related to gestational diabetes is necessary to answer the question correctly. If you had difficulty with this question, take time now to review gestational diabetes. You are likely to find a question related to this disorder on NCLEX-RN!

Level of Cognitive Ability: Analysis
Phase of Nursing Process: Evaluation
Client Needs: Physiological Integrity
Content Area: Maternity

Reference

Nichols, F., & Zwelling, E. (1997). *Maternal-newborn nursing: Theory and practice.* Philadelphia: W. B. Saunders, p. 675.

202. A post-stroke male client has left-sided hemiparesis. Which statement by the client indicates that more teaching is needed in the area of self-care activities?

1. "I got the shirt on, but the buttons are really hard to fasten."
2. "My wife cries every time she comes and sees me struggle to dress myself."
3. "I was able to use my left arm some to wash today, since I got that long-handled bath brush."
4. "I'm so proud that I did everything for the first time with my right arm."

Answer: 4

Rationale: The client often struggles with self-care management. In options 1, 2, and 3, the client has some difficulty but apparently accomplishes the task. In option 4 the client does not use the affected, weak left arm, which he should be encouraged to use for rebuilding of strength and nerve pathways.

Test-Taking Strategy: The key phrase is "left-sided hemiparesis." Option 4 indicates a misunderstanding of what should be accomplished and addresses the right arm. The nurse must know from general nursing knowledge that the affected limbs must be used even if they are slow or clumsy at first. Braces, slings, and special devices are available.

Level of Cognitive Ability: Analysis
Phase of Nursing Process: Evaluation
Client Needs: Physiological Integrity
Content Area: Adult Health/Neurological

Reference

Black, J., & Matassarin-Jacobs, E. (1997). *Medical-surgical nursing: Clinical management for continuity of care* (5th ed.). Philadelphia: W. B. Saunders, p. 803.

203. The client has received a diagnosis of an irregular heart rate. What question by the client would indicate client teaching should begin?

1. "How is an ECG interpreted?"
2. "What is it like to have a pacemaker?"
3. "Can you tell me what a diagnosis of irregular heart rate means?"
4. "What is wrong with my roommate's heart?"

Answer: 3

Rationale: A significant factor influencing learning is the learner's readiness to learn. Option 3 addresses the client's readiness because the client is directly asking about the disorder. At this point, the client is motivated to learn.

Test-Taking Strategy: Learning depends on two things: physical and emotional readiness to learn. Without one or the other, teaching can occur, but learning may not take place. There is usually a time at which the client will indicate an interest in learning. Use the process of elimination. Note the similarity of "irregular heart rate" in the question and in the correct response. Review teaching-learning principles now if you had difficulty with this question!

Level of Cognitive Ability: Analysis
Phase of Nursing Process: Evaluation
Client Needs: Psychosocial Integrity
Content Area: Adult Health/Cardiovascular

Reference

Smeltzer, S., & Bare, B. (1996). *Brunner and Suddarth's Textbook of medical-surgical nursing* (8th ed.). Philadelphia: Lippincott-Raven, p. 41.

---

204. The physician orders 20% Intralipids, an intravenous fat emulsion, for a client who will be receiving total parenteral nutrition (TPN) for several months. The nurse explains to the client that the fat solution is administered

1 To increase the amount of fluid given by intravenous route.
2 On a daily basis at the same time each day.
3 To decrease the incidence of phlebitis in the vein in which the TPN is administered.
4 To provide essential fatty acids and additional calories.

Answer: 4

Rationale: Intralipids is a brand of intravenous fat emulsion. Clients receiving their total nutrition parenterally for a prolonged period of time are at risk for developing essential fatty acid deficiency. Fat emulsions are given to meet client nonprotein caloric needs that cannot be met by glucose administration alone.

Test-Taking Strategy: The issue of the question is specific content: intravenous fat emulsion. Note the relationship between "fat emulsion" in the question and "fatty acids" in the correct option. If you had difficulty with this question, take time now to review the purpose of administering fat emulsion during TPN therapy!

Level of Cognitive Ability: Application
Phase of Nursing Process: Evaluation
Client Needs: Physiological Integrity
Content Area: Fundamental Skills

Reference

Deglin, J. H., & Vallerand, A. H. (1997). *Davis's drug guide for nurses* (4th ed.). Philadelphia: F. A. Davis, pp. 451–453.

---

205. Upon admission to the home health care agency, the nurse assesses that the elderly female client has occasional urgency and frequent stress incontinence. With this information, the nurse evaluates that

1 This is a normal physiological sign of aging.
2 This finding is caused by stress on the bladder.
3 Follow-up medical care is necessary.
4 A bladder-training program is necessary for the client.

Answer: 3

Rationale: Occasionally, women experience stress incontinence associated with aging, which is often a result of decreased perineal tone. Bladder training is premature without further assessment and work-up, chiefly with the primary care provider.

Test-Taking Strategy: This question centers on what nurses know about the normal aging process and abnormal physical findings. Evaluation in this question guides the nurse to seek medical care, knowing that it is not a normal physiological process and the nurse cannot diagnose the problem. Review the physiological process of aging now if you had difficulty with this question!

Level of Cognitive Ability: Analysis
Phase of Nursing Process: Evaluation
Client Needs: Physiological Integrity
Content Area: Adult Health/Renal

Reference

Rice, R. (1996). *Home health nursing practice: Concepts and application* (2nd ed.). St. Louis: Mosby–Year Book, p. 423.

206. The home care nurse is visiting the client who has been experiencing nosebleeds with the onset of winter months. The nurse evaluates that the client has followed the suggestion of the nurse to reduce nosebleeds if the client reports having done which of the following?

1 Having the chimney cleaned
2 Having the furnace serviced
3 Buying a humidifier
4 Starting to damp dust

Answer: 3

Rationale: Nosebleeds may occur during the winter as a result of decreased humidity in the home. The use of a humidifier helps alleviate this problem. Environmental allergens can be reduced by having the chimney cleaned and by dusting with a damp cloth. Having the furnace serviced will detect the leakage or presence of carbon monoxide, which is harmful to the client.

Test-Taking Strategy: To answer this question accurately, an understanding of the factors contributing to nosebleeds, one of which is dry air, is required. Dust and chimney soot do not typically cause nosebleeds, so options 1 and 4 may eliminated first. Of the two remaining, dry air is a more likely cause of nosebleeds than a malfunctioning or improperly serviced furnace, making the purchase of a humidifier the option of choice.

Level of Cognitive Ability: Analysis
Phase of Nursing Process: Evaluation
Client Needs: Health Promotion and Maintenance
Content Area: Adult Health/Respiratory

Reference

Black, J., & Matassarin-Jacobs, E. (1997). *Medical-surgical nursing: Clinical management for continuity of care* (5th ed.). Philadelphia: W. B. Saunders, p. 1048.

---

207. The psychiatric nurse has completed the medication teaching for a depressed client who is taking sertraline (Zoloft), 50 mg PO QD. Which of the following statements indicates that the client understands the appropriate use of this medication?

1 "I'll make certain to cut out cheese, Chianti, chocolate, and all the other foods on the list you gave me."
2 "If I experience dry mouth, I'll use sugarless hard candy."
3 "I'll make certain to get monthly blood levels."
4 "I'll take my medication on an empty stomach to speed its absorption."

Answer: 2

Rationale: Zoloft, a selective serotonin reuptake inhibitor, can cause dry mouth, which is remedied by sucking on sugarless hard candy and chewing gum. Foods such as cheese, Chianti, and chocolate contain an amino acid, tyramine, which reacts with monoamine oxidase inhibitors (MAOIs). Monthly blood levels are usually required for clients who are receiving lithium therapy. Zoloft is usually taken with meals.

Test-Taking Strategy: Knowledge that Zoloft is a selective serotonin reuptake inhibitor will assist in eliminating options 1 and 3. Of the remaining two options, if you are unsure, the best selection is option 2 because it is an appropriate statement. If you had difficulty with this question, take time now to review this medication!

Level of Cognitive Ability: Analysis
Phase of Nursing Process: Evaluation
Client Needs: Health Promotion and Maintenance
Content Area: Pharmacology

Reference

Hodgson, B., & Kizior, R. (1998). *Saunders nursing drug handbook 1998.* Philadelphia: W. B. Saunders, p. 1103.

208. The clients state, "Our son hung himself. He was the fifth teen-age suicide in our neighborhood in 6 months. The papers say that it's happening because they were hopeless about their future. In our day, the pastor or your councilman got you a good union job. We couldn't afford to send our son to college." Which of the following statements by the survivors indicates that the clients have begun to successfully integrate the suicide experience into their lives?

1 "We are so ashamed and embarrassed at church and social functions."
2 "We realize that we are angry that our son did this to us!"
3 "We have joined a neighborhood support group."
4 "We are talking more openly with our other children and our friends."

Answer: 4

Rationale: As with all loss experienced by individuals and families, opening up the communications channels is a key factor in successful grieving and surviving. Often, estrangement occurs in families because well-meaning relatives and friends do not know how to respond. This uncertainty and fear cause them to isolate when communication and an opportunity to grieve with support are crucial. Joining a support group is a positive outcome, but if the clients are not talking among themselves and their families, it is likely that they will not receive the maximum benefit from the group.

Test-Taking Strategy: Effective communication is an essential concept in all interpersonal relationships and in growth and development. Although options 1 and 2 accurately reflect the feelings of survivors, expression of such feelings alone does not demonstrate a positive outcome and/or adaptation. Although joining a support group would be considered a positive outcome, it does not mean that the clients are receiving benefit from participation. Option 4 indicates both an expression of feelings and growth in relations.

Level of Cognitive Ability: Analysis
Phase of Nursing Process: Evaluation
Client Needs: Psychosocial Integrity
Content Area: Mental Health

Reference

Antai-Otong, D. (1995). *Psychiatric nursing: Biological and behavioral concepts.* Philadelphia: W. B. Saunders, pp. 352–353.

---

209. The community health nurse visits the client at home. Warfarin sodium (Coumadin) has been prescribed for the client. The nurse teaches the client and family about the medication. Which of the following statements, if made by the client, indicates that further teaching is necessary?

1 "I'll use only an electric shaver until the anticoagulant is discontinued."
2 "I will buy a medication alert tag that indicates that I'm on anticoagulants."
3 "I will not take any over-the-counter medications except aspirin."
4 "I won't participate in games such as football anymore."

Answer: 3

Rationale: No over-the-counter medications of any kind should be ingested by clients who receive anticoagulants. This is especially true of aspirin and/or aspirin-containing products (because of the potential to cause bleeding).

Test-Taking Strategy: In option 1, electric shavers are less irritating to the skin than razors and less likely to cause a skin breakdown and bleeding. In option 2, medication alert tags are recommended in case of an emergency. In addition, all clients should be taught to carry identification cards that list all medications currently being taken. In option 4, strenuous games such as contact sports that can cause bruising and bleeding are to be strictly avoided. If you had difficulty with this question, take time now to review teaching points for clients on anticoagulants!

Level of Cognitive Ability: Analysis
Phase of Nursing Process: Evaluation
Client Needs: Health Promotion and Maintenance
Content Area: Pharmacology

Reference

Hodgson, B., & Kizior, R. (1998). *Saunders nursing drug handbook 1998.* Philadelphia: W. B. Saunders, pp. 1062–1064.

210. The postoperative client with no history of respiratory disease is still drowsy on arrival from the postanesthesia care unit. The client has an oxygen mask delivering 40% oxygen. The nurse attaches a pulse oximeter and gets a reading of 89%. The nurse evaluates that the client should be

1 Given a dose of naloxone (Narcan).
2 Aroused and nasotracheally suctioned.
3 Awakened and encouraged to breathe deeply.
4 Allowed to rest with another measurement done in 1 hour.

Answer: 3

Rationale: If values fall below a preset norm, which is usually 90%, the client should be instructed to take several deep breaths. This is especially true of a client without a respiratory history who is still under the effects of sedation. If the client did have a respiratory disease history, it may be an indication that supplemental oxygen should be put in place or increased.

Test-Taking Strategy: Eliminate option 4 first as the least therapeutic of all the options. Option 2 is discarded next because there is no evidence that the client needs suctioning; rather the low measurement seems to be a result of hypoventilation. Of the two remaining, option 3 is the better choice because Narcan would totally reverse any analgesics in the client's system and would cause the client to experience postoperative pain suddenly. Additionally, Narcan cannot be administered without a physician's order.

Level of Cognitive Ability: Analysis
Phase of Nursing Process: Evaluation
Client Needs: Physiological Integrity
Content Area: Adult Health/Respiratory

Reference

Black, J., & Matassarin-Jacobs, E. (1997). *Medical-surgical nursing: Clinical management for continuity of care* (5th ed.). Philadelphia: W. B. Saunders, pp. 1053, 1055.

211. A client has had a sputum specimen sent to the laboratory for Gram's stain and for culture and sensitivity testing. The laboratory calls back initial results within 1 hour. The nurse evaluates the laboratory findings. The nurse would prepare to telephone the physician about which of the following reports?

1 Gram's stain
2 Culture
3 Sensitivity
4 Culture and sensitivity

Answer: 1

Rationale: Gram's stain classifies the organism as gram-negative or gram-positive and may be done immediately. This gives initial information about the type of organism when initiation of antibiotic therapy is a high priority. The specimen is then incubated on a culture medium for at least 24 hours more to identify the specific organisms. The sensitivity test gives the physician precise information about which antibiotics the organism is sensitive to.

Test-Taking Strategy: Basic principles of microbiology as they are applied to client care are needed to answer this question. Knowing that a culture takes at least 24 hours for an initial report helps you eliminate options 2 and 4. Because the sensitivity testing cannot be done until the organism is identified, the only remaining option is the Gram's stain, which quickly discriminates between gram-positive and gram-negative bacteria.

Level of Cognitive Ability: Application
Phase of Nursing Process: Evaluation
Client Needs: Safe, Effective Care Environment
Content Area: Adult Health/Respiratory

Reference

Black, J., & Matassarin-Jacobs, E. (1997). *Medical-surgical nursing: Clinical management for continuity of care* (5th ed.). Philadelphia: W. B. Saunders, p. 1063.

212. The nurse enters the room of a client after being asked by the physician to assist with thoracentesis, which is to be done at the bedside. The nurse would evaluate that the client is positioned optimally if the client is found

1 Sitting upright, leaning over an overbed table.
2 Sitting erect with the bed in high Fowler's position.
3 Kneeling and facing the mattress with the bed in high Fowler's position.
4 In a side-lying position with a pillow under the head.

Answer: 1

Rationale: The optimal position for the client is upright and leaning over an overbed table. This allows pleural fluid to accumulate in the lowest part of the pleural space.

Test-Taking Strategy: The client should be positioned for this procedure to allow access to the fluid in the pleural space and also to have the client in a position in which the ribs are well separated for easier insertion of the thoracentesis needle. Using these concepts as a guide, eliminate options 2 and 3 first, because they do not enhance rib separation. You would choose option 1 over option 4 because the side-lying position would cause fluid to accumulate under the client and away from the access site, which is ineffective. Take time now to review client position during thoracentesis, if you had difficulty with this question!

Level of Cognitive Ability: Application
Phase of Nursing Process: Evaluation
Client Needs: Physiological Integrity
Content Area: Adult Health/Respiratory

Reference
Black, J., & Matassarin-Jacobs, E. (1997). *Medical-surgical nursing: Clinical management for continuity of care* (5th ed.). Philadelphia: W. B. Saunders, p. 1063.

213. The client has undergone pleural biopsy at the bedside. The nurse evaluates that the client has tolerated the procedure if the client exhibits

1 Dyspnea.
2 Mild pain.
3 Pallor.
4 Diaphoresis.

Answer: 2

Rationale: Complications after pleural biopsy include hemothorax, pneumothorax, and temporary pain from intercostal nerve injury. The nurse notes indications of these complications, such as dyspnea, excessive pain, pallor, or diaphoresis. Mild pain is expected.

Test-Taking Strategy: This question is straightforward in wording and theory. Dyspnea, pallor, and diaphoresis do not indicate tolerance of the procedure. Note the word "mild" in the correct option. If this question was difficult, take a few moments to review this procedure, and the symptoms of complications that result from it!

Level of Cognitive Ability: Analysis
Phase of Nursing Process: Evaluation
Client Needs: Physiological Integrity
Content Area: Adult Health/Respiratory

Reference
Black, J., & Matassarin-Jacobs, E. (1997). *Medical-surgical nursing: Clinical management for continuity of care* (5th ed.). Philadelphia: W. B. Saunders, p. 1064.

214. The client being seen in an ambulatory care facility has an arterial blood gas measurement. The nurse would evaluate that the client understands how to monitor the site for complications if the client stated that he or she would report

1 Formation of hematoma.
2 Warm hand temperature.
3 Pink nailbeds.
4 Positive radial pulse.

Answer: 1

Rationale: After arterial blood gas sampling, the site should be assessed for bleeding and hematoma formation, as well as injury to the artery or surrounding structures.

Test-Taking Strategy: This question is worded to seek an item that is not a normal finding. Knowledge of basic normal circulatory assessments helps you to choose the correct answer quickly and easily. The only abnormal finding is option 1!

Level of Cognitive Ability: Analysis
Phase of Nursing Process: Evaluation
Client Needs: Health Promotion and Maintenance
Content Area: Adult Health/Cardiovascular

Reference

Black, J., & Matassarin-Jacobs, E. (1997). *Medical-surgical nursing: Clinical management for continuity of care* (5th ed.). Philadelphia: W. B. Saunders, p. 1057.

---

215. The emergency room nurse has instructed the client with rib fracture about recovery time and resumption of activities before discharge. The nurse evaluates that the client understands the information if which of the following statements is made by the client?

1 "The pain should be better in 3 weeks, and I can resume full activity in a month."
2 "The pain should be better in a week, and I can resume full activity in 6 weeks."
3 "The pain should be better in 3 days, and I can resume full activity in 2 weeks."
4 "The pain should be better in 2 weeks, and I can resume full activity in 2 months."

Answer: 2

Rationale: The nurse teaches the client that the pain of fractured ribs generally lasts for about 5–7 days. Full healing takes about 6 weeks, after which full activity may be resumed.

Test-Taking Strategy: Option 3 can be eliminated first, as being too quick. Knowing that fractures of small bones heal in about 6 weeks helps you to discriminate among the other choices, eliminating options 1 and 4. Review client teaching after rib fracture if you had difficulty with this question!

Level of Cognitive Ability: Analysis
Phase of Nursing Process: Evaluation
Client Needs: Health Promotion and Maintenance
Content Area: Adult Health/Musculoskeletal

Reference

Black, J., & Matassarin-Jacobs, E. (1997). *Medical-surgical nursing: Clinical management for continuity of care* (5th ed.). Philadelphia: W. B. Saunders, p. 2526.

---

216. The nurse has taught the client with a small flail chest about measures to promote lung expansion and clearance of secretions. The nurse evaluates that the client best understands the instructions if the client

1 Demonstrates effective coughing and deep breathing independently.
2 Uses an incentive spirometer upon request.
3 Rings the nurse call bell if suctioning is needed.
4 Demonstrates correct use of a nebulizer.

Answer: 1

Rationale: Coughing and deep breathing will effectively promote lung expansion and clearance of mucus. Using an incentive spirometer is helpful, but it is most effective if the client uses it independently without coaching. The nurse may not need to suction the client if the client is not intubated. Use of a nebulizer is not indicated; rather, the client would benefit from humidified oxygen.

Test-Taking Strategy: Begin to answer this question by eliminating options 3 and 4 first because suctioning and a nebulizer are unnecessary components of care with this client. Of the two remaining, option 1 is an independent action on the part of the client and is therefore preferable to option 2, in which the nurse is the initiator of the respiratory exercise.

Level of Cognitive Ability: Analysis
Phase of Nursing Process: Evaluation
Client Needs: Health Promotion and Maintenance
Content Area: Adult Health/Respiratory

Reference

Ignatavicius, D. D., Workman, M. L., & Mishler, M. A. (1995). *Medical-surgical nursing: A nursing process approach* (2nd ed.). Philadelphia: W. B. Saunders, p. 767.

217. The home care nurse would conclude that a client was coping most effectively with a new diagnosis of heart disease if the client made which of the following statements?

1 "Someone from the American Heart Association is coming to visit me tomorrow."
2 "I'm going to ask the doctor if I can just cut down on smoking."
3 "I'll only have to take my medications until I feel better."
4 "It worries me that I may need surgery someday."

Answer: 1

Rationale: An expected outcome for a person with a cardiac disorder is that the client uses appropriate resources for support during emotionally stressful times.

Test-Taking Strategy: The phrase "most effectively" in the stem implies degrees of correct and incorrect responses. Use the process of elimination. Options 2 and 3 can be eliminated readily. Option 1 is better than option 4 because it is an adaptive response to a stressor.

Level of Cognitive Ability: Analysis
Phase of Nursing Process: Evaluation
Client Needs: Psychosocial Integrity
Content Area: Adult Health/Cardiovascular

Reference
Smeltzer, S., & Bare, B. (1996). *Brunner and Suddarth's Textbook of medical-surgical nursing* (8th ed.). Philadelphia: Lippincott-Raven, p. 644.

---

218. The nurse has conducted teaching with a client who recently received a diagnosis of Prinzmetal's (variant) angina. The nurse would evaluate the session as being successful if the client stated that this form of angina

1 Has the same risk factors as stable and unstable angina.
2 Responds readily to a low-sodium diet.
3 Is most effectively managed by beta-blocking agents.
4 Is treated with calcium channel–blocking agents.

Answer: 4

Rationale: Prinzmetal's angina results from spasm of the coronary vessels. The risk factors are unknown, and it is relatively unresponsive to nitrates. Beta-blockers may worsen the spasm. Diet therapy is not indicated. Calcium-channel blockers are prescribed for this type of angina.

Test-Taking Strategy: Variant angina results from coronary spasm, so it is a functional disorder and not due to atherosclerosis. Look for the option that is effective against spasm, which is option 4. If you are unfamiliar with this type of angina, review now!

Level of Cognitive Ability: Analysis
Phase of Nursing Process: Evaluation
Client Needs: Physiological Integrity
Content Area: Adult Health/Cardiovascular

Reference
Luckmann, J. (1997). *Saunders manual of nursing care.* Philadelphia: W. B. Saunders, p. 1038.

---

219. The nurse has counseled the client with myocardial infarction about limiting cholesterol and saturated fat in the diet. The nurse would document that the client demonstrates understanding of dietary modifications if the client selected which of the following sample meals as most appropriate?

1 Spaghetti and sweet sausage in tomato sauce, vanilla pudding (with 4% milk)
2 Pork chop, baked potato, cauliflower in cheese sauce, ice cream
3 Cheeseburger, pan-fried potatoes, whole kernel corn, sherbet
4 Baked haddock, steamed broccoli, herbed rice, sliced strawberries

Answer: 4

Rationale: To lower blood cholesterol, recommended dietary modifications include decreasing the use of fatty cuts of beef, lamb, and pork; decreasing the consumption of organ meats, sausage, hot dogs, bacon, and sardines; avoiding vegetables prepared in butter, cream, or other dairy sauces; substituting low-fat milk products for whole-milk products and cream; and decreasing the amount of commercial prepared baked goods.

Test-Taking Strategy: The phrase "most appropriate" alerts you that there are varying degrees of correctness of at least a few options. It may help you to systematically eliminate incorrect answers if you first evaluate the meat and milk food groups and then look at the quality of the vegetables, breads, and cereals. Fruits are generally good unless they are in a sweetened sauce.

Level of Cognitive Ability: Analysis
Phase of Nursing Process: Evaluation
Client Needs: Health Promotion and Maintenance
Content Area: Adult Health/Cardiovascular

Reference
Lutz, C., & Przytulski, K. (1997). *Nutrition and diet therapy* (2nd ed.). Philadelphia: F. A. Davis, pp. 372–373.

220. The nurse caring for a client with right-sided heart failure has formulated a nursing diagnosis of Fluid Volume Excess. The client has been on furosemide (Lasix) for 3 days. The nurse would evaluate that the outcome criteria have not been successfully met if the client has

1 High daytime urinary output.
2 Nocturia with daytime oliguria.
3 Serum BUN level of 20 mg/dL.
4 Serum creatinine level of 0.9 mg/dL.

Answer: 2

Rationale: With right-sided heart failure, fluid pools in the interstitial spaces of the periphery of the body. At night, with the effects of gravity eliminated, fluid reenters the blood stream and is eliminated by the kidneys, producing nocturia. This indicates that medical therapy is not yet effective.

Test-Taking Strategy: The question is looking for an incorrect item. Knowledge of normal common laboratory values eliminates 3 and 4. Knowledge that diuretic therapy, administered in the morning, results in daytime diuresis eliminates option 1.

Level of Cognitive Ability: Analysis
Phase of Nursing Process: Evaluation
Client Needs: Physiological Integrity
Content Area: Adult Health/Cardiovascular

Reference
Jaffee, M., & McVan, B. (1997). *Davis's laboratory and diagnostic test handbook.* Philadelphia: F. A. Davis, pp. 202, 350.

---

221. A client with angina pectoris has received instructions on lifestyle changes to control the disease process. The nurse would evaluate the teaching as needing reinforcement if the client stated that he or she would

1 Try to exercise at least once a week for 30 minutes.
2 Avoid using table salt with meals.
3 Use muscle relaxation to cope with stressful situations.
4 Take nitroglycerin at the first sign of chest discomfort.

Answer: 1

Rationale: Exercise is most effective when done at least 3 times a week. Other good habits include limiting salt and fat in the diet, using stress management techniques, and knowing when and how to use medications.

Test-Taking Strategy: The question asks you for an item indicating that reinforcement is needed. Options 2, 3, and 4 are indicated, which leaves option 1 as the answer. Exercise should be done at least three times a week for optimal benefit.

Level of Cognitive Ability: Analysis
Phase of Nursing Process: Evaluation
Client Needs: Health Promotion and Maintenance
Content Area: Adult Health/Cardiovascular

Reference
Smeltzer, S., & Bare, B. (1996). *Brunner and Suddarth's Textbook of medical-surgical nursing* (8th ed.). Philadelphia: Lippincott-Raven, p. 644.

---

222. The nurse is evaluating the client's ability to cope with the experience of having a myocardial infarction (MI). Which of the following statements, if made by the client, is the best indicator of positive adaptation?

1 "I still can't really believe this has all happened to me."
2 "Why me? I have my fair share of problems already."
3 "I'll have to get a second job to help pay for my medications."
4 "Since I can't smoke in the hospital, I might as well try to quit altogether."

Answer: 4

Rationale: The client progresses through stages of coping after MI, which commonly include denial, anger, and depression, before coming to acceptance. The first two statements represent denial and anger, respectively. A new, added job after MI is not a positive adaptation, because it would increase physiological stress and could harm the client. Modification of risk factors (such as smoking) is a positive step.

Test-Taking Strategy: Knowledge of the stages of grieving/coping assists you in answering this question. Options 1 and 2 can be fairly easily eliminated. Discriminate between options 3 and 4 by looking at which one promotes the client's health in a more positive manner.

Level of Cognitive Ability: Analysis
Phase of Nursing Process: Evaluation
Client Needs: Psychosocial Integrity
Content Area: Adult Health/Cardiovascular

Reference

Ignatavicius, D. D., Workman, M. L., & Mishler, M. A. (1995). *Medical-surgical nursing: A nursing process approach* (2nd ed.). Philadelphia: W. B. Saunders, p. 998.

---

223. The client with pulmonary edema is getting ready for discharge. The nurse evaluates that the client can identify preventive measures by stating the importance of

1 Weighing self at least once each week.
2 Sleeping with the head of bed elevated on 10-inch blocks.
3 Taking an extra dose of diuretic if peripheral edema is noted.
4 Taking an extra dose of digoxin (Lanoxin) if slight respiratory distress occurs.

Answer: 2

Rationale: A long-range approach to the prevention of pulmonary edema is to minimize any pulmonary congestion. During recumbent sleep, fluid (which has seeped into the interstitium by day with the assistance of the effects of gravity) is rapidly reabsorbed into the systemic circulation. Sleeping with the head of bed elevated 10 inches helps prevent circulatory overload.

Test-Taking Strategy: Eliminate options 3 and 4 first because it is unsafe for clients to regulate their own medication dosages on the basis of symptoms. Option 1 is discarded next because clients should weigh themselves on a daily, not weekly, basis. Review home care measures now if you had difficulty with this question!

Level of Cognitive Ability: Analysis
Phase of Nursing Process: Evaluation
Client Needs: Health Promotion and Maintenance
Content Area: Adult Health/Cardiovascular

References

Smeltzer, S., & Bare, B. (1996). *Brunner and Suddarth's Textbook of medical-surgical nursing* (8th ed.). Philadelphia: Lippincott-Raven, p. 663.

---

224. The nurse is evaluating the effects of therapy for the client with pulmonary edema. The nurse would consider that the interventions were most effective if the client exhibited which of the following?

1 Blood pressure (BP), 96/56; pulse, 110; respiratory rate (RR), 28; urine output, 30 mL/hour
2 BP, 88/50; pulse, 116; RR, 26; urine output, 25 mL/hour
3 BP, 108/62; pulse, 98; RR, 24; urine output, 40 mL/hour
4 BP, 116/68; pulse, 86; RR, 20; urine output, 50 mL/hour

Answer: 4

Rationale: Expected outcomes for the client with pulmonary edema include improved cardiac output, as evidenced by normal vital signs and urine output greater than 30 mL/hour.

Test-Taking Strategy: Knowledge of normal vital signs and urine output will help you systematically eliminate each of the incorrect options. Eliminate options 1 and 2 first because the urine output needs to be greater than 30 mL. In the remaining two options, examine the vital signs. Option 4 identifies the most normal BP, pulse, and RR!

Level of Cognitive Ability: Analysis
Phase of Nursing Process: Evaluation
Client Needs: Physiological Integrity
Content Area: Adult Health/Cardiovascular

Reference

Luckmann, J. (1997). *Saunders manual of nursing care.* Philadelphia: W. B. Saunders, p. 1074.

225. The nurse has taught the post–cardiac surgery client about activity limitations for the first 6 weeks after hospital discharge. The nurse would evaluate that the client has understood the instructions if the client stated that he or she would

1. Use the arms for balance, not weight support, when getting out of bed or chair.
2. Lift nothing heavier than 25 pounds.
3. Drive only if wearing lap and shoulder seat belts.
4. Resume activities that involve straining as long as they do not cause pain.

Answer: 1

Rationale: Typical discharge activity instructions for the first 6 weeks include lifting nothing heavier than 5 pounds, not driving, and avoiding any activities that cause straining. The client is taught to use the arms for balance, but not for weight support, to avoid the effects of straining. These limitations are to allow for sternal healing, which takes approximately 6 weeks.

Test-Taking Strategy: Option 4 is eliminated first because it is contraindicated in several cardiac conditions. Option 2 is excessive, so that can be eliminated next. Of the remaining options, it is common practice after many surgical procedures to prohibit driving temporarily; this leaves you with the correct option, which is 1 (this option, incidentally, helps the client avoid straining).

Level of Cognitive Ability: Analysis
Phase of Nursing Process: Evaluation
Client Needs: Health Promotion and Maintenance
Content Area: Adult Health/Cardiovascular

Reference

Black, J., & Matassarin-Jacobs, E. (1997). *Medical-surgical nursing: Clinical management for continuity of care* (5th ed.). Philadelphia: W. B. Saunders, p. 1363.

---

226. The nurse has counseled the client after cardiac surgery about when it is safe to resume sexual activities. The nurse would need to correct the client if which of the following statements was made?

1. "I should be OK when I can walk one block or can climb two flights of stairs."
2. "I should wait for 2 hours after eating or drinking alcohol."
3. "The room should be slightly chilly so I don't get overheated."
4. "A comfortable position will probably work best."

Answer: 3

Rationale: Clients can resume sexual activity on the advice of a physician, which generally is given when the client can walk one block or climb two flights of stairs without discomfort. Suggestions to minimize potential problems include waiting for 2 hours after meals or alcohol consumption, making sure that the client feels well rested, using a comfortable position, and keeping the room at a mild temperature.

Test-Taking Strategy: The question is worded to look for an incorrect statement. Use the process of elimination and knowledge regarding client teaching in this area. Quickly review these now if you had difficulty with this question!

Level of Cognitive Ability: Analysis
Phase of Nursing Process: Evaluation
Client Needs: Health Promotion and Maintenance
Content Area: Adult Health/Cardiovascular

Reference

Luckmann, J. (1997). *Saunders manual of nursing care.* Philadelphia: W. B. Saunders, p. 1077.

227. The nurse has oriented a new employee to basic procedures for continuous ECG monitoring. The nurse would need to intervene if the orientee did which of the following while initiating cardiac monitoring on a client?

1 Cleansed the skin with povidone iodine (Betadine) before applying electrodes
2 Clipped small areas of hair under the area planned for electrode placement
3 Stated the need to change the electrodes every 24 hours and inspect the skin
4 Stated the availability of hypoallergenic electrodes for clients who are sensitive

Answer: 1

Rationale: The skin is cleansed with soap and water (not Betadine), denatured with alcohol, and allowed to air dry before electrodes are applied. The other three options are correct.

Test-Taking Strategy: The word "intervene" in the stem makes you look for an incorrect item. Eliminate options 3 and 4 because they are correct. If you have trouble discriminating between the two remaining options, remember that Betadine is used to cleanse the skin, usually before some type of invasive procedure that breaks the skin barrier. ECG monitoring does not break the skin.

Level of Cognitive Ability: Analysis
Phase of Nursing Process: Evaluation
Client Needs: Safe, Effective Care Environment
Content Area: Adult Health/Cardiovascular

Reference

Black, J., & Matassarin-Jacobs, E. (1997). *Medical-surgical nursing: Clinical management for continuity of care* (5th ed.). Philadelphia: W. B. Saunders, p. 1221.

228. The client has undergone defibrillation three times with an automatic external defibrillator (AED). The nurse observes that the attempts to convert the ventricular fibrillation were unsuccessful. On the basis of an evaluation of the situation, the nurse anticipates that which of the following actions would be best?

1 Performing CPR for 1 minute, then defibrillating up to three more times at 360 joules
2 Performing CPR for 5 minutes, then defibrillating three more times at 400 joules
3 Administering sodium bicarbonate intravenously
4 Terminating the resuscitation effort

Answer: 1

Rationale: After three unsuccessful defibrillation attempts, CPR should be done for 1 minute, followed by three more shocks, each delivered at 360 joules.

Test-Taking Strategy: There is no information in the stem to indicate that life support should be terminated, so option 4 is eliminated. Sodium bicarbonate is plausible, but the question asks for the "best" next action. Thus your realistic choices are narrowed to the first two options. Giving CPR for 5 minutes may not help oxygenation to the brain and myocardium in the long run. It would be better to do CPR for 1 minute and then resume attempts to convert the rhythm to a viable one.

Level of Cognitive Ability: Analysis
Phase of Nursing Process: Evaluation
Client Needs: Physiological Integrity
Content Area: Adult Health/Cardiovascular

Reference

Ignatavicius, D. D., Workman, M. L., & Mishler, M. A. (1995). *Medical-surgical nursing: A nursing process approach* (2nd ed.). Philadelphia: W. B. Saunders, p. 879.

229. Which of the following evaluative statements indicates a positive outcome for a child with a nursing diagnosis of Altered Growth and Development related to immobilization and hospitalization?

1. The fracture heals without complications
2. The child displays age-appropriate developmental behaviors
3. The caregivers verbalize safe and effective home care
4. The child maintains normal joint and muscle integrity

Answer: 2

Rationale: Regression and inappropriate developmental behaviors may be displayed in response to immobilization and hospitalization. With individualized care planning, a positive outcome of age-appropriate behavior can be achieved. Options 1, 3, and 4 are appropriate evaluative statements for an immobilized child but do not directly address the problem statement: Altered Growth and Development.

Test-Taking Strategy: The question seeks an evaluative statement that addresses the nursing diagnosis Altered Growth and Development. By definition, Altered Growth and Development is the state in which an individual is not performing age-appropriate tasks. All options are evaluative statements, but only option 2 addresses this nursing diagnosis. Focus on the issue of the question!

Level of Cognitive Ability: Analysis
Phase of Nursing Process: Evaluation
Client Needs: Health Promotion and Maintenance
Content Area: Child Health

Reference

Ashwill, J., & Droske, S. (1997). *Nursing care of children: Principles and practice.* Philadelphia: W. B. Saunders, pp. 1105–1111.

---

230. The nurse is evaluating the parent's understanding of discharge care, including the functioning of the infant's ventricular peritoneal shunt. Which of the following statements, if made by the parent, indicates accurate assessment of shunt complications?

1. "If the baby has a high-pitched cry, I should call the doctor."
2. "I should position my baby on the side with the shunt when sleeping."
3. "My baby will pass urine more often now that the shunt is in place."
4. "I should call my doctor if my baby refuses purées."

Answer: 1

Rationale: If the shunt is broken or malfunctioning, the fluid from the ventricle part of the brain will not be diverted to the peritoneal cavity. The cerebrospinal fluid will build up in the cranial area. The result is intracranial pressure, which then causes pain, which the infant manifests with a high-pitched cry. The baby should not have pressure when on the shunt side; skin breakdown and possible compressions to the apparatus could result. This type of shunt affects the gastrointestinal system, not the genitourinary system. Option 4 is a concern only if the baby becomes malnourished or dehydrated, which could then raise the body temperature; otherwise, refusal to eat purées has no direct relationship to the shunt's functioning.

Test-Taking Strategy: Knowledge regarding a ventricular peritoneal shunt is necessary to answer the question. Use the process of elimination on the basis of this knowledge to answer the question. Remember that a high-pitched cry in an infant indicates pain or another problem. If you had difficulty with this question, take time now to review assessment findings that indicate a complication with a shunt!

Level of Cognitive Ability: Analysis
Phase of Nursing Process: Evaluation
Client Needs: Physiological Integrity
Content Area: Child Health

Reference

Ashwill, J., & Droske, S. (1997). *Nursing care of children: Principles and practice.* Philadelphia: W. B. Saunders, pp. 1237–1240.

231. The nurse is reviewing the instillation technique for cromolyn sodium (Crolom) eyedrops and an antibiotic eye ointment with the parent of a pediatric client with a diagnosis of bacterial conjunctivitis. Which of the following statements made by the parent indicates that learning has taken place?

1. "I will administer the eye ointment, then wait 5 minutes and administer the eyedrops."
2. "I will place the child on her left side to administer drops in the right eye."
3. "I will have my child blink after the instillation to encourage thorough distribution of the eyedrops."
4. "I'll be careful not to touch the eye or eyelid during administration."

Answer: 4

Rationale: Eyedrops should be administered first, then eye ointment. The child should be placed in a supine position with neck slightly hyperextended for administration. Blinking will increase the loss of medication. Touching the eye or eyelid during medication administration can contaminate the dropper and also cause eye injury.

Test-Taking Strategy: Knowledge regarding the administration of eyedrops and ointments is necessary to answer the question. Use the process of elimination looking for a correct action. Review the basic principles associated with the administration of eyedrops and ointments now if you had difficulty with this question!

Level of Cognitive Ability: Analysis
Phase of Nursing Process: Evaluation
Client Needs: Health Promotion and Maintenance
Content Area: Child Health

Reference

Ashwill, J., & Droske, S. (1997). *Nursing care of children: Principles and practice.* Philadelphia: W. B. Saunders, pp. 498, 1337.

---

232. Which activity by the family of a baby with respiratory syncytial virus (RSV) who is receiving ribavirin (Virazole) would indicate knowledge deficit regarding the management of the disease process?

1. Telling Grandpa who has asthma that he may not visit
2. The family wears a gown, gloves, mask, and hair covering when they visit the infant
3. Before leaving the infant's room, all family members wash their hands
4. The infant's pregnant aunt visits while the infant is receiving ribavirin

Answer: 4

Rationale: Whenever anyone is receiving ribavirin, there are precautions to exposure. Everyone who enters the room while the client is receiving ribavirin should wear gown, mask, gloves, and hair covering. Anyone who is pregnant or considering pregnancy and anyone with a history of respiratory problems or reactive airway disease should not care for or visit anyone who is receiving ribavirin. Good handwashing is absolutely necessary before leaving the room; handwashing prevents the spread of germs.

Test-Taking Strategy: This question evaluates the family's ability to determine who can visit their child and what they need to do while in the room. Use the process of elimination. You should easily be able to identify the correct option to this question as it is stated because of the key phrase "pregnant aunt" in the correct option.

Level of Cognitive Ability: Analysis
Phase of Nursing Process: Evaluation
Client Needs: Safe, Effective Care Environment
Content Area: Child Health

Reference

Ashwill, J., & Droske, S. (1997). *Nursing care of children: Principles and practice.* Philadelphia: W. B. Saunders, p. 844.

---

233. The nurse is caring for a child after a hernia repair. Which of these findings would indicate that the surgical repair for an inguinal hernia was effective?

1. Abdominal distention
2. Absence of inguinal swelling with crying
3. A clean, dry incision
4. An adequate flow of urine

Answer: 2

Rationale: With an inguinal hernia, inguinal swelling occurs when an infant cries or strains. Absence of this swelling would indicate resolution of this problem. Abdominal distention indicates a continuing gastrointestinal problem. A clean, dry incision reflects lack of infection in the wound after surgery. The flow of urine is not specific to an inguinal hernia.

Test-Taking Strategy: Use the process of elimination, focusing on the issue: effective inguinal hernia repair. The only option that addresses this issue is option 2. Note the similarity, the word "inguinal," in the question and in the correct option!

Level of Cognitive Ability: Analysis
Phase of Nursing Process: Evaluation
Client Needs: Physiological Integrity
Content Area: Child Health

Reference

Wong, D. (1995). *Whaley and Wong's Nursing care of infants and children* (5th ed.). St. Louis: Mosby–Year Book, pp. 492–493.

---

234. After hydrostatic reduction for intussusception, the nurse should expect to observe which of these client responses?

1 Severe, colicky-type pain with vomiting
2 Currant jelly–like stools
3 Passage of barium or water-soluble contrast material with stools
4 Severe abdominal distention

Answer: 3

Rationale: After hydrostatic reduction, the nurse observes for passage of barium or water-soluble contrast material with stools. Options 1 and 2 are clinical indicators of intussusception. Option 4 is a sign of an unresolved gastrointestinal disorder.

Test-Taking Strategy: Use knowledge regarding hydrostatic reduction and the process of elimination to answer the question. On the basis of the question, seek a response that reflects a positive outcome. Options 1, 2, and 4 identify negative outcomes. If you had difficulty with this question, take time now to review hydrostatic reduction!

Level of Cognitive Ability: Analysis
Phase of Nursing Process: Evaluation
Client Needs: Physiological Integrity
Content Area: Child Health

Reference

Wong, D., & Perry, S. (1998). *Maternal-child nursing care*. St. Louis: Mosby–Year Book, p. 1430.

---

235. A 6-year-old with diabetes mellitus comes into the clinic with the mother for a routine examination. The nurse evaluates the data collected during this visit to determine whether the child has been euglycemic since the last visit. Which information is the most significant indicator of this?

1 The daily glucose monitor log
2 A fasting blood sugar (FBS) test today
3 A glycosylated hemoglobin measurement
4 A dietary history for last week

Answer: 3

Rationale: The glycosylated hemoglobin measures the glucose molecules that attach to the hemoglobin A molecules and remain there for the life of the red blood cell, which is approximately 120 days. This is not reversible and can't be altered by human intervention. Daily glucose logs for the period are useful if they are kept regularly and accurately. They reflect the blood glucose level only at the time the test was done. A FBS done today is time limited in its scope, as is the dietary history.

Test-Taking Strategy: A key phrase in the question is "last visit." Look for the option that would evaluate long-term euglycemia. This will assist in eliminating options 1, 2, and 4 because these options reflect short-term monitoring. If you had difficulty with this question, take time now to review glycosylated hemoglobin!

Level of Cognitive Ability: Analysis
Phase of Nursing Process: Evaluation
Client Needs: Physiological Integrity
Content Area: Child Health

Reference

Wong, D. (1995). *Whaley and Wong's Nursing care of infants and children* (5th ed.). St. Louis: Mosby–Year Book, p. 1770.

236. A child's fasting blood glucose levels range between 100 and 150 mg/dL daily. The before-dinner blood glucose levels are between 120 and 130 mg/dL with no reported episodes of hypoglycemia. Mixed insulin is administered before breakfast and before dinner. The nurse evaluates that the child's

1 Dietary needs are being met for adequate growth and development.
2 Dietary intake should be increased to avoid hypoglycemic reactions.
3 Insulin doses are appropriate for food ingested and activity level.
4 Exercise should be increased to reduce blood sugar levels.

Answer: 3

Rationale: The answer reflects the awareness of the interactive triad of effective management in diabetes: diet, medication, and exercise. Blood glucose levels are a measure of the balance between the three components. Options 2 and 4 imply that the data analyzed are abnormal. There are no data in the question to determine growth and development status, such as height, weight, age, or behavior. Supporting normal growth and development is an important goal in managing diabetes in children, but that isn't what is being evaluated here.

Test-Taking Strategy: Knowledge of the blood glucose norms and the basic components of management of diabetes would assist in eliminating options 2 and 4. The only option that identifies all three components of diabetic management is option 3.

Level of Cognitive Ability: Analysis
Phase of Nursing Process: Evaluation
Client Needs: Physiological Integrity
Content Area: Child Health

Reference

Wong, D. (1995). *Whaley and Wong's Nursing care of infants and children* (5th ed.). St. Louis: Mosby–Year Book, pp. 1778–1784.

237. The nurse has completed giving discharge instructions to the client after total knee replacement with a metal prosthesis. The nurse would evaluate that the client does not fully understand the instructions if the client verbalizes that he or she will

1 Report fever, redness, or increased pain.
2 Ignore changes in the shape of the knee.
3 Report bleeding gums or tarry stools.
4 Tell future caregivers about the metal implant.

Answer: 2

Rationale: After total knee replacement, the client should report signs and the symptoms of infection and any changes in the shape of the knee. Any of these could indicate developing complications. With a metal implant, the client must be on anticoagulant therapy and should report adverse effects of this therapy, including bleeding from a variety of sources. With a metal implant, the client must notify caregivers, because magnetic resonance imaging (MRI) will need to be avoided, and the client will need antibiotic prophylaxis for invasive procedures.

Test-Taking Strategy: The stem states that there is a metal prosthesis, which indicates that anticoagulant therapy is indicated. This would make options 3 and 4 appropriate responses. It is important to report signs and symptoms of infection (option 1), so that is eliminated as the answer to this question as well. By elimination, the correct answer is option 2. The client also needs to report changes in the shape of the knee, as this could indicate developing complications with the prosthesis.

Level of Cognitive Ability: Analysis
Phase of Nursing Process: Evaluation
Client Needs: Health Promotion and Maintenance
Content Area: Adult Health/Musculoskeletal

Reference

Luckmann, J. (1997). *Saunders manual of nursing care*. Philadelphia: W. B. Saunders, p. 1610.

238. The nurse has taught the client with herniated lumbar disk about proper body mechanics and other items pertinent to low back care. The nurse evaluates that the client needs further instruction if the client verbalizes that he or she will

1 Get out of bed by sitting straight up and swinging legs over the side of the bed.
2 Increase fiber and fluids in the diet.
3 Strengthen the back muscles by swimming or walking.
4 Bend at the knees to pick up objects.

Answer: 1

Rationale: Clients are taught to get out of bed by sliding near to the edge of the mattress, then rolling onto one side and pushing up from the bed, using one or both arms. The back is kept straight, and the legs are swung over the side. Increasing fluids and dietary fiber helps prevent straining at stool, thereby preventing increases in intraspinal pressure. Walking and swimming are excellent exercises for strengthening lower back muscles. Proper body mechanics includes bending at the knees, not the waist, to lift objects.

Test-Taking Strategy: The wording of this question guides you to look for an incorrect action. Options 3 and 4 are examples of classic interventions that are indicated, and so they are eliminated as answers to this question as stated. Clients with low back pain should avoid events that increase intraspinal pressure. Option 2 prevents increases in intraspinal pressure. Option 1 causes an increase in intraspinal pressure if you think of the body mechanics involved in getting out of bed this way. Therefore, you would choose option 1 as the answer to the question as it is phrased.

Level of Cognitive Ability: Analysis
Phase of Nursing Process: Evaluation
Client Needs: Health Promotion and Maintenance
Content Area: Adult Health/Musculoskeletal

Reference

Black, J., & Matassarin-Jacobs, E. (1997). *Medical-surgical nursing: Clinical management for continuity of care* (5th ed.). Philadelphia: W. B. Saunders, p. 918.

239. The client is being discharged to home after spinal fusion with insertion of a Harrington rod. The nurse would consult with the continuing care nurse regarding the need for follow-up modification of the home environment if the client stated that

1 The bedroom and bath are on the second floor of the home.
2 The bathroom has hand railings in the shower.
3 The family has rented a commode for use by the client.
4 There are three steps to get up to the front door.

Answer: 1

Rationale: Stair climbing may be restricted or limited for several weeks after spinal fusion with instrumentation. The nurse ensures that resources are in place before discharge so that the client may sleep and perform all ADLs on a single living level.

Test-Taking Strategy: Options 2 and 3 are obviously useful to the client and can therefore be eliminated as answers to the question as stated. To discriminate between options 1 and 4 (both of which involve stairs), you would determine that option 4 is the least problematic, whereas option 1 poses a significant problem to the client who is restricted from stair climbing. Thus option 1 is the answer to the question as it is stated.

Level of Cognitive Ability: Analysis
Phase of Nursing Process: Evaluation
Client Needs: Health Promotion and Maintenance
Content Area: Adult Health/Musculoskeletal

Reference

Ignatavicius, D. D., Workman, M. L., & Mishler, M. A. (1995). *Medical-surgical nursing: A nursing process approach* (2nd ed.). Philadelphia: W. B. Saunders, p. 1181.

240. The client has just had a cast removed, and the underlying skin is yellow-brown and crusted. The nurse gives the client instructions for skin care. The nurse evaluates that the client has misunderstood the directions if the client states that he or she will

1 Soak the skin and wash it gently.
2 Scrub the skin vigorously with soap and water.
3 Apply an emollient lotion to enhance softening.
4 Use a sunscreen on the skin if exposed for a period of time.

Answer: 2

Rationale: The skin under a casted area may be discolored and crusted with dead skin layers. The client should gently soak and wash the skin for the first few days. The skin should be patted dry, and a lubricating lotion should be applied. Clients often want to scrub the dead skin away, which irritates the skin. The client should avoid overexposing the skin to the sunlight.

Test-Taking Strategy: The question is worded to make you look for an incorrect item. Option 3 is obviously helpful and therefore cannot be the answer to the question as stated. Option 4 is good advice if the skin has been covered and is eliminated next. Options 1 and 2 seem to oppose each other, which makes it likely that one of them is correct. Because vigorous scrubbing is more likely to be irritating than is gentle soaking, the former is the most likely answer to the question.

Level of Cognitive Ability: Analysis
Phase of Nursing Process: Evaluation
Client Needs: Health Promotion and Maintenance
Content Area: Adult Health/Musculoskeletal

Reference

Black, J., & Matassarin-Jacobs, E. (1997). *Medical-surgical nursing: Clinical management for continuity of care* (5th ed.). Philadelphia: W. B. Saunders, pp. 2152–2153.

---

241. The nurse is evaluating goal achievement for the client in traction with a nursing diagnosis of Impaired Physical Mobility. The nurse would evaluate that the client has not successfully met all of the goals formulated if which of the following outcomes were noted?

1 Negative Homans' sign
2 Active ROM exercises of uninvolved joints
3 Intact skin surfaces
4 Bowel movement every 4 days

Answer: 4

Rationale: Expected outcomes for the client in traction with Impaired Physical Mobility include absence of thrombophlebitis (measurable by negative Homans' sign), active baseline ROM exercises of uninvolved joints, clear lung sounds, intact skin, and bowel movement every other day.

Test-Taking Strategy: This question can be answered systematically by evaluating the degree of normalcy of each option. The only abnormal option is option 4. A bowel movement every 4 days is insufficient. Constipation is a known complication of immobility.

Level of Cognitive Ability: Analysis
Phase of Nursing Process: Evaluation
Client Needs: Physiological Integrity
Content Area: Adult Health/Musculoskeletal

Reference

Black, J., & Matassarin-Jacobs, E. (1997). *Medical-surgical nursing: Clinical management for continuity of care* (5th ed.). Philadelphia: W. B. Saunders, p. 2143.

242. The nurse has given medication instructions to the client beginning therapy with carisoprodol (Soma). The nurse evaluates that the client understands the effects of the medication if the client states that he or she will

1 Expect muscle spasticity as a side effect.
2 Take a missed dose when remembered, regardless of when next dose is due.
3 Avoid alcohol while taking this medication.
4 Drive on city streets, but avoid highway driving.

Answer: 3

Rationale: Carisoprodol, a centrally acting skeletal muscle relaxant, may cause CNS side effects of drowsiness and dizziness. For this reason, the client avoids other CNS depressants, such as alcohol, while taking this medication. Driving and other activities requiring mental alertness are also avoided until the client's reaction to the medication is known. The medication is used to reduce muscle spasticity and pain. Missed doses should be taken if remembered within 1 hour.

Test-Taking Strategy: Begin to answer this question by eliminating option 4, because driving is either indicated or not indicated. Knowing that this medication is a skeletal muscle relaxant helps you to eliminate option 1 next, because this medication relieves muscle spasms. To discriminate between the last two options, knowing that alcohol should not be taken while on any medication that affects the CNS helps you to choose option 3 over option 2 as the correct answer.

Level of Cognitive Ability: Analysis
Phase of Nursing Process: Evaluation
Client Needs: Health Promotion and Maintenance
Content Area: Pharmacology

Reference

Deglin, J. H., & Vallerand, A. H. (1997). *Davis's drug guide for nurses* (5th ed.). Philadelphia: F. A. Davis, pp. 224–225.

243. Teaching for a family of a child who is a diabetic is considered to be effective if the family

1 Gives the child a diet carbonated beverage when the child feels shaky.
2 Has the child carry Life Savers with him or her whenever he or she leaves the home.
3 Administers glucagon when the child has a fruity, acetone breath odor.
4 Takes the child to the emergency room when the child's blood glucose level is 60 mg/dL.

Answer: 2

Rationale: The family needs to have the child carry a source of glucose with him or her for an instant source of glucose for a hypoglycemic reaction. Life Savers will provide that source of glucose. A diet carbonated beverage will not provide this need. A fruity, acetone breath odor indicates that the child needs immediate care. If the child's blood glucose level is 60 mg/dL, a source of glucose may be needed, but not necessarily in the emergency room.

Test-Taking Strategy: The issue of the question is the appropriate treatment for hypoglycemia. Options 1, 3, and 4 are inaccurate measures of care for hypoglycemia. Take time now to review the treatment for hypoglycemia, if you had difficulty with this question!

Level of Cognitive Ability: Analysis
Phase of Nursing Process: Evaluation
Client Needs: Physiological Integrity
Content Area: Child Health

Reference

Wong, D. (1995). *Whaley and Wong's Nursing care of infants and children* (5th ed.). St. Louis: Mosby–Year Book, p. 1772.

244. The community health nurse visits a client with Parkinson's disease at home. Amantadine (Symmetrel), 100 mg PO BID, has been prescribed for the client. The nurse teaches the client about the medication. Which of the following statements, if made by the client, indicates that further teaching is necessary?

1. "I'll take this medication early in the morning and at bedtime."
2. "I can empty the capsules into food or fluid to make swallowing easier."
3. "I can get this medication in syrup form if I have difficulty swallowing."
4. "I should see improvement in my condition in about 7 days."

Answer: 1

Rationale: Amantadine (Symmetrel) is administered twice a day, but the last dose should not be administered near bedtime because it may cause insomnia in some clients. Options 2, 3, and 4 are correct statements.

Test-Taking Strategy: This question tests your knowledge of amantadine and the nursing implications for its administration. Options 2, 3, and 4 all reflect correct answers regarding the administration of the medication. If you had difficulty with this question, take time now to review the nursing implications associated with its administration!

Level of Cognitive Ability: Analysis
Phase of Nursing Process: Evaluation
Client Needs: Health Promotion and Maintenance
Content Area: Pharmacology

Reference

Hodgson, B., & Kizior, R. (1998). *Saunders nursing drug handbook 1998.* Philadelphia: W. B. Saunders, pp. 35–37.

---

245. The adolescent client is preparing for discharge after spinal fusion with instrumentation for treatment of scoliosis. Which of the following statements by the client indicates the need for further teaching?

1. "I should eat a well-balanced diet."
2. "I will not be able to go rollerblading for the first few weeks after surgery."
3. "I should not bend or twist at the waist for several months."
4. "I will not participate in gym class for a few months."

Answer: 2

Rationale: Activity restrictions may vary from physician to physician, but generally include *no* bike riding, rollerblading, horseback riding, lawn mowing, skiing, lifting more than 10 pounds, or bending or twisting at the waist. Activity restrictions are maintained for 6–9 months, depending on degree and type of surgery. Option 1, eating a well-balanced diet, is always a prudent choice for postoperative clients, so that can be quickly eliminated (from the need for "further teaching").

Test-Taking Strategy: Use the process of elimination. Eliminate option 1 first because this is a general and appropriate statement. The key information needed to answer this question is that activity restrictions are maintained for 6–9 months, which points to option 2 as the statement which indicates the need for further teaching. Take time now to review postoperative teaching after spinal fusion with instrumentation if you had difficulty with this question!

Level of Cognitive Ability: Analysis
Phase of Nursing Process: Evaluation
Client Needs: Health Promotion and Maintenance
Content Area: Child Health

Reference

Ashwill, J., & Droske, S. (1997). *Nursing care of children: Principles and practice.* Philadelphia: W. B. Saunders, p. 1148.

---

246. Which of the following statements by the parents of a child with a short arm cast indicates that teaching regarding cast care was not effective?

1. "Check the skin around the cast edges for irritation."
2. "Keep the extremity elevated as much as possible to reduce swelling."
3. "Use a ruler padded with gauze to scratch under the cast."
4. "Call the doctor for any unusual odor from the cast."

Answer: 3

Rationale: Do not put anything inside a cast! A cotton-tipped applicator with rubbing alcohol may be used near cast edges to relieve itching. The skin around the cast edges should be checked for redness, irritation, and blistering. The extremity should be elevated as much as possible to minimize swelling. The physician should be notified for unusual odor and/or sudden unexplained fever (indicating infection), numbness/tingling, pallor, cyanosis, and/or pain unrelieved by medication (indicating neurovascular compromise).

Test-Taking Strategy: Knowledge regarding cast care is necessary to answer the question. Use the process of elimination, remembering that any form of object should never be placed into a cast. Review cast care now if you had difficulty with this question!

Level of Cognitive Ability: Analysis
Phase of Nursing Process: Evaluation
Client Needs: Health Promotion and Maintenance
Content Area: Child Health

Reference

Ball, J., & Bindler, R. (1995). *Pediatric nursing: Caring for children.* Norwalk, CT: Appleton & Lange, p. 587.

---

247. Which of the following evaluative statements indicates a positive outcome for a child with hemophilia?

1 The child's demand for oxygen will be balanced with the body's supply
2 The child experiences no long-term complications from bleeding injury
3 The child remains free from infection
4 The child will tolerate a well-balanced diet

Answer: 2

Rationale: Because risk for injury related to prolonged bleeding is a major problem for children with hemophilia, a positive outcome is achieved if the child experiences no long-term complications from bleeding. Options 1, 3, and 4 may be appropriate but are not specific to the child with hemophilia.

Test-Taking Strategy: Use the process of elimination, considering the issue of the question, which is the child with hemophilia. Knowledge that bleeding is a major concern with hemophilia should direct you to the correct option. If you had difficulty with this question, take time now to review hemophilia!

Level of Cognitive Ability: Analysis
Phase of Nursing Process: Evaluation
Client Needs: Physiological Integrity
Content Area: Child Health

Reference

Ashwill, J., & Droske, S. (1997). *Nursing care of children: Principles and practice.* Philadelphia: W. B. Saunders, pp. 979–981.

---

248. The client is receiving sulfisoxazole. The nurse evaluates the effectiveness of the therapy by monitoring the client's

1 Blood pressure.
2 Blood glucose.
3 Red blood cell count.
4 White blood cell count.

Answer: 4

Rationale: Sulfisoxazole is an anti-infective used primarily to treat urinary tract infections. The effectiveness of the medication may be evaluated by monitoring the client's white blood cell count, which should decrease to within normal limits with therapy. The client should also experience relief of symptoms.

Test-Taking Strategy: To answer this question accurately, it is necessary to know that this medication is an anti-infective and not used as an antihypertensive (option 1), as a hypoglycemic agent (option 2), or to treat anemia (option 3). If you had difficulty with this question, take time now to review the action of this medication!

Level of Cognitive Ability: Analysis
Phase of Nursing Process: Evaluation
Client Needs: Physiological Integrity
Content Area: Pharmacology

Reference

Deglin, J. H., & Vallerand, A. H. (1997). *Davis's drug guide for nurses* (5th ed.). Philadelphia: F. A. Davis, p. 1116.

249. The client is receiving supplemental therapy with folic acid (Folvite). The nurse evaluates the effectiveness of this therapy by monitoring the results of which of the following laboratory studies?

1 Complete blood count
2 Blood urea nitrogen
3 Blood glucose
4 Alkaline phosphatase

Answer: 1

Rationale: Folic acid is necessary for red blood cell (RBC) production and is classified as a vitamin and an antianemic. The effectiveness of therapy can be measured by monitoring the results of periodic complete blood count levels, noting particularly the hematocrit level.

Test-Taking Strategy: To answer this question accurately, it is necessary to know that folic acid is a vitamin, which may be used as a supplement to treat anemia. From this point, you should be able to eliminate options 2, 3, and 4. If you are not familiar with effects of folic acid on the body, take a few moments to review these basic concepts now!

Level of Cognitive Ability: Analysis
Phase of Nursing Process: Evaluation
Client Needs: Physiological Integrity
Content Area: Pharmacology

Reference

Hodgson, B., & Kizior, R. (1998). *Saunders nursing drug handbook 1998.* Philadelphia: W. B. Saunders, pp. 445–446.

---

250. The client with a history of prostatic hypertrophy has been prescribed propantheline (Pro-Banthīne) for the treatment of peptic ulcer disease. The nurse evaluates that medication instruction has been effective if the client states that he or she will report

1 Abdominal cramping or diarrhea.
2 Excessive salivation.
3 Urinary hesitancy or retention.
4 Excessive sweating.

Answer: 3

Rationale: Propantheline is an anticholinergic medication that is used as an adjunct for therapy in peptic ulcer disease. It is also used as an antispasmodic agent. It should be used cautiously with prostatic hypertrophy because the anticholinergic effects of the medication could cause exacerbation of symptoms, including urinary retention or hesitancy. Other side effects of the medication include constipation, dry mouth, and decreased sweating. Tachycardia is a common cardiovascular side effect.

Test-Taking Strategy: Begin to answer this question by analyzing the information in the stem. The prescribed medication is an anticholinergic, which causes urinary retention. The client already has a potential problem with urinary elimination. Using this combined knowledge, you would rapidly eliminate each of the other incorrect responses. Note the relationship between "prostatic hypertrophy" in the question and "urinary hesitancy or retention" in the correct option. Review the side effects of this medication now if you had difficulty with this question!

Level of Cognitive Ability: Analysis
Phase of Nursing Process: Evaluation
Client Needs: Health Promotion and Maintenance
Content Area: Pharmacology

Reference

Deglin, J. H., & Vallerand, A. H. (1997). *Davis's drug guide for nurses* (5th ed.). Philadelphia: F. A. Davis, p. 1023.

251. The home care nurse has given instructions to the female client with cystitis about measures to prevent recurrence. The nurse evaluates that the client needs further instruction if the client verbalizes that he or she will

1. Take bubble baths for more effective hygiene.
2. Wear underwear made of cotton or with cotton panels.
3. Drink a glass of water and void after intercourse.
4. Avoid wearing pantyhose while wearing slacks.

Answer: 1

Rationale: Measures to prevent cystitis include increasing fluid intake to 3 liters/day; using an acid-ash diet; wiping front to back after urination; using showers instead of tub baths; drinking water and voiding after intercourse; avoiding bubble baths, feminine hygiene sprays, perfumed toilet tissue, and scented sanitary pads; and wearing clothes that "breathe" (cotton pants, no tight jeans, no pantyhose under slacks). Other measures include teaching pregnant women to void every 2 hours and teaching menopausal women to use estrogen vaginal creams to restore vaginal pH.

Test-Taking Strategy: The wording of the question guides you to look for an incorrect response. Options 2 and 4 are eliminated first as possible choices because they are good actions to promote circulation of air through the fabric. Knowing that drinking water and voiding after intercourse helps prevent bacteria from ascending the urinary tract helps you to eliminate this option as well. Thus the correct answer is the bubble bath. Bubble baths, tub baths, perfumes, and sprays are all avoided in the client with cystitis.

Level of Cognitive Ability: Analysis
Phase of Nursing Process: Evaluation
Client Needs: Health Promotion and Maintenance
Content Area: Adult Health/Renal

Reference

Black, J., & Matassarin-Jacobs, E. (1997). *Medical-surgical nursing: Clinical management for continuity of care* (5th ed.). Philadelphia: W. B. Saunders, p. 1573.

---

252. The client with pyelonephritis is being discharged from the hospital. The nurse gives the client discharge instructions to prevent recurrence. The nurse evaluates that the client understands the information that was given if the client states an intention to

1. Report signs and symptoms of urinary tract infection (UTI) if they persist for more than 1 week.
2. Take the prescribed antibiotics until all symptoms subside.
3. Return to the physician's office for scheduled follow-up urine cultures.
4. Modify fluid intake for the day on the basis of the previous day's output.

Answer: 3

Rationale: The client with pyelonephritis should take the full course of antibiotic therapy that has been prescribed and return to the physician's office for follow-up urine cultures if so instructed. The client should learn the signs and symptoms of UTI, and report them immediately if they occur. The client should use all measures that are used to prevent cystitis, which includes forcing fluids to 3 liters/day.

Test-Taking Strategy: Begin to answer this question by eliminating option 1 because UTI symptoms should never go unreported for a week. Option 2 is eliminated next because antibiotics should be taken for the full course of treatment for adequate elimination of the infection. Knowing that the client needs follow-up urine cultures helps you to choose option 3 over option 4, which is not done.

Level of Cognitive Ability: Analysis
Phase of Nursing Process: Evaluation
Client Needs: Health Promotion and Maintenance
Content Area: Adult Health/Renal

Reference

Black, J., & Matassarin-Jacobs, E. (1997). *Medical-surgical nursing: Clinical management for continuity of care* (5th ed.). Philadelphia: W. B. Saunders, p. 1630.

253. The nurse is evaluating the effects of care for the client with nephrotic syndrome. The nurse would evaluate that the client showed the least amount of improvement if which of the following information was obtained serially over 2 days of care?

1 Initial weight 208 pounds, down to 203 pounds
2 Daily intake/output record of 2100 mL/1900 mL and 2000 mL/2900 mL
3 Blood pressure 160/90, down to 148/85
4 Serum albumin 1.9 g/dL, up to 2.0 g/dL

Answer: 4

Rationale: The goal of therapy in nephrotic syndrome is to heal the leaking glomerular membrane. This would then control edema by stopping loss of protein in the urine. Fluid balance and albumin levels are monitored to determine effectiveness of therapy. Option 1 represents a loss of fluid that slightly exceeds 2 liters and represents a significant improvement. Option 2 represents a total fluid loss of 700 mL over the 2 days, which is also helpful. Option 3 shows improvement because both systolic and diastolic blood pressures are lower, with the diastolic pressure reentering the normal range. The least amount of improvement is in the serum albumin level, because the normal albumin level is 3.5–5.0 g/dL.

Test-Taking Strategy: The question asks for the item that indicates the least amount of clinical improvement. This implies that more than one or all of the responses are partially correct. Option 1 illustrates the greatest improvement and is eliminated first. Option 2 is also a significant improvement and is eliminated next. To discriminate between options 3 and 4, knowing that the blood pressure has reentered the normal range for the diastolic pressure may help you to choose this option over the albumin level.

Level of Cognitive Ability: Analysis
Phase of Nursing Process: Evaluation
Client Needs: Physiological Integrity
Content Area: Adult Health/Renal

Reference

Black, J., & Matassarin-Jacobs, E. (1997). *Medical-surgical nursing: Clinical management for continuity of care* (5th ed.). Philadelphia: W. B. Saunders, p. 1635.

254. The nurse has given the client with polycystic disease information about management of the disorder and about prevention and recognition of complications. The nurse evaluates that the client needs further instruction if the client states that he or she will report

1 Lowered blood pressure.
2 Onset of shortness of breath.
3 Fever.
4 Burning on urination.

Answer: 1

Rationale: The client with polycystic kidney disease should report any signs and symptoms of urinary tract infection so that treatment may begin promptly. The client should also report rises in blood pressure, as control of hypertension is essential. The client may experience heart failure as a result of hypertension, and thus any symptoms of heart failure, such as shortness of breath, are also reported.

Test-Taking Strategy: The wording of the question guides you to look for an incorrect response. Begin to answer this question by eliminating options 3 and 4 first, because signs of infection should be reported to the physician. To discriminate accurately between the remaining two options, it is necessary to know that the client with polycystic kidney disease is likely to be hypertensive. Because a complication of hypertension is heart failure, the nurse also teaches the client to report these signs and symptoms. With this in mind, you would know that shortness of breath should be reported. This leaves, option 1, lowered blood pressure, as the correct answer. Lowered blood pressure is not a complication of polycystic kidney disease, and it is an expected effect of effective antihypertensive therapy. Thus this does not need to be reported, and option 1 is the answer to the question as stated.

Level of Cognitive Ability: Analysis
Phase of Nursing Process: Evaluation
Client Needs: Health Promotion and Maintenance
Content Area: Adult Health/Renal

Reference

Black, J., & Matassarin-Jacobs, E. (1997). *Medical-surgical nursing: Clinical management for continuity of care* (5th ed.). Philadelphia: W. B. Saunders, pp. 1678–1679.

255. The nurse is discharging the client to home after cystolitholapaxy. The nurse would evaluate that the client understands instructions for prevention of recurrence of calcium oxalate stones if the client states that he or she will

1 Self-treat with cranberry juice if symptoms of urinary tract infection occur.
2 Follow a diet to keep the urine alkaline.
3 Hold the urine for 4–6 hours between voidings.
4 Take in at least 3 liters of fluid per day.

Answer: 4

Rationale: Prevention of recurrence of urinary stones is accomplished by drinking at least 3 liters of fluid per day; voiding every 2 hours; following an acid-ash diet; and notifying the physician promptly if symptoms of urinary tract infection (UTI) occur.

Test-Taking Strategy: Begin to answer this question by eliminating options 1 and 3 first. These are not the measures that are generally indicated for clients with urinary tract problems. To discriminate accurately between options 2 and 4, it is necessary to know that the diet should be acid-ash. This would allow you to choose option 4 (3 liter fluid intake per day) as the correct answer. Review client instructions for the treatment of calcium oxalate stones now if you had difficulty with this question!

Level of Cognitive Ability: Analysis
Phase of Nursing Process: Evaluation
Client Needs: Health Promotion and Maintenance
Content Area: Adult Health/Renal

Reference

Black, J., & Matassarin-Jacobs, E. (1997). *Medical-surgical nursing: Clinical management for continuity of care* (5th ed.). Philadelphia: W. B. Saunders, pp. 1597–1598.

256. The client is being discharged to home after undergoing extracorporeal shock wave lithotripsy. The nurse evaluates that the client has a good understanding of discharge instructions if the client verbalizes that he or she will report which of the following?

1 Bruising along the flank area
2 Flank pain or difficulty urinating
3 Passing of stone fragments
4 Hematuria

Answer: 2

Rationale: The client should report pain in the flank area or the bladder, because it may indicate infection or the beginning of another calculus. The client also should report difficulty urinating, as well as fever, chills, or nausea. The client is taught to expect flank bruising to remain for some weeks after the procedure and to expect hematuria for a few days. Passing of remaining calculus fragments may occur and is expected.

Test-Taking Strategy: Begin to answer this question by eliminating option 3 because this would be an obvious expected effect of the procedure. Because of the nature of the procedure and the effect of the shocks to the tissues, you may then eliminate options 1 and 4 as temporary effects. This would leave option 2 as the correct answer. Using a different train of thought, you may also select option 2 as the correct option to report by knowing that these symptoms are consistent with urinary obstruction or infection.

Level of Cognitive Ability: Analysis
Phase of Nursing Process: Evaluation
Client Needs: Physiological Integrity
Content Area: Adult Health/Renal

Reference

Black, J., & Matassarin-Jacobs, E. (1997). *Medical-surgical nursing: Clinical management for continuity of care* (5th ed.). Philadelphia: W. B. Saunders, p. 2072.

257. The client with renal cancer is being treated preoperatively with radiation therapy. The nurse evaluates that the client has an understanding of proper care of the skin over the treatment field if the client states that he or she will

1. Avoid skin exposure to direct sunlight and chlorinated water.
2. Use lanolin-based cream on the affected skin on a daily basis.
3. Remove the lines or ink marks by using a gentle soap after each treatment.
4. Use the hottest water possible to wash the treatment site twice daily.

Answer: 1

Rationale: The client undergoing radiation therapy should avoid washing the site until instructed to do so. The client should then wash with mild soap and warm or cool water and pat the area dry. No lotions, creams, alcohol, or deodorants should be placed on the skin over the treatment site. Lines or ink marks that are placed on the skin to guide the radiation therapy should be left in place. The affected skin should be protected from temperature extremes, direct sunlight, and chlorinated water (as from swimming pools).

Test-Taking Strategy: Begin to answer this question by eliminating options 2 and 4 because they are contraindicated in the care of this client. Knowing that markings used to guide therapy are to be left in place helps you to choose option 1 over option 3. Review skin care for the client undergoing radiation now if you had difficulty with this question!

Level of Cognitive Ability: Analysis
Phase of Nursing Process: Evaluation
Client Needs: Physiological Integrity
Content Area: Adult Health/Oncology

Reference

Black, J., & Matassarin-Jacobs, E. (1997). *Medical-surgical nursing: Clinical management for continuity of care* (5th ed.). Philadelphia: W. B. Saunders, pp. 571, 1673.

258. Teaching interventions to help the child and family to understand treatment for a child with acute lymphocytic leukemia (ALL), who has come out of remission twice, should be considered effective if the family states

1. "Our child will be just fine in a few days. Our child always was before."
2. "We know that a bone marrow transplant may not work; however, we will have to go ahead with the treatment as chemotherapy has not helped."
3. "There is no effective treatment for ALL now. We will have to look for alternative therapies."
4. "Fortunately, our child will not have to undergo any more treatments before the bone marrow transplant. We do not want to see our child have any more radiation or medications."

Answer: 2

Rationale: Bone marrow transplantation is the treatment of choice for ALL after the child has come out of remission twice. The prognosis for a child after bone marrow transplantation is between 25% and 50%. The child faces almost certain death if bone marrow transplantation is not done. The child will have to have extensive radiation and medications before transplantation.

Test-Taking Strategy: Knowledge regarding the treatments for ALL is necessary to answer the question. Options 1, 3, and 4 are inaccurate parent responses. Take time now to review treatments for ALL and bone marrow transplantation if you had difficulty with this question!

Level of Cognitive Ability: Analysis
Phase of Nursing Process: Evaluation
Client Needs: Physiological Integrity
Content Area: Child Health

Reference

Pillitteri, A. (1995). *Maternal and child health nursing: Care of the childbearing and childrearing family* (2nd ed.). Philadelphia: Lippincott-Raven, pp. 1372–1373.

259. A 2-month-old infant has just had the recommended immunizations at the pediatrician's office. The nurse has given the immunizations and questioned the mother about the home care instructions. Which statement by the mother would indicate that she needs further instructions?

1. "If the baby becomes fussy, I will give the baby some Tylenol."
2. "If the baby develops a high fever, I will give the baby Children's Motrin."
3. "I will not give the baby a bottle until I get home."
4. I will wash my hands well after I change the baby's diaper."

Answer: 2

Rationale: A high fever after receiving the first set of immunizations could be an indication of a severe reaction to the diphteria, pertussis, and tetanus (DPT) immunization. The mother is instructed to call her pediatrician if the infant develops a high fever.

Test-Taking Strategy: This question asks you to select the response that indicates that the mother needs further teaching. Use the process of elimination and knowledge regarding reactions to immunizations. The key phrase in the correct option is "high fever." If this occurs, the physician should be notified!

Level of Cognitive Ability: Analysis
Phase of Nursing Process: Evaluation
Client Needs: Health Promotion and Maintenance
Content Area: Child Health

Reference

Ashwill, J., & Droske, S. (1997). *Nursing care of children: Principles and practice.* Philadelphia: W. B. Saunders, p. 597.

---

260. The client is gravida 4, para 3. Ultrasonography has revealed a large fetus. Because of these risk factors, the nurse plans to promote a controlled, well-coached labor. This may prevent an augmented or difficult labor, an additional risk variable for amniotic fluid embolism. Which of the following outcomes will best indicate that the nursing strategies to meet that goal have been successful?

1. The client states, "We had too much to do to attend the birthing class reviews, but with as many children as we have, we will make it through this one."
2. A 4-hour labor culminates in an uncomplicated delivery
3. After 8 hours of labor, the physician orders oxytocin (Pitocin) augmentation, second stage is reached within an hour, and vaginal delivery completed after a half hour of pushing
4. With the assistance of the nurse, the husband attempts to coach the client throughout labor

Answer: 2

Rationale: Option 1 is not specific to the issue of the question and does not address a positive outcome. Four hours is an appropriate time for a normal labor of a multiparous woman and is not considered difficult. Eight hours of labor is not optimal. Note the phrase "husband attempts" in option 4. This also is not the most positive outcome. Optimum health potential for a childbearing family is a normal labor and delivery with a healthy mother and baby. This is the cardinal measurement of the effectiveness of risk prevention in labor.

Test-Taking Strategy: In a risk prevention (health maintenance) or health promotion question, the correct answer will describe the ideal outcome for the client. Use the process of elimination, identifying the most optimal situation. This process should direct you to option 2.

Level of Cognitive Ability: Analysis
Phase of Nursing Process: Evaluation
Client Needs: Health Promotion and Maintenance
Content Area: Maternity

Reference

Reeder, S., Martin, L., & Koniak-Griffin, D. (1997). *Maternity nursing* (18th ed.). Philadelphia: Lippincott-Raven, p. 523.

261. The client's congestive heart failure is stabilized, and the client is ready for discharge from the hospital. The nurse evaluates that the client is ready for discharge to home if the client can

1 Verbally describe the daily medications, doses, and times.
2 Get the prescriptions filled.
3 Be self-sufficient at home without any help.
4 Independently dress and put on support hose.

Answer: 1

Rationale: Medication therapy is an essential part of the therapeutic regimen for treating cardiac failure. The client must have a clear understanding of which medications to take and when to take them. Options 2 and 4 can be carried out with the assistance of someone else. Option 3 may not be realistic for the client who could maintain an acceptable level of functioning with help.

Test-Taking Strategy: Note the issue of the question: that the client is ready for discharge. Also identify the priority for home care. Options 2, 3, and 4 can be accomplished by others or with the assistance of others. It is a priority that the client understand the medication regimen.

Level of Cognitive Ability: Analysis
Phase of Nursing Process: Evaluation
Client Needs: Health Promotion and Maintenance
Content Area: Adult Health/Cardiovascular

Reference

Black, J., & Matassarin-Jacobs, E. (1997). *Medical-surgical nursing: Clinical management for continuity of care* (5th ed.). Philadelphia: W. B. Saunders, p. 1291.

262. The community health nurse visits an older female adult client at home. The client was found wandering the highway in her nightgown last night. Her daughter, who lives with her, says to the nurse, "This wandering started last week, but this is the first time she got out of the house. She always seems to do it around 10:00 P.M. What can I do?" On the basis of an evaluation of the situation, the most therapeutic response would be

1 "This is probably 'sundowners syndrome,' a common occurrence in older adults."
2 "Since this is the first time your mother has gotten away from you, what has worked before this time?"
3 "I think you need to consider a nursing home immediately. Put your mother's name in, and when an empty bed comes up, let the doctor admit her. You can't handle this alone, and she could get killed!"
4 "Try approaching her before it happens so she doesn't wander. This could be seen as neglect, and you could be prosecuted."

Answer: 2

Rationale: This question tests your knowledge of the appropriate therapeutic communication to employ with a caregiver who is puzzled and frightened by a change in her mother's behavior. The nurse is most therapeutic if an accurate assessment of this change is first made. The best response here is the one that focuses the daughter's problem solving so that the nurse can then suggest strategies to try. The nurse will want to carefully document this behavior change and visit frequently to evaluate the client more specifically.

Test-Taking Strategy: Option 1, while it may be correct, does not help at this time, and it is too early to judge (other factors may be causing confusion, which is why assessment needs to be developed further). Option 3 is histrionic and too early an intervention, according to the inadequate information. Option 4 is a fine intervention, but the nurse doesn't know what the caregiver may have tried, and it may cause resentment if the nurse assumes the caregiver did not think critically.

Level of Cognitive Ability: Application
Phase of Nursing Process: Evaluation
Client Needs: Psychosocial Integrity
Content Area: Mental Health

Reference

Antai-Otong, D. (1995). *Psychiatric nursing: Biological and behavioral concepts.* Philadelphia: W. B. Saunders, pp. 543–576.

263. The community health nurse visits an older adult client at home who says to the nurse, "I wonder if you could do a little grocery shopping for me? I usually go but I'm feeling so 'punk' that I don't think I can manage." Which of the following statements, if made by the nurse, would be the most therapeutic response?

1 "I'm sorry, but I'm not allowed to do that; it's against agency policy."
2 "Do you have any family or support systems you can call on when you're feeling 'punk'?"
3 "Professional nurses don't have the time to do these things with their heavy caseloads. Please call a grocery store with home delivery."
4 "This is a problem not having someone to help on those 'punk' days. Let's discuss how we can solve it."

Answer: 4

Rationale: The client is feeling "punk" and asks for the nurse's assistance. The nurse has two immediate tasks. The first is to set limits on what the nurse can reasonably accomplish (given a normal caseload, which is usually heavy and tightly scheduled). The second task (but really the first priority) is the nurse's commitment to helping the client. It is important that the nurse assess first and find out what feeling "punk" means. Then the nurse must find an immediate solution and a solution for the long-term problem.

Test-Taking Strategy: This question tests your knowledge of therapeutic communications for an older adult client who has asked the nurse to extend roles and responsibilities. It is not so much a lack of willingness as it is appropriate delegation of authority and assisting the client. In option 1, the nurse hides behind policy and rules, a very passive approach. In option 2, the nurse asks a closed-ended question. In addition, the nurse's question could depress the client even more. Option 3 is pompous and makes the nurse seem to be one who thinks more of status than of helping the client. Option 4 reflects the client's situation and begins to work with the client in a mutual way that preserves the client's locus of control.

Level of Cognitive Ability: Application
Phase of Nursing Process: Evaluation
Client Needs: Psychosocial Integrity
Content Area: Mental Health

References

Antai-Otong, D. (1995). *Psychiatric nursing: Biological and behavioral concepts.* Philadelphia: W. B. Saunders, pp. 543–576.

264. In care for a child with juvenile rheumatoid arthritis (JRA), which of the following is an appropriate evaluative statement indicating a positive outcome?

1 Maintain therapeutic blood levels of nonsteroidal anti-inflammatory drugs (NSAIDs) to control pain and ensure maximum comfort
2 The child will exhibit age-appropriate growth and development
3 The child experienced relief from pain, as evidenced by resting more comfortably and increased levels of self-care
4 The child will accept activity restrictions and increase joint mobility and muscle strength

Answer: 3

Rationale: An evaluative statement gives information about whether a particular outcome was achieved. Option 3 is the only statement that fits this description.

Test-Taking Strategy: Recognize that the question asks for an evaluation statement. Options 2 and 4 are expected outcomes (goals) and should be eliminated. Note the similarity in these statements: "The child will." Similarly, option 1 can be eliminated because it is not an evaluative statement. This option addresses the medical plan rather than the nursing plan.

Level of Cognitive Ability: Analysis
Phase of Nursing Process: Evaluation
Client Needs: Physiological Integrity
Content Area: Child Health

Reference

Ashwill, J., & Droske, S. (1997). *Nursing care of children: Principles and practice.* Philadelphia: W. B. Saunders, pp. 1127–1132.

265. The community health nurse visits an obese older adult client at home, and on physical examination, the nurse observes that the client has a barrel chest, dyspnea on exertion, and diminished breath sounds with intermittent wheezes and rhonchi. The client complains of bringing up large amounts of sputum. The client tells the nurse, "I've had this condition for several years." The nurse consults with the physician. Which of the following statements, if made by the nurse, indicates knowledge of the findings?

1. "Doctor, I think you will want to see this client immediately for treatment before the condition becomes chronic."
2. "Doctor, the client has dyspnea on exertion and diminished breath sounds with intermittent wheezes and rhonchi. These changes weren't present last week, so I've ordered an ambulance to take this client to the hospital emergency room as I knew you'd want to admit this client."
3. "Doctor, the client has dyspnea on exertion, diminished breath sounds with intermittent wheezes, and rhonchi. I'm concerned that there may be a chronic bronchitis that needs treatment. Do you want me to schedule the client for an appointment with you?"
4. "Doctor, this client is going into cor pulmonale before my eyes! I'm sending the client to the emergency room immediately!"

Answer: 3

Rationale: Chronic bronchitis is an inflammation of one or more bronchi (usually involving the trachea as well as the bronchi). In determining a diagnosis, the nurse would check for risk factors such as obesity, family history of cystic fibrosis, coughing with sputum production, inability to tolerate activity, recurrent respiratory infections, and a chronic, productive cough for at least 3 continuous months. Scheduling the client for an appointment is the most appropriate nursing intervention for this client. The most therapeutic communication technique is also the most professional one. The nurse describes her findings, makes a tentative nursing diagnosis, and explores effective problem solving with the colleague.

Test-Taking Strategy: Option 1 is a histrionic and unprofessional response and preempts the physician's decision making. No data that the nurse collected indicate a need to treat this condition as an emergency. Option 2 provides a professional communication when the nurse describes the findings, but then the nurse again preempts the primary care provider's decision making. As the condition does not warrant immediate attention, managed care will not pay an unnecessary expense, which will be charged to the client. Option 4, cor pulmonale, is right-sided heart failure secondary to diseased blood vessels in the lungs. The nurse has not found evidence of an enlarged right ventricle on chest x-ray. Again, the nurse preempts the primary care provider's decision making.

Level of Cognitive Ability: Application
Phase of Nursing Process: Evaluation
Client Needs: Psychosocial Integrity
Content Area: Adult Health/Respiratory

References

Antai-Otong, D. (1995). *Psychiatric nursing: Biological and behavioral concepts.* Philadelphia: W. B. Saunders, pp. 543–576.

Luckmann, J. (1997). *Saunders manual of nursing care.* Philadelphia: W. B. Saunders, pp. 941–943.

266. The community health nurse visits a client at home. Amiodarone (Cordarone) has been prescribed for the client. The nurse teaches the client about the medication. Which of the following statements, if made by the client, indicates that further teaching is necessary?

1. "I'll report any tiredness, coughing, or chest pain to my doctor."
2. "I'll be careful to use dark glasses and to avoid skin exposure to the sun."
3. "I'll take this medication with food."
4. "If I don't feel better in a couple of days, I'll notify my doctor."

Answer: 4

Rationale: Amiodarone (Cordarone), a group III antidysrhythmic agent, will probably not demonstrate therapeutic effects for 1–3 weeks. Options 1, 2, and 3 are all correct answers. This medication can cause fatigue, dyspnea, coughing, or pleuritic pain. Clients who take this medication must avoid skin exposure (photosensitivity) and wear dark glasses in the sun (photophobia). This medication is given with food to reduce any gastrointestinal distress.

Test-Taking Strategy: This question tests your knowledge of amiodarone (Cordarone) and the group III antidysrhythmic agents. Use the process of elimination. You can easily eliminate options 1 and 2. From the remaining two options, note the phrase "a couple of days" in option 4. This is a rather vague statement and the better option to select for this question as it is stated. Review this medication now if you had difficulty with this question!

Level of Cognitive Ability: Application
Phase of Nursing Process: Evaluation
Client Needs: Physiological Integrity
Content Area: Pharmacology

Reference

Clark, J., Queener, S., & Karb, V. (1997). *Pharmacologic basis of nursing practice* (5th ed.). St. Louis: Mosby–Year Book, pp. 232–249.

---

267. The nurse is caring for a client who is being treated with an IV bolus of lidocaine hydrochloride (Xylocaine) administered over a period of 2 minutes. The nurse evaluates the client's response for potential side effects by monitoring the client's

1. Respiratory status and blood pressure frequently during the infusion.
2. Urinary pH frequently during the infusion.
3. Continuous electrocardiogram (ECG) for accelerating or shortened PR interval during the infusion.
4. Temperature during the infusion.

Answer: 1

Rationale: The nurse is responsible to monitor the client's respiratory status and blood pressure while the client is being treated with an IV bolus of lidocaine hydrochloride (Xylocaine). Options 2, 3, and 4 are all incorrect and provide inaccurate information. Although cardiac monitoring is required, the nurse would monitor for prolonged PR interval and QRS complexes as a sign of excessive cardiac depression. The urinary pH and temperature are nonspecific with this medication.

Test-Taking Strategy: If you are unfamiliar with this medication, use the ABCs—airway, breathing, and circulation—to answer the question. In addition, cardiac monitoring, not continuous ECG monitoring, is required. This should direct you to the correct option, option 1. If you had difficulty with this question, take time now to review nursing responsibilities when administering lidocaine hydrochloride (Xylocaine)!

Level of Cognitive Ability: Analysis
Phase of Nursing Process: Evaluation
Client Needs: Physiological Integrity
Content Area: Pharmacology

Reference

Hodgson, B., & Kizior, R. (1998). *Saunders nursing drug handbook 1998.* Philadelphia: W. B. Saunders, pp. 591–594.

---

268. The community health nurse visits an elderly client who lives with her husband in a four-bedroom home. The client states, "I am such a bother to my husband. He has to do all the heavy work now that my arthritis has gotten worse. When I say we should move to a smaller place, he explodes." After evaluation of the client's statement, which of the following responses by the nurse would be the most therapeutic communication technique?

1. "I keep noticing bruises on your body, and a month ago you suffered a cracked rib."
2. "Sounds as if he doesn't want to sell, so why pressure him? He's the one who does all the work."
3. "A four-bedroom house! It really sounds like you need to sell to me! Why not let me speak to him?"
4. "He explodes? Does he always take his anger out on you? Tell him he'll have to deal with me next time!"

Answer: 1

Rationale: The client has verbalized feelings of being a "bother." This is often a sign of spousal abuse. It is important to note that the nurse should directly observe and verbalize the objective data that have been collected without labeling it as abuse. In Option 2, the nurse patronizes the client and also does not hear the verbal cues from the client. In option 3, the nurse uses sarcastic humor, which is belittling to the client. In addition, the nurse's suggested intervention removes control from the client and probably would add to the client's feelings of powerlessness. In option 4, the nurse again uses sarcasm and humor that belittles the client. Verbalizing the nurse's observation (reflection) back to the client without making any judgmental statements is a facilitative technique that will allow the client to share her situation, her feelings, and any fears. If the client is able to respond to the nurse, it will "open the door" for the nurse to intervene with the couple and any supportive family.

Test-Taking Strategy: This question tests your knowledge of the epidemiology of elder abuse and the appropriate assessment technique to employ for an elderly client who you suspect is suffering spousal abuse. Remember the therapeutic communication techniques when answering the question. Use the process of elimination. Option 1 is the only option that reflects a therapeutic technique!

Level of Cognitive Ability: Application
Phase of Nursing Process: Evaluation
Client Needs: Psychosocial Integrity
Content Area: Mental Health

Reference

Antai-Otong, D. (1995). *Psychiatric nursing: Biological and behavioral concepts.* Philadelphia: W. B. Saunders, pp. 543–576.

269. During a day hospital initial nursing assessment, the client tells the nurse that he or she has been doubling the daily dosage of bupropion (Wellbutrin) to aid in getting better faster. The nurse evaluates the client's statement and determines that ongoing nursing is necessary to

1 Monitor for orthostatic hypotension.
2 Monitor for seizure activity.
3 Monitor for weight gain.
4 Monitor for insomnia.

Answer: 2

Rationale: Wellbutrin, an antidepressant, does not cause significant orthostatic blood pressure changes. Seizure activity is common in dosages greater than 150 mg per dose. Wellbutrin frequently causes a drop in body weight. Insomnia is a side effect, but seizure activity poses a greater risk to the client.

Test-Taking Strategy: Knowledge regarding this medication is necessary to answer the question. If you had difficulty with this question and are unfamiliar with this medication, take time now to review the nursing implications!

Level of Cognitive Ability: Application
Phase of Nursing Process: Evaluation
Client Needs: Physiological Integrity
Content Area: Pharmacology

Reference
Hodgson, B., & Kizior, R. (1998). *Saunders nursing drug handbook 1998.* Philadelphia: W. B. Saunders, pp. 130–131.

270. When planning the discharge of a client with chronic anxiety, the nurse evaluates achievement of the discharge maintenance goals. Which of the following goals would most appropriately have been included in the plan of care requiring evaluation?

1 Continued contact with a crisis counselor
2 Identify anxiety-producing situations
3 Ignore feelings of anxiety
4 Eliminate of all anxiety from daily situations

Answer: 2

Rationale: Counselors will not be available for all anxiety-producing situations. This option does not encourage the development of internal strengths. Recognizing situations that produce anxiety allows the client to prepare to cope with anxiety or avoid specific stimuli. Ignoring feelings will not resolve anxiety. It is impossible to eliminate all anxiety from life.

Test-Taking Strategy: Use the process of elimination. Eliminate option 1 because it promotes dependence on a counselor. Eliminate options 3 and 4 because of the words "ignored" and "all" found in these options. Option 2 is the only realistic option.

Level of Cognitive Ability: Application
Phase of Nursing Process: Evaluation
Client Needs: Psychosocial Integrity
Content Area: Mental Health

Reference
Fortinash, K. M., & Holoday-Worret, P. A. (1996). *Psychiatric–mental health nursing.* St. Louis: Mosby–Year Book, p. 238.

271. The nurse conducts a relaxation exercise with a client with a diagnosis of anxiety. Which of the following would the nurse evaluate as an indicator that the client is applying relaxation techniques?

1 The client watches television with eyes closed
2 The client enters a room in which soft music is playing and breathes slowly
3 The client states, "Don't interrupt me, I'm meditating."
4 The client talks in a soft voice at all times

Answer: 2

Rationale: The client's identification of the stressor and taking action to remove the stressor indicates recognition, application, and control. The client may shut out all visual stimulus (option 1), but this does not indicate control of the environment. Interruptions by other clients and staff are common and must be dealt with by the client, but does this not indicate application of relaxation techniques. A constant soft voice does not indicate stress management. Option 2 identifies the application of a relaxation technique.

Test-Taking Strategy: Note the key phrase in the question "applying relaxation techniques." Use the process of elimination, noting that option 2 is the only option that identifies the application of a relaxation technique.

Level of Cognitive Ability: Analysis
Phase of Nursing Process: Evaluation
Client Needs: Psychosocial Integrity
Content Area: Mental Health

Reference

Fortinash, K. M., & Holoday-Worret, P. A. (1996). *Psychiatric–mental health nursing*. St. Louis: Mosby–Year Book, p. 91.

---

272. A client is discharged on phenobarbital (Luminal) 100 mg by mouth BID. Which of the following statements by the client to the nurse reflects an accurate understanding of safety precautions with this medication?

1 "I can take my medication at any time during the day."
2 "Using a daily dosing system container is critical to the prevention of an overdose."
3 "Drinking one beer may change the way my medication works."
4 "I must always take my medication on an empty stomach."

Answer: 3

Rationale: Taking medication at the same time daily is a good medication administration policy, and the client should understand this. Dose containers are helpful, but not critical, in preventing dose omissions. Barbiturates should be used with caution to prevent additive effects with other central nervous system agents such as alcohol. An empty stomach may increase the side effects of this drug.

Test-Taking Strategy: Use the process of elimination. Option 1 can be easily eliminated. Options 2 and 4 can be eliminated next because of the absolute terms "critical" and "must." Remembering that alcohol can affect the action of medications should guide you to the correct option to this question as it is stated. Review this medication now if you had difficulty with this question!

Level of Cognitive Ability: Analysis
Phase of Nursing Process: Evaluation
Client Needs: Physiological Integrity
Content Area: Pharmacology

Reference

Hodgson, B., & Kizior, R. (1998). *Saunders nursing drug handbook 1998.* Philadelphia: W. B. Saunders, pp. 815–818.

---

273. The client is being discharged from the ambulatory care unit after cataract removal. The nurse provides instructions regarding home care. Which of the following, if stated by the client, indicates effective teaching?

1 "I will take aspirin if I have any discomfort."
2 "I will sleep on the side that I was operated on."
3 "I will wear my eye shield at night and my glasses during the day."
4 "I will not lift anything if it weighs more than 10 pounds."

Answer: 3

Rationale: The client is instructed to wear a metal or plastic shield to protect the eye from accidental injury and is instructed not to rub the eye. Glasses may be worn during the day. Aspirin or medications containing aspirin are not to be administered or taken by the client; instead, the client is instructed to take acetaminophen (Tylenol) as needed for pain. The client is instructed not to sleep on the side of the body that was operated on. The client is not to lift more than 5 pounds.

Test-Taking Strategy: Use the process of elimination to answer this question. Read the stem of the question carefully, noting that the correct option indicates effective teaching. This will assist in directing you to the correct option. If you had difficulty with this question, take time now to review the discharge instructions for the client after cataract extraction!

Level of Cognitive Ability: Application
Phase of Nursing Process: Evaluation
Client Needs: Physiological Integrity
Content Area: Adult Health/Eye

Reference

Black, J., & Matassarin-Jacobs, E. (1997). *Medical-surgical nursing: Clinical management for continuity of care* (5th ed.). Philadelphia: W. B. Saunders, p. 961.

274. The nurse has completed counseling about smoking cessation with a client with coronary artery disease. The nurse evaluates that the client has understood the material best if the client states that

1 "If I quit now, I can cut my risk of cardiovascular disease to that of a nonsmoker in 3–4 years."
2 "I may try just cutting down first, because most of the damage has already been done."
3 "I'm never going to start again, because I can cut my risk to zero within a year."
4 "I don't think I want to quit, because none of the effects are reversible anyway."

Answer: 1

Rationale: The risks to the cardiovascular system from smoking are noncumulative and not permanent. Three to 4 years after cessation, a client's cardiovascular risk is similar to that of a person who never smoked.

Test-Taking Strategy: The words "zero" and "none" in options 3 and 4 are absolute, and those options should be discarded. You may eliminate option 2 because of the word "most" and because it is less precise than option 1.

Level of Cognitive Ability: Analysis
Phase of Nursing Process: Evaluation
Client Needs: Health Promotion and Maintenance
Content Area: Adult Health/Cardiovascular

Reference
Ignatavicius, D. D., Workman, M. L., & Mishler, M. A. (1995). *Medical-surgical nursing: A nursing process approach* (2nd ed.). Philadelphia: W. B. Saunders, p. 787.

---

275. The nurse has given the client recovering from cardiogenic shock simple instructions on preventing some of the complications of bed rest. Which of the following activities is contraindicated, necessitating the nurse's intervention?

1 Repositioning self from side to side
2 Deep breathing and coughing
3 Isometric exercises of the arms and legs
4 Ankle circles and plantar and dorsiflexion exercises

Answer: 3

Rationale: The client with myocardial infarction, even when uncomplicated by cardiogenic shock, should avoid activities that tense the muscles, such as isometric exercises. These increase intra-abdominal and intrathoracic pressures and can decrease the cardiac output. They can also trigger vagal stimulation, causing bradycardia.

Test-Taking Strategy: The stem of the question directly guides you to the important concept, prevention of complications of bed rest. Knowledge of this basic area helps you eliminate the incorrect options fairly easily. Remember that the question is addressing a cardiac client. Options 1, 2, and 4 are appropriate because they are basic and nonstressful exercises. Review activities related to the cardiac client now if you had difficulty with this question!

Level of Cognitive Ability: Analysis
Phase of Nursing Process: Evaluation
Client Needs: Physiological Integrity
Content Area: Adult Health/Cardiovascular

Reference
Smeltzer, S., & Bare, B. (1996). *Brunner and Suddarth's Textbook of medical-surgical nursing* (8th ed.). Philadelphia: Lippincott-Raven, p. 655.

---

276. The client is recovering from myocardial infarction complicated by cardiogenic shock. The nurse would evaluate the client's status as most satisfactory if which of the following observations were made?

1 Blood pressure (BP), 110/70; pulse (P), 86; capillary refill, 5 seconds; oxygen saturation (SaO_2), 92%
2 BP, 120/60; pulse, 80; capillary refill, 4 seconds; oxygen saturation, 94%
3 BP, 118/74; pulse, 72; capillary refill, 1 second; oxygen saturation, 98%
4 BP, 100/50; pulse, 90; capillary refill, 3 seconds; oxygen saturation, 97%

Answer: 3

Rationale: In the adult, normal systolic blood pressure is less than 140 mmHg, normal diastolic blood pressure is less than 90 mmHg, the normal heart rate ranges from 60–100 beats per minute, and capillary refill times should be within 3 seconds. Normal oxygen saturation values are 95%–100%.

Test-Taking Strategy: Knowledge of normal capillary refill and oxygen saturation measurements helps you eliminate options 1 and 2. The phrase "most satisfactory" in the stem leads you to select option 3 over option 4.

Level of Cognitive Ability: Analysis
Phase of Nursing Process: Evaluation
Client Needs: Physiological Integrity
Content Area: Adult Health/Cardiovascular

Reference

Ignatavicius, D. D., Workman, M. L., & Mishler, M. A. (1995). *Medical-surgical nursing: A nursing process approach* (2nd ed.). Philadelphia: W. B. Saunders, pp. 630, 792.

---

277. The nurse has given instructions to the family of an elderly client who seems anxious about being discharged after cardiac surgery. The nurse would need to reinforce the teaching if the family member made which of the following statements?

1 "Fatigue, discomfort, and lack of appetite occur more commonly with older people and may last for 2–5 weeks."
2 "A daily half-mile-long brisk walk generally helps people bounce back more quickly and have more of a sense of control."
3 "Recuperation after cardiac surgery is generally slower for older people."
4 "It's important to get out of bed every day, even if tired or weak at first."

Answer: 2

Rationale: The statements made in options 1, 3, and 4 are true. Clients generally increase activity by beginning a simple walking program, starting with distances of 400 feet twice daily and gradually increasing distance until they are able to walk 1/4 mile (usually at the end of the second week). Exercise has physiological and psychological benefits.

Test-Taking Strategy: The question is worded so as to seek an incorrect statement. Knowledge of concepts of both self-care and the aging process helps you eliminate options 3 and 4. If you are uncertain how to discriminate between options 1 and 2, note the words "half-mile-long brisk" in option 2. Because activity is resumed gradually, it may help you choose this as the incorrect response.

Level of Cognitive Ability: Analysis
Phase of Nursing Process: Evaluation
Client Needs: Physiological Integrity
Content Area: Adult Health/Cardiovascular

Reference

Luckmann, J. (1997). *Saunders manual of nursing care.* Philadelphia: W. B. Saunders, p. 1077.

---

278. The client with unstable ventricular tachycardia (VT) loses consciousness and becomes pulseless after initial treatment with a dose of lidocaine intravenously. The nurse evaluates that which of the following is needed immediately?

1 A second dose of lidocaine
2 A pacemaker
3 An electrocardiogram (ECG) machine
4 A defibrillator

Answer: 4

Rationale: For the client with VT who becomes pulseless, the physician or qualified advanced cardiac life support (ACLS) personnel immediately defibrillate the client if a defibrillator is available. In the absence of this equipment, cardiopulmonary resuscitation (CPR) is initiated immediately.

Test-Taking Strategy: The wording of the question tells you that there is only one correct response. Options 1 and 3 should be eliminated first, because option 1 was unsuccessful and option 3 is of no use. Choose option 4 over 2 as the piece of equipment needed "immediately" for emergency resuscitation.

Level of Cognitive Ability: Analysis
Phase of Nursing Process: Evaluation
Client Needs: Physiological Integrity
Content Area: Adult Health/Cardiovascular

Reference

Ignatavicius, D. D., Workman, M. L., & Mishler, M. A. (1995). *Medical-surgical nursing: A nursing process approach* (2nd ed.). Philadelphia: W. B. Saunders, p. 851.

279. The adult client has been defibrillated three times unsuccessfully for ventricular fibrillation, and cardiopulmonary resuscitation (CPR) is ongoing by two health care workers. The best indicator to the nurse that CPR is being performed effectively is if

1 The chest compressions are given at a depth of 1½–2 inches.
2 The ratio of compressions to ventilations given is 5:1.
3 Respirations are given at a rate of 12 breaths per minute.
4 The carotid pulse is palpable with each compression.

Answer: 4

Rationale: Correct procedure for CPR with two rescuers includes a compression-to-ventilation ratio of 5:1. With adults, compressions are performed at a depth of 1½–2 inches. The 5:1 ratio yields an effective rate of 12 breaths per minute. With effective compressions, carotid pulsations should be present. At its best, CPR produces only 30% of the normal cardiac output, so correct technique is vital.

Test-Taking Strategy: The question asks for the "best" indicator, implying that more than one option is correct. In this case, all options are correct; however, options 1, 2, and 3 are procedural and do not reflect an outcome. The word "effectively" guides you to look for an end result of the procedure, which then guides you to option 4. In addition, note the word "given" in each of the incorrect options. This reflects procedure.

Level of Cognitive Ability: Analysis
Phase of Nursing Process: Evaluation
Client Needs: Physiological Integrity
Content Area: Adult Health/Cardiovascular

Reference

Ignatavicius, D. D., Workman, M. L., & Mishler, M. A. (1995). *Medical-surgical nursing: A nursing process approach* (2nd ed.). Philadelphia: W. B. Saunders, pp. 876–878.

280. The nurse has finished suctioning the client. The nurse would use which of the following parameters to best determine the effectiveness of suctioning?

1 SaO_2 of 94% by pulse oximetry
2 Clear breath sounds
3 Client's statement of comfort
4 Arterial blood gas (ABG) oxygen level of 90 mmHg

Answer: 2

Rationale: The nurse evaluates the effectiveness of the suctioning procedure by auscultating breath sounds. This helps to determine whether the respiratory tree is clear of secretions. Options 1, 3, and 4 do not determine the effectiveness of suctioning.

Test-Taking Strategy: The key word in the stem that you would use to answer this question is the word "best." This implies that more than one or more options may be completely or partially correct. It is necessary to prioritize accurately to select the correct response. The least favorable response is the oxygen saturation of 94%, and so you would eliminate this option. Client comfort and ABG values are not the best determinant of the effectiveness of suctioning, as compared with clear breath sounds.

Level of Cognitive Ability: Analysis
Phase of Nursing Process: Evaluation
Client Needs: Physiological Integrity
Content Area: Adult Health/Cardiovascular

Reference

Taylor, C., Lillis, C., & LeMone, P. (1997). *Fundamentals of nursing: The art and science of nursing care* (3rd ed.). Philadelphia: Lippincott-Raven, p. 1351.

281. The client who underwent bronchoscopy was returned to the nursing unit 1 hour ago. The nurse evaluates that the client is experiencing complications of the procedure if the nurse notes

1 Diminished breath sounds on the left side.
2 Respiratory rate of 22 per minute.
3 Oxygen saturation of 95%.
4 Weak gag and cough reflex.

Answer: 1

Rationale: Asymmetrical breath sounds could indicate pneumothorax, and this should be reported to the physician. A weak cough and gag reflex 1 hour after the procedure is an expected finding, caused by residual effects of IV sedation and local anesthesia. A respiratory rate of 22 and oxygen saturation of 95% are acceptable measurements.

Test-Taking Strategy: Begin to answer this question by eliminating options 2 and 3, which are acceptable data. Knowing that the client is premedicated before this procedure forces you to choose option 1 over option 4, because unequal breath sounds are always abnormal. Review post-bronchoscopy complications now if you had difficulty with this question!

Level of Cognitive Ability: Analysis
Phase of Nursing Process: Evaluation
Client Needs: Physiological Integrity
Content Area: Adult Health/Respiratory

Reference
Black, J., & Matassarin-Jacobs, E. (1997). *Medical-surgical nursing: Clinical management for continuity of care* (5th ed.). Philadelphia: W. B. Saunders, p. 1062.

---

282. The client has undergone fluoroscopy-assisted aspiration biopsy of a chest lesion. The nurse evaluates that the client is experiencing complications from the procedure if the nurse notes which of the following?

1 Pulse rate is 80, up from 74 per minute
2 Skin is warm and dry
3 Absence of breath sounds in the right upper lobe
4 Oxygen saturation of 97% by pulse oximetry

Answer: 3

Rationale: Pneumothorax and bleeding are possible after this procedure. The client is observed for signs of respiratory difficulty, such as dyspnea, change in breath sounds, vital signs, pallor, and diaphoresis. Observation of the sputum for traces of blood or hemoptysis is also indicated.

Test-Taking Strategy: Begin to answer this question by eliminating options 2 and 4 first, because they indicate normal data. Option 1 is a mild change in pulse rate and may be expected with this procedure. Absence of breath sounds is always an abnormal finding, making option 3 the correct answer to this question. Review postprocedure complications after fluoroscopy-assisted aspiration biopsy now if you had difficulty with this question!

Level of Cognitive Ability: Analysis
Phase of Nursing Process: Evaluation
Client Needs: Physiological Integrity
Content Area: Adult Health/Respiratory

Reference
Black, J., & Matassarin-Jacobs, E. (1997). *Medical-surgical nursing: Clinical management for continuity of care* (5th ed.). Philadelphia: W. B. Saunders, pp. 1064–1065.

283. The client with a respiratory disorder has a nursing diagnosis of Altered Nutrition: Less Than Body Requirements related to anorexia secondary to fatigue and dyspnea while eating. The nurse evaluates that the client has followed the suggestions of the nurse to improve intake if the client

1 Selected foods that are very dry.
2 Ate the largest meal of the day at a time when most hungry.
3 Increased the use of milk products.
4 Increased the use of stimulants, such as caffeine.

Answer: 2

Rationale: The client is taught to plan the largest meal of the day at a time when the client is most likely to be hungry. It is also beneficial to eat four to six small meals per day if needed. The client avoids dry foods, which are hard to chew and swallow. The client also avoids milk and chocolate, which have a tendency to thicken saliva and secretions. Finally, the client should avoid the use of caffeine, which contributes to dehydration by promoting diuresis.

Test-Taking Strategy: Eliminate option 1 first as an obviously wrong answer. Options 3 and 4 are eliminated next because milk products thicken secretions and caffeine has a dehydrating effect. This leaves option 2 as the correct choice. Review dietary suggestions for the client with a respiratory disorder now if you had difficulty with this question!

Level of Cognitive Ability: Analysis
Phase of Nursing Process: Evaluation
Client Needs: Physiological Integrity
Content Area: Adult Health/Respiratory

Reference

Ignatavicius, D. D., Workman, M. L., & Mishler, M. A. (1995). *Medical-surgical nursing: A nursing process approach* (2nd ed.). Philadelphia: W. B. Saunders, pp. 704–705.

284. The nurse in the physician's office has instructed the client with pneumonia about measures to prevent upper respiratory tract infection. The nurse evaluates that the client did not fully understand the instructions if the client verbalized that he or she would

1 Avoid crowds, especially in the fall and winter seasons.
2 Avoid contact with persons with the flu or a cold.
3 Receive a pneumococcal vaccine yearly.
4 Receive an influenza vaccine yearly.

Answer: 3

Rationale: The pneumococcal vaccine is currently recommended to be given once in a lifetime. The influenza vaccine is recommended yearly. The client avoids contact with persons infected with colds or flu to prevent reinfection. The client also avoids exposure to crowds in the fall and winter seasons, when there is a higher prevalence of viruses. The client should also avoid exposure to irritating substances such as smoke. All of these measures, in addition to proper nutrition and adequate fluid intake, help to prevent reinfection in the client with pneumonia.

Test-Taking Strategy: The wording of the question guides you to look for an incorrect statement. Eliminate options 1 and 2 first as the most obviously appropriate responses. To discriminate between options 3 and 4, recall that the flu vaccine is given yearly, whereas the pneumococcal vaccine is only given once. This will help you to choose option 3 as the answer to the question, according to the way it is stated.

Level of Cognitive Ability: Analysis
Phase of Nursing Process: Evaluation
Client Needs: Health Promotion and Maintenance
Content Area: Adult Health/Respiratory

Reference

Ignatavicius, D. D., Workman, M. L., & Mishler, M. A. (1995). *Medical-surgical nursing: A nursing process approach* (2nd ed.). Philadelphia: W. B. Saunders, p. 717.

285. The client with acquired immunodeficiency syndrome (AIDS) has difficulty swallowing. The nurse has given the client suggestions to minimize the problem. The nurse would evaluate that the client has understood the instructions if the client verbalized that he or she would increase intake of foods such as

1 Raw fruits and vegetables.
2 Hot soup.
3 Peanut butter.
4 Noodle dishes.

Answer: 4

Rationale: The client is instructed to avoid spicy, sticky, or excessively hot or cold foods. The client is also instructed to avoid foods that are rough, such as uncooked fruits and vegetables. The client is encouraged to consume foods that are mild, nonabrasive, and easy to swallow. Examples of these include baked fish, noodle dishes, well-cooked eggs, and desserts such as ice cream or pudding. Dry grain foods such as crackers, bread, and cookies may be softened in milk or another beverage before being eaten.

Test-Taking Strategy: This question may be fairly easy to decipher by simply evaluating each of the foods listed in terms of how easily they are swallowed. The rough, hot, and sticky foods in options 1, 2, and 3, respectively, help you to choose option 4 as the correct response.

Level of Cognitive Ability: Analysis
Phase of Nursing Process: Evaluation
Client Needs: Physiological Integrity
Content Area: Adult Health/Gastrointestinal

Reference

Black, J., & Matassarin-Jacobs, E. (1997). *Medical-surgical nursing: Clinical management for continuity of care* (5th ed.). Philadelphia: W. B. Saunders, p. 635.

286. The nurse has instructed the client about the procedure for continuous ambulatory peritoneal dialysis (CAPD). The nurse evaluates that the client needs further instruction if the client

1 States that he or she will expect yellow-colored dialysate drainage.
2 Gets air in the dialysis tubing.
3 Warms the dialysate solution before infusion.
4 Plans on doing four exchanges per day.

Answer: 2

Rationale: Peritoneal dialysis tubing is flushed to avoid introducing air into the peritoneal cavity. The dialysate solution should be warmed before use. With CAPD, there are usually four exchanges planned per day, with dwell times varying according to whether an exchange is during the day or night. The dialysate solution should be slightly warmed to 37°C (98.6 F) before use. The excretion of waste products and urea cause the dialysate drainage to be yellow-tinged.

Test-Taking Strategy: The wording of the question guides you to look for an incorrect response. Knowing that metabolites discolor the drained dialysate solution helps you eliminate option 1. Knowledge of the proper procedure for CAPD helps you discriminate correctly among the three remaining options. Review the procedure for peritoneal dialysis now if you had difficulty with this question!

Level of Cognitive Ability: Analysis
Phase of Nursing Process: Evaluation
Client Needs: Health Promotion and Maintenance
Content Area: Adult Health/Renal

Reference

Black, J., & Matassarin-Jacobs, E. (1997). *Medical-surgical nursing: Clinical management for continuity of care* (5th ed.). Philadelphia: W. B. Saunders, p. 1649.

287. The client has received instructions on self-management of peritoneal dialysis. The nurse evaluates that the client needs further instruction if the client states that he or she will

1. Use a strong adhesive tape to anchor the catheter dressing.
2. Use meticulous aseptic technique for dialysate bag changes.
3. Take own vital signs daily.
4. Monitor own weight daily.

Answer: 1

Rationale: The client is at risk for impairment of skin integrity because of the presence of the catheter, exposure to moisture, and irritation from tape and cleansing solutions. The client should be instructed to use paper or nonallergenic tape to prevent skin irritation and breakdown. It is proper procedure for the client to use aseptic technique and to self-monitor vital signs and weight on a daily basis.

Test-Taking Strategy: The wording of the question guides you to look for an incorrect response. Knowing that self-monitoring of weight and vital signs is important helps you eliminate options 3 and 4 readily. To choose correctly between options 1 and 2, you should know either that meticulous technique is used to prevent the occurrence of peritonitis or that the skin needs to be protected from maceration by using a variety of methods. Note the word "strong" in the incorrect option.

Level of Cognitive Ability: Analysis
Phase of Nursing Process: Evaluation
Client Needs: Health Promotion and Maintenance
Content Area: Adult Health/Renal

Reference

Luckmann, J. (1997). *Saunders manual of nursing care.* Philadelphia: W. B. Saunders, p. 1193.

---

288. The nurse has given the client with a nephrostomy tube instructions to follow after hospital discharge. The nurse evaluates that the client understands the instructions if the client verbalizes that he or she will drink at least how many glasses of water per day?

1. 2–4
2. 6–8
3. 10–12
4. 14–16

Answer: 2

Rationale: The client with a nephrostomy tube needs to have adequate fluid intake to dilute urinary particles that could cause calculus and to provide good mechanical flushing of the kidney and tube. The nurse encourages the client to take in at least 2000 mL fluid per day, which is roughly equivalent to 6–8 glasses of water.

Test-Taking Strategy: This question can be answered most easily by knowing that the client needs at least 2 liters of fluid per day and by knowing how to convert ounces to milliliters. You would avoid options that reflect higher volumes, which could possibly cause undue distention of the renal pelvis; therefore, eliminate options 3 and 4. Of the remaining options, option 2 is the best, because 2–4 glasses is lower than a recommended amount.

Level of Cognitive Ability: Analysis
Phase of Nursing Process: Evaluation
Client Needs: Physiological Integrity
Content Area: Adult Health/Renal

Reference

Smeltzer, S., & Bare, B. (1996). *Brunner and Suddarth's Textbook of medical-surgical nursing* (8th ed.). Philadelphia: Lippincott-Raven, pp. 1169, 1173.

289. The nurse has completed nutritional counseling with an overweight client about weight reduction to modify the risk for coronary artery disease. The nurse would evaluate the teaching as most successful if the client stated a safe weight loss goal of

1 One-half pound per day.
2 Two pounds per week
3 Four pounds per week.
4 Six pounds per week.

Answer: 2

Rationale: Most people, including the mildly and moderately obese, can lose only about 2 pounds per week of weight from fat loss. Weight loss beyond that level is probably attributable to protein and water loss alone.

Test-Taking Strategy: Options 1 and 3 are very similar and may be eliminated. The word "safe" before weight loss implies an optimum value. Two pounds of weight loss per week is safer than six. Therefore, option 2 is the best option.

Level of Cognitive Ability: Analysis
Phase of Nursing Process: Evaluation
Client Needs: Physiological Integrity
Content Area: Adult Health/Cardiovascular

Reference
Lutz, C., & Przytulski, K. (1997). *Nutrition and diet therapy* (2nd ed.). Philadelphia: F. A. Davis, p. 319.

---

290. The client with myasthenia gravis describes to the nurse the use of oral neostigmine (Prostigmine). The nurse's evaluation leads to the conclusion that the client may be developing myasthenic crisis when the client comments

1. "The nurse gave me my pills late last night."
2 "I can hardly think straight today."
3 "I dropped one of my pills on the floor."
4 "I can't swallow very well today."

Answer: 4

Rationale: Because dysphagia is a classic sign of myasthenia gravis exacerbation, observing how a client is able to ingest food is a critical step in the evaluation phase of the nursing. Timing of this medication is of paramount concern. Although options 1, 2, and 3 may require further assessment, option 4 reflects the potential of myasthenic crisis.

Test-Taking Strategy: Use the process of elimination, remembering that dysphagia is a key sign of myasthenic crisis. Options 1 and 3, while significant to cause a crisis, are inconclusive (more verification is indicated). This medication does not primarily affect the central nervous system (CNS), and mentation is usually intact. Option 4 is the most confirming of classic myasthenia crisis recurrence. Review the clinical manifestations of myasthenic crisis now if you had difficulty with this question!

Level of Cognitive Ability: Analysis
Phase of Nursing Process: Evaluation
Client Needs: Physiological Integrity
Content Area: Adult Health/Neurological

Reference
Black, J., & Matassarin-Jacobs, E. (1997). *Medical-surgical nursing: Clinical management for continuity of care* (5th ed.). Philadelphia: W. B. Saunders, p. 885.

---

291. A post-gastrectomy client has the nursing diagnosis High Risk for Hyperglycemia related to uncontrolled gastric emptying of fluid/food bolus into small intestine. To evaluate the effectiveness of the nursing care plan for this nursing diagnosis, the nurse should

1 Monitor fasting blood glucose readings.
2 Monitor postprandial blood glucose readings.
3 Monitor client's daily weights.
4 Monitor calorie counts from dietary department.

Answer: 2

Rationale: Late manifestations of dumping syndrome after a gastrectomy occur 2–3 hours after eating and result from rapid entry of increased carbohydrate food into the jejunum, a rise in blood glucose levels, and excessive insulin secretion. To monitor this, the nurse checks blood glucose levels 2 hours after meals. Options 3 and 4 are unrelated to the issue of the question. A fasting blood glucose reading would not accurately determine hyperglycemia.

Test-Taking Strategy: This question is asking for the best answer. All the options are areas that may be monitored by the nurse, but only option 2 will provide information to evaluate the goal of the nursing diagnosis, which is to avoid uncontrolled gastric emptying. Use the process of elimination. Eliminate options 3 and 4 first because they are unrelated to the issue of the question. From this point, note the key phrase "emptying of fluid/food bolus into small intestine." This should assist in determining that option 2 is most accurate.

Level of Cognitive Ability: Analysis
Phase of Nursing Process: Evaluation
Client Needs: Physiological Integrity
Content Area: Adult Health/Gastrointestinal

Reference

Black, J., & Matassarin-Jacobs, E. (1997). *Medical-surgical nursing: Clinical management for continuity of care* (5th ed.). Philadelphia: W. B. Saunders, pp. 1778–1779.

---

292. A client has received instructions about an upcoming cardiac catheterization. The nurse would evaluate that the client has the best understanding of the procedure if the client knew to report which of the following items?

1 Warm, flushed feeling
2 Pressure at the insertion site
3 Chest pain
4 Urge to cough

Answer: 3

Rationale: The client is taught before cardiac catheterization to immediately report chest pain or any unusual sensations. The client is taught that a warm, flushed feeling may accompany dye injection, and occasional palpitations may occur as the catheter tip touches the cardiac muscle. The client may be asked to cough or breathe deeply from time to time during the procedure. Because local anesthetic is used, the client should feel pressure, but not pain, at the insertion site.

Test-Taking Strategy: The question asks you for a "best understanding" of what to report, indicating that you are looking for an adverse consequence. An option such as chest pain is often a good choice in questions such as these, in which the other options do not necessarily have a negative connotation. Review the cardiac catheterization procedure now if you had difficulty with this question!

Level of Cognitive Ability: Analysis
Phase of Nursing Process: Evaluation
Client Needs: Physiological Integrity
Content Area: Adult Health/Cardiovascular

Reference

Ignatavicius, D. D., Workman, M. L., & Mishler, M. A. (1995). *Medical-surgical nursing: A nursing process approach* (2nd ed.). Philadelphia: W. B. Saunders, p. 802.

---

293. The client with coronary artery disease has selected guided imagery to help cope with psychological stress. Which of the following statements, if made by the client, is the best indication that this method will be beneficial?

1 "I think this will work for me if I am alone in a quiet area."
2 "This seems to help only if I play music at the same time."
3 "I think I want to do this only when I lie down in case I fall asleep."
4 "The best thing about this is that I can use it anywhere, anytime."

Answer: 4

Rationale: Guided imagery involves the client's creation of an image in the mind, concentrating on the image, and gradually become less aware of the offending stimulus. It does not require any adjuncts, although some clients may use relaxation techniques or music with it.

Test-Taking Strategy: The question asks for the "best indication" that the method will be beneficial, implying more than one possible plausible option. In all three of the other options, limitations to the method are built into the response, which makes them less attractive as choices. Review guided imagery now if you had difficulty with this question!

Level of Cognitive Ability: Analysis
Phase of Nursing Process: Evaluation
Client Needs: Psychosocial Integrity
Content Area: Adult Health/Cardiovascular

Reference

Potter, P., & Perry, A. (1997). *Fundamentals of nursing: Concepts, process, and practice* (4th ed.). St. Louis: Mosby–Year Book, p. 1174.

294. The client, 36 hours after myocardial infarction, has ambulated for the first time. The nurse would evaluate that the client best tolerated the activity if which of the following observations were made?

1 Skin cool but slightly diaphoretic
2 Dyspnea noted only at the end of the exercise
3 Preactivity pulse rate, 86; postactivity pulse rate, 94
4 Preactivity BP, 140/84; postactivity BP, 110/72

Answer: 3

Rationale: The nurse assesses vital signs and level of fatigue with each activity. The client is not tolerating the activity if there is a drop in systolic BP of more than 20 mmHg, if there are changes in pulse rate of more than 20/minute, and if there is dyspnea or chest pain. Cool, diaphoretic skin is a sign of some degree of cardiovascular collapse.

Test-Taking Strategy: The question asks about activity tolerance, which tells you that you are looking for normal data. If you do not know which one to choose, look for normal values or the least degree of variation. Options 1 and 2 clearly identify abnormal data. Option 4 identifies a significant drop in BP, indicating an abnormal condition. An increase in pulse as reflected in option 3 is a normal expectation after exercise.

Level of Cognitive Ability: Analysis
Phase of Nursing Process: Evaluation
Client Needs: Physiological Integrity
Content Area: Adult Health/Cardiovascular

Reference

Ignatavicius, D. D., Workman, M. L., & Mishler, M. A. (1995). *Medical-surgical nursing: A nursing process approach* (2nd ed.). Philadelphia: W. B. Saunders, p. 998.

---

295. The nurse is preparing the postpartum cesarean delivery client for discharge. Which statement made by the client indicates a need for more information?

1 "I can start doing abdominal exercises as soon as I get home."
2 "I will lift nothing heavier than the baby for 2 weeks."
3 "If I develop a fever, I will call my doctor."
4 "When getting out of bed, I will turn on my side and push up with my arms."

Answer: 1

Rationale: Abdominal exercises should not be started after abdominal surgery until 3–4 weeks postoperatively, to allow for healing of the incision and decrease of client discomfort. Options 2, 3, and 4 reflect proper understanding of self-care after discharge.

Test-Taking Strategy: Read the question carefully noting that the client had cesarean delivery. Note the key words "need for more information." This should easily direct you to option 1.

Level of Cognitive Ability: Analysis
Phase of Nursing Process: Evaluation
Client Needs: Health Promotion and Maintenance
Content Area: Maternity

Reference

Nichols, F., & Zwelling, E. (1997). *Maternal-newborn nursing: Theory and practice.* Philadelphia: W. B. Saunders, pp. 1326–1327.

---

296. The home care nurse has completed client education regarding cardiac failure. The client will be discharged on digoxin (Lanoxin) and furosemide (Lasix). The nurse would document that the teaching goals have been met if the client states that he or she will report a

1 Sudden increase in appetite.
2 Weight gain of 2–3 pounds in a few days.
3 Cough that accompanies a cold.
4 High urine output during the day.

Answer: 2

Rationale: Clients with heart failure should immediately report weight gain, loss of appetite, shortness of breath with activity, edema, persistent cough, and nocturia. A high urine output is expected with these medications. A cough that accompanies a cold is normal. A sudden increase in appetite is insignificant.

Test-Taking Strategy: Use the process of elimination. Option 1 is either good or irrelevant. Option 4 is expected with diuretic therapy administered in the morning. The client should report a persistent cough, not necessarily one that accompanies a cold. Option 2 would accompany fluid retention, indicating a complication of the heart failure, and should be reported.

Level of Cognitive Ability: Analysis
Phase of Nursing Process: Evaluation
Client Needs: Physiological Integrity
Content Area: Adult Health/Cardiovascular

Reference

Smeltzer, S., & Bare, B. (1996). *Brunner and Suddarth's Textbook of medical-surgical nursing* (8th ed.). Philadelphia: Lippincott-Raven, p. 671.

---

297. The nurse is evaluating care given to the client with a small foot ulcer from thromboangiitis obliterans (Buerger's disease). The ulceration now has developed a blackened appearance, and the surrounding skin is pale and very cool. On the basis of this evaluation, the nurse would then

1 Turn up the thermostat in the client's room.
2 Report the findings to a physician.
3 Place a dry, sterile dressing over the area.
4 Irrigate the area with normal saline.

Answer: 2

Rationale: Signs and symptoms of gangrene should be reported to the physician. Turning the thermostat up will be of no assistance. Placing a dry, sterile dressing over the area can cause injury, particularly when the dressing is removed. Irrigation with normal saline should not be instituted unless prescribed by the physician.

Test-Taking Strategy: Eliminate option 1 first as being the least helpful of those mentioned. Next, eliminate option 3 because a dry sterile dressing is not used in treating ulcerations. Of the remaining two, the mention of new signs of gangrene indicates that the physician needs to be notified.

Level of Cognitive Ability: Application
Phase of Nursing Process: Evaluation
Client Needs: Physiological Integrity
Content Area: Adult Health/Cardiovascular

Reference

Black, J., & Matassarin-Jacobs, E. (1997). *Medical-surgical nursing: Clinical management for continuity of care* (5th ed.). Philadelphia: W. B. Saunders, p. 1431.

---

298. The nurse has done preoperative teaching with a client scheduled for percutaneous insertion of an inferior vena cava (IVC) filter. The nurse would evaluate that the client needs further clarification if the client stated that the procedure

1 Is rarely associated with complications.
2 Eliminates the need for anticoagulant therapy.
3 Is done with general anesthesia.
4 May cause congestion when clots get trapped at the filter.

Answer: 3

Rationale: Complications after insertion of an IVC filter are very rare. When they do occur, they include air embolism, improper placement, and filter migration. The percutaneous approach is used with local anesthesia. There is no need for anticoagulant therapy after surgery. Venous congestion can occur from accumulation of thrombi on the filter; however, the process usually occurs gradually.

Test-Taking Strategy: The question is worded to make you look for an incorrect statement. Noting the key word "percutaneous" should easily direct you to option 3. General anesthesia is not used in this procedure. Review this procedure now if you had difficulty with this question!

Level of Cognitive Ability: Analysis
Phase of Nursing Process: Evaluation
Client Needs: Physiological Integrity
Content Area: Adult Health/Cardiovascular

Reference

Lewis, S., Collier, I., & Heitkemper, M. (1996). *Medical-surgical nursing: Assessment and management of clinical problems* (4th ed.). St. Louis: Mosby–Year Book, p. 1057.

299. The client is being discharged to home with enoxaparin (Lovenox), 30 mg subcutaneously twice a day for 7 days. The nurse has instructed the client in self-administration of the medication. The nurse would evaluate that the client understands the correct procedure if the client does which of the following?

1 Flattens the skin before injection
2 Uses a 25- to 27-gauge, 5/8-inch needle
3 Aspirates before injection
4 Massages after injection

Answer: 2

Rationale: With subcutaneous injection of enoxaparin, the administration technique is the same as for heparin. Use the smallest gauge needle available (25- to 27-gauge) to prevent injection site hematoma; use a "bunching" technique or Z-track technique; inject deep into fatty abdominal tissue; do not aspirate before injecting; and do not massage the injection site. Withdraw gently to minimize bleeding, and rotate injection sites systematically.

Test-Taking Strategy: This question asks about basic nursing knowledge of injection technique. You need to know that clients may be discharged home with enoxaparin, a subcutaneously administered anticoagulant medication. Knowing this, you can select the statement that is standard subcutaneous injection technique. Review the subcutaneous procedure for injections now if you had difficulty with this question!

Level of Cognitive Ability: Analysis
Phase of Nursing Process: Evaluation
Client Needs: Physiological Integrity
Content Area: Fundamental Skills

Reference

Hodgson, B., & Kizior, R. (1998). *Saunders nursing drug handbook 1998.* Philadelphia: W. B. Saunders, pp. 365–366.

---

300. The home care nurse has completed a medication review with the elderly diet-controlled diabetic client who is also receiving furosemide (Lasix). The nurse would evaluate that the client needs further reinforcement of instructions if the client stated that he or she would

1 Report ringing in the ears or hearing loss.
2 Check blood glucose levels routinely.
3 Limit the amount of fluids taken in.
4 Sit or stand up gradually.

Answer: 3

Rationale: Elderly clients are more at risk of experiencing adverse effects of furosemide therapy, including orthostatic hypotension, ototoxicity, and elevations in blood glucose levels. Elderly clients are also more at risk for dehydration and should not limit fluid intake unless specifically prescribed to do so by the physician.

Test-Taking Strategy: This question is worded to make you look for an incorrect statement. Many diuretics, not just the loop diuretics, cause postural hypotension, which eliminates option 4. To answer this question correctly, you need to know that elderly clients are more at risk of developing adverse effects of this medication, including ototoxicity and hyperglycemia. This would guide you to the correct answer (option 3), which is also true for other types of diuretics as well. Fluid intake should not be restricted; rather, normal amounts of fluids are needed for hydration.

Level of Cognitive Ability: Analysis
Phase of Nursing Process: Evaluation
Client Needs: Physiological Integrity
Content Area: Pharmacology

Reference

Hodgson, B., & Kizior, R. (1998). *Saunders nursing drug handbook 1998.* Philadelphia: W. B. Saunders, pp. 452–454.

REFERENCES

Antai-Otong, D. (1995). *Psychiatric nursing: Biological and behavioral concepts*. Philadelphia: W. B. Saunders.

Ashwill, J., & Droske, S. (1997). *Nursing care of children: Principles and practice*. Philadelphia: W. B. Saunders.

Baer, C., & Williams, B. (1996). *Clinical pharmacology and nursing* (3rd ed.). Springhouse, PA: Springhouse.

Ball, J., & Bindler, R. (1995). *Pediatric nursing: Caring for children*. Stamford, CT: Appleton & Lange.

Bandman, E., & Bandman, B. (1995). *Nursing ethics through the life span*. Stamford, CT: Appleton & Lange.

Barry, P. (1997). *Psychosocial nursing: Care of physically ill patients and their families* (3rd ed.). Philadelphia: Lippincott-Raven.

Black, J., & Matassarin-Jacobs, E. (1997). *Medical-surgical nursing: Clinical management for continuity of care* (5th ed.). Philadelphia: W. B. Saunders.

Burrell, P., Gerlach, M., & Pless, S. (1997). *Adult nursing: Acute and community care* (2nd ed.). Stamford, CT: Appleton & Lange.

Carson, V., & Arnold, E. (1996). *Mental health nursing: The nurse-patient journey*. Philadelphia: W. B. Saunders.

Clark, J., Queener, S., & Karb, V. (1997). *Pharmacologic basis of nursing practice* (5th ed.). St. Louis: Mosby–Year Book.

Deglin, J. H., & Vallerand, A. H. (1997). *Davis's drug guide for nurses* (5th ed.). Philadelphia: F. A. Davis.

Fortinash, K. M., & Holoday-Worret, P. A. (1996). *Psychiatric–mental health nursing*. St. Louis: Mosby–Year Book.

Gorrie, T. M., McKinney, E. S., & Murray, S. S. (1994). *Foundations of maternal-newborn nursing*. Philadelphia: W. B. Saunders.

Hodgson, B., & Kizior, R. (1998). *Saunders nursing drug handbook 1998*. Philadelphia: W. B. Saunders.

Huff, J. (1997). *ECG workout: Exercises in arrhythmia interpretation* (3rd ed.). Philadelphia: Lippincott-Raven.

Ignatavicius, D. D., Workman, M. L., & Mishler, M. A. (1995). *Medical-surgical nursing: A nursing process approach* (2nd ed.). Philadelphia: W. B. Saunders.

Jaffee, M., & McVan, B. (1997). *Davis's laboratory and diagnostic test handbook*. Philadelphia: F. A. Davis.

Johnson, B. (1997). *Psychiatric mental health nursing: Adaptation and growth* (4th ed.). Philadelphia: Lippincott-Raven.

Karch, A. (1997). *1997 Lippincott's nursing drug guide*. Philadelphia: Lippincott-Raven.

Kee, J., & Hayes, E. (1997). *Pharmacology: A nursing process approach* (2nd ed.). Philadelphia: W. B. Saunders.

Kozier, B., Glenora, E., & Blais, K. (1995). *Fundamentals of nursing: Concepts, process, and practice* (5th ed.). Menlo Park, CA: Addison-Wesley.

Lammon, C. B., Foote, A. W., Leli, P. G., et al. (1995). *Clinical nursing skills*. Philadelphia: W. B. Saunders.

Lehne, R. A. (1998). *Pharmacology for nursing care* (3rd ed.). Philadelphia: W. B. Saunders.

LeMone, P., & Burke, K. M. (1996). *Medical-surgical nursing: Critical thinking in client care*. Menlo Park, CA: Addison-Wesley.

Lewis, S., Collier, I., & Heitkemper, M. (1996). *Medical-surgical nursing: Assessment and management of clinical problems* (4th ed.). St. Louis: Mosby–Year Book.

Lowdermilk, D., Perry, S., & Bobak, I. (1997). *Maternity and women's health care* (6th ed.). St. Louis: Mosby–Year Book.

Luckmann, J. (1997). *Saunders manual of nursing care*. Philadelphia: W. B. Saunders.

Lutz, C., & Przytulski, K. (1997). *Nutrition and diet therapy* (2nd ed.). Philadelphia: F. A. Davis.

Mahan, L., & Escott-Stump, S. (1996). *Krause's Food, nutrition, and diet therapy* (9th ed.). Philadelphia: W. B. Saunders.

National Council of State Boards of Nursing (1997). *Test plan for the National Council Licensure Examination for Registered Nurses*. Chicago: Author.

Nichols, F., & Zwelling, E. (1997). *Maternal-newborn nursing: Theory and practice*. Philadelphia: W. B. Saunders.

Olds, S., London, M., & Ladewig, P. (1996). *Maternal-newborn nursing: A family-centered approach* (5th ed.). Menlo Park, CA: Addison-Wesley.

Pillitteri, A. (1995). *Maternal and child health nursing: Care of the childbearing and child rearing family* (2nd ed.). Philadelphia: Lippincott-Raven.

Pinnell, N. (1996). *Nursing pharmacology*. Philadelphia: W. B. Saunders.

Polaski, A., & Tatro, S. (1996). *Luckmann's Core principles and practice of medical-surgical nursing*. Philadelphia: W. B. Saunders.

Potter, P., & Perry, A. (1997). *Fundamentals of nursing: Concepts, process, and practice* (4th ed.). St. Louis: Mosby–Year Book.

Reeder, S., Martin, L., & Koniak-Griffin, D. (1997). *Maternity nursing* (18th ed.). Philadelphia: Lippincott-Raven.

Rice, R. (1996). *Home health nursing practice: Concepts and application* (2nd ed.). St. Louis: Mosby–Year Book.

Smeltzer, S., & Bare, B. (1996). *Brunner and Suddarth's Textbook of medical-surgical nursing* (8th ed.). Philadelphia: Lippincott-Raven.

Taylor, C., Lillis, C., & LeMone, P. (1997). *Fundamentals of nursing: The art and science of nursing care* (3rd ed.). Philadelphia: Lippincott-Raven.

Varcarolis, E. M. (1998). *Foundations of psychiatric mental health nursing* (3rd ed.). Philadelphia: W. B. Saunders.

Wilson, B., Shannon, M., & Stang, C. (1996). *Nurse's drug guide*. Stamford, CT: Appleton & Lange.

Wilson, H., & Kneisl, C. (1996). *Psychiatric nursing* (5th ed.). Menlo Park, CA: Addison-Wesley.

Wong, D. L. (1995). *Whaley and Wong's Nursing care of infants and children* (5th ed.). St. Louis: Mosby–Year Book.

Wong, D. (1997). *Whaley and Wong's Essentials of pediatric nursing* (5th ed.). St. Louis: Mosby–Year Book.

Wong, D., & Perry, S. (1998). *Maternal-child nursing care*. St. Louis: Mosby–Year Book.

Zang, S., & Bailey, N. (1997). *Home care manual: Making the transition*. Philadelphia: Lippincott-Raven.

UNIT III

Client Needs

CHAPTER 10

Safe, Effective Care Environment

Safe, Effective Care Environment is a major category of Client Needs. The two subcategories of this Client Needs component are (1) Management of Care and (2) Safety and Infection and Control.

MANAGEMENT OF CARE

The Management of Care subcategory includes content related to the nurse's role in providing integrated and cost-effective care to clients. It includes the nurse's role in coordinating, supervising, and/or collaborating with members of the multidisciplinary health care team. The percentage of test questions in the Management of Care subcategory on NCLEX-RN is 7%–13%.

BOX 10–1. Management of Care

Advocacy
Ethical Practice and Legal Responsibilities
Client Rights
Advance Directives
Organ Donation
Confidentiality
Informed Consent
Incident Reports
Concepts of Management
Continuity of Care
Delegation and Supervision
Case Management
Continuous Quality Improvement
Consultation and Referrals
Resources Management

SAFETY AND INFECTION AND CONTROL

The Safety and Infection and Control subcategory includes content related to the nurse's role in protecting the client and health care personnel from environmental hazards. The percentage of test questions in the Safety and Infection and Control subcategory on NCLEX-RN is 5%–11%.

BOX 10–2. Safety and Infection and Control

Medical and Surgical Asepsis
Standard (Universal) and Other Precautions
Handling Hazardous and Infectious Materials
Error Prevention
Accident Prevention
Use of Restraints
Disaster Planning

PRACTICE TEST

1. The nurse consults with the dietician to develop a teaching plan for the child with celiac disease. The plan will advise parents to

   1 Read all label ingredients carefully to avoid hidden sources of gluten.
   2 Restrict corn and rice in diet.
   3 Restrict fresh starchy vegetables in diet.
   4 Substitute grain cereals with pasta products.

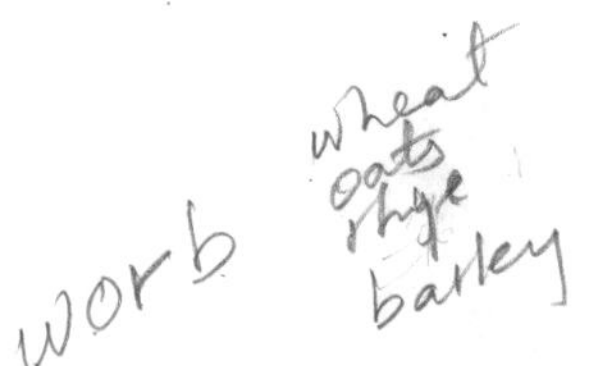

Answer: 1

Rationale: Gluten is found primarily in the grains of wheat and rye. Corn and rice become substitute foods. Gluten is added to many foods as hydrolyzed vegetable protein derived from cereal grains; therefore, labels need to be read. Corn and rice, as well as other vegetables, are acceptable in a gluten-free diet. Many pasta products contain gluten. Grains are frequently added to processed foods for thickness or as fillers.

Test-Taking Strategy: Remembering that a gluten-free diet is required for clients with celiac disease will assist in directing you to the correct option. In addition, option 1 is the most global response. If you had difficulty with this question, take time now to review the required diet in celiac disease!

Level of Cognitive Ability: Application
Phase of Nursing Process: Planning
Client Needs: Safe, Effective Care Environment
Content Area: Child Health

Reference
Wong, D., & Perry, S. (1998). *Maternal-child nursing care.* St. Louis: Mosby–Year Book, pp. 1432–1433.

---

2. When a child who is hospitalized with intussusception passes a normal brown stool, which action should the nurse take first?

   1 Report the passage of a normal brown stool to the physician immediately
   2 Prepare the child/parents for the possibility of surgery
   3 Obtain the history of the child's physical and behavior symptoms
   4 Prepare the child for hydrostatic reduction

Answer: 1

Rationale: Passage of a normal brown stool usually indicates that the intussusception has reduced itself. This is immediately reported to the physician, who may chose to alter the diagnostic/therapeutic plan of care. It is important for the nurse to document this occurrence.

Test-Taking Strategy: The key words to focus your attention on are "first" and "normal." This should provide you with the indication that the problem has resolved. In addition, note that the issue in the question is repeated in the correct option.

Level of Cognitive Ability: Application
Phase of Nursing Process: Implementation
Client Needs: Safe, Effective Care Environment
Content Area: Child Health

Reference
Wong, D., & Perry, S. (1998). *Maternal-child nursing care.* St. Louis: Mosby–Year Book, pp. 1429–1430.

---

3. The client is psychotic, pacing, agitated, and using aggressive gestures. The client's speech pattern is rapid, and affect is belligerent. On the basis of these objective data, the nurse's immediate priority of care is to

   1 Provide safety for the client and other clients on the unit.
   2 Offer the client a less stimulated area to calm down and regain self-control.
   3 Provide the clients on the unit with a sense of comfort and safety.
   4 Assist staff in caring for the client in a controlled environment.

Answer: 1

Rationale: Seclusion may be needed in order to provide safety for the client and other clients on the unit if the client is out of control. Option 1 is the only response which addresses the client and other clients' safety needs. Option 2 addresses the client's needs. Option 3 addresses other clients' needs. Option 4 is not client centered.

Test-Taking Strategy: Use Maslow's hierarchy of needs theory to prioritize. Note the words "belligerent," "agitated," and "aggressive." Safety is the key issue. Option 1 is the global response and addresses the safety of all.

Level of Cognitive Ability: Application
Phase of Nursing Process: Planning
Client Needs: Safe, Effective Care Environment
Content Area: Mental Health

Reference

Carson, V., & Arnold, E. (1996). *Mental health nursing: The nurse-patient journey.* Philadelphia: W. B. Saunders, p. 348.

---

4. The nurse is engaged in the working phase of a therapeutic relationship with the client. The client has sought counseling after trying to save a drowning nephew. In spite of the client's attempts, the client was not able to save the child. Which of the following actions would the nurse be engaged in with the client during the working phase of the relationship?

1 Exploring the client's potential for self-harm
2 Exploring the client's ability to function
3 Inquiring about the client's perception/appraisal of the drowning
4 Inquiring and examining the client's feelings that may block adaptive coping

Answer: 4

Rationale: The client must first deal with feelings and negative responses before the client is able to work through the meaning of the crisis. Option 4 pertains directly to implementation/intervention. Options 1 and 2 relate to assessment. Option 3 relates to the planning phase of nursing process and would determine the implementation. The nurse and the client must work together to establish a therapeutic and safe milieu/environment to proceed in the caring process.

Test-Taking Strategy: It is necessary to know the tasks pertaining to each nursing process phase as well as to know crisis intervention content. Within the implementation phase, the nurse works collaboratively with the client to help the client realize the potential for growth after uncovering and examining blocks to the recovery process, learn to ask for help, use adaptive coping, and focus on resolution. Review the phases of a therapeutic relationship now if you had difficulty with this question!

Level of Cognitive Ability: Application
Phase of Nursing Process: Implementation
Client Needs: Safe, Effective Care Environment
Content Area: Mental Health

Reference

Johnson, B. (1997). *Psychiatric–mental health nursing: Adaptation and growth.* Philadelphia: Lippincott-Raven, p. 798.

---

5. Magnetic resonance imaging (MRI) is ordered for a client with Bell's palsy. Which nursing action should be included in the client's plan of care to prepare for this test?

1 Keep NPO for 6 hours before the test
2 Remove all metal-containing objects from the client
3 Shave the groin for insertion of femoral catheter
4 Instruct client in inhalation techniques for radioactive gas

Answer: 2

Rationale: Radiofrequency pulses in a magnetic field are converted into pictures in MRI. All metal objects such as rings, bracelets, hairpins, and watches should be removed. In addition, a history should be taken to ascertain whether the client has any internal metallic devices such as orthopedic hardware, pacemakers, shrapnel, and so forth. For an abdominal MRI, the client is usually on NPO status. NPO status is not necessary for MRI of the head. The groin may be shaved for angiography, and inhalation of gas can be ordered with positron emission tomography (PET).

Test-Taking Strategy: Note the word "magnetic" in the stem and the word "metal" in the correct answer. If you are unfamiliar with client preparation for an MRI, review this now!

Level of Cognitive Ability: Application
Phase of Nursing Process: Planning
Client Needs: Safe, Effective Care Management
Content Area: Adult Health/Neurological

Reference

Black, J., & Matassarin-Jacobs, E. (1997). *Medical-surgical nursing: Clinical management for continuity of care* (5th ed.). Philadelphia: W. B. Saunders, p. 252.

6. The charge nurse in an intensive care unit (ICU) observes a client who is agitated and incoherent. The nurse suspects the client is having a reaction to medication. The plan developed by the nurse that will most likely result in safe care for the client is
   1 Requesting the physician to order restraints and sedation.
   2 Asking the family to stay with the client.
   3 Having a nurse observe the client continuously.
   4 Using an interdisciplinary approach to solve the problem.

Answer: 4

Rationale: In managing care for a safe, effective care environment, the nurse needs to use an approach that integrates the members of the health care team. Options 1, 2, and 3 rely on individuals to solve the problem.

Test-Taking Strategy: Option 4 is the most global response involving members of the health care team. This option is different from the other options in that options 1, 2, and 3 involve individuals. In addition, this approach provides the safest environment.

Level of Cognitive Ability: Application
Phase of Nursing Process: Planning
Client Needs: Safe, Effective Care Environment
Content Area: Fundamental Skills

Reference

Gillies, D. (1994). *Nursing management: A systems approach.* Philadelphia: W. B. Saunders, pp. 114–115.

7. The physician told the nurse to discontinue the feeding tube in a client who was in a chronic vegetative state. The request was made by the client's spouse and children. The nurse needs to be aware of the legal basis for carrying out the order. The first requirement is
   1 Court approval to discontinue the treatment.
   2 A written order by the physician to remove the tube.
   3 Authorization by the family to discontinue the treatment.
   4 Approval by the institutional Ethics Committee.

Answer: 3

Rationale: The family or a legal guardian can make treatment decisions. In general, they make decisions in collaboration with physicians, other health care workers, and other trusted advisors.

Test-Taking Strategy: The key word "first" prompts you to determine the sequence of decision making in this and other similar client care situations. Review these principles now if you had difficulty with this question!

Level of Cognitive Ability: Analysis
Phase of Nursing Process: Analysis
Client Needs: Safe, Effective Care Environment
Content Area: Fundamental Skills

Reference

Brent, N. (1997). *Nurses and the law.* Philadelphia: W. B. Saunders, pp. 275–287.

8. The doctor has just diagnosed a uterine inversion in a client who has completed an oxytocin- (Pitocin-) induced labor and birth. Which of the following, noted in the plan of care, is the priority to keep the client's environment safe during this critical time?
   1 Placing the client in a multipositional labor-delivery bed
   2 Continuous monitoring of mother and fetus
   3 Reviewing the expected events of labor with the client and support person
   4 Hanging the intravenous (IV) Pitocin drip on a Y-tubing with plain lactated Ringer's solution on the other arm of the Y-tubing

Answer: 4

Rationale: The action of Pitocin is to contract the uterus. If the cervix contracts, it will be difficult to rectify the uterine inversion. The use of the Y-tubing with a Pitocin intravenous drip allows the Pitocin to be withheld while the client can still receive fluids as necessary. In this case, the potential of hemorrhage with an inverted uterus makes the necessity of intravenous fluid replacement a priority. In any case in which a Pitocin drip is used, a Y-tubing set up with a plain infusion fluid is a standard safety procedure.

Test-Taking Strategy: Focus on the issue of the question. This is an environmental safety question related to the management of Pitocin drips and potential emergencies in which Pitocin might need to be stopped quickly to protect the client from adverse effects. Option 4 is the only option that addresses the use of Pitocin, the issue of the question!

Level of Cognitive Ability: Analysis
Phase of Nursing Process: Planning
Client Needs: Safe, Effective Care Environment
Content Area: Maternity

Reference

Lowdermilk, D., Perry, S., & Bobak, I. (1997). *Maternity and women's health care* (6th ed.). St. Louis: Mosby–Year Book, p. 784.

---

9. The nurse is assisting the physician with the insertion of a Miller-Abbott tube. The nurse understands that the procedure puts the client at risk for aspiration. Which of the following nursing actions will decrease the risk of aspiration?

1. Inserting the tube with the balloon inflated
2. Instructing the client to cough when the tube reaches the nasal pharynx
3. Placing the client in a high Fowler's position
4. Instructing the client to perform a Valsalva maneuver if the impulse to gag occurs

Answer: 3

Rationale: The Miller-Abbott tube is a nasoenteric tube that is used to decompress the intestine, as in correcting a bowel obstruction. Initial insertion of the tube is a physician's responsibility. The tube is inserted with the balloon deflated in a manner that is similar to the proper procedure for inserting a nasogastric tube. The client is usually given water to drink to facilitate passage of the tube through the nasopharynx and esophagus. A high Fowler's position decreases the risk of aspiration if vomiting occurs.

Test-Taking Strategy: The issue of the question is decreasing the risk of aspiration for the client undergoing insertion of a Miller-Abbott tube. Option 1 can be easily eliminated because a tube could not be inserted if the balloon were inflated. Coughing can cause the tube to be expelled. A Valsalva maneuver is not used if the impulse to gag occurs. Review this procedure now if you had difficulty with this question!

Level of Cognitive Ability: Application
Phase of Nursing Process: Planning
Client Needs: Safe, Effective Care Environment
Content Area: Adult Health/Gastrointestinal

Reference

Lammon, C. B., Foote, A. W., Leli, P. G., et al. (1995). *Clinical nursing skills.* Philadelphia: W. B. Saunders, pp. 418–422.

---

10. Which of the following nursing actions will decrease the risk for developing an infection in clients receiving total parenteral nutrition (TPN)?

1. Assessing vital signs at 4-hour intervals
2. Instructing the client to perform a Valsalva maneuver during intravenous tubing changes
3. Administering acetaminophen (Tylenol) before changing the central line dressing
4. Using aseptic technique in handling the TPN solution and tubing

Answer: 4

Rationale: Clients receiving TPN are at high risk for developing infection. A concentrated glucose solution is an excellent medium for bacterial growth. Using aseptic technique in handling all equipment and solutions is paramount to prevention. Option 1 will detect signs of an infection but is not a preventive measure.

Test-Taking Strategy: Note the key phrase "decrease the risk." Option 1 relates to early detection of infection, not decreasing the risk. Options 2 and 3 do not relate to the issue of the question. Aseptic technique is critical for preventing infection!

Level of Cognitive Ability: Application
Phase of Nursing Process: Implementation
Client Needs: Safe, Effective Care Environment
Content Area: Fundamental Skills

Reference

Black, J., & Matassarin-Jacobs, E. (1997). *Medical-surgical nursing: Clinical management for continuity of care* (5th ed.). Philadelphia: W. B. Saunders, pp. 1754–1756.

11. The nurse is assisting the home health care client in managing cancer pain. To ensure that the client has adequate and safe pain control, the planning strategy would include

1 Trying multiple medication modalities for pain relief to get the maximum pain relief effect.
2 Starting with low doses of medication and gradually increase to a dose that relieves pain, not exceeding the maximal daily dose.
3 Relying totally on prescription and over-the-counter medications to relieve pain.
4 Keeping a baseline level of pain so that the client does not get sedated or addicted.

Answer: 2

Rationale: The correct option is to start with low doses and work up to a dose of medication that relieves the pain. One goal in pain management is to keep the protocol simple but effective. Multiple medication interventions can be unsafe and ineffective. Option 3 does not take into account other nursing interventions that may relieve pain, such as massage, therapeutic touch, or music. Finally, keeping a baseline level of pain is not appropriate practice unless the client requests this, and this information has not been provided in the case situation.

Test-Taking Strategy: Option 1 uses the word "multiple" and option 3 uses the word "totally." Eliminate these options. Option 4 can be easily eliminated because it is inaccurate information. Focus on safety when selecting an option.

Level of Cognitive Ability: Application
Phase of Nursing Process: Planning
Client Needs: Safe, Effective Care Environment
Content Area: Adult Health/Oncology

Reference

Como, N. (1995). *Home health nursing pocket consultant.* St. Louis: Mosby–Year Book, p. 279.

12. To ensure safe administration of medication in the home, the home health care nurse

1 Demonstrates the proper procedure to take prescribed medications.
2 Allows the client to verbalize and demonstrate correct administration procedures.
3 Instructs the client that it is OK to double up on medications if a dose has been missed.
4 Conducts pill counts on each home visit.

Answer: 2

Rationale: Outcome-driven home care requires the client to verbalize and describe proper procedure and administration of medications. Demonstrating the proper procedure does not ensure that the client can safely perform this procedure. It is not acceptable to double up on medication, and conducting a pill count on each visit is not realistic or appropriate.

Test-Taking Strategy: Options 3 and 4 can be easily eliminated because these are not appropriate practices. Of the remaining options, option 2 is client centered. Review the principles of teaching and learning now if you had difficulty with this question!

Level of Cognitive Ability: Application
Phase of Nursing Process: Implementation
Client Needs: Safe, Effective Care Environment
Content Area: Fundamental Skills

Reference

Swanson, J., & Nies, M. (1997). *Community health nursing: Promoting the health of aggregates* (2nd ed.). Philadelphia: W. B. Saunders, p. 799.

13. A 45-year-old client is admitted for evaluation of recurrent runs of ventricular tachycardia seen on Holter monitoring. The client is scheduled for electrophysiology studies (EPS) the following morning. Which of the following would the nurse include in a teaching plan for this client?

1 "During the procedure, a special wire is used to increase the heart rate and produce the irregular beats that caused your signs and symptoms."
2 "You will be sedated during the procedure and will not remember what has happened."
3 "This test is a noninvasive method of determining the effectiveness of your medication regime."
4 "You will continue to take your medications until the morning of the test."

Answer: 1

Rationale: The purpose of EPS is to study the heart's electrical system. Client education is very important because this invasive procedure introduces a special wire into the heart to produce dysrhythmias. To prepare for this procedure, the client should be NPO for 6–8 hours before, and all antidysrhythmics are withheld for at least 24 hours before the test in order to study the dysrhythmias without the influence of medications. Because the client's verbal response to the rhythm changes are extremely important, heavy sedation is avoided if possible.

Test-Taking Strategy: The question requires a knowledge of client preparation for EPS. Review this procedure now if you had difficulty with this question!

Level of Cognitive Ability: Application
Phase of Nursing Process: Planning
Client Needs: Safe, Effective Care Environment
Content Area: Adult Health/Cardiovascular

Reference
VanRiper, S., & VanRiper, J. (1997). *Cardiac diagnostic tests: A guide for nurses.* Philadelphia: W. B. Saunders, pp. 310–313.

---

14. The client remains in an atrial fibrillation with rapid ventricular response, despite pharmacological intervention. Synchronous cardioversion is scheduled to convert the rapid rhythm. Which of the following is the most important nursing action to prevent complications?

1 Sedate the client before cardioversion
2 Ensure the emergency equipment is available
3 Ensure that the monitor is set on the synchronous mode
4 Cardiovert at 360 joules

Answer: 3

Rationale: Cardioversion is similar to defibrillation with two major exceptions: The countershock is synchronized to occur during ventricular depolarization (QRS complex), and less energy is used for countershock. The rationale for delivering the shock during the QRS complex is to prevent the shock from being delivered during repolarization (T wave), often termed the vulnerable period. If the shock is delivered during this period, the resulting complication is ventricular fibrillation. It is crucial that the defibrillator be set on the "synchronous" mode for a successful cardioversion.

Test-Taking Strategy: Note the word "synchronous" in the question and in the correct option. In addition, option 3 is the only option that addresses the first step of the Nursing Process, Assessment. Review this procedure now if you had difficulty with this question!

Level of Cognitive Ability: Application
Phase of Nursing Process: Planning
Client Needs: Safe, Effective Care Environment
Content Area: Adult Health/Cardiovascular

Reference
Hartshorn, J., Sole, M., & Lamborn, M. (1997). *Introduction to critical care nursing* (2nd ed.). Philadelphia: W. B. Saunders, pp. 183–184.

---

15. The client is being treated with heparin sodium therapy for a diagnosis of thrombophlebitis. In planning care, what medication should the nurse have available if the client develops a significant bleeding problem?

1 Fresh-frozen plasma
2 Protamine sulfate
3 Streptokinase
4 Vitamin K

Answer: 2

Rationale: Protamine sulfate is the antidote for heparin. Vitamin K is the antidote for warfarin (Coumadin). Fresh-frozen plasma may also be used for bleeding related to Coumadin therapy. Streptokinase is a thrombolytic agent used to dissolve blood clots.

Test-Taking Strategy: In order to give safe care, nurses must know the antidotes for commonly used medications. Such common medications include morphine, heparin, and Coumadin. Review the antidotes now if you had difficulty with this question!

Level of Cognitive Ability: Application
Phase of Nursing Process: Planning
Client Needs: Safe, Effective Care Environment
Content Area: Pharmacology

Reference

Hodgson, B., & Kizior, R. (1998). *Saunders nursing drug handbook 1998.* Philadelphia: W. B. Saunders, p. 650.

---

16. The nurse is giving instructions to the client with cardiomyopathy. Which of the following is most important in client safety?

1 Assessment of pain
2 Avoiding over-the-counter medications
3 Administration of vasodilators
4 Avoiding orthostatic changes when rising to a standing position

Answer: 4

Rationale: Orthostatic changes may occur in the client with cardiomyopathy as a result of venous return obstruction. Sudden orthostatic changes may lead to falls. Vasodilators should not be administered. Pain may not directly affect safety in all client situations. Option 2, although accurate, is not directly related to the most important issue of safety.

Test-Taking Strategy: The question is asking about safety. Use the process of elimination, focusing on this issue. The relationship between safety and standing with orthostatic changes provides the key to this question.

Level of Cognitive Ability: Application
Phase of Nursing Process: Implementation
Client Needs: Safe, Effective Care Environment
Content Area: Adult Health/Cardiovascular

Reference

Black, J., & Matassarin-Jacobs, E. (1997). *Medical-surgical nursing: Clinical management for continuity of care* (5th ed.). Philadelphia: W. B. Saunders, p. 1344.

---

17. The nurse instructs the client with endocarditis to use an electric razor. The nurse teaches the client that the reason is that

1 Any cut may cause infection.
2 Electric razors may be disinfected.
3 All conventional razors contain microbes.
4 Clients taking anticoagulants should avoid cuts.

Answer: 4

Rationale: Clients with endocarditis are placed on anticoagulants to prevent thrombus formation and possible stroke. Options 1, 2, and 3 all concern possible infection, which is not the important reason to avoid conventional razors. Accident prevention related to bleeding is the issue of the question.

Test-Taking Strategy: Recognizing that the client with valvular disease will be placed on anticoagulants will assist in selecting the correct answer. Looking at the relationship between answers is also helpful. Options 1, 2, and 3 relate to infection. Option 4 relates to bleeding.

Level of Cognitive Ability: Application
Phase of Nursing Process: Implementation
Client Needs: Safe, Effective Care Environment
Content Area: Adult Health/Cardiovascular

Reference

Ignatavicius, D. D., Workman, M. L., & Mishler, M. A. (1995). *Medical-surgical nursing: A nursing process approach* (2nd ed.). Philadelphia: W. B. Saunders, p. 910.

18. The nurse is caring for a client during the recovery phase after a myocardial infarction. A cardiac catheterization, with the femoral artery approach, is planned to assess the degree of coronary artery thrombosis. What nursing action after the procedure is unsafe for the client?

1 Placing the client's bed in the Fowler's position
2 Encouraging the client to increase fluid intake
3 Instructing the client to move the toes when checking circulation, motion, and sensation
4 Resuming prescribed precatheterization medications

Answer: 1

Rationale: Immediately after a cardiac catheterization with the femoral artery approach, the client should not flex or hyperextend the affected leg to avoid blood vessel occlusion or hemorrhage. Placing the client in the Fowler's position (flexion) increases the risk of hemorrhage or occlusion. Fluids are encouraged in order to assist in removing the contrast medium from the body. Asking the client to move the toes is done to assess motion, which could be impaired if a hematoma or thrombus were developing. The precatheterization medications are needed to treat acute and chronic conditions.

Test-Taking Strategy: Note the word "unsafe" in the stem of the question. Also note the phrase "femoral artery approach." This should assist in directing you to the unsafe option of Fowler's position. Review post–cardiac catheterization care now if you had difficulty with this question!

Level of Cognitive Ability: Application
Phase of Nursing Process: Implementation
Client Needs: Safe, Effective Care Environment
Content Area: Adult Health/Cardiovascular

Reference

Black, J., & Matassarin-Jacobs, E. (1997). *Medical-surgical nursing: Clinical management for continuity of care* (5th ed.). Philadelphia: W. B. Saunders, p. 1232.

---

19. The client has a diagnosis of heart failure. The nurse would remove which of the following items from the client's meal tray?

1 Leafy green vegetables
2 Catsup
3 Cooked cereal
4 Sherbet

Answer: 2

Rationale: Catsup is high in sodium. Leafy green vegetables, cooked cereal, and sherbet are all low in sodium. Clients with heart failure should monitor sodium intake.

Test-Taking Strategy: Use the process of elimination, noting that options 1, 3, and 4 are alike in that they are low-sodium foods. Knowledge that the client with heart failure should monitor sodium intake and the ability to identify foods high in sodium are needed to answer this question. Review this content now if you had difficulty with this question!

Level of Cognitive Ability: Application
Phase of Nursing Process: Implementation
Client Needs: Safe, Effective Care Environment
Content Area: Adult Health/Cardiovascular

Reference

Black, J., & Matassarin-Jacobs, E. (1997). *Medical-surgical nursing: Clinical management for continuity of care* (5th ed.). Philadelphia: W. B. Saunders, p. 1286.

20. The caregiver wants to maintain food and fluid intake to minimize the risk of dehydration in a frail, elderly, diabetic client with gastroenteritis. An appropriate intervention for the caregiver to perform would be to

1 Offer only water until the client is able to tolerate solid foods.
2 Withhold all fluids until vomiting has ceased for at least 4 hours.
3 Encourage the client to take 8–12 ounces of fluid every hour while awake.
4 Maintain a clear liquid diet for at least 5 days before advancing to allow inflammation of the bowel to dissipate.

Answer: 3

Rationale: The client should be offered liquids containing both glucose and electrolytes. Small amounts of fluid may be tolerated even when vomiting is present. The diet should be advanced to a regular diet when tolerated and include a minimum of 100–150 g of carbohydrates daily.

Test-Taking Strategy: Eliminate options 1 and 2 because of the words "only" and "all." In the remaining options, note the phrase "for at least 5 days" in option 4. This is rather extreme and should be eliminated.

Level of Cognitive Ability: Application
Phase of Nursing Process: Implementation
Client Needs: Safe, Effective Care Environment
Content Area: Adult Health/Gastrointestinal

Reference

Ignatavicius, D. D., Workman, M. L., & Mishler, M. A. (1995). *Medical-surgical nursing: A nursing process approach* (2nd ed.). Philadelphia: W. B. Saunders, p. 1888.

---

21. The nurse wishes to carry out a multidisciplinary research project on the effects of immobility on clients' stress levels. Which of the following is the most important principle that the nurse must attend to while planning this project?

1 Collaboration with other disciplines is essential to the successful practice of nursing
2 The Corporate Nurse Executive should be consulted because the project will take nursing time
3 All clients have the right to refuse to participate in research using human subjects
4 The cooperation of the physician staff must be ensured in order for the project to succeed

Answer: 3

Rationale: Although options 1, 2, and 4 need to be considered, they are all secondary to the legal and ethical standard of nursing practice that any client has the right to refuse to participate in research using human subjects. The proposed project is research and does include human subjects.

Test-Taking Strategy: Note the phrase "most important principle." Options 1, 2, and 4 are correct in that it is necessary for anyone carrying out a research project to gain the approval and cooperation of all involved, but the most important principle to recall is that the client has the right to refuse to participate in research. The multidisciplinary team, the Nurse Executive, and the physicians cannot force the client into participation, even if they agree to assist in facilitating the research project itself.

Level of Cognitive Ability: Application
Phase of Nursing Process: Planning
Client Needs: Safe, Effective Care Environment
Content Area: Fundamental Skills

Reference

Wywialoski, E. (1997). *Managing client care* (2nd ed.). St. Louis: Mosby–Year Book, pp. 311–312.

---

22. The nurse has an order to obtain a sputum culture from the client who does not have an artificial airway. The nurse avoids taking which of the following actions?

1 Placing the lid of the culture container face down on the bedside table
2 Obtaining the specimen early in the morning
3 Having the client brush teeth before expectoration
4 Instructing the client to take deep breaths before coughing

Answer: 1

Rationale: Placing the lid face down on the bedside table contaminates the lid and could result in inaccurate findings. The specimen is obtained early in the morning whenever possible, because a larger amount of sputum has collected in the airways during sleep. The client should rinse the mouth or brush the teeth before specimen collection, to avoid contaminating the specimen. The client should take deep breaths before expectoration for best sputum production.

Test-Taking Strategy: Note the key word in the question, which is "avoids." Begin by eliminating options 2 and 4, which are helpful in obtaining a specimen of sufficient volume. Use basic principles of aseptic technique to choose option 1 over option 3.

Level of Cognitive Ability: Application
Phase of Nursing Process: Implementation
Client Needs: Safe, Effective Care Environment
Content Area: Fundamental Skills

Reference

Monahan, F., & Neighbors, M. (1998). *Medical-surgical nursing: Foundations for clinical practice* (2nd ed.). Philadelphia: W. B. Saunders, p. 546.

---

23. The multidisciplinary health care team is planning care for a client with hyperparathyroidism. The most important outcome for the client is to

1 Describe the administration of aluminum hydroxide gel.
2 Restrict fluids to 1000 mL/day.
3 Walk down the hall for 15 minutes, 3 times a day.
4 Discuss the use of loperamide (Imodium).

Answer: 3

Rationale: Mobility of the client with hyperparathyroidism should be encouraged as much as possible because bones subjected to normal stress break down less calcium. Hypercalcemia predisposes the client to the formation of renal calculi. Fluids should not be restricted. Discussing the use of these medications is not a priority.

Test-Taking Strategy: Knowledge that the client is predisposed to the formation of renal calculi is helpful in answering the question. This will assist in eliminating option 2 first, followed by options 1 and 4. If you had difficulty with this question, take time now to review care of the client with hyperparathyroidism!

Level of Cognitive Ability: Application
Phase of Nursing Process: Planning
Client Needs: Safe, Effective Care Environment
Content Area: Adult Health/Endocrine

Reference

Luckmann, J. (1997). *Saunders manual of nursing care*. Philadelphia: W. B. Saunders, p. 1403.

---

24. The client is unable to expectorate to yield a sputum sample, and the nurse decides to use the saline inhalation method to obtain the sample. The nurse instructs the client to inhale the warm saline vapor via nebulizer by

1 Holding the nebulizer under the nose.
2 Keeping the lips closed lightly over the seal.
3 Keeping the lips closely tightly over the seal.
4 Alternating one vapor breath with one breath from room air.

Answer: 2

Rationale: The inhalation of heated vapor helps the client to cough productively because the vapor condenses on the tracheobronchial mucosa, and stimulates the production of secretions and a cough reflex. The client is told to cover the mouthpiece with the lips, but not to form a tight seal. The client inhales vaporized saline until coughing results.

Test-Taking Strategy: Familiarity with this procedure is needed to answer this question correctly. Take a few moments now to review this variation of procedure for obtaining a sputum sample if you had difficulty with the question!

Level of Cognitive Ability: Application
Phase of Nursing Process: Implementation
Client Needs: Safe, Effective Care Environment
Content Area: Adult Health/Respiratory

Reference

Monahan, F., & Neighbors, M. (1998). *Medical-surgical nursing: Foundations for clinical practice* (2nd ed.). Philadelphia: W. B. Saunders, p. 546.

25. The nurse has completed tracheostomy care for a client whose tracheostomy tube has a nondisposable inner cannula. The nurse reinserts the inner cannula into the tracheostomy immediately after

1. Suctioning the client's airway.
2. Rinsing it with sterile water.
3. Tapping it against a sterile surface to dry it.
4. Drying it thoroughly with a sterile gauze.

Answer: 3

Rationale: After washing and rinsing the inner cannula, the nurse dries it by tapping it against a sterile surface. The nurse then inserts the cannula into the tracheostomy, and turns it clockwise to lock it into place.

Test-Taking Strategy: The key words in the question are "immediately after." Eliminate option 1 because you would not suction a client without an inner cannula in place. Eliminate option 2 because a wet cannula should not be inserted. Eliminate option 4 because using a sterile gauze to dry the cannula can cause particles of the gauze to gather on the cannula. Review the procedure for tracheotomy care now if you had difficulty with this question!

Level of Cognitive Ability: Application
Phase of Nursing Process: Implementation
Client Needs: Safe, Effective Care Environment
Content Area: Adult Health/Respiratory

Reference

DeLaune, S., & Ladner, P. (1998). *Fundamentals of nursing: Standards and practice.* Albany, NY: Delmar, p. 803.

26. The nurse has inserted a nasogastric tube into the stomach of a client. The nurse would avoid using which of the following methods for checking tube placement?

1. Aspirating the tube with a 50-mL syringe for gastric contents
2. Measuring the pH of gastric aspirate
3. Placing the end of the tube in water to check for bubbling
4. Instilling 10–20 mL of air into the tube while auscultating over the stomach

Answer: 3

Rationale: The least reliable method for determining accurate placement of a nasogastric tube is to place the end of the tube in water to observe for bubbling. Each of the other methods described is acceptable, although research has shown that each of them has drawbacks. The best method of determining tube placement is to verify by x-ray.

Test-Taking Strategy: Note the word "avoid." To answer this question accurately, it is necessary to know the basic principles involved in checking nasogastric tube placement and to know the risks and benefits of each. Review this procedure now if you had difficulty with this question!

Level of Cognitive Ability: Application
Phase of Nursing Process: Implementation
Client Needs: Safe, Effective Care Environment
Content Area: Adult Health/Gastrointestinal

Reference

Monahan, F., & Neighbors, M. (1998). *Medical-surgical nursing: Foundations for clinical practice* (2nd ed.). Philadelphia: W. B. Saunders, p. 978.

27. The client receiving total parenteral nutrition (TPN) through a central venous catheter suffers an air embolism when the central line disconnects from the IV tubing. The nurse takes immediate action by turning the client to the

1. Left side, with the head higher than the feet.
2. Right side, with the head higher than the feet.
3. Left side, with the feet higher than the head.
4. Right side, with the feet higher than the head.

Answer: 3

Rationale: If the client experiences air embolism, the immediate emergency treatment by the nurse is to place the client on the left side, with the feet higher than the head. This position traps air in the right atrium. If necessary, the air can then be directly removed by intracardiac aspiration.

Test-Taking Strategy: To answer this question correctly, it is necessary to know the proper position used in the emergency management of air embolism. If needed, take a few moments to review this procedure now!

Level of Cognitive Ability: Application
Phase of Nursing Process: Implementation
Client Needs: Safe, Effective Care Environment
Content Area: Fundamental Skills

Reference

Monahan, F., & Neighbors, M. (1998). *Medical-surgical nursing: Foundations for clinical practice* (2nd ed.). Philadelphia: W. B. Saunders, p. 988.

28. An anxious client enters the emergency room seeking treatment for a laceration of the finger while using a power tool. The client's vital signs are as follows: pulse, 96; blood pressure, 148/88; respirations, 24. After the nurse cleanses the injury and reassures the client, the vital signs are as follows: pulse, 82; blood pressure, 130/80; respirations, 20. The nurse assesses that the change in vital signs is a result of

1. Reduced stimulation of the sympathetic nervous system.
2. The cooling effects of the cleansing solution.
3. The body's physical adaptation to the air conditioning.
4. Possible impending cardiovascular collapse.

Answer: 1

Rationale: Physical or emotional stress triggers a sympathetic nervous system response. Responses that are reflected in vital signs include increased pulse, increased blood pressure, and increased respiratory rate. Stress reduction thus returns these parameters to baseline.

Test-Taking Strategy: The stem tells you that the client is anxious and has an injury. These two elements guide you to think about the body's response to stress. Relate stress to the sympathetic nervous system. In addition, the wording of the stem tells you that the nurse reduced the stress, which guides you to the correct answer!

Level of Cognitive Ability: Analysis
Phase of Nursing Process: Analysis
Client Needs: Safe, Effective Care Environment
Content Area: Fundamental Skills

Reference

Black, J., & Matassarin-Jacobs, E. (1997). *Medical-surgical nursing: Clinical management for continuity of care* (5th ed.). Philadelphia: W. B. Saunders, p. 1203.

29. The nurse is scheduling multiple diagnostic procedures for the client with activity intolerance. The procedures ordered include an echocardiogram, chest x-ray, and computed axial tomography (CT) scan. Assuming all schedules are possible, which of the following plans will best meet the needs of this client?

1. Schedule the x-ray in the morning, the echocardiogram in the afternoon, and the CT scan in the morning of the following day
2. Schedule the chest x-ray and echocardiogram together in the morning and the CT scan in the afternoon of the same day
3. Schedule the echocardiogram in the morning and the chest x-ray and CT scan together in the afternoon of the same day
4. Schedule the CT scan in the morning and the chest x-ray and echocardiogram on the following morning

Answer: 1

Rationale: The key concept tested here is achieving a balance between rest and activity. Echocardiograms are done at the bedside. Chest x-rays and CT scans are done in the radiology department (unless a portable chest x-ray is ordered). The best scenario would be to have the client go to a procedure in another department in the morning (when most rested); have a rest period; have another procedure on the unit in the afternoon (when more fatigued), and go off the nursing unit again the next morning (when rested again).

Test-Taking Strategy: A client who has activity intolerance will do best when activities are spaced. This helps you eliminate options 2 and 3. An understanding of the location where these diagnostic tests are performed helps you choose option 1 over option 4.

Level of Cognitive Ability: Application
Phase of Nursing Process: Planning
Client Needs: Safe, Effective Care Environment
Content Area: Fundamental Skills

Reference

Cox, H., Hinz, M., Lubno, M., et al. (1997). *Clinical applications of nursing diagnosis: Adult, child, women's, psychiatric, gerontic, and home health considerations* (3rd ed.). Philadelphia: F. A. Davis, p. 252.

30. A client with angina pectoris is extremely anxious after being hospitalized for the first time ever. The nurse would plan to do which of the following to minimize the client's stress?

1 Admit the client to a room as far as possible from the nursing station
2 Provide as many care choices to the client as possible
3 Encourage the client to limit visitors to as few as possible
4 Keep the door open and hallway lights on at night

Answer: 2

Rationale: General interventions to minimize stress in the hospitalized client include providing information, social support, control over choices related to care, and acknowledging the client's feelings.

Test-Taking Strategy: Recall the basic elements of stress management and apply them to this question. Being far from the nursing station may or may not help reduce stress for this client, as there is no direct information about this in the stem. Limiting visitors reduces social support, and leaving the door open with hallway lights on may keep the client oriented (which is not stated as a problem) but may also interfere with sleep. This leaves option 2 as the only option that gives the client choices and control.

Level of Cognitive Ability: Application
Phase of Nursing Process: Planning
Client Needs: Safe, Effective Care Environment
Content Area: Adult Health/Cardiovascular

Reference

Ignatavicius, D. D., Workman, M. L., & Mishler, M. A. (1995). *Medical-surgical nursing: A nursing process approach* (2nd ed.). Philadelphia: W. B. Saunders, pp. 112–113.

31. The nurse is preparing to start a client with acute myocardial infarction on an intravenous nitroglycerin drip. In the absence of an invasive monitoring line, the nurse knows that which piece of equipment will be needed for use at the bedside?

1 Defibrillator
2 Pulse oximeter
3 Central venous pressure (CVP) tray
4 Noninvasive blood pressure monitor

Answer: 4

Rationale: Nitroglycerin dilates both the arteries and the veins, causing peripheral blood pooling and thus reducing preload, afterload, and myocardial work. This also accounts for the primary side effect of nitroglycerin, which is clinical hypotension. In the absence of continuous direct arterial pressure monitoring, the nurse should have an automatic noninvasive pressure monitor in use.

Test-Taking Strategy: Knowledge of the effects of nitroglycerin on the cardiovascular system helps you to easily eliminate each of the other incorrect options. Note the phrase "absence of an invasive monitoring line." This should assist in directing you to the correct option!

Level of Cognitive Ability: Analysis
Phase of Nursing Process: Analysis
Client Needs: Safe, Effective Care Environment
Content Area: Adult Health/Cardiovascular

Reference

Smeltzer, S., & Bare, B. (1996). *Brunner and Suddarth's Textbook of medical-surgical nursing* (8th ed.). Philadelphia: Lippincott-Raven, p. 650.

32. A prenatal client has acquired the sexually transmitted disease condyloma acuminatum (caused by human papillomavirus). When planning care, which of the following interventions would the nurse consider to be safe for this maternity client?

1 Laser therapy
2 Use of cytotoxic agents
3 Treatment with interferon
4 None is required

Answer: 1

Rationale: Laser therapy is the most effective destructive method of treatment that is considered safe for pregnancy. Medications for the disease are considered toxic to the fetus. The primary neonatal effect of the virus is respiratory or laryngeal papillomatosis. The exact route of perinatal transmission is unknown.

Test-Taking Strategy: Eliminate option 4 first. Next, eliminate options 2 and 3. Medication use during pregnancy is very limited and should not be the first option. If you had difficulty with this question, review care of the prenatal client who has acquired the sexually transmitted condyloma acuminatum.

Level of Cognitive Ability: Analysis
Phase of Nursing Process: Planning
Client Needs: Safe, Effective Care Environment
Content Area: Maternity

Reference

Lowdermilk, D., Perry, S., & Bobak, I. (1997). *Maternity and women's health care* (6th ed.). St. Louis: Mosby–Year Book, pp. 741–742.

33. A client in labor has a concurrent diagnosis of sickle cell anemia. During labor, the client is at high risk for sickling crisis. Which of the following would be the priority action by the nurse to assist in preventing a crisis from occurring during labor?

1 Reassure the client
2 Administer oxygen as ordered throughout labor
3 Maintain strict asepsis
4 Prevent bearing down

Answer: 2

Rationale: An intervention to prevent sickle cell crisis during labor includes administering oxygen as needed. During the labor process, the client is at high risk for being unable to meet the oxygen demands of labor and unable to prevent sickling.

Test-Taking Strategy: The question is asking what nursing action would be done first to prevent sickling crisis. Use the ABCs: airway, breathing, and circulation. Remember that in prioritizing, airway is always first. Option 2 addresses airway. Options 1, 3, and 4 are correct answers but not for the situation described in the stem.

Level of Cognitive Ability: Application
Phase of Nursing Process: Implementation
Client Needs: Safe, Effective Care Environment
Content Area: Maternity

Reference

Lowdermilk, D., Perry, S., & Bobak, I. (1997). *Maternity and women's health care* (6th ed.). St. Louis: Mosby–Year Book, pp. 846–847.

---

34. The nurse in a preschool is planning a staff education program to prevent the spread of intestinal parasitic disease. What statement expresses the nurse's priority goal?

1 Staff will practice universal precautions when changing diapers and assisting children with toileting
2 All toileting areas will be cleansed daily with soap and water
3 Only bottled water will be used for drinking
4 All food will be cooked before eating

Answer: 1

Rationale: The fecal-oral route is the mode of transmission. Option 1 interrupts the primary route of transmission in this setting. Option 2 would be more effective if a 10% bleach solution was used. Water and fresh foods can be vehicles for transmission, but municipal water sources are usually safe. Fresh foods may be used as long as they are washed well, provided that they weren't grown in soil contaminated with human feces.

Test-Taking Strategy: Note the issue of the question and the word "priority" in the stem. Option 1 addresses the issue of the question and is the most global response addressing universal precautions!

Level of Cognitive Ability: Application
Phase of Nursing Process: Planning
Client Needs: Safe, Effective Care Environment
Content Area: Child Health

Reference

Wong, D. (1997). *Whaley and Wong's Essentials of pediatric nursing* (5th ed.). St. Louis: Mosby–Year Book, p. 414.

---

35. A client has arrived at the labor and delivery unit in active labor. The nursing assessment reveals a history of recurrent genital herpes and the presence of lesions in the genital tract. The nurse should plan to

1 Prepare the client for a cesarean delivery.
2 Limit visitors and maintain reverse isolation.
3 Prepare the client for a spontaneous vaginal delivery.
4 Rupture the membranes artificially, looking for meconium-stained fluid.

Answer: 1

Rationale: A cesarean delivery can reduce neonatal infection risk with a mother in labor who has herpetic genital tract lesions or ruptured membranes. Fifty percent of infected newborns die in 6–10 days, and half the survivors have permanent ocular or neurological sequelae.

Test-Taking Strategy: Knowing that active genital herpes lesions are present and a serious risk to the newborn, you would expect the physician to perform a cesarean delivery. Intact membranes provide another barrier to transmitting the disease to the neonate. This fact should assist in eliminating options 3 and 4. There is no need to limit visitors or maintain isolation, although universal precautions should be maintained.

Level of Cognitive Ability: Application
Phase of Nursing Process: Planning
Client Needs: Safe, Effective Care Environment
Content Area: Maternity

Reference

Nichols, F., & Zwelling, E. (1997). *Maternal-newborn nursing: Theory and practice.* Philadelphia: W. B. Saunders, pp. 1495–1496.

---

36. The client is to undergo diagnostic testing to rule out renal pathology. As an essential element of care, the nurse would plan to ask the client about a history of

1. Frequent antibiotic use.
2. Long-term diuretic therapy.
3. Allergy to shellfish or iodine.
4. Familial renal disease.

Answer: 3

Rationale: The client undergoing any type of diagnostic testing should be questioned about allergy to shellfish, seafood, or iodine. This is essential to identify potential allergic reaction to contrast dye, which may be used in some diagnostic tests. This is especially important because the client may have subsequent diagnostic tests ordered, even if the original test was noninvasive. The other items are also useful as part of the health history but are not as critical as the allergy determination.

Test-Taking Strategy: Note that the stem of the question includes the phrase "essential element of care." This implies that more than one or all options may be correct; however, one of them is of highest priority. Option 4 can be eliminated first as the least pertinent to current care. Because the stem indicates that diagnostic testing is planned, the items are evaluated against their potential connection to this aspect of care. Thus you would eliminate all options except the third, because they are less essential.

Level of Cognitive Ability: Application
Phase of Nursing Process: Planning
Client Needs: Safe, Effective Care Environment
Content Area: Adult Health/Renal

Reference

Black, J., & Matassarin-Jacobs, E. (1997). *Medical-surgical nursing: Clinical management for continuity of care* (5th ed.). Philadelphia: W. B. Saunders, p. 1550.

---

37. The nurse is inserting an indwelling bladder catheter as ordered for an assigned client. Which of the following represents an incorrect action of the nurse while completing this procedure?

1. Inflating the balloon to test patency before catheter insertion
2. Advancing the catheter just until urine appears in the catheter tubing
3. Inflating the balloon with 4–5 mL more than the stated balloon capacity
4. Placing the bag lower than bladder level, with no kinks in the tubing

Answer: 2

Rationale: The catheter should be advanced for 1 to 2 more inches beyond the point where the flow of urine is first noted. This ensures that the balloon is fully in the bladder before it is inflated. Each of the other statements represents correct procedure.

Test-Taking Strategy: Options 1 and 4 are most obviously correct and are therefore eliminated as possible answers to the question as stated. To discriminate among the last two options, you need to know either that the catheter is advanced 1–2 more inches or that extra fluid is needed to fill the lumen that runs between the external port and the balloon at the tip of the catheter.

Level of Cognitive Ability: Application
Phase of Nursing Process: Implementation
Client Needs: Safe, Effective Care Environment
Content Area: Adult Health/Renal

Reference

Taylor, C., Lillis, C., & LeMone, P. (1997). *Fundamentals of nursing: The art and science of nursing care* (3rd ed.). Philadelphia: Lippincott-Raven, p. 1237.

38. The nurse has an order to obtain a 24-hour urine collection from a client with a renal disorder. The nurse would avoid which of the following to ensure proper collection of the 24-hour specimen?

1. Have the client void at the start time, and place this specimen in the container
2. Save all subsequent voidings in the 24-hour time period
3. Place the container on ice or in a refrigerator
4. Instruct the client to void at the end time, and place this specimen in the container

Answer: 1

Rationale: The nurse asks the client to void at the beginning of the collection period and discards this urine sample. All subsequent voided urine is saved in a container, which is placed on ice or refrigerated. The client is asked to void at the finish time, and this sample is added to the collection. The container is labeled, placed on fresh ice, and sent to the laboratory immediately.

Test-Taking Strategy: Options 2 and 3 are the most obviously correct of all the options, so these are eliminated, because the question asks for an item to avoid. To discriminate between the last two, think about the process. Having the client void at the finish time makes sense, because this captures the urine that the bladder has stored between the last time of voiding and the finish time for the specimen. On the other hand, if you save the first specimen, you do not know how long that urine has been stored in the bladder. Therefore, you would not be getting a true "24-hour" collection. Thus option 1 is the answer to the question as stated.

Level of Cognitive Ability: Application
Phase of Nursing Process: Implementation
Client Needs: Safe, Effective Care Environment
Content Area: Adult Health/Renal

Reference

Black, J., & Matassarin-Jacobs, E. (1997). *Medical-surgical nursing: Clinical management for continuity of care* (5th ed.). Philadelphia: W. B. Saunders, p. 1556.

39. The nurse is caring for the client in active labor. Which of the following actions by the nurse will best prevent fetal heart rate decelerations?

1. Continue oxytocin (Pitocin) to increase uterine activity
2. Encourage upright or side-lying maternal positions
3. Assess maternal and fetal vital signs every 30 minutes
4. Prepare client for a cesarean delivery

Answer: 2

Rationale: There are many nursing interventions that support the body's normal mechanism for birth. Side-lying and upright positions such as walking, standing, and squatting can improve venous return and encourage effective uterine activity. The nurse may discontinue Pitocin in the presence of fetal heart rate decelerations, thereby reducing uterine activity and increasing uteroplacental perfusion. Monitoring vital signs every 30 minutes is not relevant to this question. There are many nursing actions to prevent fetal heart rate decelerations, without necessitating surgical intervention.

Test-Taking Strategy: The question asks for the measure to "best prevent fetal heart rate decelerations." Options 1, 3, and 4 will not "prevent" fetal heart rate decelerations. Side-lying and upright positions will encourage effective uterine activity and provide a safe environment.

Level of Cognitive Ability: Application
Phase of Nursing Process: Implementation
Client Needs: Safe, Effective Care Environment
Content Area: Maternity

Reference

Nichols, F., & Zwelling, E. (1997). *Maternal-newborn nursing: Theory and practice.* Philadelphia: W. B. Saunders, p. 951.

40. A diabetic client is 36 weeks pregnant. The client has had weekly nonstress tests for the last 3 weeks that have been reactive. This week the nonstress test was nonreactive after 40 minutes. On the basis of these results, the nurse would anticipate that the client will be prepared for

1 Immediate induction of labor.
2 Hospitalization with continuous fetal monitoring.
3 A return appointment in 2–7 days to repeat the nonstress test.
4 A contraction stress test.

Answer: 4

Rationale: There are not enough data to justify the procedures in options 1 and 2 at this time. A nonreactive test needs further assessment at this time. To send the client home for 2–7 days may put the fetus in jeopardy. A contraction stress test is the next surveillance measure needed to further assess the fetal status.

Test-Taking Strategy: Options 1 and 2 can be eliminated first because they are unnecessary at this time. Option 3 can be eliminated next because repeating the test at a later time is not a safe intervention, especially in view of the fact that previous test results were reactive. Review the meanings of the test results related to a nonstress test now if you had difficulty with this question!

Level of Cognitive Ability: Analysis
Phase of Nursing Process: Planning
Client Needs: Safe, Effective Care Environment
Content Area: Maternity

Reference

Reeder, S., Martin, L., & Koniak-Griffin, D. (1997). *Maternity nursing: Family, newborn, and women's health care* (18th ed.). Philadelphia: Lippincott-Raven, p. 1075.

---

41. The nurse is administering magnesium sulfate to a client for severe pre-eclampsia. While doing so, it is important for the nurse to implement which of the following actions?

1 Assess for signs and symptoms of labor because the client's level of consciousness will be altered
2 Assess temperature every 2 hours because the client is at high risk for infection
3 Schedule a nonstress test every 4 hours to assess fetal well-being
4 Schedule a daily ultrasound examination to assess fetal movement

Answer: 1

Rationale: Option 1 is a true statement. Because of the sedative effect of the medication, the client may not perceive labor. This client is not at high risk for infection. A nonstress test may be done, but not every 4 hours. Daily ultrasound examinations are not necessary for this client.

Test-Taking Strategy: Use the Nursing Process to answer the question. Assessment is the first step; therefore, eliminate options 3 and 4. From the remaining options, knowledge that the client is not at high risk for infection will assist in directing you to option 1. Review nursing responsibilities when administering magnesium sulfate now if you had difficulty with this question!

Level of Cognitive Ability: Application
Phase of Nursing Process: Implementation
Client Needs: Safe, Effective Care Environment
Content Area: Maternity

Reference

Reeder, S., Martin, L., & Koniak-Griffin, D. (1997). *Maternity nursing: Family, newborn, and women's health care* (18th ed.). Philadelphia: Lippincott-Raven, p. 841.

---

42. The client's nasogastric feeding tube has become clogged. Which of the following is the first action that the nurse should take?

1 Flush the tube with warm water
2 Aspirate the tube
3 Flush with carbonated liquids, such as cola
4 Replace the tube

Answer: 2

Rationale: The nurse first attempts to unclog a feeding tube by aspirating the tube. If this is not successful, the nurse tries to flush the tube with warm water. Carbonated liquids, such as cola, are sometimes used to eliminate clogging, but the tube must be rinsed thoroughly to avoid stickiness. Replacement of the tube is the last step if others are unsuccessful.

Test-Taking Strategy: To answer this question correctly, it is necessary to be familiar with basic procedures for troubleshooting tube feedings. If this question was difficult, take a few moments to review this procedure at this time!

Level of Cognitive Ability: Application
Phase of Nursing Process: Implementation
Client Needs: Safe, Effective Care Environment
Content Area: Fundamental Skills

Reference

Monahan, F., & Neighbors, M. (1998). *Medical-surgical nursing: Foundations for clinical practice* (2nd ed.). Philadelphia: W. B. Saunders, p. 986.

---

43. The moderately depressed client who was admitted 2 days ago suddenly begins smiling and reporting that the crisis is over. The client says to the nurse, "Call the doctor. I'm finally cured." The nurse interprets this behavior as a cue to modify the treatment plan by

1 Allowing off-unit privileges PRN.
2 Suggesting a reduction of medication.
3 Allowing increased "in room" activities.
4 Increasing level of suicide precautions.

Answer: 4

Rationale: A client who is moderately depressed and has been in the hospital only 2 days is very unlikely to have such a dramatic cure. When a mood lifts suddenly, it is very likely that the client may have made the decision to harm self. Suicide precautions are necessary to keep the client safe.

Test-Taking Strategy: Options 1, 2, and 3 support the client's notion that a cure has occurred, and the nurse must know that if depression decreases it does so over time. Safety is of the utmost importance now; therefore, option 4 is the choice.

Level of Cognitive Ability: Analysis
Phase of Nursing Process: Planning
Client Needs: Safe, Effective Care Environment
Content Area: Mental Health

Reference

Johnson, B. (1997). *Psychiatric–mental health nursing: Adaptation and growth.* Philadelphia: Lippincott-Raven, p. 862.

---

44. When an intravenous fluid infusion is started in order to treat dehydration in a 3-year-old child, which piece of equipment is least helpful?

1 A padded arm board
2 A 20-gtt/mL intravenous set
3 A pediatric infusion pump
4 A 24-gauge intravenous catheter

Answer: 2

Rationale: A Buretrol or a Soluset device that delivers 60 microdrops per milliliter is preferred, to prevent fluid overload. The low-volume, marked fluid chamber is another safety feature because it decreases the amount of fluid that can be infused at one time if the rate is accidentally altered. Option 1 is necessary because this device helps to preserve the integrity of the IV site. Option 3 is necessary because an infusion pump is to be used on all children getting an IV infusion. Option 4 is an appropriate-sized IV catheter to use to start an IV infusion in a toddler's extremity.

Test-Taking Strategy: Note the words "least helpful" in the stem. Focus on selecting equipment that is safe for an IV infusion in a child. Option 2 is used in adult IV therapy. Option 1 may be appropriate for a child or an adult. Option 3 has the word "pediatric" in it.

Level of Cognitive Ability: Application
Phase of Nursing Process: Planning
Client Needs: Safe, Effective Care Environment
Content Area: Child Health

Reference

Wong, D. (1995). *Whaley and Wong's Nursing care of infants and children* (5th ed.). St. Louis: Mosby–Year Book, p. 1221.

45. In planning care for the suicidal clients on the unit, the nurse needs to be aware that extra precautions are warranted at which of the following times?

1 Day shift
2 Weekdays
3 7 A.M. to 10 A.M.
4 Shift change

Answer: 4

Rationale: Often at shift changes, less staff is available. The psychiatric nurse and staff should increase precautions for identified clients at those times. Weekends, not weekdays, are also times for more suicides. Suicides are more likely during the night shift rather than the day shift.

Test-Taking Strategy: Options 1, 2, and 3 are similar and can be eliminated. The nurse could anticipate that times with less supervision of the client could be times of increased risks.

Level of Cognitive Ability: Application
Phase of Nursing Process: Planning
Client Needs: Safe, Effective Care Environment
Content Area: Mental Health

Reference

Johnson, B. (1997). *Psychiatric–mental health nursing: Adaptation and growth.* Philadelphia: Lippincott-Raven, p. 862.

---

46. For the safety of the client after a surgical procedure is complete, the nursing care plan should include techniques to prevent injury to the client. Which of these statements indicates a technique that would provide safety for the client?

1 Move the client rapidly from the surgery table to a stretcher
2 Uncover the client completely before transferring to a stretcher
3 Secure the client with safety belts after transferring to a stretcher
4 Instruct the client to move self from the surgery table to a stretcher

Answer: 3

Rationale: During the transfer of the client after the surgical procedure is complete, the nurse should avoid exposure of the client because of the potential heat loss, respiratory infection, and shock. Hurried movements and rapid changes in position should be avoided because these predispose the client to hypotension. At the time of the transfer from the surgery table to the stretcher, the client is still affected by the effects of the anesthesia; therefore, care must be provided by the nurse. Safety belts can prevent the client from falling off the stretcher.

Test-Taking Strategy: Options 1 and 2 are unsafe techniques for the client. Note the word "rapidly" in option 1 and the phrase "uncover the client completely" in option 2. Option 4 is not appropriate because of the effects of the anesthesia. Option 3 is the only safe and appropriate technique for the client.

Level of Cognitive Ability: Application
Phase of Nursing Process: Planning
Client Needs: Safe, Effective Care Environment
Content Area: Fundamental Skills

Reference

Phipps, W., Cassmeyer, V., Sands, J., et al. (1995). *Medical-surgical nursing: Concepts and clinical practice* (5th ed.). Philadelphia: Mosby–Year Book, p. 596.

---

47. Which of the following nursing interventions is warranted with the hallucinating and delusional client who has been rescued from a suicide attempt?

1 Check whereabouts of client every 15 minutes
2 Suicide precautions with 30-minute checks
3 One-to-one suicide precautions
4 Ask that the client report suicidal thoughts immediately

Answer: 3

Rationale: All of these actions are appropriate for a suicidal client. In this situation, the key information is that the client is delusional and hallucinating. Both of these factors increase the unpredictable behavior, decrease judgment, and make the risk of suicide greater. The best answer is constant supervision so that the nurse may intervene as needed if the client attempted to cause harm to self.

Test-Taking Strategy: Note the key words "suicidal," "rescued," "hallucinating," and "delusional." All of these factors indicate that the highest level of suicide precautions is necessary.

Level of Cognitive Ability: Application
Phase of Nursing Process: Implementation
Client Needs: Safe, Effective Care Environment
Content Area: Mental Health

Reference

Johnson, B. (1997). *Psychiatric–mental health nursing: Adaptation and growth.* Philadelphia: Lippincott-Raven, p. 871.

48. When planning to give a tepid tub bath to a child who has hyperthermia, which of these measures should be included?

1 Obtain isopropyl alcohol to add to the bath water
2 Warm water to the same body temperature of the child
3 Have cool water available to add to the bath water
4 Allow 15 minutes for the child to soak in the tub

Answer: 3

Rationale: Adding cool water to an already warm bath allows the water temperature to slowly drop. The child is able to gradually adjust to the changing water temperature and will not experience chilling. Option 1 is incorrect because alcohol is toxic and contraindicated for tepid sponge or tub baths. Option 2 is incorrect; to achieve the best cooling results, the water temperature should be at least 2 degrees lower than the child's body temperature. Option 4 is incorrect because the child should be in a tepid tub bath for 20 to 30 minutes to achieve maximum results.

Test-Taking Strategy: Option 1 can be easily eliminated. Eliminate option 2 because water that is the same as body temperature will not reduce hyperthermia. Eliminate option 4 because of the 15-minute time frame. Review measures for hyperthermia now if you had difficulty with this question!

Level of Cognitive Ability: Application
Phase of Nursing Process: Planning
Client Needs: Safe, Effective Care Environment
Content Area: Child Health

Reference

Wong, D. (1995). *Whaley and Wong's Nursing care of infants and children* (5th ed.). St. Louis: Mosby–Year Book, p. 1162.

49. A nurse is assigned to care for a child the day after a surgical repair of a cleft lip. Which nursing intervention is most appropriate when caring for this child's surgical incision?

1 Clean the incision only when serous exudate forms
2 Rub the incision gently with a sterile cotton-tipped swab
3 Rinse incision with sterile water after using diluted peroxide
4 Replace the Logan bar carefully after cleaning the incision

Answer: 3

Rationale: When cleaned with a solution other than water or saline, the incision should be rinsed with sterile water. Option 1 is incorrect; the incision is also cleaned after every feeding. Option 2 is incorrect; rubbing alters the integrity of the suture line, and the incision should be dabbed. Option 4 is incorrect; the purpose of the Logan bar is to maintain the integrity of the suture line. Removing the Logan bar on the first postoperative day would increase tension on the surgical incision.

Test-Taking Strategy: Eliminate options 1 and 2 because of the word "only" in option 1 and "rub" in option 2. Focus on the phrase "the day after a surgical repair" in the question. This should assist in eliminating option 4. Review care of a child after surgical repair of a cleft lip, if you had difficulty with this question!

Level of Cognitive Ability: Application
Phase of Nursing Process: Implementation
Client Needs: Safe, Effective Care Environment
Content Area: Child Health

Reference

Pillitteri, A. (1995). *Maternal and child health nursing: Care of the childbearing and childrearing family* (2nd ed.). Philadelphia: Lippincott-Raven, pp. 1127–1128.

50. The multidisciplinary health care team is preparing a teaching plan for a client receiving anticoagulant agents. The priority nursing diagnosis would be

1 Fluid Volume Deficit.
2 High Risk for Activity Intolerance.
3 High Risk for Injury.
4 High Risk for Infection.

Answer: 3

Rationale: Anticoagulant therapy predisposes the client to injury because of the inhibitory effects on the body's normal blood clotting mechanism. Bruising, bleeding, and hemorrhage may occur in the course of activities of daily living and with other activities. None of the other options have a strong relationship to the situation presented in the stem.

Test-Taking Strategy: Knowledge that anticoagulants present a risk for bleeding will assist in directing you to option 3. Options 1, 2, and 4 are not directly related to this medication. If you had difficulty with this question, take time now to review the effects of anticoagulants!

Level of Cognitive Ability: Application
Phase of Nursing Process: Planning
Client Needs: Safe, Effective Care Environment
Content Area: Pharmacology

Reference

Ignatavicius, D. D., Workman, M. L., & Mishler, M. A. (1995). *Medical-surgical nursing: A nursing process approach* (2nd ed.). Philadelphia: W. B. Saunders, pp. 957, 958.

51. The client being seen in the emergency room with complaints of abdominal pain has a working diagnosis of acute abdomen. The nurse would question an order for which of the following at this time?

1 Insertion of a nasogastric tube
2 Insertion of an intravenous line
3 Administration of a narcotic analgesic
4 Institution of NPO diet status

Answer: 3

Rationale: Until a differential diagnosis is made and a decision about the need for surgery is made, the nurse would question an order to give a narcotic analgesic, because it could mask the client's symptoms. The nurse can expect the client to be placed on NPO status and to have an IV line inserted. Insertion of a nasogastric tube may help provide decompression of the stomach.

Test-Taking Strategy: Knowing that client complaints of abdominal pain could result in NPO status and insertion of a nasogastric tube, eliminate options 1 and 4 first. You could then choose option 3 over option 2 as the correct answer, because an intravenous line is a standard and accepted intervention for providing fluids for the client who is NPO.

Level of Cognitive Ability: Application
Phase of Nursing Process: Implementation
Client Needs: Safe, Effective Care Environment
Content Area: Adult Health/Gastrointestinal

Reference

Monahan, F., & Neighbors, M. (1998). *Medical-surgical nursing: Foundations for clinical practice* (2nd ed.). Philadelphia: W. B. Saunders, p. 1064.

52. The nurse is working with a family in the home to assist them in caring for a newborn receiving enteral feedings because of a congenital tracheoesophageal fistula. A woman identifying herself as a family friend telephones the nurse to inquire whether there is anything she can do to assist the parents. The best nursing action is to

1 Request that the friend come to the client's home where she can be taught to administer the feedings.
2 Inform the friend to directly contact the family and offer her assistance to them.
3 Report the friend's telephone call to the nurse manager for referral to the client's social worker.
4 Inform the caller that the family has no need for assistance at this time as the nurse is making daily visits.

Answer: 2

Rationale: The nurse is not able to give any information regarding a client's care needs to anyone not directly involved in the client's care. This is true in the home care setting as well as in the hospital. To request that the caller come for teaching is a direct violation of the client's rights to privacy. There is nothing to indicate that the client desires assistance from (or even knows) the caller. To refer the call to the nurse manager and social worker again assumes that the caller's assistance and involvement is desired by the client. The nurse must not make that assumption. Informing the caller that the nurse is visiting daily is giving the caller information that is considered confidential. Only option 2 indicates that the nurse is giving no information regarding the client's care and refers the caller to the client.

Test-Taking Strategy: It is necessary to understand the principle of confidentiality in order to answer this question. By recalling that the nurse can give no information to persons not directly involved in the care of a client, you can easily eliminate all potential answers that include giving out even the least bit of information. Even though the caller might seem well intentioned, the nurse should not assume that the client wants or needs assistance or that the caller is even who she has presented herself to be.

Level of Cognitive Ability: Application
Phase of Nursing Process: Implementation
Client Needs: Safe, Effective Care Environment
Content Area: Fundamental Skills

Reference

Wywialoski, E. (1997). *Managing client care* (2nd ed.). St. Louis: Mosby–Year Book, pp. 296, 305.

53. The nurse has been assigned to care for a young man recovering at home from a disabling lung infection. While obtaining a nursing history, the nurse learns that the infection is probably the result of human immunodeficiency virus (HIV) infection. The nurse informs the client that she or he is morally opposed to homosexuality and cannot care for him. The nurse then leaves the client's home. Which of the following is true regarding the nurse's actions?

1 The nurse has a duty to protect the self from client care situations that are morally repellent
2 The nurse has a legal right to inform the client of any barriers to providing care
3 The nurse has the right to refuse to care for any client without justifying that refusal
4 The nurse has a duty to provide competent care to assigned clients in a nondiscriminatory manner

Answer: 4

Rationale: The nurse has a duty to provide care to all clients and in a nondiscriminatory manner. Personal autonomy does not apply if it interferes with the rights of the client. There is no legal obligation to inform the client of the nurse's personal objections to the client. Refusal to provide care may be acceptable if that refusal does not put the client's safety at risk, but this is primarily associated with religious objections and is not acceptable in instances of personal objection to assumptions about lifestyle or medical diagnosis. The nurse also has an obligation to observe the principle of nonmaleficence (neither causing nor allowing harm to befall the client).

Test-Taking Strategy: The question is asking you to make a decision regarding the appropriateness of the nurse's actions. Note the key phrase "provide competent care" and the key word "nondiscriminatory" in the correct option! The only statement that is true is option 4.

Level of Cognitive Ability: Application
Phase of Nursing Process: Planning
Client Needs: Safe, Effective Care Environment
Content Area: Fundamental Skills

Reference

Deeloughery, G. (1995). *Issues and trends in nursing* (2nd ed.). St. Louis: [illegible] Year Book, pp. 231, 237.

54. The nurse is administering heparin sodium (Liquaemin), 5000 units subcutaneously (SC). Which of the following demonstrates accurate procedure?

1 Injecting within 2 inches of the umbilicus
2 Massaging the injection site after administration
3 Injecting via an infusion device
4 Changing the needle on the syringe after withdrawing the medication from the vial

Answer: 4

Rationale: Administration of heparin SC does not require an infusion device. The injection site is above the iliac crest or in the abdominal fat layer. Do not inject within 2 inches of the umbilicus or into any scar tissue. Withdraw the needle rapidly, apply prolonged pressure at the injection site, and do not massage. Injection sites are rotated. After withdrawal of heparin from the vial, the needle is changed before injection to prevent leakage along the needle tract.

Test-Taking Strategy: Knowledge regarding the administration of heparin SC is necessary to answer this question. You may easily eliminate options 2 and 3. Review this procedure now if you had difficulty with this question!

Level of Cognitive Ability: Application
Phase of Nursing Process: Implementation
Client Needs: Safe, Effective Care Environment
Content Area: Pharmacology

Reference

Hodgson, B., & Kizior, R. (1998). *Saunders nursing drug handbook 1998.* Philadelphia: W. B. Saunders, p. 489.

55. The nurse is caring for a client with cancer. The client tells the nurse that the lawyer will be arriving today to prepare a living will. The client asks the nurse to act as one of the witnesses for the will. The most appropriate nursing action is to

1 Agree to act as a witness.
2 Refuse to help the client.
3 Inform the client that a nurse caring for a client cannot serve as a witness to a living will.
4 Call the nursing supervisor.

Answer: 3

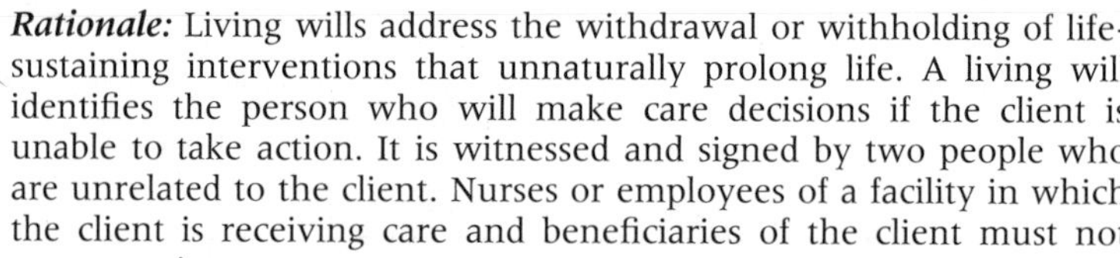

Rationale: Living wills address the withdrawal or withholding of life-sustaining interventions that unnaturally prolong life. A living will identifies the person who will make care decisions if the client is unable to take action. It is witnessed and signed by two people who are unrelated to the client. Nurses or employees of a facility in which the client is receiving care and beneficiaries of the client must not serve as witnesses.

Test-Taking Strategy: Knowledge of the procedure related to living wills will assist in answering the question. The question asks for the "most appropriate action." You can easily eliminate option 2 because of the word "refuse." Option 1 is clearly incorrect. There is no need to call the supervisor, and it is most appropriate to inform the client of the nurse's role in this procedure.

Level of Cognitive Ability: Application
Phase of Nursing Process: Implementation
Client Needs: Safe, Effective Care Environment
Content Area: Fundamental Skills

Reference

Luckmann, J. (1997). *Saunders manual of nursing care.* Philadelphia: W. B. Saunders, p. 583.

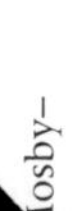

cardia.
ocaine
of 5%
using.
tion to

e, and
h
ocaine

f lido-
ns

Answer: 2

Rationale: A bolus of lidocaine can be given directly into an IV line with plain D5W because it is compatible with D5W. If D5W is the primary solution, the IV line does not need to be flushed. A new IV line is not required for the administration of this medication in this situation. There is no evidence in this question that other IV medications are being administered; therefore, option 4 is not necessary.

Test-Taking Strategy: Knowledge regarding lidocaine, its administration, and its compatibility with other substances is necessary to answer the question. Eliminate option 4 first because there are no data indicating that other medications are being administered. Eliminate option 3 next because this action is avoided if possible. Knowledge that lidocaine is compatible with D5W is necessary in order to select option 2 over option 1. Review the procedure for administering this medication now if you had difficulty with this question!

Level of Cognitive Ability: Application
Phase of Nursing Process: Implementation
Client Needs: Safe, Effective Care Environment
Content Area: Adult Health/Cardiovascular

Reference

Kee, J., & Hayes, R. (1997). *Pharmacology: A nursing process approach* (2nd ed.). Philadelphia: W. B. Saunders, pp. 112–113.

---

57. A community health nurse visits the home of a 3-year-old with chickenpox. The child's mother says that the child keeps scratching at night. She asks the nurse what she should do. The nurse tells the mother that she should

1 Apply generous amounts of a cortisone cream to prevent itching.
2 Place white cloth gloves on the child's hands at night.
3 Keep the child in a warm room at night so the covers will not cause the child to scratch.
4 Give the child a glass of warm milk at bedtime to help the child sleep.

Answer: 2

Rationale: Cloth gloves will keep the child from scratching open lesions from chickenpox. Generous amounts of any topical cream can lead to drug toxicity. A warm room will increase the child's skin temperature and make itching worse. Warm milk will have no affect on itching.

Test-Taking Strategy: Eliminate option 3 first because this action will promote itching. Option 4 should be eliminated next because it is unrelated to itching. Of the remaining two options, the phrase "generous amounts" in option 1 should provide you with the clue that this option should be avoided. White gloves are recommended, because they are free of any dyes that may be found in colored gloves.

Level of Cognitive Ability: Application
Phase of Nursing Process: Planning
Client Needs: Safe, Effective Care Environment
Content Area: Child Health

Reference

Wong, D. (1995). *Whaley and Wong's Nursing care of infants and children* (5th ed.). St. Louis: Mosby–Year Book, p. 679.

---

58. An elderly client has been identified as a victim of physical abuse. In planning of care, priority is placed on

1 Obtaining treatment for the abusing family member.
2 Adhering to the mandatory abuse reporting laws.
3 Notifying the case worker to intervene in the family situation.
4 Removing the client from any immediate danger.

Answer: 4

Rationale: Whenever the abused client remains in the abusive environment, priority must be placed on ascertaining whether the client is in any immediate danger. If so, emergency action must be taken to remove the client from the abusive situation. Options 1, 2, and 3 may be appropriate interventions but are not the priority.

Test-Taking Strategy: Use Maslow's hierarchy of needs theory, remembering that if a physiological need is not present, then safety is the priority. This guide should direct you to option 4, the only option that directly addresses client safety!

Level of Cognitive Ability: Application
Phase of Nursing Process: Planning
Client Needs: Safe, Effective Care Environment
Content Area: Mental Health

Reference

Carson, V., & Arnold, E. (1996). *Mental health nursing: The nurse-patient journey.* Philadelphia: W. B. Saunders, p. 1070.

59. A male client diagnosed with catatonic stupor evidences severe withdrawal by lying on the bed, body pulled into a fetal position. The nurse plans to

1 Leave the client alone and intermittently check on him.
2 Take the client into the dayroom with other clients so they can help watch him.
3 Sit beside him in silence with occasional open-ended questions.
4 Ask direct questions to encourage talking.

Answer: 3

Rationale: Clients who are withdrawn may be immobile and mute and require consistent, repeated approaches. Intervention includes establishment of interpersonal contact. Communication with withdrawn clients requires much patience from the nurse. The nurse facilitates communication with the client by sitting in silence, asking open-ended questions, and pausing to provide opportunities for the client to respond.

Test-Taking Strategy: Eliminate option 1 because you would not leave the client alone because of the client's clinical condition. Option 2 relies on other clients to care for this client, and this is an inappropriate expectation. Asking direct questions of this client is not therapeutic. Option 3 is the best action because it provides for client supervision and communication as appropriate.

Level of Cognitive Ability: Application
Phase of Nursing Process: Planning
Client Needs: Safe, Effective Care Environment
Content Area: Mental Health

Reference

Haber, J. (1997). *Comprehensive psychiatric nursing* (5th ed.). St. Louis: Mosby–Year Book, pp. 582, 593.

60. A client diagnosed with leukemia asks the nurse questions about preparing a living will. The nurse informs the client that the initial step in preparing this document is to

1 Consult with the American Cancer Society.
2 Talk to the hospital chaplain.
3 Contact a lawyer.
4 Discuss the request with the physician.

Answer: 4

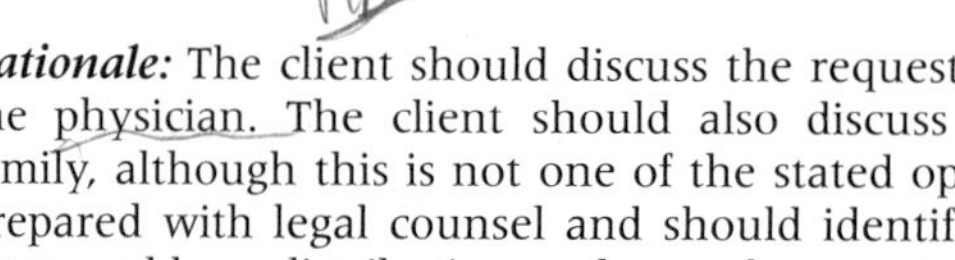

Rationale: The client should discuss the request for a living will with the physician. The client should also discuss this desire with the family, although this is not one of the stated options. Wills should be prepared with legal counsel and should identify the executor of the estate, address distribution and use of property, and specify plans for funeral arrangements. Although options 1 and 2 may be helpful, their contact would not be the initial step. The lawyer would be contacted after discussion with the physician and family.

Test-Taking Strategy: Use the process of elimination. Remembering that the physician is the primary care provider may assist in directing you to the correct option. Contacts addressed in options 1, 2, and 3 would follow the discussion with the physician.

Level of Cognitive Ability: Application
Phase of Nursing Process: Implementation
Client Needs: Safe, Effective Care Environment
Content Area: Fundamental Skills

Reference

Luckmann, J. (1997). *Saunders manual of nursing care.* Philadelphia: W. B. Saunders, p. 583.

61. The client recovering from cardiogenic shock is disoriented periodically. The most appropriate action to ensure safety for this client would be to

1 Raise the head of the bed to 45 degrees.
2 Keep side rails up at all times and call light within reach.
3 Keep the over-the-bed light on in the client's room.
4 Request only two visitors at a time.

Answer: 2

Rationale: Keeping the side rails up prevents a disoriented client from accidentally falling out of bed. Providing the call light to the client enables access to the health care team when assistance is needed. Raising the head of the bed will not ensure safety. Keeping the over-the-bed light on may be disruptive. Limiting visitors will not ensure safety.

Test-Taking Strategy: Focus on the issue of safety. Eliminate options 1 and 4 because these actions do not provide for safety for this client. Eliminate option 3 because this option may make the room more visible but leads to further disorientation with regard to time.

Level of Cognitive Ability: Application
Phase of Nursing Process: Implementation
Client Needs: Safe, Effective Care Environment
Content Area: Adult Health/Cardiovascular

Reference

Smith, S., & Duell, D. (1996). *Clinical nursing skills* (4th ed.). Stamford, CT: Appleton & Lange, p. 121.

---

62. The client with subarachnoid hemorrhage has been placed on subarachnoid (or aneurysm) precautions. The nurse ensures that the client is provided with which of the following?

1 Suction equipment
2 Bright lights
3 Television and radio
4 Enemas as needed

Answer: 1

Rationale: Subarachnoid (or aneurysm) precautions include a variety of measures designed to decrease stimuli that could increase the client's intracranial pressure. These include instituting dim lighting and reducing environmental noise and stimuli. Enemas should be avoided, but stool softeners should be provided. Straining at stool is contraindicated because it increases intracranial pressure. Suction equipment and oxygen should be available at the bedside.

Test-Taking Strategy: Use knowledge of concepts related to client safety and intracranial pressure to answer this question. Options 2 and 3 can be eliminated first because these items will stimulate the client. Eliminate option 4 because enemas will increase intracranial pressure. Considering the ABCs—airway, breathing, and circulation—will direct you to option 1.

Level of Cognitive Ability: Application
Phase of Nursing Process: Implementation
Client Needs: Safe, Effective Care Environment
Content Area: Adult Health/Neurological

Reference

Monahan, F., & Neighbors, M. (1998). *Medical-surgical nursing: Foundations for clinical practice* (2nd ed.). Philadelphia: W. B. Saunders, p. 816.

---

63. The nurse is about to give the client an intravenous dose of tobramycin (Tobrex) when the client complains to the nurse about feeling a ringing in the ears and vertigo. Which of the following is the safest action of the nurse?

1 Hang the dose immediately
2 Give a dose of droperidol (Inapsine) with this medication
3 Withhold the dose and call the physician
4 Check the client's pupillary responses

Answer: 3

Rationale: Ringing in the ears and vertigo are two symptoms that may indicate dysfunction of the eighth cranial nerve. Ototoxicity is a frequent side effect of therapy with the aminoglycosides and could result in permanent hearing loss. The nurse should withhold the dose and notify the physician.

Test-Taking Strategy: Note the key word in the question, which is "safest." Answer this question by recognizing that tobramycin is an aminoglycoside and that the nursing action is one that will keep the client from experiencing harm. Review the side effects of this medication now if you had difficulty with this question!

Level of Cognitive Ability: Application
Phase of Nursing Process: Implementation
Client Needs: Safe, Effective Care Environment
Content Area: Pharmacology

Reference

Deglin, J., & Vallerand, A. (1997). *Davis's drug guide for nurses* (5th ed.). Philadelphia: F. A. Davis, pp. 51, 53.

64. The nurse is preparing to administer amiodarone (Cordarone) intravenously. The nurse should ensure that which of the following is in use at this time?

1 Noninvasive blood pressure cuff
2 Oxygen saturation monitor
3 Oxygen therapy
4 Continuous cardiac monitoring

Answer: 4

Rationale: Amiodarone is a group III antidysrhythmic used to treat life-threatening ventricular dysrhythmias that do not respond to first-line agents. The client should have continuous cardiac monitoring in place, and the medication should be infused by intravenous pump.

Test-Taking Strategy: Knowledge that this medication is an antidysrhythmic will assist in directing you to option 4. In addition, the word "continuous" in this option should provide you with the clue that this is a correct option. If this question was difficult, take a few moments to review the classification of this medication!

Level of Cognitive Ability: Application
Phase of Nursing Process: Implementation
Client Needs: Safe, Effective Care Environment
Content Area: Pharmacology

Reference

Deglin, J., & Vallerand, A. (1997). *Davis's drug guide for nurses* (5th ed.). Philadelphia: F. A. Davis, pp. 56–58.

---

65. A client is admitted to the hospital for a bowel resection after a diagnosis of bowel tumor. During the admission assessment, the client tells the nurse that a living will was prepared 3 years ago. The client asks the nurse whether this document is still effective. The most appropriate nursing response is which of the following?

1 "Yes, it is."
2 "You will have to ask your lawyer."
3 "It should be reviewed yearly with your physician."
4 "I have no idea."

Answer: 3

Rationale: The client should discuss the living will with the physician, and it should be reviewed annually to ensure that it contains the client's current wishes and desires.

Test-Taking Strategy: Option 1 is clearly incorrect. Option 4 is not at all helpful to the client and is in fact a communication block. Although a lawyer would need to be consulted if the living will needed to be changed, the most appropriate and accurate nursing response would be to inform the client that the living will should be reviewed annually.

Level of Cognitive Ability: Application
Phase of Nursing Process: Implementation
Client Needs: Safe, Effective Care Environment
Content Area: Fundamental Skills

Reference

Luckmann, J. (1997). *Saunders manual of nursing care.* Philadelphia: W. B. Saunders, p. 584.

---

66. The home care nurse visits a client recently discharged from the hospital after an acute myocardial infarction. The client tells the nurse that a living will was prepared. The nurse would expect that a copy of the living will can be located in all of the following locations except

1 In the client's home.
2 In the physician's office.
3 In the medical record at the hospital.
4 In the hospital emergency room files.

Answer: 4

Rationale: Copies of a living will should be kept with the medical record, at the physician's office, and in the home of the client. A copy will also be maintained in the lawyer's office. The emergency room does not maintain these documents in its files.

Test-Taking Strategy: Note the key word "except." It seems reasonable that a physician would hold a copy of this document in the medical files. The client would certainly have a copy in the home because this document identifies the client's wishes. It also seems reasonable that a copy would be maintained in the client's medical record to provide guidance to care providers if during hospitalization a situation requiring referral to this document arose. It is not realistic for an emergency room to maintain such documents in its files.

Level of Cognitive Ability: Analysis
Phase of Nursing Process: Analysis
Client Needs: Safe, Effective Care Environment
Content Area: Fundamental Skills

Reference

Luckmann, J. (1997). *Saunders manual of nursing care.* Philadelphia: W. B. Saunders, p. 584.

67. A client with total parenteral nutrition (TPN) via a central intravenous (IV) line is scheduled to receive an antibiotic by the IV route. Which action by the nurse is appropriate before hanging the antibiotic solution?

1. Ensure a separate IV access for the antibiotic
2. Turn off the TPN for 30 minutes before administering the antibiotic
3. Check with the pharmacy to be sure the antibiotic can be hung through the TPN line
4. Flush the central line with 60 mL of normal saline before hanging the antibiotic

Answer: 1

Rationale: The TPN line is used only for administration of the TPN solution. Any other intravenous medication must be run though a separate IV access site.

Test-Taking Strategy: Some knowledge of TPN administration is needed. Options 2, 3, and 4 are similar in that they all involve using the TPN line for administration of the antibiotic.

Level of Cognitive Ability: Application
Phase of Nursing Process: Implementation
Client Needs: Safe, Effective Care Environment
Content Area: Fundamental Skills

Reference

Craven, R., & Hirnle, C. (1996). *Fundamentals of nursing: Human health and function* (2nd ed.). Philadelphia: Lippincott-Raven, p. 572.

68. The nurse is inserting an indwelling urinary catheter into the urethra of a male client. As the nurse inflates the balloon, the client complains of discomfort. The correct nursing action is to

1. Remove the syringe from the balloon, because discomfort is normal and temporary.
2. Aspirate the fluid, advance the catheter farther, and reinflate the balloon.
3. Aspirate the fluid, withdraw the catheter slightly, and reinflate the balloon.
4. Aspirate the fluid, remove the catheter, and reinsert a new catheter.

Answer: 2

Rationale: If the balloon is malpositioned in the urethra, inflating the balloon could produce trauma, and discomfort will occur. If this happens, the fluid should be aspirated and the catheter inserted a little farther in order to provide sufficient space to inflate the balloon. The catheter's balloon is behind the opening at the insertion tip. Inserting the catheter the extra distance will ensure that the balloon is inflated inside the bladder and not in the urethra. There is no need to remove the catheter and reinsert a new one. Pain when the balloon is inflated is not normal and will not go away.

Test-Taking Strategy: Knowledge of the proper procedure for inserting an indwelling urinary catheter is helpful in answering this question. Only option 2 will properly position the balloon in the bladder for safe balloon inflation. Option 1 is different from the other three options, but it can be eliminated because discomfort is neither normal nor temporary when caused by the balloon's being inflated when it is in the urethra. It is not necessary to withdraw the catheter and reinsert a new catheter.

Level of Cognitive Ability: Application
Phase of Nursing Process: Implementation
Client Needs: Safe, Effective Care Environment
Content Area: Fundamental Skills

Reference

Kozier, B., Erb, G., & Blais, K. (1998). *Fundamentals of nursing: Concepts, process, and practice* (5th ed.). Menlo Park, CA: Addison-Wesley, pp. 1256–1257.

69. The nurse is caring for a client immediately after a bronchoscopy. The client received light IV sedation and a topical anesthetic for the procedure. In order to provide a safe environment for this client at this time, it is most important that the nurse plan to

1 Place a padded tongue blade at the bedside in case of a seizure.
2 Check the bedside to ensure no food or fluid is within the client's reach to prevent aspiration.
3 Connect the client to a bedside electrocardiographic (ECG) monitor to detect dysrhythmias.
4 Place a water-seal chest drainage set at the bedside in case of a pneumothorax.

Answer: 2

Rationale: Nothing is given by mouth until the cough and swallow reflexes have returned, which is usually in 1–2 hours. Once the client can swallow, feeding may begin with ice chips and small sips of water. The client should be physically assessed for signs of respiratory distress, including dyspnea, changes in respiratory rate, use of accessory muscles, and changes in or absent lung sounds. Expectorated secretions are inspected for evidence of hemoptysis. Lung sounds are monitored for 24 hours. Development of asymmetrical or adventitious sounds should be reported to the physician. Pneumothorax has been noted after bronchoscopy.

Test-Taking Strategy: Look for key words in the stem of the question; note the phrase "immediately after a bronchoscopy." Other important points are that the client received IV sedation and topical anesthetic and that the nurse is planning a safe environment for this client. With this in mind, examine the options. There are no data in the question that suggest that the client is at increased risk for a seizure. A padded tongue blade would not be placed at the bedside routinely and it is not part of current practice to insert tongue blades into the mouth of a client experiencing a seizure. A pneumothorax could possibly occur, and the nurse should monitor the client for signs of distress; however, a water-seal chest drainage set would not be placed routinely at the bedside. No data are given to support that the client is at increased risk for cardiac dysrhythmias.

Level of Cognitive Ability: Application
Phase of Nursing Process: Planning
Client Needs: Safe, Effective Care Environment
Content Area: Adult Health/Respiratory

Reference

Black, J., & Matassarin-Jacobs, E. (1997). *Medical-surgical nursing: Clinical management for continuity of care* (5th ed.). Philadelphia: W. B. Saunders, pp. 1061–1062.

---

70. The client with a history of silicosis is admitted with respiratory distress and impending respiratory failure. The nurse would plan to have which of the following items readily available?

1 Chest tube and drainage system
2 Intubation tray
3 Thoracentesis tray
4 Code cart

Answer: 2

Rationale: The client with impending respiratory failure may need intubation and mechanical ventilation. The nurse ensures that an intubation tray is readily available. The other items are unnecessary.

Test-Taking Strategy: The key information in the stem is "impending respiratory failure." Knowing that the client could go into respiratory arrest, you eliminate options 1 and 3. You would choose the intubation tray over the code cart because if the client is intubated in time, the client will not experience respiratory arrest.

Level of Cognitive Ability: Application
Phase of Nursing Process: Planning
Client Needs: Safe, Effective Care Environment
Content Area: Adult Health/Respiratory

Reference

Ignatavicius, D. D., Workman, M. L., & Mishler, M. A. (1995). *Medical-surgical nursing: A nursing process approach* (2nd ed.). Philadelphia: W. B. Saunders, p. 725.

71. The client with acquired immunodeficiency syndrome (AIDS) who has cytomegalovirus- (CMV-) associated retinitis is receiving ganciclovir (Cytovene). The nurse would implement which of the following interventions in the care of this client?

1 Monitor blood glucose levels for elevation
2 Administer the medication only on an empty stomach
3 Tell the client to use a soft toothbrush and an electric razor
4 Apply pressure to venipuncture sites for 2 minutes

Answer: 3

Rationale: The most frequent side effects of ganciclovir are neutropenia and thrombocytopenia. For this reason, the nurse monitors the client for signs and symptoms of bleeding and implements the same precautions that are used for a client receiving anticoagulant therapy. Thus venipuncture sites should have pressure applied for approximately 10 minutes. The medication does not have to be taken on an empty stomach. The medication may cause hypoglycemia but not hyperglycemia.

Test-Taking Strategy: Eliminate option 4 first because this is a standard of care for any client and does not represent an individualized action based on this medication. The word "only" in option 2 makes it likely to be an incorrect choice, and thus it may be eliminated next. To discriminate correctly between options 1 and 3, it is necessary to understand that the medication can cause bleeding from thrombocytopenia. Review the nursing implications related to this medication now if you had difficulty with this question!

Level of Cognitive Ability: Application
Phase of Nursing Process: Implementation
Client Needs: Safe, Effective Care Environment
Content Area: Pharmacology

Reference

Deglin, J., & Vallerand, A. (1997). *Davis's drug guide for nurses* (5th ed.). Philadelphia: F. A. Davis, pp. 527–529.

72. The nurse is administering a first dose of pentamidine (Pentam 300) intravenously to a client. Before administering the first dose, the nurse should place the client

1 On respiratory precautions.
2 In a private room.
3 In a supine position.
4 In semi-Fowler's position.

Answer: 3

Rationale: Pentamidine can cause severe and sudden hypotension, even with administration of a single dose. The client should be lying down during administration of this medication. The blood pressure is monitored frequently during administration. Resuscitation equipment should be available for use in case it is needed.

Test-Taking Strategy: This question can be answered by using the knowledge that this medication is used to treat or prevent *Pneumocystis carinii* infection in the client who is HIV positive. With this in mind, options 1 and 2 are eliminated as unnecessary for this type of infection. Knowing that the medication causes hypotension helps you to choose option 3 over option 4. Review the nursing implications related to this medication now if you had difficulty with this question!

Level of Cognitive Ability: Application
Phase of Nursing Process: Implementation
Client Needs: Safe, Effective Care Environment
Content Area: Pharmacology

Reference

Hodgson, B., & Kizior, R. (1998). *Saunders nursing drug handbook 1998.* Philadelphia: W. B. Saunders, pp. 801–803.

73. The nurse is administering a dose of IV hydralazine (Apresoline) to a client. The nurse ensures that which of the following items is in place before injecting the medication?

1 Central line
2 Foley catheter
3 Cardiac monitor
4 Noninvasive blood pressure cuff

Answer: 4

Rationale: Hydralazine is an antihypertensive medication used in the management of moderate to severe hypertension. The blood pressure and pulse should be monitored frequently after administration, so a noninvasive blood pressure cuff is the item of choice to have in place.

Test-Taking Strategy: Knowledge of the intended effects of hydralazine is needed to answer this question correctly. The name of the medication "A*preso*line" may provide you with the clue that the medication is used to lower the blood pressure. If this question was difficult, take a few moments to review this medication now!

Level of Cognitive Ability: Application
Phase of Nursing Process: Implementation
Client Needs: Safe, Effective Care Environment
Content Area: Pharmacology

Reference

Hodgson, B., & Kizior, R. (1998). *Saunders nursing drug handbook 1998.* Philadelphia: W. B. Saunders, p. 493.

---

74. The client without history of respiratory disease has experienced sudden onset of chest pain and dyspnea, and pulmonary embolus is diagnosed. The nurse immediately implements which of the following therapeutic orders given for this client?

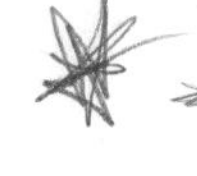

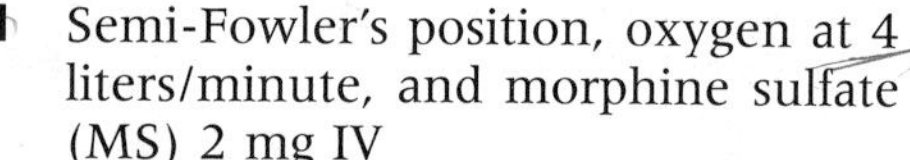

1 Semi-Fowler's position, oxygen at 4 liters/minute, and morphine sulfate (MS) 2 mg IV
2 Semi-Fowler's position, oxygen at 1 liter/minute, and meperidine (Demerol) 100 mg intramuscularly (IM)
3 High Fowler's position, oxygen at 4 liters/minute, and 2 tabs acetaminophen with codeine (Tylenol #3)
4 High Fowler's position, oxygen at 1 liter/minute, and MS 10 mg IV

Answer: 1

Rationale: Standard therapeutic intervention for the client with pulmonary embolus includes proper positioning, oxygen, and intravenous analgesics. The head of the bed is placed in semi-Fowler's position. High Fowler's is avoided because extreme hip flexure slows venous return from the legs and increases risk of new thrombi. The client without preexisting respiratory disorders can tolerate oxygen at levels exceeding 2–3 liters/minute. The usual analgesic of choice is MS administered IV. This medication reduces pain, alleviates anxiety, and can diminish congestion of blood in the pulmonary vessels because it also causes peripheral venous dilatation.

Test-Taking Strategy: The key phrase "without history of respiratory disease" should indicate that the client can tolerate a high oxygen flow. If you know that semi-Fowler's is the position of choice, the selection is limited to options 1 and 2. If you know that this client can tolerate 4 liters/minute oxygen, the selection is limited to options 1 and 3. If you know that the medication of choice is morphine sulfate, the selection is limited to options 1 and 4; from here you can proceed in either of two ways. Knowing that the dose of MS IV is 2 mg causes you to choose in favor of option 1. Option 1 is the only option that appears in all the groupings. In either case, option 1 is clearly the answer.

Level of Cognitive Ability: Application
Phase of Nursing Process: Implementation
Client Needs: Safe, Effective Care Environment
Content Area: Adult Health/Respiratory

Reference

Black, J., & Matassarin-Jacobs, E. (1997). *Medical-surgical nursing: Clinical management for continuity of care* (5th ed.). Philadelphia: W. B. Saunders, p. 1129.

---

75. The nurse is caring for the client who has undergone left pneumonectomy. The nurse plans to do which of the following immediately after transfer from the postanesthesia care unit?

1 Place the IV on a pump
2 Assist the client to sit in the bedside chair
3 Position the client to be supine
4 Position the client on the left side

Answer: 1

Rationale: After pneumonectomy, the fluid status of the client is monitored to prevent fluid overload, because the size of the pulmonary vascular bed has been reduced with lung resection. The client should be positioned on the right side to prevent shifting of the mediastinum, remaining lung, and heart. The head of bed should be elevated to promote lung expansion. The client should remain on bed rest in the immediate postoperative period.

Test-Taking Strategy: Begin to answer this question by eliminating options 3 and 4 first, because the client should not lie flat and should not lie on the affected side. Because the client should not be sitting in a chair immediately after a surgery such as this, you could choose option 1 by the process of elimination. Using another approach, if you know that a complication of this procedure is pulmonary edema from an easily induced fluid overload, you would immediately eliminate all of the other options in favor of putting the IV on a pump, which helps to avoid sudden infusion of fluid.

Level of Cognitive Ability: Application
Phase of Nursing Process: Planning
Client Needs: Safe, Effective Care Environment
Content Area: Adult Health/Respiratory

Reference

Black, J., & Matassarin-Jacobs, E. (1997). *Medical-surgical nursing: Clinical management for continuity of care* (5th ed.). Philadelphia: W. B. Saunders, pp. 1159, 1161.

---

76. The client being seen in the emergency room is being evaluated for possible pleurisy. The nurse is preparing the client for preliminary diagnostic testing. The nurse would plan to

1. Ask the client to remove a neck chain being worn.
2. Ask the client about the time of last food intake.
3. Scrub the chest with povidone-iodine (Betadine).
4. Determine whether the client has any metallic implants.

Answer: 1

Rationale: The client is initially evaluated with a chest x-ray, for which all jewelry or metal objects being worn are removed. The client does not need to have food or fluid restricted before chest x-ray, and no surface preparation is required. Subsequent diagnostic tests that may be ordered for pleurisy include sputum examination, thoracentesis, and pleural biopsy. Notation of metallic implants is required before MRI, but MRI is not used to diagnose pleurisy.

Test-Taking Strategy: To answer this question, you should recall that a common diagnostic test used to initially evaluate many lung conditions is the chest x-ray. With this in mind, you can eliminate each of the incorrect options systematically.

Level of Cognitive Ability: Application
Phase of Nursing Process: Planning
Client Needs: Safe, Effective Care Environment
Content Area: Adult Health/Respiratory

Reference

Smeltzer, S., & Bare, B. (1996). *Brunner and Suddarth's Textbook of medical-surgical nursing* (8th ed.). Philadelphia: Lippincott-Raven, p. 502.

---

77. The nurse has administered diazepam (Valium), 5 mg IV, to a client. The nurse should plan to maintain the client on bed rest for at least

1. Thirty minutes.
2. One hour.
3. Three hours.
4. Eight hours.

Answer: 3

Rationale: The client should remain in bed for at least 3 hours after a parenteral dose of diazepam. The medication is a centrally acting skeletal muscle relaxant and also has antianxiety, sedative-hypnotic, and anticonvulsant properties. Cardiopulmonary side effects of the drug include apnea, hypotension, bradycardia, and cardiac arrest. For this reason, resuscitative equipment is also kept nearby.

Test-Taking Strategy: Knowledge of the effects of diazepam administered intravenously would help you eliminate the 30- and 60-minute time frames as too brief. Eight hours, on the other hand, is excessive, which leaves the 3-hour time frame as the correct answer. This is a prudent choice. Review the nursing implications related to this medication now if you had difficulty with this question!

Level of Cognitive Ability: Application
Phase of Nursing Process: Planning
Client Needs: Safe, Effective Care Environment
Content Area: Pharmacology

Reference

Hodgson, B., & Kizior, R. (1998). *Saunders nursing drug handbook 1998.* Philadelphia: W. B. Saunders, pp. 307–309.

78. The client is having the dosage of clonazepam (Klonopin) adjusted. The nurse should plan to

1 Monitor blood glucose levels.
2 Institute seizure precautions.
3 Weigh the client daily.
4 Observe for ecchymoses.

Answer: 2

Rationale: Clonazepam is a benzodiazepine that is used as an anticonvulsant. During initial therapy and during periods of dosage adjustment, the nurse should initiate seizure precautions for the client.

Test-Taking Strategy: Because the medication is an anticonvulsant, the natural choice for the answer would be the seizure precautions. The key information in the stem that leads you to this is the information about the dosage being adjusted. This could put the client at risk for return of seizure activity and makes it the only reasonable choice, in view of the wording of the question. Review the nursing implications related to this medication now if you had difficulty with this question!

Level of Cognitive Ability: Application
Phase of Nursing Process: Planning
Client Needs: Safe, Effective Care Environment
Content Area: Pharmacology

Reference

Hodgson, B., & Kizior, R. (1998). *Saunders nursing drug handbook 1998.* Philadelphia: W. B. Saunders, pp. 238–240.

79. A client who recently experienced myocardial infarction is scheduled to undergo percutaneous transluminal coronary angioplasty (PTCA). The nurse would plan to teach the client that during this procedure, a balloon-tipped catheter will

1 Cut away the plaque from the coronary vessel wall with the use of a cutting blade.
2 Be used to compress the plaque against the coronary blood vessel wall.
3 Inflate a mesh-like device that will spring open and keep the plaque against the coronary vessel wall.
4 Be positioned in a coronary artery to take pressure measurements in the vessel.

Answer: 2

Rationale: Option 1 describes coronary atherectomy; option 2 describes PTCA; option 3 describes placement of a coronary stent; option 4 describes part of the process used in cardiac catheterization.

Test-Taking Strategy: This question involves definitions of procedures. If necessary, look at the name of the procedure, and break it down into its component parts. "Angioplasty" refers to repair of a blood vessel, which should help narrow your choices to options 1 and 2. Usually a procedure that cuts something away would have the suffix "-ectomy," which leaves you with the correct answer, which is 2.

Level of Cognitive Ability: Application
Phase of Nursing Process: Planning
Client Needs: Safe, Effective Care Environment
Content Area: Adult Health/Cardiovascular

Reference

Ignatavicius, D. D., Workman, M. L., & Mishler, M. A. (1995). *Medical-surgical nursing: A nursing process approach* (2nd ed.). Philadelphia: W. B. Saunders, p. 1002.

80. A client is being discharged from the hospital after an occurrence of hyperglycemic hyperosmolar nonketotic (HHNK) syndrome. The nurse should be sure that the client knows

1 Not to exercise for 2–3 days.
2 Signs and symptoms of dehydration.
3 To keep follow-up appointments.
4 How to control diet.

Answer: 2

Rationale: Clients with propensity for HHNK syndrome should immediately report signs and symptoms of dehydration to health care providers. Dehydration is usually severe and may progress rapidly.

Test-Taking Strategy: Knowledge regarding the factors that indicate the development of HHNK syndrome and the ability to prioritize are necessary to answer the question. Option 1 can be easily eliminated because of the importance of exercise. Options 3 and 4 are important; however, in view of Maslow's hierarchy of needs theory, option 2 identifies the physiological need.

Level of Cognitive Ability: Application
Phase of Nursing Process: Planning
Client Needs: Safe, Effective Care Environment
Content Area: Adult Health/Endocrine

Reference

Burrell, L., Gerlach, M., & Pless, B. (1997). *Adult nursing: Acute and community care* (2nd ed.). Stamford, CT: Appleton & Lange, pp. 1166–1168.

81. The client has been placed in Buck's extension traction. The nurse can provide for countertraction to reduce shear and friction by

1 Slightly elevating the head of the bed.
2 Slightly elevating the foot of the bed.
3 Providing an overhead trapeze.
4 Using a footboard.

Answer: 2

Rationale: The part of the bed under an area in traction is usually elevated to aid in countertraction. For the client in Buck's extension traction (which is applied to a leg), the foot of the bed is elevated.

Test-Taking Strategy: To answer this question accurately, you need to understand the principles of traction and countertraction and to be familiar with Buck's extension traction. Option 3 is not used for the purpose of countertraction and is thus eliminated as a possible answer. Knowing that Buck's extension traction is applied to the leg helps you eliminate option 1. Of the two remaining choices, option 4 places undue pressure on the client's unaffected foot. Furthermore, a footboard is not used for the purpose of providing countertraction. Option 2 provides a force that opposes the traction force effectively without harming the client and is thus the answer to the question.

Level of Cognitive Ability: Application
Phase of Nursing Process: Implementation
Client Needs: Safe, Effective Care Environment
Content Area: Adult Health/Musculoskeletal

Reference

Black, J., & Matassarin-Jacobs, E. (1997). *Medical-surgical nursing: Clinical management for continuity of care* (5th ed.). Philadelphia: W. B. Saunders, p. 2137.

82. The nurse has inserted a nasogastric tube (NGT) to the level of the oropharynx and has repositioned the client's head in a flexed-forward position. The client has been asked to begin dry swallowing. The nurse starts to slowly advance the nasogastric tube with each swallow. The client begins to cough, gag, and choke. Which of the following nursing actions would be the least likely to result in proper tube insertion and promote client relaxation?

1 Continue to advance the tube to the desired distance
2 Pull the tube back slightly
3 Check the back of the pharynx, using a tongue blade and a flashlight
4 Instruct the client to breathe slowly and take sips of water (if not contraindicated by physician's order)

Answer: 1

Rationale: Two nursing actions during nasogastric tube insertion are (1) helping the client relax to reduce the gag response and (2) assessing for proper tube insertion and making corrections as needed. The flexed position of the head closes off the upper airway to the trachea and opens the esophagus. Swallowing closes the epiglottis over the trachea and helps move the tube into the esophagus. Swallowing water eases gagging. Because the tube may enter the larynx and obstruct the airway, pulling the tube back slightly will remove it from the larynx; advancing the tube might position it in the trachea. The tube may coil around itself in the back of the throat, stimulating the gag reflex. Slow breathing helps the client relax, to reduce the gag response. The tube may be advanced after the client relaxes.

Test-Taking Strategy: This question asks to identify the nursing action that would be least likely to result in proper tube insertion and promote client relaxation. Options 2, 3, and 4 all aim at assessing and promoting relaxation, whereas option 1 could result in an unsafe malposition of the nasogastric tube into the trachea. The tube may be advanced to the desired distance after the client relaxes. Review this procedure now if you had difficulty with this question!

Level of Cognitive Ability: Application
Phase of Nursing Process: Implementation
Client Needs: Safe, Effective Care Environment
Content Area: Adult Health/Gastrointestinal

Reference

Potter, P., & Perry, A. (1997). *Fundamentals of nursing: Concepts, process, and practice* (4th ed.). St. Louis: Mosby–Year Book, p. 1406.

83. The nurse is planning to obtain an arterial blood gas (ABG) measurement from a client with chronic obstructive pulmonary disease (COPD). The nurse will need to plan time for which activity after the radial arterial stick is complete?

1 Holding a warm compress over the site for 5 minutes
2 Applying pressure to the site by applying 2 × 2 inch gauze over the site for 5 minutes
3 Encouraging the client to open and close the hand rapidly for 2 minutes
4 Having the client keep the radial pulse puncture site in a dependent position for 5 minutes

Answer: 2

Rationale: Applying pressure over the site reduces the risk of hematoma formation and damage to the artery. A cold compress would aid in limiting blood flow. Keeping the extremity still and out of a dependent position will aid in the formation of a clot at the puncture site.

Test-Taking Strategy: Use the process of elimination in answering this question. Preventing bleeding is the issue of the question. Options 1, 3, and 4 would promote bleeding. Option 2 would aid in the prevention of bleeding into the surrounding tissues. Review nursing responsibilities after ABG measurements now if you had difficulty with this question!

Level of Cognitive Ability: Application
Phase of Nursing Process: Planning
Client Needs: Safe, Effective Care Environment
Content Area: Adult Health/Respiratory

Reference

Potter, P., & Perry, A. (1997). *Fundamentals of nursing: Concepts, process, and practice* (4th ed.). St. Louis: Mosby–Year Book, p. 1289.

---

84. The nurse is planning care for the client with heart failure. The nurse would ask the dietary department to remove which item from all meal trays before delivering them to the client?

1 Salt packets
2 1% milk cartons
3 Light margarine
4 Decaffeinated tea

Answer: 1

Rationale: The client with heart failure typically has some degree of sodium restriction in the diet to reduce sodium and water retention and improve cardiac efficiency.

Test-Taking Strategy: A standard dietary modification for the client with heart failure is sodium restriction. Options 2 and 3 are modifications of cholesterol. Option 4 refers to caffeine restriction. Whereas all the incorrect responses may be helpful in any cardiac condition, only option 1 deals with sodium restriction.

Level of Cognitive Ability: Application
Phase of Nursing Process: Planning
Client Needs: Safe, Effective Care Environment
Content Area: Adult Health/Cardiovascular

Reference

Black, J., & Matassarin-Jacobs, E. (1997). *Medical-surgical nursing: Clinical management for continuity of care* (5th ed.). Philadelphia: W. B. Saunders, p. 1286.

85. The nurse recognizes that special safety precautions are needed when caring for an infant with spina bifida (meningomyelocele type). The gibbus (sac on the back containing cerebrospinal fluid, the meninges, and the spinal cord) has been surgically removed. Which of the following types of care would the nurse plan for in the postoperative period to maintain the infant's safety?

1 Elevate the head with the infant in the prone position
2 Cover the back dressing with a binder
3 Place the infant in a head-down position
4 Strap the infant in an infant seat sitting up

Answer: 1

Rationale: Elevating the head will decrease the chance that cerebrospinal fluid will collect in the cranial cavity. The fluid amount will take several weeks to decrease in volume after the gibbus reservoir is removed. The infant needs to be in a prone position for several days to decrease pressure on the surgical site on the back. Binders and a baby seat should not be used because of the pressure they would exert on the surgical site.

Test-Taking Strategy: Preventing pressure on the back surgical site and preventing intracranial cerebrospinal fluid collection are the main foci for the postoperative period. Use the process of elimination to answer the question. Option 1 is the only correct answer. Option 2 and 4 would increase pressure on the surgical site, and option 3 would not promote a drainage of cerebrospinal fluid from the cranial cavity. Review postoperative nursing care now if you had difficulty with this question!

Level of Cognitive Ability: Application
Phase of Nursing Process: Planning
Client Needs: Safe, Effective Care Environment
Content Area: Child Health

Reference

Wong, D., & Whaley, L. (1996). *Clinical manual of pediatric nursing* (4th ed.). St. Louis: Mosby–Year Book, pp. 469–470.

86. The nurse is administering iron dextran (InFed) to the client intravenously. The nurse checks that which of the following medications is available for use if needed as an antidote to iron?

1 Deferoxamine (Desferal)
2 Dirithromycin (Dynabac)
3 Ferrous fumarate (Feostat)
4 Ferrous sulfate (Slow Fe)

Answer: 1

Rationale: The antidote to iron dextran is deferoxamine, which is a heavy metal antagonist. This medication chelates unbound iron in the circulation and forms a water-soluble complex that can be eliminated by the kidneys. Dirithromycin is a macrolide anti-infective. Ferrous sulfate and ferrous fumarate are forms of iron supplements.

Test-Taking Strategy: Specific medication knowledge is needed to answer this question accurately. Memorize the antidote now. If this question was difficult, take a few moments to review this medication!

Level of Cognitive Ability: Application
Phase of Nursing Process: Implementation
Client Needs: Safe, Effective Care Environment
Content Area: Pharmacology

Reference

Deglin, J., & Vallerand, A. (1997). *Davis's drug guide for nurses* (5th ed.). Philadelphia: F. A. Davis, pp. 333, 388, 658.

87. The client with pulmonary edema has oxygen via nasal cannula at 6 liters/minute. Blood gas results indicate that the pH is 7.29, arterial carbon dioxide tension (PCO_2) is 49 mmHg, arterial oxygen tension (PO_2) is 58 mmHg, and bicarbonate (HCO_3^-) is 18 mEq/liter. The nurse anticipates which order for respiratory support?

1 Lowering the oxygen to 4 liters/minute via nasal cannula
2 Keeping the oxygen at 6 liters/minute via nasal cannula
3 Adding a partial rebreather mask to the current order
4 Intubation and mechanical ventilation

Answer: 4

Rationale: If respiratory failure occurs, endotracheal intubation and mechanical ventilation are necessary. The client is exhibiting respiratory acidosis, metabolical acidosis, and persistent hypoxemia.

Test-Taking Strategy: Knowledge of interpretation of blood gases is necessary to answer this question. Review these now if needed. However, just knowing that the oxygen level is low would help you to eliminate options 1 and 2. Knowing that the PCO_2 is high would eliminate option 3, as a partial rebreather mask will raise CO_2 levels even further. Thus option 4 is correct.

Level of Cognitive Ability: Analysis
Phase of Nursing Process: Analysis
Client Needs: Safe, Effective Care Environment
Content Area: Adult Health/Respiratory

Reference

Jaffe, M., & McVan, B. (1997). *Davis's laboratory and diagnostic test handbook.* Philadelphia: F. A. Davis, pp. 195–196.

88. Two nurses are on the pediatric unit discussing client care. One nurse is caring for three children who are receiving chemotherapy. The second nurse is about to discharge two infants who need their immunizations before they are discharged. Which immunization should the nurse not give to the two infants?

1 HBV (hepatitis B virus vaccine)
2 DPT (diphtheria, tetanus, pertussis)
3 HIB (*Haemophilus influenzae* type b)
4 OPV (oral poliovirus vaccine)

Answer: 4

Rationale: Chemotherapeutic medications cause immunosuppression. Immunosuppressed children cannot be exposed to live viruses as they can cause a serious illness for the immunosuppressed child.

Test-Taking Strategy: Do not read into this question. Knowledge of immunizations and the type of vaccines available is necessary for this question. You need to know that a child receiving chemotherapy is immunosuppressed and cannot be in an environment where someone has received a live or attenuated vaccine. By the process of elimination, the only correct option is option 4!

Level of Cognitive Ability: Application
Phase of Nursing Process: Planning
Client Needs: Safe, Effective Care Environment
Content Area: Child Health

Reference

Wong, D. (1995). *Whaley and Wong's Nursing care of infants and children* (5th ed.). St. Louis: Mosby–Year Book, pp. 549, 550, 551, 1627.

89. The nurse is planning to teach the elderly diabetic client about self-management of the disease. The nurse should focus on which of the following items to enhance client safety during the process?

1 Use of videotapes to show insulin administration to ensure competence
2 Ability of the client to read label markings on syringes and on blood glucose–monitoring equipment
3 Developing structured menus for adherence to diet
4 Encouraging dependence to prepare the client for the chronicity of the disease

Answer: 2

Rationale: Adults are "hands-on" learners, which eliminates option 1. The question asks for a safety-related focus, which is exemplified in option 2. Flexibility in the diet regimen improves compliance, making option 3 incorrect. Self-care is encouraged as appropriate, making option 4 incorrect.

Test-Taking Strategy: Use the process of elimination. Note also that the stem contains the key word "safety." Option 2 most closely correlates with promoting safety in diabetic self-management.

Level of Cognitive Ability: Application
Phase of Nursing Process: Planning
Client Needs: Safe, Effective Care Environment
Content Area: Adult Health/Endocrine

Reference

Ignatavicius, D. D., Workman, M. L., & Mishler, M. A. (1995). *Medical-surgical nursing: A nursing process approach* (2nd ed.). Philadelphia: W. B. Saunders, p. 1888.

90. The client with an arteriovenous (AV) shunt in place for hemodialysis is at risk for bleeding. The nurse would do which of the following as a priority action to prevent this complication from occurring?

1 Check the results of partial thromboplastin time (PTT) tests as they are ordered
2 Observe the site once per shift
3 Check the shunt for presence of bruit and thrill
4 Ensure that small clamps are attached to the AV shunt dressing

Answer: 4

Rationale: An AV shunt is a less common form of access site, and it carries a risk for bleeding when it is used. This is because two ends of a cannula are tunneled subcutaneously into an artery and a vein, and the ends of the cannula are joined. If accidental disconnection occurs, the client could lose blood rapidly. For this reason, small clamps are attached to the dressing that covers the insertion site for use if needed. The shunt site should also be observed at least every 4 hours.

Test-Taking Strategy: Begin to answer this question by eliminating option 1, which is an assessment, not an action. Option 3, as worded, addresses patency, not bleeding, and is therefore incorrect. The frequency of observation in option 2 is substandard and is eliminated. This leaves option 4, which is completely correct.

Level of Cognitive Ability: Application
Phase of Nursing Process: Implementation
Client Needs: Safe, Effective Care Environment
Content Area: Adult Health/Renal

Reference

Ignatavicius, D. D., Workman, M. L., & Mishler, M. A. (1995). *Medical-surgical nursing: A nursing process approach* (2nd ed.). Philadelphia: W. B. Saunders, pp. 2136–2137.

91. The client is due in hydrotherapy for a burn dressing change. To ensure that the procedure is most tolerable for the client, the nurse should take which of the following actions?

1 Send dressing supplies with the client to hydrotherapy
2 Ensure that the client has a robe and slippers
3 Administer an analgesic 20 minutes before therapy
4 Administer intravenous antibiotic 30 minutes before therapy

Answer: 3

Rationale: The client should receive pain medication approximately 20 minutes before a burn dressing change. This will help the client to tolerate an otherwise painful procedure. Antibiotics are timed evenly around the clock and not necessarily in relation to timing of burn dressing changes. Dressing supplies are generally available in the hydrotherapy area and do not need to be sent with the client. A robe and slippers are beneficial for the client's comfort if traveling by wheelchair, but pain medication is more essential.

Test-Taking Strategy: Use Maslow's hierarchy of needs theory to answer this question. Note the key phrase in the stem, which is "most tolerable." This guides you to select pain relief measures as the highest priority of the available options.

Level of Cognitive Ability: Application
Phase of Nursing Process: Implementation
Client Needs: Safe, Effective Care Environment
Content Area: Adult Health/Integumentary

Reference

Smeltzer, S., & Bare, B. (1996). *Brunner and Suddarth's Textbook of medical-surgical nursing* (8th ed.). Philadelphia: Lippincott-Raven, p. 1565.

92. The client with heart failure has a magnesium level of 1.5 mg/dL. The nurse should

1 Encourage increased intake of phosphate antacids.
2 Monitor the client for dysrhythmias.
3 Administer ordered magnesium in normal saline.
4 Encourage the client to eat foods such as ground beef, eggs, and chicken breast.

Answer: 2

Rationale: Phosphate use should be limited in the presence of hypomagnesemia because it worsens the state. The client should be monitored for dysrhythmias, because the client is predisposed especially to ventricular dysrhythmias. Magnesium sulfate is not given in saline solutions. Ground beef, eggs, and chicken breast are examples of foods that are low in magnesium.

Test-Taking Strategy: To answer this question accurately, it is necessary to have a basic understanding of this electrolyte value, the implications of abnormalities, and its treatment measures. From this point, use the process of elimination. If this question was difficult, take a few moments to review this electrolyte disorder and its treatment now!

Level of Cognitive Ability: Application
Phase of Nursing Process: Implementation
Client Needs: Safe, Effective Care Environment
Content Area: Fundamental Skills

Reference

Black, J., & Matassarin-Jacobs, E. (1997). *Medical-surgical nursing: Clinical management for continuity of care* (5th ed.). Philadelphia: W. B. Saunders, p. 324.

---

93. The nurse is admitting to the nursing unit for hemodialysis a client who has an arteriovenous (AV) fistula in the right arm. The nurse would best plan to prevent injury to the site by

1 Putting a large note about the access site on the front of the medical record.
2 Applying an allergy bracelet to the right arm, indicating the presence of the fistula.
3 Placing a sign at the bedside: "No BP [blood pressure] measurements or venipunctures in the right arm."
4 Telling the client to inform all caregivers who enter the room about the presence of the access site.

Answer: 3

Rationale: There should be no venipunctures or blood pressure measurements in the limb with a hemodialysis access device. This is commonly communicated to all caregivers by placing a sign at the bedside. As part of routine client teaching, the client is also taught to tell future caregivers to avoid venipuncture and BP measurements in the limb. However, the wording of option 4 is excessive; it is not necessary to inform everyone entering the room about the access site. Options 1 and 2 are not part of standard practice.

Test-Taking Strategy: Note that the question asks for the "best" plan on the part of the nurse. This requires you to prioritize your answer. Knowing that options 1 and 2 are the least optimal guides you to eliminate them first. Knowing that option 3 is the most prudent allows you to choose this over option 4. You could also determine that option 4 is not the optimal answer by realizing the responsibility that this would place on an acutely ill client, who could forget or have some degree of cognitive impairment.

Level of Cognitive Ability: Application
Phase of Nursing Process: Planning
Client Needs: Safe, Effective Care Environment
Content Area: Adult Health/Renal

Reference

Black, J., & Matassarin-Jacobs, E. (1997). *Medical-surgical nursing: Clinical management for continuity of care* (5th ed.). Philadelphia: W. B. Saunders, p. 1659.

---

94. When preparing a client for a parathyroidectomy, it would be essential for the nurse to prepare for which of the following anticipated postoperative orders?

1 Place in a flat position with the head and neck immobilized
2 Take a rectal temperature until the client is discharged
3 Maintain endotracheal tube (ETT) for 24 hours
4 Administer continuous misting of room air or oxygen

Answer: 4

Rationale: Humidification of air oxygen helps to liquefy mucus secretions and promotes easier breathing. Pooling of thick mucus secretions in the trachea, bronchi, and lungs will cause respiratory obstruction. The results could be atelectasis and pneumonia.

Test-Taking Strategy: Remember your ABCs (Airway, Breathing, Circulation) when answering this question. A patent airway is most important; therefore, the client must be instructed in measures to keep secretions liquefied. The position of choice after a parathyroidectomy is semi-Fowler's; this assists in lung expansion, and thus option 1 is incorrect. Option 2 is incorrect because tympanic temperatures may be taken instead. Option 3 must also be eliminated because an endotracheal tube must be kept at the bedside. A client usually does not have one present for 24 hours.

Level of Cognitive Ability: Application
Phase of Nursing Process: Planning
Client Needs: Safe, Effective Care Environment
Content Area: Adult Health/Endocrine

Reference

Ignatavicius, D. D., Workman, M. L., & Mishler, M. A. (1995). *Medical-surgical nursing: A nursing process approach* (2nd ed.). Philadelphia: W. B. Saunders, p. 1853.

95. In developing a nursing care plan for a client with hyperglycemia as evidenced by a serum glucose reading of 700 mg/dL, the nurse plans for the IV insulin to be

1 Infused via an electronic infusion pump.
2 Mixed in a solution of 5% dextrose in water.
3 Changed every 6 hours.
4 Titrated according to the client's urine glucose levels.

Answer: 1

Rationale: Insulin is given via an infusion pump to prevent inadvertent overdose and subsequent hypoglycemia. Dextrose is added to the IV once the serum glucose reaches 250 mg/dL, to prevent rebound hypoglycemia. Administering glucose to a client with a serum glucose of 700 would counteract the beneficial effects of insulin in reducing the glucose level. Glycosuria is not a reliable indicator of actual serum glucose levels, since there are many factors that affect the renal threshold for glucose loss in the urine.

Test-Taking Strategy: Be alert to safety needs of the client. This client will be receiving insulin intravenously, which has the potential of causing severe hypoglycemia if too much is infused. Therefore, an electronic infusion pump is mandatory. Eliminate the three incorrect distracters by process of elimination. You would not want to give a client additional glucose when serum levels are already extremely elevated. There is no rationale for changing an IV solution every 6 hours. Urine glucose readings are not accurate enough to guide titration of treatment.

Level of Cognitive Ability: Application
Phase of Nursing Process: Planning
Client Needs: Safe, Effective Care Environment
Content Area: Adult Health/Endocrine

Reference

Polaski, A., & Tatro, S. (1996). *Luckmann's Core principles and practice of medical-surgical nursing.* Philadelphia: W. B. Saunders, p. 1192.

96. In planning care for a client with acute diabetic ketoacidosis (DKA), the nurse knows that it is important to

1 Maintain side rails in the upright position at all times.
2 Ambulate the client every 2 hours.
3 Assess for fluid overload.
4 Limit family visitation.

Answer: 1

Rationale: A client's sensorium may be diminished secondary to acidosis. Safety becomes a priority for any client with a decreased level of consciousness (LOC), thus mandating the use of side rails to prevent fall injuries. The client may be too ill to ambulate and will demonstrate fluid loss rather than overload. Family visitation is helpful for both client and family to help with psychosocial adaptation.

Test-Taking Strategy: Eliminate options 2 and 4 first. For the remaining two options, recalling that dehydration is an issue in DKA and that mental status changes occur will direct you to option 1 as the measure that will meet the need for safety in this client!

Level of Cognitive Ability: Application
Phase of Nursing Process: Planning
Client Needs: Safe, Effective Care Environment
Content Area: Adult Health/Endocrine

Reference

Lewis, S., Collier, I., & Heitkemper, M. (1996). *Medical-surgical nursing: Assessment and management of clinical problems* (4th ed.). St. Louis: Mosby–Year Book, pp. 1076, 1085, 1465.

97. Which of the following nursing interventions would not be appropriate when planning care for a client with severe hyperglycemic hyperosmolar nonketotic (HHNK) syndrome?

1 Cardiac monitoring
2 Hourly intake and output
3 Frequent oral fluids
4 Maintenance of side rails in up position

Answer: 3

Rationale: A client with severe
demonstrate neurological impai
would subject the client to potent
because the client is at risk for
lemia. Option 2 is appropriate be
imbalance. Option 4 is appropriate
injury secondary to confusion.

Test-Taking Strategy: The key word "not" in the stem of the question tells the reader that the answer must be a false statement. Also note the descriptor "severe" in regard to the diagnosis of HHNK syndrome. This alerts you to recall that decreased level of consciousness is present in the client with HHNK syndrome and directs you to option 3.

Level of Cognitive Ability: Application
Phase of Nursing Process: Planning
Client Needs: Safe, Effective Care Environment
Content Area: Adult Health/Endocrine

Reference

Lewis, S., Collier, I., & Heitkemper, M. (1996). *Medical-surgical nursing: Assessment and management of clinical problems* (4th ed.). St. Louis: Mosby–Year Book, p. 1466.

---

98. The client asks the nurse to demonstrate how to administer insulin. The order is for Regular Insulin, 10 units, and NPH Insulin, 30 units, every morning. The nurse will instruct the client to

1 Draw up each insulin in a separate syringe.
2 Draw up the Regular Insulin and then the NPH Insulin in the same syringe.
3 Draw up the NPH Insulin and then the Regular Insulin in the same syringe.
4 Demonstrate technique.

Answer: 2

Rationale: Regular Insulin is clear, whereas other insulin preparations are cloudy (with sediments). It is recommended that the clear formulation (Regular Insulin) be drawn up first, followed by the cloudy formulation (NPH Insulin). When Regular and NPH Insulation are to be administered, they are not drawn into separate syringes. It is not appropriate to ask the client to demonstrate technique at this time. The client is seeking information, which the nurse needs to provide. Option 4 may cause anxiety in the client.

Test-Taking Strategy: When administering Regular and NPH Insulin, remember "RN": Regular Insulin is drawn before NPH. Review this procedure now if you had difficulty with this question!

Level of Cognitive Ability: Application
Phase of Nursing Process: Implementation
Client Needs: Safe, Effective Care Environment
Content Area: Adult Health/Endocrine

Reference

Burrell, L., Gerlach, M., & Pless, B. (1997). *Adult nursing: Acute and community care* (2nd ed.). Stamford, CT: Appleton & Lange, p. 1160.

---

99. The client with carbon monoxide poisoning is to receive hyperbaric oxygen therapy. Which of the following nursing interventions is the priority during the procedure?

1 Assessing that oxygen is being delivered
2 Maintenance of intravenous access
3 Administration of sedation to prevent claustrophobia
4 Checking that the pressure seal on the chamber is intact

Answer: 1

Rationale: Hyperbaric oxygen therapy is a process by which 100% oxygen is administered at greater than normal pressure. In carbon monoxide poisoning, this therapy causes an increase in alveolar oxygen pressure and forces the carbon monoxide, attached to the hemoglobin, to be replaced by oxygen. Because the client is placed in a closed chamber, the administration of oxygen is of primary importance.

Test-Taking Strategy: Using the ABCs—airway, breathing, and circulation—you can establish breathing as the highest priority option. Note the phrase "hyperbaric oxygen therapy" in the question. This should direct you to the correct option!

Level of Cognitive Ability: Application
Phase of Nursing Process: Implementation
Client Needs: Safe, Effective Care Environment
Content Area: Adult Health/Respiratory

Reference

Luckmann, J. (1997). *Saunders manual of nursing care*. Philadelphia: W. B. Saunders, p. 221.

100. The nurse has an order to place the client, who is on bed rest with herniated lumbar intervertebral disk, in Williams position to minimize the pain. The nurse plans to put the bed

1. In high Fowler's position with the foot of bed flat.
2. In semi-Fowler's position with the knee gatch slightly raised.
3. In semi-Fowler's position with the foot of bed flat.
4. Flat with the knee gatch raised.

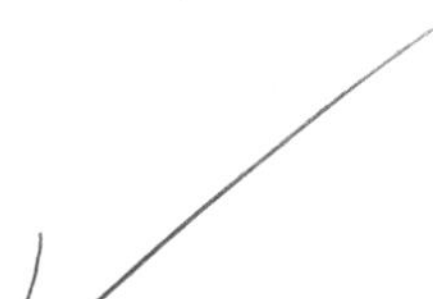

Answer: 2

Rationale: Clients with low back pain are often more comfortable when placed in Williams position. The bed is placed in semi-Fowler's position with the knee gatch raised sufficiently to flex the knees. This relaxes the muscles of the lower back and relieves pressure on the spinal nerve root.

Test-Taking Strategy: Knowledge of this specific position helps you to answer this question quickly and easily. If you are not familiar with it, however, look at the information in the stem. The client has back pain with a ruptured intervertebral disk. Keeping the foot of the bed flat will enhance extension of the spine, so options 1 and 3 should be eliminated first. Option 4 would excessively stretch the lower back and would also put the client at risk for thrombophlebitis. By the process of elimination, the correct answer is option 2.

Level of Cognitive Ability: Application
Phase of Nursing Process: Planning
Client Needs: Safe, Effective Care Environment
Content Area: Adult Health/Neurological

Reference

Ignatavicius, D. D., Workman, M. L., & Mishler, M. A. (1995). *Medical-surgical nursing: A nursing process approach* (2nd ed.). Philadelphia: W. B. Saunders, p. 1172.

---

101. The nurse is scheduling a client for diagnostic studies of the gastrointestinal (GI) system. Which of the following studies, if ordered, should the nurse schedule last?

1. Abdominal scan
2. Ultrasonography
3. Colonoscopy
4. Barium enema study

Answer: 4

Rationale: Barium is instilled into the lower GI tract during a barium enema study and may take up to 72 hours to clear the GI tract. The presence of barium could cause interference with obtaining clear visualization and accurate results of the other tests listed, if those are performed before the client has fully excreted the barium. For this reason, diagnostic studies that involve barium contrast are scheduled at the conclusion of other diagnostic studies.

Test-Taking Strategy: Note the key word in the question is "last." Recalling that barium shows up on x-ray as opaque, you could reason that this substance would impair visualization during other tests. With this in mind, you could easily eliminate each of the other incorrect options.

Level of Cognitive Ability: Application
Phase of Nursing Process: Planning
Client Needs: Safe, Effective Care Environment
Content Area: Adult Health/Gastrointestinal

Reference

Black, J., & Matassarin-Jacobs, E. (1997). *Medical-surgical nursing: Clinical management for continuity of care* (5th ed.). Philadelphia: W. B. Saunders, p. 1714.

---

102. The client has an order for a stool culture. The nurse avoids doing which of the following when carrying out this order?

1. Wearing sterile gloves
2. Using a sterile container
3. Refrigerating the specimen
4. Sending the specimen directly to the laboratory

Answer: 3

Rationale: Storing a stool specimen in a refrigerator is contraindicated because it can retard the growth of organisms. A stool specimen is obtained with the use of sterile gloves and a sterile container. After the specimen is obtained, the stool is sent immediately to the laboratory.

Test-Taking Strategy: Note the key word in the question, which is "avoids." This indicates that the correct answer will be a wrong action on the part of the nurse. Knowledge that a culture is done to identify organisms will assist you in realizing that options 1, 2, and 4 must be carried out to ensure accuracy of results.

Level of Cognitive Ability: Application
Phase of Nursing Process: Implementation
Client Needs: Safe, Effective Care Environment
Content Area: Adult Health/Gastrointestinal

Reference
Black, J., & Matassarin-Jacobs, E. (1997). *Medical-surgical nursing: Clinical management for continuity of care* (5th ed.). Philadelphia: W. B. Saunders, p. 1712.

---

103. The nurse is caring for a client who is scheduled to undergo a liver biopsy. Before this procedure, it is most important for the nurse to assess the client's

1 History of nausea and vomiting.
2 Tolerance for pain.
3 Allergy to iodine or shellfish.
4 Ability to lie still and hold breath.

Answer: 4

Rationale: It is most important for the nurse to assess the client's ability to lie still and hold the breath for the procedure. This helps the physician to avoid complications, such as puncturing the lung or other organs. Assessment of allergy to iodine or shellfish is unnecessary for this procedure because no contrast dye is used. History related to nausea and vomiting is generally part of assessment of the GI system, but it has no bearing on the current procedure. The client's tolerance for pain is a useful item to know; however, the area will receive a local anesthetic, and pain tolerance is less important than the client's ability to cooperate during the procedure.

Test-Taking Strategy: Use basic knowledge related to diagnostic studies to eliminate options 1 and 3. Use prioritizing skills to choose option 4 over option 2. Take time now to review this procedure if you had difficulty with this question!

Level of Cognitive Ability: Application
Phase of Nursing Process: Assessment
Client Needs: Safe, Effective Care Environment
Content Area: Adult Health/Gastrointestinal

Reference
Black, J., & Matassarin-Jacobs, E. (1997). *Medical-surgical nursing: Clinical management for continuity of care* (5th ed.). Philadelphia: W. B. Saunders, p. 1855.

---

104. The client is being transferred to the nursing unit from the postanesthesia care unit after spinal fusion with Harrington rod insertion. The nurse would prepare to transfer the client from the stretcher to the bed by using

1 A bath blanket and the assistance of three people.
2 A bath blanket and the assistance of four people.
3 A slider board and the assistance of two people.
4 A slider board and the assistance of four people.

Answer: 4

Rationale: After spinal fusion, with or without instrumentation, the client is transferred from stretcher to bed with the use of a slider board and the assistance of four people. This permits optimal stabilization and support of the spine, while allowing the client to be moved smoothly and gently.

Test-Taking Strategy: This question can be answered by analyzing the level of comfort and stability provided to the client's spine with the amounts of assistance given in each option. Using this approach, you can systematically eliminate each of the incorrect options. Review care of the client after Harrington rod insertion now if you had difficulty with this question!

Level of Cognitive Ability: Application
Phase of Nursing Process: Planning
Client Needs: Safe, Effective Care Environment
Content Area: Adult Health/Neurological

Reference
Black, J., & Matassarin-Jacobs, E. (1997). *Medical-surgical nursing: Clinical management for continuity of care* (5th ed.). Philadelphia: W. B. Saunders, p. 923.

105. The nurse is caring for the client with pneumonia. The nurse would plan which of the following as the best time to take the client for a short walk?

1 After the client uses the metered-dose inhaler
2 After recording oxygen saturation on the bedside flow sheet
3 After the client eats lunch
4 After the client has a brief nap

Answer: 1

Rationale: The nurse should schedule activities for the client with pneumonia after the client has received respiratory treatments or medications. After administration of bronchodilators (often administered by metered-dose inhaler), the client has the best air exchange possible and would tolerate the activity best.

Test-Taking Strategy: Begin to answer this question by eliminating options 2 and 3 as the least plausible options. Discriminate between options 1 and 4 by noting that although a brief nap would make the client feel more rested, the use of bronchodilator medication would widen the air passages, allowing for more air to enter the client's lungs. This makes option 1 a better choice than option 4.

Level of Cognitive Ability: Application
Phase of Nursing Process: Planning
Client Needs: Safe, Effective Care Environment
Content Area: Adult Health/Respiratory

Reference

Black, J., & Matassarin-Jacobs, E. (1997). *Medical-surgical nursing: Clinical management for continuity of care* (5th ed.). Philadelphia: W. B. Saunders, p. 1138.

---

106. The nurse is preparing to nasotracheally suction the client with acquired immunodeficiency syndrome (AIDS) who has had blood-tinged sputum with previous suctioning. The nurse should plan to use which of the following items as part of universal precautions for this client?

1 Gloves, mask, and protective eyewear
2 Gloves, gown, and mask
3 Gown, mask, and protective eyewear
4 Gloves, gown, and protective eyewear

Answer: 1

Rationale: Universal precautions include use of gloves whenever there is actual or potential contact with blood or body fluids. During procedures that aerosolize blood, the nurse wears a mask and protective eyewear or a face shield. Impervious gowns are worn in instances when it is anticipated that there will be contact with a large amount of blood.

Test-Taking Strategy: Note that the question addresses suctioning, so expect airborne secretions and possibly airborne particles of blood with this procedure. Basic knowledge of universal precautions, then, forces you to look for an option that includes mask, protective eyewear, and gloves. The only option that contains these three items is option 1. If you did not answer this question correctly, stop and review universal precautions now.

Level of Cognitive Ability: Application
Phase of Nursing Process: Planning
Client Needs: Safe, Effective Care Environment
Content Area: Fundamental Skills

Reference

Black, J., & Matassarin-Jacobs, E. (1997). *Medical-surgical nursing: Clinical management for continuity of care* (5th ed.). Philadelphia: W. B. Saunders, p. 620.

107. The nurse is inserting an indwelling urinary catheter into a male client. As the catheter is inserted into the urethra, urine begins to flow into the tubing. At this point, the nurse

1. Immediately inflates the balloon.
2. Withdraws the catheter approximately 1 inch and inflates the balloon.
3. Inserts the catheter until resistance is met and inflates the balloon.
4. Inserts the catheter 2.5–5 cm and inflates the balloon.

Answer: 4

Rationale: The catheter's balloon is behind the opening at the insertion tip. The catheter is inserted 2.5–5 cm after urine begins to flow in order to provide sufficient space to inflate the balloon. Inserting the catheter the extra distance will ensure that the balloon is inflated inside the bladder and not in the urethra. Inflating the balloon in the urethra could produce trauma.

Test-Taking Strategy: Knowledge of the proper procedure for inserting an indwelling urinary catheter will assist you in answering this question. Take time now to review the procedure for inserting a urinary catheter into a male now if you had difficulty with this question!

Level of Cognitive Ability: Application
Phase of Nursing Process: Implementation
Client Needs: Safe, Effective Care Environment
Content Area: Fundamental Skills

Reference

Kozier, B., Erb, G., & Blais, K. (1998). *Fundamentals of nursing: Concepts, process, and practice* (5th ed.). Menlo Park, CA: Addison-Wesley, pp. 1256–1257.

108. The nurse has just inserted an indwelling catheter into the bladder of a postoperative client who has not voided for 6 hours and has a distended bladder. After the tubing is secured and the collection bag is hung on the bed frame, the nurse notices that 750 mL of urine has drained into the collection bag. The most appropriate nursing action for the safety of the client is to

1. Clamp the tubing for 30 minutes and then release.
2. Provide suprapubic pressure to maintain steady flow of urine.
3. Check the specific gravity of the urine.
4. Raise the collection bag high enough to slow the rate of drainage.

Answer: 1

Rationale: Rapid emptying of a large volume of urine may cause engorgement of pelvic blood vessels and hypovolemic shock. Clamping the tubing for 30 minutes allows for equilibration to prevent complications. Option 2 would increase the flow of urine, which would lead to hypovolemic shock. Option 3 would be an assessment and would not affect the flow of urine or prevent the possible hypovolemic shock. Option 4 could cause backflow of urine. Infection is likely to develop if urine is allowed to flow back into the bladder.

Test-Taking Strategy: Knowledge of the procedure for inserting an indwelling urinary catheter and the physiology of the hemodynamic changes after the rapid collapse of an over-distended bladder will assist you in answering this question. Option 3 is different from the other three options. It is an assessment action rather than an action that affects the amount of urine drainage. Slowing the rate of urine drainage is the issue; therefore, options 2 and 3 can be ruled out. Option 1 is the only option that safely prevents hypovolemic shock. Urinary collection bags should never be elevated above the level of the bladder.

Level of Cognitive Ability: Application
Phase of Nursing Process: Implementation
Client Needs: Safe, Effective Care Environment
Content Area: Fundamental Skills

Reference

Potter, P., & Perry, A. (1997). *Fundamentals of nursing: Concepts, process, and practice* (4th ed.). St. Louis: Mosby–Year Book, p. 1324.

109. The nurse is preparing to administer oxygen to the client with carbon dioxide narcosis who has a history of chronic airflow limitation (CAL). The nurse checks to see that the oxygen flow rate is at

1. 2–3 liters/minute.
2. 4–5 liters/minute.
3. 6–8 liters/minute.
4. 8–10 liters/minute.

Answer: 1

Rationale: The nurse administers oxygen to the client with carbon dioxide narcosis very cautiously. This is because the client's respiratory center is insensitive to carbon dioxide levels as the respiratory stimulant and instead relies on oxygen levels. If oxygen is given too freely, the client loses the respiratory drive, and respiratory failure results. Thus the nurse checks the flow of oxygen to see that it does not exceed 2–3 liters/minute.

Test-Taking Strategy: This question tests the fundamental concept of safe oxygen levels for the client with an altered respiratory drive. If this question was difficult in any way, take a few moments now to review the concerns related to the administration of oxygen to a client with CAL!

Level of Cognitive Ability: Application
Phase of Nursing Process: Implementation
Client Needs: Safe, Effective Care Environment
Content Area: Adult Health/Respiratory

Reference

Smeltzer, S., & Bare, B. (1996). *Brunner and Suddarth's Textbook of medical-surgical nursing* (8th ed.). Philadelphia: Lippincott-Raven, p. 235.

---

110. The nurse has an order to administer amphotericin B intravenously to the client with histoplasmosis. The nurse plans to do which of the following during administration of the medication?

1 Monitor for hypothermia
2 Give a concurrent fluid challenge
3 Assess the intravenous infusion site
4 Monitor for an excessive urine output

Answer: 3

Rationale: Amphotericin B is a toxic medication that can produce symptoms during administration such as chills, fever, headache, vomiting, and impaired renal function. The medication is also very irritating to the IV site, commonly causing thrombophlebitis. The nurse administering this medication watches for all of these problems.

Test-Taking Strategy: Knowledge of this potent medication is needed to answer this question accurately. Knowing that fever and chills can occur helps you eliminate option 1. Knowing that the medication can be toxic to the kidneys helps you eliminate option 4. Because there is no rationale for giving concurrent fluids, the answer is to monitor the IV site. You would be especially sure of this answer if you know that this medication is very irritating to the blood vessels. Review nursing care related to the administration of this medication now if you had difficulty with this question!

Level of Cognitive Ability: Application
Phase of Nursing Process: Planning
Client Needs: Safe, Effective Care Environment
Content Area: Pharmacology

Reference

Black, J., & Matassarin-Jacobs, E. (1997). *Medical-surgical nursing: Clinical management for continuity of care* (5th ed.). Philadelphia: W. B. Saunders, p. 1147.

---

111. The client with repeated pleural effusions from inoperable lung cancer is to undergo pleurodesis. The nurse anticipates doing which of the following after the physician injects the sclerosing agent through the chest tube?

1 Clamping the chest tube
2 Ambulating the client
3 Asking the client to cough and deep breathe
4 Asking the client to remain in one position only

Answer: 1

Rationale: After injection of the sclerosing agent, the nurse clamps the chest tube to prevent the agent from draining back out of the pleural space. A repositioning schedule is used by some physicians, but its usefulness in dispersing the substance is controversial. Ambulation, coughing, and deep breathing have no specific purpose in the immediate period after injection.

Test-Taking Strategy: Option 2 seems the least plausible after the client has undergone a procedure such as this and may be eliminated first. On the other hand, there is no logical reason to keep the client in the same position, so option 4 may be eliminated next. To discriminate between the last two, it seems more plausible to clamp the chest tube so that the sclerosing agent cannot flow back out of the tube, so you would choose this over the coughing and deep breathing option, which has no specific purpose in this situation. Review this procedure now if you had difficulty with this question!

Level of Cognitive Ability: Analysis
Phase of Nursing Process: Planning
Client Needs: Safe, Effective Care Environment
Content Area: Adult Health/Respiratory

Reference

Ignatavicius, D. D., Workman, M. L., & Mishler, M. A. (1995). *Medical-surgical nursing: A nursing process approach* (2nd ed.). Philadelphia: W. B. Saunders, p. 742.

112. The client with bladder injury has had surgical repair of the injured area and placement of a suprapubic catheter. The nurse plans to do which of the following to prevent complications of this procedure?

1 Monitor urine output every shift
2 Encourage a high intake of oral fluids
3 Prevent kinking of the catheter tubing
4 Measure specific gravity once a shift

Answer: 3

Rationale: A complication after surgical repair of the bladder is disruption of sutures caused by tension on them from urine buildup. The nurse prevents this from happening by ensuring that the catheter is able to drain freely. This involves basic catheter care, including keeping the tubing free from kinks, keeping tubing below the level of the bladder, and monitoring the flow of urine frequently. Measurement of urine specific gravity and high oral fluid intake do not prevent complications of bladder surgery. Monitoring of urine output every shift is insufficient to detect decreased flow from catheter kinking.

Test-Taking Strategy: Begin to answer this question by eliminating option 4 first. Specific gravity measurement is not a preventive action. Using the same reasoning, eliminate option 1 next, because once-a-shift measurement is not a preventive action and is also insufficient in frequency. To discriminate between the last two items, knowing that high oral fluid intake will not prevent complications from this procedure will allow you to choose option 3 as correct. Knowing that a key principle of catheter management is to prevent kinking of the tubing would also allow you to choose option 3 over option 2.

Level of Cognitive Ability: Application
Phase of Nursing Process: Planning
Client Needs: Safe, Effective Care Environment
Content Area: Adult Health/Renal

Reference

Black, J., & Matassarin-Jacobs, E. (1997). *Medical-surgical nursing: Clinical management for continuity of care* (5th ed.). Philadelphia: W. B. Saunders, p. 1619.

113. The client undergoes a subtotal thyroidectomy for thyroid storm. It would be a priority for the nurse to have which of the following items at the client's bedside upon arrival from the operating room?

1 An apnea monitor
2 A blood transfusion warmer
3 A suction unit and oxygen
4 An ampule of phytonadione (vitamin K)

Answer: 3

Rationale: After thyroidectomy, respiratory distress can occur from tetany, tissue swelling, or hemorrhage. It is important to have oxygen and suction equipment readily available and in working order in case of such an emergency. Apnea is not a problem associated with thyroidectomy unless the client suffers respiratory arrest. Blood transfusions can be administered without a warmer if necessary. Vitamin K would not be administered for a client hemorrhaging unless deficiencies in clotting factors warrant its administration.

Test-Taking Strategy: When answering this question, use the principles associated with prioritizing. Recall the anatomical location of the thyroid gland and its close proximity to the trachea. Remember the ABCs: airway, breathing, and circulation. Knowing the location of the incision as well as the possible postoperative complications associated with the surgical procedure, you will determine that option 3 is the correct answer.

Level of Cognitive Ability: Application
Phase of Nursing Process: Planning
Client Needs: Safe, Effective Care Environment
Content Area: Adult Health/Endocrine

Reference

Ignatavicius, D. D., Workman, M. L., & Mishler, M. A. (1995). *Medical-surgical nursing: A nursing process approach* (2nd ed.). Philadelphia: W. B. Saunders, pp. 1841–1842.

114. The client has multiple traumatic musculoskeletal injuries. The nurse prepares a nursing care plan for the client, and in the planning, the nurse understands that a life-threatening complication of fat embolism syndrome (FES) can occur within 24–48 hours after injury. The essential component of the care plan should include

1 Anticipating possible use of mechanical ventilation with positive end-expiratory pressure (PEEP).
2 Preparing to administer IV anticoagulants.
3 Having the client sign a permit for surgery.
4 Measuring client for antiembolic stockings.

Answer: 1

Rationale: FES (fat embolism syndrome) includes direct damage to the lung, which results in pulmonary hypertension. The nurse must have a high index of suspicion for FES. The classic picture of FES includes altered mental status, tachypnea, tachycardia, petechiae, and fever. The pathophysiological process is similar to that of adult respiratory distress syndrome (ARDS). Mechanical ventilation with PEEP would be necessary.

Test-Taking Strategy: Use knowledge regarding the manifestations associated with FES to answer the question. Recalling that the syndrome is similar to ARDS will assist in directing you to the correct option. Review this syndrome now if you had difficulty with this question!

Level of Cognitive Ability: Application
Phase of Nursing Process: Planning
Client Needs: Safe, Effective Care Environment
Content Area: Adult Health/Musculoskeletal

Reference

Black, J., & Matassarin-Jacobs, E. (1997). *Medical-surgical nursing: Clinical management for continuity of care* (5th ed.). Philadelphia: W. B. Saunders, p. 2140.

115. The client with benign prostatic hyperplasia undergoes transurethral resection of the prostate (TURP). The nurse plans to ensure that which of the following solutions is available postoperatively for continuous bladder irrigation?

1 Sterile water
2 Sterile normal saline
3 Sterile Dakin's solution
4 Sterile water with 5% dextrose

Answer: 2

Rationale: Continuous bladder irrigation is done after TURP with sterile normal saline, which is isotonic. Sterile water is not used because the solution could be absorbed systemically, precipitating hemolysis and possibly renal failure. Dakin's solution contains hypochlorite and is used only for wound irrigation in selected circumstances. Solutions containing dextrose are not introduced into the bladder.

Test-Taking Strategy: Begin to answer this question by eliminating options 3 and 4. These are the least likely substances to be introduced into the bladder postoperatively. To discriminate between options 1 and 2, it is necessary to know that sterile saline is isotonic, whereas sterile water is hypotonic. Because an isotonic solution is needed, sterile saline is the correct option.

Level of Cognitive Ability: Application
Phase of Nursing Process: Planning
Client Needs: Safe, Effective Care Environment
Content Area: Adult Health/Renal

Reference

Black, J., & Matassarin-Jacobs, E. (1997). *Medical-surgical nursing: Clinical management for continuity of care* (5th ed.). Philadelphia: W. B. Saunders, p. 2358.

116. The nurse places a hospitalized client with active tuberculosis in a private, well-ventilated room. In addition, which of the following actions is most appropriate for the nurse to use before entering the room?

1 Proper handwashing technique
2 High-efficiency particulate air (HEPA) respirator and proper handwashing
3 The nurse needs no special precautions, but the client should cover his or her mouth and nose when coughing or sneezing, followed by proper handwashing.
4 Gowning, gloving, and proper handwashing

Answer: 2

Rationale: The nurse wears a HEPA respirator when caring for a client with active or "suspected" tuberculosis. Hands are always thoroughly washed before and after caring for the client. Option 1 is not complete and therefore not the most appropriate. Option 3 is an incorrect statement. Option 4 is also inaccurate because gowning is indicated only when there is a possibility of contaminating clothing.

Test-Taking Strategy: Knowledge about acid-fast bacteria isolation precautions is necessary to answer this question. The question asks you which of the actions is the most appropriate. Option 1 contains an appropriate action, but option 2 is most appropriate. Review these respiratory isolation precautions now if you had difficulty with this question!

Level of Cognitive Ability: Application
Phase of Nursing Process: Implementation
Client Needs: Safe, Effective Care Environment
Content Area: Adult Health/Respiratory

Reference

Ignatavicius, D. D., Workman, M. L., & Mishler, M. A. (1995). *Medical-surgical nursing: A nursing process approach* (2nd ed.). Philadelphia: W. B. Saunders, p. 720.

---

117. The client with AIDS is being admitted for treatment of *Pneumocystis carinii* infection. Which of the following activities does the nurse plan to include in the care of this client that assist in maintaining comfort?

1 Assess respiratory rate, rhythm, and depth and breath sounds every 8 hours
2 Evaluate blood gas results
3 Keep the head of the bed elevated
4 Monitor vital signs every hour

Answer: 3

Rationale: Clients with respiratory difficulties are often more comfortable with the head of the bed elevated. Options 1, 2, and 4 are appropriate measures for evaluating respiratory function and avoiding complications. Option 3 is the only response that addresses planning for client comfort.

Test-Taking Strategy: All responses are appropriate nursing measures for the client with *P. carinii* infection, but the question specifically addresses comfort. Also, you can use the strategy of selecting the response that is different. Options 1, 2, and 4 are all measures for evaluating respiratory function, whereas option 3 is not.

Level of Cognitive Ability: Application
Phase of Nursing Process: Planning
Client Needs: Safe, Effective Care Environment
Content Area: Adult Health/Respiratory

Reference

Ignatavicius, D. D., Workman, M. L., & Mishler, M. A. (1995). *Medical-surgical nursing: A nursing process approach* (2nd ed.). Philadelphia: W. B. Saunders, p. 510.

---

118. An adolescent is returning home after an acute psychiatric hospitalization for a suicide attempt. Which of the following would be least effective in preparing the client to return to a safe, effective care environment?

1 Identify the family's strengths and weaknesses
2 Suggest that the mother's boyfriend move out of the home
3 Provide and offer the family options and resources
4 Encourage sharing of feelings

Answer: 2

Rationale: Option 2 is clearly the least effective response because there is no information in the stem that leads us to believe that the boyfriend's involvement has anything to do with the suicide attempt. Options 1, 2, and 4 are open-ended and offer helpful ways to enhance the family processes.

Test-Taking Strategy: The stem asks for the "least" effective option. Avoid reading into the question. There is no information in the stem that leads you to believe there is a problem with the boyfriend that led the adolescent to attempt suicide. It is important that a nurse remain nonjudgmental when dealing with clients. In addition, options 1, 3, and 4 identify positive measures that will ensure a safe environment for the client!

Level of Cognitive Ability: Application
Phase of Nursing Process: Implementation
Client Needs: Safe, Effective Care Environment
Content Area: Mental Health

Reference

Antai-Otong, D. (1995). *Psychiatric nursing: Biological and behavioral concepts.* Philadelphia: W. B. Saunders, p. 147.

---

119. In planning care for a hospitalized toddler, the highest priority should be directed toward

1 Protecting the toddler from injury.
2 Adapting the toddler to the hospital routine.
3 Allowing the toddler to participate in play and divisional activities.
4 Providing a consistent caregiver.

Answer: 1

Rationale: The toddler is at high risk for injury as a result of limited abilities related to developmental age, and an unfamiliar environment with many potential hazards. Although adaptation, diversion, and consistency are important, protection from injury is the highest priority.

Test-Taking Strategy: The key words in the stem of the question are "highest priority." According to Maslow's hierarchy of needs theory, physiological needs come first, followed by safety. Because no physiological needs are addressed, the safety option of preventing injury takes priority.

Level of Cognitive Ability: Application
Phase of Nursing Process: Planning
Client Needs: Safe, Effective Care Environment
Content Area: Child Health

Reference

Wong, D. (1997). *Whaley and Wong's Essentials of pediatric nursing* (5th ed.). St. Louis: Mosby–Year Book, p. 652.

---

120. The client is to undergo pleural biopsy at the bedside. Knowing the potential complications of the procedure, the nurse would plan to have which of the following items available at the bedside?

1 Chest tube and drainage system
2 Intubation tray
3 Portable chest x-ray machine
4 Morphine sulfate injection

Answer: 1

Rationale: Complications after pleural biopsy include hemothorax, pneumothorax, and temporary pain from intercostal nerve injury. The nurse has a chest tube and drainage system available at the bedside for use if hemothorax or pneumothorax develops. An intubation tray is not indicated. The client should be premedicated before the procedure, or a local anesthetic is used. A portable chest x-ray machine would be called for to verify placement of a chest tube if one was inserted, but it is unnecessary to have at the bedside before the procedure.

Test-Taking Strategy: This question tests the knowledge of hemothorax and pneumothorax as potential complications of this procedure. Knowing this forces you to choose option 1 as the item needed for possible immediate use at the bedside. If this question was problematic, take a few moments now to review this procedure and its complications!

Level of Cognitive Ability: Application
Phase of Nursing Process: Planning
Client Needs: Safe, Effective Care Environment
Content Area: Adult Health/Respiratory

Reference

Black, J., & Matassarin-Jacobs, E. (1997). *Medical-surgical nursing: Clinical management for continuity of care* (5th ed.). Philadelphia: W. B. Saunders, p. 1064.

121. The client with painful respiration and significant flail chest has arterial blood gas measurements that reveal an arterial oxygen tension (PaO_2) of 68 and an arterial carbon dioxide tension ($PaCO_2$) of 51. Two hours ago, the PaO_2 was 82 and the $PaCO_2$ was 44. The nurse should plan to have which of the following items available at the bedside?

1. Injectable lidocaine (Xylocaine)
2. Portable chest x-ray machine
3. Intubation tray
4. Chest tube insertion set

Answer: 3

Rationale: The client with flail chest has painful, rapid, shallow respirations while experiencing severe dyspnea. The effort of breathing and the paradoxical chest movement have the net effect of producing hypoxia and hypercapnea. The client develops respiratory failure and requires intubation and mechanical ventilation, usually with PEEP. Therefore, an intubation tray is necessary.

Test-Taking Strategy: To answer this question quickly and easily, recall that a falling arterial oxygen level and a rising carbon dioxide level indicate respiratory failure. The usual treatment for respiratory failure is intubation, which makes option 3 the appropriate response.

Level of Cognitive Ability: Application
Phase of Nursing Process: Planning
Client Needs: Safe, Effective Care Environment
Content Area: Adult Health/Respiratory

Reference

Black, J., & Matassarin-Jacobs, E. (1997). *Medical-surgical nursing: Clinical management for continuity of care* (5th ed.). Philadelphia: W. B. Saunders, p. 2527.

---

122. An 11-year-old child scheduled for a procedure will have an IV line inserted and will receive an IM injection. Effective preparation includes

1. Teaching the parents so that they can explain everything to their child.
2. Using pictures, concrete words, and demonstrations to describe what will happen.
3. Telling the child not to worry because the doctors take care of everything.
4. Reassuring the child that he or she will not feel any pain.

Answer: 2

Rationale: The school-age child understands best with visual aids and concrete language. Option 1 inappropriately delegates the responsibility for teaching to the parents. Options 3 and 4 devalue the child's feelings by reassuring and telling the client how to feel. Option 4 is also a false statement.

Test-Taking Strategy: Recognizing that reassuring and telling are blocks to communication will assist in eliminating options 3 and 4. In option 1, a nursing responsibility is inappropriately delegated to parents.

Level of Cognitive Ability: Application
Phase of Nursing Process: Implementation
Client Needs: Safe, Effective Care Environment
Content Area: Child Health

Reference

Wong, D. (1997). *Whaley and Wong's Essentials of pediatric nursing* (5th ed.). St. Louis: Mosby–Year Book, pp. 652–653.

---

123. The nurse is preparing a client for a transbronchial lung biopsy. Which of the following nursing actions is the most important at this time?

1. Instructing the client that food and fluid will be withheld for several hours after the procedure
2. Leading the client in breathing exercises
3. Ensuring that the client signed the consent form for the procedure
4. Making sure the client has a clean hospital gown

Answer: 3

Rationale: The transbronchial lung biopsy is an invasive procedure. A consent form is signed before the procedure. The nurse provides explanations and clarifies questions that the client may have.

Test-Taking Strategy: Note the key word "preparing" and the phrase "most important." Option 1 is important but could be reinforced in the postprocedure period. Option 2 is more applicable in situations in which the client is at risk for shallow breathing. Option 3 is more important than option 4 because it protects the client (and hospital) from unwarranted procedures and is done after the client has been provided information and had the opportunity to ask questions.

Level of Cognitive Ability: Application
Phase of Nursing Process: Implementation
Client Needs: Safe, Effective Care Environment
Content Area: Adult Health/Respiratory

Reference

Black, J., & Matassarin-Jacobs, E. (1997). *Medical-surgical nursing: Clinical management for continuity of care* (5th ed.). Philadelphia: W. B. Saunders, p. 1064.

124. The nurse is about to begin hemodialysis. Which of the following measures would the nurse plan to avoid in the care of the client?

1 Putting on a mask and giving one to the client to wear during connection to the machine
2 Wearing full protective clothing such as goggles, mask, apron, and gloves
3 Covering the connection site with a bath blanket to enhance extremity warmth
4 Using sterile technique for needle insertion

Answer: 3

Rationale: Infection is a major concern with hemodialysis. For that reason, the use of sterile technique and the application of a face mask for both nurse and client are extremely important. It is also imperative that universal precautions be followed, which includes the use of goggles, mask, gloves, and apron. The connection site should not be covered; it should be visible so that the nurse can assess for bleeding, ischemia, and infection at the site during the hemodialysis procedure.

Test-Taking Strategy: The wording of the question guides you to look for an incorrect statement. Being able to recognize proper actions for infection control and universal precautions allows you to eliminate each of the incorrect responses systematically. You could also choose correctly if you know that the access site should remain visible to detect bleeding as well as signs of ischemia and infection.

Level of Cognitive Ability: Application
Phase of Nursing Process: Planning
Client Needs: Safe, Effective Care Environment
Content Area: Adult Health/Renal

Reference

Luckmann, J. (1997). *Saunders manual of nursing care*. Philadelphia: W. B. Saunders, p. 1194.

125. The nurse is going to suction an adult client with a tracheostomy who has copious amounts of secretions. The nurse would do which of the following to accomplish this procedure safely and effectively for the client?

1 Hyperoxygenate the client, using an Ambu bag
2 Set the suction pressure range between 160 and 180 mmHg
3 Occlude the Y-port of the catheter while advancing it into the tracheostomy
4 Apply continuous suction in the airway for up to 15 seconds

Answer: 1

Rationale: To perform suctioning correctly, the nurse hyperoxygenates the client, using a manual resuscitation bag or the sigh mechanism if the client is on a mechanical ventilator. The safe suction range for an adult is 100–120 mmHg. The nurse advances the catheter into the tracheostomy without occluding the Y-port; suction is never applied while introducing the catheter because it would traumatize mucosa and remove oxygen from the respiratory tract. The nurse uses intermittent suction in the airway for up to 10–15 seconds.

Test-Taking Strategy: The wording of this question guides you to look for an appropriate nursing action. Knowing that suction is applied intermittently and on catheter withdrawal only, you would eliminate options 3 and 4 automatically. To discriminate between options 1 and 2, knowing that hyperoxygenation of the client is a good action may help you to choose this as the correct answer, even without recalling specific suction pressures.

Level of Cognitive Ability: Application
Phase of Nursing Process: Implementation
Client Needs: Safe, Effective Care Environment
Content Area: Adult Health/Respiratory

Reference

Taylor, C., Lillis, C., & LeMone, P. (1997). *Fundamentals of nursing: The art and science of nursing care* (3rd ed.). Philadelphia: Lippincott-Raven, pp. 1352–1353.

126. The client with empyema is to have a thoracentesis at the bedside. Because of the nature of the client's problem, the nurse plans to have which of the following available if the procedure is not effective?

1 Code cart
2 Chest tube and drainage system
3 Extra large drainage bottle
4 A small-bore needle

Answer: 2

Rationale: If the empyema is too thick for drainage during thoracentesis, the client may require placement of a chest tube to adequately drain the purulent effusion.

Test-Taking Strategy: Note the key word "empyema." In this condition the exudate is often very thick. Knowing that the purpose of thoracentesis is to provide drainage of the pleura, look for an alternative method for accomplishing this goal as you evaluate each of the options. The only response that has to do with pleural drainage is the chest tube with drainage system, making it the only plausible option.

Level of Cognitive Ability: Application
Phase of Nursing Process: Planning
Client Needs: Safe, Effective Care Environment
Content Area: Adult Health/Respiratory

Reference

Smeltzer, S., & Bare, B. (1996). *Brunner and Suddarth's Textbook of medical-surgical nursing* (8th ed.). Philadelphia: Lippincott-Raven, p. 503.

---

127. The nurse is administering a dose of fentanyl (Sublimaze) to the client via an epidural catheter after nephrectomy. Before administering the medication, the nurse would plan to

1 Aspirate to ensure that there is a cerebrospinal fluid (CSF) return.
2 Ensure that naloxone (Narcan) is readily available.
3 Place the head of the bed flat.
4 Flush the catheter with 6 mL sterile water.

Answer: 2

Rationale: Epidural analgesia is used for clients with high levels of expected postoperative pain. The nurse carefully checks the medication, notes the client's level of sedation, and makes sure that the head of bed is elevated 30 degrees unless contraindicated. The nurse aspirates to make sure there is no CSF return. If CSF returns with aspiration, the catheter has migrated from the epidural space into the subarachnoid space. The catheter is not flushed with 6 mL of sterile water. Naloxone should be readily available for use if respiratory depression should occur.

Test-Taking Strategy: Begin to answer this question by eliminating option 4 first. Flushing 6 mL of sterile water through an epidural catheter is the least plausible and most dangerous option. Option 1 is eliminated next, because CSF aspiration should not occur with an epidural catheter. To discriminate between the last two options, you would choose option 2 as the correct answer if you knew that the antidote to fentanyl is naloxone. Or, you would choose option 2 by the process of elimination if you knew that the head of the bed should be elevated at least 30 degrees.

Level of Cognitive Ability: Application
Phase of Nursing Process: Planning
Client Needs: Safe, Effective Care Environment
Content Area: Pharmacology

Reference

Black, J., & Matassarin-Jacobs, E. (1997). *Medical-surgical nursing: Clinical management for continuity of care* (5th ed.). Philadelphia: W. B. Saunders, pp. 383, 1673.

128. The nurse has just collected a sputum specimen by expectoration for a culture for a client who has a productive cough. The nurse will plan to implement all of the following nursing prescriptions. Which of the following nursing actions should the nurse identify as most important?

1 Give the client mouthwash
2 Check to see that the sputum basin is clean
3 Send the sputum specimen to the laboratory immediately
4 Provide tissues for expectoration

Answer: 3

Rationale: Sputum specimens for culture should be labeled and transported immediately to the laboratory. Identification of the organism is critical in determining the appropriate treatment for the client. If the sputum sample is not transported immediately for culture, organisms will collect and the potential for contamination of the sample exists, which, if it occurs, will then alter results. Options 1, 3, and 4 are important, but option 3 identifies the most important action.

Test-Taking Strategy: Knowledge that microorganisms will multiply when specimens are left at the bedside for long periods is necessary, given the implications that this multiplication has for a sputum culture. Using critical thinking, all of the nursing prescriptions are important, but option 3 would have the most significant implications.

Level of Cognitive Ability: Application
Phase of Nursing Process: Planning
Client Needs: Safe, Effective Care Environment
Content Area: Fundamental Skills

Reference

Bolander, V. (1994). *Sorensen and Luckmann's Basic nursing: A psychophysiologic approach* (3rd ed.). Philadelphia: W. B. Saunders, pp. 1214–1215.

---

129. The post–myocardial infarction client is scheduled for a multiple-gated acquisition scan (MUGA). The nurse would assess to make sure which item is in place before the procedure?

1 Signed consent for cardiac catheterization
2 Notation of allergies to iodine or shellfish
3 An intravenous line
4 A Foley catheter

Answer: 3

Rationale: MUGA is a radionuclide study used to detect myocardial infarction, decreased myocardial blood flow, and left ventricular function. The radioisotope is injected intravenously. The procedure is not the same as cardiac catheterization and does not use radiopaque dye. A Foley catheter is not required.

Test-Taking Strategy: Options 1 and 2 can be eliminated, because option 1 necessitates that 2 is also correct. Knowledge that the procedure involves injection of a radioisotope guides you to select option 3. Option 4 is irrelevant. Review preparation for this procedure now if you had difficulty with this question!

Level of Cognitive Ability: Application
Phase of Nursing Process: Assessment
Client Needs: Safe, Effective Care Environment
Content Area: Adult Health/Cardiovascular

Reference

Smeltzer, S., & Bare, B. (1996). *Brunner and Suddarth's Textbook of medical-surgical nursing* (8th ed.). Philadelphia: Lippincott-Raven, p. 610.

---

130. The nurse is planning care for the client with a chest tube attached to a Pleur-Evac drainage system. The nurse would plan to avoid which of the following activities to prevent tension pneumothorax?

1 Adding water to the suction chamber as it evaporates
2 Taping the connection between the chest tube and the drainage system
3 Raising the collection chamber above the client's waist
4 Clamping the chest tube

Answer: 4

Rationale: To avoid causing tension pneumothorax, the nurse avoids clamping the chest tube unless specifically ordered. In most instances, clamping of the chest tube is contraindicated and forbidden by agency policy. Adding water to the suction control chamber is an appropriate nursing action that is done as needed to maintain the full suction level ordered. Taping the connection between chest tube and system is also indicated to prevent accidental disconnection. Raising the system above waist level is contraindicated, but not because of risk of tension pneumothorax; rather, this would allow fluid to reenter the pleural space. Air cannot reenter because of the water seal in the system. It is air that would cause a tension pneumothorax.

Test-Taking Strategy: Recall that tension pneumothorax occurs when air is trapped in the pleural space and has no exit. Therefore, it is necessary to evaluate each of the options in terms of relative risk for air trapping in the pleural space. Using this line of reasoning, you would automatically eliminate options 1 and 2. Option 3 would allow fluid to flow back into the client's chest (and is contraindicated), but air could not reenter unless the water seal was disrupted. Thus, the only alternative is option 4. Clamping the chest tube could trap air in the pleural space and should be avoided by the nurse. Review tension pneumothorax now if you had difficulty with this question!

Level of Cognitive Ability: Application
Phase of Nursing Process: Planning
Client Needs: Safe, Effective Care Environment
Content Area: Adult Health/Respiratory

Reference

Black, J., & Matassarin-Jacobs, E. (1997). *Medical-surgical nursing: Clinical management for continuity of care* (5th ed.). Philadelphia: W. B. Saunders, p. 1165.

---

131. In developing a nursing care plan for a client with severe Alzheimer's disease, the nurse recognizes that the priority of care will be

1 Impaired communication.
2 Disturbance in role performance.
3 High risk for injury.
4 Social isolation.

Answer: 3

Rationale: Clients who have Alzheimer's disease have significant cognitive impairment and are therefore at high risk for injury. It is critical for the nurse to maintain a safe environment, particularly as the client's judgment becomes increasingly impaired. Options 1, 2, and 4 may be appropriate, but the highest priority is directed toward safety.

Test-Taking Strategy: Use Maslow's hierarchy of needs theory to answer this question. When a physiological need is not addressed, safety needs receive priority!

Level of Cognitive Ability: Application
Phase of Nursing Process: Implementation
Client Needs: Safe, Effective Care Environment
Content Area: Adult Health/Neurological

Reference

Black, J., & Matassarin-Jacobs, E. (1997). *Medical-surgical nursing: Clinical management for continuity of care* (5th ed.). Philadelphia: W. B. Saunders, p. 868.

---

132. A client with a diagnosis of major depression, recurrent, with psychotic features is admitted to the unit. In an attempt to create a safe environment for the client, it is most important that the nurse devise a plan of care that deals specifically with the client's

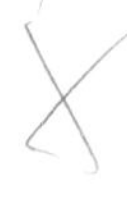

1 Altered thought processes.
2 Altered nutrition.
3 Self-care deficit.
4 Knowledge deficit.

Answer: 1

Rationale: The diagnosis major depression, recurrent, with psychotic features alerts the nurse that in addition to the criteria that designate the diagnosis of major depression, the nurse must also deal with a client's psychosis. Psychosis is defined as a state in which a person's mental capacity to recognize reality and communicate with and relate to others is impaired, thus interfering with the person's capacity to deal with life's demands. Altered thought processes generally indicates a state of increased anxiety in which hallucinations and delusions prevail.

Test-Taking Strategy: All of the nursing diagnoses listed may be appropriate for a client diagnosed with major depression. The key to the answer lies with the specifier "psychotic features" in which the client often suffers from altered thought processes, such as hallucinations and delusions. Altered thought processes present a risk related to safety.

Level of Cognitive Ability: Application
Level of Nursing Process: Planning
Client Needs: Safe, Effective Care Environment
Content Area: Mental Health

Reference

Antai-Otong, D. (1995). *Psychiatric nursing: Biological and behavioral concepts.* Philadelphia: W. B. Saunders, pp. 241, 249.

133. The nurse is assisting a client with a chest tube in getting out of bed. The tubing accidentally gets caught in the bed rail and disconnects from the chest. As the nurse seeks to reestablish the connection, the Pleur-Evac drainage system falls over and cracks. The nurse should first

1 Call the physician.
2 Immerse the chest tube in a bottle of sterile saline.
3 Apply a petrolatum gauze over the end of the chest tube.
4 Clamp the chest tube.

Answer: 2

Rationale: If a chest tube accidentally disconnects from the tubing of the drainage apparatus, the nurse should first reestablish under-water seal to prevent tension pneumothorax and mediastinal shift. This can be accomplished by reconnecting the chest tube or, in this case, immersing the chest tube in a bottle of sterile normal saline or water. The physician should be notified after the nurse takes corrective action. If the physician is called first, tension pneumothorax has time to develop. Clamping the chest tube could also cause tension pneumothorax. A petrolatum gauze would be applied to the skin over the chest tube insertion site if the entire chest tube was accidentally removed.

Test-Taking Strategy: This question tests the concept that a chest tube requires a water seal at all times to prevent pneumothorax. Evaluate each of the options in light of this concept, and note that the question asks for the "first" action. You would eliminate option 1 as too time consuming to be the logical "first" action. Options 3 and 4 would create a tension pneumothorax, because they do not reestablish an under-water seal, and prevent air release on exhalation. This leaves option 2 as the correct answer. Option 1 would be the next action, in terms of priority.

Level of Cognitive Ability: Application
Phase of Nursing Process: Implementation
Client Needs: Safe, Effective Care Environment
Content Area: Adult Health/Respiratory

Reference

Black, J., & Matassarin-Jacobs, E. (1997). *Medical-surgical nursing: Clinical management for continuity of care* (5th ed.). Philadelphia: W. B. Saunders, p. 1165.

134. A client has a medical diagnosis of Cushing's syndrome. The nurse should have which of the following available to detect a potential complication of this medical condition?

1 Glucometer
2 BP cuff
3 Oxygen saturation monitor
4 Specific gravity manometer

Answer: 1

Rationale: Increased levels of glucocorticoids can result in hyperglycemia and signs and symptoms of diabetes mellitus. The client's blood glucose levels should be monitored periodically. Each of the other responses is incorrect.

Test-Taking Strategy: Knowledge of clinical manifestations and complications of this medical condition will assist you in choosing the correct answer. Review the clinical manifestations associated with Cushing's syndrome now if you had difficulty with this question!

Level of Cognitive Ability: Application
Phase of Nursing Process: Planning
Client Needs: Safe, Effective Care Environment
Content Area: Adult Health/Endocrine

Reference

LeMone, P., & Burke, K. (1996). *Medical-surgical nursing: Critical thinking in client care*. Menlo Park, CA: Addison-Wesley, pp. 692, 694.

135. The client undergoing hemodialysis becomes suddenly short of breath and complains of chest pain. The client is tachycardic, pale, and anxious. The nurse suspects air embolism. The nurse should

1. Continue dialysis at a slower rate after checking the lines for air.
2. Discontinue dialysis and notify the physician.
3. Monitor vital signs every 15 minutes for the next hour.
4. Administer a bolus to the client with 500 mL normal saline to break up the air embolus.

Answer: 2

Rationale: If the client experiences air embolus during hemodialysis, the nurse should terminate dialysis immediately, notify the physician, and administer oxygen as needed. All other actions are incorrect.

Test-Taking Strategy: To answer this question accurately, recall that air embolus is an emergency situation that affects the cardiopulmonary system suddenly and profoundly. With this in mind, all options except option 2 would be eliminated quickly.

Level of Cognitive Ability: Application
Phase of Nursing Process: Implementation
Client Needs: Safe, Effective Care Environment
Content Area: Adult Health/Renal

Reference

Luckmann, J. (1997). *Saunders manual of nursing care.* Philadelphia: W. B. Saunders, p. 1195.

---

136. A nurse determines that a client with aldosteronism is experiencing a complication of the disorder. The nurse immediately obtains which of the following items to use in client assessment?

1. Cardiac monitor
2. BP cuff
3. Foley catheter
4. Glucometer

Answer: 1

Rationale: Aldosteronism can lead to hypokalemia, which in turn can cause life-threatening dysrhythmias. These are detected by placing the client on a cardiac monitor. Options 2, 3, and 4 are not immediate priorities for this client.

Test-Taking Strategy: To answer this question accurately, it is necessary to be familiar with this disorder and its complications. If needed, take a few moments to review it now!

Level of Cognitive Ability: Application
Phase of Nursing Process: Planning
Client Needs: Safe, Effective Care Environment
Content Area: Adult Health/Endocrine

Reference

Black, J., & Matassarin-Jacobs, E. (1997). *Medical-surgical nursing: Clinical management for continuity of care* (5th ed.). Philadelphia: W. B. Saunders, pp. 2055, 2056.

---

137. The nurse is monitoring the results of serial blood gas measurements for the client who has suffered carbon monoxide poisoning. The client does not want to keep the oxygen mask in place. The nurse evaluates that the oxygen may be safely removed once the carboxyhemoglobin level decreases to less than

1. 5%.
2. 10%.
3. 15%.
4. 25%.

Answer: 1

Rationale: Oxygen may be removed safely from the client with carbon monoxide poisoning once carboxyhemoglobin levels are less than 5%.

Test-Taking Strategy: Knowledge regarding carbon monoxide levels is necessary to answer this question. If you are unsure, it would be best to select the lowest level of carbon monoxide as identified in option 1. If this question was difficult, take a few moments to briefly review this content area now!

Level of Cognitive Ability: Analysis
Phase of Nursing Process: Evaluation
Client Needs: Safe, Effective Care Environment
Content Area: Adult Health/Respiratory

Reference

Smeltzer, S., & Bare, B. (1996). *Brunner and Suddarth's Textbook of medical-surgical nursing* (8th ed.). Philadelphia: Lippincott-Raven, p. 2025.

138. The nurse is teaching a pregnant client about nutrition. What information must the nurse include in this client's teaching plan to promote safe and adequate fetal development?

1 The nutritional status of the mother significantly influences fetal growth and development
2 All mothers are at high risk for nutritional deficiencies
3 Calcium is not important until the third trimester
4 Iron supplements are not necessary unless the mother has iron-deficiency anemia

Answer: 1

Rationale: Poor nutrition during pregnancy can negatively influence fetal growth and development. Although pregnancy poses some nutritional risk for the mother, not all clients are at high risk. Calcium is critical during the third trimester, but calcium intake must be increased from the onset of pregnancy. Intake of dietary iron is insufficient for the majority of pregnant women, and iron supplements are routinely encouraged.

Test-Taking Strategy: Option 2 uses the absolute "all"; therefore eliminate this option. Options 3 and 4 offer specific time frames or conditions for interventions, which are not mentioned in the stem. Option 1 is a general or global statement that is true for any stage of pregnancy.

Level of Cognitive Ability: Application
Phase of Nursing Process: Planning
Client Needs: Safe, Effective Care Environment
Content Area: Maternity

Reference
Potter, P., & Perry, A. (1997). *Fundamentals of nursing: Concepts, process, and practice* (4th ed.). St. Louis: Mosby–Year Book, p. 1104.

---

139. The nurse is formulating a plan of care for a client receiving enteral feedings. Which nursing diagnosis is the highest priority for this client?

1 Altered Nutrition, Less than Body Requirements
2 High Risk for Aspiration
3 High Risk for Fluid Volume Deficit
4 Diarrhea

Answer: 2

Rationale: Any condition in which gastrointestinal motility is slowed or esophageal reflux is possible places a client at risk for aspiration. Although options 1, 3, and 4 may be a concern, these are not the priority.

Test-Taking Strategy: Use the ABCs: airway, breathing, circulation. Option 2 addresses airway management. Options 1, 3, and 4 are possible problems but not as high a priority as airway maintenance.

Level of Cognitive Ability: Application
Phase of Nursing Process: Planning
Client Needs: Safe, Effective Care Environment
Content Area: Fundamental Skills

Reference
Burrell, L., Gerlach, M., & Pless, B. (1997). *Adult nursing: Acute and community care* (2nd ed.). Stamford, CT: Appleton & Lange, pp. 1345–1346.

---

140. The client is being admitted to the nursing unit after receiving a radium implant for bladder cancer. The nurse would take which of the following priority actions in the care of this client?

1 Encourage the client to take frequent rest periods
2 Admit the client to a private room
3 Encourage the family to visit
4 Place the client in reverse isolation

Answer: 2

Rationale: The client who has a radium implant is placed in a private room and has limited visitors. This reduces the exposure of others to the radiation. Frequent rest periods are a helpful general intervention but are not a priority for the client in this situation. Reverse isolation is unnecessary.

Test-Taking Strategy: Begin to answer the question by eliminating option 4 first as an unnecessary action. Option 1 is helpful but is not considered a priority and may be eliminated next. To discriminate between options 2 and 3, it is necessary to know that other individuals should have limited exposure to clients with radium implants. This would allow you to choose option 2 over option 3.

Level of Cognitive Ability: Application
Phase of Nursing Process: Implementation
Client Needs: Safe, Effective Care Environment
Content Area: Adult Health/Oncology

Reference

Black, J., & Matassarin-Jacobs, E. (1997). *Medical-surgical nursing: Clinical management for continuity of care* (5th ed.). Philadelphia: W. B. Saunders, p. 1585.

---

141. A client is admitted to the hospital with a diagnosis of Cushing's syndrome. What symptoms should the nurse plan to address first to maintain client safety?

1 Fluid volume deficit
2 Hypoglycemia
3 Respiratory distress
4 Mental status changes

Answer: 4

Rationale: When Cushing's syndrome develops, the normal function of the glucocorticoids becomes exaggerated, and the classic picture of the syndrome emerges. This exaggerated physiological action can cause mental status changes, including memory loss, poor concentration and cognition, euphoria, and depression. Mental status changes place the client at risk for injury. The disorder can also cause persistent hyperglycemia along with sodium and water retention, producing edema and hypertension.

Test-Taking Strategy: This question asks you to identify symptoms that pose a risk to the client with Cushing's syndrome. This is a difficult question because there are no similar distracters; however, you can probably eliminate option 1 because fluid volume deficit is not a symptom. If you know the physiological action of glucocorticoids, you can predict that an excess of glucocorticoids can produce mental status changes.

Level of Cognitive Ability: Application
Phase of Nursing Process: Planning
Client Needs: Safe, Effective Care Environment
Content Area: Adult Health/Endocrine

Reference

Polaski, A., & Tatro, S. (1996). *Luckmann's Core principles and practice of medical-surgical nursing.* Philadelphia: W. B. Saunders, p. 1237.

---

142. The physician is performing direct visualization of the larynx to rule out laryngeal cancer. The nurse would plan to tell the client to do which of the following to decrease the gag reflex during the procedure?

1 Try to swallow
2 Hold the breath
3 Breathe in and out quickly (pant)
4 Roll the tongue to the back of the mouth

Answer: 3

Rationale: The client is instructed to pant, or breathe in and out quickly, to decrease gagging during the procedure. The tongue cannot be moved back; if it could, it would occlude the airway. Swallowing cannot be done with the instrument in place. The procedure takes longer than the time the client would be able to hold the breath, and holding the breath is ineffective anyway.

Test-Taking Strategy: Option 4 is eliminated first because it is not possible to move the tongue back with the instrument in place. It would also cause the airway to become occluded. In view of the length of time needed for the procedure, the client could not realistically hold the breath, so option 2 may be eliminated next. Trying to swallow would actually cause the larynx to move against the instrument and could cause gagging. By the process of elimination, panting, or breathing in and out quickly, is the answer, because it provides for the least movement of the larynx and trachea.

Level of Cognitive Ability: Application
Phase of Nursing Process: Planning
Client Needs: Safe, Effective Care Environment
Content Area: Adult Health/Oncology

Reference

Black, J., & Matassarin-Jacobs, E. (1997). *Medical-surgical nursing: Clinical management for continuity of care* (5th ed.). Philadelphia: W. B. Saunders, p. 1084.

143. The client is to undergo weekly intravesical chemotherapy for bladder cancer for the next 8 weeks. The nurse interprets that the client understands management of the urine as a biohazard if the client states that he or she will

1. Disinfect the urine and toilet with bleach for 6 hours after a treatment.
2. Have one bathroom strictly set aside for the client's use for the next 2 months.
3. Purchase extra bottles of scented disinfectant for daily bathroom cleansing.
4. Void into a bedpan and then emptying the urine into the toilet.

Answer: 1

Rationale: After intravesical chemotherapy, the client treats the urine as a biohazard. This involves disinfecting the urine and the toilet with household bleach for 6 hours. Scented disinfectants are of no particular use. The client does not need to have a separate bathroom for personal use. There is no value in using a bedpan for voiding.

Test-Taking Strategy: Option 4 is the least plausible of all the options for this question and may be eliminated first. Because scented disinfectants have no obvious value, option 3 is eliminated next. Knowing that the urine needs special treatment for only 6 hours after each session allows you to choose option 1 over option 2. Also, option 2 is unnecessary and may be unrealistic for a number of clients.

Level of Cognitive Ability: Analysis
Phase of Nursing Process: Evaluation
Client Needs: Safe, Effective Care Environment
Content Area: Adult Health/Oncology

Reference

Black, J., & Matassarin-Jacobs, E. (1997). *Medical-surgical nursing: Clinical management for continuity of care* (5th ed.). Philadelphia: W. B. Saunders, p. 1585.

144. The male client who is admitted for an unrelated medical problem is diagnosed with urethritis caused by chlamydial infection. The nursing assistant assigned to the client asks the nurse which measures are necessary to prevent contraction of the infection during care. The nurse tells the assistant that

1. Enteric precautions should be instituted for the client.
2. Contact isolation should be initiated, because the disease is highly contagious.
3. Universal precautions are quite sufficient, because the disease is transmitted sexually.
4. Gloves and mask should be used when in the client's room.

Answer: 3

Rationale: Chlamydia is a sexually transmitted disease and in the male client is frequently called nongonococcal urethritis. No special precautions are required other than universal precautions. Caregivers cannot acquire the disease during administration of care, and using universal precautions is the only measure that needs to be used.

Test-Taking Strategy: This question is straightforward in nature. A basic knowledge of infection control and disease transmission guides you to select option 3 as correct. If this question was difficult for you, take a few moments to review transmission of this disorder and universal precautions!

Level of Cognitive Ability: Application
Phase of Nursing Process: Implementation
Client Needs: Safe, Effective Care Environment
Content Area: Fundamental Skills

Reference

Black, J., & Matassarin-Jacobs, E. (1997). *Medical-surgical nursing: Clinical management for continuity of care* (5th ed.). Philadelphia: W. B. Saunders, p. 2470.

145. Which of the following information should be included in the teaching plan for a client being prepared to undergo a bilateral adrenalectomy for treatment of an adrenal tumor that is producing excessive aldosterone?

1. "You will most likely need to undergo chemotherapy after surgery."
2. "You will need to take hormone replacements for the rest of your life."
3. "You will need to wear an abdominal binder after surgery."
4. "You will not require any special long-term treatment after surgery."

Answer: 2

Rationale: The major cause of primary hyperaldosteronism is an aldosterone-secreting tumor called an aldosteronoma. Surgery is the treatment of choice. Clients undergoing a bilateral adrenalectomy will need permanent replacement of adrenal hormones.

Test-Taking Strategy: Note the key word "bilateral" in the question. Knowing that the glucocorticoids and mineralocorticoids are essential to sustain life should lead you to the correct answer of option 2. Review care after bilateral adrenalectomy now if you had difficulty with this question!

Level of Cognitive Ability: Application
Phase of Nursing Process: Planning
Client Needs: Safe, Effective Care Environment
Content Area: Adult Health/Endocrine

Reference

Black, J., & Matassarin-Jacobs, E. (1997). *Medical-surgical nursing: Clinical management for continuity of care* (5th ed.). Philadelphia: W. B. Saunders, p. 2056.

146. The client is in extreme pain from scrotal swelling that is caused by epididymitis. The nurse administers an intramuscular narcotic analgesic in the left arm to relieve the pain. The nurse should plan to take which of the following actions next?

1. Tell the client to do range-of-motion (ROM) exercises with the left arm to absorb the medication into the blood stream
2. Check the name bracelet of the client
3. Put the side rails up on the bed
4. Dim the lights in the room

Answer: 3

Rationale: The client who receives a narcotic analgesic should immediately have the side rails raised on the bed, to prevent injury once the medication has taken effect. Dimming the light in the room is the next most helpful action. The name bracelet should have been checked before the medication was administered. It is unnecessary to perform ROM exercises in the site of injection.

Test-Taking Strategy: Begin to answer this question by eliminating option 2, because this should have been done before medication administration. Option 1 is not necessary and may be eliminated next. To discriminate between options 3 and 4, note that the question asks you for the action to be taken "next." With this in mind, you would choose option 3 over option 4. Although option 4 is a correct answer, it would be done when the nurse leaves the room. As part of protecting the client's safety after administration of a narcotic analgesic, you would put the side rails up first.

Level of Cognitive Ability: Application
Phase of Nursing Process: Planning
Client Needs: Safe, Effective Care Environment
Content Area: Pharmacology

Reference

Black, J., & Matassarin-Jacobs, E. (1997). *Medical-surgical nursing: Clinical management for continuity of care* (5th ed.). Philadelphia: W. B. Saunders, p. 2381.

147. In order to prevent the development of Addison's crisis, which of the following medications would the nurse prepare to administer in the immediate preoperative period before an adrenalectomy?

1. Spironolactone (Aldactone), intramuscularly
2. Cortisol, intravenously
3. Prednisone, orally
4. Fludrocortisone (Florinef), subcutaneously

Answer: 2

Rationale: A glucocorticoid preparation will be administered intravenously or intramuscularly in the immediate preoperative period for an adrenalectomy. A water-soluble cortisol preparation may be given throughout the surgical procedure. Cortisol protects the client from developing acute adrenal insufficiency during an adrenalectomy.

Test-Taking Strategy: Knowledge of the action and uses of these medications is needed to assist you in answering this question. The question asks about Addisonian crisis in a surgical client and such a situation requires immediate intervention. Knowing that medications that are administered intravenously are absorbed most rapidly, you should be able to select option 2, which is a glucocorticoid administered intravenously.

Level of Cognitive Ability: Application
Phase of Nursing Process: Planning
Client Needs: Safe, Effective Care Environment
Content Area: Adult Health/Endocrine

Reference

Black, J., & Matassarin-Jacobs, E. (1997). *Medical-surgical nursing: Clinical management for continuity of care* (5th ed.). Philadelphia: W. B. Saunders, pp. 2052–2053.

---

148. The nurse observes a withdrawn client blocking the hallway, walking three steps forward and then two steps backward. Other clients are agitated in trying to get past. The nurse intervenes in this problem by

1 Standing along side of client and saying, "You're very anxious today."
2 Stopping the behavior and saying, "You're going to get exhausted."
3 Having the client taken to the TV lounge and saying, "Relax and watch television now."
4 Walking along side of client and saying, "You're not going anywhere very fast doing this."

Answer: 1

Rationale: An important consideration when working with clients who are withdrawn is the maintenance of safety in the environment. Negative symptoms might precipitate a dangerous situation. Anxiety occurs when a person feels threatened, and a prime consideration is alleviating the anxiety by encouraging the client to recognize the meaning of the experience in terms of identifying the threat.

Test-Taking Strategy: Eliminate options 2 and 3 because they do not address the increased anxiety and need for control underlying the behavior, and may escalate the behavior. Option 4 does not raise the client to a functioning level. Review measures related to the care of a withdrawn client now if you had difficulty with this question!

Level of Cognitive Ability: Application
Phase of Nursing Process: Implementation
Client Needs: Safe, Effective Care Environment
Content Area: Mental Health

Reference

Haber, J. (1997). *Comprehensive psychiatric nursing* (5th ed.). St. Louis: Mosby–Year Book, pp. 589, 595–596.

---

149. The nurse is preparing the client's morning NPH Insulin dose. The nurse notices a clumpy precipitate inside the insulin vial. The most appropriate nursing action would be to

1 Draw up and administer the dose.
2 Shake the vial in an attempt to disperse the clumps.
3 Draw the dose from a new vial.
4 Warm the bottle under running water to dissolve the clump.

Answer: 3

Rationale: The person preparing insulin for injection should always inspect the vial before use for changes that may signify loss of potency. NPH Insulin normally is uniformly cloudy. Clumping, frosting, and precipitates are signs of insulin damage; thus, because potency is questionable, it is safer to discard the vial and draw up the dose from a new vial.

Test-Taking Strategy: Remember that NPH Insulin is cloudy but not clumpy. If you did not know this, you could select the best answer from the options by selecting the safest action for the client. When in doubt, throw it out!

Level of Cognitive Ability: Application
Phase of Nursing Process: Implementation
Client Needs: Safe, Effective Care Environment
Content Area: Pharmacology

Reference

Ignatavicius, D. D., Workman, M. L., & Mishler, M. A. (1995). *Medical-surgical nursing: A nursing process approach* (2nd ed.). Philadelphia: W. B. Saunders, p. 1884.

150. A nurse is preparing the bedside for a client immediately after parathyroidectomy. Which piece of medical equipment would be routinely appropriate for anticipating the safety needs of this client?

1 Under-water seal chest drainage
2 Tracheotomy set
3 Intermittent gastric suction
4 Cardiac monitor

Answer: 2

Rationale: Respiratory distress resulting from hemorrhage and from swelling with compression of the trachea is a paramount concern for the nurse managing the care of a client immediately after parathyroidectomy. Thus an emergency tracheotomy set is always routinely placed at the bedside of the client after this type of surgery.

Test-Taking Strategy: The key phrase in this question is "routinely appropriate." Although all of the equipment cited could be used, the tracheotomy set would be routinely used in preparing the bedside for a parathyroidectomy client. If you didn't know this, think about the location of the surgical incision and which potential problems might occur in that location. Review care after parathyroidectomy now if you had difficulty with this question!

Level of Cognitive Ability: Application
Phase of Nursing Process: Planning
Client Needs: Safe, Effective Care Environment
Content Area: Adult Health/Endocrine

Reference
Ignatavicius, D. D., Workman, M. L., & Mishler, M. A. (1995). *Medical-surgical nursing: A nursing process approach* (2nd ed.). Philadelphia: W. B. Saunders, p. 1853.

---

151. The nurse prepares a nursing care plan for a client with Graves' disease who is to receive radioactive iodine therapy (RAI). Which of the following statements would be most appropriate for the nurse to include in the teaching plan?

1 "The radioactive iodine is designed to destroy the entire thyroid gland with just one dose."
2 "It takes 6–8 weeks after treatment with RAI to experience relief from the symptoms of the disease."
3 "The high levels of radioactivity prohibit contact with family for 4 weeks after initial treatment."
4 "After the initial dose of RAI, subsequent treatments with RAI must continue lifelong."

Answer: 2

Rationale: After treatment with RAI, a decrease in thyroid hormone level should be noted; this would help alleviate symptoms, although relief does not occur until 6–8 weeks after initial treatment. RAI therapy is not designed to destroy the entire gland; rather, some of the cells that synthesize thyroid hormone will be destroyed by the local radiation. The nurse needs to reassure the client and family that unless the dosage of RAI is extremely high, clients are not required to observe radiation precautions. The rationale for this is that the radioactivity quickly dissipates. Occasionally, a client may require a second or third dose of RAI, but this treatment is never lifelong.

Test-Taking Strategy: Knowledge regarding treatment with RAI will assist you in answering this question correctly. Read each response and eliminate the answers that are inaccurate regarding initial dose of RAI. Options 1 and 4 can be eliminated immediately. Because there is no mention in the stem that the dose is exceptionally high, your best option is to select option 2.

Level of Cognitive Ability: Application
Phase of Nursing Process: Planning
Client Needs: Safe, Effective Care Environment
Content Area: Adult Health/Endocrine

Reference
Ignatavicius, D. D., Workman, M. L., & Mishler, M. A. (1995). *Medical-surgical nursing: A nursing process approach* (2nd ed.). Philadelphia: W. B. Saunders, p. 1840.

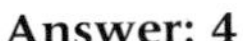

152. A client presents to the emergency room with upper GI bleeding and is in moderate distress. In the planning of priorities for the care of this client, which nursing action would be the first priority for this client?

1 Thorough investigation of precipitating events
2 Insertion of a nasogastric tube and testing emesis for blood
3 Complete abdominal physical examination
4 Determination of vital signs.

Answer: 4

Rationale: An initial nursing assessment should be performed while the client is getting ready for initial treatment. The immediate determination of vital signs indicates whether the client is in shock from blood loss and also provides a baseline blood pressure and pulse by which to monitor the progress of treatment. Signs and symptoms of shock include low blood pressure; rapid, weak pulse; increased thirst; cold, clammy skin; and restlessness. Vital signs should be monitored every 10 to 15 minutes, and the physician should be informed of any significant changes. The client may not be able to provide subjective data until the immediate physical needs are met.

Test-Taking Strategy: Although all the choices are important components of a complete nursing assessment for this client, use principles of prioritization when answering this question. A client with acute upper GI bleeding is at risk for shock. Monitoring vital signs is the nursing action that will assess circulation, provide information about the client's circulating volume status, and alert the nurse to early stages of shock.

Level of Cognitive Ability: Application
Phase of Nursing Process: Planning
Client Needs: Safe, Effective Care Environment
Content Area: Adult Health/Gastrointestinal

Reference

Luckmann, J. (1997). *Saunders manual of nursing care.* Philadelphia: W. B. Saunders, p. 1723.

153. The client with acute renal failure is ordered to be on fluid restriction of 1500 mL/day. The nurse could best plan to assist the client with maintaining the restriction by

1 Prohibiting beverages with sugar to minimize thirst.
2 Using mouthwash with alcohol for mouth care.
3 Asking the client to calculate IV fluids into the total daily allotment.
4 Removing the water pitcher from the bedside.

Answer: 4

Rationale: The nurse can help the client maintain fluid restriction through a variety of means. One way is to give frequent mouth care; however, alcohol-based products should be avoided because they dry mucous membranes. Beverages that the client enjoys are provided and are not restricted on the basis of sugar content. The water pitcher should be removed from the bedside to aid in compliance. The client is not asked to keep track of IV fluid intake; this is the responsibility of the nurse. The use of ice chips and the application of lip ointments are other interventions that may be helpful to the client on fluid restriction. Putting allotted water into a spray bottle may help to spread out the amount taken.

Test-Taking Strategy: Begin to answer this question by eliminating option 3, because this is a nursing responsibility. Discard option 2 next, because alcohol-containing products dry oral mucous membranes and could exacerbate thirst. Good nursing judgment would guide you to choose option 4 over option 1 as the "best" nursing action.

Level of Cognitive Ability: Application
Phase of Nursing Process: Planning
Client Needs: Safe, Effective Care Environment
Content Area: Adult Health/Renal

Reference

Black, J., & Matassarin-Jacobs, E. (1997). *Medical-surgical nursing: Clinical management for continuity of care* (5th ed.). Philadelphia: W. B. Saunders, p. 1640.

154. The nurse has administered approximately half of a high cleansing enema when the client complains of pain and cramping. Which of the following nursing actions is the most appropriate?

1 Raise the enema bag so that the solution can be completed quickly
2 Clamp the tubing for 30 seconds and restart the flow at a slower rate
3 Reassure the client and continue the flow
4 Discontinue the enema and notify the physician

Answer: 2

Rationale: The enema fluid should be administered slowly. If the client complains of fullness or pain, stop the flow for 30 seconds and restart at a slower rate. Slow enema administration and stopping the flow temporarily, if necessary, will decrease the likelihood of intestinal spasm and premature ejection of the solution. The higher the solution container is held above the rectum, the faster is the flow and the greater is the force in the rectum. Pain and cramping are usually caused by intestinal spasm and subside when the enema is stopped briefly, after which the enema may be resumed. There is no need to discontinue the enema and notify the physician at this time.

Test-Taking Strategy: The issue of the question is alleviating pain and cramping. Eliminate option 4 first. Options 1 and 3 are similar; therefore, eliminate these options. Review the procedure for enema administration now if you had difficulty with this question.

Level of Cognitive Ability: Application
Phase of Nursing Process: Implementation
Client Needs: Safe, Effective Care Environment
Content Area: Fundamental Skills

Reference

Kozier, B., Erb, G., & Blais, K. (1998). *Fundamentals of nursing: Concepts, process, and practice* (5th ed.). Menlo Park, CA: Addison-Wesley, pp. 1203, 1205.

155. The client with chronic renal failure who is scheduled for hemodialysis this morning is to receive a daily dose of enalapril (Vasotec). The nurse should plan to administer this medication

1 Just before dialysis.
2 During dialysis.
3 Upon return from dialysis.
4 The day after dialysis.

Answer: 3

Rationale: Antihypertensive medications such as enalapril are given to the client after hemodialysis. This prevents the client from becoming hypotensive during dialysis and also from having the medication removed from the blood stream by dialysis. There is no rationale for waiting a full day to resume the medication. This would lead to ineffective control of the blood pressure.

Test-Taking Strategy: Begin to answer this question by recalling the effects of an antihypertensive medication on the blood pressure when fluid is being removed from the body. Because hypotension is much more likely to occur in this circumstance, you would eliminate options 1 and 2 as possible answers. Most clients undergo hemodialysis three times a week. If the medication was held for dialysis until the following day, the client would miss three of the seven doses that would usually be given in a week. This would lead to ineffective blood pressure control. Thus option 4 is incorrect, leaving option 3 as correct. The medication is administered after return from hemodialysis.

Level of Cognitive Ability: Application
Phase of Nursing Process: Planning
Client Needs: Safe, Effective Care Environment
Content Area: Pharmacology

Reference

Black, J., & Matassarin-Jacobs, E. (1997). *Medical-surgical nursing: Clinical management for continuity of care* (5th ed.). Philadelphia: W. B. Saunders, p. 1654.

156. The nurse is preparing to administer a high cleansing enema. The nurse positions the client in the

1. Left lateral position with the right leg acutely flexed.
2. Supine position with the legs elevated.
3. Dorsal recumbent position.
4. Right lateral position with the left leg acutely flexed.

Answer: 1

Rationale: The sigmoid and descending colon are located on the left side. Therefore, the left lateral position uses gravity to facilitate the flow of solution into the sigmoid and descending colon. Acute flexion of the right leg allows for adequate exposure of the anus. Options 2, 3, and 4 are incorrect.

Test-Taking Strategy: Knowledge of anatomy and the procedure for administering a high cleansing enema will assist you in answering this question. The sigmoid and descending colon are anatomically located on the left side. Gravity will facilitate the solution's flow into the sigmoid and descending colon if the client is positioned in the left lateral position. The right leg is acutely flexed for ease in visualizing the anal area.

Level of Cognitive Ability: Application
Phase of Nursing Process: Implementation
Client Needs: Safe, Effective Care Environment
Content Area: Fundamental Skills

Reference
Kozier, B., Erb, G., & Blais, K. (1998). *Fundamentals of nursing: Concepts, process, and practice* (5th ed.). Menlo Park, CA: Addison-Wesley, p. 1204.

---

157. While planning for the arrival of a subtotal thyroidectomy client from the operating room, the nurse should anticipate the need for which of the following items to be used at the bedside?

1. Emergency tracheostomy kit
2. Ampule of saturated solution of potassium iodide (SSKI)
3. Hypothermia blanket
4. Magnesium sulfate in a ready-to-inject vial

Answer: 1

Rationale: One of the severe complications that could develop after a thyroidectomy is respiratory distress. This complication results from postoperative swelling, tetany, or laryngeal stridor. In the event that symptoms of this complication are present, the nurse would want an emergency tracheostomy kit easily available, preferably at the bedside. SSKI is typically given preoperatively to block thyroid hormone synthesis and release, as well as for placing the client in a euthyroid state. Iodine makes the thyroid gland less vascular before surgery. Surgery on the thyroid does not alter the heat control mechanism of the body. Magnesium sulfate would not be indicated because hypomagnesemia is not a common problem after thyroidectomy.

Test-Taking Strategy: Knowledge regarding the complications that develop in the postoperative stage and recall of the anatomical location of the thyroid gland will assist you in answering this question correctly. Also, remember to use the ABCs: airway, breathing, and circulation. Maintaining a patent airway is critical!

Level of Cognitive Ability: Application
Phase of Nursing Process: Planning
Client Needs: Safe, Effective Care Environment
Content Area: Adult Health/Endocrine

Reference
Ignatavicius, D. D., Workman, M. L., & Mishler, M. A. (1995). *Medical-surgical nursing: A nursing process approach* (2nd ed.). Philadelphia: W. B. Saunders, pp. 1840–1842.

158. The nurse has an order to administer foscarnet (Foscavir), intravenously, to a client with AIDS. Before administering this medication, the nurse would plan to

1 Place the solution on an infusion pump.
2 Obtain folic acid as an antidote.
3 Ensure that liver enzymes have been measured as baseline.
4 Obtain a sputum culture.

Answer: 1

Rationale: Foscarnet is an antiviral agent used to treat cytomegalovirus (CMV) retinitis in clients with AIDS. Because of the potential toxicity of the medication, it is administered with the use of a controlled infusion device. It is very toxic to the kidneys, and serum creatinine levels are measured frequently during therapy. Folic acid is not an antidote.

Test-Taking Strategy: Begin to answer this question by eliminating option 4, because the medication is usually indicated in the treatment of CMV retinitis and not respiratory infection. Option 2 is eliminated next, because folic acid is not an antidote. To discriminate between the last two options, it is necessary to know that the medication is very toxic and cannot be infused too quickly. This would allow you to choose option 1 as correct. You may also choose correctly if you knew that the medication is toxic to the kidneys, not to the liver. Review this medication now if you had difficulty with this question!

Level of Cognitive Ability: Application
Phase of Nursing Process: Planning
Client Needs: Safe, Effective Care Environment
Content Area: Pharmacology

Reference

Deglin, J., & Vallerand, A. (1997). *Davis's drug guide for nurses* (5th ed.). Philadelphia: F. A. Davis, pp. 522–523.

---

159. The client is scheduled for gallbladder surgery in the morning. The client is mentally impaired and is unable to communicate. Which of the following nursing interventions would be appropriate for the nurse to perform?

1 Ensure that the family has signed the informed consent
2 Ensure that the client has signed the informed consent
3 Inform the family about the advance directive process
4 Inform the family about the process of a living will

Answer: 1

Rationale: The informed consent process occurs when competent clients can be in dialogue with loved ones and the persons providing care. The primary responsibility for informing the client rests with the physician. A living will lists the medical treatment that a person chooses to omit or refuse if the person becomes unable to make decisions and is terminally ill. Advance directives are forms of communication in which persons can give direction on how they wish to be treated when they cannot speak for themselves.

Test-Taking Strategy: The client is scheduled for a surgical procedure. The key phrase is "mentally impaired." Knowledge that informed consent is required will enable you to eliminate options 3 and 4. Knowledge that a client must be mentally alert to sign a consent form will help you eliminate option 2. Review the process of informed consent now if you had difficulty with this question!

Level of Cognitive Ability: Application
Phase of Nursing Process: Implementation
Client Needs: Safe, Effective Care Environment
Content Area: Fundamental Skills

Reference

Potter, P., & Perry, A. (1997). *Fundamentals of nursing: Concepts, process, and practice* (4th ed.). St. Louis: Mosby–Year Book, pp. 327, 328, 1393.

160. The client diagnosed with tuberculosis is scheduled to have x-rays. Which of the following nursing interventions would be appropriate for the nurse to perform?

1 Apply a mask to the client
2 Apply a mask and gown to the client
3 Apply mask, gown, and gloves to the client
4 Notify the x-ray department personnel so they can be sure to wear a mask when the client arrives

Answer: 1

Rationale: Clients known to have or suspected of having tuberculosis should wear a mask when out of their room. A high efficiency particulate air (HEPA) respirator (mask) is worn by the nurse when caring for the client with tuberculosis.

Test-Taking Strategy: Remembering that the route of transmission of tuberculosis pathogens is airborne will assist in answering the question. The issue relates to when the client is out of his or her room. Common sense tells you that it would be impossible for everyone outside of the client's room to wear a mask; therefore, eliminate option 4. Again, recalling the route of transmission, eliminate options 2 and 3. Review the transmission associated with tuberculosis now if you had difficulty with this question.

Level of Cognitive Ability: Application
Phase of Nursing Process: Implementation
Client Needs: Safe, Effective Care Environment
Content Area: Adult Health/Respiratory

Reference
Potter, P., & Perry, A. (1997). *Fundamentals of nursing: Concepts, process, and practice* (4th ed.). St. Louis: Mosby–Year Book, p. 762.

---

161. The nurse is taking care of a client on contact isolation. After the nursing care has been performed, which protective items worn during client care would the nurse remove first, upon leaving the room?

1 Gloves
2 Mask
3 Eyewear
4 Gown

Answer: 3

Rationale: Remove eyewear (goggles), untie the gown at the waist, remove one glove by grasping the cuff and pulling the glove inside out over the hand, and discard the glove. With the ungloved hand, tuck a finger inside the cuff of the remaining glove and pull it off, inside out. Untie mask strings next, and drop the mask into a trash receptacle. Untie the neck strings of the gown and allow the gown to fall from your shoulders. Remove your hands from the sleeves, without touching the outside of the gown. Hold the gown inside at the shoulder seams, and fold inside out. Discard in a laundry bag and wash your hands.

Test-Taking Strategy: Using knowledge of universal precautions and the methods of contaminating items, attempt to visualize the correct process of removing contaminated clothing and items after caring for a client. This visualization should direct you to the correct option. Review this procedure now if you had difficulty with this question!

Level of Cognitive Ability: Application
Phase of Nursing Process: Implementation
Client Needs: Safe, Effective Care Environment
Content Area: Fundamental Skills

Reference
Potter, P., & Perry, A. (1997). *Fundamentals of nursing: Concepts, process, and practice* (4th ed.). St. Louis: Mosby–Year Book, p. 766.

---

162. The client requests pain medication from the nurse. After administration of the IM injection, the nurse would do which of the following first?

1 Recap the needle
2 Assist the client to a comfortable position
3 Massage injection site with alcohol
4 Place syringe in needle box container

Answer: 3

Rationale: Massage the skin lightly after an IM injection to assist in medication absorption. Do not massage the skin after a subcutaneous injection of heparin or insulin or after an intradermal (ID) injection. Then assist the client to a comfortable position. Discard the uncapped needle or the needle enclosed in a safety shield in the appropriately labeled receptacle. Then remove disposable gloves and wash hands.

Test-Taking Strategy: The question is asking for the first nursing action. Attempt to visualize the scenario, read each option, and consider what the nurse would do first. Remember, the issue relates to an IM injection. Review this procedure now if you had difficulty with this question!

Level of Cognitive Ability: Application
Phase of Nursing Process: Implementation
Client Needs: Safe, Effective Care Environment
Content Area: Fundamental Skills

Reference

Potter, P., & Perry, A. (1997). *Fundamentals of nursing: Concepts, process, and practice* (4th ed.). St. Louis: Mosby–Year Book, p. 832.

---

163. The nurse is in the process of giving the client a bed bath. In the middle of the procedure, the unit secretary calls the nurse on the intercom to tell the nurse that there is an emergency phone call. What should the nurse's next action be?

1 Leave the door open so that client can be monitored and answer the phone call
2 Finish the bath before answering the phone call
3 Walk out of the room and answer the phone call
4 Put the call light within reach and answer the phone call

Answer: 4

Rationale: Because the call is an emergency call, the nurse may need to answer it. The other appropriate action is to ask another nurse to accept the call. This, however, is not one of the options. To maintain safety, place the call light within the client's reach if it is necessary to leave the room temporarily. The door should be closed or room curtains pulled around the bathing area, to provide privacy.

Test-Taking Strategy: Note the key phrase "emergency phone call." This should assist in eliminating option 2. Once it has been determined that the nurse needs to answer the phone call, the only option that addresses client safety and comfort is option 4.

Level of Cognitive Ability: Application
Phase of Nursing Process: Implementation
Client Needs: Safe, Effective Care Environment
Content Area: Fundamental Skills

Reference

Potter, P., & Perry, A. (1997). *Fundamentals of nursing: Concepts, process, and practice* (4th ed.). St. Louis: Mosby–Year Book, p. 1024.

---

164. The nursing manager is reviewing with the nursing staff the purpose for applying restraints. Which of the following would not be a part of the review because it is not an indication for the use of a restraint?

1 To prevent falls
2 To restrict client movement
3 To prevent the client from pulling out IV lines and catheters
4 To prevent the violent client from injuring staff

Answer: 1

Rationale: Restraints do not necessarily prevent falls or injury. In fact, it has been shown that clients incur fewer severe injuries if left unrestrained. Restraints are devices used to restrict the client's movement in situations when it is necessary to immobilize a limb or other body part. They are applied to keep the client from self-inflicted injury or from injuring others; from pulling out intravenous lines, catheters, or tubes; or from removing dressings. Restraints also may be used to keep children still and from injuring themselves during treatments and diagnostic procedures. Restraints should not be used as a form of punishment.

Test-Taking Strategy: Note the key word "not" in the stem of the question and carefully read the options. You can easily eliminate options 3 and 4. From the remaining two options, remember that there are guidelines for the use of restraints. Although the phrase "to restrict mobility" seems like a harsh one, think about the many clinical situations that necessitate temporary restraint for mobility restriction of a body part. This should direct you to option 1. Take time now to review the use of restraints, if you had difficulty with this question!

Level of Cognitive Ability: Analysis
Phase of Nursing Process: Analysis
Client Needs: Safe, Effective Care Environment
Content Area: Fundamental Skills

Reference

Lammon, C. B., Foote, A. W., Leli, P. G., et al. (1995). *Clinical nursing skills.* Philadelphia: W. B. Saunders, p. 287.

165. The client has an order for valproic acid (Depakene), 250 mg once daily. To maximize the client's safety, the nurse should plan to schedule the medication

1 At bedtime.
2 Before breakfast.
3 After breakfast.
4 With lunch.

Answer: 1

Rationale: Valproic acid is an anticonvulsant that causes central nervous system (CNS) depression. For this reason, the side effects of the drug include sedation, dizziness, ataxia, and confusion. When the client is taking this medication as a single daily dose, administering it at bedtime negates the risk of injury from sedation and enhances client safety.

Test-Taking Strategy: Begin to answer this question by recalling that this medication is an anticonvulsant with CNS depressant properties. This train of thought leads you to think of sedation as a key side effect. Bedtime administration would allow the sedative effects of the medication to occur at a time when the client is sleeping, with less likelihood that the client will become injured as a result of drug effects.

Level of Cognitive Ability: Application
Phase of Nursing Process: Planning
Client Needs: Safe, Effective Care Environment
Content Area: Pharmacology

Reference
Deglin, J., & Vallerand, A. (1997). *Davis's drug guide for nurses* (5th ed.). Philadelphia: F. A. Davis, pp. 1201–1202.

166. The mother of a teenage client with an anxiety disorder is concerned about her daughter's progress upon discharge. She states that her daughter "stashes food," "eats all the wrong things that make her hyperactive," and "hangs out with the wrong crowd." In helping the mother prepare for her daughter's discharge, you would instruct her to

1 Restrict the daughter's socializing time with her friends.
2 Consider taking time from work to help her daughter readjust to the home environment.
3 Restrict the amount of chocolate and caffeine products in the home.
4 Keep her daughter out of school until she can adjust to the school environment.

Answer: 3

Rationale: It is strongly recommended that clients with anxiety disorder abstain from or limit their intake of caffeine, chocolate, and alcohol. These products have the potential of increasing anxiety. Options 1 and 4 are unreasonable and are unhealthy approaches. It may not be realistic for a family member to take time off from work.

Test-Taking Strategy: Eliminate similar distracters. Options 1, 2, and 4 are concerned with monitoring or curtailing the client's physical activities, whereas option 3 addresses preparation of the environment. Option 3 also focuses on the concern or issue expressed in the question.

Level of Cognitive Ability: Application
Phase of Nursing Process: Planning
Client Needs: Safe, Effective Care Environment
Content Area: Mental Health

Reference
Fontaine, K., & Fletcher, J. (1995). *Essentials of mental health nursing* (3rd ed.). Redwood City, CA: Addison-Wesley, pp. 177–178.

167. The client in cardiogenic shock has an order for sodium nitroprusside (Nipride) for preload and afterload reduction. The nurse would plan to do which of the following when preparing to administer this medication?

1 Protect the solution from light
2 Add potassium to the infusion
3 Give it only through a central line
4 Obtain a baseline thiocyanate level

Answer: 1

Rationale: Sodium nitroprusside becomes unstable when exposed to light and must be shielded from light. No other medications are added to the infusion, which must be remixed every 4 hours. It can be given through a peripheral line. The level of thiocyanate (a nitroprusside metabolite, similar to cyanide) is usually measured if the client is maintained on this therapy for several days.

Test-Taking Strategy: Options 2 and 3 can be eliminated without much hesitation, even with no knowledge of this medication, because they are relatively implausible. Usually, levels of any medication or their by-products are measured after administration has been ongoing, so eliminate option 4. Review this medication now if you had difficulty with this question!

Level of Cognitive Ability: Application
Phase of Nursing Process: Planning
Client Needs: Safe, Effective Care Environment
Content Area: Pharmacology

Reference

Clark, J., Queener, S., & Karb, V. (1997). *Pharmacologic basis of nursing practice* (5th ed.). St. Louis: Mosby–Year Book, p. 158.

---

168. The nurse is encouraging the client to cough and breathe deeply after cardiac surgery. The nurse would ensure that which of the following items is available to maximize the effectiveness of this procedure?

1 Ambu bag
2 Incisional splinting device
3 Suction equipment
4 Nebulizer

Answer: 2

Rationale: The use of an incisional splint such as a "cough pillow" can ease discomfort during coughing and deep breathing, which are indicated every 1–2 hours. The client who is comfortable will perform deep breathing and coughing exercises more effectively. Use of an incentive spirometer is also indicated. Options 1, 3, and 4 will not encourage the client to cough and breathe deeply.

Test-Taking Strategy: The content of this question is part of basic nursing care and may likely be encountered in some form. The question asks for an item that will help the client, which eliminates options 1 and 3, which are used by the nurse. A nebulizer (option 4) delivers medication, leaving option 2 as the correct answer.

Level of Cognitive Ability: Application
Phase of Nursing Process: Assessment
Client Needs: Safe, Effective Care Environment
Content Area: Adult Health/Respiratory

Reference

Black, J., & Matassarin-Jacobs, E. (1997). *Medical-surgical nursing: Clinical management for continuity of care* (5th ed.). Philadelphia: W. B. Saunders, p. 1361.

---

169. The client with an acute respiratory infection is admitted with sinus tachycardia. The nurse would plan to minimize this symptom by

1 Providing the client with short, frequent walks.
2 Measuring the client's pulse each shift.
3 Eliminating sources of caffeine from meal trays.
4 Limiting oral and intravenous fluids.

Answer: 3

Rationale: Sinus tachycardia is often caused by fever, physical and emotional stress, heart failure, hypovolemia, certain medications, nicotine, caffeine, and exercise.

Test-Taking Strategy: The question asks for the action that will minimize this symptom. Eliminate options 1 and 4 first; exercise and fluid restriction will not alleviate tachycardia. Option 2 is a good measure, but it is an assessment, not an action to decrease the heart rate.

Level of Cognitive Ability: Application
Phase of Nursing Process: Planning
Client Needs: Safe, Effective Care Environment
Content Area: Adult Health/Cardiovascular

Reference

Black, J., & Matassarin-Jacobs, E. (1997). *Medical-surgical nursing: Clinical management for continuity of care* (5th ed.). Philadelphia: W. B. Saunders, p. 1298.

170. The nurse has an order to obtain a specimen for urinalysis from a client with an indwelling urinary catheter. The nurse would plan to avoid which of the following, which could contaminate the specimen?

1 Obtaining the specimen from the urinary drainage bag
2 Clamping the tubing of the drainage bag
3 Aspirating a sample from the port on the drainage bag
4 Wiping the port with an alcohol swab before inserting the syringe

Answer: 1

Rationale: A urine specimen is not taken from the urinary drainage bag. Urine undergoes chemical changes while sitting in the bag and does not necessarily reflect current client status. In addition, it may become contaminated with bacteria from opening the system.

Test-Taking Strategy: This question tests a core principle of asepsis. Use the process of elimination, bearing in mind the issue of preventing contamination. This thought process should assist in directing you to the correct option. If this question was difficult in any way, take a few moments now to review this key area of nursing practice.

Level of Cognitive Ability: Application
Phase of Nursing Process: Planning
Client Needs: Safe, Effective Care Environment
Content Area: Fundamental Skills

Reference

Black, J., & Matassarin-Jacobs, E. (1997). *Medical-surgical nursing: Clinical management for continuity of care* (5th ed.). Philadelphia: W. B. Saunders, pp. 1555–1556.

---

171. Before administering an intermittent tube feeding through a nasogastric tube, the nurse assesses for gastric residual. The nurse aspirates the stomach contents and withdraws 40 mL of undigested formula. What is the rationale for assessing gastric residual before administering the tube feeding?

1 To confirm proper nasogastric tube placement
2 To observe digestion of formula
3 To assess fluid and electrolyte status
4 To evaluate absorption of the last feeding

Answer: 4

Rationale: All the stomach contents are aspirated and measured before a tube feeding is administered. This procedure measures the gastric residual. The gastric residual is assessed in order to confirm whether undigested formula from a previous feeding remains and thereby enables the nurse to evaluate the absorption of the last feeding. It is important to assess gastric residual because administration of a tube feeding to a full stomach could result in overdistention, thus predisposing the client to regurgitation and possible aspiration.

Test-Taking Strategy: Carefully note the wording in each option. Option 1 can be eliminated because the description in the question does not concern tube placement. Option 3 can be eliminated because fluid and electrolyte status is not determined by this method. Select option 4 over option 2 because you cannot observe digestion. Rather, you would evaluate absorption of a feeding.

Level of Cognitive Ability: Analysis
Phase of Nursing Process: Assessment
Client Needs: Safe, Effective Care Environment
Content Area: Fundamental Skills

Reference

Luckmann, J. (1997). *Saunders manual of nursing care.* Philadelphia: W. B. Saunders, p. 316.

---

172. The client with tension pneumothorax begins to exhibit marked dyspnea and tracheal deviation. After calling the physician, the nurse would take which of the following actions as the next priority of care?

1 Call for a portable chest x-ray
2 Call the central supply room for a chest tube
3 Bring the code cart to the client's room
4 Bring an 18-gauge needle to the bedside

Answer: 4

Rationale: As an emergency measure, a tension pneumothorax may be converted to an open pneumothorax, which is a less serious problem. An 18-gauge needle is inserted into the affected pleural space at the second intercostal space, midclavicular line. This is a potentially life-saving measure, which results in immediate release of the tension pneumothorax, lung reexpansion, and correction of mediastinal shift. Once emergency treatment has been accomplished, a chest tube is inserted and attached to a closed chest drainage system.

Test-Taking Strategy: The key concept to recall in answering this question is what will need to be done to immediately release the tension pneumothorax. Using this line of reasoning, eliminate options 1 and 3 first. You would choose option 4 over option 2 because its use will provide an immediate benefit to the client. In addition, someone else could be asked to call for the chest tube.

Level of Cognitive Ability: Application
Phase of Nursing Process: Implementation
Client Needs: Safe, Effective Care Environment
Content Area: Adult Health/Respiratory

Reference

Black, J., & Matassarin-Jacobs, E. (1997). *Medical-surgical nursing: Clinical management for continuity of care* (5th ed.). Philadelphia: W. B. Saunders, p. 2526.

---

173. The client is being started on first-line antituberculosis medication. Which of the following antituberculosis medications would require the nurse to assess the client periodically for renal and auditory impairment?

1 Isoniazid (INH)
2 Rifampin (Rifadin)
3 Streptomycin
4 Ethambutol (Myambutol)

Answer: 3

Rationale: The aminoglycosides, which include streptomycin, are recognized for causing nephrotoxicity and auditory damage. A hallmark side effect of isoniazid is neuritis. With rifampin, the nurse must consider hepatic side effects. Ethambutol is associated with optic neuritis.

Test-Taking Strategy: Knowledge of the actions and uses of these medications is necessary to assist you in answering this question. If you are unfamiliar with the medications addressed in this question, it would be important to review them now!

Level of Cognitive Ability: Analysis
Phase of Nursing Process: Analysis
Client Needs: Safe, Effective Care Environment
Content Area: Pharmacology

Reference

Smeltzer, S., & Bare, B. (1996). *Brunner and Suddarth's Textbook of medical-surgical nursing* (8th ed.). Philadelphia: Lippincott-Raven, p. 498.

---

174. The nurse is caring for a client scheduled to undergo a renal biopsy. To help minimize the risk of postprocedure complications, the nurse plans to ensure that the results of which of the following laboratory studies is available and reported as necessary before the procedure?

1 Blood urea nitrogen (BUN) level, 25 mg/dL
2 Serum creatinine level, 1.9 mg/dL
3 Bleeding time, 13 minutes
4 Potassium level, 3.8 mEq/liter

Answer: 3

Rationale: Postprocedure hemorrhage is a significant complication of this procedure. Because of this, clotting times are assessed before the procedure. The nurse should plan to ensure that these results are available and to report abnormalities promptly.

Test-Taking Strategy: When a client is to have a biopsy, remember that bleeding is a concern. Begin to answer this question by eliminating option 4, because this is a normal value. To discriminate among the remaining options, it is necessary to know that bleeding is a complication after this procedure and that the bleeding time is prolonged. A prolonged bleeding time automatically places the client at increased risk. This would allow you to choose the correct option over the two slightly elevated renal function values.

Level of Cognitive Ability: Analysis
Phase of Nursing Process: Planning
Client Needs: Safe, Effective Care Environment
Content Area: Adult Health/Renal

Reference

Black, J., & Matassarin-Jacobs, E. (1997). *Medical-surgical nursing: Clinical management for continuity of care* (5th ed.). Philadelphia: W. B. Saunders, p. 1569.

175. The client was involved in a house fire, and an inhalation injury is suspected. Which of the following would be monitored for carbon monoxide poisoning?

1 Pulse oximetry
2 Urine myoglobin
3 Sputum carbon levels
4 Serum carboxyhemoglobin levels

Answer: 4

Rationale: Serum carboxyhemoglobin levels provide the most direct measure of carbon monoxide poisoning and would indicate the level of poisoning and thus determine the appropriate treatment measures. The carbon monoxide molecule's affinity for binding with hemoglobin is 200 times greater than that of an oxygen molecule, causing decreased availability of oxygen to the cells. Clients are treated with 100% oxygen.

Test-Taking Strategy: Knowledge of the method for determining carboxyhemoglobin levels is necessary to answer this question. Note the term "serum" in the correct option. This should provide you with the clue that this is the correct option. Take time now to review carbon monoxide poisoning, if you had difficulty with this question!

Level of Cognitive Ability: Analysis
Phase of Nursing Process: Assessment
Client Needs: Safe, Effective Care Environment
Content Area: Adult Health/Respiratory

Reference
Black, J., & Matassarin-Jacobs, E. (1997). *Medical-surgical nursing: Clinical management for continuity of care* (5th ed.). Philadelphia: W. B. Saunders, p. 2237.

---

176. The client with cystitis also has an indwelling urinary catheter. The nurse would plan to ensure that the nursing assistant does not

1 Use soap and water to cleanse the perineal area.
2 Keep the drainage bag below the level of the bladder.
3 Use the drainage tubing port to obtain urine samples.
4 Let the drainage tubing rest under the leg.

Answer: 4

Rationale: Proper care of an indwelling catheter is especially important for preventing prolonged infection or reinfection in the client with cystitis. The nurse and all caregivers must use strict aseptic technique when emptying the drainage bag or obtaining urine specimens. The perineal area is cleansed thoroughly using mild soap and water at least twice a day and after the client has a bowel movement. The drainage bag is kept below the level of the bladder to prevent urine from being trapped in the bladder, and for the same reason, the drainage tubing is not placed under the client's leg. The tubing must drain freely at all times.

Test-Taking Strategy: Eliminate option 1 first because this is a basic standard of care for the client with an indwelling catheter. Option 3 is also consistent with principles of asepsis and is eliminated next. To discriminate between options 2 and 4, recall that option 2 promotes drainage, whereas option 4 could impede drainage. Thus the answer to the question is option 4, according to the wording of the question.

Level of Cognitive Ability: Application
Phase of Nursing Process: Planning
Client Needs: Safe, Effective Care Environment
Content Area: Fundamental Skills

Reference
Black, J., & Matassarin-Jacobs, E. (1997). *Medical-surgical nursing: Clinical management for continuity of care* (5th ed.). Philadelphia: W. B. Saunders, p. 1573.

177. When caring for a woman with pre-eclampsia, the nurse should initiate which of the following actions?

1 Turning off room lights and drawing the window shades
2 Fluid and sodium restrictions
3 Measuring vital signs every 4 hours
4 Encouraging visits from family and friends for psychosocial support

Answer: 1

Rationale: Clients with pre-eclampsia are at risk of developing eclampsia (convulsion). Bright lights and sudden loud noises may bring about convulsions. A woman with pre-eclampsia is placed in a dim, quiet, private room. The nurse maintains a quiet, low-stimulus environment. Visitors are limited to allow for rest and to prevent overstimulation. Clients with pre-eclampsia have less plasma volume than normal, and therefore fluid and sodium restrictions are not recommended. Adequate fluid and sodium intake is necessary to maintain fluid volume and tissue perfusion. If magnesium sulfate therapy is instituted, fluid intake is closely monitored to prevent fluid overload. Vital signs are monitored closely when pre-eclampsia is present.

Test-Taking Strategy: Eliminate option 4 because physiological needs take priority over psychosocial needs in the client at risk for complications of a condition. Eliminate option 3 because vital signs need to be monitored more frequently than every 4 hours. For the remaining two options, knowing that seizures may be precipitated by sudden loud noises and bright lights will assist you in selecting the correct answer.

Level of Cognitive Ability: Application
Phase of Nursing Process: Implementation
Client's Needs: Safe, Effective Care Environment
Content Area: Maternity

Reference

Nichols, F., & Zwelling, E. (1997). *Maternal-newborn nursing: Theory and practice.* Philadelphia: W. B. Saunders, p. 651.

178. In planning care for the client with hypertonic labor contractions, the nurse understands the importance of conserving energy and promoting rest. This can be facilitated by

1 Avoiding the use of uncomfortable procedures such as intravenous infusions or epidural anesthesia.
2 Assisting the client with breathing and relaxation techniques.
3 Keeping the room brightly lit so the client can watch her monitor.
4 Keeping the television or radio on to provide distraction.

Answer: 2

Rationale: Breathing and relaxation techniques aid the client in coping with the discomfort of labor and in conserving energy. Maternal exhaustion is a risk with the severe discomfort of hypertonic contractions, which generally occur during the early or latent phase of labor. Intravenous or epidural pain relief can be useful. Intravenous hydration can increase perfusion and oxygenation of maternal and fetal tissues and provide glucose for energy needs. Noise and light stimulation do not promote rest; a quiet, dim environment would be more advantageous.

Test-Taking Strategy: The case situation states the importance of conserving energy and promoting rest for the client. Remember Maslow's hierarchy of needs theory to prioritize: meet physiological needs first. Option 2 is the only option that addresses the physiological issue of the question.

Level of Cognitive Ability: Application
Phase of Nursing Process: Planning
Client Needs: Safe, Effective Care Environment
Content Area: Maternity

Reference

Nichols, F., & Zwelling, E. (1997). *Maternal-newborn nursing: Theory and practice.* Philadelphia: W. B. Saunders, p. 778.

179. The client with acute pyelonephritis has nausea and vomiting and is scheduled for intravenous pyelography. The nurse should plan to take which of the following actions as the highest priority?

1 Monitor intake and output hourly
2 Request an order for IV therapy from the physician
3 Ask the client to sign the informed consent
4 Explain the procedure thoroughly to the client

Answer: 2

Rationale: The highest priority of the nurse should be to obtain an order for IV therapy. This is needed to replace fluid lost with vomiting and will be necessary for dye injection for the procedure. The intake and output should be measured, but this will not yield optimal results if the client becomes dehydrated from vomiting. Explanation of the procedure and obtaining the signed consent are done once the client's physiological needs are met.

Test-Taking Strategy: The question asks for the option that has the highest priority, which implies that more than one of the actions are correct. Option 4 has the lowest priority because the client is in distress, and it is therefore eliminated first. Monitoring the client's intake and output is helpful but does not actively assist the client; therefore, you would eliminate option 1 next. Options 2 and 3 compete for priority. However, knowing that an access route is needed to replace fluid losses and avoid dehydration helps you choose option 2 over option 3 as the correct answer.

Level of Cognitive Ability: Application
Phase of Nursing Process: Planning
Client Needs: Safe, Effective Care Environment
Content Area: Adult Health/Renal

Reference

Black, J., & Matassarin-Jacobs, E. (1997). *Medical-surgical nursing: Clinical management for continuity of care* (5th ed.). Philadelphia: W. B. Saunders, p. 1629.

---

180. In planning care for a client with a T3 spinal cord injury, the nurse is aware that autonomic dysreflexia is a possible complication. Which of the following interventions should be included in the plan?

1 Assess vital signs, observing for hypotension, tachycardia, and tachypnea
2 Teach the client that this condition is relatively minor with few symptoms
3 Assist client in developing a daily bowel routine to prevent constipation
4 Administer dexamethasone (Decadron) as per physician's order

Answer: 3

Rationale: Autonomic dysreflexia may be triggered by bowel distention. A daily bowel program eliminates this trigger. A client with autonomic dysreflexia would be hypertensive and bradycardic. Autonomic dysreflexia is potentially life-threatening if intervention does not occur. Removal of the stimuli results in prompt resolution of the signs and symptoms. Option 4 is unrelated to this specific condition.

Test-Taking Strategy: Knowledge about autonomic dysreflexia is necessary to correctly answer this question. Remembering that this condition may be triggered by bowel distention will assist in directing you to the correct option. If you are unfamiliar with this syndrome, it would be important to review!

Level of Cognitive Ability: Application
Phase of Nursing Process: Planning
Client Needs: Safe, Effective Care Environment
Content Area: Adult Health/Musculoskeletal

Reference

Burrell, L., Gerlach, M., & Pless, B. (1997). *Adult nursing: Acute and community care* (2nd ed.). Stamford, CT: Appleton & Lange, p. 959.

181. The client is scheduled for bronchoscopy. The nurse should plan for which of the following measures as the highest priority item?

1 Restricting the diet to clear liquids on the day of the test
2 Asking the client about allergies to shellfish
3 Obtaining informed consent for an invasive procedure
4 Administration of preprocedure antibiotics prophylactically

Answer: 3

Rationale: Bronchoscopy requires that informed consent be obtained from the client before the procedure. The client is kept on NPO status for at least 6 hours before the procedure. It is unnecessary to inquire about allergies to shellfish before this procedure because no contrast dye is injected. There is also no need for prophylactic antibiotics.

Test-Taking Strategy: This question can be answered quickly and correctly just by knowing that bronchoscopy is an invasive procedure and, as such, requires completion of an informed consent specific for this procedure. If this question was difficult, review this procedure briefly!

Level of Cognitive Ability: Application
Phase of Nursing Process: Planning
Client Needs: Safe, Effective Care Environment
Content Area: Adult Health/Respiratory

Reference

Smeltzer, S., & Bare, B. (1996). *Brunner and Suddarth's Textbook of medical-surgical nursing* (8th ed.). Philadelphia: Lippincott-Raven, p. 455.

---

182. The client in cardiogenic shock has an order for an intravenous nitroglycerin (Nitrostat) drip for control of chest pain and to increase myocardial tissue perfusion. The nurse knows that the nitroglycerin must be prepared by mixing the medication

1 In solution that is in a plastic bag.
2 In solution that is in a glass bottle.
3 Every 2 hours because it is unstable.
4 Under a laminar flow hood.

Answer: 2

Rationale: Intravenous nitroglycerin is prepared only in glass bottles, with the administration sets provided. Standard plastic (polyvinyl chloride) tubings will cause nitroglycerin to adsorb, thus reducing the potency and reliability of the infusion. It should also be protected from extremes of light and temperature. It should be remixed every 4 hours. It does not require mixture under a laminar flow hood.

Test-Taking Strategy: Options 1 and 2 provide two opposite methods of administration, which should provide a clue that one of these methods may be accurate. Remembering that standard plastic tubings will cause nitroglycerin to adsorb, thus reducing the potency and reliability of the infusion, will assist in directing you to the correct option!

Level of Cognitive Ability: Analysis
Phase of Nursing Process: Implementation
Client Needs: Safe, Effective Care Environment
Content Area: Pharmacology

Reference

Hodgson, B., & Kizior, R. (1998). *Saunders nursing drug handbook 1998.* Philadelphia: W. B. Saunders, p. 750.

---

183. A client had a cervical cord transection 2 months ago and is now in a rehabilitation center. Which of the following instructions is most appropriate for the nurse to give to the assistant as they are planning the client's care?

1 Insert an indwelling catheter if the client cannot void
2 Keep the client in supine position
3 Keep the side rails up while the client is in bed
4 Give the client an enema if the client cannot defecate

Answer: 3

Rationale: In cord-injured clients, spasticity develops when spinal cord shock subsides, about 3–6 weeks after the injury. Leg spasms may be strong enough to cause a fall from the bed. Therefore, the side rails must be up. Additional instructions should include turning the client side to side every 2 hours while the client is in bed and implementing bowel and bladder retraining, such as intermittent catheterization and digital stimulation of the bowel.

Test-Taking Strategy: Pay close attention to time frameworks when they are included in the question. In this case, the time frame of 2 months indicates that paralysis is spastic rather than flaccid. Eliminate options 1 and 4 because they require the use of invasive techniques. Of the remaining two options, option 2 addresses the issue of safety.

Level of Cognitive Ability: Application
Phase of Nursing Process: Planning
Client Needs: Safe, Effective Care Environment
Content Area: Adult Health/Neuromuscular

Reference

Smeltzer, S., & Bare, B. (1996). *Brunner and Suddarth's Textbook of medical-surgical nursing* (8th ed.). Philadelphia: Lippincott-Raven, pp. 1800, 1808.

---

184. The nurse has given a subcutaneous injection to the client with acquired immunodeficiency syndrome (AIDS). The nurse disposes of the used needle and syringe by

1 Placing the uncapped needle and syringe in a labeled, rigid plastic container.
2 Recapping the needle and discarding the syringe in the disposal unit.
3 Breaking the needle before discarding it.
4 Placing the uncapped needle and syringe in a labeled cardboard box.

Answer: 1

Rationale: Universal precautions include specific guidelines for handling of needles. Needles should not be recapped, bent, broken, or cut after use. They should be disposed of in a labeled, impermeable container specific for this purpose. Needles should not be discarded in cardboard boxes, because such boxes are not impervious. Needles should never be left lying around after use.

Test-Taking Strategy: This question tests fundamental and vitally important concepts related to the handling of sharps. If this question was problematic in any way, take a few moments now to review these principles.

Level of Cognitive Ability: Application
Phase of Nursing Process: Implementation
Client Needs: Safe, Effective Care Environment
Content Area: Fundamental Skills

Reference

Black, J., & Matassarin-Jacobs, E. (1997). *Medical-surgical nursing: Clinical management for continuity of care* (5th ed.). Philadelphia: W. B. Saunders, p. 620.

---

185. The client has a left pleural effusion that has not yet been treated. The nurse plans to have which of the following items available for immediate use?

1 Thoracentesis tray
2 Paracentesis tray
3 Intubation tray
4 Central line insertion tray

Answer: 1

Rationale: The client with a significant pleural effusion is usually treated by thoracentesis. This procedure allows drainage of the fluid, which is then analyzed to determine the precise cause of the effusion. The nurse ensures that a thoracentesis tray is readily available, in case the client's symptoms rapidly become more severe. A paracentesis tray is needed for the removal of abdominal effusion. Options 3 and 4 are not specifically indicated for this procedure.

Test-Taking Strategy: To answer this question accurately, it is necessary to know the usual treatment for pleural effusion. Noting the word "pleural" in the question may assist you in determining the relationship to option 1. If this question was difficult, take a few moments now to review thoracentesis and pleural effusion!

Level of Cognitive Ability: Application
Phase of Nursing Process: Planning
Client Needs: Safe, Effective Care Environment
Content Area: Adult Health/Respiratory

Reference

Smeltzer, S., & Bare, B. (1996). *Brunner and Suddarth's Textbook of medical-surgical nursing* (8th ed.). Philadelphia: Lippincott-Raven, p. 503.

186. The nurse is caring for the client with acute glomerulonephritis. The nurse instructs the nursing assistant to do which of the following to provide a safe environment for the client?

1. Monitor the temperature every 2 hours
2. Remove the water pitcher from the bedside
3. Ambulate the client frequently
4. Encourage a diet that is high in protein

Answer: 2

Rationale: The client with acute glomerulonephritis commonly experiences fluid volume excess and fatigue. Interventions include fluid restriction, as well as monitoring weight and monitoring intake and output. The client is placed on bed rest, or at least encouraged to rest, because proteinuria and hematuria are directly correlated with increased activity levels. The diet is high in calories but low in protein. It is unnecessary to monitor the temperature as frequently as every 2 hours.

Test-Taking Strategy: The stem of the question does not tell you about the client's actual temperature, so option 1 may be eliminated first. Knowing that the client needs rest enables you to eliminate option 3. To choose correctly between the two remaining options, it is necessary to know either that fluids are restricted or to know that protein is limited. Knowledge of either concept would enable you to choose option 2. Review interventions related to this condition now if you had difficulty with this question!

Level of Cognitive Ability: Application
Phase of Nursing Process: Planning
Client Needs: Safe, Effective Care Environment
Content Area: Adult Health/Renal

Reference

Black, J., & Matassarin-Jacobs, E. (1997). *Medical-surgical nursing: Clinical management for continuity of care* (5th ed.). Philadelphia: W. B. Saunders, p. 1632.

187. Which nursing implementation should be used during the spinal shock phase to prepare a client with a C6 spinal cord injury for sitting in a chair?

1. Teaching the client to lock the knees during the pivoting stage of the transfer
2. Giving a vasodilator before the client sits, in order to improve circulation of lower limbs
3. Raising the head of the bed slowly to decrease orthostatic hypotensive episodes
4. Applying knee splints to stabilize the joints during transfer

Answer: 3

Rationale: Spinal shock is often accompanied by vasodilation of lower limbs, which results in a fall in blood pressure when the client rises. The client may have dizziness and feel faint. The nurse should provide for a gradual progression in head elevation while monitoring the blood pressure. Thigh-length elastic stocking and vasopressors can be used as well.

Test-Taking Strategy: This question requires knowledge of the effect of spinal cord injuries on blood pressure. Vasodilation is the physiological problem, which would be exacerbated by vasodilators; therefore, eliminate option 2. Clients with cervical cord injuries cannot lock their knees, and the use of braces would impair the transfer. This should assist you in eliminating options 1 and 4.

Level of Cognitive Ability: Application
Phase of Nursing Process: Implementation
Client Needs: Safe, Effective Care Environment
Content Area: Adult Health/Musculoskeletal

Reference

Smeltzer, S., & Bare, B. (1996). *Brunner and Suddarth's Textbook of medical-surgical nursing* (8th ed.). Philadelphia: Lippincott-Raven, pp. 1803–1804.

188. Early ambulation is encouraged to avoid cardiovascular and respiratory complications. As the nurse assists the client in progressing from a lying position to ambulation, safety should be a primary concern. Which of the following actions would be most appropriate to maintain the safety of the client?

1 Assisting the client to move quickly from the lying position to the sitting position
2 Assessing the client for signs of dizziness and hypotension in the sitting position
3 Elevating the head of the bed quickly to assist the client to a sitting position
4 Allowing the client to rise from the bed to a standing position unassisted

Answer: 2

Rationale: Early ambulation should not exceed the client's tolerance. The client is assisted in rising from the lying position to the sitting position gradually until any evidence of dizziness has subsided. This position can be achieved by raising the head of the bed slowly. After sitting, the client may be assisted to a standing position. The nurse should be at the client's side to give physical support and encouragement.

Test-Taking Strategy: By the process of elimination determine that option 2 would provide the greatest degree of safety for the client. Options 1, 3, and 4 contain unsafe activities such as moving quickly and not assisting the client.

Level of Cognitive Ability: Application
Phase of Nursing Process: Implementation
Client Needs: Safe, Effective Care Environment
Content Area: Adult Health/Cardiovascular

Reference

Smeltzer, S., & Bare, B. (1996). *Brunner and Suddarth's Textbook of medical-surgical nursing* (8th ed.). Philadelphia: Lippincott-Raven, p. 401.

---

189. The client is taking procainamide (Pronestyl), 500 mg PO q 6 hr. The nurse prepares to give the medication. Which of the following should be the first action the nurse takes before giving the medication?

1 Nothing, because this is a nontoxic drug
2 Assessing the client for side effects of the medication
3 Scheduling the client for a drug level 1 hour after the first dose
4 Monitoring vital signs and electrocardiogram continuously

Answer: 2

Rationale: This medication may cause such side effects as diarrhea, nausea and vomiting, and heart failure; therefore, the client should be assessed before the administration of the medication. Although vital signs need to be monitored, continuous monitoring is not necessary. Option 1 is inappropriate, and option 3 is not an action taken before administration of the medication.

Test-Taking Strategy: Options 1 and 3 are inappropriate options. Both options 2 and 4 are appropriate; however, option 4 is not the best option because that action will take place after the medication is given. Side effects of a medication will need to be brought to the physician's attention if present. The physician then decides whether the medication should be given. Review this medication now if you had difficulty with this question!

Level of Cognitive Ability: Application
Phase of Nursing Process: Planning
Client Needs: Safe, Effective Care Environment
Content Area: Pharmacology

Reference

Luckmann, J. (1997). *Saunders manual of nursing care.* Philadelphia: W. B. Saunders, p. 1014.

---

190. The client with urolithiasis is being evaluated to determine the type of stone that is being formed. The nurse would plan to keep which of the following items available in the client's room to assist in this process?

1 A calorie count sheet
2 A strainer
3 An intake and output record
4 A vital signs graphic sheet

Answer: 2

Rationale: The urine is strained during the waiting period until stones are obtained and analyzed. Strainers will catch small stones that may be sent to the laboratory for analysis. Once the type of stone is determined, an individualized plan of care and prevention is developed.

Test-Taking Strategy: Note that the stem of the question asks for an item that will help to determine the type of stone. Therefore, even if several of the options may be appropriate for use with the client with urolithiasis, you must select the one that is specific for this purpose. Begin by eliminating options 3 and 4 because these items give information about vital signs and fluid balance but will not provide data that will help determine the type of calculus. Of the remaining two, you would choose option 2 over option 1 if you knew that straining the urine would enable possible capture of crystals or small calculi, which could then be sent to the laboratory for analysis.

Level of Cognitive Ability: Application
Phase of Nursing Process: Planning
Client Needs: Safe, Effective Care Environment
Content Area: Adult Health/Renal

Reference

Luckmann, J. (1997). *Saunders manual of nursing care.* Philadelphia: W. B. Saunders, p. 1217.

---

191. The nurse caring for a client with bilateral wheezes, orthopnea, tachypnea, and 2+ pitting edema suspects pulmonary edema and notifies the physician. What nursing action while waiting for the physician would be unsafe for the client?

1 Obtaining morphine sulfate (MS) IV
2 Placing the client in high Fowler's position
3 Elevating the client's legs
4 Obtaining IV nitroprusside (Nipride)

Answer: 3

Rationale: Elevating the client's legs would rapidly increase venous return to the right side of the heart and worsen the client's condition. The feet should be in the horizontal position, or they could dangle at the bedside if the client's condition permits. Morphine reduces anxiety; anxiety causes an increase in the oxygen demands on the heart. A high Fowler's position increases the thoracic capacity, allowing for improved ventilation. Nitroprusside (Nipride) is the drug of choice for treating client's with pulmonary edema. It is a potent vasodilator that reduces preload and afterload.

Test-Taking Strategy: Knowledge of the pathophysiology of acute pulmonary edema and the care of the client is necessary to answer this question. Knowing that the pulmonary system is congested will assist in directing you to option 3 as being unsafe because this action would cause further congestion of the pulmonary system!

Level of Cognitive Ability: Application
Phase of Nursing Process: Implementation
Client Needs: Safe, Effective Care Environment
Content Area: Adult Health/Cardiovascular

Reference

Black, J., & Matassarin-Jacobs, E. (1997). *Medical-surgical nursing: Clinical management for continuity of care* (5th ed.). Philadelphia: W. B. Saunders, p. 1283.

---

192. The nurse is caring for a client who has had a ureterolithotomy. The nurse has a PRN order to irrigate the ureteral catheter. The nurse would plan to avoid which of the following in the management of this catheter?

1 Irrigating, using gentle force
2 Irrigating, using gravity
3 Clamping the tube
4 Using a separate drainage bag for that catheter

Answer: 3

Rationale: A ureteral tube is never clamped, because the renal pelvis can hold only about 5 mL at a time. The nurse who has an order to irrigate the tube may do so by using gravity or gentle force only. A drainage bag for that specific catheter alone is used so that urine flow can be accurately measured.

Test-Taking Strategy: Because the question asks for an item that is to be avoided, you would look for an item that would be contraindicated. Eliminate option 4 first, because drainage from a ureteral catheter may often be monitored. Irrigation of a gentle nature, such as in options 1 and 2, is also acceptable, and thus they are eliminated next. This leaves option 3 as the item to avoid. Ureteral catheters are never clamped.

Level of Cognitive Ability: Application
Phase of Nursing Process: Planning
Client Needs: Safe, Effective Care Environment
Content Area: Adult Health/Renal

Reference

Black, J., & Matassarin-Jacobs, E. (1997). *Medical-surgical nursing: Clinical management for continuity of care* (5th ed.). Philadelphia: W. B. Saunders, p. 1598.

193. A nurse is caring for a client with cardiac tamponade. In planning for the client's safety, the nurse does not leave the client unattended. The most important reason for this is

1 The client may suffer infarction.
2 The client may have a cerebral vascular accident (CVA).
3 The client may panic and be injured.
4 The client is at risk for hemorrhage.

Answer: 3

Rationale: As fluid rapidly accumulates in the pericardium, the client may suddenly have a sense of impending doom or panic. Cardiac tamponade is a medical emergency, and the client should not be left unattended. Options 1, 2, and 4 are medical complications.

Test-Taking Strategy: The issue of the question relates to safety considerations for the client. Option 3 deals directly with the client's safety. Note the key word "safety" in the question and "injured" in the correct option.

Level of Cognitive Ability: Analysis
Phase of Nursing Process: Planning
Client Needs: Safe, Effective Care Environment
Content Area: Adult Health/Cardiovascular

Reference

Black, J., & Matassarin-Jacobs, E. (1997). *Medical-surgical nursing: Clinical management for continuity of care* (5th ed.). Philadelphia: W. B. Saunders, p. 1337.

194. A client's lithium level is 3.9 mEq/L. The highest priority nursing intervention for this client includes

1 Determining visual acuity.
2 Balancing intake and output.
3 Keeping side rails up.
4 Instituting seizure precautions.

Answer: 4

Rationale: The therapeutic regimen is designed to attain a serum lithium level of 1.0–1.5 mEq/L during acute mania and levels of 0.6–1.4 mEq/L for maintenance treatment. A level of 3.9 mEq/L is within the toxic range, and one of the complications is the possibility of seizures. Seizures may occur at levels of 3.5 mEq/L and higher. The other interventions are necessary but not, however, a priority.

Test-Taking Strategy: The question asks for a priority action; therefore, all choices are probably correct. When all choices seem to be correct, select the one option that is the most critical and relates to the issue of the question. Option 4 is the most global response and is therefore correct. Review toxicity related to lithium and the manifestations that occur as a result of toxicity now if you had difficulty with this question!

Level of Cognitive Ability: Analysis
Phase of Nursing Process: Implementation
Client Needs: Safe, Effective Care Environment
Content Area: Pharmacology

Reference

Hodgson, B., & Kizior, R. (1998). *Saunders nursing drug handbook 1998*. Philadelphia: W. B. Saunders, pp. 598–600.

195. The client with a diagnosis of anorexia nervosa, who is in a state of starvation, is in a two-bed room. A newly admitted client will be assigned to this client's room. Which of the following would be the worst choice for this client's roommate?

1 A client with pneumonia
2 A client with a fractured leg
3 A client who could benefit from the client's assistance at mealtime
4 A client who thrives on managing others

Answer: 1

Rationale: The client who has been starving has a compromised immune system. Having a roommate with pneumonia would put the client at risk for infection. The client with a fractured leg is an acceptable roommate. The client should not be put in a position in which he or she is able to focus on the nutritional needs of others or being managed by others, because this may contribute to sublimation and suppression of his or her own hunger. However, such roommates are not as dangerous as one with pneumonia.

Test-Taking Strategy: The key phrase is "in a state of starvation." Use Maslow's hierarchy of needs to answer the question. The priority needs of the client with anorexia nervosa are physiological. The plan of care involves keeping the client free from opportunistic infections. This should direct you to option 1.

Level of Cognitive Ability: Application
Phase of Nursing Process: Planning
Client Needs: Safe, Effective Care Environment
Content Area: Mental Health

Reference

Wilson, H., & Kneisl, C. (1996). *Psychiatric nursing* (5th ed.). Menlo Park, CA: Addison-Wesley, pp. 427, 443.

---

196. A child is hospitalized with an undiagnosed exanthema (rash) profusely covering the trunk and sparsely on the extremities. The child was exposed to varicella 2 weeks ago. The most appropriate nursing intervention will be

1 Allowing the client to play in the playroom until you can contact the physician.
2 Placing client in a private room on strict isolation.
3 Immediately admitting the client to any available bed.
4 Assessing the progression of the exanthema and reporting it to physician.

Answer: 2

Rationale: The client with undiagnosed exanthema needs to be placed in strict isolation. Varicella causes a profuse rash on the trunk with a sparse rash on the extremities. The incubation period is 14–21 days. It is important to prevent the spread of this communicable disease by placing the client in isolation until further diagnosis is made and treatment is instituted.

Test-Taking Strategy: Option 2 prevents the client from exposing other children to varicella and keeps staff, visitors, and other people at minimal risk. Option 1 exposes other children or the environment unnecessarily to varicella. Admitting the child to "any" room is inappropriate. Assessing the progression of the exanthema is correct, but it is not the most appropriate immediate intervention.

Level of Cognitive Ability: Application
Phase of Nursing Process: Implementation
Client Needs: Safe, Effective Care Environment
Content Area: Child Health

Reference

Wong, D. (1997). *Whaley and Wong's Essentials of pediatric nursing* (5th ed.). St. Louis: Mosby–Year Book, pp. 401, 403.

---

197. The nurse has aspirated 40 mL of undigested formula from the client's nasogastric tube before administering an intermittent tube feeding. The nurse understands that before administering the tube feeding, the 40 mL of gastric aspirate should be

1 Discarded properly and recorded as output on the client's input and output record.
2 Poured into the nasogastric tube through a syringe with the plunger removed.
3 Mixed with the formula and poured into the nasogastric tube through a syringe without a plunger.
4 Diluted with water and injected into the nasogastric tube by putting pressure on the plunger.

Answer: 2

Rationale: After checking residual feeding contents, reinstill the gastric contents into the stomach by removing the syringe bulb or plunger, and pour the gastric contents via the syringe into the nasogastric tube. Gastric contents should be reinstilled in order to maintain the client's electrolyte balance. The gastric contents should be poured into the nasogastric tube. The aspirate of the gastric contents does not need to be mixed with water; it should not be discarded; and it should not be injected by pushing on the plunger.

Test-Taking Strategy: Remembering that the removal of the gastric contents could disturb the client's electrolyte balance will assist in eliminating option 1. Eliminate option 4 because of the word "pressure." Knowledge that gastric contents aspirated should be immediately replaced will assist in directing you to the correct option. Review this procedure now if you had difficulty with this question!

Level of Cognitive Ability: Application
Phase of Nursing Process: Implementation
Client Needs: Safe, Effective Care Environment
Content Area: Fundamental Skills

Reference

Kozier, B., Erb, G., & Blais, K. (1998). *Fundamentals of nursing: Concepts, process, and practice* (5th ed.). Menlo Park, CA: Addison-Wesley, p. 1050.

198. The nurse is caring for the client with suspected carbon monoxide poisoning, who is an otherwise healthy 25-year-old person. The nurse assists in implementing the following interventions; which is of highest priority?

1 Requesting a building inspection from the local health department
2 Drawing blood for measuring carboxyhemoglobin levels
3 Frequently observing the client
4 Administering 100% oxygen

Answer: 4

Rationale: One hundred percent oxygen is administered at atmospheric pressure or hyperbaric pressure to speed up the elimination of carbon monoxide from the hemoglobin and to reverse hypoxia. The next most important action is constant observation of the client. After resuscitation, the client may exhibit a variety of symptoms resulting from central nervous system damage, which include ataxia, spastic paralysis, visual disturbances, personality changes, and psychoses. Blood is drawn serially to monitor carboxyhemoglobin levels; once they drop under 5%, oxygen may be removed. If the episode was unintentional and precipitated by conditions in a dwelling, the Health Department is notified.

Test-Taking Strategy: Begin to answer this question by eliminating options 1 and 2, which are of the lowest immediate priority. To discriminate between options 3 and 4, knowing that the client requires oxygen therapy helps you to choose this over the alternative of observing the client frequently. From another perspective, knowing that the client needs continuous, not frequent, supervision would also lead you to the correct answer.

Level of Cognitive Ability: Application
Phase of Nursing Process: Implementation
Client Needs: Safe, Effective Care Environment
Content Area: Adult Health/Respiratory

Reference

Smeltzer, S., & Bare, B. (1996). *Brunner and Suddarth's Textbook of medical-surgical nursing* (8th ed.). Philadelphia: Lippincott-Raven, p. 2025.

---

199. The nurse is observing a second nurse who is performing hemodialysis on a client. The second nurse is drinking coffee and eating a doughnut next to the hemodialysis machine, while talking with the client about the events of the client's week. The first nurse should

1 Appreciate what a wonderful therapeutic relationship this nurse and client have.
2 Disregard this behavior as unprofessional.
3 Ask the client if he or she would like a cup of coffee also.
4 Ask the nurse to refrain from eating and drinking in that area.

Answer: 4

Rationale: A potential complication with hemodialysis is the acquisition of dialysis-associated hepatitis B. This is a concern for clients (who may carry the virus), clients' families (at risk from contact with client and with environmental surfaces), and staff (who may acquire the virus from contact with the client's blood). This risk is minimized by use of universal precautions, appropriate handwashing and sterilization procedures, and the prohibition of eating, drinking, smoking, or other hand-to-mouth activity in the hemodialysis unit. The first nurse should ask the second nurse to stop eating and drinking in the work area.

Test-Taking Strategy: To answer this question correctly, you need to have an understanding of the potential complications of hemodialysis and their prevention. Using the process of elimination and the principles related to universal precautions will assist in directing you to the correct option. If needed, take a few moments now to review this material!

Level of Cognitive Ability: Application
Phase of Nursing Process: Implementation
Client Needs: Safe, Effective Care Environment
Content Area: Adult Health/Renal

Reference

Potter, P., & Perry, A. (1997). *Fundamentals of nursing: Concepts, process, and practice* (4th ed.). St. Louis: Mosby–Year Book, p. 755.

200. The client with adult respiratory distress syndrome has an order to be placed on a continuous positive airway pressure (CPAP) face mask. The nurse would make sure to do which of the following for this procedure to be most effective?

1 Apply the mask to the face with a snug fit
2 Obtain baseline arterial blood gas measurements
3 Obtain baseline arterial oxygen saturation level measurements
4 Allow the client to remove the mask frequently for coughing

Answer: 1

Rationale: The face mask must be applied over the nose and mouth with a tight fit, which is necessary to maintain positive pressure in the client's airways. The nurse does obtain baseline respiratory assessments and arterial blood gas measurements to evaluate the effectiveness of therapy, but these do not increase the effectiveness of the procedure, as the question asks. A disadvantage of the CPAP face mask is that the client must remove it for coughing, eating, or drinking. This removes benefit of positive pressure in the airway each time it is removed.

Test-Taking Strategy: The question asks about a nursing action that will make the procedure most effective. Options 2 and 3 are good nursing actions, but they do not make the therapy more effective, and so they are eliminated. To discriminate between the remaining options, knowing that positive pressure must be maintained to be effective helps you to choose the tight fitting mask over removing it frequently.

Level of Cognitive Ability: Application
Phase of Nursing Process: Planning
Client Needs: Safe, Effective Care Environment
Content Area: Adult Health/Respiratory

Reference
Luckmann, J. (1997). *Saunders manual of nursing care.* Philadelphia: W. B. Saunders, p. 966.

---

201. The client with obsessive-compulsive disorder spends many hours during the day and night washing hands. When initially planning for a safe environment, the nurse allows the client to continue this behavior because

1 It relieves the client's anxiety.
2 It decreases the chance of infection.
3 It gives the client a feeling of self-control.
4 It increases self-esteem.

Answer: 1

Rationale: The compulsive act provides immediate relief from anxiety and is used to cope with psychic stress, conflict, or pain. Although the client may feel the need to increase self-esteem, that is not the primary goal.

Test-Taking Strategy: Knowledge regarding the behavior associated with compulsive disorders is necessary to answer the question. If you are unfamiliar with this content, take time now to review this important disorder!

Level of Cognitive Ability: Analysis
Phase of Nursing Process: Planning
Client Needs: Safe, Effective Care Environment
Content Area: Mental Health

Reference
Carson, V., & Arnold, E. (1996). *Mental health nursing: The nurse-patient journey.* Philadelphia: W. B. Saunders, p. 702.

202. A client is scheduled to undergo cardiac catheterization for the first time. Which of the following points would the nurse plan to include in preprocedure teaching?

1 The procedure is performed in the operating room, with the personnel wearing scrub gowns and masks
2 The client may feel fatigue and have various aches, because it is necessary to lie quietly on a hard x-ray table for about 4 hours
3 The client may feel certain sensations at various points during the procedure, such as a fluttery feeling, a flushed, warm feeling, a desire to cough, or palpitations
4 The initial catheter insertion is quite painful; after that, there is little or no pain

Answer: 3

Rationale: Preprocedure teaching points include that the procedure is done in a darkened cardiac catheterization room and that ECG leads are attached to the limbs. A local anesthetic is used, so there is little to no pain with catheter insertion, and the x-ray table is hard and may be tilted periodically. The procedure may take up to 2 hours, and the client may feel various sensations with catheter passage and dye injection.

Test-Taking Strategy: The wording of the question makes you look for a correct statement. The operating room location (option 1) is incorrect; the duration of the procedure in option 2 (4 hours) is incorrect; and the phrase "quite painful" in option 4 is incorrect. If you had difficulty with this question, take time now to review the client preparation for this procedure!

Level of Cognitive Ability: Application
Phase of Nursing Process: Planning
Client Needs: Safe, Effective Care Environment
Content Area: Adult Health/Cardiovascular

Reference

Black, J., & Matassarin-Jacobs, E. (1997). *Medical-surgical nursing: Clinical management for continuity of care* (5th ed.). Philadelphia: W. B. Saunders, p. 1231.

---

203. The nurse has inserted an indwelling Foley catheter, inflates the balloon, and releases the hold on the catheter. The client immediately complains of pain. Which of the following represents the best plan by the nurse?

1 Tell the client that the discomfort will pass
2 Withdraw 1 mL from the balloon of the catheter
3 Deflate the balloon and push it further into the bladder
4 Deflate the balloon and replace it with another catheter

Answer: 4

Rationale: The appropriate procedure if the client complains of pain after insertion is to remove the catheter after deflating the balloon and replace it with another catheter. This is preferred to option 3, which could put the client more at risk for developing urinary tract infection, because the catheter would be advanced after part of it was resting against the client's external genitalia. Options 1 and 2 are totally incorrect.

Test-Taking Strategy: Options 1 and 2 are the least plausible and should be eliminated first. You would be able to discriminate correctly between options 3 and 4 by using principles of aseptic technique. Review this procedure now if you had difficulty with this question!

Level of Cognitive Ability: Application
Phase of Nursing Process: Planning
Client Needs: Safe, Effective Care Environment
Content Area: Fundamental Skills

Reference

Taylor, C., Lillis, C., & LeMone, P. (1997). *Fundamentals of nursing: The art and science of nursing care* (3rd ed.). Philadelphia: Lippincott-Raven, p. 1237.

204. The client with AIDS will be receiving aerosolized pentamidine isethionate (NebuPent) prophylactically once every 4 weeks. The public health nurse visits and instructs the client about the drug. Which of the following statements would not be a component of the teaching plan?

1. "If you develop a cough or shortness of breath after receiving pentamidine inhalation therapy, let a doctor or nurse know."
2. "If you have any visual disturbances, let the doctor know."
3. "There are no known side effects of aerosolized pentamidine."
4. "You may experience some nausea with aerosolized pentamidine."

Answer: 3

Rationale: The nurse needs to provide the client with accurate information so that safety is ensured with administration and monitoring of this medication. Options 1, 2, and 4 are correct statements.

Test-Taking Strategy: Knowledge about the side effects of pentamidine would help you answer this question. Options 1, 2, and 4 are all specific side effects of this medication. If you were unfamiliar with this medication, note that option 3, the only option without specific side effects, is therefore different and most likely to be the correct answer. Review this medication now if you had difficulty with this question!

Level of Cognitive Ability: Application
Phase of Nursing Process: Planning
Client Needs: Safe, Effective Care Environment
Content Area: Pharmacology

Reference

Hodgson, B., & Kizior, R. (1998). *Saunders nursing drug handbook 1998.* Philadelphia: W. B. Saunders, p. 801.

---

205. The nurse is caring for the client who is going to undergo arthrography with a contrast medium. Which of the following assessments by the nurse would be of highest priority?

1. Allergy to iodine or shellfish
2. Ability of the client to remain still during the procedure
3. Whether the client has any remaining questions about the procedure
4. Whether the client wishes to void before the procedure

Answer: 1

Rationale: Because of the risk of allergy to contrast dye, the nurse places highest priority on assessing whether the client has an allergy to iodine or shellfish. The nurse also reinforces information about the test, tells the client about the need to remain still during the procedure, and encourages the client to void before the procedure for comfort.

Test-Taking Strategy: Note that this question asks which option is of the "highest priority." This tells you that more than one or all of the options are correct (in fact, they all are). Although options 2, 3, and 4 all are important, only option 1 obviously concerns medical risk. The consequence of possible anaphylactic shock (physiological risk) makes this the correct choice.

Level of Cognitive Ability: Analysis
Phase of Nursing Process: Assessment
Client Needs: Safe, Effective Care Environment
Content Area: Adult Health/Musculoskeletal

Reference

Black, J., & Matassarin-Jacobs, E. (1997). *Medical-surgical nursing: Clinical management for continuity of care* (5th ed.). Philadelphia: W. B. Saunders, p. 2094.

---

206. The client with possible rib fracture has never had a chest x-ray. The nurse would plan to tell the client which of the following items about the procedure?

1. The x-rays stimulate a small amount of pain
2. It is necessary to remove jewelry and any other metal objects
3. The client will be asked to breathe in and out during the x-ray
4. The x-ray technologist will stand next to the client during the x-ray

Answer: 2

Rationale: An x-ray leaves a photographic image of a part of the body on a special film, which is used to diagnose a wide variety of conditions. The x-ray itself is painless; any discomfort would arise from repositioning a painful part for filming. The nurse may want to premedicate a client who is at risk for pain. Any radiopaque objects such as jewelry or other metal must be removed. The client is asked to breathe in deeply and then hold the breath while the chest x-ray is taken. To minimize risk of radiation exposure, the x-ray technologist stands in a separate area protected by a lead wall. The client also wears a lead shield over the gonads.

Test-Taking Strategy: Options 1 and 4 are obviously incorrect and are eliminated first. Of the two remaining, option 3 is incorrect because the client needs to be still during the x-ray. Option 2 is the better choice and is the correct answer to this question.

Level of Cognitive Ability: Application
Phase of Nursing Process: Planning
Client Needs: Safe, Effective Care Environment
Content Area: Adult Health/Musculoskeletal

Reference

Black, J., & Matassarin-Jacobs, E. (1997). *Medical-surgical nursing: Clinical management for continuity of care* (5th ed.). Philadelphia: W. B. Saunders, p. 250.

---

207. The nurse admits a client with myocardial infarction to the coronary care unit (CCU). The nurse would plan to do which of the following in delivering care to this client?

1 Administer oxygen at a rate of 6 liters/minute by nasal cannula
2 Infuse intravenous fluid at a rate of 150 mL/hour
3 Begin a continuous heparin drip at a rate of 2000 units/hour
4 Place the client on continuous cardiac monitoring

Answer: 4

Rationale: Standard interventions upon admittance to CCU as they relate to this question include continuous cardiac monitoring, oxygen at a rate of 2 liters/minute unless otherwise ordered, and IV line insertion with a keep-vein-open (KVO) rate or heparin lock (to prevent fluid overload and heart failure). Heparin drip may be instituted according to protocol, but a rate of 2000 units per hour is excessive.

Test-Taking Strategy: Look at options 1, 2, and 3. You will note that the values in the distracters related to oxygen, IV fluid, and heparin therapy are on the high side and could jeopardize some or all clients. Review care to the client after myocardial infarction now if you had difficulty with this question!

Level of Cognitive Ability: Application
Phase of Nursing Process: Planning
Client Needs: Safe, Effective Care Environment
Content Area: Adult Health/Cardiovascular

Reference

Smeltzer, S., & Bare, B. (1996). *Brunner and Suddarth's Textbook of medical-surgical nursing* (8th ed.). Philadelphia: Lippincott-Raven, p. 652.

---

208. The client has just had skeletal traction pins inserted. The weights have been attached to the pins with the use of a wire bow and a rope pulley system. Which of the following nursing interventions should the nurse plan once assessment of the traction setup is complete?

1 Cover the ends of the traction pins with cork or tape
2 Perform pin site care
3 Provide for distraction such as television
4 Teach the client about pin care

Answer: 1

Rationale: After insertion of skeletal traction pins, the ends are covered with tape or cork to prevent injury to the client and to health care personnel. The other options are appropriate at a later time.

Test-Taking Strategy: Eliminate option 3 first because it is the least plausible. Option 4 is not timely, so that is eliminated also. Performing pin site care is not the priority at this time. This leaves option 1 as correct. Covering traction pins provides for the protection of clients and staff. Review care to the client after skeletal traction pin insertion now if you had difficulty with this question!

Level of Cognitive Ability: Application
Phase of Nursing Process: Planning
Client Needs: Safe, Effective Care Environment
Content Area: Adult Health/Musculoskeletal

Reference

Smeltzer, S., & Bare, B. (1996). *Brunner and Suddarth's Textbook of medical-surgical nursing* (8th ed.). Philadelphia: Lippincott-Raven, p. 1862.

209. The nurse is planning discharge teaching for the client with a spinal cord injury. To provide for a safe environment regarding home care, which of the following would be the priority in the plan of care?

1. What the physician has indicated needs to be taught
2. Follow-up laboratory and diagnostic tests
3. Assisting the client to deal with long-term care placement
4. Including the significant others in the teaching session

Answer: 4

Rationale: Involving the client's significant others in discharge teaching is a priority in planning for the client with a spinal cord injury. The client will need the support of the significant others. Knowledge and understanding of what to expect will help both the client and the significant other deal with the limitations. A physician's order is not necessary for discharge planning and teaching; this is an independent nursing action. Laboratory and diagnostic testing are inappropriate discharge instructions for this client. Long-term placement is not the only appropriate environment for clients with spinal cord injury.

Test-Taking Strategy: Eliminate option 3 first because long-term placement is not the only appropriate environment. Eliminate option 1 next because although the physician's orders need to be addressed, teaching is an independent nursing action. From the remaining options, consider the client's diagnosis. Home care and support will be needed. Use your nursing knowledge. Therefore, select option 4 over option 2.

Level of Cognitive Ability: Application
Phase of Nursing Process: Planning
Client Needs: Safe, Effective Care Environment
Content Area: Adult Health/Neurological

Reference

Luckmann, J. (1997). *Saunders manual of nursing care.* Philadelphia: W. B. Saunders, p. 195.

---

210. A nurse is trying to evaluate an electrocardiogram rhythm strip on an assigned client and asks another nurse how much time each little box on the ECG paper represents. The second nurse would respond that each small box measures

1. 0.02 second.
2. 0.04 second.
3. 0.20 second.
4. 0.40 second.

Answer: 2

Rationale: Standard ECG graph paper measurements are 0.04 seconds for each small box on the horizontal axis (measuring time) and 1 mm (measuring voltage) for each small box on the vertical axis.

Test-Taking Strategy: Items such as these are probably not abundant on NCLEX-RN, but knowledge of such basics may be required to assist in answering questions related to dysrhythmias. Review these basics now, if necessary!

Level of Cognitive Ability: Application
Phase of Nursing Process: Implementation
Client Needs: Safe, Effective Care Environment
Content Area: Adult Health/Cardiovascular

Reference

Ignatavicius, D. D., Workman, M. L., & Mishler, M. A. (1995). *Medical-surgical nursing: A nursing process approach* (2nd ed.). Philadelphia: W. B. Saunders, p. 824.

---

211. The nurse is applying ECG electrodes to a diaphoretic client. The nurse would do which of the following to keep the electrodes from coming loose?

1. Secure the electrodes with adhesive tape
2. Place clear, transparent dressings over the electrodes
3. Apply lanolin to the skin before applying the electrodes
4. Apply a little benzoin to the skin before applying the electrodes

Answer: 4

Rationale: Tincture of benzoin is commonly used with a diaphoretic client to help the electrodes adhere to the skin. Adhesive tape or a clear dressing over the electrodes does not help the adhesive gel of the actual electrode make better contact with the diaphoretic skin. Lanolin or any other lotion makes the skin slippery and prevents good initial adherence.

Test-Taking Strategy: You can easily eliminate option 3. Note that option 1 and 2 are similar in that both provide an external form of providing security of the electrodes. Option 4 is the only option that addresses direct contact with the skin.

Level of Cognitive Ability: Application
Phase of Nursing Process: Implementation
Client Needs: Safe, Effective Care Environment
Content Area: Adult Health/Cardiovascular

Reference

Smeltzer, S., & Bare, B. (1996). *Brunner and Suddarth's Textbook of medical-surgical nursing* (8th ed.). Philadelphia: Lippincott-Raven, p. 606.

---

212. The nurse has developed a plan of care for a client with a diagnosis of anterior cord syndrome. Which of the following interventions would be included in that plan of care?

1 Assess client for pain before physical therapy
2 Remind client to change positions slowly
3 Assess sensation of touch and vibration above the level of injury
4 Teach client with regard to loss of motor function and temperature sensation

Answer: 4

Rationale: Clinical findings related to anterior cord syndrome include loss of motor function and temperature sensation below the level of injury. The syndrome is not painful and does not affect sensations of touch, motion, position, and vibration above the level of the injury.

Test-Taking Strategy: Knowledge of anterior cord syndrome is necessary to correctly answer this question. If you are unfamiliar with this syndrome, take time now to review the important nursing interventions related to the disorder!

Level of Cognitive Ability: Application
Phase of Nursing Process: Planning
Client Needs: Safe, Effective Care Environment
Content Area: Adult Health/Neurological

Reference

Burrell, L., Gerlach, M., & Pless, B. (1997). *Adult nursing: Acute and community care* (2nd ed.). Stamford: Appleton & Lange, p. 951.

---

213. The nurse is caring for a client with high thoracic spinal cord injury. As part of the nursing care plan, the nurse monitors for spinal shock. In the event that spinal shock occurs, the nurse would anticipate that the most likely IV therapy to be prescribed would be

1 5% dextrose in water (D5W).
2 Dextran.
3 5% dextrose in normal saline (D5NS).
4 0.9% normal saline (NS).

Answer: 4

Rationale: NS, 0.9%, is an isotonic crystalloid that remains primarily in the intravascular space, increasing intravascular volume. This intervention would increase the client's blood pressure. Dextran is rarely used in spinal shock because isotonic fluid administration is usually sufficient. In addition, dextran has potentially serious side effects. D5W is a hypotonic solution that pulls fluid out of the intravascular space and is not indicated for shock. D5NS is hypertonic and indicated for shock resulting from hemorrhage or burns.

Test-Taking Strategy: Knowledge of the treatment for spinal shock is necessary to answer the question. Review the IV therapy associated with this disorder now if you had difficulty with this question!

Level of Cognitive Ability: Analysis
Phase of Nursing Process: Analysis
Client Needs: Safe, Effective Care Environment
Content Area: Adult Health/Neurological

Reference

Lewis, S., Collier, I, & Heitkemper, M. (1996). *Medical-surgical nursing: Assessment and management of clinical problems* (4th ed.). St. Louis: Mosby–Year Book, p. 130.

214. The client with myocardial infarction is experiencing new, multiform premature ventricular contractions (PVCs). The nurse would plan to have which one of the following medications available for immediate use?

1 Digoxin (Lanoxin)
2 Metoprolol (Lopressor)
3 Verapamil (Isoptin)
4 Lidocaine hydrochloride (Xylocaine HCl)

Answer: 4

Rationale: Lidocaine hydrochloride is a class 1 antidysrhythmic that is the medication of choice used to treat ventricular dysrhythmias with acute myocardial ischemia or infarction. Other frequently ordered medications include procainamide (Pronestyl), bretylium tosylate (Bretylol), and magnesium sulfate (magnesium sulfate injection). Digoxin is a cardiac glycoside; metoprolol is a beta-adrenergic blocking agent; verapamil is a calcium channel–blocking agent.

Test-Taking Strategy: Medication knowledge is needed to accurately answer this question. If you are not familiar with these medications and their uses, review these first-line antidysrhythmic agents now.

Level of Cognitive Ability: Application
Phase of Nursing Process: Planning
Client Needs: Safe, Effective Care Environment
Content Area: Pharmacology

Reference

Ignatavicius, D. D., Workman, M. L., & Mishler, M. A. (1995). *Medical-surgical nursing: A nursing process approach* (2nd ed.). Philadelphia: W. B. Saunders, p. 850.

---

215. A nurse observes a client wringing his or her hands and looking frightened. The client reports feeling out of control. Which approach by the nurse is most appropriate to maintain a safe environment?

1 Administer the ordered PRN anxiety medication immediately
2 Move the client to a quiet room and talk about his or her feelings
3 Isolate the client in a "time-out" room
4 Observe client in an ongoing manner but do not intervene

Answer: 2

Rationale: The anxiety symptoms demonstrated by this client require some form of intervention. Moving the client to a quiet room decreases environmental stimulus. Talking gives the nurse an opportunity to assess the cause of these feelings and to identify appropriate interventions. Isolation is appropriate if client is a danger to self or others. There is no indication in the stem of the question that the client poses a threat to others. Medication is used only when other noninvasive approaches have been unsuccessful.

Test-Taking Strategy: A key word in the stem of this question is "frightened." Eliminate options 1 and 4 first. Of the remaining two options, select option 2 over option 3 because it addresses the client's feelings.

Level of Cognitive Ability: Application
Phase of Nursing Process: Implementation
Client Needs: Safe, Effective Care Environment
Content Area: Mental Health

Reference

Fortinash, K., & Holoday-Worret, P. (1996). *Psychiatric–mental health nursing.* St. Louis: Mosby–Year Book, p. 231.

---

216. The client has Buck's extension traction applied to the right leg. The nurse would plan which of the following interventions to prevent complications of the device?

1 Massage the skin of the right leg with lotion every 8 hours
2 Give pin care once a shift
3 Inspect the skin on the right leg at least once every 8 hours
4 Release the weights on the right leg for range-of-motion exercises daily

Answer: 3

Rationale: Buck's extension traction is a type of skin traction. The nurse inspects the skin of the limb in traction at least once every 8 hours for irritation or inflammation. Massaging the skin with lotion is not indicated. The nurse never releases the weights of traction unless specifically ordered by the physician. There are no pins to care for with skin traction.

Test-Taking Strategy: A baseline knowledge of Buck's extension traction allows you to eliminate options 2 and 4 easily. There are no pins, and the nurse never removes weights without a specific order to do so. Because the apparatus would have to be removed to apply lotion, which is unnecessary, the answer is to assess the skin integrity. Review care to the client in Buck's traction now if you had difficulty with this question!

Level of Cognitive Ability: Application
Phase of Nursing Process: Planning
Client Needs: Safe, Effective Care Environment
Content Area: Adult Health/Musculoskeletal

Reference

Ignatavicius, D. D., Workman, M. L., & Mishler, M. A. (1995). *Medical-surgical nursing: A nursing process approach* (2nd ed.). Philadelphia: W. B. Saunders, pp. 1462–1463.

---

217. The client with urolithiasis is scheduled for extracorporeal shock wave lithotripsy. The nurse assesses to ensure that which of the following items are in place or maintained before sending the client for the procedure?

1 Signed consent, clear liquid restriction, Foley catheter
2 Signed consent, NPO status, IV line
3 IV line, clear liquid restriction, Foley catheter
4 IV line, NPO status, Foley catheter

Answer: 2

Rationale: Extracorporeal shock wave lithotripsy is done with the client under epidural or general anesthesia. The client must sign a special consent form for the procedure and must be on NPO status for the procedure. The client needs an IV line for the procedure as well. A Foley catheter is not needed.

Test-Taking Strategy: Begin to answer this question by eliminating options 3 and 4, because the client must sign a special consent for this procedure. To discriminate between options 1 and 2, it is necessary to know that the procedure is done under general or epidural anesthesia. With this in mind, you would realize that the client must be on NPO status, and choose option 2 over option 1.

Level of Cognitive Ability: Application
Phase of Nursing Process: Assessment
Client Needs: Safe, Effective Care Environment
Content Area: Adult Health/Renal

Reference

Black, J., & Matassarin-Jacobs, E. (1997). *Medical-surgical nursing: Clinical management for continuity of care* (5th ed.). Philadelphia: W. B. Saunders, p. 2070.

---

218. The nurse is in the room of the monitored client who goes into ventricular fibrillation (VF). The nurse calls for help, knowing that which of the following items will be needed immediately?

1 Pacemaker insertion tray
2 Ventilator
3 Defibrillator
4 Lidocaine (Xylocaine)

Answer: 3

Rationale: A physician or a nurse certified in advanced cardiac life support (ACLS) must immediately defibrillate the client to convert VF to an organized rhythm. If a defibrillator is not readily available, the properly trained nurse may administer a precordial thump, followed by cardiopulmonary resuscitation until help arrives.

Test-Taking Strategy: Eliminate options 1 and 2 first because they will do nothing to convert the deadly dysrhythmia. To discriminate between 3 and 4, remember that lidocaine is given with ventricular tachycardia (an organized although potentially deadly rhythm). Defibrillation is always needed to convert VF.

Level of Cognitive Ability: Application
Phase of Nursing Process: Planning
Client Needs: Safe, Effective Care Environment
Content Area: Adult Health/Cardiovascular

Reference

Ignatavicius, D. D., Workman, M. L., & Mishler, M. A. (1995). *Medical-surgical nursing: A nursing process approach* (2nd ed.). Philadelphia: W. B. Saunders, pp. 852–853.

219. The nurse is assisting at a code, and the physician is going to defibrillate. Of the following items, which is the only one that the nurse does not need to plan to remove from the bedside just before the client is defibrillated?

1 Backboard
2 Oxygen
3 Nitroglycerin patch
4 Ventilator

Answer: 1

Rationale: Flammable materials and metal devices or liquids (which are capable of carrying electricity) are removed from the client and bed before the paddles of the defibrillator are discharged.

Test-Taking Strategy: Options 2 and 4 are similar and therefore are eliminated. Of the remaining two options, the nitroglycerin patch has a metallic backing and should be removed. The backboard is needed to resume cardiopulmonary resuscitation immediately if defibrillation is unsuccessful.

Level of Cognitive Ability: Application
Phase of Nursing Process: Planning
Client Needs: Safe, Effective Care Environment
Content Area: Adult Health/Cardiovascular

Reference

Black, J., & Matassarin-Jacobs, E. (1997). *Medical-surgical nursing: Clinical management for continuity of care* (5th ed.). Philadelphia: W. B. Saunders, p. 1311.

---

220. The nurse is planning the discharge instructions from the emergency room for an adult client who is a victim of family violence. The discharge plans must include

1 Instructions to call the police next time the abuse occurs.
2 Exploration of the pros and cons of remaining with the abusive family member.
3 Specific information regarding "safe havens" or shelters in the client's neighborhood.
4 Specific information about self-defense classes.

Answer: 3

Rationale: Tertiary prevention of family violence includes assisting the victim once the abuse has already occurred. This includes helping the victim understand where to find help. Assisting the victim of family violence in devising a specific plan for removing self from the abuser should this situation recur is essential. Specific information about escape, safe havens, hot lines, and so forth is essential.

Test-Taking Strategy: Any of the options might be included at some point if long-term therapy or a long-term relationship with the nurse is established. The question specifies an emergency room setting. The most important prevention education for known victims of abuse is to assist them in devising a plan for how to remove themselves from harmful situations should they arise again. An abused person is usually reluctant to call the police. Teaching the victim to fight back (as in the use of self-defense) is not the best response when dealing with a violent person.

Level of Cognitive Ability: Application
Phase of Nursing Process: Planning
Client Needs: Safe, Effective Care Environment
Content Area: Mental Health

Reference

Carson, V., & Arnold, E. (1996). *Mental health nursing: The nurse-patient journey.* Philadelphia: W. B. Saunders, p. 1059–1061.

---

221. The nurse is caring for a client with fresh application of a plaster leg cast. The nurse would plan to prevent the development of compartment syndrome by instructing the licensed practical nurse to

1 Elevate the limb and apply ice to the affected leg.
2 Elevate the limb and cover the limb with bath blankets.
3 Place the leg in a slightly dependent position and apply ice.
4 Keep the leg horizontal and apply heat to the affected leg.

Answer: 1

Rationale: Compartment syndrome is prevented by controlling edema. This is achieved most optimally with elevation and application of ice.

Test-Taking Strategy: Knowing that edema is controlled or prevented with limb elevation helps you to eliminate options 3 and 4 as possible choices. To discriminate between the last two choices, look at the effects of ice versus bath blankets. Ice will further control edema, while bath blankets will produce heat and prevent air circulation needed for the cast to dry. This comparison helps you to choose option 1 over option 2.

Level of Cognitive Ability: Application
Phase of Nursing Process: Planning
Client Needs: Safe, Effective Care Environment
Content Area: Adult Health/Musculoskeletal

Reference

Smeltzer, S., & Bare, B. (1996). *Brunner and Suddarth's Textbook of medical-surgical nursing* (8th ed.). Philadelphia: Lippincott-Raven, p. 1917.

---

222. An 8-year-old is admitted to the health care facility. The child has a recent history of sexual abuse by an adult family member. The child is withdrawn and appears frightened. Which of the following describes the best plan for the initial nursing encounter to convey concern and support?

1 Introduce self, explain role, and ask the child to act out the sexual encounter with the abuser, using art therapy
2 Introduce self, then ask the child to express how he or she feels about the events leading up to this admission
3 Introduce self and explain to the child that he or she is safe now that he or she is in the hospital
4 Introduce self and tell the child that the nurse would like to sit with him or her for a little while

Answer: 4

Rationale: Victims of sexual abuse may exhibit fear and anxiety over what has just occurred. In addition, they may fear that the abuse could be repeated. On initiating contact with a child victim of sexual abuse who demonstrates fear of others, it is best to convey a willingness to spend time and move slowly to initiate activities that may be perceived as threatening. Once rapport is established, the nurse may explore the child's feelings or use various therapeutic modalities to encourage recounting the offensive experience.

Test-Taking Strategy: The initial role of the nurse working with an abused victim is to establish trust. Trust is established when the nurse conveys a nonthreatening, consistent, and safe environment. Establishing trust takes time. Answer 4 conveys a plan for an initial encounter that establishes trust by sitting with the child in a nonthreatening atmosphere without a hurried appearance. Options 1 and 2 may be asked once trust and rapport is established. Option 3 is a good statement but does not convey concern and support by the nurse.

Level of Cognitive Ability: Application
Phase of Nursing Process: Planning
Client Needs: Safe, Effective Care Environment
Content Area: Child Health

Reference

Carson, V., & Arnold, E. (1996). *Mental health nursing: The nurse-patient journey.* Philadelphia: W. B. Saunders, p. 1050.

---

223. The physician is about to defibrillate a client in ventricular fibrillation and says in a loud voice, "Clear!" The nurse immediately

1 Shuts off the IV infusion going into the client's arm.
2 Shuts off the mechanical ventilator.
3 Steps away from the bed and makes sure all others have done the same.
4 Places the conductive gel pads for defibrillation on the client's chest.

Answer: 3

Rationale: For the safety of all personnel, when the defibrillator paddles are being discharged, all personnel must stand back and be clear of all contact with the client and the client's bed. It is the primary responsibility of the person defibrillating to communicate the "clear" message loudly enough for all to hear, and ensure their compliance. All personnel must immediately comply with this command.

Test-Taking Strategy: The gel pads should have been placed on the client's chest before the defibrillator paddles were applied, so option 4 is eliminated first. A ventilator is not in use during a code—rather, an Ambu bag is used—so option 2 is also incorrect. Of the remaining two options, shutting off the infusion has no useful purpose. Stepping back from the bed prevents the nurse from being defibrillated along with the client, which makes option 3 clearly the correct choice.

Level of Cognitive Ability: Application
Phase of Nursing Process: Implementation
Client Needs: Safe, Effective Care Environment
Content Area: Adult Health/Cardiovascular

Reference

Black, J., & Matassarin-Jacobs, E. (1997). *Medical-surgical nursing: Clinical management for continuity of care* (5th ed.). Philadelphia: W. B. Saunders, p. 1311.

224. The client with chronic renal failure has an indwelling catheter for peritoneal dialysis in the abdomen. The client spills water on the dressing while bathing. The nurse should plan to immediately

1 Reinforce the dressing.
2 Change the dressing.
3 Flush the peritoneal dialysis catheter.
4 Scrub the catheter with povidone iodine.

Answer: 2

Rationale: Clients with peritoneal dialysis catheters are at high risk for infection. A dressing that is wet is a conduit for bacteria to reach the catheter insertion site. The nurse ensures that the dressing is kept dry at all times. Reinforcing the dressing is not a safe practice to prevent infection in this circumstance. Flushing the catheter is not indicated. Scrubbing the catheter with povidone iodine is done at the time of connection or disconnection of peritoneal dialysis.

Test-Taking Strategy: The issue of the question is that the dressing is wet. The correct option would focus on the dressing, not the catheter. This eliminates options 3 and 4. Knowing that it is better to change a wet dressing than reinforce it, you would choose option 2 as the correct answer.

Level of Cognitive Ability: Application
Phase of Nursing Process: Planning
Client Needs: Safe, Effective Care Environment
Content Area: Adult Health/Renal

Reference

Black, J., & Matassarin-Jacobs, E. (1997). *Medical-surgical nursing: Clinical management for continuity of care* (5th ed.). Philadelphia: W. B. Saunders, p. 1658.

225. A female victim of a sexual assault is being seen in the crisis center for a third visit. She states that although the rape occurred nearly 2 months ago, she still feels "as though the rape just happened yesterday." The nurse's best response might be

1 "What can you do to alleviate some of your fears about being assaulted again?"
2 "Tell me more about those aspects of the rape that cause you to feel like the rape just occurred."
3 "In time, our goal will be to help you move on from these strong feelings about your rape."
4 "In reality, the rape did not just occur. It has been over 2 months now."

Answer: 2

Rationale: This response allows for the client to express her ideas and feelings more fully and reflects an unhurried, nonjudgmental, supportive attitude. Clients need to be reassured that their feelings are normal and that they may freely express their concerns in a safe care environment.

Test-Taking Strategy: The client is seeking help. Option 1 places the problem solving totally on the client. Option 3 places the client's feelings on hold. Although option 4 is true, it immediately blocks communication. Always address the client's feelings first!

Level of Cognitive Ability: Application
Phase of Nursing Process: Implementation
Client Needs: Safe, Effective Care Environment
Content Area: Mental Health

Reference

Carson, V., & Arnold, E. (1996). *Mental health nursing: The nurse-patient journey.* Philadelphia: W. B. Saunders, p. 1096.

226. A client is scheduled for elective cardioversion to treat chronic high-rate atrial fibrillation. The nurse assesses that the client is not yet ready for the procedure after determining that

1 The client's digoxin has been withheld for the last 48 hours.
2 The client has received a dose of midazolam (Versed) intravenously.
3 The client is wearing a nasal cannula delivering oxygen at 2 liters per minute.
4 The defibrillator has the synchronizer turned on and is set at 50 joules.

Answer: 3

Rationale: Digoxin may be withheld for up to 48 hours before cardioversion because it increases ventricular irritability and may cause ventricular dysrhythmias after countershock. The client typically receives a dose of an IV sedative or antianxiety agent. The defibrillator is switched to synchronizer mode to time the delivery of the electrical impulse to coincide with the QRS and avoid the T wave, which could cause ventricular fibrillation. Energy level is typically set at 50–100 joules. During the procedure, any oxygen is removed temporarily because oxygen supports combustion.

Test-Taking Strategy: The question is worded to prompt you to look for an incorrect item. A review of the key differences between cardioversion and defibrillation is needed to select the correct answer. The concept of oxygen combustion may prove useful in questions related to either cardioversion or defibrillation. Review this procedure now if you had difficulty with this question!

Level of Cognitive Ability: Analysis
Phase of Nursing Process: Assessment
Client Needs: Safe, Effective Care Environment
Content Area: Adult Health/Cardiovascular

Reference

Black, J., & Matassarin-Jacobs, E. (1997). *Medical-surgical nursing: Clinical management for continuity of care* (5th ed.). Philadelphia: W. B. Saunders, p. 1313.

---

227. The client is admitted to the unit with a diagnosis of schizophrenia. A nursing diagnosis formulated for the client is Altered Thought Process, secondary to paranoia. In formulating a nursing care plan with the team, the nurse includes instruction to the staff to

1. Avoid laughing or whispering in front of the client.
2. Increase socialization of the client with peers.
3. Have the client sign a release of information to appropriate parties so that adequate data can be obtained for assessment purposes.
4. Begin to educate the client about social supports in the community.

Answer: 1

Rationale: Altered thought process secondary to paranoia is the client's problem, and the plan of care must respond to this. The client is experiencing paranoia, which is distrust and suspiciousness of others. The treatment team needs to establish rapport with the client and the client's trust. Hence, laughing or whispering in front of the client would be counterproductive.

Test-Taking Strategy: Use knowledge regarding this disorder to answer the question. Options 2, 3, and 4 ask the client to trust on a multitude of levels. These options are actions that are too intrusive for a client who is paranoid. Review this disorder now if you had difficulty with this question!

Level of Cognitive Ability: Application
Phase of Nursing Process: Implementation
Client Needs: Safe, Effective Environment
Content Area: Mental Health

Reference

Antai-Otong, D. (1995). *Psychiatric nursing: Biological and behavioral changes.* Philadelphia: W. B. Saunders, p. 301.

---

228. In planning activities for the depressed client, especially during the early stages of hospitalization, which of the following actions is most appropriate?

1. Provide an activity that is quiet and solitary in nature, such as working on a puzzle or reading a book, to avoid increased fatigue
2. Plan nothing until the client asks to participate in milieu
3. Offer the client a menu of daily activities and insist the client participate in all of them
4. Provide a structured daily program of activities and encourage the client to participate

Answer: 4

Rationale: A depressed person is often withdrawn. Also, the person experiences difficulty concentrating, loss of interest or pleasure, low energy, fatigue, and feelings of worthlessness and poor self-esteem. The plan of care needs to provide successful experiences in a stimulating and yet structured environment.

Test-Taking Strategy: The depressed client requires a structured and stimulating program. Options 1 and 2 are too "restrictive" and offer little or no structure and stimulation. Option 3 is eliminated because of the high demands it places on the client. Option 4 is the only reasonable option that will provide an effective care environment!

Level of Cognitive Ability: Application
Phase of Nursing Process: Planning
Client Needs: Safe, Effective Care Environment
Content Area: Mental Health

Reference

Antai-Otong, D. (1995). *Psychiatric nursing: Biological and behavioral concepts.* Philadelphia: W. B. Saunders, pp. 170, 184.

229. The nurse is caring for an elderly client who had a hip pinned for a fractured hip. In planning nursing care, which of the following would the nurse avoid to minimize the chance for further injury?

1 Side rails in the "up" position
2 Use of nightlight in hospital room and bathroom
3 Call bell placed within reach
4 Delays in responding to call light

Answer: 4

Rationale: Safe nursing actions intended to prevent injury to the client include keeping side rails up, keeping the bed in a low position, and providing a call bell that is within the client's reach. Responding promptly to the client's use of the call light minimizes the chance that the client will try to get up alone, which could result in a fall.

Test-Taking Strategy: The wording of this question asks you to identify an incorrect or potentially harmful item. Because options 1 and 3 (side rails up and call bell in reach) are standard nursing actions, they are eliminated. Use of a nightlight would help prevent falls, which is also helpful, and so option 2 can be eliminated. This leaves option 4 as the correct answer. Delays will give the client reason to try to get up unattended, and risk another fall and possible injury.

Level of Cognitive Ability: Application
Phase of Nursing Process: Planning
Client Needs: Safe, Effective Care Environment
Content Area: Fundamental Skills

Reference

Smeltzer, S., & Bare, B. (1996). *Brunner and Suddarth's Textbook of medical-surgical nursing* (8th ed.). Philadelphia: Lippincott-Raven, p. 1930.

---

230. The nurse is assisting in the care of a client who is to undergo cardioversion. The nurse plans to set the defibrillator to which of the following starting energy levels, depending on the specific physician order?

1 50–100 joules
2 150–200 joules
3 250–300 joules
4 350–400 joules

Answer: 1

Rationale: The capacitor on the defibrillator is charged to the energy level ordered by the physician, usually starting at 50–100 joules. The amount varies according to the predicated amount of electrical impedance to the current.

Test-Taking Strategy: This question may be difficult if you are relatively unfamiliar with the procedure. In general, however, remember that cardioversion is used for an underlying cardiac rhythm that needs only to be converted to a better rhythm. Therefore, the lowest voltages are the better option. Review this procedure now if you had difficulty with this question!

Level of Cognitive Ability: Application
Phase of Nursing Process: Planning
Client Needs: Safe, Effective Care Environment
Content Area: Adult Health/Cardiovascular

Reference

Black, J., & Matassarin-Jacobs, E. (1997). *Medical-surgical nursing: Clinical management for continuity of care* (5th ed.). Philadelphia: W. B. Saunders, p. 1313.

231. The nurse has an order to get the client out of bed to a chair on the first postoperative day after total knee replacement. The nurse would plan to do which of the following to protect the knee joint?

1 Apply a knee immobilizer before getting the client up, and elevate the client's surgical leg while the client is sitting
2 Apply an Ace wrap around the dressing, and put ice on the knee while the client is sitting
3 Lift the client to the bedside chair, leaving the continuous passive motion (CPM) machine in place
4 Obtain a walker to minimize weight bearing by the client on the affected leg

Answer: 1

Rationale: On the first postoperative day, the nurse assists the client in getting out of bed after putting a knee immobilizer on the affected joint for stability. The surgeon orders the weight-bearing limits on the affected leg. The leg is elevated while the client is sitting in the chair, to minimize edema.

Test-Taking Strategy: A compression dressing should already be in place on the wound, so option 2 should be eliminated first. Because the CPM machine is used only while the client is in bed, option 3 is incorrect and is eliminated also. To discriminate between the last two options, knowing that ambulation is not started until the second postoperative day would help you choose correctly. The knee immobilizer should be a natural choice when you are answering a question about protecting a knee joint.

Level of Cognitive Ability: Application
Phase of Nursing Process: Planning
Client Needs: Safe, Effective Care Environment
Content Area: Adult Health/Musculoskeletal

Reference

Smeltzer, S., & Bare, B. (1996). *Brunner and Suddarth's Textbook of medical-surgical nursing* (8th ed.). Philadelphia: Lippincott-Raven, p. 1877.

---

232. The client undergoing hemodialysis becomes hypotensive. Which of the following nursing actions is contraindicated?

1 Administering albumin
2 Administering a 250-mL normal saline bolus
3 Increasing the blood flow into the dialyzer
4 Raising the client's legs and feet

Answer: 3

Rationale: To treat hypotension during hemodialysis, it is accepted practice to raise the client's feet and legs to enhance cardiac return. A normal saline bolus of up to 500 mL may be given to increase circulating volume. Albumin may be given as per protocol to increase colloid oncotic pressure. Finally, the transmembrane hydrostatic pressure or the blood flow rate into the dialyzer is decreased. All of these measures should improve the circulating volume and blood pressure.

Test-Taking Strategy: The stem tells you that the client is hypotensive, which means that the question as stated is asking about which measure would aggravate the low blood pressure. With this in mind, each of the incorrect responses may be eliminated systematically according to basic concepts of fluid and electrolyte balance. Review the treatment for this complication of dialysis, if you had difficulty with this question!

Level of Cognitive Ability: Analysis
Phase of Nursing Process: Analysis
Client Needs: Safe, Effective Care Environment
Content Area: Adult Health/Renal

Reference

Luckmann, J. (1997). *Saunders manual of nursing care*. Philadelphia: W. B. Saunders, p. 1194.

233. A client is admitted to the psychiatric unit after a suicidal attempt by hanging. The nurse's most important aspect of care is to maintain client safety. This is accomplished best by

1. Assigning a staff member to the client who will remain with the client at all times.
2. Admitting client to a seclusion room in which all potentially dangerous articles are removed.
3. Removing the client's clothing and placing the client in a hospital gown.
4. Requesting that a peer remain with the client at all times.

Answer: 1

Rationale: Hanging is a serious suicide attempt. The plan of care must reflect the action that will promote the client's safety. Constant observation status with a staff member who is never less than an arm's length away is the best selection.

Test-Taking Strategy: Eliminate option 4 first because it is not a peer's responsibility to safeguard a client. Eliminate option 3 next because removing clothing does not maximize all possible safety strategies. From the remaining two options, select option 1 over option 2 because the correct option provides a constant supervision in this critical situation!

Level of Cognitive Ability: Analysis
Phase of Nursing Process: Planning
Client Needs: Safe, Effective Care Environment
Content Area: Mental Health

Reference

Carson, V., & Arnold, E. (1996). *Mental health nursing: The nurse-patient journey.* Philadelphia: W. B. Saunders, p. 939.

---

234. The nurse is preparing a client for cardioversion with anterolateral paddle placement. The nurse would place the conductive gel pads at which areas on the client's chest?

1. Right second intercostal space and left fifth intercostal space at anterior axillary line
2. Left second intercostal space and left fifth intercostal space at midaxillary line
3. Right fourth intercostal space and left fifth intercostal space at anterior axillary line
4. Left fourth intercostal space and left fifth intercostal space at midaxillary line

Answer: 1

Rationale: Anterolateral paddle placement for external countershock involves placing one paddle at the second right intercostal space and at the other in the fifth intercostal space at the anterior axillary line.

Test-Taking Strategy: This question may look complicated on the surface because of the length of description, but it is fairly easy to work through. You must position the paddles so that the electric shock travels through as much myocardium as possible. Imagine each of the placements as described, using your knowledge of cardiothoracic landmarks, and remember the position of the heart in the chest. In doing so, you will eliminate each of the incorrect options.

Level of Cognitive Ability: Application
Phase of Nursing Process: Implementation
Client Needs: Safe, Effective Care Environment
Content Area: Adult Health/Cardiovascular

Reference

Black, J., & Matassarin-Jacobs, E. (1997). *Medical-surgical nursing: Clinical management for continuity of care* (5th ed.). Philadelphia: W. B. Saunders, p. 1312.

---

235. A nurse receives a telephone call from a male client who states that he wants to kill himself and has a loaded gun on the table. The best nursing intervention that can be made is to

1. Insist that the client give you his name and address so that you can get the police there immediately.
2. Keep the client talking and allow the client to ventilate feelings.
3. Use therapeutic communications, especially the reflection of feelings.
4. Keep the client talking, and signal to another staff member to trace the call so that appropriate help can be sent.

Answer: 4

Rationale: In a crisis, the nurse must take an authoritative, active role to promote the client's safety. A loaded gun in a client's home who verbalizes that he wants to kill himself is a "crisis." The client's safety is of prime concern. Keeping the client on the phone and getting help to the client is the best intervention.

Test-Taking Strategy: The action of "insisting" may anger the client, and he might hang up. Option 2 lacks the authoritative action stance of securing the client's safety. Using therapeutic communication is important, but overuse of "reflection" may sound uncaring or superficial and does not provide direction or solutions to the immediate problem of the client's safety. Option 4 is the most global response and encompasses the necessary action.

Level of Cognitive Ability: Application
Phase of Nursing Process: Implementation
Client Needs: Safe, Effective Care Environment
Content Area: Mental Health

Reference

Carson, V., & Arnold, E. (1996). *Mental health nursing: The nurse-patient journey.* Philadelphia: W. B. Saunders, pp. 936–937.

---

236. After initial assessment, the nurse determines the need to place a vest restraint on a client. The client does not want the vest restraint applied. What would be the best nursing action?

1 Apply the restraint anyway
2 Obtain a physician's order
3 Medicate the client with a sedative and then apply the restraint
4 Reach a compromise with the client to use wrist restraints

Answer: 2

Rationale: The use of restraints should be avoided if possible. If the nurse determines that a restraint is necessary, this should be discussed with the family, and an order needs to be obtained from the physician. The physician's order protects the nurse from liability. The nurse should explain carefully to the client and family the reasons why the restraint is necessary, the type of restraint selected, and anticipated duration of restraint.

Test-Taking Strategy: Eliminate option 1 first; if the nurse applied the restraint on a client who was refusing it, the nurse could be charged with battery. Eliminate option 3 next because, again, the nurse could be charged with battery. Option 4 could be unsafe and ineffective if the vest restraint was deemed necessary initially.

Level of Cognitive Ability: Application
Phase of Nursing Process: Implementation
Client Needs: Safe, Effective Care Environment
Content Area: Fundamental Skills

Reference

Potter, P., & Perry, A. (1997). *Fundamentals of nursing: Concepts, process, and practice* (4th ed.). St. Louis: Mosby–Year Book, p. 886.

---

237. A client is being discharged and will receive oxygen therapy at home. The nurse is teaching the client and family about oxygen safety measures while at home. Which of the following statements indicates that the client needs further teaching?

1 "I realize that I should check the oxygen level of the portable tank on a consistent basis."
2 "I will keep my scented candles within 5 feet of my oxygen tank."
3 "I will not sit in front of my fireplace (wood-burning) with my oxygen on."
4 "I will call the physician if I experience any shortness of breath."

Answer: 2

Rationale: Oxygen is a highly combustible gas, although it will not spontaneously burn or cause an explosion. It can easily cause a fire to ignite in a client's room if it contacts a spark from a cigarette or electrical equipment. Oxygen in high concentrations has a great combustion potential and fuels fire readily.

Test-Taking Strategy: Remembering that oxygen is a highly combustible gas will assist in answering the question. Option 4 can be eliminated first because it is unrelated to oxygen therapy. Options 1 and 3 can then be eliminated. If you had difficulty with this question, take time now to review teaching points related to home care and oxygen!

Level of Cognitive Ability: Analysis
Phase of Nursing Process: Evaluation
Client Needs: Safe, Effective Care Environment
Content Area: Fundamental Skills

Reference

Potter, P., & Perry, A. (1997). *Fundamentals of nursing: Concepts, process, and practice* (4th ed.). St. Louis: Mosby–Year Book, p. 1233.

238. A home health nurse visits a client receiving IV therapy via an IV pump. The nurse notes that the electrical cord coming from the wall to the IV pump has only two prongs. Which of the following is the most appropriate action?

1 Use the plug anyway
2 Pull the plug, using the cord
3 Run the plug under the carpet
4 Obtain a three-prong grounded plug

Answer: 4

Rationale: Electrical equipment must be maintained in good working order and should be grounded. The third prong in an electrical plug is the longest and is the ground prong. Theoretically, the ground prong carries any stray electrical current back to the ground; hence its name. The other two prongs carry the power to the piece of electrical equipment. Never run electrical wiring under carpets. Never pull a plug by using the cord; always grasp the plug.

Test-Taking Strategy: Principles of basic electrical safety should assist in directing you to the correct option. Note the key phrase "only two prongs" in the question. This should assist in directing you to the correct option. Review these principles now if you had difficulty with this question!

Level of Cognitive Ability: Analysis
Phase of Nursing Process: Implementation
Client Needs: Safe, Effective Care Environment
Content Area: Fundamental Skills

Reference

Potter, P., & Perry, A. (1997). *Fundamentals of nursing: Concepts, process, and practice* (4th ed.). St. Louis: Mosby–Year Book, pp. 885, 889.

239. Upon entering the client's house, the home health nurse assesses the environment for potential hazards. Which of the following observations is an indication that the client needs instruction about safety?

1 Skid-resistant small area rugs in the living room
2 Clothes hamper at the end of the hallway
3 Area rug at bottom of the stairs
4 Stair carpeting secured with carpet tacks

Answer: 3

Rationale: Area rugs and runners should not be used on or near stairs. Any carpeting on the stairs should be secured with carpet tacks. Injuries in the home frequently result from objects, including small rugs on the stairs and floor, wet spots on the floor, and clutter on bedside tables, closet shelves, the top of the refrigerator, and bookshelves. Care should also be taken to ensure that end tables are secure and have stable, straight legs. Nonessential items should be placed in drawers to eliminate clutter.

Test-Taking Strategy: Using the principles related to home safety should assist in directing you to the correct option. You can easily eliminate options 2 and 4. Read the remaining options carefully. Note that option 1 addresses skid-resistant small area rugs. This can be eliminated, leaving option 3. Review these principles now if you had difficulty with this question!

Level of Cognitive Ability: Analysis
Phase of Nursing Process: Evaluation
Client Needs: Safe, Effective Care Environment
Content Area: Fundamental Skills

Reference

Potter, P., & Perry, A. (1997). *Fundamentals of nursing: Concepts, process, and practice* (4th ed.). St. Louis: Mosby–Year Book, p. 872.

240. A hospitalized client with a history of alcohol abuse tells the nurse, "I am leaving now. I have to go. I don't want any more treatment. I have things that I have to do right away." The client has not been discharged. In fact, the client is scheduled for an important diagnostic test to be performed in 1 hour. After discussing the client's concerns with the nurse, the client dresses and begins to walk out of the hospital room. The most appropriate nursing action is to

1 Restrain the client until the physician can be reached.
2 Call security to block all exit areas.
3 Tell the client that he or she cannot return to this hospital again if he or she leaves now.
4 Call the nursing supervisor.

Answer: 4

Rationale: A nurse can be charged with false imprisonment if a client is made to wrongfully believe that he or she cannot leave the hospital. Most health care facilities have documents that clients are asked to sign that relate to their responsibilities when they leave against medical advice (AMA). The client should be asked to sign this document before leaving. The nurse should request that the client wait to speak to the physician before leaving, but if the client refuses to do so, the nurse cannot hold the client against the client's will. Restraining the client and calling security to block exits constitutes false imprisonment. Any client has a right to health care and cannot be told otherwise.

Test-Taking Strategy: Keeping the concept of false imprisonment in mind, eliminate options 1 and 2 because they are similar. Eliminate option 3, knowing that any client has a right to health care. Of the options presented, the best action is option 4. Review the points related to false imprisonment now if you had difficulty with this question!

Level of Cognitive Ability: Application
Phase of Nursing Process: Implementation
Client Needs: Safe, Effective Care Environment
Content Area: Fundamental Skills

Reference

DeLaune, S., & Ladner, P. (1998). *Fundamentals of nursing: Standards and practice.* Albany, NY: Delmar, p. 233.

---

241. Two nurses are in the cafeteria having lunch in a quiet, secluded area. A physical therapist from the physical therapy (PT) department joins the nurses. During lunch, the nurses discuss a client who was physically abused. After lunch, the physical therapist provides therapy prescribed for the client and asks the client questions about the physical abuse. The client discovers that the nurses told the therapist about the abuse situation and is emotionally harmed. The ramifications associated with the nurses' discussion about the client are most appropriately associated with which of the following?

1 None, because they were in a quiet, secluded area
2 They can be charged with slander
3 They can be charged with libel
4 None, because the physical therapist is involved in the client's care

Answer: 2

Rationale: Defamation occurs when information is communicated to a third party that causes damage to someone else's reputation either in writing (libel) or verbally (slander). The most common examples are giving out inaccurate or inappropriate information from the medical record; discussing clients, families, or visitors in public areas; or speaking negatively about coworkers. This situation can cause emotional harm to the client, and the nurses could be charged with slander. This situation also violates the client's right to confidentiality.

Test-Taking Strategy: Knowledge regarding the law and legal responsibilities of the nurse in protecting the client is necessary to answer the question. Eliminate options 1 and 4 first. For the remaining two options, it is necessary to know that slander is defined as verbal discussion regarding a client. Review this legal responsibility now if you had difficulty with this question.

Level of Cognitive Ability: Analysis
Phase of Nursing Process: Analysis
Client Needs: Safe, Effective Care Environment
Content Area: Fundamental Skills

Reference

DeLaune, S., & Ladner, P. (1998). *Fundamentals of nursing: Standards and practice.* Albany, NY: Delmar, p. 233.

242. A nurse arrives at work and is told that the intensive care unit (ICU) is in need of assistance. The nurse is told by the supervisor that the assignment today is to work in the ICU. The nurse has never worked in the ICU and shares concerns with the supervisor regarding the unfamiliarity with the technological equipment used in that unit. The nurse is again told to report to the ICU. The most appropriate action by the nurse is to

1 Refuse to go to the ICU.
2 Go to the ICU and tell the charge nurse that he or she is ill and needs to go home.
3 Call the hospital lawyer.
4 Go to the ICU and inform the charge nurse of the tasks that cannot be performed.

Answer: 4

Rationale: Legally, a nurse cannot refuse to float unless a union contract guarantees that nurses can work only in a specified area or the nurse can prove the lack of knowledge for the performance of assigned tasks. When encountered with this situation, nurses should set priorities and identify potential areas of harm to the client. All pertinent facts related to client care problems and safety issues should be documented. The nurse should perform only the tasks in which the nurse has received training. It is the nurse's responsibility to clearly describe these responsibilities.

Test-Taking Strategy: Eliminate option 1; if a nurse refuses to care for a client, the nurse can be charged with abandonment. Eliminate option 2 because it is similar to option 1 and is ethically unsound. Of the remaining two options, the best is option 4. Report to the ICU, provide assistance with client care, and be clear about the tasks that are unfamiliar and would jeopardize client safety.

Level of Cognitive Ability: Application
Phase of Nursing Process: Implementation
Client Needs: Safe, Effective Care Environment
Content Area: Fundamental Skills

Reference
Brent, N. (1997). *Nurses and the law.* Philadelphia: W. B. Saunders, p. 391.

243. The registered nurse (RN) asks the licensed practical nurse (LPN) to change the colostomy bag on a client. The LPN tells the RN that although the LPN received complete inservice training for this procedure, the LPN never performed it on a client. The most appropriate action by the RN is

1 Request that the LPN review the materials from the inservice before performing the procedure.
2 Request that the LPN review the procedure in the hospital manual and to bring the written procedure into the client's room for guidance during the procedure.
3 Request that another LPN observe the procedure when it is performed.
4 Perform the procedure with the LPN.

Answer: 4

Rationale: The nurse leader must remember that even though a task may be delegated to someone, the nurse who delegates maintains accountability for the overall nursing care of the client. Only the task, not the ultimate accountability, may be delegated to another. The RN is responsible for ensuring that competent and accurate care is delivered to the client. Requesting that another LPN observe the procedure does not ensure that the procedure will be done correctly. Because this is a new procedure for this LPN, the RN should accompany the LPN, provide guidance, and answer questions after the procedure.

Test-Taking Strategy: Eliminate options 1 and 2 first. Although it may be important for the LPN to review inservice materials and the hospital procedure manual, these options are not complete. Of the remaining two options, option 3 does not ensure that the LPN will perform this procedure safely. In addition, it is the RN's responsibility to educate.

Level of Cognitive Ability: Application
Phase of Nursing Process: Implementation
Client Needs: Safe, Effective Care Environment
Content Area: Fundamental Skills

Reference
DeLaune, S., & Ladner, P. (1998). *Fundamentals of nursing: Standards and practice.* Albany, NY: Delmar, p. 237.

244. The client is in suspected ventricular fibrillation, and an automatic external defibrillator is available. In planning to use this equipment, the nurse knows that the client must be placed on a

1 Water mattress.
2 Stretcher.
3 Non-electric bed.
4 Firm, dry surface.

Answer: 4

Rationale: The client must be placed on a firm, dry surface (as for any other form of defibrillation). The American Heart Association has been promoting the use of automatic external defibrillators by lay people and emergency medical technicians since 1992.

Test-Taking Strategy: You can begin to answer this question by eliminating the water mattress, because water disperses the electrical current, and so it does not get to the myocardium as effectively. The non-electric bed is unnecessary because beds are unplugged just before electric shock is delivered. A stretcher is one type of firm, dry surface, but this option is too narrow for any number of cardiac arrest scenarios. This leads you to the correct response, which also happens to be the most global: the firm, dry surface.

Level of Cognitive Ability: Application
Phase of Nursing Process: Planning
Client Needs: Safe, Effective Care Environment
Content Area: Adult Health/Cardiovascular

Reference

Ignatavicius, D. D., Workman, M. L., & Mishler, M. A. (1995). *Medical-surgical nursing: A nursing process approach* (2nd ed.). Philadelphia: W. B. Saunders, p. 879.

---

245. The nurse has applied the patch electrodes of an automatic external defibrillator (AED) to the chest of a client. The defibrillator has interpreted the rhythm to be ventricular fibrillation. The client is pulseless. The nurse then

1 Orders any personnel away from the client, charges the machine, and defibrillates through the console.
2 Performs cardiopulmonary resuscitation (CPR) for 1 minute before defibrillating.
3 Charges the machine and immediately pushes the "discharge" buttons on the console.
4 Administers rescue breathing during the defibrillation.

Answer: 1

Rationale: If the AED advises to defibrillate, the rescuer orders all persons away from the client, charges the capacitor, and pushes both of the "discharge" buttons on the console at the same time. The charge is delivered through the patch electrodes, so this method is known as "hands off" defibrillation, which is safer for the rescuer. The sequence of charges (up to three consecutive attempts at 200, 300, and 360 joules) is similar to that of conventional defibrillation.

Test-Taking Strategy: Option 4 is contraindicated, for the safety of any rescuer. There would be no benefit to the myocardium by delaying the defibrillation attempt, which eliminates option 2 as well. The two remaining options are very similar, but the correct response has a first step that the other doesn't, which is the order to "clear."

Level of Cognitive Ability: Application
Phase of Nursing Process: Implementation
Client Needs: Safe, Effective Care Environment
Content Area: Adult Health/Cardiovascular

Reference

Ignatavicius, D. D., Workman, M. L., & Mishler, M. A. (1995). *Medical-surgical nursing: A nursing process approach* (2nd ed.). Philadelphia: W. B. Saunders, p. 879.

---

246. The nurse is planning care for the client diagnosed with deep vein thrombosis (DVT) of the left leg. Which of the following interventions would the nurse avoid in the care of this client?

1 Application of moist heat to the left leg
2 Administration of acetaminophen (Tylenol)
3 Elevation of the left leg
4 Ambulation in the hall once per shift

Answer: 4

Rationale: Standard management of the client with DVT includes bed rest for 5 to 7 days; limb elevation; relief of discomfort with warm moist heat and analgesics as needed; anticoagulant therapy; and monitoring for signs of pulmonary embolism. Ambulation is contraindicated, as it increases the likelihood of dislodgment of the tail of the thrombus, which would travel to the lungs as a pulmonary embolism.

Test-Taking Strategy: This question is worded to make you look for an incorrect action, as noted by the word "avoid" in the stem. Application of heat and limb elevation are indicated to reduce inflammation and edema, so these options are not the correct answers. Tylenol relieves discomfort and is also indicated. This leaves ambulation, which could lead to pulmonary embolism. This is the dangerous action and is the correct answer for this item.

Level of Cognitive Ability: Application
Phase of Nursing Process: Planning
Client Needs: Safe, Effective Care Environment
Content Area: Adult Health/Cardiovascular

Reference

Black, J., & Matassarin-Jacobs, E. (1997). *Medical-surgical nursing: Clinical management for continuity of care* (5th ed.). Philadelphia: W. B. Saunders, p. 1435.

247. The nurse is planning care for a client scheduled for venography. The nurse knows that which of the following actions does not have to be implemented before this procedure?

1 Notation of allergies to iodine or shellfish
2 Signed consent form
3 Determining location and strength of peripheral pulses
4 NPO after midnight

Answer: 4

Rationale: Venography is similar to arteriography except it evaluates the venous system. A radiopaque dye is injected into selected veins to evaluate patency and blood flow characteristics. The client signs a special consent form, because it is an invasive procedure. Allergies to shellfish or iodine must be noted. Peripheral pulses are assessed so that comparisons can be made after the procedure. The client is usually given clear liquids for 3–4 hours before the procedure to help with dye excretion afterward.

Test-Taking Strategy: Because venography is an invasive procedure with the use of a contrast agent, options 1 and 2 are necessary; therefore, they are the wrong answers. Option 3 may be confusing, because it is an arterial measurement, not a venous one, but it is also necessary for assessing postprocedure complications. This leaves option 4, the correct choice, because NPO status will promote dehydration rather than dye clearance.

Level of Cognitive Ability: Application
Phase of Nursing Process: Planning
Client Needs: Safe, Effective Care Environment
Content Area: Adult Health/Cardiovascular

Reference

Black, J., & Matassarin-Jacobs, E. (1997). *Medical-surgical nursing: Clinical management for continuity of care* (5th ed.). Philadelphia: W. B. Saunders, p. 1385.

248. The nurse is caring for a client with severe pre-eclampsia. The client is receiving an IV infusion of magnesium sulfate. Of the following items, which item is considered to be of highest priority to have available?

1 Percussion hammer
2 Tongue blade
3 Potassium chloride injection
4 Calcium gluconate injection

Answer: 4

Rationale: Toxic effects of magnesium sulfate may cause loss of deep tendon reflexes, heart block, respiratory paralysis, and cardiac arrest. The antidote is 10–20 mL of 10% calcium gluconate (5–10 mEq of calcium). A percussion hammer may be important for assessing reflexes but is not the highest priority item. An airway rather than a tongue blade is appropriate but also is not the highest priority. Potassium chloride is not related to the issue in this question.

Test-Taking Strategy: Eliminate option 3 first because this is an unrelated item. Eliminate option 2 next. From the remaining two options, note the key phrase "highest priority." The percussion hammer would identify the decrease in deep tendon reflexes, but the calcium gluconate is necessary to treat the life-threatening condition that can occur!

Level of Cognitive Ability: Application
Phase of Nursing Process: Planning
Client Needs: Safe, Effective Care Environment
Content Area: Pharmacology

Reference

Hodgson, B., & Kizior, R. (1998). *Saunders nursing drug handbook 1998.* Philadelphia: W. B. Saunders, p. 618.

249. The nurse administers the morning dose of digoxin (Lanoxin) to the client. When the nurse charts the medication, the nurse discovers that a dose of 0.25 mg was administered rather than the prescribed dose of 0.125 mg. Which of the following actions will the nurse take?

1 Administer the additional 0.125 mg
2 Tell the client that the dose administered was not the total amount and administer the additional dose
3 Tell the client that too much medication was administered and an error was made
4 Complete an incident report

Answer: 4

Rationale: In accord with agency's policies, nurses are required to file incident reports when a situation arises that could or did cause client harm. If a dose of 0.125 mg was prescribed and a dose of 0.25 mg was administered, then the client received too much medication. Additional medication is not required and in fact could be detrimental. The client should be informed when an error has occurred but in a professional manner so as not to cause great fear and concern. In many situations, the physician will discuss this with the client.

Test-Taking Strategy: Simple math calculation will assist in eliminating both options 1 and 2. From the remaining two options, select option 4 because it is the nurse's responsibility to complete this form.

Level of Cognitive Ability: Application
Phase of Nursing Process: Implementation
Client Needs: Safe, Effective Care Environment
Content Area: Fundamental Skills

Reference

DeLaune, S., & Ladner, P. (1998). *Fundamentals of nursing: Standards and practice.* Albany, NY: Delmar, p. 237.

250. The nurse teaches a client about home care for a peripherally inserted central catheter (PICC). Which of the following would not be included in the plan of care?

1 "The catheter should be able to stay in place for several months."
2 "You should not lift heavy weights."
3 "If you notice slight redness around the site, the line will need to be discontinued."
4 "You should avoid pulling on the PICC."

Answer: 3

Rationale: Slight redness around the PICC site can be normal and often is relieved by placing warm compresses around the site and elevating the site. All of the other options reflect correct teaching for a client with a PICC line. Weight lifting can cause malpositioning of the PICC or damage to the PICC. The PICC can stay in place for months if complications do not occur. It should not be pulled on.

Test-Taking Strategy: Read the stem of the question carefully to determine that the option that would not be included in the teaching plan is the correct option. Basic knowledge of PICC care is essential for choosing the correct answer. Review this content now if you have difficulty answering this question!

Level of Cognitive Ability: Application
Phase of Nursing Process: Planning
Client Needs: Safe, Effective Care Environment
Content Area: Fundamental Skills

Reference

Phillips, L. (1997). *Manual of IV therapeutics* (2nd ed.). Philadelphia: F. A. Davis, pp. 402, 410.

251. The physician writes an order to obtain a 12-lead electrocardiogram (ECG) on a client. The nurse informs the client of the procedure. Which of the following would indicate that the client understands the procedure?

1 "I cannot breathe while the ECG is running."
2 "When the ECG begins, I must take a deep breath."
3 "I need to lie still while the ECG is being done."
4 "If I move when the ECG begins I will be shocked."

Answer: 3

Rationale: Good contact between the skin and electrode is necessary to obtain a clear 12-lead ECG printout. Therefore, the electrodes are placed on the flat surfaces of the skin just above the ankles and wrists. Movement may cause a disruption in that contact. The client does not need to hold the breath or take a deep breath during the procedure. The client needs to be reassured that a shock will not be received.

Test-Taking Strategy: While a 12-lead ECG is being done, it is best if the client does not move the extremity. This will aid in obtaining a clear ECG. Options 1, 2, and 4 are inappropriate statements. Review the procedure for obtaining an ECG now if you had difficulty with this question!

Level of Cognitive Ability: Analysis
Phase of Nursing Process: Evaluation
Client Needs: Safe, Effective Care Environment
Content Area: Adult Health/Cardiovascular

Reference

Smeltzer, S., & Bare, B. (1996). *Brunner and Suddarth's Textbook of medical-surgical nursing* (8th ed.). Philadelphia: Lippincott-Raven, p. 616.

---

252. When planning the discharge of a client with chronic anxiety, the nurse directs the goals at promoting a safe environment at home. The most appropriate maintenance goal should focus on which of the following?

1 Continued contact with a crisis counselor
2 Identifying anxiety-producing situations
3 Ignoring feelings of anxiety
4 Eliminating all anxiety from daily situations

Answer: 2

Rationale: Recognizing situations that produce anxiety allows the client to prepare to cope with anxiety or avoid specific stimuli. Counselors will not be available for all anxiety-producing situations. This option does not encourage the development of internal strengths. Ignoring feelings will not resolve anxiety. It is impossible to eliminate all anxiety from life.

Test-Taking Strategy: Eliminate option 4 first because of the word "all." Eliminate option 3 next because feelings should not be ignored. Of the remaining two options, select option 2 over option 1 because this option is more client centered and provides the preparation for the client to deal with anxiety should it occur.

Level of Cognitive Ability: Application
Phase of Nursing Process: Planning
Client Needs: Safe, Effective Care Environment
Content Area: Mental Health

Reference

Fortinash, K., & Holoday-Worret, P. (1996). *Psychiatric–mental health nursing.* St. Louis: Mosby–Year Book, p. 238.

---

253. The nurse is planning to instruct the client with chronic vertigo about safety measures to prevent exacerbation of symptoms or injury. The nurse plans to teach the client that it is important to

1 Drive at times when the client does not feel dizzy.
2 Go to the bedroom and lie down when vertigo is experienced.
3 Remove throw rugs and clutter in the home.
4 Turn the head slowly when spoken to.

Answer: 3

Rationale: The client with chronic vertigo should avoid driving and using public transportation. The sudden movements involved in each could precipitate an attack. To further prevent vertigo attacks, the client should change position slowly and should turn the entire body, not just the head, when spoken to. If vertigo does occur, the client should immediately sit down or grasp the nearest piece of furniture. The client should maintain the home in a state that is free of clutter and has throw rugs removed, because the effort of trying to regain balance after slipping could trigger the onset of vertigo.

Test-Taking Strategy: Begin to answer this question by eliminating options 1 and 2 first, because they put the client at greatest risk of injury secondary to vertigo. Choose option 3 over option 4 because it is the safer intervention of the two.

Level of Cognitive Ability: Application
Phase of Nursing Process: Planning
Client Needs: Safe, Effective Care Environment
Content Area: Adult Health/Neurological

Reference

Burrell, P., Gerlach, M., & Pless, B. (1997). *Adult nursing: Acute and community care* (2nd ed.). Stamford, CT: Appleton & Lange, p. 1933.

254. A client receiving heparin therapy for acute myocardial infarction has an activated partial thromboplastin time (APTT) value of 100 seconds. Before reporting the results to the physician, the nurse may verify that which of the following is available for use?

1 Protamine sulfate
2 Vitamin K (Synkayvite)
3 Vitamin B_{12} (cyanocobalamin)
4 Methylene blue (Urolene Blue)

Answer: 1

Rationale: Therapeutic values of APTT for clients on heparin range between 60 and 70 seconds. A value of 100 seconds indicates that the client has received too much heparin. The antidote for heparin overdosage is protamine sulfate. Vitamin K is the antidote for warfarin sodium overdosage. Methylene blue is an antidote for cyanide poisoning. Vitamin B_{12} is used to treat clients with pernicious anemia.

Test-Taking Strategy: Knowledge of the normal APTT values and the significance of abnormally prolonged values is necessary to answer the question. Eliminate options 3 and 4, knowing that options 1 and 2 are the antidotes for anticoagulants. From this point, it is necessary to know that protamine sulfate is the antidote for heparin.

Level of Cognitive Ability: Analysis
Phase of Nursing Process: Planning
Client Needs: Safe, Effective Care Environment
Content Area: Pharmacology

Reference

Wilson, B., Shannon, M., & Stang, C. (1997). *Nurse's drug guide.* Stamford, CT: Appleton & Lange, p. 1178.

---

255. A suicidal male client is being discharged home to family. Which of the following statements by family members might constitute criteria for delaying discharge?

1 The client's wife asks, "Does he know that I've already moved out and filed for a divorce?"
2 The client's son states, "One of his friends visited last week to tell us Dad's union is out on strike."
3 The client's daughter states, "I've decided to postpone my wedding until Dad's feeling better."
4 The client's brother asks, "Will my brother be able to continue as executor of our parent's trust?"

Answer: 1

Rationale: Among single, divorced, and widowed persons, suicide rates are four to five times higher than those among persons who are married. Although the situation of the strike is stressful, the client will probably receive a portion of his wages and can derive hope and a sense of belonging from being a member of the union. Although the client might feel responsible for his daughter's postponement of the wedding, if presented as an action to include him, the client will feel loved and cared for. Although being suicidal may reduce the ability to concentrate, if the client perceives the executorship positively, taking the role away reinforces the client's low self-esteem and self-worth. This statement by the client's brother indicates a need for the client's brother to be educated about depressive illness.

Test-Taking Strategy: The issue of the question is the presence of a safe environment at home. Eliminate options 2, 3, and 4. Option 1 reveals that the client's wife has left him and filed for divorce without telling him. To expose the client to this situation without preparation would set him up for emotional trauma as soon as he returned home.

Level of Cognitive Ability: Analysis
Phase of Nursing Process: Evaluation
Client Needs: Safe, Effective Care Environment
Content Area: Mental Health

Reference

Carson, V., & Arnold, E. (1996). *Mental health nursing: The nurse-patient journey.* Philadelphia: W. B. Saunders, p. 930.

256. Which of the following is most important to assess before ambulating a client with Parkinson's disease who has recently started L-dopa (Levodopa) therapy?

1 Assistive devices used by the client
2 The degree of intention tremors exhibited by the client
3 The client's history of falls
4 The client's postural vital signs

Answer: 4

Rationale: Clients with Parkinson's disease are at risk for postural (orthostatic) hypotension from the disease. This problem is exacerbated with the introduction of L-dopa, which can also cause postural hypotension, thus increasing the client's risk for falls. Although knowledge of the client's use of assistive devices and history of falls is helpful, it is not the most important piece of assessment data, according to the wording of this question. Clients with Parkinson's disease generally have resting, not intention, tremors.

Test-Taking Strategy: The stem of the question asks for the most important assessment parameter before ambulation for the client on L-dopa. Postural hypotension presents the largest safety risk to the client. Remember your ABCs—airway, breathing, and circulation—when prioritizing answers. Checking postural vital signs is one way to assess circulation!

Level of Cognitive Ability: Analysis
Phase of Nursing Process: Assessment
Client Needs: Safe, Effective Care Environment
Content Area: Pharmacology

Reference

Deglin, J., & Vallerand, A. (1997). *Davis's drug guide for nurses* (5th ed.). Philadelphia: F. A. Davis, pp. 693–694.

257. The nurse is giving a bed bath to a client who is on strict bed rest. In order to increase venous return, the nurse bathes the client's extremities by using

1 Long, firm strokes from distal to proximal areas.
2 Firm circular strokes from proximal to distal areas.
3 Short, patting strokes from distal to proximal areas.
4 Smooth, light strokes back and forth from proximal to distal areas.

Answer: 1

Rationale: Long, firm strokes in the direction of venous flow promote venous return when the extremities are bathed. Circular strokes are used on the face. Short, patting strokes and light strokes are not as comfortable for the client and do not promote venous return.

Test-Taking Strategy: Knowledge of the procedure for bathing a client will assist you in answering this question. Eliminate options 2 and 4 first because a stroke from proximal to distal will not promote venous return. Select option 1 over option 3 because long, firm strokes will promote venous return and client comfort.

Level of Cognitive Ability: Application
Phase of Nursing Process: Implementation
Client Needs: Safe, Effective Care Environment
Content Area: Fundamental Skills

Reference

Kozier, B., Erb, G., & Blais, K. (1998). *Fundamentals of nursing: Concepts, process, and practice* (5th ed.). Menlo Park, CA: Addison-Wesley, pp. 740–741.

258. The nurse is preparing to give an intramuscular (IM) injection that is irritating to the subcutaneous tissues. The drug reference recommends that it be given with the Z-track technique. Which of the following procedural steps would cause tracking of the medication through the subcutaneous tissues?

1. Preparing a 0.2-mL air lock in the syringe after drawing up the medication
2. Massaging the site after injecting the medication
3. Attaching a new sterile needle to the syringe after drawing up the medication
4. Retracting the skin to the side before piercing the skin with the needle

Answer: 2

Rationale: The Z-track variation of the standard IM technique is used to administer IM medications that are highly irritating to subcutaneous and skin tissues. A new sterile needle is attached so that the new needle will not have any medication adhering to the outside that could be irritating to the tissues. Preparing an air lock keeps the needle clean of medication on insertion, and as the air is injected behind the medication, it provides a seal at the point of insertion to prevent tracking of the medication. Retracting the skin provides a seal over the injected medication to prevent tracking through the subcutaneous tissues. The site should not be massaged because this can lead to tissue irritation.

Test-Taking Strategy: Options 1, 3, and 4 are procedural steps for Z-track injection. Option 2 is incorrect; Z-track injections are not massaged because this could lead to tissue irritation. Review this procedure for administering medications now if you had difficulty with this question!

Level of Cognitive Ability: Application
Phase of Nursing Process: Implementation
Client Needs: Safe, Effective Care Environment
Content Area: Fundamental Skills

Reference

Kozier, B., Erb, G., & Blais, K. (1998). *Fundamentals of nursing: Concepts, process, and practice* (5th ed.). Menlo Park, CA: Addison-Wesley, pp. 1331–1332.

259. The nurse is preparing to transfer an average-sized client with right-sided hemiplegia from the bed to the wheelchair. The client is able to support weight on the unaffected side. The nurse plans to use the hemiplegic transfer technique. The client is sitting up in bed with the legs dangling over the side. For the safest transfer, the wheelchair should be positioned

1. Near the client's right leg.
2. Next to either leg.
3. As space in the room permits.
4. Near the client's left leg.

Answer: 4

Rationale: Space in the room is an important consideration for placement of the wheelchair for a transfer; however, when the client has an affected lower extremity, movement should always occur toward the client's unaffected (strong) side. For example, if the client's right leg is involved, and the client is sitting on the edge of the bed, position the wheelchair next to the client's left side. This wheelchair position allows the client to use the unaffected leg effectively and safely.

Test-Taking Strategy: The question asks you to select the option that will provide the safest transfer for the client. Although option 3 is a consideration for wheelchair position, it is not the safest answer. Option 4 will provide the safest transfer because positioning the wheelchair next to the client's unaffected leg allows the client to use the stronger leg more effectively for a safe transfer.

Level of Cognitive Ability: Application
Phase of Nursing Process: Implementation
Client Needs: Safe, Effective Care Environment
Content Area: Fundamental Skills

Reference

Kozier, B., Erb, G., & Blais, K. (1998). *Fundamentals of nursing: Concepts, process, and practice* (5th ed.). Menlo Park, CA: Addison-Wesley, pp. 923–926.

260. The nurse is preparing to suction a client's tracheostomy. In order to promote deep breathing and coughing, the client should ideally be positioned in the

1. Supine position.
2. Lateral position.
3. High Fowler's position.
4. Semi-Fowler's position.

Answer: 4

Rationale: If it is not contraindicated because of health, the client before suctioning of a tracheostomy is placed in semi-Fowler's position to promote deep breathing, maximum lung expansion, and productive coughing. With the client in this position, gravity pulls downward on the diaphragm, which allows greater chest expansion and lung volume.

Test-Taking Strategy: Knowledge of the procedure for suctioning a tracheostomy will assist you in answering this question. You can easily eliminate options 1 and 2 first. From the remaining two options, eliminate option 3 because the high Fowler's position would not allow for easy visualization of the tracheostomy or easy access of the suction catheter. The semi-Fowler's position promotes deep breathing, maximum lung expansion, and productive coughing. Review this procedure now if you had difficulty with this question!

Level of Cognitive Ability: Application
Phase of Nursing Process: Implementation
Client Needs: Safe, Effective Care Environment
Content Area: Fundamental Skills

Reference

Kozier, B., Erb, G., & Blais, K. (1998). *Fundamentals of nursing: Concepts, process, and practice* (5th ed.). Menlo Park, CA: Addison-Wesley, p. 1164.

---

261. The pregnant client is at full term. The fetal heart rate (FHR) is being monitored for a baseline rate. The nurse is satisfied with the results and tells the client that the baby's heart rate is within normal limits. This is based on which of the following data?

1. FHR of 90–100 beats per minute
2. FHR of 140–150 beats per minute
3. FHR of 80–90 beats per minute
4. FHR of 170–180 beats per minute

Answer: 2

Rationale: The average FHR at term is 140 beats per minute. The normal range is 110–160 beats per minute; therefore, option 2 is the only correct answer.

Test-Taking Strategy: Knowledge of the normal fetal heart rate is necessary to answer this question. If you are unfamiliar with this content take the time now to review it.

Level of Cognitive Ability: Analysis
Phase of Nursing Process: Evaluation
Client Needs: Safe, Effective Care Environment
Content Area: Maternity

Reference

Nichols, F., & Zwelling, E. (1997). *Maternal-newborn nursing: Theory and practice.* Philadelphia: W. B. Saunders, p. 1068.

---

262. The nurse is caring for a client with a grave clinical condition who is a potential organ donor. Before approaching the family to discuss organ donation, the nurse reviews the client's medical record for contraindications to organ donation, which would include

1. Allergy to penicillin-type antibiotics.
2. Age of 38 years.
3. Hepatitis B infection.
4. Negative rapid plasma reagin (RPR) laboratory result.

Answer: 3

Rationale: A potential organ donor must meet age eligibility requirements, which vary by organ. For example, age must not exceed 65 for kidney donation, 55 for pancreas and liver, or 40 for heart. The client should be free of communicable disease, such as HIV and hepatitis, and the involved organ may not be diseased. Another contraindication to transplantation is malignancy, with the exception of noninvolved skin and cornea.

Test-Taking Strategy: The key word in the stem is "contraindicated." With this in mind, you would eliminate option 2 first. Because allergies are not part of decision-making criteria, you would eliminate option 1 next. Option 4 indicates an absence of syphilis (a communicable disease), which leaves option 3 (hepatitis B) as the correct choice.

Level of Cognitive Ability: Application
Phase of Nursing Process: Analysis
Client Needs: Safe, Effective Care Environment
Content Area: Fundamental Skills

Reference

Black, J., & Matassarin-Jacobs, E. (1997). *Medical-surgical nursing: Clinical management for continuity of care* (5th ed.). Philadelphia: W. B. Saunders, p. 646.

---

263. The nurse is evaluating the ongoing care given to the potential organ donor who has received a diagnosis of brain death. The nurse evaluates that the standard of care has been maintained if which of the following data is observed?

1 Urine output, 45 mL/hour
2 Capillary refill, 5 seconds
3 Serum pH, 7.32
4 Blood pressure, 90/48 mmHg

Answer: 1

Rationale: Adequate perfusion must be maintained to all vital organs in order for the organs to remain viable for donation. A urine output of 45 mL/hour indicates adequate renal perfusion. Low blood pressure and delayed capillary refill time are circulatory system indicators of inadequate perfusion. A serum pH of 7.32 is acidotic, which adversely affects all body tissues.

Test-Taking Strategy: Eliminate options 2, 3, and 4 because they are abnormal values. If this question was difficult, take a few moments to review normal values for physical assessment measurements!

Level of Cognitive Ability: Analysis
Phase of Nursing Process: Evaluation
Client Needs: Safe, Effective Care Environment
Content Area: Fundamental Skills

Reference

Black, J., & Matassarin-Jacobs, E. (1997). *Medical-surgical nursing: Clinical management for continuity of care* (5th ed.). Philadelphia: W. B. Saunders, p. 647.

---

264. The client who suffered a severe head injury has had vigorous treatment to control cerebral edema. Brain death has now been determined. The nurse prepares to carry out which of the following orders to maintain viability of the kidneys before organ donation?

1 Monitoring of temperature
2 Administration of IV fluids
3 Assessment of lung sounds
4 Frequent range of motion to extremities

Answer: 2

Rationale: Perfusion to the kidney is affected by blood pressure, which is in turn affected by blood vessel tone and fluid volume. Therefore, the client who was previously dehydrated in order to control intracranial pressure is now in need of rehydration to maintain perfusion to the kidneys. Thus the nurse prepares to infuse IV fluids as ordered and continues to monitor urine output.

Test-Taking Strategy: Note the key words in the question, which are "maintain viability." This implies an action orientation, guiding you to look for options that are interventions rather than assessments. With this in mind, you would eliminate options 1 and 3 first. You would choose the correct answer of the remaining two by comparing them in terms of their benefit to the kidneys.

Level of Cognitive Ability: Application
Phase of Nursing Process: Planning
Client Needs: Safe, Effective Care Environment
Content Area: Fundamental Skills

Reference

Black, J., & Matassarin-Jacobs, E. (1997). *Medical-surgical nursing: Clinical management for continuity of care* (5th ed.). Philadelphia: W. B. Saunders, p. 647.

265. The nurse is working in the emergency room of a small local hospital when a client with multiple gunshot wounds arrives by ambulance. Which of the following actions by the nurse is contraindicated in the proper care of handling legal evidence?

1 Cutting clothing along seams, avoiding bullet holes
2 Initiating a chain-of-custody log
3 Placing personal belongings in a labeled, sealed paper bag
4 Giving clothing and wallet to the family

Answer: 4

Rationale: Basic rules for handling evidence include limiting the number of people with access to the evidence; initiating a chain-of-custody log to track handling and movement of evidence; and careful removal of clothing to avoid destroying evidence. This usually includes cutting clothes along seams, while avoiding areas where there are obvious holes or tears. Potential evidence is never released to the family to take home.

Test-Taking Strategy: The key word in this question is "contraindicated." Use knowledge of basic emergency nursing principles to eliminate each of the incorrect options. You should easily be directed toward option 4 because giving these belongings to the family may be giving up evidence. If this question was difficult, review these core principles at this time.

Level of Cognitive Ability: Application
Phase of Nursing Process: Implementation
Client Needs: Safe, Effective Care Environment
Content Area: Fundamental Skills

Reference

Luckmann, J. (1997). *Saunders manual of nursing care.* Philadelphia: W. B. Saunders, p. 1791.

266. The nurse working on a medical nursing unit during an external disaster is called to assist with care for clients coming into the emergency room. Using principles of triage, the nurse initiates care for a client with which of the following injuries?

1 Bright red bleeding from a neck wound
2 Penetrating abdominal injury
3 Fractured tibia
4 Open severe head injury with deep coma

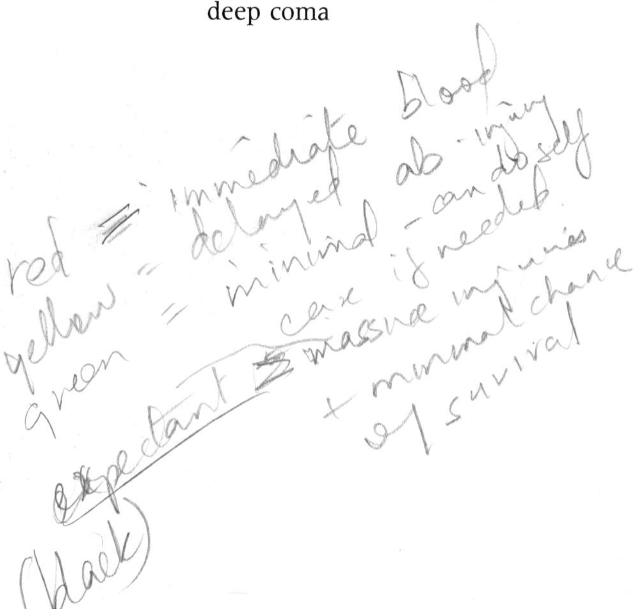

Answer: 1

Rationale: The client with arterial bleeding from a neck wound is in "immediate" need of treatment to save the client's life. A client in this classification would wear a color tag of red from the triage process. The client with a penetrating abdominal injury would be tagged yellow and classified as "delayed," requiring intervention within 30 to 60 minutes. A green or "minimal" designation would be given to the client with a fractured tibia, who requires intervention but who can provide self-care if needed. A designation of "expectant" would be applied to the client with massive injuries and minimal chance of survival. This client would be color coded "black" in the triage process. These clients are given supportive care and pain management, but are given definitive treatment last.

Test-Taking Strategy: To answer this question accurately, you must be able to apply principles of triage to the clients identified in the case. Eliminate options 2 and 3 first, because they are least in need of immediate care. Discriminate between options 1 and 4 by determining which client has the better chance of a positive outcome from intervention.

Level of Cognitive Ability: Analysis
Phase of Nursing Process: Implementation
Client Needs: Safe, Effective Care Environment
Content Area: Fundamental Skills

Reference

Luckmann, J. (1997). *Saunders manual of nursing care.* Philadelphia: W. B. Saunders, p. 1792.

267. The nurse working on an adult nursing unit is told to review the client census to determine which clients could be discharged if there are a large number of admissions from a newly declared disaster. The nurse interprets that the client with which of the following problems would not be able to be discharged, even if support was available at home?

1 Laparoscopic cholecystectomy (same day)
2 Ongoing ventricular dysrhythmias while on procainamide (Procan-Bid)
3 Diabetes with blood glucose at 180 mg/dL
4 Fractured hip pinned 5 days ago

Answer: 2

Rationale: The client with ongoing ventricular dysrhythmias requires ongoing medical evaluation and treatment, because of potentially lethal consequences of the problem. Each of the other problems listed may be managed at home with appropriate agency referrals for home care services and with support from the family at home.

Test-Taking Strategy: Use principles of triage to answer this question accurately. Severity of illness usually guides the determination of who requires ongoing monitoring and care. Use the ABCs: airway, breathing, and circulation. With this in mind, you may eliminate each of the other incorrect responses.

Level of Cognitive Ability: Analysis
Phase of Nursing Process: Analysis
Client Needs: Safe, Effective Care Environment
Content Area: Fundamental Skills

Reference

Luckmann, J. (1997). *Saunders manual of nursing care.* Philadelphia: W. B. Saunders, p. 1698.

268. The nurse is orienting a nursing assistant to the clinical nursing unit. The nurse would intervene if the nursing assistant did which of the following during a routine handwashing procedure?

1 Kept hands lower than elbows
2 Used 3–5 mL soap from dispenser
3 Washed continuously for 10–15 seconds
4 Dried from forearm down to fingers

Answer: 4

Rationale: Proper handwashing procedure involves wetting hands and wrists and keeping hands lower than forearms so water flows toward fingertips. The nurse uses 3–5 mL of soap and scrubs for 10–15 seconds, using rubbing and circular motions. The hands are rinsed and then dried, moving from fingers to forearms. The paper towel is then discarded, and a second one is used to turn off the faucet to avoid hand contamination.

Test-Taking Strategy: Note that the wording of the question guides you to look for an incorrect response. Use basic principles of medical asepsis to answer this question. If you answered incorrectly, review this fundamental nursing procedure at this time!

Level of Cognitive Ability: Application
Phase of Nursing Process: Implementation
Client Needs: Safe, Effective Care Environment
Content Area: Fundamental Skills

Reference

Taylor, C., Lillis, C., & LeMone, P. (1997). *Fundamentals of nursing: The art and science of nursing care* (3rd ed.). Philadelphia: Lippincott-Raven, pp. 564–565.

269. The client who is immunosuppressed is being admitted with neutropenic precautions. The nurse plans to ensure that which of the following does not occur in the care of the client?

1 Placing a mask on client if the client leaves the room
2 Removal of a vase with fresh flowers left by a previous client
3 Admitting the client to a semiprivate room
4 Placing a sign on the door to the room

Answer: 3

Rationale: The client who is on neutropenic precautions is immunosuppressed and is admitted to a single room on the nursing unit. A sign indicating neutropenic precautions have been initiated should be placed on the door to the client's room. Removal of sources of standing water and fresh flowers is done to decrease microorganism count. The client should wear a mask whenever leaving the room to be protected from exposure to microorganisms.

Test-Taking Strategy: The wording of the question guides you to look for an option that is an incorrect nursing action. Knowing that neutropenic precautions are instituted when the client is at risk for infection because of impaired immune function, you would eliminate each of the incorrect options systematically. If this question was difficult, take a few moments to review this type of infection control precaution at this time!

Level of Cognitive Ability: Application
Phase of Nursing Process: Planning
Client Needs: Safe, Effective Care Environment
Content Area: Adult Health/Oncology

Reference

Taylor, C., Lillis, C., & LeMone, P. (1997). *Fundamentals of nursing: The art and science of nursing care* (3rd ed.). Philadelphia: Lippincott-Raven, p. 572.

---

270. The client who received a dose of chemotherapy 12 hours ago is incontinent of urine while in bed. The nurse should plan to wear which of the following when cleaning the client?

1. Mask and gloves
2. Gown and gloves
3. Mask, gown, and gloves
4. Gown, gloves, and eyewear

Answer: 2

Rationale: The client who has received chemotherapy within the last 48 hours will have antineoplastic agents or their metabolites in body fluids and excreta. For this reason, the nurse should wear protection from likely sources of contamination. In this instance, the nurse should wear gloves and gown, to protect the hands and uniform from contamination.

Test-Taking Strategy: Begin to answer this question by reasoning that the potential source of contamination in this situation is the client's urine. Because urine present on the hospital gown and bedclothes is not likely to splash, you may eliminate the options involving a mask or eyewear. This leaves only option 2, which is the correct answer.

Level of Cognitive Ability: Application
Phase of Nursing Process: Planning
Client Needs: Safe, Effective Care Environment
Content Area: Adult Health/Oncology

Reference

Black, J., & Matassarin-Jacobs, E. (1997). *Medical-surgical nursing: Clinical management for continuity of care* (5th ed.). Philadelphia: W. B. Saunders, p. 576.

---

271. The client receiving chemotherapy has infiltration of the intravenous line and extravasation at the site. The nurse would avoid doing which of the following in the management of this situation?

1. Stopping the drug administration
2. Leaving the needle in place and aspirating any residual medication
3. Administering an available antidote
4. Applying direct manual pressure to the site

Answer: 4

Rationale: General recommendations for managing extravasation of a chemotherapeutic agent include stopping the infusion; leaving the needle in place and attempting to aspirate any residual drug from the site and tubing; administering an antidote if available; and assessment of the site for complications. Direct pressure is not applied to the site because it could further injure tissues exposed to the chemotherapeutic drug.

Test-Taking Strategy: The wording of the question guides you to look for an action that the nurse would avoid. A review of each of the options should allow you to eliminate the options that reflect correct actions systematically. Review treatment measures for extravasation now if you had difficulty with this question!

Level of Cognitive Ability: Application
Phase of Nursing Process: Implementation
Client Needs: Safe, Effective Care Environment
Content Area: Adult Health/Oncology

Reference

Black, J., & Matassarin-Jacobs, E. (1997). *Medical-surgical nursing: Clinical management for continuity of care* (5th ed.). Philadelphia: W. B. Saunders, p. 576.

272. The nurse receives a call that a client who will undergo implantation of a sealed internal radiation source is being admitted. The nurse contacts the admissions clerk to ensure that which of the following beds is booked for the client?

1 A single room at the distant end of the hall
2 A single room near the nurse's station
3 A semiprivate room between two isolation rooms
4 A semiprivate room near the nurse's station

Answer: 1

Rationale: The client receiving an implantation of a sealed radiation source should be placed in a single room in an area that reduces the risk of exposure to others. For this reason, rooms that are at the end of a hall or near a stairwell are often used.

Test-Taking Strategy: To answer this question accurately, use the principle of shielding related to radiation therapy. This would guide you to eliminate options 3 and 4 first, because they do not provide distance to protect other clients. The nurse would use the same principle to choose option 1 over option 2.

Level of Cognitive Ability: Application
Phase of Nursing Process: Implementation
Client Needs: Safe, Effective Care Environment
Content Area: Adult Health/Oncology

Reference

Black, J., & Matassarin-Jacobs, E. (1997). *Medical-surgical nursing: Clinical management for continuity of care* (5th ed.). Philadelphia: W. B. Saunders, pp. 572–573.

273. The nurse is assessing the corneal reflex on an unconscious client. The nurse would use which of the following as the safest stimulus to touch the client's cornea?

1 Wisp of cotton
2 Sterile drop of saline
3 Sterile glove
4 Tip of a 1-mL syringe

Answer: 2

Rationale: The client who is unconscious is at great risk of corneal abrasion. For this reason, the safest way to test the corneal reflex is by using a drop of sterile saline.

Test-Taking Strategy: Remember that options that are similar are not likely to be correct. In this case, each of the incorrect options is a solid substance, whereas the correct answer is a liquid.

Level of Cognitive Ability: Application
Phase of Nursing Process: Implementation
Client Needs: Safe, Effective Care Environment
Content Area: Adult Health/Neurological

Reference

Black, J., & Matassarin-Jacobs, E. (1997). *Medical-surgical nursing: Clinical management for continuity of care* (5th ed.). Philadelphia: W. B. Saunders, pp. 726–727.

274. The nurse is preparing to assist the client from bed to chair, using a hydraulic lift. The nurse would do which of the following to move the client correctly with this device?

1 Have three staff members available to assist
2 Position the client in the center of the sling
3 Have the client grasp the chains attaching the sling to the lift
4 Lower the client rapidly once he or she is positioned over the chair

Answer: 2

Rationale: One person may operate a hydraulic lift, although two people are better. The client is positioned in the center of the sling, which is then attached to chains or straps that attach the sling to the lift. The client's hands and arms are crossed over the chest, and the client is raised from the bed into a sitting position. The client is also raised off the mattress with the lift and is lowered slowly once the sling is positioned over the chair.

Test-Taking Strategy: Familiarity with this basic procedure is necessary to answer this question correctly. If needed, take a few moments to review this procedure now!

Level of Cognitive Ability: Application
Phase of Nursing Process: Implementation
Client Needs: Safe, Effective Care Environment
Content Area: Fundamental Skills

Reference

Taylor, C., Lillis, C., & LeMone, P. (1997). *Fundamentals of nursing: The art and science of nursing care* (3rd ed.). Philadelphia: Lippincott-Raven, p. 1048.

275. The nurse is caring for the client who has an intracranial pressure monitor in place. The nurse observes a dampened wave form on the screen and begins to obtain inaccurate readings. The nurse interprets that which of the following could not be responsible for this problem?

1 Transducer placed at the level of the device
2 Presence of a leak in the system
3 Valsalva maneuver by the client
4 Obstruction in the tubing

Answer: 1

Rationale: A dampened wave form and inaccurate readings could be attributed to leaks or kinks in the system, differences between transducer height and the device, or a Valsalva maneuver by the client. If a dampened wave form occurs, a preliminary action would be to flush the system.

Test-Taking Strategy: To answer this question accurately, use principles related to monitoring of closed systems, similar to monitoring with central venous pressure or intra-arterial lines. This should allow you to eliminate each of the incorrect options systematically.
Level of Cognitive Ability: Analysis
Phase of Nursing Process: Analysis
Client Needs: Safe, Effective Care Environment
Content Area: Adult Health/Neurological

Reference

Black, J., & Matassarin-Jacobs, E. (1997). *Medical-surgical nursing: Clinical management for continuity of care* (5th ed.). Philadelphia: W. B. Saunders, p. 777.

---

276. The elderly client in a long-term care facility has a nursing diagnosis of Risk for Injury related to confusion. The client's gait is stable. Which of the following methods of restraint would be best used by the nurse to prevent injury to the client?

1 Vest restraint
2 Waist restraint
3 Chair with locking lap tray
4 Alarm-activating bracelet

Answer: 4

Rationale: If the client is confused and has a stable gait, the least intrusive method of restraint is the use of an alarm-activating bracelet, or "wandering bracelet." This allows the client to move about the residence freely while preventing the client from leaving the premises.

Test-Taking Strategy: To answer this question accurately, it is necessary to be familiar with the various restraint methods and the ethical and legal ramifications of restraint. This knowledge will allow you to eliminate each of the incorrect options. The use of the phrase "stable gait" is also a guide in your selection.

Level of Cognitive Ability: Application
Phase of Nursing Process: Planning
Client Needs: Safe, Effective Care Environment
Content Area: Fundamental Skills

Reference

Black, J., & Matassarin-Jacobs, E. (1997). *Medical-surgical nursing: Clinical management for continuity of care* (5th ed.). Philadelphia: W. B. Saunders, p. 767.

---

277. The nurse is suctioning the airway of a client with a tracheostomy. To properly perform the procedure, the nurse

1 Turns on wall suction to 180 mmHg.
2 Inserts the catheter until coughing or resistance is felt.
3 Withdraws the catheter while suctioning.
4 Reinserts the catheter into the tracheostomy after suctioning the mouth.

Answer: 2

Rationale: The wall suction unit is usually set to 80–120 mmHg of pressure. This allows adequate removal of secretions while protecting the airway from trauma. The nurse inserts the catheter until resistance is felt and then withdraws it 1 cm to move away from mucosa. The nurse suctions intermittently and does not reinsert the catheter into the tracheostomy after suctioning the client's mouth.

Test-Taking Strategy: Familiarity with this common procedure is needed to answer this question accurately. From this knowledge, use the process of elimination. If needed, take a few moments to review this procedure now!

Level of Cognitive Ability: Application
Phase of Nursing Process: Implementation
Client Needs: Safe, Effective Care Environment
Content Area: Adult Health/Respiratory

Reference

Potter, P., & Perry, A. (1997). *Fundamentals of nursing: Concepts, process, and practice* (4th ed.). St. Louis: Mosby–Year Book, pp. 1223–1225.

278. Furosemide (Lasix), 40 mg PO, has been prescribed for the client. The nurse administers Lasix, 80 mg, to the client at 10:00 A.M. After discovery of the error, the nurse completes an incident report. Which of the following would the nurse document on this report?

1. Lasix, 80 mg, was given to the client instead of 40 mg
2. The wrong dose of medication was given to the client at 10:00 A.M.
3. I meant to give 40 mg of Lasix but I was rushed to get to another client who needed me and I gave the wrong dose
4. Lasix, 80 mg, administered at 10:00 A.M.

Answer: 4

Rationale: When filing an incident report, the nurse should state the fact clearly. Assumptions, opinions, judgments, or conclusions about what occurred should not be recorded. The nurse should not assign blame or suggest how to prevent an occurrence of a similar incident.

Test-Taking Strategy: Read the occurrence as stated in the question. Using the process of elimination, select the response that clearly and most directly states what has occurred. Option 1 is eliminated first because it contains unnecessary information. Option 2 is incorrect because it assigns blame to the nurse. Option 3 provides a judgment. Option 4 clearly and simply states the occurrence.

Level of Cognitive Ability: Application
Phase of Nursing Process: Implementation
Client Needs: Safe, Effective Care Environment
Content Area: Fundamental Skills

Reference
DeLaune, S., & Ladner, P. (1998). *Fundamentals of nursing: Standards and practice.* Albany, NY: Delmar, pp. 236, 502.

---

279. The nurse leader on the night shift assists the staff member in completing an incident report for a client who was found sitting on the floor. After completion of the report, which of the following would the nurse leader not instruct the staff member to do?

1. Document in the nurse's notes that an incident report was filed
2. Forward the incident report to the Continuous Quality Improvement Department
3. Ask the unit secretary to call the physician
4. Notify the nursing supervisor

Answer: 1

Rationale: Nurses are advised not to document the filing of an incident report in their notes. Information in the medical record can be considered evidence, and the record can be obtained by subpoena if a lawsuit is filed by the client. Incident reports inform the facility's administration of the incident so that risk management personnel can consider changes to prevent similar occurrences in the future. Incident reports also alert the facility's insurance company to a potential claim and the need for further investigation. Options 2, 3, and 4 are accurate interventions.

Test-Taking Strategy: Use the process of elimination. Note the word "not" in the stem of the question. Note that options 2, 3, and 4 are related to notification of key individuals or departments. Option 1 relates to inappropriate documentation. Review the concepts that surround incident reports now if you had difficulty with this question!

Level of Cognitive Ability: Application
Phase of Nursing Process: Implementation
Client Needs: Safe, Effective Care Environment
Content Area: Fundamental Skills

Reference
DeLaune, S., & Ladner, P. (1998). *Fundamentals of nursing: Standards and practice.* Albany, NY: Delmar, p. 502.

---

280. During a visit to a client on the nursing unit, the physician is called to another nursing unit to assess a client in extreme pain. The physician states to the nurse, "I'm in a hurry. Can you write the order to decrease the atenolol (Tenormin) to 25 mg daily?" Which of the following is the most appropriate nursing action?

1. Write the order as stated
2. Call the nursing supervisor to write the order
3. Ask the physician to return to the nursing unit to write the order
4. Inform the client of the change of medication

Answer: 3

Rationale: Nurses are encouraged not to accept verbal orders from the physician because of the risks of error. The only exception to this may be in an emergency situation, and then the agency policy and procedure must be adhered to. Although the client will be informed of the change in the treatment plan, this is not the most appropriate action at this time. The physician needs to write the new order.

Test-Taking Strategy: Knowledge that verbal orders are not acceptable will assist in selecting the correct option. Options 1 and 2 are similar; therefore, eliminate these options. Option 4 is appropriate but not at this time. Option 3 clearly identifies the nurse's responsibility in this situation. Review these principles now if you had difficulty with this question!

Level of Cognitive Ability: Application
Phase of Nursing Process: Implementation
Client Needs: Safe, Effective Care Environment
Content Area: Fundamental Skills

Reference

DeLaune, S., & Ladner, P. (1998). *Fundamentals of nursing: Standards and practice.* Albany, NY: Delmar, p. 237.

---

281. The nurse is preparing the client for a gallium scan. Which of the following should the nurse plan to include in preprocedure instructions to the client?

1 All metal objects must be removed
2 The client must not be allergic to iodine
3 There is no need for signed consent
4 There is absolutely no pain involved

Answer: 1

Rationale: A gallium scan uses an IV injection of the radioisotope gallium citrate. Tumors and inflammations take up the gallium, as do many organs. It is often used to differentiate tumor from pulmonary embolus when x-ray is unclear. No iodine is involved, but there is local pain at the injection site. Serial scans are completed at 24, 48, and 72 hours. The client must remove all metal for the procedure, although it may be completed with clothing on. A signed consent is necessary for injection of the radioisotope.

Test-Taking Strategy: To answer this question accurately, it is necessary to know that gallium is a radioisotope. With this in mind, you may eliminate options 2 and 3. You would choose option 1 over option 4 by recalling that the substance may cause discomfort during injection.

Level of Cognitive Ability: Application
Phase of Nursing Process: Planning
Client Needs: Safe, Effective Care Environment
Content Area: Adult Health/Respiratory

Reference

Black, J., & Matassarin-Jacobs, E. (1997). *Medical-surgical nursing: Clinical management for continuity of care* (5th ed.). Philadelphia: W. B. Saunders, p. 1061.

---

282. The nurse is taking a 1-minute pulse on a client with a permanent-demand ventricular pacemaker set at a rate of 72 beats/minute. The nurse notes the client's pulse to be 67. Which of the following is the most important action by the nurse?

1 Document the pulse on the medical record
2 Recheck the pulse in 4 hours
3 Check the life span of the pacemaker battery
4 Notify the physician

Answer: 4

Rationale: A client who has a pacemaker rate that is lower than the preset rate is experiencing some form of pacemaker failure. This may occur due to conditions such as low voltage, battery failure, sensing malfunction, or disconnected or broken lead wire. The physician should be notified.

Test-Taking Strategy: To answer this question correctly, note the key phrase in this question, which is "most important." This tells you that you must prioritize your answer. Begin to answer the question by eliminating option 2 first. Options 1 and 3 are done, but they are ultimately less important than option 4, which is of utmost importance.

Level of Cognitive Ability: Application
Phase of Nursing Process: Implementation
Client Needs: Safe, Effective Care Environment
Content Area: Adult Health/Cardiovascular

Reference

Black, J., & Matassarin-Jacobs, E. (1997). *Medical-surgical nursing: Clinical management for continuity of care* (5th ed.). Philadelphia: W. B. Saunders, p. 1321.

283. The nurse has prepared the client for intravenous pyelography. The nurse evaluates that the client is knowledgeable about the procedure if the client states that he or she will report which of the following sensations immediately?

1 Nausea
2 Difficulty breathing
3 Warm, flushed feeling in the body
4 Salty taste in the mouth

Answer: 2

Rationale: Intravenous pyelography is a contrast study of the kidneys to determine a variety of disorders of the kidneys, ureters, and bladder. Normal sensations during injection of the iodine-based radiopaque dye include a warm, flushed feeling; salty taste in the mouth; and transient nausea. Hives, itching, wheezing, and difficulty breathing signal an allergic response and should be reported immediately. This complication is prevented by inquiring about allergies to iodine or shellfish before the procedure.

Test-Taking Strategy: To answer this question correctly, it is necessary to know that this diagnostic test involves injection of an iodine-based contrast medium. Differentiate between the normal expectations and the symptom that would indicate a reaction. With this in mind, you may eliminate each of the incorrect options systematically.

Level of Cognitive Ability: Analysis
Phase of Nursing Process: Evaluation
Client Needs: Safe, Effective Care Environment
Content Area: Adult Health/Renal

Reference

Black, J., & Matassarin-Jacobs, E. (1997). *Medical-surgical nursing: Clinical management for continuity of care* (5th ed.). Philadelphia: W. B. Saunders, pp. 1562–1563.

284. The 15-year-old pregnant client is being treated for acne. Which of the following will most likely be avoided with this client?

1 Topical erythromycin
2 Exfoliation
3 Cleansing with antibacterial soap
4 Oral tetracycline

Answer: 4

Rationale: The use of tetracycline is contraindicated during pregnancy. The medication readily crosses the placenta and may produce permanent teeth discoloration/enamel hypoplasia.

Test-Taking Strategy: Focus on the safety factor for the unseen client (fetus). Knowledge regarding medications and safety during pregnancy is necessary to answer the question. Note the word "avoid" in the question. Look at the options. The only option that addresses oral use of a medication is option 4. This would present the greatest risk to the fetus.

Level of Cognitive Ability: Analysis
Phase of Nursing Process: Analysis
Client Needs: Safe, Effective Care Environment
Content Area: Maternity

Reference

Wilson, B., Shannon, M., & Stang, C. (1997). *Nurse's drug guide.* Stamford, CT: Appleton & Lange, p. 1305.

285. The client with a bone infection is to undergo indium imaging. The client asks the nurse to explain how the procedure is done. The nurse's response is based on the understanding that

1. Indium is injected into the blood stream and collects in normal bone, but not in infected areas.
2. Indium is injected into the blood stream and highlights the vascular supply to the bone.
3. A sample of the client's leukocytes is tagged with indium and will subsequently accumulate in infected bone.
4. A sample of the client's red blood cells (RBCs) is tagged with indium and will highlight normal bone.

Answer: 3

Rationale: A sample of the client's blood is collected, and the leukocytes are tagged with indium. The leukocytes are then reinjected into the client. They accumulate in infected areas of bone and can be detected with scanning. No special preparation or aftercare is necessary.

Test-Taking Strategy: This question is difficult if you are not familiar with the procedure. Look at the information. The client has a bone infection. With any type of infection, leukocytes migrate to the area (and bone is not a highly vascular area). This might suggest option 3 to you as the correct choice in answering this question.

Level of Cognitive Ability: Analysis
Phase of Nursing Process: Analysis
Client Needs: Safe, Effective Care Environment
Content Area: Fundamental Skills

Reference

Black, J., & Matassarin-Jacobs, E. (1997). *Medical-surgical nursing: Clinical management for continuity of care* (5th ed.). Philadelphia: W. B. Saunders, pp. 2094–2095.

---

286. The client on the nursing unit has an order for dextroamphetamine (Dexedrine), 25 mg PO daily. The nurse collaborates with the dietician to limit the amount of which of the following items on the client's dietary trays?

1. Starch
2. Caffeine
3. Protein
4. Fat

Answer: 2

Rationale: Dextroamphetamine is a central nervous system (CNS) stimulant. Caffeine is also a stimulant and should be limited in the client taking this medication. The client should be taught to limit his or her own caffeine intake as well.

Test-Taking Strategy: To answer this question quickly and accurately, you should remember that this medication is a CNS stimulant. You would then evaluate each of the options in terms of the additive stimulation provided by the items listed as options. Knowing that caffeine is also a stimulant would help you to choose this as the item to be limited.

Level of Cognitive Ability: Application
Phase of Nursing Process: Implementation
Client Needs: Safe, Effective Care Environment
Content Area: Pharmacology

Reference

Deglin, J., & Vallerand, A. (1997). *Davis's drug guide for nurses* (5th ed.). Philadelphia: F. A. Davis, p. 341.

---

287. The nurse is planning an exercise program for clients in the rehabilitation facility with peripheral arterial disease. The client who would benefit most from this program would be the one who has

1. Cellulitis of the lower third of the leg.
2. Hair loss on the legs with brittle nails.
3. Gangrene on the tips of the toes.
4. Arterial leg ulcer.

Answer: 2

Rationale: Clients with leg ulcers, cellulitis, or gangrene have such a critical impairment of circulation that the metabolical needs of the body cannot be met even at rest. These clients should be maintained on bed rest. Trophic changes (hair loss, dry scaly skin, brittle toenails) are expected findings in the client with peripheral arterial disease caused by chronic tissue malnutrition.

Test-Taking Strategy: The question asks you to identify the client who would "benefit most." In questions such as these, the answer may be the client whose disease is at an early stage, in which symptoms are reversible or can be controlled with appropriate intervention. Because each of the incorrect responses indicates a critical level of tissue ischemia, the answer is option 2, which indicates only milder signs.

Level of Cognitive Ability: Analysis
Phase of Nursing Process: Analysis
Client Needs: Safe, Effective Care Environment
Content Area: Adult Health/Cardiovascular

Reference

Smeltzer, S., & Bare, B. (1996). *Brunner and Suddarth's Textbook of medical-surgical nursing* (8th ed.). Philadelphia: Lippincott-Raven, p. 729.

---

288. The client with repeated episodes of pulmonary emboli from thromboembolism is scheduled for insertion of an inferior vena cava (IVC) filter. The nurse assesses that the client has an adequate understanding of the procedure if the client makes which of the following statements?

1. "The filter will keep new blood clots from forming in my legs."
2. "I don't mind having a filter in my artery if it means I don't have any more trouble."
3. "The filter will be like a catcher's mitt and keep the clots from going to my lungs."
4. "It's too bad I have to continue anticoagulant therapy after the surgery."

Answer: 3

Rationale: Insertion of an IVC filter is indicated for clients with recurrent deep vein thrombosis and/or pulmonary emboli who do not respond to medical therapy and who cannot tolerate anticoagulant therapy. The filter device, or "umbrella," is inserted percutaneously in the IVC, where it springs open and attaches itself to the vena caval wall. The device has holes to allow blood flow but traps larger clots, thus preventing pulmonary emboli.

Test-Taking Strategy: Eliminate option 2 first because placement is not in an artery. Option 1 describes anticoagulant therapy, not the filter, so that is eliminated next. You would choose option 3 over option 4 because the procedure is indicated for clients who cannot tolerate anticoagulants.

Level of Cognitive Ability: Analysis
Phase of Nursing Process: Assessment
Client Needs: Safe, Effective Care Environment
Content Area: Adult Health/Cardiovascular

Reference

Ignatavicius, D. D., Workman, M. L., & Mishler, M. A. (1995). *Medical-surgical nursing: A nursing process approach* (2nd ed.). Philadelphia: W. B. Saunders, p. 957.

---

289. The nurse is planning preoperative care for the client scheduled for insertion of an inferior vena cava (IVC) filter. The nurse would want to question the physician about withholding which of the following regularly scheduled medications the day before surgery?

1. Furosemide (Lasix)
2. Potassium chloride (K-Dur)
3. Docusate (Colace)
4. Heparin sodium (Liquaemin)

Answer: 4

Rationale: The nurse should consult with the physician in the preoperative period before IVC filter insertion about the discontinuation of heparin to avoid hemorrhage.

Test-Taking Strategy: You would evaluate this question by analyzing which of the medications could cause the client harm if administered up until the time of surgery. Heparin is the only medication that meets this criterion, since it could cause bleeding or hemorrhage during and after surgery.

Level of Cognitive Ability: Analysis
Phase of Nursing Process: Planning
Client Needs: Safe, Effective Care Environment
Content Area: Adult Health/Cardiovascular

Reference

Ignatavicius, D. D., Workman, M. L., & Mishler, M. A. (1995). *Medical-surgical nursing: A nursing process approach* (2nd ed.). Philadelphia: W. B. Saunders, p. 957.

290. The hospitalized client with hypertension has been started on captopril (Capoten). The nurse would ensure that the client does which of the following with regard to this medication to ensure client safety?

1 Eat foods that are high in potassium
2 Take in sufficient amounts of high-fiber foods
3 Sit up and stand slowly while on this medication
4 Drink plenty of water while on this medication

Answer: 3

Rationale: Orthostatic hypotension is a real concern for clients taking antihypertensive medications. Clients are advised to avoid standing in one position for lengthy amounts of time, to change positions slowly, and avoid extreme warmth (in showers, baths, weather). Clients are also taught to recognize the symptoms of orthostatic hypotension, including dizziness, lightheadedness, weakness, and syncope.

Test-Taking Strategy: Knowledge of medications is necessary to answer this question. If you know that captopril is an antihypertensive, then option 3 is a good choice, because the risk of orthostatic hypotension is present with all types of antihypertensives!

Level of Cognitive Ability: Application
Phase of Nursing Process: Implementation
Client Needs: Safe, Effective Care Environment
Content Area: Adult Health/Cardiovascular

Reference
Clark, J., Queener, S., & Karb, V. (1997). *Pharmacologic basis of nursing practice* (5th ed.). St. Louis: Mosby–Year Book, p. 157.

291. The physician's order reads heparin sodium (Liquaemin) 25,000 units in 250 mL of 5% dextrose in water (D5W) continuously at a rate of 800 units/hour IV. The nurse would plan on setting the intravenous pump to how many milliliters per hour?

1 8 mL/hour
2 32 mL/hour
3 40 mL/hour
4 80 mL/hour

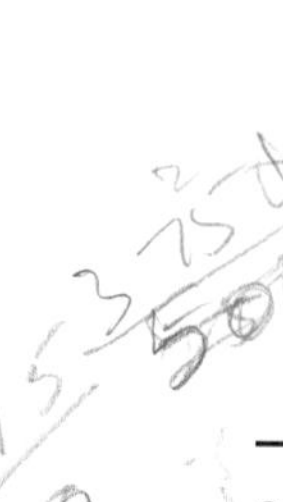

Answer: 1

Rationale: The desired infusion rate is 800 units/hour. The amount of heparin available is 25,000 units/250 mL of D5W. First, divide the 25,000 units by the 250 mL to give an effective concentration of 100 units/mL. Next, divide 800 units/hour by 100 units/mL, which is 8 mL/hour. Thus the nurse would set the pump at 8 mL/hour.

Test-Taking Strategy: This question looks more complicated on the surface than it is. Use the regular "desired/have available" formula, and you will get the correct answer. Think about the answer to be sure it makes sense. Options 2, 3, and 4 are relatively high figures.

Level of Cognitive Ability: Application
Phase of Nursing Process: Planning
Client Needs: Safe, Effective Care Environment
Content Area: Fundamental Skills

Reference
Clark, J., Queener, S., & Karb, V. (1997). *Pharmacologic basis of nursing practice* (5th ed.). St. Louis: Mosby–Year Book, pp. 75–83.

292. The nurse is planning care for the client who is scheduled for admission after femoral-popliteal bypass grafting. The nurse would not plan to have which of the following available at the bedside to enhance circulation to the affected extremity?

1 Sheepskin
2 Bed cradle
3 Lightweight blanket
4 Ace wraps

Answer: 4

Rationale: Sheepskin, bed cradle, and the use of lightweight blankets can promote warmth in the extremity and protect it from harm. Ace wraps, if ordered, would be used when the client is out of bed to reduce edema, but remember that they could impair wound healing. Frequently the surgical limb is left unwrapped for assessment and not covered by TED hoses or pneumatic boots. These may be placed on the alternate extremity.

Test-Taking Strategy: The surgical limb needs frequent assessment, warmth, and protection. Remembering these concepts as you evaluate each option helps you find the correct answer readily.

Level of Cognitive Ability: Application
Phase of Nursing Process: Planning
Client Needs: Safe, Effective Care Environment
Content Area: Adult Health/Cardiovascular

Reference
Black, J., & Matassarin-Jacobs, E. (1997). *Medical-surgical nursing: Clinical management for continuity of care* (5th ed.). Philadelphia: W. B. Saunders, pp. 1416–1417.

293. The client is admitted with infective endocarditis caused by *Streptococcus viridans*. The client asks the nurse about the antibiotic therapy that will be given. Knowing that the client has no medication allergies, the nurse responds that the client will most likely receive

1. Penicillin intravenously (IV) for 10 days, followed by oral doses for 2 more weeks.
2. Penicillin IV for 4–6 weeks, continuing at home after hospital discharge.
3. Amphotericin B IV for 10 days, followed by oral doses for 3 more weeks.
4. Amphotericin B IV for 4–6 weeks, continuing at home after hospital discharge.

Answer: 2

Rationale: Penicillin is frequently the medication of choice in treating endocarditis of bacterial origin. The standard duration of therapy is 4–6 weeks, with home care support after hospital discharge, which is usually after only 7–10 days. Amphotericin B is an antifungal agent.

Test-Taking Strategy: Knowledge of amphotericin B as an antifungal agent helps you eliminate options 3 and 4. The severity and nature of the infection makes continued IV therapy necessary, and therefore option 2 is a better choice than option 1. Review the treatment for this disorder now if you had difficulty with this question!

Level of Cognitive Ability: Analysis
Phase of Nursing Process: Implementation
Client Needs: Safe, Effective Care Environment
Content Area: Adult Health/Cardiovascular

Reference

Ignatavicius, D. D., Workman, M. L., & Mishler, M. A. (1995). *Medical-surgical nursing: A nursing process approach* (2nd ed.). Philadelphia: W. B. Saunders, p. 913.

---

294. The nurse is working with a newly hired nurse, and they are caring for a post–coronary artery bypass client who develops cardiac tamponade. The orientee asks the nurse why the client is returning to the operating room, instead of undergoing pericardiocentesis. In formulating a response, the nurse incorporates the knowledge that

1. The infection rate is lowest if done in the operating room.
2. The blood may have clotted in the pericardium.
3. It is the safest environment if the client should code.
4. The pericardium is torn and needs surgical repair.

Answer: 2

Rationale: After cardiac surgery, pericardiocentesis may not be appropriate for clients because the blood in the pericardial sac may have clotted.

Test-Taking Strategy: Option 4 can be immediately discounted, because cardiac tamponade results from rapid accumulation of blood or fluid in the pericardium, which holds it in and causes pressure. Options 1 and 3 are both arguable, whereas option 2 makes the most sense because clots cannot be easily aspirated out of a 16- or 18-gauge needle and because this option is most specific to the issue of the question.

Level of Cognitive Ability: Analysis
Phase of Nursing Process: Analysis
Client Needs: Safe, Effective Care Environment
Content Area: Adult Health/Cardiovascular

Reference

Ignatavicius, D. D., Workman, M. L., & Mishler, M. A. (1995). *Medical-surgical nursing: A nursing process approach* (2nd ed.). Philadelphia: W. B. Saunders, p. 1010.

---

295. The nurse is doing a dressing change on a venous stasis ulcer that is clean and has a growing bed of granulation tissue. The nurse would safeguard wound integrity by avoiding the use of which of the following dressing materials on this wound?

1. Wet-to-dry saline dressing
2. Wet-to-wet saline dressing
3. Hydrocolloid dressing
4. Vaseline gauze dressing

Answer: 1

Rationale: The use of wet-to-dry saline dressings provides nonselective mechanical débridement, whereby both devitalized and viable tissue are removed. This method should never be used on a clean, granulating wound. Granulation tissue in a venous stasis ulcer is protected through the use of wet-to-wet saline dressings, Vaseline gauze, or moist occlusive dressings, such as hydrocolloid dressings.

Test-Taking Strategy: Read the stem carefully. It specifically tells you that the wound is clean with granulation tissue (which needs protection). Next, look at your options and evaluate them comparatively. You will see that options 2, 3, and 4 all have one thing in common: continuous moisture. This helps you to draw the conclusion that the wet-to-dry saline dressing is the incorrect choice, because it is the only one that could disrupt this healing tissue.

Level of Cognitive Ability: Application
Phase of Nursing Process: Implementation
Client Needs: Safe, Effective Care Environment
Content Area: Fundamental Skills

Reference

Black, J., & Matassarin-Jacobs, E. (1997). *Medical-surgical nursing: Clinical management for continuity of care* (5th ed.). Philadelphia: W. B. Saunders, p. 1438.

---

296. The nurse is preparing to admit to the nursing unit an elderly client who has severe digitalis toxicity from accidental ingestion of a week's supply of the medication. The nurse should plan to see whether which medication can be brought to the nursing unit?

1 Digoxin immune Fab (Digibind)
2 Potassium chloride (K-Dur)
3 Protamine sulfate (Protamine)
4 Furosemide (Lasix)

Answer: 1

Rationale: Digibind is an antidote for severe digitalis toxicity. It uses an antibody produced in sheep that antigenically binds any unbound digitalis in the serum and removes it. As more digoxin reenters the blood stream from the tissues, it binds that also for excretion by the kidneys.

Test-Taking Strategy: Probably the name of the medication will help you with this one! From a logical standpoint, however, potassium chloride and furosemide are other medications commonly used with cardiac conditions in conjunction with digoxin, so they should be eliminated first. Knowing that protamine is the antidote for heparin leads you to the only option left, which is digoxin immune Fab.

Level of Cognitive Ability: Application
Phase of Nursing Process: Planning
Client Needs: Safe, Effective Care Environment
Content Area: Pharmacology

Reference

Deglin, J., & Vallerand, A. (1997). *Davis's drug guide for nurses* (5th ed.). Philadelphia: F. A. Davis, p. 372.

---

297. The client receiving lisinopril (Prinivil) has a white blood cell (WBC) count of 3,800/mm^3. The nurse would plan to do which of the following in the care of this client?

1 Follow aseptic technique diligently
2 Request prophylactic antibiotics from the physician
3 Place the client in respiratory isolation
4 Use antibacterial soap when bathing the client

Answer: 1

Rationale: The client taking angiotensin converting enzyme (ACE) inhibitors such as lisinopril is at risk of developing neutropenia. These clients require the use of good aseptic technique by the nurse. The client should also be taught to report signs and symptoms of infection, such as sore throat and fever, to the physician. The WBC count with differential may be monitored monthly for up to 6 months in clients deemed at risk.

Test-Taking Strategy: This question is fairly straightforward and can be correctly answered even without knowing that ACE inhibitors cause neutropenia, as long as you can recognize abnormally low WBC values. This question is an example of the benefits of knowing the normal reference ranges for commonly ordered laboratory tests.

Level of Cognitive Ability: Application
Phase of Nursing Process: Planning
Client Needs: Safe, Effective Care Environment
Content Area: Pharmacology

Reference

Deglin, J., & Vallerand, A. (1997). *Davis's drug guide for nurses* (5th ed.). Philadelphia: F. A. Davis, p. 92.

298. The nurse is taking a client's temperature with a glass thermometer. The nurse shakes down the thermometer and drops the thermometer on the floor. Which of the following actions will the nurse take?

1 Carefully wipe up the spill, avoiding getting cut from the glass
2 Use a mop and dust pan to clean up the spill, avoiding contact with the glass and mercury
3 Notify the Environmental Services Department of the spill
4 Call the housekeeping department to clean up the spill and broken glass

Answer: 3

Rationale: Mercury is a hazardous material. Accidental breakage of a mercury-in-glass thermometer is a health hazard to the client, nurse, and health care worker. Mercury droplets are not to be touched. If a breakage or spill occurs, the Environmental Services Department is called, and a mercury spill kit is used to clean up the spill.

Test-Taking Strategy: Remembering that mercury is a hazardous material will assist in directing you to eliminate options 1, 2, and 4. Be sure to review the principles associated with mercury spills now if you had difficulty with this question!

Level of Cognitive Ability: Application
Phase of Nursing Process: Implementation
Client Needs: Safe, Effective Care Environment
Content Area: Fundamental Skills

Reference

Potter, P., & Perry, A. (1997). *Fundamentals of nursing: Concepts, process, and practice* (4th ed.). St. Louis: Mosby–Year Book, p. 609.

---

299. A nurse is called to a client's room by another nurse. When the nurse arrives at the room, the nurse discovers that a fire has occurred in the client's waste basket. The first nurse has removed the client from the room. What is the second nurse's next action?

1 Evacuate the unit
2 Extinguish the fire
3 Confine the fire
4 Activate the fire alarm

Answer: 4

Rationale: Remember the acronym RACE to set priorities if a fire occurs: R stands for rescue; A stands for alarm; C stands for confine; and E stands for extinguish. In this situation, the client has been rescued from the immediate vicinity of the fire. The next action is to activate the fire alarm.

Test-Taking Strategy: Use the RACE acronym to set priorities and answer the question. If you had difficulty with this question, take time now to review fire safety!

Level of Cognitive Ability: Application
Phase of Nursing Process: Implementation
Client Needs: Safe, Effective Care Environment
Content Area: Fundamental Skills

Reference

Potter, P., & Perry, A. (1997). *Fundamentals of nursing: Concepts, process, and practice* (4th ed.). St. Louis: Mosby–Year Book, p. 884.

---

300. The nurse is caring for a client with cervical cancer. The client has an internal radiation implant. Which of the following items would the nurse ensure is kept in the client's room during this treatment?

1 A bedside commode
2 A lead shield
3 Long-handled forceps and a lead container
4 A No. 16 Foley catheter

Answer: 3

Rationale: In the case of dislodgment of an internal radiation implant, the radioactive source is never touched with the bare hands. It is retrieved with long-handled forceps and placed in the lead container kept in the client's room. In many situations, the client has a Foley catheter inserted and is on bed rest during treatment to prevent dislodgment. A lead apron, although one may be in the room, is not the required item. Nurses wear a dosimeter badge while in the client's room to measure the exposure to radiation.

Test-Taking Strategy: Use knowledge regarding radioactive materials and care of the client with a radiation implant to answer the question. Eliminate options 1 and 4 because they are similar and relate to urinary output. Of the remaining two options, select option 3 over option 2, keeping in mind the risk of dislodgment that can occur. Review these principles now if you had difficulty with this question!

Level of Cognitive Ability: Application
Phase of Nursing Process: Implementation
Client Needs: Safe, Effective Care Environment
Content Area: Fundamental Skills

Reference

Ignatavicius, D. D., Workman, M. L., & Mishler, M. A. (1995). *Medical-surgical nursing: A nursing process approach* (2nd ed.). Philadelphia: W. B. Saunders, p. 569.

REFERENCES

Antai-Otong, D. (1995). *Psychiatric nursing: Biological and behavioral concepts.* Philadelphia: W. B. Saunders.

Black, J., & Matassarin-Jacobs, E. (1997). *Medical-surgical nursing: Clinical management for continuity of care* (5th ed.). Philadelphia: W. B. Saunders.

Bolander, V. (1994). *Sorensen and Luckmann's Basic nursing: A psychophysiologic approach* (3rd ed.). Philadelphia: W. B. Saunders.

Brent, N. (1997). *Nurses and the law.* Philadelphia: W. B. Saunders.

Burrell, L., Gerlach, M., & Pless, B. (1997). *Adult nursing: Acute and community care* (2nd ed.). Stamford, CT: Appleton & Lange.

Carson, V., & Arnold, E. (1996). *Mental health nursing: The nurse-patient journey.* Philadelphia: W. B. Saunders.

Clark, J., Queener, S., & Karb, V. (1997). *Pharmacologic basis of nursing practice* (5th ed.). St. Louis: Mosby–Year Book.

Como, N. (1995). *Home health nursing pocket consultant.* St. Louis: Mosby–Year Book.

Cox, H., Hinz, M., Lubno, M., et al. (1997). *Clinical applications of nursing diagnosis: Adult, child, women's, psychiatric, gerontic, and home health considerations* (3rd ed.). Philadelphia: F. A. Davis.

Craven, R., & Hirnle, C. (1996). *Fundamentals of nursing human health and function* (2nd ed.). Philadelphia: Lippincott-Raven.

Deeloughery, G. (1995). *Issues and trends in nursing* (2nd ed.). St. Louis: Mosby–Year Book.

Deglin, J., & Vallerand, A. (1997). *Davis's drug guide for nurses* (5th ed.). Philadelphia: F. A. Davis.

DeLaune, S., & Ladner, P. (1998). *Fundamentals of nursing: Standards and practice.* Albany, NY: Delmar.

Fontaine, K., & Fletcher, J. (1995). *Essentials of mental health nursing* (3rd ed.). Redwood City, CA: Addison-Wesley.

Fortinash, K., & Holoday-Worret, P. (1996). *Psychiatric–mental health nursing.* St. Louis: Mosby–Year Book.

Gillies, D. (1994). *Nursing management: A systems approach.* Philadelphia: W.B. Saunders.

Haber, J. (1997). *Comprehensive psychiatric nursing* (5th ed.). St. Louis: Mosby–Year Book.

Hartshorn, J., Sole, M., & Lamborn, M. (1997). *Introduction to critical care nursing* (2nd ed.). Philadelphia: W. B. Saunders.

Hodgson, B., & Kizior, R. (1998). *Saunders nursing drug handbook 1998.* Philadelphia: W. B. Saunders.

Ignatavicius, D. D., Workman, M. L., & Mishler, M. A. (1995). *Medical-surgical nursing: A nursing process approach* (2nd ed.). Philadelphia: W. B. Saunders.

Jaffe, M., & McVan, B. (1997). *Davis's laboratory and diagnostic test handbook.* Philadelphia: F. A. Davis, pp. 195–196.

Johnson, B. (1997). *Psychiatric–mental health nursing: Adaptation and growth* (4th ed.). Philadelphia: Lippincott-Raven.

Kee, J., & Hayes, R. (1997). *Pharmacology: A nursing process approach* (2nd ed.). Philadelphia: W.B. Saunders.

Kozier, B., Erb, G., & Blais, K. (1998). *Fundamentals of nursing: Concepts, process, and practice* (5th ed.). Menlo Park, CA: Addison-Wesley.

Lammon, C. B., Foote, A. W., Leli, P. G., et al. (1995). *Clinical nursing skills.* Philadelphia: W. B. Saunders.

LeMone, P., & Burke, K. (1996). *Medical-surgical nursing: Critical thinking in client care.* Menlo Park, CA: Addison-Wesley, pp. 692, 694.

Lewis, S., Collier, I., & Heitkemper, M. (1996). *Medical-surgical nursing: Assessment and management of clinical problems* (4th ed.). Philadelphia: Mosby–Year Book.

Lowdermilk, D., Perry, S., & Bobak, I. (1997). *Maternity and women's health care* (6th ed.). St. Louis: Mosby–Year Book.

Luckmann, J. (1997). *Saunders manual of nursing care.* Philadelphia: W. B. Saunders.

Monahan, F., & Neighbors, M. (1998). *Medical-surgical nursing: Foundations for clinical practice* (2nd ed.). Philadelphia: W. B. Saunders.

National Council of State Boards of Nursing. (1997). *Plan for the National Council Licensure Examination for Registered Nurses.* Chicago: Author.

Nichols, F., & Zwelling, E. (1997). *Maternal-newborn nursing: Theory and practice.* Philadelphia: W. B. Saunders.

Phillips, L. (1997). *Manual of IV therapeutics* (2nd ed.). Philadelphia: F. A. Davis.

Phipps, W., Cassmeyer, V., Sands, J., et al. (1995). *Medical-surgical nursing: Concepts and clinical practice* (5th ed.). Philadelphia: Mosby–Year Book.

Pillitteri, A. (1995). *Maternal and child health nursing: Care of the childbearing and childrearing family* (2nd ed.). Philadelphia: Lippincott-Raven.

Polaski, A., & Tatro, S. (1996). *Luckmann's core principles and practice of medical-surgical nursing.* Philadelphia: W. B. Saunders.

Potter, P., & Perry, A. (1997). *Fundamentals of nursing: Concepts, process, and practice* (4th ed.). Philadelphia: Mosby–Year Book.

Reeder, S., Martin, L., & Koniak-Griffin, D. (1997). *Maternity nursing: Family, newborn, and women's health care* (18th ed.). Philadelphia: Lippincott-Raven.

Smeltzer, S., & Bare, B. (1996). *Brunner and Suddarth's Textbook of medical-surgical nursing* (8th ed.). Philadelphia: Lippincott-Raven.

Smith, S., & Duell, D. (1996). *Clinical nursing skills* (4th ed.). Stamford, CT: Appleton & Lange.

Swanson, J., & Nies, M. (1997). *Community health nursing: Promoting the health of aggregates* (2nd ed.). Philadelphia: W. B. Saunders.

Taylor, C., Lillis, C., & LeMone, P. (1997). *Fundamentals of nursing: The art and science of nursing care* (3rd ed.). Philadelphia: Lippincott-Raven.

VanRiper, S., & VanRiper, J. (1997). *Cardiac diagnostic tests: A guide for nurses.* Philadelphia: W. B. Saunders.

Wilson, B., Shannon, M., & Stang, C. (1997). *Nurse's drug guide.* Stamford, CT: Appleton & Lange.

Wilson, H., & Kneisl, C. (1996). *Psychiatric nursing* (5th ed.). Menlo Park, CA: Addison-Wesley.

Wong, D. (1995). *Whaley and Wong's Nursing care of infants and children* (5th ed.). St. Louis: Mosby–Year Book.

Wong, D. (1997). *Whaley and Wong's essentials of pediatric nursing* (5th ed.). St. Louis: Mosby–Year Book.

Wong, D., & Perry, S. (1998). *Maternal-child nursing care.* St. Louis: Mosby–Year Book.

Wong, D., & Whaley, L. (1996). *Clinical manual of pediatric nursing* (4th ed.). St. Louis: Mosby–Year Book.

Wywialoski, E. (1997). *Managing client care* (2nd ed.). St. Louis: Mosby–Year Book.

CHAPTER 11

Physiological Integrity

Physiological Integrity is a major category of Client Needs. There are four subcategories of Physiological Integrity: Basic Care and Comfort, Pharmacological and Parenteral Therapies, Reduction of Risk Potential, and Physiological Adaptation.

BASIC CARE AND COMFORT

The Basic Care and Comfort subcategory includes content concerning the nurse's role in providing comfort and assistance to the client in the performance of activities of daily living. The proportion of test questions in this subcategory of the National Council Licensure Examination for Registered Nurses (NCLEX-RN) is 7%–13%.

PHARMACOLOGICAL AND PARENTERAL THERAPIES

The Pharmacological and Parenteral Therapies subcategory includes content concerning the nurse's role in managing and providing care related to the administration of medications and parenteral therapies. The proportion of test questions in this subcategory of NCLEX-RN is 5%–11%.

REDUCTION OF RISK POTENTIAL

The Reduction of Risk Potential subcategory includes content concerning the nurse's role in reducing the likelihood that clients will develop complications or health problems related to existing conditions, treatments, or procedures. The proportion of test questions in this subcategory of NCLEX-RN is 12%–18%.

BOX 11–1. Basic Care and Comfort

- Personal hygiene
- Nutrition and oral hydration
- Elimination
- Rest and sleep
- Nonpharmacological comfort interventions
- Mobility and immobility
- Assistive devices

BOX 11–2. Pharmacological and Parenteral Therapies

- Administration of blood and blood products
- Intravenous therapy
- Central venous access devices
- Parenteral fluids
- Total parenteral nutrition
- Medication administration
- Pharmacological agents
- Pharmacological actions
- Chemotherapy
- Expected effects of medication and intravenous therapy
- Side effects of medication and intravenous therapy
- Untoward effects of medication and intravenous therapy

BOX 11–3. Reduction of Risk Potential

- Pathophysiology
- Alterations in body systems
- Laboratory values
- Diagnostic tests
- Therapeutic procedures
- Potential complications of diagnostic tests, procedures, surgery, and health alterations

PHYSIOLOGICAL ADAPTATION

The Physiological Adaptation subcategory includes content concerning the nurse's role in managing and providing care to clients with acute, chronic, or life-threatening physical health conditions. The proportion of test questions in this subcategory of NCLEX-RN is 12%–18%.

BOX 11-4. Physiological Adaptation

Pathophysiology
Alterations in body systems
Fluid and electrolyte imbalances
Hemodynamics
Medical emergencies
Infectious diseases
Respiratory care
Radiation therapy
Unexpected response to therapies

PRACTICE TEST

1. When a client has been raped, which action should a nurse take during the examination in the emergency room?
   1 Try to avoid talking about what the client can expect to allay anxiety
   2 Provide the person who accompanies the victim to the emergency room with a description of the procedures
   3 Give the victim a concise description of the usual steps for a rape examination
   4 Explain every assessment procedure and why it is being done

Answer: 4

Rationale: The client who has been raped needs to trust the nurse in the emergency room. The client must receive an explanation of the procedures and, importantly, why these are being completed. Option 2 does not address the client. Avoidance of talking and providing a concise description do not provide support and reassurance to the client.

Test-Taking Strategy: Use the process of elimination. Eliminate option 2 first because it does not address the client of the question. Eliminate option 1 next because the nurse would not avoid talking to the client. Eliminate option 3 next because a "concise description" may increase anxiety.

Level of Cognitive Ability: Application
Phase of Nursing Process: Implementation
Client Needs: Physiological Integrity
Content Area: Mental Health

Reference
Townsend, M. C. (1996). *Psychiatric-mental health nursing: Concepts of care* (2nd ed.). Philadelphia: F. A. Davis, p. 770.

---

2. When assessing a client who has a nursing diagnosis of Risk for Self-Directed Violence related to feelings of hopelessness, the client says, "You won't have to worry about me much longer." The nurse should prioritize this statement as
   1 The expression of hopelessness.
   2 An expression of depression.
   3 An intention for self-mutilation.
   4 The intention of suicide.

Answer: 4

Rationale: The suicidal client who says he or she will not be around much longer is making an expression of suicidal intent. The nurse's assessment concludes this as priority assessment data. An individual who is depressed is frequently suicidal. The individual with suicidal tendencies frequently does self-mutilating acts. The client's statement that he or she will not be around, however, is a direct comment about the act.

Test-Taking Strategy: Focus on the client's statement. Because all the options could be correct, the comment about not being around much longer indicates an intent is evident. This eliminates options 1, 2, and 3 and easily directs you to option 4.

Level of Cognitive Ability: Analysis
Phase of Nursing Process: Analysis
Client Needs: Physiological Integrity
Content Area: Mental Health

Reference
Townsend, M. C. (1996). *Psychiatric–mental health nursing: Concepts of care* (2nd ed.). Philadelphia: F. A. Davis, p. 254.

3. A child with celiac disease asks how long a special diet is necessary. Which of these responses would be appropriate for a nurse to make?

   1 "A gluten-free diet will need to be followed for life"
   2 "Adequate nutritional status will help prevent celiac crisis"
   3 "Supplemental vitamins, iron, and folate will prevent complications"
   4 "A lactose-free diet will need to be followed temporarily"

Answer: 1

Rationale: The main nursing consideration with celiac disease is helping the child adhere to dietary management. Treatment of celiac disease consists primarily of dietary management with a gluten-free diet. Options 2, 3, and 4 are all true statements but do not answer the question the child is asking. Children with untreated celiac disease may have lactose intolerance, which usually improves with gluten withdrawal. Nutritional deficiencies resulting from malabsorption are treated with appropriate supplements.

Test-Taking Strategy: Focus on the issue of the question: "the length of time a special diet is necessary." This focus directs you to the correct option. If you had difficulty with this question, take time now to review dietary requirements for celiac disease.

Level of Cognitive Ability: Application
Phase of Nursing Process: Implementation
Client Needs: Physiological Integrity
Content Area: Child Health

Reference

Wong, D., & Perry, S. (1998). *Maternal-child nursing care.* St. Louis: Mosby–Year Book, pp. 1432–1433.

4. When providing the health history, the parents report their 6-month-old boy has been screaming and drawing the knees up to the chest and now has passed stools that are mixed with blood and mucus and are jelly-like. A nurse should recognize these signs and symptoms as indicative of

   1 Hirschsprung's disease.
   2 Peritonitis.
   3 Intussusception.
   4 Appendicitis.

Answer: 3

Rationale: The classic signs and symptoms of intussusception are acute colicky abdominal pain with currant jelly–like stools. Clinical manifestations of Hirschsprung's disease include constipation; abdominal distention; and ribbon-like, foul-smelling stools. Peritonitis is a serious complication that may follow intestinal obstructions and perforation. The most common symptom of appendicitis is colicky periumbilical or lower abdominal pain in the right quadrant.

Test-Taking Strategy: Eliminate the options you know are incorrect as options 2 and 4. Knowing that in Hirschsprung's disease the stools are ribbon-like may assist in eliminating option 1. If you had difficulty with this question, take time now to review the clinical manifestations of intussusception.

Level of Cognitive Ability: Analysis
Phase of Nursing Process: Assessment
Client Needs: Physiological Integrity
Content Area: Child Health

Reference

Ashwill, J., & Droske, S. (1997). *Nursing care of children: Principles and practice.* Philadelphia: W. B. Saunders, pp. 749–751.

5. The client has been placed in seclusion. The nurse is responsible for providing and documenting care for the client. Which of the following most completely identifies the component requiring documentation?

1 Vital signs, toileting, and checking client on the basis of protocol time frame such as every 15 minutes
2 Ambulating, toileting, and checking client on the basis of protocol time frame such as every 15 minutes
3 Vital signs, toileting, feeding and fluid intake, and checking client on the basis of protocol time frame such as every 15 minutes
4 Vital signs, reason for the procedure, documentation of date and time

Answer: 3

Rationale: Option 3 addresses the client's basic needs during seclusion. Options 1 and 2 are not complete in terms of identification of physiological needs. Option 4 contains client documentation that would follow the care during the seclusion.

Test-Taking Strategy: Use Maslow's hierarchy of needs theory to prioritize and the process of elimination. Vital signs should be checked and recorded regularly according to protocol. The client should be toileted according to protocol. Food and fluid are served on paper plates with plastic utensils and cups and should be monitored. If you had difficulty with this question, take time now to review seclusion/isolation content and nursing care.

Level of Cognitive Ability: Application
Phase of Nursing Process: Implementation
Client Needs: Physiological Integrity
Content Area: Mental Health

Reference

Carson, V., & Arnold, E. (1996). *Mental health nursing: The nurse-patient journey.* Philadelphia: W. B. Saunders, p. 348.

6. During the admission assessment, the nurse asks the client to run the heel of one foot down the lower anterior surface of the other leg. The nurse notices rhythmic tremors of the leg being tested and concludes that the client has an interference in the area of

1 Muscle strength and flexibility.
2 Balance and coordination.
3 Sensation and reflexes.
4 Bowel and bladder function.

Answer: 2

Rationale: The nurse is performing one test of cerebellar function, in this case for ataxia. Examples of interferences in this area could be Parkinson's disease, multiple sclerosis, or cerebrovascular accident.

Test-Taking Strategy: Note that the stem contains information about the leg tremors. Using your nursing knowledge, try to think of interferences that might contain that sign or symptom. Note the relationship between tremors and coordination in option 2. If you had difficulty with this question, take time now to review assessment techniques for coordination.

Level of Cognitive Ability: Analysis
Phase of Nursing Process: Analysis
Client Needs: Physiological Integrity
Content Area: Adult Health/Neurological

Reference

Smeltzer, S., & Bare, B. (1996). *Brunner and Suddarth's Textbook of medical-surgical nursing* (8th ed.). Philadelphia: Lippincott-Raven, pp. 1690, 1728, 1767, 1772.

7. The intracranial pressure (ICP) of a client with a head injury is being monitored. The cerebrospinal fluid (CSF) pressure is averaging 25 mmHg. The nurse analyzes these results as

1 Normal.
2 Compensation, indicating adequate brain adaptation.
3 Borderline elevation, indicating the initial stage of decompensation.
4 Increased, indicating a serious compromise in cerebral perfusion.

Answer: 4

Rationale: The normal CSF pressure is 5–15 mmHg, and pressures in excess of 20 mmHg are considered increased and serious.

Test-Taking Strategy: This question asks you for specific information related to a numerical value. Use the process of elimination. Options 2 and 3 are basically stating the same idea; therefore it is likely that they are incorrect. You can narrow your choices to normal or elevated. Review the terms "compensation" and "decompensation" and "ICP" and "normal pressure" if you had difficulty with this question.

Level of Cognitive Ability: Analysis
Phase of Nursing Process: Analysis
Client Needs: Physiological Integrity
Content Area: Adult Health/Neurological

Reference
Black, J., & Matassarin-Jacobs, E. (1997). *Medical-surgical nursing: Clinical management for continuity of care* (5th ed.). Philadelphia: W. B. Saunders, pp. 771, 772.

---

8. The nurse is starting blood transfusions on two assigned clients. The highest priority nursing action is to

1. Make sure the right blood is obtained from the blood bank.
2. Ask the client or family if there were previous transfusions.
3. Check the client's vital signs every 1/2 hour and record them.
4. Check the blood with another nurse to ensure correctness.

Answer: 4

Rationale: Implementation requires the nurse to check the blood with another nurse to ensure it is correct. That is the highest priority. Options 1, 2, and 3 are all nursing actions that are done but are not the highest priority of the options presented.

Test-Taking Strategy: Note the key phrase, "highest priority." Note the word "correctness" in the correct option. If you had difficulty with this question, take time now to review the nurse's responsibility when administering blood.

Level of Cognitive Ability: Application
Phase of Nursing Process: Implementation
Client Needs: Physiological Integrity
Content Area: Fundamental Skills

Reference
Brent, N. (1997). *Nurses and the law.* Philadelphia: W. B. Saunders, p. 149.

---

9. During an emergency delivery, the ventilator tubing did not fit the endotracheal tube and an Ambu bag was not available for the infant. The infant survived but had multiple medical problems. A lawsuit was filed against the hospital, physician, and nurse. The nurse could have avoided charges of professional misconduct by

1. Asking the physician what was needed before the delivery.
2. Checking with the charge nurse about the equipment.
3. Making sure that the malpractice insurance covered the situation.
4. Assessing all the equipment before the delivery.

Answer: 4

Rationale: Nurses are required to provide safe care for clients. The nurse has the responsibility for ensuring that the delivery room equipment and supplies are available and in working order.

Test-Taking Strategy: Options 1 and 2 do not directly address the responsibility of the nurse in this situation. They rely on someone else to solve the problem. Option 3 is important but does not directly address how the nurse could have avoided this problem. Option 4 focuses directly on the action the nurse should have taken to avoid problems. It is a general response that would fit all situations related to procedures.

Level of Cognitive Ability: Application
Phase of Nursing Process: Assessment
Client Needs: Physiological Integrity
Content Area: Maternity

Reference
Brent, N. (1997). *Nurses and the law.* Philadelphia: W. B. Saunders, pp. 49–50.

10. The client has just been given a preliminary diagnosis of amniotic fluid embolism after experiencing cyanosis, dyspnea, hypotension, and tachypnea immediately after a difficult labor and delivery. Which of the following actions should the nurse take to ensure adequate maternal circulation in this situation?

1 Maintain the intravenous fluid rate at 125 mL/hour
2 Place the client in a modified Sims' position
3 Administer the oxygen at no more than 2 liters by nasal cannula
4 Monitor fluids carefully using an intravenous infusion pump and a Foley catheter attached to a calibrated urine collection bag

Answer: 4

Rationale: Amniotic fluid contains small particles of matter, such as lanugo, vernix caseosa, and sometimes meconium, which can form emboli. Amniotic emboli occlude the pulmonary capillaries if they reach the lungs and cause intense vasospasm leading to right-sided heart failure and pulmonary edema, clinically manifested by respiratory distress. Because of these complications, fluids are restricted, and intake and output are meticulously monitored. An infusion pump allows intravenous fluids to be controlled to avoid additional stress on the circulatory system, which would worsen the pulmonary edema. An indwelling Foley catheter with a calibrated urine collection bag enables the nurse to observe hourly urine output.

Test-Taking Strategy: Carefully consider the pathophysiological factors underlying the case situation. Answers that are inconsistent with improving the situation, such as low-dose oxygen for a client in respiratory distress, can be eliminated. Similarly, intravenous fluids at a rate of 125 mL/hour are inconsistent with decreasing the load on a heart already in failure. A modified Sims' position would not assist the client. If you had difficulty with this question, take time now to review care of the client with amniotic fluid embolism.

Level of Cognitive Ability: Application
Phase of Nursing Process: Implementation
Client Needs: Physiological Integrity
Content Area: Maternity

Reference

Reeder, S., Martin L., & Koniak-Griffin, D. (1997). *Maternity nursing* (18th ed.). Philadelphia: Lippincott-Raven, p. 1002.

11. A woman 32 weeks pregnant is brought into the emergency room after an automobile accident. The client is bleeding vaginally, and fetal assessment indicates moderate fetal distress. Which of the following will the nurse do first in an attempt to reduce the stress on the fetus?

1 Start intravenous fluids at a keep open rate
2 Administer oxygen with a face mask at 7–10 liters/minute
3 Elevate the bed to a semi-Fowler's position
4 Set up for an immediate cesarean section delivery

Answer: 2

Rationale: Administering oxygen increases the amount of oxygen for transport to the fetus, partially compensating for the loss of circulating blood volume. This action can be done quickly and easily and is essential regardless of the cause or amount of bleeding. Options 1, 3, and 4 do not provide immediate intervention to the fetus.

Test-Taking Strategy: In the obstetrical couplet of pregnant woman and fetus, determine which is the primary focus of the question. In this question, the client is the fetus. Note the word "first" in the stem, which indicates a priority choice among several options that may be appropriate for the situation. Using the ABCs (airway, breathing, circulation) guides you to select the correct response.

Level of Cognitive Ability: Application
Phase of Nursing Process: Implementation
Client Needs: Physiological Integrity
Content Area: Maternity

Reference

Olds, S., London, M., & Ladewig, P. (1996). *Maternal-newborn nursing* (5th ed.). Menlo Park, CA: Addison-Wesley, p. 730.

12. A client with a Sengstaken-Blakemore tube in place is admitted from the emergency room. The nurse understands that the purpose of this tube is to

1 Control bleeding from gastritis.
2 Apply pressure to esophageal varices.
3 Control ascites.
4 Remove ammonia-forming bacteria from the gastrointestinal tract.

Answer: 2

Rationale: A Sengstaken-Blakemore tube is inserted in cirrhosis clients with ruptured esophageal varices. It has esophageal and gastric balloons. The esophageal balloon exerts pressure on the ruptured esophageal varices and stops the bleeding. The gastric balloon holds the tube in correct position and prevents migration of the esophageal balloon, which would harm the client.

Test-Taking Strategy: The issue of this question is specific content: the purpose of a Sengstaken-Blakemore tube. Option 2 correctly defines the purpose. All other options describe correct treatment goals for clients with ruptured esophageal varices. Take the time now to review the concepts related to this type of tube if you are unfamiliar with them.

Level of Cognitive Ability: Analysis
Phase of Nursing Process: Analysis
Client Needs: Physiological Integrity
Content Area: Adult Health/Gastrointestinal

Reference

Black, J., & Matassarin-Jacobs, E. (1997). *Medical-surgical nursing: Clinical management for continuity of care* (5th ed.). Philadelphia: W. B. Saunders, p. 1885.

13. The physician orders the deflation of the esophageal balloon of a Sengstaken-Blakemore tube in a client. The nurse monitors the client after the deflation because the client may be at risk for

1 Increased ascites.
2 Esophageal necrosis.
3 Hemorrhaging again from the esophageal varices.
4 Esophageal rupture.

Answer: 3

Rationale: A Sengstaken-Blakemore tube is inserted in cirrhosis clients with ruptured esophageal varices. The esophageal balloon exerts pressure on the ruptured esophageal varices and stops the bleeding. The pressure of the esophageal balloon is released at intervals to decrease the risk of trauma to the esophageal tissues, which can lead to esophageal rupture or necrosis. When the balloon is deflated, the client may begin to bleed again from the esophageal varices.

Test-Taking Strategy: The issue of this question is specific content: Identify the risk factor for a client who has a Sengstaken-Blakemore tube in place with the esophageal balloon deflated. Remembering that the esophageal balloon exerts pressure on the ruptured esophageal varices and stops the bleeding can assist in directing you to the correct option. Take the time now to review the complications associated with this type of tube if you are unfamiliar with them.

Level of Cognitive Ability: Analysis
Phase of Nursing Process: Analysis
Client Needs: Physiological Integrity
Content Area: Adult Health/Gastrointestinal

Reference

Black, J., & Matassarin-Jacobs, E. (1997). *Medical-surgical nursing: Clinical management for continuity of care* (5th ed.). Philadelphia: W. B. Saunders, p. 1885.

14. The home health care nurse is instructing the client with chronic obstructive pulmonary disease (COPD) in breathing techniques. Breathing techniques incorporate which of the following modalities?

1 Pursed-lip breathing
2 Intercostal chest expansion
3 Abdominal breathing
4 Chest physical therapy

Answer: 1

Rationale: Pursed-lip breathing allows the client to exhale carbon dioxide slowly while keeping the airways open. Intercostal chest expansion is not a technique. Abdominal breathing is recommended for clients with dyspnea and is not to be confused with diaphragmatic breathing techniques. Chest physical therapy is not a breathing technique.

Test-Taking Strategy: The nurse needs to differentiate between breathing techniques and appropriate interventions specific to COPD clients. Eliminate options 2 and 4 first because these are not breathing techniques. Remembering that pursed-lip breathing is associated with the

COPD client can assist in directing you to the correct option. Review pursed-lip breathing if you are unfamiliar with the purpose and technique.

Level of Cognitive Ability: Analysis
Phase of Nursing Process: Analysis
Client Needs: Physiological Integrity
Content Area: Adult Health/Respiratory

Reference
Black, J., & Matassarin-Jacobs, E. (1997). *Medical-surgical nursing: Clinical management for continuity of care* (5th ed.). Philadelphia: W. B. Saunders, pp. 1120–1122.

---

15. The physician has ordered a partial rebreathing face mask for the home care client who has terminal lung cancer. The home health care nurse knows that the mask

1 Delivers accurate FIO_2 to the client.
2 Conserves oxygen by having the client rebreathe his or her own exhaled air.
3 Requires that the reservoir bag be deflated to work effectively.
4 Requires a low liter flow to prevent rebreathing of carbon dioxide.

Answer: 2

Rationale: Rebreathing masks have a reservoir bag that conserves oxygen and requires a high liter flow to achieve concentrations of 40%–60%. It does not deliver accurate FIO_2 to the client. The bag should not deflate during inspiration. The rebreathing bags do conserve oxygen by having the client rebreathe his or her own exhaled air.

Test-Taking Strategy: This question requires application of basic knowledge of oxygen therapy. Note the relationship of the phrase "partial rebreathing" in the question and "rebreathe his or her own exhaled air" in the answer. Review oxygen delivery systems now if you had difficulty with this question.

Level of Cognitive Ability: Analysis
Phase of Nursing Process: Analysis
Client Needs: Physiological Integrity
Content Area: Adult Health/Respiratory

Reference
Lewis, S., Collier, I., & Heitkemper, M. (1996). *Medical-surgical nursing: Assessment and management of clinical problems* (4th ed.). St. Louis: Mosby–Year Book, p. 648.

---

16. A client presents with a slow, regular pulse. On the monitor, the nurse notes regular QRS complexes with no associated P waves and a ventricular rate of 50 beats/minute. The nurse suspects that there is a problem at which part of the cardiac conduction system?

1 Sinoatrial (SA) node
2 Atrioventricular (AV) node
3 Bundle of His
4 Left ventricle

Answer: 1

Rationale: A normal P wave indicates that the impulse that depolarized the atrium was initiated in the SA node. A change in the form or the absence of a P wave can indicate a problem at this part of the conduction system with the resulting impulse originating from an alternate site lower in the conduction pathway.

Test-Taking Strategy: Use the process of elimination. Option 4 can be eliminated because it does not identify a mechanism of the conduction system. The case study also identifies a normal QRS complex and a rate of 50 beats/minute indicating an intact AV node; thus the problem lies higher in the conduction system. Correlate P wave with the SA node. If you had difficulty with this question, take time now to review the conduction system of the heart.

Level of Cognitive Ability: Analysis
Phase of Nursing Process: Analysis
Client Needs: Physiological Integrity
Content Area: Adult Health/Cardiovascular

Reference
Hartshorn, J., Sole, M., & Lamborn, M. (1997). *Introduction to critical care nursing* (2nd ed.). Philadelphia: W. B. Saunders, p. 42.

17. The nurse finds a client lying tense in bed staring at the cardiac monitor. The client states, "There sure are a lot of wires around there. I sure hope we don't get hit by lightning." The most appropriate nursing response would be

1 "Would you like a mild sedative to help you relax?"
2 "Oh, don't worry, the weather is supposed to be sunny and clear today."
3 "Yes, all those wires must be a little scary. Did someone explain what the cardiac monitor was for?"
4 "Your family can stay tonight if they wish."

Answer: 3

Rationale: Clients admitted to critical care units face many stressors, which can affect physiological integrity. Within the critical care unit (CCU) setting, the client is powerless to control even the basic activities of daily living. The client's comment regarding the telemetry wire may be in response to this anxiety and loss of control. The nurse should respond initially to validate the client's concern, then to assess the client's knowledge level of the cardiac monitor. This gives the nurse an opportunity to do client education if necessary. Bringing in the family, friends, or chaplain as an alternate resource may provide the client with additional psychological support. Pharmacological interventions should be considered only if necessary.

Test-Taking Strategy: The key words in this stem are "most appropriate." Because the client is the first priority, the focus of the nurse's concern should be the client's feelings related to the procedure. Option 3 validates the client's anxiety and goes a step further to assess why the client might be anxious. Remember to address the client's feelings first and explain the purpose of the treatment.

Level of Cognitive Ability: Application
Phase of Nursing Process: Implementation
Client Needs: Physiological Integrity
Content Area: Adult Health/Cardiovascular

Reference

Hartshorn, J., Sole, M., & Lamborn, M. (1997). *Introduction to critical care nursing* (2nd ed.). Philadelphia: W. B. Saunders, pp. 8–10.

---

18. The client is hospitalized with thrombophlebitis and is being treated with heparin therapy. About 24 hours after the infusion has begun, the nurse notes that the client's partial thromboplastin time (PTT) is 100 seconds (control is 60–70 seconds). What is the most appropriate initial action by the nurse?

1 Discontinue the heparin infusion
2 Do nothing; the client is adequately anticoagulated
3 Notify the physician of the laboratory results
4 Prepare to administer protamine sulfate

Answer: 2

Rationale: The effectiveness of heparin therapy is monitored through the use of PTT. Desired ranges for therapeutic anticoagulation are 1.5–2.5 times the control. A PTT of greater than 175 seconds would indicate that too much heparin is being given, putting the client at high risk of serious spontaneous bleeding.

Test-Taking Strategy: Avoid options that tell the nurse to call the physician unless the situation is a life-threatening one. Although they are sometimes the correct response, be certain that an independent nursing action is not a more appropriate choice. Remembering that the desired ranges for therapeutic anticoagulation are 1.5–2.5 times the control can assist in answering this question. Learn this now. You are likely to find a similar question on NCLEX-RN.

Level of Cognitive Ability: Application
Phase of Nursing Process: Implementation
Client Needs: Physiological Integrity
Content Area: Pharmacology

Reference

Black, J., & Matassarin-Jacobs, E. (1997). *Medical-surgical nursing: Clinical management for continuity of care* (5th ed.). Philadelphia: W. B. Saunders, pp. 1434–1435.

19. A 48-year-old man is brought to the emergency room complaining of chest pain. His vital signs are blood pressure (BP), 150/90 mmHg; pulse, 88 beats/minute; and respirations, 20 breaths/minute. The nurse administers nitroglycerin, 0.4 mg sublingually. To evaluate the effectiveness of this medication, the nurse should expect which of the following changes in the vital signs?

1 BP, 160/100; pulse, 120; respirations, 16
2 BP, 150/90; pulse, 70; respirations, 24
3 BP, 100/60; pulse, 96; respirations, 20
4 BP, 100/60; pulse, 70; respirations, 24

Answer: 3

Rationale: Nitroglycerin dilates both arteries and veins causing blood to pool in the periphery. This causes a reduced preload and therefore a drop in cardiac output. This vasodilation causes BP to fall. The drop in cardiac output causes the sympathetic nervous system to respond and attempt to maintain cardiac output by increasing the pulse. Beta-blockers such as propranolol (Inderal) are often used in conjunction with nitroglycerin to prevent this rise in heart rate.

Test-Taking Strategy: Knowing that nitroglycerin is a vasodilator and that it causes the BP to drop can assist in eliminating options 1 and 2. Also, if chest pain is reduced and cardiac workload is reduced, the client will be more comfortable, and therefore a rise in respirations should not be seen. This should assist in directing you to the only possible correct option. If you had difficulty with this question, take time now to review the effects of nitroglycerin.

Level of Cognitive Ability: Analysis
Phase of Nursing Process: Evaluation
Client Needs: Physiological Integrity
Content Area: Pharmacology

Reference

Hodgson, B., & Kizior, R. (1998). *Saunders nursing drug handbook 1998.* Philadelphia: W. B. Saunders, pp. 750–753.

20. The client who has had an abdominal aortic aneurysm repair is 1 day postoperative. The nurse notes the absence of bowel sounds. The nurse's best action is to

1 Call physician immediately.
2 Remove the nasogastric tube.
3 Feed the client.
4 Continue to assess for bowel sounds.

Answer: 4

Rationale: Bowel sounds may be absent for 3–4 days postoperatively because of bowel manipulation during surgery. The nurse should continue to monitor the client, the nasogastric tube should stay in place, and the client should be kept NPO (nothing by mouth) until after the onset of bowel sounds. There is no need to call the physician immediately at this time.

Test-Taking Strategy: Note the key phrase "1 day postoperative." Knowledge that bowel sounds may not return for 3–4 days postoperatively can assist in answering this question. If you had difficulty with this question, take time now to review normal postoperative assessment findings.

Level of Cognitive Ability: Application
Phase of Nursing Process: Implementation
Client Needs: Physiological Integrity
Content Area: Adult Health/Cardiovascular

Reference

Ignatavicius, D. D., Workman, M. L., & Mishler, M. A. (1995). *Medical-surgical nursing: A nursing process approach* (2nd ed.). Philadelphia: W. B. Saunders, p. 910.

21. Which complication should the nurse be particularly alert for when monitoring a client with pregnancy-induced hypertension (PIH) during labor?

1 Grand mal convulsions
2 Placenta previa
3 Hallucinations
4 Altered respiratory status

Answer: 1

Rationale: The major complication of PIH is grand mal seizures. Placenta previa, hallucinations, and altered respiratory status are not directly associated with PIH.

Test-Taking Strategy: Use the process of elimination. Remembering that convulsions are a concern with PIH can assist in directing you to the correct option. If you had difficulty with this question, take time now to review PIH.

Level of Cognitive Ability: Analysis
Phase of Nursing Process: Assessment
Client Needs: Physiological Integrity
Content Area: Maternity

Reference

Olds, S., London, M., & Ladewig, P. (1996). *Maternal-newborn nursing* (5th ed.). Menlo Park, CA: Addison-Wesley, pp. 40–41.

---

22. Which statement by the mother of a newly circumcised infant indicates a knowledge of necessary postcircumcision care?

1. "I need to check for bleeding every hour for the first 12 hours"
2. "I need to clean the penis every hour with baby wipes"
3. "I need to wrap the penis completely in dry sterile gauze, making sure it is dry, when I change his diaper"
4. "The baby will not urinate because of swelling for the next 24 hours"

Answer: 1

Rationale: The mother needs to be taught to observe for bleeding, assessing the site hourly, for the next 8–12 hours. Voiding needs to be assessed. The mother should call the physician if the infant has not urinated within 24 hours. Swelling or damage may obstruct urine output. When the diaper is changed, petroleum jelly (Vaseline) gauze should be reapplied. Frequent diaper changing prevents contamination of the site. Water is used for cleaning because soap or baby wipes may irritate the area and cause discomfort.

Test-Taking Strategy: Use the process of elimination. Baby wipes cause stinging in the newly circumcised penis. The area of the circumcision should be wrapped with Vaseline gauze. Gauze sticks to the penis if it is completely dry. Penile swelling that prevents voiding needs to be reported to the physician. Review postcircumcision care now if you had difficulty answering the question.

Level of Cognitive Ability: Analysis
Phase of Nursing Process: Evaluation
Client Needs: Physiological Integrity
Content Area: Maternity

Reference

Nichols, F., & Zwelling, E. (1997). *Maternal-newborn nursing: Theory and practice.* Philadelphia: W. B. Saunders, p. 1167–1168.

---

23. The nurse is evaluating the outcomes of care for a client who experienced an acute myocardial infarction. Which of the following findings indicate that one of the expected outcomes for the nursing diagnosis of Decreased Cardiac Output has been met?

1. Cardiac output is 3 liters/minute when measured with a pulmonary artery catheter
2. The cardiac monitor shows a heart rate of 50 beats/minute after the client has eaten dinner
3. The client identifies symptoms that require immediate action after client teaching
4. The client reports absence of dyspnea and angina with activity

Answer: 4

Rationale: Dyspnea and angina are signs of altered cardiac output. The absence of these with activity indicates that cardiac output is adequate. Normal adult cardiac output is 4–8 liters/minute. This reading is low. Large meals may increase myocardial workload, causing vagal stimulation and dysrhythmias. Because the cardiac output is determined by stroke volume × heart rate, a low heart rate affects cardiac output. The client's rate should be between 60 and 100 beats/minute. Identifying symptoms that require immediate action is an outcome criterion for knowledge deficit.

Test-Taking Strategy: Use the ABCs. Note the key phrase "absence of dyspnea and angina" in the correct option. If you had difficulty with this question, take time now to review normal cardiac output and heart rate.

Level of Cognitive Ability: Analysis
Phase of Nursing Process: Evaluation
Client Needs: Physiological Integrity
Content Area: Adult Health/Cardiovascular

Reference

Black, J., & Matassarin-Jacobs, E. (1997). *Medical-surgical nursing: Clinical management for continuity of care* (5th ed.). Philadelphia: W. B. Saunders, p. 1271.

24. The nurse analyzed a 6-second electrocardiogram (ECG) strip for a client with left-sided heart failure as follows: atrial rate, no identifiable P waves; baseline irregular ventricular rate, 160 beats/minute; rhythm, irregular PR interval and indiscernible; QRS at 0.08. The nurse interprets the rhythm strip as

1. Sinus dysrhythmia.
2. Atrial fibrillation.
3. Ventricular fibrillation.
4. Third-degree heart block.

Answer: 2

Rationale: Atrial fibrillation is characterized by rapid, chaotic atrial depolarization, with ventricular rates ranging from 160 to 180 beats/minute. The ECG reveals erratic or no identifiable P waves and a baseline that appears to be irregular and undulating. A sinus dysrhythmia has a normal P wave, PR interval, and QRS complex. The P-P interval is irregular. In ventricular fibrillation, there are no identifiable P waves, QRS complexes, or T waves. In third-degree heart block, the atria and ventricles beat independently. The ventricular rate is between 40 and 60 beats/minute.

Test-Taking Strategy: Knowledge that in atrial fibrillation the P wave is absent can assist in answering the question. If you are unfamiliar with these cardiac dysrhythmias, review them now.

Level of Cognitive Ability: Analysis
Phase of Nursing Process: Analysis
Client Needs: Physiological Integrity
Content Area: Adult Health/Cardiovascular

Reference

Black, J., & Matassarin-Jacobs, E. (1997). *Medical-surgical nursing: Clinical management for continuity of care* (5th ed.). Philadelphia: W. B. Saunders, p. 1301.

---

25. The nurse has been caring for a client with multiple myeloma. The nurse has been administering intravenous hydration at 100 mL/hour. Which of the following findings would indicate a positive response to the treatment plan?

1. Weight increase of 1 kg
2. White blood cell (WBC) count of 6000/mm^3
3. Respirations of 18 breaths/minute
4. Creatinine of 1.0

Answer: 4

Rationale: In multiple myeloma, hydration is essential to prevent renal damage resulting from the Bence-Jones protein precipitating in the renal tubules and from excessive calcium and uric acid in the blood. Creatinine is the most accurate measure of renal status.

Test-Taking Strategy: Knowledge that renal failure is a concern in multiple myeloma is required to answer the question. Eliminate options 2 and 3 because hydration does not relate to WBC count or respirations. Weight gain is not a positive sign when concerned with renal status, eliminating option 1. If you had difficulty with this question, take time now to review care of the client with multiple myeloma.

Level of Cognitive Ability: Analysis
Phase of Nursing Process: Evaluation
Client Needs: Physiological Integrity
Content Area: Adult Health/Oncology

Reference

Smeltzer, S., & Bare, B. (1996). *Brunner and Suddarth's Textbook of medical-surgical nursing* (8th ed.). Philadelphia: Lippincott-Raven, p. 798.

---

26. Which of the following discharge instructions is essential to give to a client with testicular cancer after testicular surgery?

1. "Report any elevation in temperature to your physician"
2. "You will be unable to drive for 6 weeks"
3. "You cannot be fitted for a prosthesis for 6 months"
4. "Refrain from sitting for long periods"

Answer: 1

Rationale: For the client who has had testicular surgery, the nurse should emphasize the importance of notifying the physician if chills, fever, drainage, redness, or discharge occurs. These symptoms may indicate the presence of an infection. One week after testicular surgery, clients may drive, and often a prosthesis is inserted during surgery. Sitting needs to be avoided with prostate surgery because of hemorrhage, but the risk is not as high with testicular surgery.

Test-Taking Strategy: Use Maslow's hierarchy of needs theory. Infection is the priority. After any surgical procedure, elevation of temperature could signal an infection and should be reported. Review post-testicular surgical teaching points now if you had difficulty with this question.

Level of Cognitive Ability: Analysis
Phase of Nursing Process: Implementation
Client Needs: Physiological Integrity
Content Area: Adult Health/Oncology

Reference

Ignatavicius, D. D., Workman, M. L., & Mishler, M. A. (1995). *Medical-surgical nursing: A nursing process approach* (2nd ed.). Philadelphia: W. B. Saunders, pp. 1069–1070.

---

27. A comatose client is admitted to the intensive care unit (ICU). Laboratory values are as follows: blood glucose, 368 mg/dL; arterial pH, 7.2; arterial bicarbonate, 14 mEq/liter; and positive serum ketones. The client's admitting diagnosis is diabetic ketoacidosis (DKA). During the initial assessment, which of the following will the nurse not expect to note?

1 Hypertension.
2 Dry, cracked mucous membranes.
3 "Fruity" breath odor.
4 Rapid, deep breathing.

Answer: 1

Rationale: Diabetic ketoacidotic coma is usually preceded by a day or more of polyuria and polydipsia associated with marked fatigue, nausea, and vomiting. All of the options are evidence of dehydration and metabolized fatty acids except hypertension. The client with dehydration would be hypotensive.

Test-Taking Strategy: Knowledge that rapid, deep breathing and fruity breath and dehydration are associated with DKA can assist in eliminating options 2, 3, and 4. If you had difficulty with this question, take time now to review DKA.

Level of Cognitive Ability: Analysis
Phase of Nursing Process: Assessment
Client Needs: Physiological Integrity
Content Area: Adult Health/Endocrine

Reference

Black, J., & Matassarin-Jacobs, E. (1997). *Medical-surgical nursing: Clinical management for continuity of care* (5th ed.). Philadelphia: W. B. Saunders, p. 1983.

---

28. Which of the following statements by the spouse of a home care client with end-stage liver failure indicates the need for additional interventions by the multidisciplinary team for the management of pain?

1 "If the pain increases, I must let the nurse know immediately"
2 "I should have my husband try the breathing exercises to help control pain"
3 "This narcotic will cause very deep sleep, which is what my husband needs"
4 "If constipation is a problem, increased fluids will help"

Answer: 3

Rationale: Changes in level of consciousness are a potential indicator of narcotic overdose as well as indicative of numerous fluid, electrolyte, and oxygenation deficits. It is necessary to clarify with the spouse to be certain that the differences in sleep related to relief of pain and changes in neurological status related to these deficits are understood. Option 3 is therefore the correct answer. Options 1, 2, and 4 all are indicative of an understanding of appropriate steps to be taken in the management of discomforts that occur with liver failure.

Test-Taking Strategy: Note the key phrases "additional interventions" and "management of pain" in the question. Option 1 is an accurate statement. Even though the client is end stage, increases in pain level must be noted and interventions taken to relieve that pain. Option 2 is also correct because nonpharmacological interventions are useful in relief of pain. Option 4 is correct and relates to a general principle.

Level of Cognitive Ability: Analysis
Phase of Nursing Process: Evaluation
Client Needs: Physiological Integrity
Content Area: Adult Health/Gastrointestinal

Reference

Barry, P. (1996). *Psychosocial nursing: Care of physically ill patients and their families* (3rd ed.). Philadelphia: Lippincott-Raven, pp. 397–400.

29. The registered nurse (RN) has delegated care of a newly postoperative client to a licensed practical nurse (LPN). The LPN notifies the RN that the client's vital signs are elevated and the client is complaining of pain and dyspnea. Which of the following is the most appropriate action of the RN?

1 The RN need not carry out further action because the LPN is experienced and trustworthy
2 The RN requests that the LPN offer the client a narcotic analgesic that has been ordered postoperatively
3 The RN places a call to the attending surgeon and reports that the client is having pain
4 The RN checks the client's surgical notes and gathers additional data before calling the surgeon

Answer: 4

Rationale: The RN must not depend exclusively on the judgment of an LPN because the RN is responsible for supervising those to whom client care has been delegated. Option 1 is therefore incorrect. The client has recently had surgery, and there is the potential for complications, which may be signaled by alterations in vital signs and respiratory status. An analgesic may not be advisable, but to make that determination, the RN must have more information; therefore 2 is incorrect. A call to the surgeon may be warranted, but the RN has insufficient data at this time, making option 3 incorrect. To provide the client with the degree of care required, the RN must gather additional information and analyze that information before notifying the surgeon, making option 4 the correct choice.

Test-Taking Strategy: Eliminate options 1 and 2 because they are similar indicating that the RN does not gather any additional data, even though the client is newly postoperative. From the remaining two options, option 4 reflects the process of assessment and gathering data and therefore is the best option. Review the role of the RN in delegating and supervising tasks delegated to others if you had difficulty with this question.

Level of Cognitive Ability: Application
Phase of Nursing Process: Implementation
Client Needs: Physiological Integrity
Content Area: Fundamental Skills

Reference

Potter, P., & Perry, A. (1997). *Fundamentals of nursing: Concepts, process, and practice* (4th ed.). St. Louis: Mosby–Year Book, pp. 62–63.

30. An outbreak of illness has occurred in a community and is suspected to be related to food ingestion. One of the first assessment activities of the community health nurse is to

1 Determine what common food item was ingested by those affected.
2 Review the signs and symptoms related to the *Salmonella* bacteria.
3 Involve the Centers for Disease Control and Prevention.
4 Teach the basic methods for preventing food contamination to those affected.

Answer: 1

Rationale: The first step is to determine or assess what food has been ingested. Option 2 involves teaching and is not the appropriate first step. Options 3 and 4 involve potential interventions.

Test-Taking Strategy: The key phrase is "first assessment." Use the nursing process to answer the question. The only option that addresses assessment is option 1.

Level of Cognitive Ability: Application
Phase of Nursing Process: Assessment
Client Needs: Physiological Integrity
Content Area: Fundamental Skills

Reference

Spradley, B., & Allender, J. (1996). *Community health nursing: Concepts and practice* (4th ed.). Philadelphia: Lippincott-Raven, pp. 129–130.

31. On receiving the antenatal history of a client in early labor, the labor room nurse recognizes which of the following factors as having the greatest potential for causing neonatal sepsis after delivery?

1 Adequate prenatal care
2 Appropriate maternal nutrition and weight gain
3 Spontaneous rupture of membranes 2 hours ago
4 History of substance abuse during pregnancy

Answer: 4

Rationale: Risk factors for neonatal sepsis can arise from maternal, intrapartal, or neonatal conditions. Maternal risk factors before delivery include low socioeconomic status, poor prenatal care and nutrition, and a history of substance abuse during pregnancy. Premature rupture of membranes or prolonged rupture of membranes greater than 18 hours before birth is also a risk factor for neonatal acquisition of infection.

Test-Taking Strategy: Use the process of elimination. Options 1 and 2 are optimal findings and give no additional risk. Knowledge of risk factors helps you accurately discriminate between options 3 and 4. Additionally note the phrase "2 hours ago," which should assist in eliminating option 3. If you had difficulty with this question, take time now to review potential maternal physiological and psychosocial risk factors that may cause neonatal infections.

Level of Cognitive Ability: Analysis
Phase of Nursing Process: Assessment
Client Needs: Physiological Integrity
Content Area: Maternity

Reference

Lowdermilk, D., Perry, S., & Bobak, I. (1997). *Maternity and women's health care* (6th ed.). St. Louis: Mosby–Year Book, pp. 1083, 1084.

---

32. The client who uses alcohol frequently is in the first trimester of pregnancy. The nurse initiates interventions to assist the client to reduce or cease alcohol consumption to

1 Promote the normal psychosocial adaptation of the mother to pregnancy.
2 Reduce the potential for fetal growth restriction in utero.
3 Minimize the potential for placental abruptions during the intrapartum period.
4 Reduce the risk of teratogenic effects to developing fetal organs, tissues, and structures.

Answer: 4

Rationale: The first trimester, "organogenesis," is characterized by the differentiation and development of fetal organs, systems, and structures. The effects of alcohol on the developing fetus during this crucial period depend not only on the amount of alcohol consumed, but also on the interaction of quantity, frequency, and type of alcohol and other drugs that may be abused during this period by the pregnant woman. Reducing consumption during this time may promote normal fetal organ development.

Test-Taking Strategy: Option 4 specifically relates to the issue of the question. Options 1, 2, and 3 are nursing actions that reflect global guidelines appropriate for all antenatal clients. If you had difficulty with this question, take time now to review the effects of alcohol on the fetus in the first trimester of pregnancy.

Level of Cognitive Ability: Application
Phase of Nursing Process: Implementation
Client Needs: Physiological Integrity
Content Area: Maternity

Reference

Lowdermilk, D., Perry, S., & Bobak, I. (1997). *Maternity and women's health care* (6th ed.). St. Louis: Mosby–Year Book, pp. 1094–1095.

33. A mother infected with human immunodeficiency virus (HIV) brings her 5-year-old into the clinic to get routine immunizations according to the recommended schedule. Which immunization is contraindicated because of the mother's status?

1 MMR (measles, mumps, and rubella)
2 DTP (diphtheria, tetanus, and pertussis)
3 HIB (*Haemophilus influenzae* type B)
4 OPV (oral polio vaccine)

Answer: 4

Rationale: The OPV is the vaccine made from a live virus, which could be transmitted to an immunocompromised household member. Inactive polio vaccine (IPV) would be substituted. The other vaccines have inactive organisms. HIB is not recommended for this age.

Test-Taking Strategy: Knowing the recommended immunization schedule is helpful. Option 3 could be eliminated because it is not age appropriate. If you are unsure of the correct option, note that options 1, 2, and 3 are injectable vaccines, and option 4 is oral and therefore different. If you had difficulty with this question, take time now to review the contraindications to immunizations.

Level of Cognitive Ability: Analysis
Phase of Nursing Process: Analysis
Client Needs: Physiological Integrity
Content Area: Child Health

Reference

Wong, D. (1997). *Whaley and Wong's Essentials of pediatric nursing* (5th ed.). St. Louis: Mosby–Year Book, pp. 314, 318, 320.

34. A teenage girl is seen for the third time in 6 months for the treatment of vaginal candidal infections. The nurse is aware that additional tests may be indicated to identify an undiagnosed underlying chronic disease. Which test would the nurse anticipate would most likely be prescribed?

1 Papanicolaou (Pap) smear
2 Blood culture
3 Throat culture
4 Blood glucose level

Answer: 4

Rationale: A blood glucose level is an indicator of diabetes. Type I diabetes mellitus is an autoimmune disease, which if untreated provides an ideal environment for frequent infections. In females, monilial infections of the genitourinary tract are the most common manifestation. Pap smears are specific for cancer of the cervix, which is usually asymptomatic. A throat culture may show a candidal infection, but it is not usually chronic or asymptomatic. An infection of the blood is systemic and with apparent symptoms. It isn't a likely result of frequent vaginal infections.

Test-Taking Strategy: The key phrase in the question is "chronic disease." Options 1, 2, and 3 do not necessarily identify chronic disease. If you had difficulty with this question, take time now to review the clinical manifestations associated with diabetes mellitus.

Level of Cognitive Ability: Analysis
Phase of Nursing Process: Analysis
Client Needs: Physiological Integrity
Content Area: Child Health

Reference

Wong, D. (1995). *Whaley and Wong's Nursing care of infants and children* (5th ed.). St. Louis: Mosby–Year Book, p. 1768.

35. When a nurse is admitting a client with a diagnosis of myxedema, which of the following physical assessment techniques provide data that are necessary to support the admitting diagnosis?

1 Inspection of facial features
2 Palpation of the adrenal glands
3 Percussion of the thyroid gland
4 Auscultation of lung sounds

Answer: 1

Rationale: Inspection of facial features reveals the characteristic coarse features, presence of edema around the eyes and face, and blank expression that are characteristic of hypothyroidism. The other assessment techniques in options 2, 3, and 4 do not reveal any data that would support the diagnosis of myxedema.

Test-Taking Strategy: Use the process of elimination. Eliminate options 2 and 4 because they do not relate to the thyroid gland. Palpation, rather than percussion, of the thyroid is the preferred assessment technique when evaluating the thyroid gland, so option 3 can be eliminated. The only remaining option is 1. If you had difficulty with this question, take time now to review the clinical manifestations associated with hypothyroidism.

Level of Cognitive Ability: Application
Phase of Nursing Process: Assessment
Client Needs: Physiological Integrity
Content Area: Adult Health/Endocrine

Reference

Ignatavicius, D. D., Workman, M. L., & Mishler, M. A. (1995). *Medical-surgical nursing: A nursing process approach* (2nd ed.). Philadelphia: W. B. Saunders, p. 1846.

---

36. The nurse is teaching a client with COPD how to do pursed-lip breathing. Which of the following instructions by the nurse would be correct?

1 Inform the client that inhalation should be twice as long as exhalation
2 Instruct the client to loosen the abdominal muscles while breathing out
3 Inform the client that exhalation should be twice as long as inhalation
4 Encourage the client to inhale with pursed lips and to exhale with the mouth open wide

Answer: 3

Rationale: Prolonging the time for exhaling reduces air trapping because of airway narrowing or collapse in COPD. Tightening the abdominal muscles aids in expelling air. Exhaling through pursed lips increases the intraluminal pressure and prevents the airways from collapsing.

Test-Taking Strategy: A basic understanding of the physiological purpose of pursed-lip breathing is needed to answer this question. Knowing that a major purpose of pursed-lip breathing is to prevent air trapping during exhalation can lead you to the correct answer. Review the principles of pursed-lip breathing if you are unfamiliar with this technique.

Level of Cognitive Ability: Application
Phase of Nursing Process: Implementation
Client Needs: Physiological Integrity
Content Area: Adult Health/Respiratory

Reference

Burrell, L., Gerlach, M., & Pless, B. (1997). *Adult nursing: Acute and community care* (2nd ed.). Stamford, CT: Appleton & Lange, pp. 666–667.

---

37. The nurse is caring for the pregnant client with a history of HIV. Which nursing diagnosis, if formulated by the nurse, has the highest priority for this client?

1 Self-Care Deficit
2 Risk for Infection
3 Nutritional Deficit
4 Activity Intolerance

Answer: 2

Rationale: Clients with HIV often show some evidence of immune dysfunction and may have increased vulnerability to common infections. Options 1 and 4 can be easily eliminated. Although nutritional deficit is a concern, infection is specifically related to HIV and is a priority.

Test-Taking Strategy: Not every client with HIV has problems with activity, self-care, or nutrition. HIV infection impairs cellular and humoral immune function. Individuals with HIV are vulnerable to common bacterial infections. If you had difficulty with this question, take time now to review the risks associated with HIV infection.

Level of Cognitive Ability: Analysis
Phase of Nursing Process: Analysis
Client Needs: Physiological Integrity
Content Area: Maternity

Reference

Nichols, F., & Zwelling, E. (1997). *Maternal-newborn nursing: Theory and practice.* Philadelphia: W. B. Saunders, pp. 1497–1501.

38. A 44-year-old is taking lithium carbonate (Lithium) for treatment of bipolar disorder. Which of the following assessment questions should be asked to determine signs of early drug toxicity?

1. "Have you been experiencing seizures over the past few days?"
2. "Do you have frequent headaches?"
3. "Have you been experiencing any nausea, vomiting, or diarrhea?"
4. "Have you noted excessive urination?"

Answer: 3

Rationale: One of the most common early signs of lithium toxicity is gastrointestinal disturbances, such as nausea, vomiting, or diarrhea. The assessment questions in options 1, 2, and 4 are unrelated to lithium toxicity.

Test-Taking Strategy: The question asked for the early signs of lithium toxicity. The key word "toxicity" should assist in directing you to the correct option. Review these signs now because it is likely that you will find a question related to lithium toxicity on NCLEX-RN.

Level of Cognitive Ability: Application
Phase of Nursing Process: Assessment
Client Needs: Physiological Integrity
Content Area: Pharmacology

Reference

Carson, V., & Arnold, E. (1996). *Mental health nursing: The nurse-patient journey.* Philadelphia: W. B. Saunders, p. 547.

39. The physician's order reads "meperidine hydrochloride (Demerol), 125 mg IM." The medication is available in a 100 mg/mL preparation. How many milliliters of the medication would the nurse draw into the syringe for injection?

1. 1.5 mL
2. 1.8 mL
3. 1.75 mL
4. 1.25 mL

Answer: 4

Rationale: Desired amount = 125 mg; available amount = 1 mL = 100 mg; ratio = 125 mg:x mL::100 mg:1 mL; therefore, 125 = 100x = 1.25 mL.

Test-Taking Strategy: When reading math calculation questions, identify the dosage or concentration on hand and the dosage or concentration needed. Once these are identified, set up the mathematical problem and solve for x. Make sure that the answer makes sense.

Level of Cognitive Ability: Application
Phase of Nursing Process: Implementation
Client Needs: Physiological Integrity
Content Area: Pharmacology

Reference

Kee, J., & Hayes, E. (1997). *Pharmacology: A nursing process approach* (2nd ed.). Philadelphia: W. B. Saunders, p. 55.

40. While doing a prenatal examination on a client in the third trimester, the nurse begins an abdominal examination including Leopold maneuvers. After performing the first maneuver, the nurse determines

1. Fetal lie and presentation.
2. Fetal descent.
3. Strength of uterine contractions.
4. Placenta previa.

Answer: 1

Rationale: The first maneuver is to determine the contents of the fundus (either fetal head or breech) and thereby the fetal lie (cephalic or breech). Leopold maneuvers should not be performed during a contraction. Placenta previa is diagnosed by ultrasound and not by palpation. Fetal descent is determined with the fourth maneuver.

Test-Taking Strategy: Knowledge of this specific maneuver is needed to answer this question correctly. If necessary, take a few moments now to review this procedure.

Level of Cognitive Ability: Application
Phase of Nursing Process: Assessment
Client Needs: Physiological Integrity
Content Area: Maternity

Reference

Nichols, F., & Zwelling, E. (1997). *Maternal-newborn nursing: Theory and practice.* Philadelphia: W. B. Saunders, pp. 433–436.

41. Assessment of which physiological parameter provides the nurse with the best information about recovery from spinal shock?

1. BP
2. Pulse rate
3. Reflexes
4. Temperature

Answer: 3

Rationale: Areflexia characterizes spinal shock, and therefore reflexes provide the best information. Vital sign changes are not consistently affected by spinal shock.

Test-Taking Strategy: The stem asks for the best sign of recovery from shock. Because vital signs are affected by many factors, they do not give reliable information about spinal shock recovery. BP would provide good information about recovery from other types of shock but not spinal shock. Note that options 1, 2, and 4 are all vital signs. Option 3 is the different option. Take time now to review spinal shock if you are unfamiliar with this content.

Level of Cognitive Ability: Analysis
Phase of Nursing Process: Assessment
Client Needs: Physiological Integrity
Content Area: Adult Health/Neurological

Reference

Smeltzer, S., & Bare, B. (1996). *Brunner and Suddarth's Textbook of medical-surgical nursing* (8th ed.). Philadelphia: Lippincott-Raven, p. 1800.

---

42. A client is admitted for repair of an unruptured cerebral aneurysm. Which assessment finding would be seen first if the aneurysm ruptures?

1. Widened pulse pressure
2. Unilateral slowing of pupil response
3. Unilateral motor weakness
4. A decline in the level of consciousness

Answer: 4

Rationale: Rupture of a cerebral aneurysm usually results in increased intracranial pressure (ICP). The first sign of increased ICP is a change in the level of consciousness. This change in consciousness can be as subtle as drowsiness or restlessness. Because centers that control BP are located lower in the brain stem than those that control consciousness, pulse pressure alteration is a later sign. Options 2 and 3 are not early signs of increased ICP.

Test-Taking Strategy: Note the key word "first." Remember that changes in level of consciousness are the first indication of increased ICP. Review the clinical manifestations associated with ICP if you had difficulty with this question.

Level of Cognitive Ability: Analysis
Phase of Nursing Process: Assessment
Client Needs: Physiological Integrity
Content Area: Adult Health/Neurological

Reference

Smeltzer, S., & Bare, B. (1996). *Brunner and Suddarth's Textbook of medical-surgical nursing* (8th ed.). Philadelphia: Lippincott-Raven, pp. 1713, 1766.

---

43. The emergency room staff calls the mental health unit and tells the nurse that a severely depressed client is being transported to the unit. The nurse expects which of the following when performing the assessment for this client?

1. Weight gain, hypersomnia, blunted affect
2. Increased crying spells, normal weight, and normal sleep
3. Hesitancy to participate but no change in affect
4. Weight loss, insomnia, decreased crying spells

Answer: 4

Rationale: In the severely depressed client, loss of weight is typical, whereas the mildly depressed client may experience a gain in weight. Sleep is generally affected in a similar way, with hypersomnia in the mildly depressed client and insomnia in the severely depressed client. The severely depressed client may report that no tears are left for crying.

Test-Taking Strategy: Options 2 and 3 identify some degree of normalcy and can be eliminated, leaving only two options remaining. Option one indicates some degree of normalcy with the term "blunted affect"; therefore eliminate this option. This leaves option 4 as the best answer. Review assessment findings associated with the severely depressed client if you had difficulty with this question.

Level of Cognitive Ability: Analysis
Phase of Nursing Process: Assessment
Client Needs: Physiological Integrity
Content Area: Mental Health

Reference

Johnson, B. (1997). *Psychiatric–mental health nursing: Adaptation and growth* (4th ed.). Philadelphia: Lippincott-Raven, p. 546.

---

44. The client with a prior history of suicide attempts is admitted with the diagnosis of depression. The therapist reports to the nurse on the telephone that the client had called earlier and was having severe suicidal thoughts. Keeping this information in mind, the nurse must assess

1 Presence of suicidal thoughts now.
2 Interaction with peers.
3 Food intake for past 24 hours.
4 Past treatment regimen.

Answer: 1

Rationale: The most crucial presenting information from the therapist's report is that the client is having frequent thoughts of self-harm; therefore, the nurse needs further information about present thoughts of suicide, so that the treatment plan may be as appropriate as possible. The nurse and the health care facility must make sure the client is safe. Other items should be assessed; however, assessment of suicide potential is most important.

Test-Taking Strategy: Note the relationship between "severe suicidal thoughts" in the question and in the correct option. In addition, option 1 is the priority assessment.

Level of Cognitive Ability: Application
Phase of Nursing Process: Assessment
Client Needs: Physiological Integrity
Content Area: Mental Health

Reference

Johnson, B. (1997). *Psychiatric–mental health nursing: Adaptation and growth* (4th ed.). Philadelphia: Lippincott-Raven, p. 865.

---

45. The home care nurse finds the client in the bedroom, unconscious, with a pill bottle in hand. The pill bottle contained the selective serotonin reuptake inhibitor sertraline (Zoloft). What assessment does the nurse perform first?

1 BP
2 Respirations
3 Pulse
4 Urinary output

Answer: 2

Rationale: In the emergency situation, the nurse should determine breathlessness first, then pulselessness. BP is assessed after these assessments are determined. Urinary output is important also but not the priority at this time.

Test-Taking Strategy: The ABCs should serve as the guide for answering this question. Respirations specifically relate to breathing and airway.

Level of Cognitive Ability: Application
Phase of Nursing Process: Assessment
Client Needs: Physiological Integrity
Content Area: Fundamental Skills

Reference

Hodgson, B., & Kizior, R. (1998). *Saunders nursing drug handbook 1998.* Philadelphia: W. B. Saunders, pp. 926–927.

---

46. The nurse is checking a unit of blood and notices that there are gas bubbles in the bag. The nurse should take which of the following actions?

1 Add 10 mL normal saline to the bag
2 Agitate bag gently to mix contents
3 Add 100 units of heparin to the bag
4 Return the bag to the blood bank

Answer: 4

Rationale: The nurse should return the unit of blood to the blood bank. The presence of gas bubbles in the bag indicates possible bacterial growth, and the unit is considered contaminated.

Test-Taking Strategy: To answer this question correctly, it is necessary to be familiar with the process of checking blood and what to do if abnormalities are found. When in doubt, consult with the blood bank. Review concepts related to transfusion of blood if this question was difficult.

Level of Cognitive Ability: Application
Phase of Nursing Process: Implementation
Client Needs: Physiological Integrity
Content Area: Fundamental Skills

Reference

Monahan, F., & Neighbors, M. (1998). *Medical-surgical nursing: Foundations for clinical practice* (2nd ed.). Philadelphia: W. B. Saunders, p. 457.

---

47. The nurse has an order to infuse a unit of blood. The nurse checks the client's intravenous line to make sure that the gauge of the intravenous catheter is

1 14 gauge or larger.
2 19 gauge or larger.
3 22 gauge or larger.
4 24 gauge or larger.

Answer: 2

Rationale: An intravenous line used to infuse blood should be 19 gauge or larger. This allows infusion of the blood elements without clogging the line.

Test-Taking Strategy: Specific knowledge related to blood transfusion techniques is needed to answer this question correctly. Options 3 and 4 can be eliminated first. From the remaining two options, familiarity with intravenous catheters should assist in directing you to option 2. If needed, take a few moments to review intravenous lines and blood transfusions.

Level of Cognitive Ability: Application
Phase of Nursing Process: Implementation
Client Needs: Physiological Integrity
Content Area: Fundamental Skills

Reference

Monahan, F., & Neighbors, M. (1998). *Medical-surgical nursing: Foundations for clinical practice* (2nd ed.). Philadelphia: W. B. Saunders, p. 457.

---

48. The client began receiving a unit of blood 30 minutes ago. The client rings the call bell and complains of difficulty breathing, itching, and a tight sensation in the chest. Which of the following is the first action of the nurse?

1 Recheck the unit of blood for compatibility
2 Check the client's temperature
3 Stop the transfusion
4 Call the physician

Answer: 3

Rationale: The symptoms reported by the client are compatible with transfusion reaction. The first action of the nurse when a transfusion reaction is suspected is to discontinue the transfusion. The intravenous line is kept open with normal saline. The physician is notified. Depending on agency protocol, the nurse may then obtain a urinalysis, draw a sample of blood, and return blood and tubing to the blood bank. The nurse also institutes supportive care for the client, which may include administration of antihistamines, crystalloids, epinephrine, or vasopressors.

Test-Taking Strategy: Knowledge of the specific sequence of events to be followed with transfusion reaction is needed to answer this question correctly. Note that the question asks for the "first action." This should direct you to option 3. If you answered incorrectly, review this standard nursing procedure. You are likely to find a question related to this procedure on NCLEX-RN.

Level of Cognitive Ability: Application
Phase of Nursing Process: Implementation
Client Needs: Physiological Integrity
Content Area: Fundamental Skills

Reference

Monahan, F., & Neighbors, M. (1998). *Medical-surgical nursing: Foundations for clinical practice* (2nd ed.). Philadelphia: W. B. Saunders, pp. 460–461.

49. The client has not eaten or had anything to drink for 4 hours after two episodes of nausea and vomiting. Which of the following items would be best to offer the client who is ready to try resuming oral intake?

1 Ginger ale
2 Gelatin
3 Toast
4 Dry cereal

Answer: 1

Rationale: Clear liquids are tolerated first after episodes of nausea and vomiting. If the client tolerates sips (20–30 mL at a time) of clear liquids, such as water or ginger ale, the amounts may be increased, and gelatin, tea, and broth may be added. Once these are tolerated, solid foods, such as toast, cereal, chicken, and other easily digested foods, may be tried.

Test-Taking Strategy: Begin to answer this question by eliminating options 3 and 4, which identify solid foods and are less well tolerated than liquids. Choose ginger ale over gelatin because it is a liquid at all temperatures.

Level of Cognitive Ability: Application
Phase of Nursing Process: Implementation
Client Needs: Physiological Integrity
Content Area: Adult Health/Gastrointestinal

Reference

Monahan, F., & Neighbors, M. (1998). *Medical-surgical nursing: Foundations for clinical practice* (2nd ed.). Philadelphia: W. B. Saunders, p. 960.

---

50. The client has just undergone an upper gastrointestinal series. The nurse provides which of the following on the client's return to the unit as an important part of routine postprocedure care?

1 Increased fluids
2 Bland diet
3 Liquid diet
4 Laxative

Answer: 4

Rationale: Barium sulfate, which is used as contrast material during an upper gastrointestinal series, is a constipating material. If it is not eliminated from the gastrointestinal tract, it can cause obstruction. Therefore laxatives or cathartics are administered. Option 1 is helpful; options 2 and 3 are unnecessary.

Test-Taking Strategy: To answer this question accurately, it is necessary to know that barium is administered during this test and what its side effects are. This allows you to eliminate each of the incorrect options systematically. Review care after an upper gastrointestinal series now if you had difficulty with this question.

Level of Cognitive Ability: Application
Phase of Nursing Process: Implementation
Client Needs: Physiological Integrity
Content Area: Adult Health/Gastrointestinal

Reference

Monahan, F., & Neighbors, M. (1998). *Medical-surgical nursing: Foundations for clinical practice* (2nd ed.). Philadelphia: W. B. Saunders, p. 970.

---

51. The nurse has an order to discontinue the nasogastric tube of an assigned client. After explaining the procedure to the client, the nurse raises the bed to a semi-Fowler's position, places a towel across the chest, clears the tube with normal saline, clamps the tube, and removes the tube

1 During inspiration.
2 During expiration.
3 After inspiration but before expiration.
4 After expiration but before inspiration.

Answer: 2

Rationale: A nasogastric tube is removed during expiration, so that air and the tube are moving in the same direction.

Test-Taking Strategy: To answer the question correctly, it is necessary to be familiar with this basic nursing procedure. If this question was difficult, review this procedure briefly at this time.

Level of Cognitive Ability: Application
Phase of Nursing Process: Implementation
Client Needs: Physiological Integrity
Content Area: Adult Health/Gastrointestinal

Reference

Monahan, F., & Neighbors, M. (1998). *Medical-surgical nursing: Foundations for clinical practice* (2nd ed.). Philadelphia: W. B. Saunders, p. 980.

52. The nurse is caring for a client who has an order to receive an intravenous intralipid infusion. Which of the following actions does the nurse take as part of proper procedure before hanging the emulsion?

1 Add 100 mL normal saline to the bottle
2 Attach an in-line filter
3 Remove the bottle from the refrigerator
4 Check the solution for separation or oily appearance

Answer: 4

Rationale: Intralipid solutions should not be refrigerated. There should be no additives placed in the bottle because this could affect the stability of the solution. The emulsion should be checked for separation or oily appearance. If found, it should not be used. An in-line filter is not used because it could disturb the emulsion or become clogged.

Test-Taking Strategy: Familiarity with the basic steps of hanging an intralipid infusion is necessary to answer this question accurately. If you are not familiar with this procedure, take time now to review it.

Level of Cognitive Ability: Application
Phase of Nursing Process: Implementation
Client Needs: Physiological Integrity
Content Area: Fundamental Skills

Reference

Monahan, F., & Neighbors, M. (1998). *Medical-surgical nursing: Foundations for clinical practice* (2nd ed.). Philadelphia: W. B. Saunders, p. 990.

53. The nurse is administering continuous tube feedings to a client. The nurse takes which of the following actions as part of routine care for this client?

1 Check the residual every 4 hours
2 Change the feeding bag and tubing every 12 hours
3 Pour additional feeding into the bag when 25 mL are left
4 Hold the feeding if greater than 200 mL are aspirated

Answer: 1

Rationale: The placement of a nasogastric feeding tube and residual are checked at least every 4 hours when administering continuous tube feedings. It is checked before each bolus with intermittent feedings. The feeding should be withheld for 30–60 minutes if the residual is greater than 30 mL. The bag and tubing are completely changed every 24 hours. The bag should be rinsed before adding new formula to the bag that is hanging.

Test-Taking Strategy: The key phrase is "continuous tube feedings." Use the nursing process to answer the question. Option 1 is the only option that addresses assessment. If you had difficulty with this question, take time now to review the nursing care associated with this procedure.

Level of Cognitive Ability: Application
Phase of Nursing Process: Implementation
Client Needs: Physiological Integrity
Content Area: Fundamental Skills

Reference

Monahan, F., & Neighbors, M. (1998). *Medical-surgical nursing: Foundations for clinical practice* (2nd ed.). Philadelphia: W. B. Saunders, p. 985.

54. The physician is inserting a chest tube. The nurse selects which of the following materials to be used as the first layer of the dressing at the chest tube insertion site?

1 Sterile 4 × 4 gauze pad
2 Absorbent Kerlix dressing
3 Gauze impregnated with povidone-iodine
4 Vaseline gauze

Answer: 4

Rationale: The first layer of the chest tube dressing is Vaseline gauze, which allows for an occlusive seal at the chest tube insertion site. Additional layers of gauze cover this layer, and the dressing is secured with a strong adhesive tape or Elastoplast tape.

Test-Taking Strategy: The key words in this question are "first layer." To answer this question correctly, you should know that it is imperative to have an occlusive seal at the site and which dressing material will help you achieve that end. Option 4 is the only option that can achieve that occlusive seal.

Level of Cognitive Ability: Application
Phase of Nursing Process: Implementation
Client Needs: Physiological Integrity
Content Area: Adult Health/Respiratory

Reference

Monahan, F., & Neighbors, M. (1998). *Medical-surgical nursing: Foundations for clinical practice* (2nd ed.). Philadelphia: W. B. Saunders, p. 577.

---

55. The client being seen in the physician's office for follow-up 2 weeks after pneumonectomy complains of numbness and tenderness at the surgical site. The nurse tells the client that this is

1 A severe problem, and the client will probably be rehospitalized.
2 Often the first sign of wound infection and checks the client's temperature.
3 Probably due to permanent nerve damage as a result of surgery.
4 Not likely to be permanent but may last for some months.

Answer: 4

Rationale: Clients who undergo pneumonectomy may experience numbness, altered sensation, or tenderness in the area that surrounds the incision. These sensations may last for months. It is not considered to be a severe problem and is not indicative of wound infection.

Test-Taking Strategy: Eliminate option 1 because of the word "severe." Eliminate option 2 because numbness and tenderness are not signs of infection. Eliminate option 3 because of the word "permanent." Take a few moments to review this surgical procedure if you are not familiar with it.

Level of Cognitive Ability: Application
Phase of Nursing Process: Implementation
Client Needs: Physiological Integrity
Content Area: Adult Health/Respiratory

Reference

Monahan, F., & Neighbors, M. (1998). *Medical-surgical nursing: Foundations for clinical practice* (2nd ed.). Philadelphia: W. B. Saunders, pp. 581–582.

---

56. The client scheduled for pneumonectomy tells the nurse that a friend had chest surgery and asks how long the chest tubes will be in place. The nurse responds

1 "They will be in for 24–48 hours."
2 "They will be removed after 3–4 days."
3 "They usually function for a full week after surgery."
4 "There will be no chest tubes in place after surgery."

Answer: 4

Rationale: Pneumonectomy involves removal of the entire lung, usually because of extensive disease, such as bronchogenic carcinoma, unilateral tuberculosis, or lung abscess. Chest tubes are not inserted because the cavity is left to fill with serosanguineous fluid, which later solidifies. The phrenic nerve is severed or crushed to elevate the diaphragm, further decreasing the size of the chest cavity on the operative side.

Test-Taking Strategy: To answer this question accurately, it is necessary to know that the entire lung is removed with this procedure. This would guide you to reason that chest tubes are unnecessary because there is no lung remaining to reinflate to fill the pleural space.

Level of Cognitive Ability: Application
Phase of Nursing Process: Implementation
Client Needs: Physiological Integrity
Content Area: Adult Health/Respiratory

Reference

Monahan, F., & Neighbors, M. (1998). *Medical-surgical nursing: Foundations for clinical practice* (2nd ed.). Philadelphia: W. B. Saunders, p. 581.

57. The nurse is caring for the client with a dissecting abdominal aortic aneurysm. The nurse would avoid doing which of the following?

1 Turn the client to the side to look for ecchymoses on the lower back
2 Auscultate the arteries for bruits
3 Perform deep palpation of the abdomen
4 Tell the client to report back, shoulder, or neck pain

Answer: 3

Rationale: The nurse avoids deep palpation in the client in whom a dissecting aneurysm is known or suspected. Doing so could place the client at risk for rupture. The nurse does look for ecchymoses on the lower back to determine aneurysm leaking and tells the client to report back, neck, shoulder, or extremity pain. The nurse may auscultate the arteries for bruits.

Test-Taking Strategy: Note the key word "avoid" in the stem. This tells you that the correct answer is an incorrect nursing action or one that is contraindicated. With the diagnosis presented, the only option that could cause harm is the option related to deep palpation. Review care to the client with a dissecting abdominal aortic aneurysm if you had difficulty with this question.

Level of Cognitive Ability: Application
Phase of Nursing Process: Implementation
Client Needs: Physiological Integrity
Content Area: Adult Health/Cardiovascular

Reference

Monahan, F., & Neighbors, M. (1998). *Medical-surgical nursing: Foundations for clinical practice* (2nd ed.). Philadelphia: W. B. Saunders, p. 372.

58. The client has undergone angioplasty of the iliac artery. The nurse best detects bleeding from angioplasty in this region by

1 Measuring abdominal girth every 4 hours.
2 Auscultating over the area with a Doppler monitor every 4 hours.
3 Asking the client about the presence of mild pain.
4 Palpating the pedal pulses every 4 hours.

Answer: 1

Rationale: Bleeding after iliac artery angioplasty causes blood to accumulate in the retroperitoneal area. This can be detected most directly by measuring abdominal girth. Palpation and auscultation of pulses determines patency and may be of some value with assessing bleeding. Pulses will diminish because of reduced circulating volume. Assessment of pain is routinely done, and mild regional discomfort is expected.

Test-Taking Strategy: The key words in this question are "bleeding," "iliac artery," and "best detects." The use of the word "best" tells you that more than one or all of the options may be partially or totally correct. Recalling the anatomical location of the iliac artery (peritoneal cavity) will assist in directing you to option 1, the option that addresses abdominal assessment.

Level of Cognitive Ability: Application
Phase of Nursing Process: Implementation
Client Needs: Physiological Integrity
Content Area: Adult Health/Cardiovascular

Reference

Monahan, F., & Neighbors, M. (1998). *Medical-surgical nursing: Foundations for clinical practice* (2nd ed.). Philadelphia: W. B. Saunders, p. 344.

59. The client is scheduled for a right femoral-popliteal bypass graft. The client has a nursing diagnosis of Altered Peripheral Tissue Perfusion. The nurse takes which of the following actions before surgery to address this nursing diagnosis?

1 Completes a preoperative checklist
2 Marks the location of pedal pulses on the right leg
3 Has the client void before surgery
4 Reviews the results of any baseline coagulation studies

Answer: 2

Rationale: The client scheduled for femoral-popliteal bypass grafting is likely to have diminished peripheral pulses. It is important to mark the location of any pulses that are palpated or auscultated. This provides a baseline for comparison in the postoperative period. The other options are part of routine preoperative care.

Test-Taking Strategy: The key words in the question are "to address this nursing diagnosis." Focusing on the nursing diagnosis will direct you to option 2. Note that options 1, 3, and 4 are actions that are part of routine preoperative care and are not specific to this nursing diagnosis.

Level of Cognitive Ability: Application
Phase of Nursing Process: Implementation
Client Needs: Physiological Integrity
Content Area: Adult Health/Cardiovascular

Reference

Monahan, F., & Neighbors, M. (1998). *Medical-surgical nursing: Foundations for clinical practice* (2nd ed.). Philadelphia: W. B. Saunders, p. 347.

---

60. The client who underwent peripheral arterial bypass surgery 16 hours ago complains of increasing pain in the leg at rest, which worsens with movement and is accompanied by paresthesias. The nurse should take which of the following actions?

1 Administer a narcotic analgesic
2 Apply warm, moist heat for comfort
3 Apply ice to minimize any developing swelling
4 Call the physician

Answer: 4

Rationale: The classic signs of compartment syndrome are pain at rest that intensifies with movement and the development of paresthesias. Compartment syndrome is characterized by increased pressure within a muscle compartment because of bleeding or excessive edema. It compresses the nerves in the area and can cause vascular compromise. The physician is notified immediately because the client could require an emergency fasciotomy.

Test-Taking Strategy: The signs and symptoms described in the case situation indicate a new problem. Note that the surgery was 16 hours ago. These factors should indicate that the physician needs to be notified.

Level of Cognitive Ability: Application
Phase of Nursing Process: Implementation
Client Needs: Physiological Integrity
Content Area: Adult Health/Cardiovascular

Reference

Monahan, F., & Neighbors, M. (1998). *Medical-surgical nursing: Foundations for clinical practice* (2nd ed.). Philadelphia: W. B. Saunders, p. 347.

---

61. In an ambulatory care clinic, the nurse measures the client's blood pressure (BP) in the left arm as 200/118. The first action of the nurse is to

1 Notify the physician.
2 Inquire about the presence of kidney disorders.
3 Check the BP in the right arm.
4 Recheck the pressure in the same arm within 30 seconds.

Answer: 3

Rationale: On getting an initially high reading, the nurse takes the pressure in the opposite arm to see if the BP is elevated in one extremity only. The nurse would also recheck the BP in the same arm but would wait at least 2 minutes between readings. The nurse would inquire about the presence of kidney disorders, which could contribute to elevated BP, but this is not the first action. The nurse would notify the physician because immediate treatment is required, but this would not be done without obtaining verification of the elevation.

Test-Taking Strategy: Note the key word in the question is "first." This tells you that more than one or all of the options may be partially or totally correct. In this instance, eliminate option 4 first because it is incorrect. Choose option 3 over the others because it provides verification of the initial reading.

Level of Cognitive Ability: Application
Phase of Nursing Process: Implementation
Client Needs: Physiological Integrity
Content Area: Adult Health/Cardiovascular

Reference

Monahan, F., & Neighbors, M. (1998). *Medical-surgical nursing: Foundations for clinical practice* (2nd ed.). Philadelphia: W. B. Saunders, p. 375.

62. The hospitalized client has received a diagnosis of thrombophlebitis. The nurse would avoid doing which of the following during the care of this client?

1 Maintaining the client on bed rest
2 Applying moist heat to the leg
3 Elevating the feet above heart level
4 Placing a pillow under the client's knees

Answer: 4

Rationale: The nurse avoids placing a pillow under the knees of a client with thrombophlebitis because it obstructs venous return to the heart and exacerbates impairment of blood flow. The client is maintained on bed rest for 3–7 days after a diagnosis of thrombophlebitis is made to prevent occurrence of pulmonary embolus. The feet are elevated above heart level to aid in venous return, and warm, moist heat may be used to aid in comfort and reduce venospasm.

Test-Taking Strategy: Note the key word in the question is "avoid." This tells you that the correct response is an incorrect nursing action. Use principles related to gravity and relief of inflammation to answer this question. This should direct you to the action to avoid.

Level of Cognitive Ability: Application
Phase of Nursing Process: Implementation
Client Needs: Physiological Integrity
Content Area: Adult Health/Cardiovascular

Reference

Monahan, F., & Neighbors, M. (1998). *Medical-surgical nursing: Foundations for clinical practice* (2nd ed.). Philadelphia: W. B. Saunders, p. 387.

---

63. A new prenatal client is 6 months pregnant. On the first prenatal visit, the nurse notes that the client is gravida 4, para 0, aborta 3. The client is 5 feet 6 inches tall, weighs 130 pounds, and is 25 years old. The client states, "I get really tired after working all day and I can't keep up with my housework." Which factor in the data given would lead the nurse to suspect gestational diabetes?

1 Fatigue
2 Obesity
3 Maternal age
4 Previous fetal demise

Answer: 4

Rationale: Fatigue is a normal occurrence during pregnancy. At 5 feet 6 inches tall, 130 pounds, the client does not meet the criteria of 20% over ideal weight; therefore the client is not obese. To be at high risk for gestational diabetes, the maternal age should be greater than 30 years. A previous history of unexplained stillbirths or miscarriages puts the client at high risk for gestational diabetes.

Test-Taking Strategy: Option 1 can be easily eliminated. Options 2, 3, and 4 are all risk factors for gestational diabetes. When rereading the stem of the question, however, options 2 and 3 do not apply to this client. If you had difficulty with this question, take time now to review the risk factors associated with gestational diabetes.

Level of Cognitive Ability: Analysis
Phase of Nursing Process: Analysis
Client Needs: Physiological Integrity
Content Area: Maternity

Reference

Lowdermilk, D., Perry, S., & Bobak, I. (1997). *Maternity and women's health care* (6th ed.). St. Louis: Mosby–Year Book, pp. 813–814.

---

64. When a client progresses from preeclampsia to eclampsia, the nurse's first action should be to

1 Administer intravenous magnesium sulfate.
2 Assess the BP and fetal heart tones.
3 Clear and maintain an open airway.
4 Administer oxygen by face mask.

Answer: 3

Rationale: Options 1, 2, and 4 are all procedures that should be done but are not the first action. It is important as a first action to keep an open airway and prevent injuries to the client.

Test-Taking Strategy: Note the question asks for the "first action." All of the options are correct procedures for this client. A certain order ought to be followed for the client's safety, however. Use the ABCs to answer the question.

Level of Cognitive Ability: Application
Phase of Nursing Process: Implementation
Client Needs: Physiological Integrity
Content Area: Maternity

Reference

Lowdermilk, D., Perry, S., & Bobak, I. (1997). *Maternity and women's health care* (6th ed.). St. Louis: Mosby–Year Book, p. 715.

---

65. The nurse in the emergency room admits a client who is bleeding from a scalp laceration obtained during a fall from a stepladder when the client was doing outdoor home repair. The nurse would take which of the following actions first in the care of this wound?

1 Ask the client about timing of last tetanus vaccination
2 Cleanse the wound with sterile normal saline
3 Prepare for suturing the area
4 Administer a prophylactic antibiotic

Answer: 2

Rationale: The initial nursing action is to cleanse the wound thoroughly with sterile normal saline. This removes dirt or foreign matter in the wound and allows visualization of the size of the wound. Direct pressure is applied as needed to control bleeding. If suturing is necessary, the surrounding hair may be shaved. Prophylactic antibiotics are often ordered. The date of the client's last tetanus shot is determined, and prophylaxis is given if needed.

Test-Taking Strategy: The key words in the question are "care of the wound" and "first." The key word "first" implies that more than one or all of the options may be partially or totally correct. In this instance, all of the options are reasonable. Therefore your answer should be the first action that focuses on actual care of the wound, which is option 2.

Level of Cognitive Ability: Application
Phase of Nursing Process: Implementation
Client Needs: Physiological Integrity
Content Area: Adult Health/Integumentary

Reference

Monahan, F., & Neighbors, M. (1998). *Medical-surgical nursing: Foundations for clinical practice* (2nd ed.). Philadelphia: W. B. Saunders, p. 817.

---

66. The client was admitted to the nursing unit with a closed head injury 6 hours ago. After report, the nurse finds the client has vomited, is confused, and complains of dizziness and headache. The nurse should do which of the following as the most important nursing action?

1 Administer an antiemetic
2 Change the client's gown and bed linens
3 Reorient the client to surroundings
4 Notify the physician

Answer: 4

Rationale: The client with a closed head injury is at risk of developing increased ICP. This is evidenced by symptoms such as headache, dizziness, confusion, weakness, and vomiting. Because of the implications of the symptoms, the most important nursing action is to notify the physician. Other nursing actions that are appropriate include physical care of the client and reorientation to surroundings.

Test-Taking Strategy: Note that the key words in the question are "most important." This directs you to prioritize the possible nursing actions. Note that the question does not ask what the "first" or "initial" action would be. Considering the closed head injury and the developing signs and symptoms, the nurse should suspect increased ICP. The physician needs to be notified.

Level of Cognitive Ability: Application
Phase of Nursing Process: Implementation
Client Needs: Physiological Integrity
Content Area: Adult Health/Neurological

Reference

Monahan, F., & Neighbors, M. (1998). *Medical-surgical nursing: Foundations for clinical practice* (2nd ed.). Philadelphia: W. B. Saunders, p. 819.

67. The client is being brought into the emergency room after suffering a head injury. The first action by the nurse is to determine the client's

1 Respiratory rate and depth.
2 Pulse and BP.
3 Level of consciousness.
4 Ability to move extremities.

Answer: 1

Rationale: The first action of the nurse is to ensure that the client has an adequate airway and respiratory status. In rapid sequence, the client's circulatory status is evaluated, followed by evaluation of the neurological status.

Test-Taking Strategy: In emergency situations, remember the ABCs. The correct answer is most often the option that deals with the client's airway. Respiratory rate and depth supports this action.

Level of Cognitive Ability: Application
Phase of Nursing Process: Implementation
Client Needs: Physiological Integrity
Content Area: Adult Health/Neurological

Reference

Monahan, F., & Neighbors, M. (1998). *Medical-surgical nursing: Foundations for clinical practice* (2nd ed.). Philadelphia: W. B. Saunders, p. 821.

68. The client with spinal cord injury is at risk of developing footdrop. The nurse uses which of the following as the most effective preventive measure?

1 Heel protectors
2 Posterior splints
3 Pneumatic boots
4 Foot board

Answer: 2

Rationale: The most effective means of preventing footdrop are the use of posterior splints or high-top sneakers. A foot board prevents plantar flexion but also places the client more at risk for developing pressure ulcers of the feet. Pneumatic boots prevent deep vein thrombosis but not footdrop. Heel protectors protect the skin but do not prevent footdrop.

Test-Taking Strategy: Note that the focus of the question is on the "prevention" of footdrop. This guides you to select the option that immobilizes the foot in a functional position while protecting the skin of the extremities. Review the purposes of these devices if you had difficulty with this question.

Level of Cognitive Ability: Application
Phase of Nursing Process: Implementation
Client Needs: Physiological Integrity
Content Area: Adult Health/Neurological

Reference

Monahan, F., & Neighbors, M. (1998). *Medical-surgical nursing: Foundations for clinical practice* (2nd ed.). Philadelphia: W. B. Saunders, p. 826.

69. The client is ambulatory and wearing a halo vest after cervical spine fracture. The nurse tells the client to avoid which of the following because the client has a risk for injury?

1 Bending at the waist
2 Using a walker
3 Wearing rubber-soled shoes
4 Scanning the environment

Answer: 1

Rationale: The client with a halo vest should avoid bending at the waist because the halo vest is heavy, and the client's trunk is limited in flexibility. It is helpful for the client to scan the environment visually because the client's peripheral vision is diminished from keeping the neck in a stationary position. Use of a walker and rubber-soled shoes may help prevent falls and injury, and therefore these devices are also helpful.

Test-Taking Strategy: Note the key word "avoid" in the stem. This guides you to look for an action that could put the client at risk for injury. A review of each of the possible options allows you to eliminate each of the incorrect responses systematically. Attempt to visualize each of the items or actions in the options to assist in identifying how injury could be prevented.

Level of Cognitive Ability: Application
Phase of Nursing Process: Implementation
Client Needs: Physiological Integrity
Content Area: Adult Health/Neurological

Reference

Monahan, F., & Neighbors, M. (1998). *Medical-surgical nursing: Foundations for clinical practice* (2nd ed.). Philadelphia: W. B. Saunders, p. 826.

---

70. The nurse is caring for the client who has undergone transsphenoidal resection of a pituitary adenoma. The nurse measures which of the following to detect occurrence of the most common complication of this surgery?

1 Pulse rate
2 Temperature
3 Urine output
4 Oxygen saturation

Answer: 3

Rationale: The most common complication of surgery on the pituitary gland is temporary diabetes insipidus. This results from deficiency in antidiuretic hormone (ADH) secretion as a result of surgical trauma. The nurse measures the client's urine output to determine whether this complication is occurring.

Test-Taking Strategy: To answer this question correctly, recall that the pituitary gland is responsible for the production of ADH. This allows you to eliminate each of the incorrect responses systematically and directs you to option 3. Review the complications of this surgical procedure if you had difficulty with this question.

Level of Cognitive Ability: Application
Phase of Nursing Process: Implementation
Client Needs: Physiological Integrity
Content Area: Adult Health/Neurological

Reference

Monahan, F., & Neighbors, M. (1998). *Medical-surgical nursing: Foundations for clinical practice* (2nd ed.). Philadelphia: W. B. Saunders, pp. 1267, 1275.

---

71. The nurse is sending an arterial blood gas specimen to the laboratory for analysis. The nurse does not need to write which of the following pieces of information on the laboratory requisition?

1 The date and time the specimen was drawn
2 A list of client allergies
3 Any supplemental oxygen the client is receiving
4 The client's temperature

Answer: 2

Rationale: An arterial blood gas requisition usually contains information about the date and time the specimen was drawn, the client's temperature, whether the specimen was drawn on room air or using supplemental oxygen, and the ventilator settings if the client is on a mechanical ventilator.

Test-Taking Strategy: To answer this question most easily, review the options from the viewpoint of the relevance of the item to the client's airway status or oxygen utilization. With this in mind, you would be able to eliminate each of the incorrect options. The client's allergies do not have a direct bearing on the laboratory results.

Level of Cognitive Ability: Application
Phase of Nursing Process: Implementation
Client Needs: Physiological Integrity
Content Area: Adult Health/Respiratory

Reference

Monahan, F., & Neighbors, M. (1998). *Medical-surgical nursing: Foundations for clinical practice* (2nd ed.). Philadelphia: W. B. Saunders, p. 543.

72. To promote a successful postoperative recovery for a client who had one adrenal gland removed, discharge instructions should include

1. The need for lifelong replacement of all adrenal hormones.
2. Instructions about early signs of a wound infection.
3. The reason for maintaining a diabetic diet.
4. Teaching proper application of an ostomy pouch.

Answer: 2

Rationale: A client who is undergoing a unilateral adrenalectomy is placed on corticosteroids temporarily to avoid a cortisol deficiency. These medications are gradually weaned in the postoperative period. Because of the anti-inflammatory properties of corticosteroids, clients who undergo adrenalectomies are at increased risk of developing wound infections. Because of this increased risk of infection, it is important for the client to know measures to prevent infection, early signs of infection, and what to do if an infection seems to be present.

Test-Taking Strategy: This question asks you to identify teaching needs of a client undergoing an adrenalectomy. In reading the stem, it is essential to notice that only one adrenal gland was removed. Knowing that the hormones from the adrenal glands are needed for proper immune system function should narrow your choices to options 1 or 2. Also recognizing that one gland can take over the function of two adrenal glands should allow you to select option 2 as the correct answer.

Level of Cognitive Ability: Application
Phase of Nursing Process: Planning
Client Needs: Physiological Integrity
Content Area: Adult Health/Endocrine

Reference

Burrell, L., Gerlach, M., & Pless, B. (1997). *Adult nursing: Acute and community care* (2nd ed.). Stamford, CT: Appleton & Lange, p. 1106.

---

73. The client has undergone transsphenoidal surgery for a pituitary adenoma. The nurse teaches the client to

1. Remove the nasal packing after 48 hours.
2. Cough and deep breathe hourly.
3. Take acetaminophen (Tylenol) for severe headache.
4. Report frequent swallowing or postnasal drip.

Answer: 4

Rationale: The client should report frequent swallowing or postnasal drip after transsphenoidal surgery because it could indicate CSF leakage. The surgeon removes the nasal packing, usually after 24 hours. The client should deep breathe, but coughing is contraindicated because it could cause increased ICP. The client should also report severe headache because it could indicate increased ICP.

Test-Taking Strategy: Knowledge of the anatomical location related to this surgery can assist in providing the clue that the concern is increased ICP and symptoms of CSF leak. Option 1 can be easily eliminated. Options 2 and 3 can be eliminated next. Coughing can cause increased ICP, and severe headache is an indication of such.

Level of Cognitive Ability: Application
Phase of Nursing Process: Implementation
Client Needs: Physiological Integrity
Content Area: Adult Health/Neurological

Reference

Monahan, F., & Neighbors, M. (1998). *Medical-surgical nursing: Foundations for clinical practice* (2nd ed.). Philadelphia: W. B. Saunders, p. 1269.

---

74. The client is receiving desmopressin (DDAVP) intranasally. The nurse would not use which of the following measurements to determine the effectiveness of this medication?

1. Urine output
2. Pupillary response
3. Presence of edema
4. Daily weight

Answer: 2

Rationale: Desmopressin is an analog of vasopressin (antidiuretic hormone). It is used in the management of diabetes insipidus. The nurse monitors the client's fluid balance to determine the effectiveness of the medication. Fluid status can be evaluated by noting intake, urine output, daily weight, and presence of edema.

Test-Taking Strategy: Remember that options that are similar are not likely to be correct. In this case, each of the incorrect options relates to fluid balance. The response that is different, the pupillary response, is the answer to the question as stated.

Level of Cognitive Ability: Application
Phase of Nursing Process: Implementation
Client Needs: Physiological Integrity
Content Area: Pharmacology

Reference

Hodgson, B., & Kizior, R. (1998). *Saunders nursing drug handbook 1998.* Philadelphia: W. B. Saunders, pp. 293–295.

---

75. As the nurse brings the 10 A.M. doses of furosemide (Lasix) and nifedipine (Procardia) into the room of an assigned client, the client asks the nurse for a dose of aluminum hydroxide gel, which is ordered on a PRN basis for dyspepsia. Which of the following actions by the nurse would be best?

1 Administer all three medications at this time
2 Ask the client if it is possible to wait 1 hour for the aluminum hydroxide
3 Give the nifedipine and aluminum hydroxide now and the furosemide in 1 hour
4 Give the furosemide and aluminum hydroxide now and the nifedipine in 1 hour

Answer: 2

Rationale: Antacids such as aluminum hydroxide often interfere with the absorption of other medications. For this reason, antacids should be separated from other medications by at least 1 hour. Because of the diuretic action of the furosemide and the antihypertensive action of the nifedipine, it is more important to receive them on time, if the client can tolerate waiting for the aluminum hydroxide.

Test-Taking Strategy: To answer this question accurately, it is necessary to understand that antacids interfere with absorption of other medications. With this in mind, option 1 may be eliminated easily. Knowledge that the diuretic and antihypertensive medication should be administered on time can assist in directing you to option 2.

Level of Cognitive Ability: Application
Phase of Nursing Process: Implementation
Client Needs: Physiological Integrity
Content Area: Pharmacology

Reference

Deglin, J., & Vallerand, A. (1997). *Davis's drug guide for nurses* (5th ed.). Philadelphia: F. A. Davis, p. 39.

---

76. The client has been placed on medication therapy with amitriptyline (Elavil). The nurse monitors the client for which common side effect of this medication?

1 Drowsiness and fatigue
2 Diarrhea
3 Hypertension
4 Polyuria

Answer: 1

Rationale: Common side effects of medication therapy with amitriptyline (a tricyclic antidepressant) are the central nervous system effects of drowsiness, fatigue, lethargy, and sedation. Other common side effects include dry mouth or eyes, blurred vision, hypotension, and constipation. The nurse monitors the client for response to therapy.

Test-Taking Strategy: Knowledge of this medication and its common side effects is needed to answer this question correctly. Take a few moments to review this medication if needed.

Level of Cognitive Ability: Application
Phase of Nursing Process: Assessment
Client Needs: Physiological Integrity
Content Area: Pharmacology

Reference

Hodgson, B., & Kizior, R. (1998). *Saunders nursing drug handbook 1998.* Philadelphia: W. B. Saunders, pp. 49–51.

77. A nurse working in a newborn nursery assesses that which of the following infants is most likely to show signs and symptoms of respiratory distress syndrome (RDS)?

1. Male, intrauterine growth retardation, blood glucose of 40
2. Female, preterm, 1 week old, intraventricular hemorrhage
3. Male, preterm, lecithin-sphingomyelin (L/S) ratio 1:1, temperature 97.4°F axillary
4. Female, dizygotic twin, trisomy 21

Answer: 3

Rationale: Males are affected with RDS more than females (2:1). Preterm infants lack the maturity of the respiratory system, including insufficient surfactants. The L/S ratio should be 2:1 to show adequate lung maturity, and a low temperature would put a preterm infant at risk of cold stress. A blood glucose of 40 is normal, and trisomy 21 or dizygotic twin does not predispose to RDS. RDS typically is seen in the first 2–3 days of life.

Test-Taking Strategy: This question requires that you know and understand which infants are at risk for RDS. In the elimination process, take out females because males are 2:1 more likely to have RDS. Also a preterm infant is most at risk. Select an answer that contains both male and preterm, which is option 3. If you had difficulty with this question, review newborns at risk for RDS.

Level of Cognitive Ability: Analysis
Phase of Nursing Process: Assessment
Client Needs: Physiological Integrity
Content Area: Maternity

Reference

Nichols, F., & Zwelling, E. (1997). *Maternal-newborn nursing: Theory and practice.* Philadelphia: W. B. Saunders, pp. 1340–1345.

---

78. The client has been admitted to the psychiatric unit on a voluntary basis. The client has reported a history of depression over the past 5 years. Which of the following comments by the nurse would help gain the most assessment data regarding the recent sleeping patterns of the client?

1. "Have you been having trouble sleeping at home?"
2. "How did you sleep last night?"
3. "Tell me about your sleeping patterns."
4. "You look as if you could use some sleep."

Answer: 3

Rationale: Option 3 allows the client to take this statement and say what is most relevant and important at the time. It is open ended and does not suggest a particular response. Option 1 could lead to a one-word answer, and that is not the desired response for adequate assessment. One night of sleep does not tell the nurse how the pattern has been over time. Anyone may or may not sleep well for one night, and that sleep or loss of sleep does not indicate a problem. Option 4 could be interpreted by the depressed person as a negative statement and could close further communication needed for a thorough assessment.

Test-Taking Strategy: When answering communication-type questions, usually the item that allows the client to take the lead in the conversation is the better answer. Be careful not to close communication, and usually options that allow only one-word answers are incorrect.

Level of Cognitive Ability: Application
Phase of Nursing Process: Assessment
Client Needs: Physiological Integrity
Content Area: Mental Health

Reference

Johnson, B. (1997). *Psychiatric-mental health nursing: Adaptation and growth* (4th ed.). Philadelphia: Lippincott-Raven, pp. 68–73.

79. The newly admitted bipolar client is trying to organize a dance with the other clients and is planning an on-unit supper. To lessen stimulation, the nurse should encourage the client to

1 Engage the help of other clients on the unit to accomplish the task.
2 Seek assistance from other staff members.
3 Postpone the dance and work on writing a short story.
4 Firmly tell the client that this task is inappropriate.

Answer: 3

Rationale: Because the bipolar client is easily stimulated by the environment, sedentary activities are the best outlets for energy. The writing task is appropriate. An activity such as the one mentioned by the client might be appropriate at some point but not for the newly admitted client who has impaired judgment and short attention span.

Test-Taking Strategy: Note the key phrase "to lessen stimulation." Options 1 and 2 encourage activity and should be eliminated. Option 4 simply tells the client that the activity is inappropriate, and this could result in an angry outburst because the affect of the bipolar client is labile. Only option 3 limits activity. If you had difficulty with this question, review appropriate activities for the bipolar client.

Level of Cognitive Ability: Application
Phase of Nursing Process: Implementation
Client Needs: Physiological Integrity
Content Area: Mental Health

Reference

Johnson, B. (1997). *Psychiatric-mental health nursing: Adaptation and growth* (4th ed.). Philadelphia: Lippincott-Raven, pp. 558–560.

80. The nurse is admitting a client who has a history of bipolar disorder, and the physician has indicated that the client is currently in the manic phase. In assessing the client for rest needs, the nurse knows that the most reliable information may be obtained by

1 Asking the client how many hours of sleep were obtained last night.
2 Observing the facial appearance of the client.
3 Asking the significant other about the sleep patterns.
4 Asking the night shift to record hours of sleep tonight.

Answer: 3

Rationale: Option 3 provides the most reliable information because the client may not be able to report sleep accurately. The client may report that sleep has not been a problem when in fact only minimal hours of sleep have been obtained for the last several days. Rest needs are important because the manic client may be at the point of exhaustion by the time hospitalization occurs. Facial expressions may be an indicator of fatigue, but they are not quantifiable. Asking the night shift for assessment data is not in the best interest of the client.

Test-Taking Strategy: The answer that is likely to give the most quantifiable data is the clear choice. In this situation, the significant other is the only one that can give information about the past few days or weeks. Waiting for assessment data from the night shift will delay planning care.

Level of Cognitive Ability: Application
Phase of Nursing Process: Assessment
Client Needs: Physiological Integrity
Content Area: Mental Health

Reference

Johnson, B. (1997). *Psychiatric-mental health nursing: Adaptation and growth* (4th ed.). Philadelphia: Lippincott-Raven, pp. 544–546.

81. Which nursing intervention is appropriate when caring for a child after a tepid tub bath to treat hyperthermia?

1 Place the child in bed and cover with a blanket
2 Leave the child uncovered for 15 minutes
3 Assist the child to put on a cotton sleep shirt
4 Take the child's axillary temperature in 1 hour

Answer: 3

Rationale: Cotton is a lightweight material that protects the child from becoming chilled after the bath. Option 1 is incorrect because a blanket is heavy and may increase the child's body temperature and further increase metabolism. Option 2 is incorrect because the child should not be left uncovered. Option 4 is incorrect because the child's temperature should be reassessed 1/2 hour after the bath.

Test-Taking Strategy: Use the process of elimination and knowledge regarding bathing for hyperthermia to answer the question. Eliminate option 1 because of the word "blanket." Eliminate option 2 because the child should not be left uncovered. Eliminate option 4 because the child's temperature should be reassessed 1/2 hour after the bath. If you had difficulty with this question, review care of a child with hyperthermia.

Level of Cognitive Ability: Application
Phase of Nursing Process: Implementation
Client Needs: Physiological Integrity
Content Area: Child Health

Reference

Wong, D. (1995). *Whaley and Wong's Nursing care of infants and children* (5th ed.). St. Louis: Mosby–Year Book, p. 1162.

---

82. A nurse is caring for an infant who has diarrhea. Which of these clinical manifestations should a nurse recognize as the earliest symptom of dehydration?

1. Apical pulse rate of 200 beats/minute
2. Capillary refill of 2 seconds
3. Gray, mottled skin
4. Cool extremities

Answer: 1

Rationale: Dehydration causes interstitial fluid to shift to the vascular compartment in an attempt to maintain fluid volume. When the body is unable to compensate for fluid lost, circulatory failure occurs. The BP decreases, and the pulse increases. This is followed by peripheral symptoms. Options 2, 3, and 4 are incorrect. These assessment findings reflect diminished peripheral circulation.

Test-Taking Strategy: Focus on the key word "earliest." This question asks the reader to determine which symptom happens first. Option 1 is most directly related to the ABCs. If you had difficulty with this question, review the signs of dehydration.

Level of Cognitive Ability: Analysis
Phase of Nursing Process: Assessment
Client Needs: Physiological Integrity
Content Area: Child Health

Reference

Wong, D. (1995). *Whaley and Wong's Nursing care of infants and children* (5th ed.). St. Louis: Mosby–Year Book, p. 1210.

---

83. The nurse administers acetylsalicylic acid (aspirin) before a percutaneous transluminal coronary angioplasty (PTCA) for coronary artery disease to

1. Prevent postprocedure hyperthermia.
2. Relieve postprocedure pain.
3. Prevent thrombus formation.
4. Prevent inflammation of puncture site.

Answer: 3

Rationale: Before PTCA, the client is usually given an anticoagulant, commonly aspirin, to help reduce the risk of occlusion of the artery during the procedure. Options 1, 2, and 4 are unrelated to the purpose of administering aspirin to this client.

Test-Taking Strategy: Knowledge regarding the action and properties of aspirin can assist in directing you to the correct option. In addition, awareness of the potential complications of a PTCA and nursing measures to prevent these complications can assist in answering the question. If you had difficulty with this question, take time now to review the action and uses of aspirin and the complications associated with PTCA.

Level of Cognitive Ability: Application
Phase of Nursing Process: Implementation
Client Needs: Physiological Integrity
Content Area: Adult Health/Cardiovascular

Reference

Hodgson, B., & Kizior, R. (1998). *Saunders nursing drug handbook 1998.* Philadelphia: W. B. Saunders, pp. 75–77.

84. The nurse gives acetaminophen (Tylenol) before the administration of topical nitrates because

1 Headache is a common side effect of nitrates.
2 Acetaminophen potentiates the therapeutic effects of nitrates.
3 Acetaminophen does not interfere with platelet action as aspirin (acetylsalicylic acid) does.
4 Fever usually accompanies myocardial infarction.

Answer: 1

Rationale: Headache occurs as a side effect of nitroglycerin. Acetaminophen may be given before nitrates to prevent headaches or minimize the discomfort from the headaches.

Test-Taking Strategy: The key elements of the stem are a medication and a specific nursing action. Knowledge that headache is a common side effect of nitrates can assist in directing you to the correct option. Eliminate option 2 first because this is an incorrect statement. Although options 3 and 4 are true statements, they do not address the issue of the question. If you had difficulty with this question, review the side effects of nitrates and the purpose of administering acetaminophen before these medications.

Level of Cognitive Ability: Application
Phase of Nursing Process: Implementation
Client Needs: Physiological Integrity
Content Area: Pharmacology

Reference

Ignatavicius, D. D., Workman, M. L., & Mishler, M. A. (1995). *Medical-surgical nursing: A nursing process approach* (2nd ed.). Philadelphia: W. B. Saunders, p. 996.

---

85. The nurse develops a plan of care for a newly admitted client with an acute myocardial infarction. The priority nursing diagnosis in the acute phase would be

1 Anxiety.
2 Altered Family Processes.
3 Altered Comfort.
4 Impaired Tissue Integrity.

Answer: 3

Rationale: Pain is the prevailing symptom of acute myocardial infarction. Relief of pain is a priority. Pain stimulates the autonomic nervous system increasing myocardial oxygen demand. Although options 1, 2, and 4 are also appropriate nursing diagnoses, the presence of pain impacts on these additional nursing diagnoses.

Test-Taking Strategy: All four options may be a part of the illness experience of the client with acute myocardial infarction. Using Maslow's hierarchy of needs, physiological needs are the priority, and options 1 and 2 can be eliminated. From the remaining two options, comfort is certainly the priority over tissue "integrity."

Level of Cognitive Ability: Analysis
Phase of Nursing Process: Analysis
Client Needs: Physiological Integrity
Content Area: Adult Health/Cardiovascular

Reference

Black, J., & Matassarin-Jacobs, E. (1997). *Medical-surgical nursing: Clinical management for continuity of care* (5th ed.). Philadelphia: W. B. Saunders, pp. 1262–1263.

---

86. The nurse is caring for a male client with urolithiasis. Important care and teaching includes which of the following?

1 Turn, cough, and deep breathe every 2 hours
2 Restrict physical activities
3 Strain all urine from each voiding
4 Weigh the client daily

Answer: 3

Rationale: Obstruction of the urinary tract is the primary problem associated with urolithiasis. Stones recovered from straining urine can be analyzed and can provide direction for prevention of further stone formation. Activities should not be restricted. Options 1 and 4 are not specifically related to the issue of the question.

Test-Taking Strategy: In this question, use the process of elimination and select the response that is associated most commonly with the client with urolithiasis. In this situation, straining all urine is the most common or typical intervention. If you had difficulty with this question, take time now to review care of the client with urolithiasis.

Level of Cognitive Ability: Application
Phase of Nursing Process: Implementation
Client Needs: Physiological Integrity
Content Area: Adult Health/Renal

Reference

LeMone, P., & Burke, K. (1996). *Medical-surgical nursing: Critical thinking in client care.* Menlo Park, CA: Addison-Wesley, p. 904.

---

87. The nurse is caring for a newly delivered breast-feeding infant. Which of the following interventions performed by the nurse would best prevent jaundice in this infant?

1. Encouraging the mother to offer a formula supplement after each breast-feeding session
2. Keeping the infant NPO until the second period of reactivity
3. Placing the infant under phototherapy
4. Requesting that the mother breast-feed the infant every 2–3 hours

Answer: 4

Rationale: To help facilitate a decrease in breast-feeding jaundice, the mother should feed the infant frequently in the immediate birth period because colostrum is a natural laxative and helps promote the passage of meconium. In option 1, offering the infant a formula supplement causes nipple confusion. Breast-feeding should begin as soon as possible after birth while the infant is in the first period of reactivity. Delaying breast-feeding decreases the production of prolactin, which decreases the mother's milk production. Phototherapy requires a physician's order and is not implemented until bilirubin levels are 12 mg/dL or higher in the healthy term infant.

Test-Taking Strategy: Knowledge of nursing interventions used to prevent jaundice in the breast-feeding infant must be applied to answer this question. If you had difficulty with this question, review these important nursing interventions now.

Level of Cognitive Ability: Application
Phase of Nursing Process: Implementation
Client Needs: Physiological Integrity
Content Area: Maternity

Reference

Pillitteri, A. (1995). *Maternal and child health nursing: Care of the childbearing and childrearing family* (2nd ed.). Philadelphia: Lippincott-Raven, pp. 688–689, 691–692.

---

88. A nurse is reviewing a rhythm strip and discovers a client is having frequent premature ventricular contractions (PVCs), trigeminal in nature. The nurse recognizes that which of the following is the cause of this disturbance?

1. There is a conduction defect from the SA node to the AV node
2. The client is moving about too briskly
3. The electrodes have come loose and need replacing
4. There is an irritable ventricular focus causing this disturbance

Answer: 4

Rationale: PVCs are usually caused by the firing of an irritable focus in the ventricle. Ventricular dysrhythmias result from an ectopic focus in any portion of the ventricular myocardium. There are numerous causes of PVCs.

Test-Taking Strategy: "Irritable" is the key word in the correct option. Also note the word "ventricular" in the question and in the correct option. If you are unfamiliar with the physiological event associated with PVCs, review this information now.

Level of Cognitive Ability: Analysis
Phase of Nursing Process: Analysis
Client Needs: Physiological Integrity
Content Area: Adult Health/Cardiovascular

Reference

Black, J., & Matassarin-Jacobs, E. (1997). *Medical-surgical nursing: Clinical management for continuity of care* (5th ed.). Philadelphia: W. B. Saunders, p. 1266.

89. The nurse is caring for a client scheduled for arthroscopy. In the postoperative period, the priority nursing action would include which of the following?

1 Monitor intake and output
2 Monitor for numbness or tingling
3 Assess the complete blood count results
4 Assess the tissue at the surgical site

Answer: 2

Rationale: The priority nursing action is to monitor the affected area for numbness or tingling. Options 1, 3, and 4 are also a component of postoperative care but considering the options presented are not the priority.

Test-Taking Strategy: Use the ABCs to answer the question. This can assist in directing you to option 2. If you had difficulty with this question, take time now to review nursing care after arthroscopy.

Level of Cognitive Ability: Application
Phase of Nursing Process: Implementation
Client Needs: Physiological Integrity
Content Area: Adult Health/Musculoskeletal

Reference

Black, J., & Matassarin-Jacobs, E. (1997). *Medical-surgical nursing: Clinical management for continuity of care* (5th ed.). Philadelphia: W. B. Saunders, pp. 2095–2096.

---

90. The nurse is caring for a client with active tuberculosis who has started medication therapy that includes rifampin (Rifadin). Which of the following would be an expected observation?

1 Orange secretions
2 Bilious urine
3 Yellow sclera
4 Clay-colored stools

Answer: 1

Rationale: Secretions are orange in color when the client is taking rifampin. The client should be instructed that the secretions will be orange in color and will permanently discolor soft contact lenses. Options 2, 3, and 4 are not expected observations.

Test-Taking Strategy: Knowledge of the side effects of rifampin is necessary to answer this question. Options 2, 3, and 4 are not expected observations. If you look at these three options, you will find a similarity in that they are all symptoms of intrahepatic obstruction as seen in viral hepatitis. If you had difficulty with this question, take time now to review this important medication.

Level of Cognitive Ability: Analysis
Phase of Nursing Process: Assessment
Client Needs: Physiological Integrity
Content Area: Pharmacology

Reference

Hodgson, B., & Kizior, R. (1998). *Saunders nursing drug handbook 1998.* Philadelphia: W. B. Saunders, pp. 904–905.

---

91. The nurse sends a sputum specimen for culture from a client with suspected active tuberculosis. The results report that *Mycobacterium tuberculosis* is cultured. The nurse analyzes these results as

1 Positive for active tuberculosis.
2 Inconclusive until a repeat sputum specimen is sent.
3 Not reliable unless the client has also had a positive Mantoux test.
4 Positive for a less virulent strain of tuberculosis.

Answer: 1

Rationale: Culture of *M. tuberculosis* from sputum or other body secretions or tissue is the only method of confirming the diagnosis. Options 2 and 4 are incorrect statements. The Mantoux test is used in making the diagnosis but does not confirm active disease.

Test-Taking Strategy: In this case, you need to know that *M. tuberculosis* is the bacterium responsible for tuberculosis and that culture of the bacteria from sputum confirms the diagnosis. Because tuberculosis affects the respiratory system, it would make sense that the bacteria would be found in the sputum if the client had active disease, therefore confirming the diagnosis. If you had difficulty with this question, review the diagnostic tests associated with active tuberculosis.

Level of Cognitive Ability: Analysis
Phase of Nursing Process: Analysis
Client Needs: Physiological Integrity
Content Area: Adult Health/Respiratory

Reference

Black, J., & Matassarin-Jacobs, E. (1997). *Medical-surgical nursing: Clinical management for continuity of care* (5th ed.). Philadelphia: W. B. Saunders, pp. 1144–1145.

92. The CCU nurse is caring for a client admitted with acute myocardial infarction. In planning care, the nurse prepares for the most common complication of

1 Cardiogenic shock.
2 Cardiac dysrhythmias.
3 Congestive heart failure.
4 Recurrent myocardial infarction.

Answer: 2

Rationale: Dysrhythmias are the major cause of death after a myocardial infarction accounting for 40%–50% of deaths after myocardial infarction. Cardiogenic shock, congestive heart failure, and recurrent myocardial infarction are also complications of myocardial infarction but occur less frequently.

Test-Taking Strategy: Knowledge of the most common complication after myocardial infarction is required to answer this question. If you were unsure of the answer to this question, take time to review this content.

Level of Cognitive Ability: Application
Phase of Nursing Process: Planning
Client Needs: Physiological Integrity
Content Area: Adult Health/Cardiovascular

Reference

Black, J., & Matassarin-Jacobs, E. (1997). *Medical-surgical nursing: Clinical management for continuity of care* (5th ed.). Philadelphia: W. B. Saunders, pp. 1266, 1267.

93. Dietary modifications are being planned for a client with urolithiasis. The nurse should include which of the following in the plan of care?

1 Restrict fluid intake to only 1000 mL/day
2 Increase intake of calcium and vitamin D–enriched foods
3 Increase intake of purine-rich foods
4 Increase intake of acid ash foods

Answer: 4

Rationale: Increased fluid intake of 2.5–3 liters/day ensures the production of approximately 2–2.5 liters of urine per day, which prevents stone-forming salts from becoming concentrated enough to precipitate. For calcium stones, dietary calcium and vitamin D–enriched foods are restricted. Stones composed of uric acid require a restriction in purine-rich foods. Increasing the amount of acid ash foods lowers the pH of the urine, as more alkaline urine promotes calcium stone and urinary tract infections.

Test-Taking Strategy: Eliminate option 1 first because restriction of fluid is not recommended with urolithiasis. Use basic principles related to physiology and nutrition to select the correct option. It is helpful if you can remember that many renal stones are made up of calcium or uric acid. This assists in eliminating options 2 and 3. Remembering that acidic urine assists in preventing infection and stone formation directs you to option 4.

Level of Cognitive Ability: Application
Phase of Nursing Process: Planning
Client Needs: Physiological Integrity
Content Area: Adult Health/Renal

Reference

LeMone, P., & Burke, K. (1996). *Medical-surgical nursing: Critical thinking in client care.* Menlo Park, CA: Addison-Wesley, pp. 899–900.

94. The nurse is planning for admission of a large-for-gestational-age (LGA) infant. In getting ready to care for this infant, the nurse prepares equipment for which diagnostic test?

1 Indirect and direct bilirubin levels
2 Rh and ABO blood typing
3 Heel stick blood glucose
4 Serum insulin level

Answer: 3

Rationale: After birth, the most common problem in the LGA infant is hypoglycemia, especially with a diabetic mother. At delivery when the umbilical cord is clamped and cut, the maternal blood glucose supply is lost. The newborn continues to produce large amounts of insulin, which depletes the infant's blood glucose within the first hours after birth. If immediate identification and treatment of hypoglycemia is not performed, the newborn may suffer central nervous system damage because of inadequate circulation of glucose to the brain. Indirect and direct bilirubin levels are usually ordered after the first 24 hours because jaundice is usually seen at 48–72 hours after birth. There is no rationale for ordering an Rh and ABO blood type unless the maternal blood type is O or Rh negative. Serum insulin levels are not helpful because there is no intervention to decrease these levels to prevent hypoglycemia.

Test-Taking Strategy: This question tests your understanding of the complications associated with the LGA infant. Options 2 is unncessary, and option 1 can be eliminated because this laboratory test is not required immediately after birth. Option 4 is not helpful. Review care to the LGA infant if you had difficulty with this question.

Level of Cognitive Ability: Application
Phase of Nursing Process: Planning
Client Needs: Physiological Integrity
Content Area: Maternity

Reference

Olds, S., London, M., & Ladewig, P. (1996). *Maternal-newborn nursing* (5th ed.). Menlo Park, CA: Addison-Wesley, p. 930.

---

95. The nurse is caring for a 30-week gestation client in preterm labor. The physician orders betamethasone (Celestone). The client asks the nurse why she is receiving steroids. The nurse tells the client that the betamethasone will

1 "Help your baby's lungs mature faster."
2 "Prevent your membranes from rupturing."
3 "Decrease the incidence of fetal infection."
4 "Help stop your labor contractions."

Answer: 1

Rationale: RDS is the most common cause of morbidity and mortality in preterm infants. Betamethasone, a corticosteroid, is given to enhance fetal lung maturity in 24- to 34-week gestations. The medication's optimal benefits begin 24 hours after initial therapy. Options 2 and 3 are incorrect. Betamethasone can actually mask signs of infection when the client has premature rupture of the membranes with preterm labor. Betamethasone does not prevent rupture of the membranes. Even though betamethasone may be given during the time that tocolytic agents are administered, it does not inhibit preterm labor.

Test-Taking Strategy: The word "preterm" may assist you in recalling that this medication is given to enhance fetal lung maturity. Review the action of this important medication if you had difficulty with this question.

Level of Cognitive Ability: Application
Phase of Nursing Process: Implementation
Client Needs: Physiological Integrity
Content Area: Pharmacology

Reference

Reeder, S., Martin, L., & Koniak-Griffin, D. (1997). *Maternity nursing: Family, newborn, and women's health care* (18th ed.). Philadelphia: Lippincott-Raven, p. 981.

---

96. When planning for care of a client with a stage III ruptured cerebral aneurysm, the nurse would consider which of the following?

1 Provide frequent auditory and visual stimuli and reassess orientation every 2 hours
2 Keep environment calm and quiet, and avoid situations that may be emotionally upsetting to the client
3 Encourage client to cough and deep breathe
4 Position client in semi-Fowler's position with head turned to side

Answer: 2

Rationale: Clients with ruptured cerebral aneurysms, which are not surgically repaired, are at serious risk for recurrent rupture in 7–10 days after original hemorrhage. Aneurysm precautions involve controlling the environment and reducing stimuli. Lights should be dim, and visitors should be kept to a minimum. Interventions aimed at preventing increased ICP should also be implemented. Options 3 and 4 both increase ICP.

Test-Taking Strategy: Use your nursing knowledge regarding ICP and cerebral bleeding. Options 1, 3, and 4 increase ICP. Only option 2 does not increase ICP. If you had difficulty with this question, take time now to review aneurysm precautions.

Level of Cognitive Ability: Application
Phase of Nursing Process: Planning
Client Needs: Physiological Integrity
Content Area: Adult Health/Neurological

Reference

Hartshorn, J., Lamborn, M., & Sole, M. (1997). *Introduction to critical care nursing* (2nd ed.). Philadelphia: W. B. Saunders, pp. 288, 289.

97. A client receiving total parenteral nutrition (TPN) has a history of congestive heart failure. The physician has ordered furosemide (Lasix), 40 mg daily, to prevent fluid overload. Which laboratory value should be closely monitored by the nurse to prevent adverse effects from treatment?

1 Glucose
2 Sodium
3 Potassium
4 Magnesium

Answer: 3

Rationale: Furosemide is a non–potassium-sparing diuretic, and insufficient replacement may lead to hypokalemia.

Test-Taking Strategy: Some knowledge of the action of furosemide is needed. As a non–potassium-sparing diuretic, the most critical laboratory value to watch with its use is the potassium level. The case addresses the issue that furosemide is ordered to prevent fluid overload. This is the key to suggesting that this medication is a diuretic.

Level of Cognitive Ability: Analysis
Phase of Nursing Process: Assessment
Client Needs: Physiological Integrity
Content Area: Fundamental Skills

Reference
Craven, R., & Hirnle, C. (1996). *Fundamentals of nursing: Human health and function* (2nd ed.). Philadelphia: Lippincott-Raven, p. 575.

---

98. A client receiving TPN suddenly develops chest pain, dyspnea, tachycardia, cyanosis, and decreased level of consciousness. Which complication of TPN should the nurse suspect?

1 Hyperglycemia
2 Catheter-related sepsis
3 Allergic reaction to the TPN catheter
4 Air embolism

Answer: 4

Rationale: Symptoms of air embolism include decreased level of consciousness, tachycardia, dyspnea, anxiety, feelings of impending doom, chest pain, cyanosis, and hypotension. Options 1, 2, and 3 are incorrect.

Test-Taking Strategy: Note the similar words in the question and option. Key words in the question are "dyspnea" and "cyanosis," which would indicate a respiratory system problem. Option 4 contains the word "air."

Level of Cognitive Ability: Analysis
Phase of Nursing Process: Evaluation
Client Needs: Physiological Integrity
Content Area: Fundamental Skills

Reference
Craven, R., & Hirnle, C. (1996). *Fundamentals of nursing: Human health and function* (2nd ed.). Philadelphia: Lippincott-Raven, p. 572.

---

99. The client has a nursing diagnosis of Fluid Volume Excess. After assessing the client, the nurse records which of the following data in the medical record, which supports continued use of this nursing diagnosis?

1 Bibasilar crackles
2 Weak pulse
3 Decreased BP
4 Flat neck veins with head of bed at 45 degrees

Answer: 1

Rationale: Signs of fluid volume excess include bounding pulse, elevated BP, crackles or other adventitious breath sounds, edema of sacrum or lower extremities, and neck vein distention with head of bed positioned at a 45-degree angle.

Test-Taking Strategy: Note the key phrase in the question, "supports continued use." This tells you that the correct answer is consistent with fluid volume excess. Use basic nursing knowledge of the effects of volume on the cardiovascular and respiratory systems to eliminate incorrect choices.

Level of Cognitive Ability: Application
Phase of Nursing Process: Implementation
Client Needs: Physiological Integrity
Content Area: Adult Health/Cardiovascular

Reference
Black, J., & Matassarin-Jacobs, E. (1997). *Medical-surgical nursing: Clinical management for continuity of care* (5th ed.). Philadelphia: W. B. Saunders, p. 288.

100. The client is suffering acute cardiac and cerebral symptoms related to fluid volume excess. The nurse should take which of the following measures to increase the client's comfort until specific therapy is ordered by the physician?

1 Begin oxygen at 4 liters/minute by nasal cannula
2 Elevate the client's head of bed to at least 45 degrees
3 Measure urine output on an hourly basis
4 Record intravenous and oral fluid intake

Answer: 2

Rationale: Elevating the head of the bed to 45 degrees decreases venous return to the heart from the lower body, thus reducing the volume of blood that has to be pumped. It also promotes venous drainage from the brain, reducing cerebral symptoms. Oxygen is a medication and is not administered without an order. Intake and output should be monitored and recorded to provide current information about the client's volume status. Options 3 and 4 are extremely valuable as assessment measures, but they do not improve the state of the client.

Test-Taking Strategy: Note the key words in this question, "increase the client's comfort." This tells you that the correct answer is one that directly involves care delivery to the client. With this in mind, options 3 and 4 are eliminated first because they are assessment measures and do not improve the condition of the client. Basic respiratory knowledge guides you to choose option 2 over option 1.

Level of Cognitive Ability: Application
Phase of Nursing Process: Implementation
Client Needs: Physiological Integrity
Content Area: Adult Health/Cardiovascular

Reference

Black, J., & Matassarin-Jacobs, E. (1997). *Medical-surgical nursing: Clinical management for continuity of care* (5th ed.). Philadelphia: W. B. Saunders, pp. 288–289.

101. The client is receiving daunorubicin (Cerubidine) intravenously. The nurse monitors the client for

1 Hypertension.
2 Polycythemia.
3 Nausea and vomiting.
4 Hypovolemia.

Answer: 3

Rationale: Daunorubicin is an antineoplastic medication. The major gastrointestinal side effects include nausea, vomiting, stomatitis, and esophagitis. Cardiovascular side effects include congestive heart failure and dysrhythmias. Other frequently occurring side effects are alopecia and bone marrow depression. Hypertension and hypovolemia are not directly related to this medication.

Test-Taking Strategy: To answer this question correctly, it is necessary to know that the medication is an antineoplastic. Knowing that antineoplastic medications commonly cause gastrointestinal side effects, you could eliminate each of the other responses fairly easily.

Level of Cognitive Ability: Application
Phase of Nursing Process: Assessment
Client Needs: Physiological Integrity
Content Area: Pharmacology

Reference

Hodgson, B., & Kizior, R. (1998). *Saunders nursing drug handbook 1998*. Philadelphia: W. B. Saunders, pp. 286–289.

102. The home health nurse is visiting a client who was discharged to home with orders for continued administration of enoxaparin (Lovenox), 30 mg twice a day subcutaneously. The nurse questions the client about which of the following highest priority items?

1 Fear of needles
2 Bleeding gums or bruising
3 Constipation
4 Nausea or vomiting

Answer: 2

Rationale: Enoxaparin is an anticoagulant. A common side effect of anticoagulant therapy is bleeding. Because of this, the nurse questions the client about symptoms that could indicate bleeding, such as bleeding gums, bruising, hematuria, or dark tarry stools.

Test-Taking Strategy: To answer this question accurately, it is necessary to know that the medication is an anticoagulant. This enables you to eliminate options 3 and 4 first. Note the key phrase "highest priority" in the stem. This guides you to choose option 2 over option 1 as the correct response.

Level of Cognitive Ability: Application
Phase of Nursing Process: Implementation
Client Needs: Physiological Integrity
Content Area: Pharmacology

Reference

Hodgson, B., & Kizior, R. (1998). *Saunders nursing drug handbook 1998.* Philadelphia: W. B. Saunders, pp. 365–366.

---

103. The client has been given a prescription for sulfasalazine (Azulfidine) for the treatment of ulcerative colitis. While conducting medication teaching, the nurse asks the client if he or she has a history of allergy to

1 Salicylates or acetaminophen.
2 Sulfonamides or salicylates.
3 Shellfish or calcium channel blockers.
4 Histamine receptor antagonists or beta-blockers.

Answer: 2

Rationale: The client who has been prescribed sulfasalazine should be checked for history of allergy to either sulfonamides or salicylates because of the chemical composition of the medication. The other options are incorrect.

Test-Taking Strategy: Specific medication knowledge is needed to answer this question accurately. Note the relationship of "sulfasalazine" in the question and "sulfonamides" in the correct option. If needed, take a few moments to review information about this medication.

Level of Cognitive Ability: Application
Phase of Nursing Process: Implementation
Client Needs: Physiological Integrity
Content Area: Pharmacology

Reference

Hodgson, B., & Kizior, R. (1998). *Saunders nursing drug handbook 1998.* Philadelphia: W. B. Saunders, pp. 953–955.

---

104. The nurse is caring for the hypernatremic client with a nursing diagnosis of Altered Oral Mucous Membranes. The nurse would avoid using which of the following items when giving mouth care to this client?

1 Nonalcoholic mouthwash
2 Soft toothbrush
3 Lip moistener
4 Lemon-glycerin swabs

Answer: 4

Rationale: The nurse avoids using lemon-glycerin swabs for the client with altered oral mucous membranes because they dry the membranes further and could cause pain. Items that are helpful include a soft toothbrush to prevent trauma, lip moistener to prevent lip cracking, and soothing cleansing rinses, such as nonalcoholic mouthwash and 1:1 saline and peroxide mixture.

Test-Taking Strategy: To answer this question accurately, evaluate each of the options in terms of the likelihood of causing trauma to at-risk tissue. This approach guides you to eliminate each of the incorrect options easily.

Level of Cognitive Ability: Application
Phase of Nursing Process: Implementation
Client Needs: Physiological Integrity
Content Area: Fundamental Skills

Reference

Black, J., & Matassarin-Jacobs, E. (1997). *Medical-surgical nursing: Clinical management for continuity of care* (5th ed.). Philadelphia: W. B. Saunders, p. 304.

---

105. The nurse has an order to administer 20 mEq of potassium to the client with a potassium level of 3.1 mEq/liter. The nurse draws up this medication knowing it will be administered

1 After dilution in an intravenous solution.
2 Directly by intravenous push.
3 Intramuscularly.
4 Subcutaneously.

Answer: 1

Rationale: Potassium chloride may be administered by the intravenous route when the client has moderate-to-severe hypokalemia. It is always diluted in intravenous solution; administration by intravenous push could cause death by cardiac arrest. It is not administered intramuscularly or subcutaneously. A cardiac monitor should also be in use when administering intravenous potassium for moderate-to-severe hypokalemia.

Test-Taking Strategy: Use basic knowledge of electrolyte replacement and medication administration to answer this question. Recalling the physiology of the cardiac conduction system and the effects of potassium on the heart can assist in directing you to the correct option. If this question was difficult, take a few moments to review this critically important concept immediately.

Level of Cognitive Ability: Application
Phase of Nursing Process: Implementation
Client Needs: Physiological Integrity
Content Area: Pharmacology

Reference

Black, J., & Matassarin-Jacobs, E. (1997). *Medical-surgical nursing: Clinical management for continuity of care* (5th ed.). Philadelphia: W. B. Saunders, p. 306.

---

106. The client has asymptomatic hypocalcemia from decreased dietary intake. The nurse giving the client an oral calcium supplement should administer this medication with

1 Water.
2 Milk.
3 Fruit juice.
4 Any product that is lactose-free.

Answer: 2

Rationale: Calcium supplements are best absorbed when administered with milk 30 minutes before a meal. The vitamin D in the milk promotes absorption of the calcium. An exception to this is the client who is hypoparathyroid. In this case, the client is given vitamin D in pill form to avoid the phosphates in milk.

Test-Taking Strategy: Knowledge of principles of nutrition is needed to answer this question accurately. It would seem reasonable, however, that milk would be the likely answer because the client is hypocalcemic and milk contains calcium. If needed, take a few moments to review the administration of oral calcium.

Level of Cognitive Ability: Application
Phase of Nursing Process: Implementation
Client Needs: Physiological Integrity
Content Area: Pharmacology

Reference

Black, J., & Matassarin-Jacobs, E. (1997). *Medical-surgical nursing: Clinical management for continuity of care* (5th ed.). Philadelphia: W. B. Saunders, p. 318.

---

107. The nurse has an order to administer two ophthalmic medications to the client who has undergone eye surgery. The nurse waits for how many minutes after the first medication before giving the second?

1 1
2 2
3 5
4 10

Answer: 3

Rationale: The nurse waits for 5 minutes between administration of the two separate ophthalmic medications. This allows for adequate ocular absorption of the medication, and prevents the second medication from flushing out the first.

Test-Taking Strategy: Specific knowledge of time frames for administration of ocular medications is needed to answer this question. Take a few moments to review principles of ocular medication administration if you had difficulty with this question.

Level of Cognitive Ability: Application
Phase of Nursing Process: Implementation
Client Needs: Physiological Integrity
Content Area: Adult Health/Eye

Reference

Luckmann, J. (1997). *Saunders manual of nursing care*. Philadelphia: W. B. Saunders, p. 766.

108. The client has hypercalcemia according to serum levels. The nurse avoids doing which of the following, which would aggravate the condition?

1 Limit sodium intake
2 Encourage increased fluid intake
3 Withhold calcium carbonate antacids
4 Encourage increased intake of high-fiber foods

Answer: 1

Rationale: Sodium should not be limited for the client with hypercalcemia, unless contraindicated (such as with heart failure). Retention of sodium promotes loss of calcium by the kidneys. Fluid intake is increased to help flush calcium from the body, calcium-containing medications are withheld, and calcium-containing foods are limited. High-fiber foods prevent constipation, which can occur with hypercalcemia.

Test-Taking Strategy: Note that the key word in this question is "avoid." This tells you that the correct answer is an incorrect treatment option for hypercalcemia. Use your nursing knowledge to eliminate each of the incorrect options systematically. Review the treatment for hypercalcemia if you had difficulty with this question.

Level of Cognitive Ability: Application
Phase of Nursing Process: Implementation
Client Needs: Physiological Integrity
Content Area: Fundamental Skills

Reference
Black, J., & Matassarin-Jacobs, E. (1997). *Medical-surgical nursing: Clinical management for continuity of care* (5th ed.). Philadelphia: W. B. Saunders, p. 322.

---

109. The client has a pH of 7.51 with a bicarbonate level of 29 mEq/liter. The nurse administers which of the following medications, which would be ordered to treat this acid-base disorder?

1 Sodium bicarbonate
2 Furosemide (Lasix)
3 Acetazolamide (Diamox)
4 Spironolactone (Aldactone)

Answer: 3

Rationale: Acetazolamide is a diuretic used in the treatment of metabolic alkalosis. This medication causes excretion of sodium, potassium, bicarbonate, and water by inhibiting the action of carbonic anhydrase. Administration of sodium bicarbonate aggravates the already existing condition and is contraindicated. Furosemide and spironolactone are loop and potassium-sparing diuretics. These are of no value when there is a need to excrete bicarbonate.

Test-Taking Strategy: Begin to answer this question by interpreting the acid-base disorder as metabolic alkalosis. Eliminate option 1 first on the basis of this conclusion. Knowing which of the three diuretics is used to excrete bicarbonate can help you choose correctly among the remaining three options.

Level of Cognitive Ability: Application
Phase of Nursing Process: Implementation
Client Needs: Physiological Integrity
Content Area: Fundamental Skills

Reference
Black, J., & Matassarin-Jacobs, E. (1997). *Medical-surgical nursing: Clinical management for continuity of care* (5th ed.). Philadelphia: W. B. Saunders, p. 338.

---

110. The client is admitted in metabolic acidosis caused by diabetic ketoacidosis (DKA). The nurse administers which of the following medications as a primary treatment for this problem?

1 Sodium bicarbonate
2 Calcium gluconate
3 Potassium
4 Insulin

Answer: 4

Rationale: The primary treatment for any acid-base imbalance is treatment of the underlying disorder that caused the problem. In this case, the underlying cause of the metabolic acidosis is anaerobic metabolism as a result of lack of ability to use circulating glucose. Administration of insulin corrects this problem.

Test-Taking Strategy: The key words in the question are "primary" and "diabetic." This should assist in directing you to option 4. Knowledge of causes and treatments for various acid-base disorders guides you to eliminate each of the incorrect responses systematically.

Level of Cognitive Ability: Application
Phase of Nursing Process: Implementation
Client Needs: Physiological Integrity
Content Area: Adult health/Endocrine

Reference

Smeltzer, S., & Bare, B. (1996). *Brunner and Suddarth's Textbook of medical-surgical nursing* (8th ed.). Philadelphia: Lippincott-Raven, p. 234.

---

111. The client is in respiratory alkalosis induced by gram-negative sepsis. The nurse carries out which of the following measures as the most effective means to treat the problem?

1 Administer prescribed antibiotics
2 Administer PRN antipyretics
3 Have the client breathe into a paper bag
4 Request an order for a partial rebreather oxygen mask

Answer: 1

Rationale: The most effective way to treat an acid-base disorder is to treat the underlying disorder. In this case, the problem is sepsis, which is most effectively treated with antibiotic therapy. Antipyretics control fever secondary to sepsis but do nothing to control acid-base balance. The paper bag and partial rebreather mask assist the client to rebreathe exhaled carbon dioxide, but these do not treat the primary cause of the imbalance.

Test-Taking Strategy: Note the key words in the stem of the question, "most effective" and "sepsis." Knowing that the most effective treatment of acid-base imbalances involves treatment of the primary problem, you would choose the correct answer by knowing that sepsis is a systemic infection.

Level of Cognitive Ability: Application
Phase of Nursing Process: Implementation
Client Needs: Physiological Integrity
Content Area: Fundamental Skills

Reference

Smeltzer, S., & Bare, B. (1996). *Brunner and Suddarth's Textbook of medical-surgical nursing* (8th ed.). Philadelphia: Lippincott-Raven, p. 235.

---

112. The client receiving lithium therapy is noted to be drowsy, with slurred speech, and experiencing muscle twitching and impaired coordination. Which of the following actions should be taken by the nurse?

1 Double the next lithium dose
2 Increase fluids to 2000 mL/day
3 Hold one dose of lithium
4 Call the physician

Answer: 4

Rationale: Signs and symptoms of lithium toxicity include vomiting and diarrhea and nervous system changes such as slurred speech, incoordination, drowsiness, muscle weakness, or twitching. Before administering any further doses, the physician should be notified. As long as there are no contraindications, the client should routinely take in 2000–3000 mL of fluid per day while taking this medication.

Test-Taking Strategy: To answer this question accurately, it is necessary to be familiar with the symptoms of lithium overdose. You may be able to narrow the possible choices, however, by realizing that it is not common practice either to hold one dose or to double a medication dose without a specific order. Review the signs of toxicity of this important medication if you had difficulty with this question.

Level of Cognitive Ability: Application
Phase of Nursing Process: Implementation
Client Needs: Physiological Integrity
Content Area: Pharmacology

Reference

Deglin, J., & Vallerand, A. (1997). *Davis's drug guide for nurses* (5th ed.). Philadelphia: F. A. Davis, p. 704.

113. The client has been started on medication therapy with metoclopramide (Reglan). The nurse monitors which of the following to determine effectiveness of therapy?

1 Urine output
2 Breath sounds
3 Complaints of headache
4 Episodes of vomiting

Answer: 4

Rationale: Metoclopramide is an antiemetic. The nurse would monitor to see whether the client has experienced a decrease or absence of vomiting to determine the effectiveness of therapy.

Test-Taking Strategy: Familiarity with this medication is needed to choose the correct response. If you are unfamiliar with this medication, take time now to review it.

Level of Cognitive Ability: Application
Phase of Nursing Process: Evaluation
Client Needs: Physiological Integrity
Content Area: Pharmacology

Reference

Deglin, J., & Vallerand, A. (1997). *Davis's drug guide for nurses* (5th ed.). Philadelphia: F. A. Davis, p. 782.

114. A victim of child abuse admits to the nurse that before this admission he or she has used repression to cope with past life experiences. The nurse implements an appropriate plan of care that includes

1 Placing the child on medications that will help the client forget the incidents.
2 Having the child talk about the abuse in detail during the first therapy session.
3 Encouraging the child to use play therapy to act out past experiences.
4 Advising the child to let the past go and concentrate on the present and future.

Answer: 3

Rationale: Play therapy is a nonthreatening avenue through which the client can use artwork, dolls, or puppets to act out frightening life experiences. Options 1 and 4 devalue the child and force the child to repress further harmful past experiences rather than facing them and moving on. Option 2 would be extremely threatening to the child and nontherapeutic.

Test-Taking Strategy: Note the relationship of "past life experiences" in the question and "past experiences" in the correct option. You can easily eliminate options 1 and 2. From the remaining two options, select option 3 over option 4 because option 4 encourages the child to repress further harmful past experiences rather than facing them.

Level of Cognitive Ability: Application
Phase of Nursing Process: Implementation
Client Needs: Physiological Integrity
Content Area: Child Health

Reference

Wong, D. (1997). *Whaley and Wong's Essentials of pediatric nursing*. St. Louis: Mosby–Year Book, p. 645.

115. A mother comes to the pediatric clinic because her previously continent 6-year-old son has resumed bedwetting. After discovering that there is a new baby in the home, the nurse evaluates the information and explains to the mother that the son is using the defense mechanism of

1 Identification.
2 Regression.
3 Rationalization.
4 Repression.

Answer: 2

Rationale: The defense mechanism of regression is characterized by returning to an earlier form of expressing an impulse. Option 1 occurs when a person models behavior after someone else. Option 3 occurs when a person unconsciously falsifies an experience by giving a "rational" explanation. Option 4 is characterized by blocking a wish or desire from conscious expression.

Test-Taking Strategy: To answer this question, you must recognize that the issue of the question is knowing the definition of each of the defense mechanisms and being able to use the behavioral information to evaluate which one the child is exhibiting. Review defense mechanisms now if you had difficulty with this question.

Level of Cognitive Ability: Analysis
Phase of Nursing Process: Evaluation
Client Needs: Physiological Integrity
Content Area: Child Health

Reference

Carson, V., & Arnold, E. (1996). *Mental health nursing: The nurse-patient journey*. Philadelphia: W. B. Saunders, p. 697.

116. The best site to select for an intramuscular injection in a 2-year-old is the

1 Ventral gluteal muscle.
2 Dorsal gluteal muscle.
3 Deltoid muscle.
4 Vastus lateralis muscle.

Answer: 4

Rationale: The vastus lateralis muscle is well developed at birth. It is the best choice for all age groups but should always be used in children younger than 3 years. This muscle is able to tolerate larger volumes and is not located near vital structures such as nerves and blood vessels.

Test-Taking Strategy: The key word "best" requires prioritizing. Because options 1 and 2 are similar distracters, neither is likely to be the one right answer. The deltoid is a smaller muscle close to important nerves and is generally not a preferred site for intramuscular injection. If you had difficulty with this question, take time now to review the procedure for administering intramuscular injections in a 2-year-old.

Level of Cognitive Ability: Application
Phase of Nursing Process: Implementation
Client Needs: Physiological Integrity
Content Area: Fundamental Skills

Reference

Ashwill, J., & Droske, S. (1997). *Nursing care of children: Principles and practice.* Philadelphia: W. B. Saunders, p. 494.

117. An appropriate expected outcome for a school-age child with a knowledge deficit related to use of inhalers and peak flow meters is the child will

1 Express feelings of mastery and competence with breathing devices.
2 Have regular respirations at a rate of 18 to 22 breaths/minute.
3 Deny shortness of breath or difficulty breathing.
4 Watch the educational video and read printed information provided.

Answer: 1

Rationale: School-age children strive for mastery and competence to achieve the developmental task of industry and accomplishment. Options 2 and 3 do not relate to the knowledge deficit, which is the issue of the test item. Option 4 is an intervention rather than an outcome.

Test-Taking Strategy: Careful reading of all options reveals that 2 and 3 have similar concepts, so neither can be the one correct answer. Knowledge of the nursing process eliminates option 4 because it is not an expected outcome as required by the stem. Option 1 is the age-appropriate outcome that is related directly to the issue in the stem. If you had difficulty with this question, review developmental tasks of the school-age child.

Level of Cognitive Ability: Analysis
Phase of Nursing Process: Planning
Client Needs: Physiological Integrity
Content Area: Child Health

Reference

Wong, D. (1997). *Whaley and Wong's Essentials of pediatric nursing* (5th ed.). St. Louis: Mosby–Year Book, p. 554.

118. Which statement by an adolescent during a health history indicates a need for follow-up assessment and intervention?

1 "I find myself very moody—happy one minute and crying the next"
2 "I can't seem to wake up in the morning. I would sleep until noon if I could"
3 "I don't eat anything with fat in it and I've lost 8 pounds in 2 weeks"
4 "When I get stressed out about school, I just like to be alone"

Answer: 3

Rationale: Undereating is a common problem in teenagers, and there is heightened awareness of body image and peer pressure to go on excessively restrictive diets. The extreme limitation of omitting all fat and major weight loss during a time of growth suggest inadequate nutrition and a possible eating disorder.

Test-Taking Strategy: Note the key phrase "need for follow-up." Select the answer that indicates a problem or abnormality. Options 1, 2, and 4 are common and normal behaviors or feelings during adolescence. If you had difficulty with this question, take time now to review the developmental stage of the adolescent.

Level of Cognitive Ability: Application
Phase of Nursing Process: Assessment
Client Needs: Physiological Integrity
Content Area: Child Health

Reference

Ball, J., & Bindler, R. (1995). *Pediatric nursing: Caring for children.* Stamford, CT: Appleton & Lange, p. 70.

---

119. The nurse is caring for a client who has bipolar disorder and is in a manic episode. The most appropriate menu choice for this client would be which of the following?

1 Scrambled eggs, orange juice, coffee with cream and sugar
2 Cheeseburger, banana, milk
3 Beef stew, fruit salad, tea
4 Macaroni and cheese, apple, milk

Answer: 2

Rationale: The client in a manic state often has inadequate food and fluid intake because of physical agitation. Foods that the client can eat "on the run" are indicated because the client is too active to sit at meals and use utensils.

Test-Taking Strategy: This strategy represents selection of an option that is different. Option 2 is the only option that identifies finger foods. In addition, clients in a manic state should not have caffeine-containing products. Therefore, eliminate options 1 and 3. Then remember the concept of "finger foods" with these clients.

Level of Cognitive Ability: Application
Phase of Nursing Process: Implementation
Client Needs: Physiological Integrity
Content Area: Mental Health

Reference

Carson, V., & Arnold, E. (1996). *Mental health nursing: The nurse-patient journey.* Philadelphia: W. B. Saunders, p. 771.

---

120. The nurse is caring for a client who is receiving lithium. The lithium level is 1.8 mEq/liter. The nurse analyzes this as

1 Within normal limits.
2 Higher than normal limits, indicating toxicity.
3 Lower than normal limits.
4 Insignificant.

Answer: 2

Rationale: The therapeutic level for lithium is 0.8–1.2 mEq/liter. A level of 1.8 indicates toxicity and requires that the medication be withheld and the blood work repeated.

Test-Taking Strategy: Knowing the therapeutic level of lithium is required to answer this question. This medication has a small range between therapeutic dose and toxic dose. The nurse must be able to identify levels of toxicity and nursing interventions that are indicated when toxicity is present. Review this information now because toxicity is an important area with which to be familiar.

Level of Cognitive Ability: Analysis
Phase of Nursing Process: Analysis
Client Needs: Physiological Integrity
Content Area: Pharmacology

Reference

Hodgson, B., & Kizior, R. (1998). *Saunders nursing drug handbook 1998.* Philadelphia: W. B. Saunders, pp. 598–600.

121. The client calls the ambulatory clinic to say that she found an area that looks like the peel of an orange when performing breast self-examination (BSE) but she found no other changes. The nurse should

1 Tell the client there is nothing to worry about.
2 Arrange for the client to be seen at the clinic as soon as possible.
3 Tell the client to take her temperature and call back if she has a fever.
4 Tell the client to point the area out to the physician at her next regularly scheduled appointment.

Answer: 2

Rationale: Peau d'orange or the orange peel appearance of the skin over the breast is associated with late breast cancer. Realizing that this is what the client is describing, you would have her come to the clinic at the earliest time possible. Peau d'orange is not indicative of an infection; therefore you would not have the client take her temperature.

Test-Taking Strategy: Knowledge of the signs of breast cancer is needed to answer this question. Knowing that peau d'orange is a sign can assist in directing you to option 2. If you had difficulty with this question, review the signs of breast cancer.

Level of Cognitive Ability: Analysis
Phase of Nursing Process: Implementation
Client Needs: Physiological Integrity
Content Area: Adult Health/Oncology

Reference
Smeltzer, S., & Bare, B. (1996). *Brunner and Suddarth's Textbook of medical-surgical nursing* (8th ed.). Philadelphia: Lippincott-Raven, p. 1304.

122. Which of the following client statements indicates inaccurate information regarding BSE?

1 "I don't need to do that, I'm too old for that."
2 "I do BSE 7 days after I get my period."
3 "I examine my breasts in the shower."
4 "I lie on my back to examine my breasts."

Answer: 1

Rationale: BSE should still be done even after menopause. No one is too old to get breast cancer. The other answers each reflect a correct component of proper monthly BSE.

Test-Taking Strategy: Knowledge regarding the correct procedure for BSE is required to answer this question. If you had difficulty with this question or are unfamiliar with the procedure, take time now to review.

Level of Cognitive Ability: Analysis
Phase of Nursing Process: Evaluation
Client Needs: Physiological Integrity
Content Area: Fundamental Skills

Reference
Smeltzer, S., & Bare, B. (1996). *Brunner and Suddarth's Textbook of medical-surgical nursing* (8th ed.). Philadelphia: Lippincott-Raven, pp. 1305–1307.

123. The client has carcinoma classified by the surgeon as T4, N4, M1. The nurse analyzes this information as

1 The client is dying of cancer.
2 The tumor is very large.
3 Four lymph nodes were involved.
4 The tumor has not metastasized.

Answer: 2

Rationale: T refers to the tumor size; T0 indicates no primary tumor found, and T1 to T4 refer to progressively larger tumors. TIS is used to indicate a carcinoma in situ. N refers to regional lymph node involvement; N0 indicates normal regional nodes, and N1 to N4 indicate increasingly abnormal regional lymph nodes. M refers to metastasis; M0 means no known distant metastasis, and M1 means distant metastasis found. The TNM classification system for staging tumors is widely used.

Test-Taking Strategy: Knowledge of the TNM classification system for staging tumors is required to answer this question. If you had difficulty with this question, take time now to review this classification system.

Level of Cognitive Ability: Analysis
Phase of Nursing Process: Analysis
Client Needs: Physiological Integrity
Content Area: Adult Health/Oncology

Reference
Smeltzer, S., & Bare, B. (1996). *Brunner and Suddarth's Textbook of medical-surgical nursing* (8th ed.). Philadelphia: Lippincott-Raven, pp. 273, 276.

124. A client with Cushing's syndrome is being instructed by the nurse on follow-up care. Which of these statements, if made by the client, would indicate a need for further instruction?

1 "I should avoid contact sports."
2 "I need to avoid foods rich in potassium."
3 "I should check my ankles for swelling."
4 "I need to check my blood sugar regularly."

Answer: 2

Rationale: Hypokalemia is a common feature of this condition. Clients experience activity intolerance, osteoporosis, and frequent bruising. Fluid volume excess results from water and sodium retention. Hyperglycemia is caused by an increased cortisol secretion.

Test-Taking Strategy: Beware of the key words "need for further instruction" in the stem. From this point, knowledge regarding the clinical manifestations associated with Cushing's syndrome is required to answer this question. If you had difficulty with this question, take time now to review this disorder.

Level of Cognitive Ability: Analysis
Phase of Nursing Process: Evaluation
Client Needs: Physiological Integrity
Content Area: Adult Health/Endocrine

Reference
LeMone, P., & Burke, K. (1996). *Medical-surgical nursing: Critical thinking in client care.* Menlo Park, CA: Addison-Wesley, pp. 691, 693, 694.

---

125. A client with aldosteronism is being treated with spironolactone (Aldactone). Which of the following parameters indicates to the nurse that the treatment is effective?

1 A decrease in BP
2 A decrease in sodium excretion
3 A decrease in plasma potassium
4 A decrease in body metabolism

Answer: 1

Rationale: Spironolactone antagonizes the effect of aldosterone, decreasing circulating volume by inhibiting tubular reabsorption of sodium and water. It increases excretion of sodium and plasma potassium. It has no effect on body metabolism.

Test-Taking Strategy: A key word in the stem is "effective." Therefore the correct answer is the one that indicates a desired action of this medication. Knowledge of the effects of this medication and its use in aldosteronism is helpful to answer this question. If, however, you can recall that this medication is also used in hypertensive conditions, you would easily be able to answer this question correctly. If you had difficulty with this question, take time to review the effects of spironolactone.

Level of Cognitive Ability: Analysis
Phase of Nursing Process: Evaluation
Client Needs: Physiological Integrity
Content Area: Adult Health/Endocrine

Reference
Black, J., & Matassarin-Jacobs, E. (1997). *Medical-surgical nursing: Clinical management for continuity of care.* Philadelphia: W. B. Saunders, pp. 2055, 2056.

---

126. A nurse is assessing a postoperative adrenalectomy client. Which of the following assessment data should the nurse monitor for in this client?

1 Signs and symptoms of hypocalcemia
2 Peripheral edema
3 Signs and symptoms of hypovolemia
4 Bilateral exophthalmus

Answer: 3

Rationale: Aldosterone, secreted by the adrenal cortex, plays a major role in fluid volume balance by retaining sodium and water. A deficiency of adrenocortical hormones does not cause the clinical manifestations noted in options 1, 2, and 4.

Test-Taking Strategy: Knowledge of adrenal hypofunction is required to answer this question. You must use your knowledge of the action of adrenocortical hormones to assist in answering this question. If you had difficulty with this question, take time now to list signs and symptoms related to hypofunction and hyperfunction of these hormones.

Level of Cognitive Ability: Application
Phase of Nursing Process: Assessment
Client Needs: Physiological Integrity
Content Area: Adult Health/Endocrine

Reference

LeMone, P., & Burke, K. M. (1996). *Medical-surgical nursing: Critical thinking in client care.* Menlo Park, CA: Addison-Wesley, p. 693.

---

127. A client with cancer tells the nurse that the food on the meal tray tastes "funny." Which intervention by the nurse is appropriate?

1 Keep the client NPO
2 Administer an antiemetic as ordered
3 Provide oral hygiene care
4 Obtain an order for TPN

Answer: 3

Rationale: Cancer treatments may cause distortion of taste. Frequent oral hygiene aids in preserving taste function. Keeping a client NPO increases nutritional risks. Antiemetics are used when nausea and vomiting are a problem. TPN is used when oral intake is not possible.

Test-Taking Strategy: The issue of the question is taste sensation. Only option 3 addresses this issue. A similar thought relationship can be made with "taste" and "oral hygiene care." If you had difficulty with this question, take time now to review the effects of cancer treatments.

Level of Cognitive Ability: Application
Phase of Nursing Process: Implementation
Client Needs: Physiological Integrity
Content Area: Adult Health/Oncology

Reference

Potter, P., & Perry, A. (1997). *Fundamentals of nursing: Concepts, process, and practice* (4th ed.). St. Louis: Mosby–Year Book, p. 1050.

---

128. The nurse notes redness, warmth, and a yellowish drainage at the insertion site of a central venous catheter in a client receiving TPN. What is the rationale for immediate notification of the physician?

1 Infections of a central catheter site can lead to septicemia
2 The client is experiencing an allergy to the TPN solution
3 The TPN solution has infiltrated and must be stopped
4 The client is allergic to the dressing material covering the site

Answer: 1

Rationale: Redness, warmth, and purulent drainage are signs of an infection, not an allergic reaction. Infiltration causes the surrounding tissue to become cool and pale.

Test-Taking Strategy: The issue of this question is to identify signs of infection. Key words in the question are "redness," "warmth," and "drainage." Option 1 addresses septicemia, which can be life-threatening to the client. If you had difficulty with this question, review nursing interventions related to monitoring for complications of TPN.

Level of Cognitive Ability: Analysis
Phase of Nursing Process: Analysis
Client Needs: Physiological Integrity
Content Area: Fundamental Skills

Reference

Ignatavicius, D. D., Workman, M. L., & Mishler, M. A. (1995). *Medical-surgical nursing: A nursing process approach* (2nd ed.). Philadelphia: W. B. Saunders, pp. 284–285.

---

129. A common finding in the history of a client with chronic pancreatitis is

1 Abdominal pain relieved with food or antacids.
2 Exposure to occupational chemicals.
3 Weight gain.
4 Use of alcohol.

Answer: 4

Rationale: Chronic pancreatitis is found most often in alcoholics. Abstinence from alcohol is important to prevent the client from developing chronic pancreatitis. Clients usually have malabsorption with weight loss. Pain is not relieved with food or antacids. Chemical exposure is associated with cancer of the pancreas.

Test-Taking Strategy: Knowledge of the causes and common assessment data associated with chronic pancreatitis is needed to answer this question. Look for key words in the stem of the question to help focus your attention. If you had difficulty with this question, review the causes of pancreatitis.

Level of Cognitive Ability: Analysis
Phase of Nursing Process: Assessment
Client Needs: Physiological Integrity
Content Area: Adult Health/Gastrointestinal

Reference

Lewis, S., Collier, I., & Heitkemper, M. (1996). *Medical-surgical nursing: Assessment and management of clinical problems* (4th ed.). St. Louis: Mosby–Year Book, p. 1294.

---

130. A client has been taking steroids to control rheumatoid arthritis. What abnormal laboratory value is the client at risk for as a result of taking this medication?

1 Increased serum potassium
2 Decreased serum sodium
3 Increased serum glucose
4 Increased WBCs

Answer: 3

Rationale: Glucocorticoid medications have three primary uses: replacement therapy for adrenal insufficiency, immunosuppressive therapy, and anti-inflammatory therapy. Exogenous glucocorticoids cause the same effects on cellular activity as the naturally produced glucocorticoids; however, exogenous glucocorticoids may produce undesired clinical outcomes. The glucocorticoids stimulate appetite and increase caloric intake. They also increase the availability of glucose for energy. These combined effects cause the blood glucose levels to rise, making clients prone to hyperglycemia.

Test-Taking Strategy: This question asks to interpret laboratory data in relation to medication administration. Knowledge of commonly experienced side effects of glucocorticoids can help to answer this question. A similarity exists between options 1 and 2 because they are both electrolytes. If a similarity exists in the options, neither one is likely to be the correct option. Glucocorticoids are a frequently used medication. If you are unfamiliar with these medications, their uses, side effects, and contraindications, it is important to review them.

Level of Cognitive Ability: Analysis
Phase of Nursing Process: Analysis
Client Needs: Physiological Integrity
Content Area: Pharmacology

Reference

Pinnell, N. (1996). *Nursing pharmacology.* Philadelphia: W. B. Saunders, p. 526.

---

131. A client with Cushing's syndrome is undergoing a dexamethasone suppression test. Which of the following steps are taken during this test?

1 1 mg of dexamethasone is taken orally at night, and serum cortisol levels are measured the next morning and evening
2 After an injection of dexamethasone, a 24-hour urine specimen is collected to measure serum cortisol levels
3 Blood samples are drawn before and after exercise to evaluate the effect of exercise on serum cortisol levels
4 An injection of adrenocorticotropic hormone (ACTH) is given 30 minutes before drawing blood to measure serum cortisol levels

Answer: 1

Rationale: The dexamethasone suppression test is performed to evaluate the function of the adrenal cortex. The procedure for this test is to give 1 mg of dexamethasone at 11 P.M. to suppress ACTH formation in time for an 8 A.M. and 8 P.M. phlebotomy to measure serum cortisol levels.

Test-Taking Strategy: The question asks you to select the option that indicates correct procedure for a dexamethasone suppression test. Cushing's syndrome is a disorder caused by excessive amounts of cortisol. Because the test is a dexamethasone suppression test, you would expect that something is given to suppress cortisol production. Keeping this in mind, options 2 and 3 can be eliminated. You then need to make a choice between options 1 and 4. Knowledge of the procedure is needed to answer the question correctly. If you had difficulty with this question, take time now to review this test.

Level of Cognitive Ability: Application
Phase of Nursing Process: Implementation
Client Needs: Physiological Integrity
Content Area: Adult Health/Endocrine

Reference

Black, J., & Matassarin-Jacobs, E. (1997). *Medical-surgical nursing: Clinical management for continuity of care* (5th ed.). Philadelphia: W. B. Saunders, p. 2045.

---

132. The nurse is performing an abdominal assessment on a client. The nurse interprets that which of the following findings should be reported to the physician?

1 Concave, midline umbilicus
2 Pulsation between the umbilicus and pubis
3 Bowel sound frequency of 15 sounds/minute
4 Absence of bruit

Answer: 2

Rationale: The umbilicus should be in the midline, with a concave appearance. The presence of pulsation between the umbilicus and the pubis could indicate abdominal aortic aneurysm and should be reported to the physician. Bruits are not normally present. Bowel sounds vary according to timing of last meal and usually range in frequency from 5 to 35 per minute.

Test-Taking Strategy: Use basic nursing knowledge related to physical assessment to answer this question. The wording of the question guides you to look for an abnormal finding. Review abdominal assessment if you had difficulty with this question.

Level of Cognitive Ability: Analysis
Phase of Nursing Process: Analysis
Client Needs: Physiological Integrity
Content Area: Adult Health/Gastrointestinal

Reference
Black, J., & Matassarin-Jacobs, E. (1997). *Medical-surgical nursing: Clinical management for continuity of care* (5th ed.). Philadelphia: W. B. Saunders, p. 1707.

---

133. The nurse is performing cardiovascular assessment on a client. Which of the following would the nurse assess to gain the best information about the client's left-sided heart function?

1 Breath sounds
2 Peripheral edema
3 Jugular vein distention
4 Hepatojugular reflux

Answer: 1

Rationale: The client with heart failure may present with different symptoms depending on whether the right or the left side of the heart is failing. Peripheral edema, jugular vein distention, and hepatojugular reflux are all indicators of right-sided heart function. Breath sounds are an accurate indicator of left-sided heart function.

Test-Taking Strategy: Blood flow is impaired in the circulation behind the area of heart failure. The client with left-sided heart failure can also have right-sided symptoms if failure is severe. The question asks for the best information about left-sided heart function, which indicates more than one correct response. The correct option then is one that reflects only the left side, which is breath sounds.

Level of Cognitive Ability: Application
Phase of Nursing Process: Assessment
Client Needs: Physiological Integrity
Content Area: Adult Health/Cardiovascular

Reference
Smeltzer, S., & Bare, B. (1996). *Brunner and Suddarth's Textbook of medical-surgical nursing* (8th ed.). Philadelphia: Lippincott-Raven, pp. 600, 604.

---

134. The nurse is caring for the following group of clients on the clinical nursing unit. The nurse interprets that which of them is most at risk for development of pulmonary embolism?

1 A 65-year-old man out of bed 1 day after prostate resection
2 A 73-year-old woman who has just had pinning of a hip fracture
3 A 25-year-old woman with diabetic ketoacidosis (DKA)
4 A 38-year-old man with pulmonary contusion after an auto accident

Answer: 2

Rationale: Clients frequently at risk for pulmonary embolism include those who are immobilized. This is especially true in the immobilized postoperative client. Other clients at risk include those with conditions that are characterized by hypercoagulability, endothelial disease, and advancing age.

Test-Taking Strategy: These options can best be compared by evaluating the degree of immobility that each client has as well as the age of the client, which is given in each option. The clients in options 1 and 3 have the least long-term anticipated immobility, and therefore those options should be eliminated first. Of the two remaining, the younger client with the lung contusion would be expected to be less immobile than the elderly woman with hip fracture, leaving option 2 as the answer.

Level of Cognitive Ability: Analysis
Phase of Nursing Process: Analysis
Client Needs: Physiological Integrity
Content Area: Adult Health/Respiratory

Reference
Smeltzer, S., & Bare, B. (1996). *Brunner and Suddarth's Textbook of medical-surgical nursing* (8th ed.). Philadelphia: Lippincott-Raven, p. 526.

---

135. A graduate nurse is assigned to admit a client with the diagnosis of anorexia nervosa. The nurse preceptor would remind the graduate nurse that objective assessment findings may indicate

1 Elevated potassium levels.
2 Low blood urea nitrogen (BUN).
3 Weight loss of at least 4% of original weight over a short period.
4 That the client has extensive knowledge of nutrition.

Answer: 4

Rationale: Potassium is usually low and BUN is usually high in clients with anorexia nervosa. Clients lose at least 15% of their original body weight in a short period of time. They are knowledgeable about nutrition and the caloric value of food.

Test-Taking Strategy: Use your nursing knowledge to answer this question. The small amount of weight loss may not be a cause of concern for too many people, and options 1 and 2 do not occur in starvation or fluid/electrolyte deficiency typical of anorexia nervosa. The only alternative is option 4.

Level of Cognitive Ability: Analysis
Phase of Nursing Process: Assessment
Client Needs: Physiological Integrity
Content Area: Mental Health

Reference
Luckmann, J. (1997). *Saunders manual of nursing care*. Philadelphia: W. B. Saunders, p. 324.

---

136. The physician has inserted a nasoenteric tube for the treatment of intestinal obstruction. The nurse tells the client to lie in which position to help the tube advance into the duodenum through the pyloric sphincter?

1 Supine with head of bed flat
2 Supine with head elevated 30 degrees
3 On the right side
4 On the left side

Answer: 3

Rationale: The client is instructed to lie on the right side to aid in passage of the tube from the stomach into the duodenum, past the pyloric sphincter.

Test-Taking Strategy: Use knowledge of basic anatomy and the position of the stomach in the abdomen to help you eliminate each of the incorrect responses. Knowledge of this position can be applied to the management of a client with any type of nasoenteric tube.

Level of Cognitive Ability: Application
Phase of Nursing Process: Implementation
Client Needs: Physiological Integrity
Content Area: Adult Health/Gastrointestinal

Reference
Black, J., & Matassarin-Jacobs, E. (1997). *Medical-surgical nursing: Clinical management for continuity of care* (5th ed.). Philadelphia: W. B. Saunders, p. 1750.

---

137. A client with coronary artery disease suddenly complains of palpitations and an irregular "heartbeat." The nurse would assess for which of the following to determine an inadequacy of stroke volume?

1 Pulse pressure
2 Pulse deficit
3 Pulsus alternans
4 Water hammer pulse

Answer: 2

Rationale: Palpitations are often a subjective complaint that accompanies dysrhythmias. Irregular rhythms produce varying strengths of stroke volume as a result of irregular ventricular filling times, and therefore arterial pulsations may become weakened or intermittently absent. The nurse determines this by assessing an apical radial pulse. An apical rate that is greater than the radial rate is called a "pulse deficit." The pulse pressure is an indirect indicator of overall cardiac output. A water hammer pulse may accompany events that produce an increased cardiac output. Pulsus alternans has a regular rhythm accompanied by pulse volume that alternates strong with weak.

Test-Taking Strategy: Remember that "stroke volume × heart rate = cardiac output." Measures that give a general indication of cardiac output are not specific enough to answer this question, which eliminates pulse pressure and water hammer pulse. Pulsus alternans occurs with a regular rhythm, which eliminates this option.

Level of Cognitive Ability: Analysis
Phase of Nursing Process: Assessment
Client Needs: Physiological Integrity
Content Area: Adult Health/Cardiovascular

Reference

Smeltzer, S., & Bare, B. (1996). *Brunner and Suddarth's Textbook of medical-surgical nursing* (8th ed.). Philadelphia: Lippincott-Raven, pp. 598–599.

---

138. The nurse is listening to the client's breath sounds and hears a creaking, grating sound on inspiration and expiration over the posterior right lower lobe. The nurse assesses that this client has

1 Crackles.
2 Wheezes.
3 Rhonchi.
4 Pleural friction rub.

Answer: 4

Rationale: The nurse is hearing a pleural friction rub, which is characterized by sounds that are described as creaking, groaning, or grating in quality. The sounds are localized over an area of inflammation of the pleura, and may be heard in both the inspiratory and expiratory phases of the respiratory cycle. Crackles have the sound that is heard when a few strands of hair are rubbed together near the ear and indicate fluid in the alveoli. Wheezes are musical noises heard on inspiration, expiration, or both. They are the result of narrowed air passages. Rhonchi are usually heard on expiration when there is excessive production of mucus, which accumulates in the air passages.

Test-Taking Strategy: The adjectives "creaking" and "grating" are the key to answering this question. The image called to mind by these sounds is most compatible with the words "friction rub," and that may be sufficient to help you answer the question correctly. In addition, knowing that these sounds are not the classic descriptors for crackles, wheezes, or rhonchi helps you to eliminate each of the other options.

Level of Cognitive Ability: Analysis
Phase of Nursing Process: Assessment
Client Needs: Physiological Integrity
Content Area: Adult Health/Respiratory

Reference

Black, J., & Matassarin-Jacobs, E. (1997). *Medical-surgical nursing: Clinical management for continuity of care* (5th ed.). Philadelphia: W. B. Saunders, p. 1046.

---

139. The nurse is assessing the renal function of the client. After directly noting urine volume and characteristics, the nurse assesses which of the following items as the best indirect indicator of renal status?

1 Bladder distention
2 Level of consciousness
3 Pulse rate
4 Blood pressure (BP)

Answer: 4

Rationale: The kidneys normally receive 20%–25% of the cardiac output, even under conditions of rest. For kidney function to be optimal, adequate renal perfusion is necessary. Perfusion can best be estimated by the BP, which is an indirect reflection of the adequacy of cardiac output. The pulse rate indicates cardiac output but can be altered by factors unrelated to kidney function. Bladder distention reflects a problem or obstruction that is most often distal to the kidneys. Level of consciousness is an unrelated item.

Test-Taking Strategy: Eliminate level of consciousness first as the item most unrelated to kidney function. Because bladder distention can be affected by a number of other factors besides renal function, this is eliminated next. To choose between pulse and BP, remember that BP is the more global factor and the item more directly related to kidney perfusion, which makes 4 the better option.

Level of Cognitive Ability: Application
Phase of Nursing Process: Assessment
Client Needs: Physiological Integrity
Content Area: Adult Health/Renal

Reference

Black, J., & Matassarin-Jacobs, E. (1997). *Medical-surgical nursing: Clinical management for continuity of care* (5th ed.). Philadelphia: W. B. Saunders, p. 1537.

---

140. The nurse notes that the infusion bag of a client receiving TPN has become empty. The nurse calls the pharmacy, but the next bag will not be delivered for another 30 minutes. The nurse should plan to hang which of the following solutions until the TPN arrives?

1 5% dextrose in water
2 10% dextrose in water
3 50% dextrose in saline
4 5% lactated Ringer's

Answer: 2

Rationale: If a TPN solution bag stops running or goes dry, the nurse should hang an infusion of 10% dextrose in water until another TPN solution arrives. This minimizes the chance that the client will develop hypoglycemia because the body produces more insulin in the presence of the high TPN glucose load.

Test-Taking Strategy: Knowledge of the glucose concentration of both TPN and regular intravenous infusions is needed to answer this question. Eliminate option 3 because there is no such solution. Remember that options that are similar are not likely to be correct. This guides you to eliminate options 1 and 4, since the percentage is the same.

Level of Cognitive Ability: Application
Phase of Nursing Process: Planning
Client Needs: Physiological Integrity
Content Area: Adult Health/Gastrointestinal

Reference

Black, J., & Matassarin-Jacobs, E. (1997). *Medical-surgical nursing: Clinical management for continuity of care* (5th ed.). Philadelphia: W. B. Saunders, p. 1756.

---

141. The client who has ascites and slight jaundice is seen in the ambulatory care clinic. The nurse assesses the client for a history of chronic use of which of the following medications?

1 Acetaminophen (Tylenol)
2 Acetylsalicylic acid (Aspirin)
3 Ibuprofen (Advil)
4 Ranitidine (Zantac)

Answer: 1

Rationale: Acetaminophen is a potentially hepatotoxic medication. Use of this medication and other hepatotoxic agents should be investigated whenever a client presents with symptoms compatible with liver disease (such as ascites and jaundice).

Test-Taking Strategy: To answer this question correctly, it is first necessary to know that these symptoms are compatible with liver disease. With this in mind, you may evaluate each of the options in relation to their relative ability to be toxic to the liver. Review these medications now if you are unfamiliar with them.

Level of Cognitive Ability: Analysis
Phase of Nursing Process: Assessment
Client Needs: Physiological Integrity
Content Area: Pharmacology

Reference

Black, J., & Matassarin-Jacobs, E. (1997). *Medical-surgical nursing: Clinical management for continuity of care* (5th ed.). Philadelphia: W. B. Saunders, p. 1844.

142. The nurse is assigned to care for a client who has just undergone eye surgery. The nurse plans to instruct the client that which of the following activities is permitted in the postoperative period?

1 Reading
2 Watching television
3 Bending over
4 Lifting objects

Answer: 2

Rationale: The client is taught to avoid doing activities that raise intraocular pressure and could cause complications in the postoperative period. The client is also taught to avoid activities that cause rapid eye movements that are irritating in the presence of postoperative inflammation. For these reasons, the client is taught to avoid bending over, lifting heavy objects, straining, sneezing, making sudden movements, or reading. Watching television is permissible because the eye does not need to move rapidly with this activity, and it does not increase the intraocular pressure.

Test-Taking Strategy: Think about the issue of intraocular pressure when answering this question. Eliminate options 3 and 4 first because they obviously increase intraocular pressure. Choose option 2 over option 1 because reading is less taxing to the eyes.

Level of Cognitive Ability: Application
Phase of Nursing Process: Planning
Client Needs: Physiological Integrity
Content Area: Adult Health/Eye

Reference

Burrell, P., Gerlach, M., & Pless, B. (1997). *Adult nursing: Acute and community care* (2nd ed.). Stamford, CT: Appleton & Lange, p. 1874.

143. The nurse is listening to the lungs of a client who has left lower lobe pneumonia. The nurse interprets that the pneumonia is resolving if which of the following is heard over the affected lung area?

1 Bronchophony
2 Egophony
3 Vesicular breath sounds
4 Whispered pectoriloquy

Answer: 3

Rationale: Vesicular breath sounds are normal sounds that are heard over peripheral lung fields where the air enters the alveoli. A return of breath sounds to normal is consistent with a resolving pneumonia. Bronchophony is an abnormal finding with lung consolidation and is identified if the nurse can clearly hear the client say "ninety-nine" through the stethoscope. (Normally the client's words are unintelligible if heard through a stethoscope). Egophony occurs when the sound of the letter "e" is heard as an "a" with auscultation and also indicates lung consolidation. Finally, whispered pectoriloquy is present if the nurse hears the client when "one-two-three" is whispered. This is an abnormal finding, again heard over an area of consolidation. Consolidation typically occurs with pneumonia.

Test-Taking Strategy: To answer this question accurately and quickly, it is necessary to know the differences among these assessment findings. Knowing the areas where bronchial, vesicular, and bronchovesicular breath sounds are heard, however, is sufficient to answer this question as stated. Review these types of breath sounds now if you had difficulty with this question.

Level of Cognitive Ability: Analysis
Phase of Nursing Process: Analysis
Client Needs: Physiological Integrity
Content Area: Adult Health/Respiratory

Reference

Black, J., & Matassarin-Jacobs, E. (1997). *Medical-surgical nursing: Clinical management for continuity of care* (5th ed.). Philadelphia: W. B. Saunders, pp. 1046–1047.

144. The female client with a history of chronic infection in the urinary system complains of burning and urinary frequency. To determine whether the current problem is of renal origin, the nurse would assess whether the client has pain or discomfort in the

1 Suprapubic area.
2 Right or left costovertebral angle.
3 Urinary meatus.
4 Labium.

Answer: 2

Rationale: Pain or discomfort from a problem that originates in the kidney is felt at the costovertebral angle on the affected side. Ureteral pain is felt in the ipsilateral labium in the female client or the ipsilateral scrotum in the male client. Bladder infection is often accompanied by suprapubic pain and pain or burning at the urinary meatus when voiding.

Test-Taking Strategy: To answer this question accurately, you should know the areas in which pain is felt or referred when it originates in the urinary tract. Knowing that the kidneys sit higher than the level of the bladder and retroperitoneally, you may be able to eliminate each incorrect option using concepts related to anatomy.

Level of Cognitive Ability: Analysis
Phase of Nursing Process: Assessment
Client Needs: Physiological Integrity
Content Area: Adult Health/Renal

Reference

Black, J., & Matassarin-Jacobs, E. (1997). *Medical-surgical nursing: Clinical management for continuity of care* (5th ed.). Philadelphia: W. B. Saunders, pp. 1548–1549.

145. During a routine visit to the physician's office for monitoring of diabetic control, the elderly client complains to the nurse of vision changes. The client describes blurring of the vision, with difficulty in reading and with driving at night. Given the client's history, the nurse interprets that the client is probably developing

1 Detached retina.
2 Papilledema.
3 Glaucoma.
4 Cataracts.

Answer: 4

Rationale: Although the incidence of cataracts increases with age, the elderly client with diabetes is at greater risk for developing cataracts. The most frequent complaint is of blurred vision that is not accompanied by pain. The client may also experience difficulty with reading, night driving, and glare.

Test-Taking Strategy: Specific knowledge related to the risks for and signs and symptoms of common eye disorders is needed to answer this question. If this question was difficult, take a few moments now to review the signs and symptoms of cataracts.

Level of Cognitive Ability: Analysis
Phase of Nursing Process: Analysis
Client Needs: Physiological Integrity
Content Area: Adult Health/Eye

Reference

Burrell, P., Gerlach, M., & Pless, B. (1997). *Adult nursing: Acute and community care* (2nd ed.). Stamford, CT: Appleton & Lange, p. 1878.

146. The nurse inquires about smoking history while conducting a hospital admission assessment with a client with coronary artery disease. The most important item for the nurse to assess is the

1 Number of pack-years.
2 Brand of cigarettes used.
3 Desire to quit smoking.
4 Number of past attempts to quit smoking.

Answer: 1

Rationale: The number of cigarettes smoked daily and the duration of the habit are used to calculate the number of pack-years, which is the standard method of documenting smoking history. The brand of cigarettes may give a general indication of tar and nicotine levels, but the information has no immediate clinical use. Desire to quit and number of past attempts to quit smoking may be useful when the nurse develops a smoking cessation plan with the client.

Test-Taking Strategy: The question directs you to identify the most important item. This indicates that more than one option is correct. The option that would most closely predict the degree of added risk of coronary artery disease is the number of pack-years.

Level of Cognitive Ability: Analysis
Phase of Nursing Process: Assessment
Client Needs: Physiological Integrity
Content Area: Adult Health/Cardiovascular

Reference

Ignatavicius, D. D., Workman, M. L., & Mishler, M. A. (1995). *Medical-surgical nursing: A nursing process approach* (2nd ed.). Philadelphia: W. B. Saunders, p. 787.

---

147. The client with primary open-angle glaucoma has been prescribed timolol (Timoptic) ophthalmic drops. The client asks the nurse how this medication works. The nurse tells the client that the medication lowers intraocular pressure by

1 Reducing intracranial pressure (ICP).
2 Increasing contractions of the ciliary muscle.
3 Constricting the pupil.
4 Reducing production of aqueous humor.

Answer: 4

Rationale: Beta-adrenergic blocking agents such as timolol reduce intraocular pressure by decreasing the production of aqueous humor. Miotic agents (such as pilocarpine) increase contractions of the ciliary muscle and constrict the pupil, thereby increasing the outflow of aqueous humor.

Test-Taking Strategy: Specific knowledge about the action of this medication is needed to answer this question. If needed, take a few moments to review this medication now.

Level of Cognitive Ability: Application
Phase of Nursing Process: Implementation
Client Needs: Physiological Integrity
Content Area: Pharmacology

Reference

Burrell, P., Gerlach, M., & Pless, B. (1997). *Adult nursing: Acute and community care* (2nd ed.). Stamford, CT: Appleton & Lange, p. 1882.

---

148. The client is complaining of knee pain. The knee is swollen, reddened, and warm to the touch. The nurse interprets that the client's signs and symptoms are not compatible with

1 Inflammation.
2 Degenerative disease.
3 Infection.
4 Recent injury.

Answer: 2

Rationale: Redness and heat are associated with musculoskeletal inflammation, infection, or a recent injury. Degenerative disease is accompanied by pain, but there is no redness. Swelling may or may not occur.

Test-Taking Strategy: Swelling, redness, and warmth are signs of inflammation. The body's inflammatory response is triggered by inflammation, infection, and injury. This should easily direct you to the correct option.

Level of Cognitive Ability: Analysis
Phase of Nursing Process: Analysis
Client Needs: Physiological Integrity
Content Area: Adult Health/Musculoskeletal

Reference

Black, J., & Matassarin-Jacobs, E. (1997). *Medical-surgical nursing: Clinical management for continuity of care* (5th ed.). Philadelphia: W. B. Saunders, p. 2084.

149. The client seeks treatment in the emergency room for a lower leg injury. There is visible deformity to the lower aspect of the leg, and the injured leg appears shorter than the other. The area is painful, swollen, and beginning to become ecchymotic. The nurse interprets that this client has experienced a

1 Contusion.
2 Fracture.
3 Sprain.
4 Strain.

Answer: 2

Rationale: Typical signs and symptoms of fracture include pain, loss of function in the area, deformity, shortening of the extremity, crepitus, swelling, and ecchymosis. A contusion results from a blow to soft tissue and causes pain, swelling, and ecchymosis. A sprain is an injury to a ligament caused by a wrenching or twisting motion. Symptoms include pain, swelling, and inability to use the joint or bear weight normally. A strain results from a pulling force on the muscle. Symptoms include soreness and pain with muscle use.

Test-Taking Strategy: Within the list of signs and symptoms in the question, note the one that states one leg is shorter than another. Only a fractured bone (which shortens with displacement) could cause this sign. This makes it easy to eliminate each of the other incorrect options.

Level of Cognitive Ability: Analysis
Phase of Nursing Process: Analysis
Client Needs: Physiological Integrity
Content Area: Adult Health/Musculoskeletal

Reference
Smeltzer, S., & Bare, B. (1996). *Brunner and Suddarth's Textbook of medical-surgical nursing* (8th ed.). Philadelphia: Lippincott-Raven, pp. 1908, 1910.

150. The client presents to the emergency room with a chemical burn of the left eye. The first action of the nurse is immediately to

1 Flush the eye continuously with a sterile solution.
2 Apply a cold compress to the injured eye.
3 Apply a nonocclusive bandage to the eye.
4 Determine the nature of the chemical agent.

Answer: 1

Rationale: When the client has suffered a chemical burn of the eye, the nurse immediately flushes the site with a sterile solution continuously for 15 minutes. If a sterile eye irrigation solution is not available, running water may be used. Determining the nature of the chemical is helpful but is not the priority action. Applying compresses or bandages is incorrect because they do not rid the eye of the damaging chemical. Cold compresses are used for blows to the eye, whereas light bandages may be placed over cuts of the eye or eyelid.

Test-Taking Strategy: Begin to answer this question by eliminating options 2 and 3 first because they are the least plausible of the options. Use knowledge related to prioritizing to choose option 1 over option 4. Review emergency care related to chemical burns to the eye if you had difficulty with this question.

Level of Cognitive Ability: Application
Phase of Nursing Process: Implementation
Client Needs: Physiological Integrity
Content Area: Adult Health/Eye

Reference
Burrell, P., Gerlach, M., & Pless, B. (1997). *Adult nursing: Acute and community care* (2nd ed.). Stamford, CT: Appleton & Lange, p. 1895.

151. The client tells the nurse about a pattern of getting a strong urge to void, which is followed by incontinence before the client can get to the bathroom. The nurse formulates which of the following nursing diagnoses for this client?

1 Reflex Incontinence
2 Stress Incontinence
3 Urge Incontinence
4 Total Incontinence

Answer: 3

Rationale: Urge Incontinence occurs when the client has urinary incontinence soon after experiencing urgency. Reflex Incontinence occurs when incontinence occurs at rather predictable times that correspond to when a certain bladder volume is attained. Stress Incontinence occurs when the client voids in increments that are less than 50 mL and has increased abdominal pressure. Total Incontinence occurs when there is an unpredictable and continuous loss of urine.

Test-Taking Strategy: Eliminate option 4 first as having the least degree of "fit" with the information in the question. It is necessary to understand the definitions of each of the remaining nursing diagnoses to differentiate among them most accurately. Notice, however, that the question includes the word "urge," which helps you to choose option 3. With similar questions, look for adjectives in the question that will guide you in your selection.

Level of Cognitive Ability: Analysis
Phase of Nursing Process: Analysis
Client Needs: Physiological Integrity
Content Area: Adult Health/Renal

Reference

Cox, H., Hinz, M., Lubno, M., et al. (1997). *Clinical applications of nursing diagnosis: Adult, child, women's, psychiatric, gerontic, and home health considerations* (3rd ed.). Philadelphia: F. A. Davis, p. 229.

---

152. A 52-year-old male client is seen in the physician's office for a physical examination after experiencing unusual fatigue over the last several weeks. Height is 5 feet, 8 inches, with a weight of 220 pounds. Vital signs are as follows: temperature, 98°F oral; pulse, 86 beats/minute; respirations, 18 breaths/minute; and BP, 184/96 mmHg. Random blood glucose is 122 mg/dL. Which of the following questions should the nurse ask the client next?

1 "Do you exercise regularly?"
2 "Are you considering trying to lose weight?"
3 "Is there a history of diabetes in your family?"
4 "When was the last time you had your BP checked?"

Answer: 4

Rationale: The client is hypertensive, which is a known major modifiable risk factor for coronary artery disease. The client is overweight, which is a contributing risk factor. The client's nonmodifiable risk factors are age and gender. Because the client presents with several risk factors, the nurse places priority of attention on the client's major modifiable risk factors.

Test-Taking Strategy: Options 1 and 2 are similar and can therefore be eliminated. The question asks you to prioritize your assessment because of the word "next" in the stem. Option 4 supersedes option 3 because of the obviously greater degree of abnormality.

Level of Cognitive Ability: Analysis
Phase of Nursing Process: Assessment
Client Needs: Physiological Integrity
Content Area: Adult Health/Cardiovascular

Reference

Black, J., & Matassarin-Jacobs, E. (1997). *Medical-surgical nursing: Clinical management for continuity of care* (5th ed.). Philadelphia: W. B. Saunders, p. 1239.

---

153. The nurse is instilling an otic solution into the adult client's left ear. The nurse would avoid doing which of the following as part of this procedure?

1 Warming the solution to room temperature
2 Placing the client in a side-lying position with ear facing up
3 Pulling the auricle backward and upward
4 Placing the tip of the dropper on the edge of the ear canal

Answer: 4

Rationale: The dropper is not allowed to touch any object or any part of the client's skin. The solution is warmed before use. The client is placed on the side with the affected ear directed upward. The nurse pulls the auricle backward and upward and instills the medication by holding the dropper about 1 cm above the ear canal.

Test-Taking Strategy: Basic knowledge of proper procedure for administering otic solutions is needed to answer this question correctly. If this question was difficult, take a few moments now to review this basic nursing procedure.

Level of Cognitive Ability: Application
Phase of Nursing Process: Implementation
Client Needs: Physiological Integrity
Content Area: Adult Health/Ear

Reference

Burrell, P., Gerlach, M., & Pless, B. (1997). *Adult nursing: Acute and community care* (2nd ed.). Stamford, CT: Appleton & Lange, p. 1926.

154. Levothyroxine sodium (Synthroid or Levothyroid) is administered to a hospitalized child with congenital hypothyroidism. The child vomits 45 minutes after administration of the dose. The most appropriate nursing action is to

1 Repeat the prescribed dose.
2 Give two doses of the prescribed medication in the morning.
3 Administer the usual dose intramuscularly.
4 Hold the dose for today.

Answer: 1

Rationale: Synthetic levothyroxine sodium is the medication of choice for hypothyroidism. The most significant factor adversely affecting the eventual intelligence of children born with congenital hypothyroidism is inadequate treatment. Therefore compliance with the medication regimen is essential. If the infant or child vomits within 1 hour of taking medication, the dose should be given again.

Test-Taking Strategy: Levothyroxine is a commonly prescribed medication for all age groups experiencing hypothyroidism. If you are unfamiliar with the medication addressed in this question, it is important to review it. Recognizing the significance of avoiding undermedication, option 1 should be selected. If you had difficulty with this question, review the administration of this medication in congenital hypothyroidism.

Level of Cognitive Ability: Application
Phase of Nursing Process: Implementation
Client Needs: Physiological Integrity
Content Area: Child Health

Reference

Ashwill, J., & Droske, S. (1997). *Nursing care of children: Principles and practice.* Philadelphia: W. B. Saunders, p. 1176.

---

155. A client with a diagnosis of catatonic excitement has been pacing rapidly nonstop for several hours, not eating or drinking. The nurse recognizes that in this situation

1 There is an urgent need for physical and medical control.
2 There is an urgent need for restraint.
3 There is a need to encourage verbalization of feelings.
4 The client will soon become catatonic stuporous.

Answer: 1

Rationale: Catatonic excitement is manifested by a state of extreme psychomotor agitation. Clients urgently require physical and medical control because they are often destructive and violent to others, and their excitement can cause them to injure themselves or to collapse from complete exhaustion.

Test-Taking Strategy: Use Maslow's hierarchy of needs theory to answer the question. Physiological needs come first; select an answer that addresses them.

Level of Cognitive Ability: Analysis
Phase of Nursing Process: Assessment
Client Needs: Physiological Integrity
Content Area: Mental Health

Reference

Townsend, M. (1996). *Psychiatric–mental health nursing: Concepts of care* (2nd ed.). Philadelphia: F. A. Davis, p. 411.

---

156. Which of the following laboratory data would indicate a potential complication associated with type 1 insulin-dependent diabetes?

1 Blood glucose level of 112 mg/dL
2 Ketonuria
3 BUN level of 18 mg/dL
4 Potassium level of 4.2 mEq

Answer: 2

Rationale: Ketonuria is an abnormal finding in the diabetic client indicating ketosis. Ketosis is a metabolic effect from the lack of insulin on fat metabolism and occurs in type 1 diabetes. It is associated with the severe complication of DKA (hyperglycemia, ketosis, and acidosis). Options 1, 3, and 4 are all normal laboratory findings.

Test-Taking Strategy: Knowledge of the normal range of laboratory values can assist in answering the question. Eliminate options 3 and 4 first. Options 1 and 2 are related to insulin-dependent diabetes. From these two options, option 2 indicates an abnormal finding. If you had difficulty with this question, review the complications of insulin-dependent diabetes.

Level of Cognitive Ability: Analysis
Phase of Nursing Process: Analysis
Client Needs: Physiological Integrity
Content Area: Adult Health/Endocrine

Reference

Black, J., & Matassarin-Jacobs, E. (1997). *Medical-surgical nursing: Clinical management for continuity of care* (5th ed.). Philadelphia: W. B. Saunders, p. 1982.

---

157. The nurse in an outpatient diabetes clinic is caring for a client on insulin pump therapy. Which statement, if made by the client, indicates that a knowledge deficit exists regarding insulin pump therapy?

1 "If my blood sugars are elevated, I can bolus myself with additional insulin as ordered"
2 "I'll need to check my blood sugars before meals in case I need a premeal insulin bolus"
3 "Now that I have this pump, I don't have to worry about insulin reactions or ketoacidosis ever happening again"
4 "I still need to follow a diet and exercise plan even though I don't inject myself daily anymore"

Answer: 3

Rationale: All of the statements are correct in regard to insulin pump therapy except option 3. Hypoglycemic reactions can occur if there is an error in calculating the insulin dose or if the pump malfunctions. Ketoacidosis can occur if too little insulin is used or if there is an increase in metabolic need. The pump does not have a built-in blood glucose monitoring feedback system, so the client is subject to the usual complications associated with insulin administration without the use of a pump.

Test-Taking Strategy: Knowledge of the basics of insulin therapy is helpful to answer this question even if you know little about insulin pump therapy. Options 1, 2, and 4 are logical statements regarding the use of endogenous insulin. Option 3, however, presumes a guarantee from the usual complication of insulin therapy. No biomedical equipment is capable of being 100% safe. Additionally the option contains the word "ever," which is an absolute.

Level of Cognitive Ability: Analysis
Phase of Nursing Process: Evaluation
Client Needs: Physiological Integrity
Content Area: Adult Health/Endocrine

Reference

Black, J., & Matassarin-Jacobs, E. (1997). *Medical-surgical nursing: Clinical management for continuity of care* (5th ed.). Philadelphia: W. B. Saunders, pp. 1969–1970.

---

158. The client with Graves' disease has exophthalmos and is experiencing photophobia. Which of the following interventions would best enable the nurse to assist the client with this problem?

1 Administer methimazole (Tapazole) every 8 hours around the clock
2 Lubricate the eyes with tap water every 2–4 hours
3 Instruct the client to avoid straining or heavy lifting because this can increase eye pressure
4 Obtain dark glasses for the client

Answer: 4

Rationale: Medical therapy for Graves' disease doesn't help to alleviate the clinical manifestation of exophthalmos. Because photophobia (light intolerance) accompanies this disorder, dark glasses are helpful in alleviating the symptom. Other interventions may be used to relieve the drying that occurs from not being able to close the eyes completely; however, the question is asking what the nurse can do for photophobia. Tap water, which is hypotonic, could actually cause more swelling to the eye because it could pull fluid into the interstitial space. In addition, the client is at risk for developing an eye infection because the solution is not sterile. There is no need to prevent straining with exophthalmos.

Test-Taking Strategy: Identify key words in the stem, such as "would best enable." Knowledge of what photophobia means can help you to answer the question. Begin to eliminate options that do not apply, such as options 1, 2, and 3. Focus on the issue of photophobia. Tapazole, a medical treatment for Graves' disease, does not affect the progression of exophthalmos or alleviate the photophobia. Likewise, options 2 and 3 do not relieve the photophobia.

Level of Cognitive Ability: Application
Phase of Nursing Process: Implementation
Client Needs: Physiological Integrity
Content Area: Adult Health/Endocrine

Reference

Ignatavicius, D. D., Workman, M. L., & Mishler, M. A. (1995). *Medical-surgical nursing: A nursing process approach* (2nd ed.). Philadelphia: W. B. Saunders, p. 1843.

---

159. A priority nursing diagnosis for a postoperative subtotal thyroidectomy client would most likely include which of the following?

1 Fluid Volume Deficit related to triiodothyronine and thyroxine deficits promoting sodium and water loss
2 High Risk for Infection related to high glucose levels after removal of the thyroid
3 High Risk for Decreased Cardiac Output related to hemorrhage
4 High Risk for Altered Patterns of Urinary Elimination related to hypercalcemia and renal calculi formation

Answer: 3

Rationale: Hemorrhage is one of the most severe complications that can occur postthyroidectomy. The nurse must assess the neck dressing for bleeding and monitor vital signs frequently to detect early signs of hemorrhage that could lead to shock. Triiodothyronine and thyroxine do not regulate fluid volumes in the body. Removal of the thyroid may affect glucose levels indirectly but does not put the client at risk for infection. This is a problem more likely to be seen with an uncontrolled diabetic. Hypercalcemia and renal calculi are associated with hyperparathyroidism.

Test-Taking Strategy: Focus on the key words "priority," "most likely," and "postoperative subtotal thyroidectomy." Knowledge of thyroid function can assist to eliminate options 1, 2, and 4. Remember the ABCs. Circulation is affected if hemorrhage develops. If you had difficulty with this question, review the complications associated with thyroidectomy.

Level of Cognitive Ability: Analysis
Phase of Nursing Process: Analysis
Client Needs: Physiological Integrity
Content Area: Adult Health/Endocrine

Reference

Ignatavicius, D. D., Workman, M. L., & Mishler, M. A. (1995). *Medical-surgical nursing: A nursing process approach* (2nd ed.). Philadelphia: W. B. Saunders, pp. 1840–1841, 1851.

---

160. The nurse is caring for a client with pneumonia who suddenly becomes restless and has a PaO_2 of 60 mmHg. Which of the following nursing diagnoses would be most appropriate for this client?

1 Fatigue related to debilitated state
2 Impaired Gas Exchange related to increased pulmonary secretions
3 Ineffective Airway Clearance related to dilated bronchioles
4 Impaired Gas Exchange related to pneumonia

Answer: 2

Rationale: Restlessness and low PaO_2 are hallmark signs of impaired gas exchange. Although many clients with pneumonia experience fatigue, this diagnosis is not the most appropriate in light of inadequate oxygen intake. Dilation of bronchioles is a goal for treatment and not part of the problem. Pneumonia is a medical diagnosis.

Test-Taking Strategy: Knowledge of pneumonia and its treatment can help you answer this question. Eliminate option 4 because it is a medical diagnosis. Eliminate option 1 next because it is unrelated to the specific issue. From the remaining two options, knowing that the bronchioles are not dilated in pneumonia can assist in directing you to option 2. Be careful with questions addressing nursing diagnoses. Remember, NCLEX is a nursing examination: Avoid nursing diagnoses that address a medical diagnosis.

Level of Cognitive Ability: Analysis
Phase of Nursing Process: Analysis
Client Needs: Physiological Integrity
Content Area: Adult Health/Respiratory

Reference

Thompson, J., McFarland, G., Hirsch, J., & Tucker, S. (1997). *Mosby's clinical nursing* (4th ed.). St. Louis: Mosby–Year Book, p. 178.

161. A client with tuberculosis is to be started on rifampin (Rifadin). Which of the following teaching actions by the nurse is appropriate?

1 Tell the client not to worry about jaundice because an orange discoloration is common
2 Tell the client to wear glasses instead of soft contact lens
3 Tell the client always to take the medication on an empty stomach
4 Tell the client that as soon as the cultures come back negative the medication may be stopped

Answer: 2

Rationale: Soft contacts may be permanently damaged by the orange discoloration that rifampin causes in body fluids. Any sign of jaundice should always be reported. If rifampin is not tolerated on an empty stomach, it may be taken with food. The client may be on the medication for 12 months even if cultures are negative.

Test-Taking Strategy: Knowledge of the actions and uses of rifampin is needed to assist you in answering this question. If you are unfamiliar with this medication, review it now.

Level of Cognitive Ability: Application
Phase of Nursing Process: Implementation
Client Needs: Physiological Integrity
Content Area: Pharmacology

Reference

Hodgson, B., & Kizior, R. (1998). *Saunders nursing drug handbook 1998.* Philadelphia: W. B. Saunders, pp. 906–908.

---

162. All of the following have been ordered for a client with Guillain-Barré syndrome. Which order should the nurse question?

1 Assess vital signs every 2–4 hours
2 Clear liquid diet
3 Passive range-of-motion exercises three times per day
4 Bilateral calf measurements three times per day

Answer: 2

Rationale: Clients with Guillain-Barré syndrome have dysphagia. Clients with dysphagia are more likely to aspirate clear liquids than thick or semisolid foods. Clients with Guillain-Barré syndrome are at risk for hypotension and hypertension, bradycardia, and respiratory depression and require frequent monitoring of vital signs. Passive range-of-motion exercises can help prevent contractures, and assessing calf measurements can help detect deep vein thrombosis, for which clients are at risk.

Test-Taking Strategy: Even if you were unaware of the problems with Guillain-Barré syndrome and dysphagia, options 1, 3, and 4 are generally part of routine nursing care. Review the manifestations associated with this disorder if you had difficulty with this question.

Level of Cognitive Ability: Analysis
Phase of Nursing Process: Implementation
Client Needs: Physiological Integrity
Content Area: Adult Health/Neurological

Reference

Black, J., & Matassarin-Jacobs, E. (1997). *Medical-surgical nursing: Clinical management for continuity of care* (5th ed.). Philadelphia: W. B. Saunders, p. 877.

---

163. A client with myasthenia gravis presents to the emergency room in crisis. The physician plans to administer edrophonium (Tensilon) to differentiate between myasthenic and cholinergic crisis. If the client has cholinergic crisis, which of the following should the nurse be prepared to administer?

1 Atropine sulfate
2 Morphine sulfate
3 Pyridostigmine bromide (Mestinon)
4 Isoproterenol (Isuprel)

Answer: 1

Rationale: Clients with cholinergic crisis have too much medication in their system. Tensilon exacerbates symptoms in cholinergic crisis to the point where clients may need intubation and mechanical ventilation. Atropine is used to reverse the effects of these anticholinesterase medications. Morphine, pyridostigmine bromide, and neostigmine worsen the symptoms of cholinergic crisis. Isoproterenol is not indicated for cholinergic crisis.

Test-Taking Strategy: Knowledge of the antidote for anticholinesterase medications is necessary to answer this question. Memorize this antidote now if you had difficulty with this question.

Level of Cognitive Ability: Application
Phase of Nursing Process: Planning
Client Needs: Physiological Integrity
Content Area: Adult Health/Neurological

Reference

Ignatavicius, D. D., Workman, M. L., & Mishler, M. A. (1995). *Medical-surgical nursing: A nursing process approach* (2nd ed.). Philadelphia: W. B. Saunders, p. 1228.

---

164. The nurse is completing a health history on a diabetic client who has been taking insulin for many years. At present, the client states he or she is experiencing periods of hypoglycemia followed by periods of hyperglycemia. The most likely cause for this occurrence would be

1 Injecting insulin at the site of lipodystrophy.
2 Adjusting insulin according to blood glucose.
3 Eating snacks between meals.
4 Initiating the use of the insulin pump.

Answer: 1

Rationale: Tissue hypertrophy (lipodystrophy) involves thickening of the subcutaneous tissue at the injection sites. This can interfere with the absorption of insulin, resulting in erratic blood glucose levels. Because the client has been on insulin for many years, this is most likely the cause of poor control.

Test-Taking Strategy: To answer this question, you must know the principles of insulin administration and the complications. The phrase "taking insulin for many years" indicates that you must consider a long-term complication of insulin administration, such as lipodystrophy. Options 2, 3, and 4 are actually appropriate techniques to use to regulate blood glucose levels.

Level of Cognitive Ability: Analysis
Phase of Nursing Process: Analysis
Client Needs: Physiological Integrity
Content Area: Adult Health/Endocrine

Reference

Potter, P., & Perry, A. (1997). *Fundamentals of nursing: Concepts, process, and practice* (4th ed.). St. Louis: Mosby–Year Book, p. 828.

---

165. The nurse is conducting an antenatal visit for the client with a twin pregnancy. Which of the following signs should alert the nurse to a potential problem specifically related to the twin pregnancy?

1 Hypertension
2 Uterine size is large for gestational age
3 Elevated blood glucose
4 Rh-negative mother

Answer: 1

Rationale: The mother with a multiple-gestation pregnancy is at three to five times increased risk for pre-eclampsia than if she had a singleton pregnancy. Maternal well-being should be monitored for signs and symptoms of pre-eclampsia and preterm labor. A classic sign of pre-eclampsia is hypertension.

Test-Taking Strategy: Knowledge of the signs and symptoms of pre-eclampsia is required to answer this question. The primary maternal health risks in multiple pregnancy are pre-eclampsia and preterm labor. Elevated serum glucose and Rh sensitization are serious health risks, but they are not unique to a multiple pregnancy. Review the risks associated with multiple pregnancies if you had difficulty with this question.

Level of Cognitive Ability: Analysis
Phase of Nursing Process: Assessment
Client Needs: Physiological Integrity
Content Area: Maternity

Reference

Nichols, F., & Zwelling, E. (1997). *Maternal-newborn nursing: Theory and practice.* Philadelphia: W. B. Saunders, p. 639.

166. The nurse receives a report at the beginning of the shift regarding a client with an intrauterine fetal demise. Which of the following symptoms should the nurse expect to find during client assessment?

1. Elevated BP, proteinuria, and edema
2. Regression of pregnancy symptoms and absence of fetal heart tones
3. Uterine size greater than expected for gestational age
4. Intractable vomiting and dehydration

Answer: 2

Rationale: Symptoms of a fetal demise include decrease in fetal movement, no change or a decrease in fundal height, and absent fetal heart tones. Many symptoms of pregnancy may diminish, such as breast size and tenderness.

Test-Taking Strategy: "Fetal demise" means fetal death, which is confirmed by the absence of fetal heart tones and absence of fetal movement on ultrasonography. The symptoms listed in option 1 are associated with pre-eclampsia, and the symptoms listed in option 4 are associated with hyperemesis gravidarum. Option 3 is also incorrect. Review the signs associated with fetal demise if you had difficulty with this question.

Level of Cognitive Ability: Analysis
Phase of Nursing Process: Assessment
Client Needs: Physiological Integrity
Content Area: Maternity

Reference

Nichols, F., & Zwelling, E. (1997). *Maternal-newborn nursing: Theory and practice.* Philadelphia: W. B. Saunders, p. 635.

167. A client has a halo vest that was applied after a C6 spinal cord injury. Which assessment technique is most important in assisting the nurse to determine when the client is ready to begin sitting up?

1. Put both of the client's hip joints through full range of motion
2. Measure pulse and BP with bed flat and again with head of bed elevated
3. Loosen the vest to determine the client's strength of trunk support
4. Inspect the halo pin sites for drainage, redness, and pain

Answer: 2

Rationale: Clients with cervical cord injuries may lose control over peripheral vasoconstriction, causing postural (orthostatic) hypotension when upright. A drop of 15 mmHg in the systolic pressure or 10 mmHg in the diastolic pressure accompanied by an increase in heart rate when the head is elevated may indicate autonomic insufficiency that can cause dizziness or syncope in the upright position. Assessment of skin integrity of pin sites is important but does not affect sitting readiness. Hip range of motion is not affected initially in cord injury. The halo vest is not loosened by the nurse. The vest provides trunk stability for sitting.

Test-Taking Strategy: This question asks not only for an assessment technique, but also for a specific technique associated with sitting readiness. Option 3 can be easily eliminated. Options 1 and 4 are assessment techniques the nurse uses in the care of cord-injured clients, but only option 2 pertains to sitting readiness.

Level of Cognitive Ability: Application
Phase of Nursing Process: Assessment
Client Needs: Physiological Integrity
Content Area: Adult Health/Neurological

Reference

Smeltzer, S., & Bare, B. (1996). *Brunner and Suddarth's Textbook of medical-surgical nursing* (8th ed.). Philadelphia: Lippincott-Raven, pp. 1802–1804.

168. A client admitted from the emergency room has a C4 spinal cord injury. Which of the following assessments should the nurse perform first when admitting the client to the intensive care unit?

1 Take the temperature
2 Assess extremity muscle strength
3 Observe for dyskinesias
4 Listen to breath sounds

Answer: 4

Rationale: Because compromise of respiration is a leading cause of death in cervical cord injury, respiratory assessment is the highest priority. Assessment of temperature and strength can be done after adequate oxygenation is ensured. Dyskinesias occur in cerebellar disorders and are not as important in cord-injured clients, unless head injury is suspected.

Test-Taking Strategy: Remembering that a cord injury, particularly at the level of C4, can affect respiratory status can assist in directing you to the correct option. The ABCs can guide assessment priorities in this situation. Breath sounds are diminished if respiratory muscles are weakened or paralyzed.

Level of Cognitive Ability: Application
Phase of Nursing Process: Assessment
Client Needs: Physiological Integrity
Content Area: Adult Health/Neurological

Reference

Smeltzer, S., & Bare, B. (1996). *Brunner and Suddarth's Textbook of medical-surgical nursing* (8th ed.). Philadelphia: Lippincott-Raven, pp. 1685, 1797–1798.

169. In positioning a client for a surgical procedure, the nurse knows that the respiratory system is most vulnerable to which of the following positions?

1 Lithotomy
2 Supine
3 Lateral
4 Kidney (lateral)

Answer: 1

Rationale: The thoracic cage normally expands in all directions except posteriorly. In this position, the expansion of the lungs is restricted at the ribs or sternum, and there is a reduction in the ability of the diaphragm to push down against the abdominal muscles. Respiratory function is impaired because of this interference with normal movements. The volume of air that can be inspired is reduced.

Test-Taking Strategy: Options 3 and 4 are similar; therefore eliminate these options. From the remaining two options, attempt to visualize each of these positions and their effect on the process of respiration. The supine position would not interfere with the expansion of the lungs, as the lithotomy position would. Review these positions now if you had difficulty with this question.

Level of Cognitive Ability: Analysis
Phase of Nursing Process: Assessment
Client Needs: Physiological Integrity
Content Area: Fundamental Skills

Reference

Phipps, W., Cassmeyer, V., Sands, J., et al. (1995). *Medical-surgical nursing: Concepts and clinical practice* (5th ed.). St. Louis: Mosby–Year Book, pp. 619–621.

170. The client has frequent runs of ventricular tachycardia. The physician has prescribed flecainide (Tambocor), a potent antidysrhythmic medication. Which of the following actions by the nurse indicates awareness of the effects of the medications?

1. The nurse assesses the client for neurological problems
2. The nurse monitors the client's vital signs and ECG frequently
3. The nurse tells the client the bed rails have to stay up
4. The nurse monitors the client's urinary output

Answer: 2

Rationale: Flecainide is an antidysrhythmic medication that slows conduction and decreases excitability, conduction velocity, and automaticity. The nurse needs to monitor for the development of a new or worsening dysrhythmia. Options 1, 3, and 4 are components of standard care.

Test-Taking Strategy: Of significant importance with this medication is the further cardiac problems it can induce, hence the appropriate option is 2. If these problems occur, they are an indication or reason for discontinuance of the medication. Note the relationship of antidysrhythmic medication and the action in the correct option. Option 2 is the only option that relates to cardiac status monitoring. Review this medication now if you had difficulty with this question.

Level of Cognitive Ability: Analysis
Phase of Nursing Process: Evaluation
Client Needs: Physiological Integrity
Content Area: Pharmacology

Reference

Luckmann, J. (1997). *Saunders manual of nursing care.* Philadelphia: W. B. Saunders, p. 1014.

---

171. The nurse is monitoring a client with frequent PVCs of more than six PVCs per minute. The nurse is preparing to administer a bolus of lidocaine (Xylocaine), 100 mg intravenously. The nurse should monitor the client for

1. Skin temperature and neurological changes.
2. Vital signs, ECG, and neurological changes.
3. Kidney and liver function and ECG.
4. Visual changes and kidney and liver function.

Answer: 2

Rationale: Lidocaine can cause AV block with conduction defects. It also can cause paresthesia, numbness, disorientation, and agitation.

Test-Taking Strategy: Read questions with "and" in the option carefully. Remember that all parts of the option must be correct for it to be the most appropriate option. For this question, look at the entire statement. Remember this question states only that a bolus is being given, not a continuous infusion, hence option 2 is the most appropriate choice. Remember vital signs and ABCs as the first priority.

Level of Cognitive Ability: Application
Phase of Nursing Process: Implementation
Client Needs: Physiological Integrity
Content Area: Pharmacology

Reference

Hartshorn, J., Sole, M., & Lamborn, H. (1997). *Introduction to critical care nursing* (2nd ed.). Philadelphia: W. B. Saunders, p. 253.

---

172. To help reduce preload and afterload for a client with acute pulmonary edema, the nurse can expect to administer

1. Digoxin (Lanoxin).
2. Nitroprusside sodium (Nipride).
3. Morphine sulfate.
4. Furosemide (Lasix).

Answer: 2

Rationale: Intravenous nitroprusside is a potent vasodilator that reduces preload and afterload. It is the medication of choice for the client with pulmonary edema. Digoxin is a cardiac glycoside, which increases cardiac contractility. Morphine sulfate is a narcotic analgesic. Furosemide is a loop diuretic. Furosemide can diminish preload by enhancing the renal excretion of sodium and water, which reduces circulating blood volume.

Test-Taking Strategy: Knowledge of medications and their actions is needed to answer this question. Care must be taken when reading the question stem, which contains the word "and." Look for the medication that reduces both preload and afterload. Review these medications now if you had difficulty with this question.

Level of Cognitive Ability: Application
Phase of Nursing Process: Implementation
Client Needs: Physiological Integrity
Content Area: Pharmacology

Reference

Black, J., & Matassarin-Jacobs, E. (1997). *Medical-surgical nursing: Clinical management for continuity of care* (5th ed.). Philadelphia: W. B. Saunders, p. 1286.

---

173. Streptokinase (Streptase) is being administered to a client in the CCU after an acute inferior myocardial infarction. The nurse understands that the primary purpose of streptokinase is to

1 Inhibit further clot formation.
2 Reduce myocardial oxygen demand.
3 Prevent platelet aggregation.
4 Dissolve the thrombus.

Answer: 4

Rationale: Streptokinase is a thrombolytic medication that causes lysis of blood clots. Anticoagulants prevent further clot formation. Beta-blockers, nitrates, and calcium channel blockers are used to reduce myocardial oxygen demand. Streptokinase does not prevent platelet aggregation. Antiplatelet aggregation medications include aspirin (acetylsalicylic acid) and dipyridamole (Persantine).

Test-Taking Strategy: Knowledge of thrombolytic medications and their action is needed to answer this question. Remembering that streptokinase can dissolve a clot can assist in answering questions similar to this one. Review this medication now if you had difficulty with this question.

Level of Cognitive Ability: Analysis
Phase of Nursing Process: Analysis
Client Needs: Physiological Integrity
Content Area: Pharmacology

Reference

Black, J., & Matassarin-Jacobs, E. (1997). *Medical-surgical nursing: Clinical management for continuity of care* (5th ed.). Philadelphia: W. B. Saunders, pp. 1255, 1264.

---

174. For a client with pulmonary edema, the nurse establishes a goal to have the client participate in activities that reduce cardiac workload. Which of the following client actions will contribute to this goal?

1 Elevating the legs when in bed
2 Sleeping in the supine position
3 Seasoning food with AcCent
4 Using a bedside commode for stools

Answer: 4

Rationale: Using a bedside commode decreases the work of getting to the bathroom or struggling to use the bedpan. Elevating the client's legs increases venous return to the heart, increasing cardiac workload. The supine position increases respiratory effort and decreases oxygenation. This increases cardiac workload. AcCent is high in sodium.

Test-Taking Strategy: Option 2 can be eliminated because generally the supine position is not an appropriate position for a cardiac or pulmonary client. For the remaining options, note the key word "activities" in the question. Only options 1 and 4 are activities. Therefore option 3 can be eliminated. Knowledge of the effects of elevating the legs can help you to eliminate option 1, leaving option 4 as the only correct answer.

Level of Cognitive Ability: Application
Phase of Nursing Process: Planning
Client Needs: Physiological Integrity
Content Area: Adult Health/Cardiovascular

Reference

Black, J., & Matassarin-Jacobs, E. (1997). *Medical-surgical nursing: Clinical management for continuity of care* (5th ed.). Philadelphia: W. B. Saunders, pp. 1286–1289.

175. A child is sent to the school nurse by the teacher. As the nurse is assessing the child, the nurse observes that the child has a rash. The nurse suspects that the child has erythema infectiosum (fifth disease). The skin assessment that is typical of fifth disease is

1. A discrete rose-pink maculopapular rash on the trunk.
2. A highly pruritic, profuse macule-to-papule rash on the trunk.
3. A discrete pinkish red maculopapular rash that spreads rapidly to the trunk.
4. An erythema on the face that has a "slapped face" appearance.

Answer: 4

Rationale: The classic rash of erythema infectiosum, or fifth disease, is the erythema on the face. The discrete rose-pink maculopapular rash is the rash of exanthema subitum (roseola). The highly pruritic profuse macule-to-papule rash is the rash of varicella (chickenpox). The discrete pinkish red maculopapular rash is the rash of rubella (German measles).

Test-Taking Strategy: Knowledge of the characteristics associated with erythema infectiosum is required to answer the question. If you were unfamiliar with this disorder, note that in options 1, 2, and 3, a similarity exists in that the rash is mentioned on the trunk in all cases. Option 4 addresses a rash on the face. Review this disorder if you had difficulty with this question.

Level of Cognitive Ability: Analysis
Phase of Nursing Process: Assessment
Client Needs: Physiological Integrity
Content Area: Child Health

Reference

Wong, D. (1997). *Whaley and Wong's Essentials of pediatric nursing* (5th ed.). St. Louis: Mosby–Year Book, p. 405.

---

176. The client is taking a monoamine oxidase (MAO) inhibitor. Nursing assessments are based on the knowledge that

1. These medications increase the amount of MAO in the liver.
2. Hypotensive crisis may be precipitated by foods rich in tyramine and tryptophan.
3. Headache, hypertension, and nausea and vomiting may indicate toxicity.
4. Increased salivation is an expected side effect.

Answer: 3

Rationale: Headache, hypertension, tachycardia, and nausea and vomiting are precursors to hypertensive crisis brought about by the ingestion of foods rich in tyramine and tryptophan while a client is taking MAO inhibitors. These medications act by decreasing the amount of MAO in the liver, which is necessary for the breakdown and utilization of tyramine and tryptophan. Hypertensive crisis may lead to circulatory collapse, intracranial hemorrhage, and death.

Test-Taking Strategy: Knowledge of the action and side effects of MAO inhibitors is necessary to answer this question. Review the actions and side effects of the MAO inhibitors if you had difficulty with this question. You are likely to find questions related to these medications on NCLEX-RN.

Level of Cognitive Ability: Application
Phase of Nursing Process: Assessment
Client Needs: Physiological Integrity
Content Area: Pharmacology

Reference

Carson, V., & Arnold, E. (1996). *Mental health nursing: The nurse-patient journey.* Philadelphia: W. B. Saunders, p. 542.

---

177. The client has returned to the nursing unit after abdominal hysterectomy. To assess the client, who is lying supine, completely for postoperative bleeding, the nurse should do which of the following?

1. Check the abdominal dressing
2. Check the perineal pad
3. Ask the client about sensation of moistness
4. Roll client to one side after checking pad and dressing

Answer: 4

Rationale: The nurse should roll the client to one side after checking the perineal pad and abdominal dressing. This allows the nurse to check the rectal area, where blood may pool by gravity if the client is lying supine.

Test-Taking Strategy: Eliminate option 3 first as being the least plausible of all the possible options. Choose option 4 over the others because it is a more comprehensive and global assessment. The key word in the stem is "supine." This key word should assist in directing you to the correct option.

Level of Cognitive Ability: Application
Phase of Nursing Process: Assessment
Client Needs: Physiological Integrity
Content Area: Fundamental Skills

Reference

Burrell, P., Gerlach, M., & Pless, B. (1997). *Adult nursing: Acute and community care* (2nd ed.). Stamford, CT: Appleton & Lange, p. 1730.

---

178. The nurse is caring for the client who returned to the nursing unit after suprapubic prostatectomy. The nurse monitors the continuous bladder irrigation to detect which of the following signs of catheter blockage?

1 Drainage that is pale pink
2 Drainage that is bright red
3 Urine leakage around the three-way catheter at the meatus
4 True urine output of 50 mL/hour

Answer: 3

Rationale: Catheter blockage or occlusion by clots after prostatectomy can result in urine backup and leakage around the urethral meatus. This would be accompanied by a stoppage of outflow through the catheter into the drainage bag. Drainage that is bright red indicates that the irrigant is running too slowly; drainage that is pale pink indicates sufficient flow. A true urine output of 50 mL/hour indicates catheter patency.

Test-Taking Strategy: Eliminate options 1 and 2 first because of the word "drainage." This implies catheter patency. To discriminate between the last two options, apply basic principles related to Foley catheter management. A leakage around the catheter at the meatus indicates blockage.

Level of Cognitive Ability: Application
Phase of Nursing Process: Assessment
Client Needs: Physiological Integrity
Content Area: Adult Health/Renal

Reference

Burrell, P., Gerlach, M., & Pless, B. (1997). *Adult nursing: Acute and community care* (2nd ed.). Stamford, CT: Appleton & Lange, p. 1784.

---

179. The nurse is assigned to a client returning from the post–anesthesia care unit after transurethral prostatectomy. The nurse avoids doing which of the following after this procedure?

1 Reporting signs of confusion
2 Administering B&O (belladonna and opium) suppository at room temperature
3 Removing the traction tape on the three-way catheter
4 Monitoring hourly urine output

Answer: 3

Rationale: The nurse avoids removing the traction tape applied by the surgeon in the operating room. The purpose of this tape is to place pressure on the prostate and reduce hemorrhage. B&O suppositories, ordered on a PRN basis for bladder spasm, should be warmed to room temperature before administration. The nurse routinely monitors hourly urine output because the client has a three-way bladder irrigation running. The nurse also assesses for confusion, which could result from hyponatremia secondary to hypotonic irrigant used during the surgical procedure.

Test-Taking Strategy: The key word in the question is "avoid." Eliminate options 1 and 4 first because they are part of routine nursing care and would not be contraindicated in the care of this client. Choose correctly between the remaining options either through knowledge of bladder antispasmodics or through knowledge of this specific surgical procedure.

Level of Cognitive Ability: Application
Phase of Nursing Process: Implementation
Client Needs: Physiological Integrity
Content Area: Adult Health/Renal

Reference

Burrell, P., Gerlach, M., & Pless, B. (1997). *Adult nursing: Acute and community care* (2nd ed.). Stamford, CT: Appleton & Lange, p. 1784.

180. The client is due for a dose of bumetanide (Bumex). The nurse would temporarily withhold the dose and notify the physician if which of the following laboratory results was found?

1 Sodium, 137 mEq/liter
2 Potassium, 2.9 mEq/liter
3 Magnesium, 2.5 mEq/liter
4 Chloride, 106 mEq/liter

Answer: 2

Rationale: Bumetanide is a loop diuretic, which is not potassium sparing. The value given for potassium is below the therapeutic range of 3.5–5.0 mEq/liter for this electrolyte. The nurse should notify the physician before giving the dose.

Test-Taking Strategy: This question tests a basic concept related to the effect of loop diuretics on potassium level. In addition, knowledge of the normal potassium level directs you to the correct option. Review this medication now if you had difficulty with this question.

Level of Cognitive Ability: Application
Phase of Nursing Process: Implementation
Client Needs: Physiological Integrity
Content Area: Pharmacology

Reference

Deglin, J., & Vallerand, A. (1997). *Davis's drug guide for nurses* (5th ed.). Philadelphia: F. A. Davis, p. 393.

---

181. The client with heart failure is receiving furosemide and digoxin (Lanoxin) daily. The client complains of anorexia, nausea, and yellow vision when the nurse enters the room to administer the morning medication doses. The nurse should plan to do which of the following first?

1 Administer the medications
2 Give the digoxin only
3 Check the morning serum potassium level
4 Check the morning serum digoxin level

Answer: 4

Rationale: The nurse should check for the result of the digoxin level that was drawn because the symptoms are compatible with digoxin toxicity. Knowing that a low potassium level may contribute to digoxin toxicity, checking the serum potassium level may give useful additive information. The digoxin should be withheld until the level is known, making options 1 and 2 incorrect.

Test-Taking Strategy: Note that the key word in this question is "first." Eliminate options 1 and 2 first because it is not prudent to administer the medication(s) without doing further investigation. Use knowledge of the mechanisms of digoxin toxicity to choose correctly between options 3 and 4. Review the signs of digoxin toxicity if you had difficulty with this question.

Level of Cognitive Ability: Application
Phase of Nursing Process: Planning
Client Needs: Physiological Integrity
Content Area: Pharmacology

Reference

Hodgson, B., & Kizior, R. (1998). *Saunders nursing drug handbook 1998.* Philadelphia: W. B. Saunders, pp. 452–454.

---

182. The nurse is administering an oral dose of erythromycin (E-Mycin) to an assigned client. The nurse gives this medication with

1 A full glass of milk.
2 A full glass of water.
3 A sip of orange juice.
4 Any noncitrus beverage.

Answer: 2

Rationale: Erythromycin is a macrolide antibiotic that should be taken with a full glass of water. Sufficient volume is needed to obtain maximal effect of the medication. Depending on the specific type of erythromycin, it may need to be administered on an empty stomach, with meals, or regardless of timing of meals. The nurse should verify the best method of administration for the type ordered.

Test-Taking Strategy: Eliminate options 3 and 4 first as being the least plausible. Specific knowledge of this medication is needed to discriminate between the final two options. Take a few moments to review this medication if you had difficulty with this question.

Level of Cognitive Ability: Application
Phase of Nursing Process: Implementation
Client Needs: Physiological Integrity
Content Area: Pharmacology

Reference

Deglin, J., & Vallerand, A. (1997). *Davis's drug guide for nurses* (5th ed.). Philadelphia: F. A. Davis, p. 441.

---

183. The nurse has given the client a dose of intravenous hydralazine (Apresoline). The nurse evaluates the effectiveness of the medication by monitoring which of the following client parameters?

1 Blood pressure (BP)
2 Cardiac rhythm
3 Urine output
4 Blood glucose level

Answer: 1

Rationale: Hydralazine is an antihypertensive medication used in the management of moderate-to-severe hypertension. It is a vasodilator medication that decreases afterload. The BP needs to be monitored.

Test-Taking Strategy: Note the name of the medication: A*pres*oline. This focus should direct you to option 1. If the medication is unfamiliar to you, review it now.

Level of Cognitive Ability: Analysis
Phase of Nursing Process: Evaluation
Client Needs: Physiological Integrity
Content Area: Pharmacology

Reference

Hodgson, B., & Kizior, R. (1998). *Saunders nursing drug handbook 1998.* Philadelphia: W. B. Saunders, pp. 493–494.

---

184. The client with a fractured femur who has had an open reduction–internal fixation is receiving ketorolac (Toradol). The nurse evaluates the effectiveness of the medication by monitoring the client's

1 Serum calcium level.
2 WBC count.
3 Temperature.
4 Pain rating.

Answer: 4

Rationale: Ketorolac is a nonopioid analgesic and nonsteroidal anti-inflammatory drug (NSAID). It acts by inhibiting prostaglandin synthesis and produces analgesia that is peripherally mediated. The nurse evaluates the effectiveness of this medication by using the pain rating scale with the client.

Test-Taking Strategy: Familiarity with this medication is needed to answer this question accurately. The diagnosis of the client, fractured femur, may provide you with the clue that this medication is an analgesic. Review this medication if needed.

Level of Cognitive Ability: Analysis
Phase of Nursing Process: Evaluation
Client Needs: Physiological Integrity
Content Area: Pharmacology

Reference

Hodgson, B., & Kizior, R. (1998). *Saunders nursing drug handbook 1998.* Philadelphia: W. B. Saunders, pp. 568–570.

---

185. The client receiving a dose of intravenous vancomycin (Vancocin) develops chills, tachycardia, syncope, and flushing of the face and trunk. The nurse interprets that

1 The client is allergic to the medication.
2 The medication has interacted with another medication the client is receiving.
3 The medication is infusing too rapidly.
4 The client is experiencing upper airway obstruction.

Answer: 3

Rationale: The client is experiencing signs and symptoms of what is called "red man" or "red neck" syndrome. This is a response caused by histamine release with rapid or bolus injection. The client may experience chills; fever; flushing of the face, trunk, or both; tachycardia; syncope; tingling; and an unpleasant taste in the mouth. The corrective action is to administer the medication more slowly. An antihistamine such as diphenhydramine (Benadryl) may be administered as well.

Test-Taking Strategy: This question may be difficult, and you may want to quickly select option 1. Knowledge regarding this specific medication is necessary to answer the question. Remember that options that are similar are not likely to be correct. For this reason, begin to answer this question by eliminating options 1 and 4 first. Use medication knowledge to differentiate between the two remaining options, and if you had difficulty with the question, take the time now to review.

Level of Cognitive Ability: Analysis
Phase of Nursing Process: Analysis
Client Needs: Physiological Integrity
Content Area: Pharmacology

Reference

McKenry, L., & Salerno, E. (1998). *Mosby's pharmacology in nursing* (20th ed.). St. Louis: Mosby–Year Book, p. 914.

---

186. The client has an order to be given beclomethasone by intranasal route. The client also has an order for a nasal decongestant. Which of the following methods of administration by the nurse is correct?

1 Administer the beclomethasone 15 minutes before the decongestant
2 Administer the decongestant 15 minutes before the beclomethasone
3 Administer the beclomethasone immediately before the decongestant
4 Administer the decongestant immediately before the beclomethasone

Answer: 2

Rationale: The nasal decongestant should be administered 15 minutes before the beclomethasone (a glucocorticoid) to clear the nasal passages and enhance absorption of the medication.

Test-Taking Strategy: Use the same principles in answering this question that you would when administering bronchodilators and corticosteroids together. These principles can help you choose the correct option easily.

Level of Cognitive Ability: Application
Phase of Nursing Process: Implementation
Client Needs: Physiological Integrity
Content Area: Pharmacology

Reference

Deglin, J., & Vallerand, A. (1997). *Davis's drug guide for nurses* (5th ed.). Philadelphia: F. A. Davis, pp. 537, 541.

---

187. The client has received atropine sulfate intravenously during a surgical procedure. The nurse monitors the client for which of the following effects of atropine in the immediate postoperative period?

1 Bradycardia
2 Excessive salivation
3 Diarrhea
4 Urinary retention

Answer: 4

Rationale: Atropine is an anticholinergic medication that causes tachycardia, drowsiness, blurred vision, dry mouth, constipation, and urinary hesitancy. The nurse monitors the client for any of these effects in the immediate postoperative period.

Test-Taking Strategy: Specific knowledge of the action and effects of this medication is needed to answer this question accurately. Review the side effects of this important medication if you had difficulty with this question.

Level of Cognitive Ability: Application
Phase of Nursing Process: Assessment
Client Needs: Physiological Integrity
Content Area: Pharmacology

Reference

Hodgson, B., & Kizior, R. (1998). *Saunders nursing drug handbook 1998.* Philadelphia: W. B. Saunders, pp. 82–85.

188. The client is receiving tobramycin (Tobrex). The nurse evaluates that the client is responding well to the medication therapy if which of the following laboratory results is noted?

1 WBC count of 8000/mm^3 and creatinine concentration of 0.9 mg/dL
2 WBC count of 15,000/mm^3 and BUN concentration of 38 mg/dL
3 Sodium level of 140 mEq/liter and potassium level of 3.9 mEq/liter
4 Sodium level of 145 mEq/liter and chloride level of 106 mEq/liter

Answer: 1

Rationale: Tobramycin is an antibiotic (aminoglycoside) that causes nephrotoxicity and ototoxicity. The medication is working if the WBC count drops back into the normal range and the kidney function remains normal. Option 2 indicates an abnormal WBC count, and options 3 and 4 are unrelated to this medication.

Test-Taking Strategy: Begin to answer this question by eliminating options 3 and 4 first knowing that tobramycin is an antibiotic. Knowing that aminoglycosides cause nephrotoxicity, you would then choose option 1 over option 2 as correct, using laboratory values as your guide. Review this medication and normal laboratory values if you had difficulty with this question.

Level of Cognitive Ability: Analysis
Phase of Nursing Process: Evaluation
Client Needs: Physiological Integrity
Content Area: Pharmacology

Reference
Hodgson, B., & Kizior, R. (1998). *Saunders nursing drug handbook 1998*. Philadelphia: W. B. Saunders, pp. 998–1000.

189. Nursing interventions for the client taking maintenance dosages of lithium carbonate (Eskalith) include

1 Monitoring daily serum lithium levels.
2 Performing weekly ECG.
3 Observing for remission of depressive states.
4 Monitoring intake and output.

Answer: 4

Rationale: Lithium is used to treat manic disorders, not depression. Side effects of lithium are nausea, tremors, polyuria, and polydipsia. Serum lithium concentration is assessed approximately every 2–4 days during initial therapy and at longer intervals thereafter. Toxic levels of lithium may induce ECG changes; however, there is no need to perform weekly ECGs if maintenance levels are maintained.

Test-Taking Strategy: Eliminate options 1 and 2 first because of the words "daily" and "weekly." Knowledge of the side effects and the use of the medication can direct you to the correct option. If you had difficulty with this question, take time now to review.

Level of Cognitive Ability: Application
Phase of Nursing Process: Implementation
Client Needs: Physiological Integrity
Content Area: Pharmacology

Reference
Hodgson, B., & Kizior, R. (1998). *Saunders nursing drug handbook 1998*. Philadelphia: W. B. Saunders, pp. 598–600.

190. In assessing the client with neuroleptic malignant syndrome (NMS) resulting from the use of antipsychotic medications, the nurse would expect to find

1 Bradycardia.
2 Dysphagia.
3 Hypotension.
4 Hyperpyrexia.

Answer: 4

Rationale: Hyperpyrexia up to 107°F may be present in NMS. Symptoms develop suddenly and may include respiratory distress and muscle rigidity. As the condition progresses, there is evidence of tachycardia, hypertension, increasing respiratory distress, confusion, and delirium.

Test-Taking Strategy: Consider the physiological responses that occur in NMS to answer this question. Options 1 and 3 normally occur in conjunction with each other, and because there can be only one response, they can be eliminated. The term "malignant" in the case situation can be associated with hyperthermia, making option 4 the most likely response. Review the physiological manifestations that occur in NMS if you had difficulty with this question.

Level of Cognitive Ability: Analysis
Phase of Nursing Process: Assessment
Client Needs: Physiological Integrity
Content Area: Pharmacology

Reference

Townsend, M. (1996). *Psychiatric–mental health nursing: Concepts of care* (2nd ed.). Philadelphia: F. A. Davis, p. 286.

---

191. The nurse is performing an admission assessment on a newborn admitted with the diagnosis of subdural hematoma after a difficult vaginal delivery. The nurse assesses for major symptoms associated with subdural hematoma when the nurse

1. Tests for contractures of the extremities.
2. Tests for equality of extremities when stimulating reflexes.
3. Monitors for urinary output pattern.
4. Monitors urine for blood.

Answer: 2

Rationale: A subdural hematoma can cause pressure on a specific area of the cerebral tissue. This can, especially if actively bleeding, cause changes in the stimulus responses in the extremities on the opposite side of the body. Option 1 is not correct because contractures would not occur this soon after delivery. Options 3 and 4 are incorrect. An infant after delivery would normally be incontinent of urine, and blood in the urine would indicate abdominal trauma and not be a result of the subdural hematoma.

Test-Taking Strategy: The method of assessing for complications and active bleeding into the cranial cavity is a neurological assessment. Checking newborn reflexes is a basic neurological assessment. Some prioritizing is needed when answering this question because contractures of extremities could occur as residual effects but not immediately at the time of injury. You would then choose option 2 as the only correct answer.

Level of Cognitive Ability: Application
Phase of Nursing Process: Assessment
Client Needs: Physiological Integrity
Content Area: Maternity

Reference

Nichols, F., & Zwelling, E. (1997). *Maternal-newborn nursing: Theory and practice*. Philadelphia: W. B. Saunders, p. 1114.

---

192. The nurse is performing an admission assessment on a client admitted with a diagnosis of Raynaud's disease. Assessment for the symptoms associated with Raynaud's disease is performed when the nurse

1. Observes for softening of the nails or nail beds.
2. Palpates for diminished or absent peripheral pulses.
3. Checks for rash on the digits.
4. Palpates for rapid or irregular peripheral pulses.

Answer: 2

Rationale: Raynaud's disease produces closure of the small arteries in the distal extremities in response to cold, vibration, or external stimuli. Palpation for diminished or absent peripheral pulses checks for interruption of circulation. The nails grow slowly, become brittle or deformed, and heal poorly around nail beds when infected. Skin changes include hair loss, thinning or tightening of the skin, and delayed healing of cuts or injuries. Peripheral pulses may be normal, absent, or diminished.

Test-Taking Strategy: Knowledge of the physiological occurrences in Raynaud's disease can assist in answering the question. Using the ABCs assists in directing you to the correct option. Review the manifestations associated with this disorder if you had difficulty with this question.

Level of Cognitive Ability: Application
Phase of Nursing Process: Assessment
Client Needs: Physiological Integrity
Content Area: Adult Health/Cardiovascular

Reference

Luckmann, J. (1997). *Saunders manual of nursing care*. Philadelphia: W. B. Saunders, pp. 1115–1116.

193. A depressed client is found unconscious on the floor in the room. The nurse sees several empty bottles of a prescribed tricyclic antidepressant lying near the client. The immediate action of the nurse is to

1. Call a "code" because this incident presents a medical emergency.
2. Induce vomiting then notify the physician for further orders.
3. Call Poison Control.
4. Try to figure out the number of pills taken.

Answer: 1

Rationale: Tricyclic antidepressants can be fatal when taken as an overdose regardless of the amount ingested. Serious, life-threatening symptoms can develop after an overdose. Immediate emergency medical attention and cardiac monitoring is necessary with an overdose of tricylics.

Test-Taking Strategy: "Immediate" is the key word to answer this question and alludes to a quick, effective response. Eliminate options 3 and 4 because these measures delay immediate treatment. The client is unconscious; therefore the nurse is not to induce vomiting because of the risk of aspiration.

Level of Cognitive Ability: Application
Phase of Nursing Process: Implementation
Client Needs: Physiological Integrity
Content Area: Mental Health

Reference
Carson, V., & Arnold, E. (1996). *Mental health nursing: The nurse-patient journey.* Philadelphia: W. B. Saunders, p. 539.

---

194. The client is admitted with acute exacerbation of COPD. Which of the following blood gas results would the nurse most likely expect to note?

1. PO_2 of 68 and PCO_2 of 40
2. PO_2 of 55 and PCO_2 of 40
3. PO_2 of 70 and PCO_2 of 50
4. PO_2 of 60 and PCO_2 of 50

Answer: 4

Rationale: During an acute exacerbation, the arterial blood gases deteriorate with decreasing PO_2 and increasing PCO_2. In early stages of COPD, arterial blood gases demonstrate mild-to-moderate hypoxemia with the PO_2 in the high 60s to high 70s (mmHg) and normal arterial PCO_2. As the condition advances, hypoxemia increases, and hypercapnia may result.

Test-Taking Strategy: Knowledge regarding the physiological manifestations that occur in COPD is required to answer the question. Remembering that in COPD a low PO_2 and an elevated PCO_2 is the likely occurrence can assist in directing you to the correct option. Review the clinical manifestations that are likely to occur if you had difficulty with this question.

Level of Cognitive Ability: Analysis
Phase of Nursing Process: Analysis
Client Needs: Physiological Integrity
Content Area: Adult Health/Respiratory

Reference
Black, J., & Matassarin-Jacobs, E. (1997). *Medical-surgical nursing: Clinical management for continuity of care* (5th ed.). Philadelphia: W. B. Saunders, pp. 1108, 1113.

---

195. The nurse monitors the respiratory status of the client being treated for acute exacerbation of COPD. Which of the following assessment findings would indicate a deterioration in ventilation?

1. Cyanosis
2. Rapid, shallow respirations
3. Hyperinflated chest
4. Coarse crackles bilaterally

Answer: 2

Rationale: An increase in the rate of respirations and a decrease in the depth of respirations indicates a deterioration in ventilation. Cyanosis is not a good indicator of oxygenation in the client with COPD and may be present with some clients but not all clients. A hyperinflated chest (barrel-chest) and hypertrophy of the accessory muscles of the upper chest and neck may normally be found in clients with severe COPD. During an exacerbation, coarse crackles are expected to be heard bilaterally throughout the lungs.

Test-Taking Strategy: Note the key phrase "deterioration in ventilation." Keeping in mind the normal clinical signs seen in COPD and during an exacerbation, you can eliminate options 3 and 4. Because cyanosis is not a good indicator of oxygenation in the client with COPD, eliminate option 1. Review the clinical manifestations associated with COPD if you had difficulty with this question.

Level of Cognitive Ability: Analysis
Phase of Nursing Process: Assessment
Client Needs: Physiological Integrity
Content Area: Adult Health/Respiratory

Reference

Black, J., & Matassarin-Jacobs, E. (1997). *Medical-surgical nursing: Clinical management for continuity of care* (5th ed.). Philadelphia: W. B. Saunders, pp. 1109–1110.

---

196. Which of the following most appropriately determines the effectiveness of postural drainage and chest physiotherapy in the client with COPD?

1 The client expectorates large amounts of sputum
2 The client's cough is suppressed
3 The client is able to maintain the necessary position for postural drainage and chest physiotherapy
4 The client's expiration time becomes less prolonged

Answer: 1

Rationale: Postural drainage and chest physiotherapy aid in improving airway clearance by mobilizing secretions to make them easier to expectorate. It is necessary for the client to cough effectively to expectorate secretions. The ability to maintain the necessary position for these respiratory treatments does not evaluate the effectiveness of the treatment. It is a normal expectation that clients with even stable COPD will demonstrate a prolonged expiration time that exceeds 4 seconds.

Test-Taking Strategy: Note the key phrase "determines the effectiveness." Keeping this in mind as well as the purpose of chest physiotherapy and postural drainage can assist in directing you to the correct option. Options 2 and 3 do not determine effectiveness. Option 4 is a normal expectation and has no relationship to these respiratory treatments.

Level of Cognitive Ability: Analysis
Phase of Nursing Process: Evaluation
Client Needs: Physiological Integrity
Content Area: Adult Health/Respiratory

Reference

Lammon, C. B., Foote, A. W., Leli, P. G., et al. (1995). *Clinical nursing skills.* Philadelphia: W. B. Saunders, pp. 529–533.

---

197. During the administration of a blood transfusion to a client, the nurse suspects circulatory overload. Which of the following is not a clinical indication of circulatory overload?

1 Decreased central venous pressure
2 Lumbar pain
3 Crackles in the lung bases
4 Distended neck veins

Answer: 1

Rationale: Chest or lumbar pain, cyanosis, dyspnea, moist productive cough, crackles (rales) in lung bases, distended neck veins, and an increase in central venous pressure are clinical indications of circulatory overload caused from excessive infusion amounts or too rapid an infusion rate. The blood should be discontinued.

Test-Taking Strategy: The key words are "not" and "overload." This should assist in eliminating options 3 and 4. From the remaining two options, recall that decreased central venous pressure is noted in circulatory volume deficit. This concept can direct you to the correct option. Review the signs of circulatory overload and deficit if you had difficulty with this question.

Level of Cognitive Ability: Analysis
Phase of Nursing Process: Assessment
Client Needs: Physiological Integrity
Content Area: Fundamental Skills

Reference

Black, J., & Matassarin-Jacobs, E. (1997). *Medical-surgical nursing: Clinical management for continuity of care* (5th ed.). Philadelphia: W. B. Saunders, p. 1529.

198. Diazepam (Valium) is prescribed for the client with anxiety. The nurse should instruct the client to expect which side effect?

1 Ataxia
2 Cough
3 Tinnitus
4 Hypertension

Answer: 1

Rationale: Valium, a benzodiazepine, can cause motor incoordination and ataxia, and safety precautions should be instituted for clients taking this medication. Options 2, 3, and 4 are unrelated to this medication.

Test-Taking Strategy: Knowledge of the side effects of this medication is required to answer the question. Recalling that many of the medications used to treat anxiety can cause incoordination can assist in answering the question. Review the side effects of this medication if you had difficulty with this question.

Level of Cognitive Ability: Application
Phase of Nursing Process: Implementation
Client Needs: Physiological Integrity
Content Area: Pharmacology

Reference

Hodgson, B., & Kizior, R. (1998). *Saunders nursing drug handbook 1998.* Philadelphia: W. B. Saunders, pp. 307–309.

---

199. The client receives oxytocin (Pitocin) to induce labor. During the administration of Pitocin, it is most important for the nurse to monitor the

1 Urinary output.
2 Fetal heart rate.
3 Central venous pressure.
4 Maternal blood glucose.

Answer: 2

Rationale: Pitocin produces uterine contractions. Uterine contractions can cause fetal anoxia. Monitor fetal heart rate and notify the physician of any significant changes. Options 1, 3, and 4 are unrelated to the administration of this medication.

Test-Taking Strategy: Use the ABCs to answer the question. Review the actions and nursing implications associated with the administration of this medication if you had difficulty with this question.

Level of Cognitive Ability: Application
Phase of Nursing Process: Assessment
Client Needs: Physiological Integrity
Content Area: Pharmacology

Reference

Hodgson, B., & Kizior, R. (1998). *Saunders nursing drug handbook 1998.* Philadelphia: W. B. Saunders, pp. 781–783.

---

200. Drug toxicity is more likely to occur in the neonate because

1 The lungs are immature.
2 The kidneys are smaller.
3 Cerebral function is not fully developed.
4 The liver is not fully developed.

Answer: 4

Rationale: The liver is not fully developed in the neonate and cannot detoxify many drugs.

Test-Taking Strategy: Knowledge regarding the physiological maturity normally associated with the neonate is required to answer the question. Knowledge that the liver is associated with the detoxification of medications can assist in directing you to the correct option. Take time now to review the normal physiological findings in the neonate if you had difficulty with this question.

Level of Cognitive Ability: Analysis
Phase of Nursing Process: Analysis
Client Needs: Physiological Integrity
Content Area: Maternity

Reference

Clark, J., Queener, S., & Karb, V. (1997). *Pharmacologic basis of nursing practice.* St. Louis: Mosby–Year Book, p. 16.

201. The client is hospitalized for ingesting an overdose of acetaminophen (Tylenol). The nurse prepares to administer which specific antidote for this medication overdose?

1. Protamine sulfate
2. Naloxone (Narcan)
3. Acetylcysteine sodium (Mucomyst)
4. Vitamin K

Answer: 3

Rationale: Acetylcysteine sodium restores sulfhydryl groups that are depleted by acetaminophen metabolism. Vitamin K is the antidote for warfarin (Coumadin). Naloxone reverses respiratory depression. Protamine sulfate is the antidote for heparin.

Test-Taking Strategy: Knowledge regarding the specific antidotes for overdose is required to answer this question. Recalling the specific antidotes for both heparin and warfarin can assist in eliminating options 1 and 4. Recalling that naloxone reverses respiratory depression can assist in eliminating option 2. Review these antidotes now if you had difficulty with this question.

Level of Cognitive Ability: Analysis
Phase of Nursing Process: Planning
Client Needs: Physiological Integrity
Content Area: Pharmacology

Reference

Hodgson, B., & Kizior, R. (1998). *Saunders nursing drug handbook 1998.* Philadelphia: W. B. Saunders, pp. 6–8.

---

202. A mother arrives at the emergency room with her child stating that she just found the child sitting on the floor next to an empty bottle of aspirin. On assessment, the nurse notes that the child is drowsy but conscious. The nurse prepares to administer

1. Ipecac syrup.
2. Activated charcoal.
3. Magnesium citrate.
4. Magnesium sulfate.

Answer: 1

Rationale: Ipecac is administered to induce vomiting. In this scenario, the child is conscious and the ingested poison will not damage the esophagus or lungs; therefore the safest and most appropriate measure is to administer ipecac syrup. Activated charcoal may be used as an antidote in some poisons, but its action is to absorb ingested toxic substances. Options 3 and 4 are unrelated to treatment for this occurrence.

Test-Taking Strategy: You can easily eliminate options 3 and 4. From the remaining two options, note that the child is conscious. Also determine the effect that the specific poison may have on the esophagus if vomited. Noting that the question states that the child was "just" found and considering that this ingestion will not harm the esophagus should assist in directing you to option 1. Review measures to treat aspirin poisoning if you had difficulty with this question.

Level of Cognitive Ability: Application
Phase of Nursing Process: Planning
Client Needs: Physiological Integrity
Content Area: Pharmacology

Reference

Clark, J., Queener, S., & Karb, V. (1997). *Pharmacologic basis of nursing practice.* St. Louis: Mosby–Year Book, p. 369.

203. The nurse evaluates the correct use of the walker by the client. When evaluating, the nurse would expect to note which of the following?

1 The client puts all four points of the walker flat on the floor, puts weight on the hand pieces, and then walks into it
2 The client puts weight on the hand pieces, moves the walker forward, and then walks into it
3 The client puts weight on the hand pieces, slides the walker forward, and then walks into it
4 The client walks into the walker, puts weight on the hand pieces, and then puts all four points of the walker flat on the floor

Answer: 1

Rationale: When the client uses a walker, stand adjacent to the affected side. Instruct the client to put all four points of the walker 2 feet forward flat on the floor before putting weight on the hand pieces. This ensures client safety and prevents stress cracks in the walker. Instruct the client to move the walker forward and walk into it.

Test-Taking Strategy: Attempt to visualize each of the options. Options 2 and 3 can be eliminated because putting weight on the hand pieces initially would cause an unsafe situation. From the remaining two options, recalling that the walker is placed on all four points first can assist in directing you to option 1. Review this procedure now if you had difficulty with this question.

Level of Cognitive Ability: Analysis
Phase of Nursing Process: Evaluation
Client Needs: Physiological Integrity
Content Area: Fundamental Skills

Reference

Lammon, C. B., Foote, A. W., Leli, P. G., et al. (1995). *Clinical nursing skills.* Philadelphia: W. B. Saunders, pp. 245–247.

---

204. When evaluating for the correct height of crutches, the nurse would expect to note which of the following?

1 The client is able to rest the axillae on the axillary bars
2 The nurse is able to place two fingers comfortably between the axillae and the axillary bars
3 The client is able to maintain the arms in a straight position when standing with the crutches
4 The nurse is able to place four fingers comfortably between the axillae and the axillary bars

Answer: 2

Rationale: With the client's elbows flexed 20–30 degrees, the shoulders in a relaxed position, and the crutches placed approximately 15 cm (6 inches) anterolateral from the toes, the nurse should be able to place two fingers comfortably between the axillae and the axillary bars. Adjust the crutches if there is too much or too little space at the axillary area. Advise the client never to rest the axillae on the axillary bars because this could injure the brachial plexus (the nerves in the axillae that supply the arm and shoulder area). Terminate ambulation and recheck the crutch height if the client complains of numbness or tingling in the hands or arms.

Test-Taking Strategy: Knowledge regarding the safe use of crutches is required to answer the question. Attempt to visualize each of the options and eliminate those that are not reasonable and would not provide safety. Take time now to review this important procedure if you had difficulty with this question.

Level of Cognitive Ability: Analysis
Phase of Nursing Process: Evaluation
Client Needs: Physiological Integrity
Content Area: Fundamental Skills

Reference

Lammon, C. B., Foote, A. W., Leli, P. G., et al. (1995). *Clinical nursing skills.* Philadelphia: W. B. Saunders, p. 240.

---

205. A client with myasthenia gravis is admitted to the hospital. The nursing history reveals that the client is taking pyridostigmine (Mestinon). The nurse assesses the client for adverse effects of the medication, which would include

1 Muscle cramps.
2 Mouth ulcers.
3 Depression.
4 Unexplained weight gain.

Answer: 1

Rationale: Mestinon is an acetylcholinesterase inhibitor. Muscle cramps and small muscle contractions are side effects and occur as a result of overstimulation of neuromuscular receptors.

Test-Taking Strategy: Knowledge that myasthenia gravis is a neuromuscular disorder can assist in directing you to the option that is most closely associated with this disorder, option 1. Take time to review the side effects associated with this medication if you had difficulty with this question.

Level of Cognitive Ability: Analysis
Phase of Nursing Process: Assessment
Client Needs: Physiological Integrity
Content Area: Pharmacology

Reference

Hodgson, B., & Kizior, R. (1998). *Saunders nursing drug handbook 1998.* Philadelphia: W. B. Saunders, pp. 888–890.

---

206. A client with a fractured right ankle has a short leg plaster cast applied. During discharge teaching, the nurse should provide which of the following information to prevent complications?

1. Keep the right ankle elevated above the heart with pillows for 24–48 hours
2. Bear weight on the right leg only after the cast is dry
3. Expect burning and tingling sensations under the cast for 3–4 days
4. Trim the rough edges of the cast after it is dry

Answer: 1

Rationale: Leg elevation is important to increase venous return and decrease edema, which can cause compartment syndrome, a major complication of fractures and casting. Option 2 is incorrect because weight bearing on a fractured extremity is determined by the physician during follow-up examination after x-ray. Although the client may feel heat after the cast is applied, burning or tingling sensation indicates nerve damage and ischemia and is not expected; burning or tingling should be reported immediately. Option 4 is incorrect because any cast modifications need to be done by trained personnel under medical supervision. The client or family may be taught how to "petal" the cast to prevent skin irritation and breakdown.

Test-Taking Strategy: Knowledge of cast care and complications of casting is essential to answer this question correctly. Skin breakdown, compartment syndrome, cast damage, and venous thrombosis are all potential complications associated with casting. Use the ABCs. Option 1 is associated with maintenance of circulation.

Level of Cognitive Ability: Application
Phase of Nursing Process: Implementation
Client Needs: Physiological Integrity
Content Area: Adult Health/Musculoskeletal

Reference

Lammon, C. B., Foote, A. W., Leli, P. G., et al. (1995). *Clinical nursing skills.* Philadelphia: W. B. Saunders, p. 279.

---

207. An older female client with a fractured left tibia has a long leg cast and is using crutches to ambulate. In caring for the client, the nurse should be alert for which of the following signs and symptoms of complications associated with crutch walking?

1. Forearm muscle weakness
2. Left leg paresthesias
3. Tricep muscle spasms
4. Weak biceps brachii

Answer: 1

Rationale: Forearm muscle weakness is a sign of radial nerve injury caused by crutch pressure on the axillae. When clients lack upper body strength, especially in the flexor and extensor muscles of the arms, they frequently allow their weight to rest on their axillae instead of their arms while ambulating with crutches. Older women tend to have poor upper body strength. Option 2 is a sign of compartment syndrome, a complication of fractures, not crutch walking. Option 3 is incorrect because it might occur as a result of increased muscle use but is not a complication of crutch walking. Option 4 is a common physical assessment finding in older adults, especially women, and is not a complication of crutch walking.

Test-Taking Strategy: Knowledge of anatomy and correct crutch walking is helpful in answering this question. When asked about a complication of the use of crutches, think about nerve injury caused by crutch pressure on the axillae. Review this complication now if you had difficulty with this question.

Level of Cognitive Ability: Application
Phase of Nursing Process: Assessment
Client Needs: Physiological Integrity
Content Area: Adult Health/Musculoskeletal

Reference

Lammon, C. B., Foote, A. W., Leli, P. G., et al. (1995). *Clinical nursing skills.* Philadelphia: W. B. Saunders, p. 243.

208. A client with myasthenia gravis is experiencing prolonged periods of weakness. The physician orders a test dose of edrophonium (Tensilon), and the client becomes weaker. The result of the test dose can be interpreted as

1 Normal.
2 Positive.
3 Myasthenia crisis.
4 Cholinergic crisis.

Answer: 4

Rationale: Tensilon is administered to differentiate overdose of medication (cholinergic crisis) from worsening symptoms of the disease (myasthenic crisis). Worsening of the symptoms after the medication is administered indicates a cholinergic crisis, or negative Tensilon test.

Test-Taking Strategy: Knowledge regarding the Tensilon test and the interpretation of the results is required to answer the question. It is important to be familiar with this test and to distinguish between cholinergic and myasthenic crisis. You are likely to find questions related to this test on NCLEX-RN.

Level of Cognitive Ability: Analysis
Phase of Nursing Process: Analysis
Client Needs: Physiological Integrity
Content Area: Adult Health/Neurological

Reference

Clark, J., Queener, S., & Karb, V. (1997). *Pharmacologic basis of nursing practice.* St. Louis: Mosby–Year Book, pp. 449–450.

---

209. The nurse notes an isolated PVC on the cardiac monitor. On the basis of the assessment of this rhythm, the nurse's action is to

1 Continue to monitor the rhythm.
2 Notify the physician immediately.
3 Prepare for defibrillation.
4 Administer the ordered lidocaine.

Answer: 1

Rationale: As an isolated occurrence, the PVC is not life-threatening. In this situation, the client should be monitored. Frequent PVCs, however, may be precursors of more life-threatening rhythms, such as ventricular tachycardia and ventricular fibrillation. If this occurs, the physician needs to be notified.

Test-Taking Strategy: Note the key word "isolated." This should assist in directing you to the option that addresses continual monitoring. If you had difficulty with this question, take time now to review the implications of PVCs and the associated interventions.

Level of Cognitive Ability: Analysis
Phase of Nursing Process: Implementation
Client Needs: Physiological Integrity
Content Area: Adult Health/Cardiovascular

Reference

Black, J., & Matassarin-Jacobs, E. (1997). *Medical-surgical nursing: Clinical management for continuity of care* (5th ed.). Philadelphia: W. B. Saunders, p. 1305.

---

210. The nurse is caring for a client admitted with the diagnosis of active tuberculosis. The nurse has determined that this diagnosis is confirmed by a

1 Positive Mantoux test.
2 Positive sputum culture.
3 Positive tine test.
4 Positive chest x-ray.

Answer: 2

Rationale: Sputum culture of *M. tuberculosis* confirms the diagnosis of tuberculosis. Usually three sputum samples are obtained for the acid-fast smear. After the start of therapy, sputum samples are obtained again to determine the effectiveness of therapy. A positive tine or Mantoux test indicates exposure to tuberculosis but does not confirm the presence of *M. tuberculosis.* A positive chest x-ray may indicate the presence of tuberculosis lesions but again does not confirm active disease.

Test-Taking Strategy: Note the key word "confirmed" in the stem of the question. Active tuberculosis can be confirmed only by the presence of the acid-fast bacilli. The sputum culture is the only method of determining the presence of this organism.

Level of Cognitive Ability: Analysis
Phase of Nursing Process: Assessment
Client Needs: Physiological Integrity
Content Area: Adult Health/Respiratory

Reference

Black, J., & Matassarin-Jacobs, E. (1997). *Medical-surgical nursing: Clinical management for continuity of care* (5th ed.). Philadelphia: W. B. Saunders, p. 1142.

---

211. The nurse assesses the fundal height in a client in the second trimester of pregnancy. When measuring fundal height on the client, the nurse will most likely expect

1. The measurement to correlate with gestational age.
2. The measurement to be greater than gestational age.
3. The measurement to be lesser than gestational age.
4. The measurement to have no correlation to gestational age.

Answer: 1

Rationale: Up until the third trimester, the measurement of fundal height, on average, correlates with the gestational age.

Test-Taking Strategy: Note the key phrase "second trimester." Use this key phrase and knowledge regarding fundal height and gestational age to answer the question. If you had difficulty with this question, review this prenatal assessment now.

Level of Cognitive Ability: Analysis
Phase of Nursing Process: Assessment
Client Needs: Physiological Integrity
Content Area: Maternity

Reference

Nichols, F., & Zwelling, E. (1997). *Maternal-newborn nursing: Theory and practice.* Philadelphia: W. B. Saunders, p. 429.

---

212. The pregnant client tells the nurse that she felt wetness on her peri-pad and that she found some clear fluid. The nurse immediately inspects the perineum and notes the presence of a prolapsed cord. The nurse's initial action is to

1. Notify the physician.
2. Monitor fetal heart rate.
3. Transfer the client to the labor room.
4. Place the client in Trendelenburg's position and push the presenting part upward.

Answer: 4

Rationale: On inspection of the perineum, if it is noted that the cord is compressed by the presenting part, place the client immediately into Trendelenburg's position while pushing the presenting part upward to relieve the cord compression. Maintain this position while the physician evaluates the client further.

Test-Taking Strategy: The key phrase is "prolapsed cord," which indicates an immediate action on the nurse's part to relieve cord compression. The only action that achieves this is option 4. The physician is notified after positioning the client.

Level of Cognitive Ability: Application
Phase of Nursing Process: Implementation
Client Needs: Physiological Integrity
Content Area: Maternity

Reference

Nichols, F., & Zwelling, E. (1997). *Maternal-newborn nursing: Theory and practice.* Philadelphia: W. B. Saunders, p. 884.

---

213. The nurse admits a neonate to the nursery. On assessment, the nurse palpates the anterior fontanel of the neonate and notes it as feeling soft. This assessment is indicative of

1. Increased ICP.
2. Dehydration.
3. Decreased ICP.
4. A normal finding.

Answer: 4

Rationale: The anterior fontanel is normally 2–3 cm in width, 3–4 cm in length, and diamond-like in shape. It can be described as soft, which is normal, or full and bulging, which could be indicative of increased ICP. Conversely a depressed fontanel could mean that the neonate is dehydrated.

Test-Taking Strategy: Knowledge of the normal findings in a neonate is required to answer this question. Review the findings related to the fontanels if you had difficulty with this question.

Level of Cognitive Ability: Analysis
Phase of Nursing Process: Assessment
Client Needs: Physiological Integrity
Content Area: Maternity

Reference

Ashwill, J., & Droske, S. (1997). *Nursing care of children: Principles and practice.* Philadelphia: W. B. Saunders, p. 57.

---

214. A client with acquired immunodeficiency syndrome (AIDS) is admitted for chills, fever, nonproductive cough, and pleuritic chest pain. A diagnosis of *Pneumocystis carinii* pneumonia is made, and the client is started on intravenous pentamidine (NebuPent). Which of the following nursing actions is most important when administering this medication?

1 Infuse over 1 hour with the client in a supine position
2 Infuse over 30 minutes with the client in a reclining position
3 Infuse over 1 hour and the client may be ambulatory
4 Infuse over 15 minutes with the client in a supine position

Answer: 1

Rationale: Intravenous pentamidine is infused over 1 hour with the client supine to minimize severe hypotension and dysrhythmias. Options 2, 3, and 4 are inaccurate in either length of time pentamidine is administered or the client's position.

Test-Taking Strategy: To answer the question, you need to know that pentamidine is administered in the supine position over 1 hour and adverse effects include hypotension and dysrhythmias. Eliminate option 4 first because this time frame is short for an intravenous medication. Eliminate option 3 next because although a client may ambulate with an intravenous line, it is less likely to be the correct option from those remaining options. Of the remaining options, it is best to select the option that addresses the longer time frame. Review this medication if you had difficulty with this question.

Level of Cognitive Ability: Application
Phase of Nursing Process: Implementation
Client Needs: Physiological Integrity
Content Area: Pharmacology

Reference

Hodgson, B., & Kizior, R. (1998). *Saunders nursing drug handbook 1998.* Philadelphia: W. B. Saunders, pp. 801–802.

---

215. The nurse is caring for a client who has returned to a surgical unit from a critical care unit after having a pelvic exenteration. The client complains of pain in the calf. The nurse would

1 Administer PRN meperidine (Demerol) as ordered.
2 Observe the calf for temperature, color, and size.
3 Lightly massage the area to relieve muscle pain.
4 Ask the client to walk and observe the gait.

Answer: 2

Rationale: The nurse monitors for postoperative complications, such as deep vein thrombosis, pulmonary emboli, and wound infection. Pain in the calf could indicate a deep vein thrombosis. Change in color, temperature, or size of client's calf could also indicate this complication. Options 3 and 4 could result in an embolus if, in fact, this client had a deep vein thrombosis. Pain medication for this client complaint is not the appropriate nursing action. An assessment needs to be obtained.

Test-Taking Strategy: Remember that assessment is the first step of the Nursing Process. Option 2 is the only option that addresses assessment. Review postoperative complications and appropriate interventions if you had difficulty with this question.

Level of Cognitive Ability: Application
Phase of Nursing Process: Implementation
Client Needs: Physiological Integrity
Content Area: Fundamental Skills

Reference

Smeltzer, S., & Bare, B. (1996). *Brunner and Suddarth's Textbook of medical-surgical nursing* (8th ed.). Philadelphia: Lippincott-Raven, pp. 2250–2255.

216. The nurse reviews the electrolyte values of a client with congestive heart failure. The potassium level is low, and the physician orders intravenous potassium. When administering intravenous potassium solutions, it is critical to

1 Inject it as a bolus.
2 Dilute it as instructed.
3 Use a filter.
4 Apply cool compresses to the intravenous site.

Answer: 2

Rationale: Potassium is irritating to the vein and needs to be diluted to prevent phlebitis. Potassium is never administered as a bolus injection. A filter is not necessary for potassium solutions. Cool compresses would vasoconstrict the intravenous site, which could possibly be more irritating to the vein.

Test-Taking Strategy: The use of the word "critical" in the stem shows that the answer must be something that is to be completed whenever administering potassium. Knowledge that potassium is irritating to the veins and that it is never administered by direct intravenous push is required to answer this question correctly. Review this important medication if you had difficulty with this question. You are likely to find a question related to administering potassium on NCLEX-RN.

Level of Cognitive Ability: Application
Phase of Nursing Process: Implementation
Client Needs: Physiological Integrity
Content Area: Pharmacology

Reference
Phillips, L. (1997). *Manual of intravenous therapeutics* (2nd ed.). Philadelphia: F. A. Davis, p. 83.

217. The nurse is preparing to access an implanted vascular port to administer chemotherapy. Which of the following identifies the correct technique for port access?

1 Anchor the port with the dominant hand
2 Palpate the port to locate the center of the septum
3 Place a warm pack over the area for several minutes to alleviate possible discomfort
4 Clean the area with alcohol working from the outside in

Answer: 2

Rationale: Before accessing an implanted port, the nurse must palpate the port to locate the center of the septum. The port should then be anchored with the nondominant hand. Cool compresses over the site can help to alleviate pain on entry. The site should be cleansed with alcohol working from the inside out to prevent introducing germs into the access site.

Test-Taking Strategy: Remembering the principles of cool application and aseptic technique can assist in eliminating options 3 and 4. From the remaining two options, select option 2 over option 1 because it does not make sense to anchor the port with the dominant hand. The nurse needs the dominant hand to perform the access. Review the concepts related to implanted vascular ports if you had difficulty answering this question.

Level of Cognitive Ability: Application
Phase of Nursing Process: Implementation
Client Needs: Physiological Integrity
Content Area: Fundamental Skills

Reference
Phillips, L. (1997). *Manual of intravenous therapeutics* (2nd ed.). Philadelphia: F. A. Davis, p. 419.

218. The nurse is evaluating the patency of a peripheral intravenous site and suspects an infiltration. Which of the following is the correct way to determine whether the intravenous line has infiltrated?

1 Gently palpate the surrounding tissue for edema and coolness
2 Strip the tubing quickly while assessing for a rapid blood return
3 Increase the intravenous flow rate and observe the site for immediate tightening of tissue
4 Assess the area around the intravenous site for discomfort, redness, and warmth

Answer: 1

Rationale: When assessing an intravenous site for signs and symptoms of infiltration, it is important to assess the site for edema and coolness, which signify leakage of the intravenous fluid into the surrounding tissues. Stripping the tubing does not cause a blood return but forces intravenous fluids into the vein or surrounding tissues, which could cause more tissue damage. Increasing the flow rate may be damaging to the tissues if the intravenous line has infiltrated. The intravenous site feels cool if the intravenous fluid has infiltrated into the surrounding tissues.

Test-Taking Strategy: Although option 4 is appealing because of requiring further assessment, by carefully reading the entire option, note that the signs and symptoms presented in the option are not signs and symptoms of infiltration. Remember that the entire option must be correct, not just part of it. Review the signs of infiltration if you had difficulty with this question.

Level of Cognitive Ability: Analysis
Phase of Nursing Process: Implementation
Client Needs: Physiological Integrity
Content Area: Fundamental Skills

Reference

Kozier, B., Glenora, E., & Blais, K. (1995). *Fundamentals of nursing: Concepts, process, and practice* (5th ed.). Menlo Park, CA: Addison-Wesley, p. 1104.

219. A client is brought into the emergency room after being in a car accident. A suspected neck injury is possible. The client is unresponsive and pulseless. The nurse prepares to open the client's airway by which of the following methods?

1 Head tilt/chin lift
2 Lift head up, place two pillows under the head, and attempt to ventilate
3 Jaw thrust maneuver
4 Keep client flat and grasp the tongue

Answer: 3

Rationale: In suspected neck injuries, the most appropriate way to open the airway is the jaw thrust maneuver. If a neck injury is present, this maneuver prevents further injury.

Test-Taking Strategy: The key phrase is "suspected neck injury." Knowledge regarding airway management should assist in eliminating options 2 and 4. From the remaining two options, eliminate option 1 because this method would cause further damage to a neck injury. Review basic life support measures if you had difficulty with this question.

Level of Cognitive Ability: Application
Phase of Nursing Process: Implementation
Client Needs: Physiological Integrity
Content Area: Fundamental Skills

Reference

Lammon, C. B., Foote, A. W., Leli, P. G., et al. (1995). *Clinical nursing skills.* Philadelphia: W. B. Saunders, p. 45.

220. The nurse is caring for a child with Reye's syndrome. The nurse assesses for the major symptom associated with Reye's syndrome when the nurse notes

1 Persistent vomiting.
2 Protein in the urine.
3 A history of a staphylococcus infection.
4 Symptoms of hyperglycemia.

Answer: 1

Rationale: Persistent vomiting is a major symptom associated with ICP. ICP and encephalopathy are major symptoms of Reye's syndrome. Options 2, 3, and 4 are incorrect.

Test-Taking Strategy: This question asks you to select the response that identifies the characteristic symptom of ICP, common to Reye's syndrome. Use the process of elimination to answer the question. The nurse should monitor feeding tolerance and for vomiting episodes. If you had difficulty with this question, take time now to review the symptoms of Reye's syndrome and the signs of ICP.

Level of Cognitive Ability: Application
Phase of Nursing Process: Assessment
Client Needs: Physiological Integrity
Content Area: Child Health

Reference

O'Toole, M. (Ed.). (1997). *Miller-Keane Encyclopedia and dictionary of medicine, nursing, and allied health* (6th ed.). Philadelphia: W. B. Saunders, p. 1411.

---

221. The nurse is caring for an adolescent client with conjunctivitis. Which of the following instructions will the nurse include in the plan of care?

1 "Avoid using all eye makeup to avoid possible reinfection."
2 "Apply warm compresses to lessen irritation."
3 "Contact lenses will need to be replaced."
4 "Stay home for 3 days after starting antibiotic eye drops to avoid the spread of infection."

Answer: 3

Rationale: Eye makeup should be replaced but can still be worn. Cool compresses decrease pain and irritation. Isolation for 24 hours after antibiotics are initiated is necessary. All contact lenses should be replaced.

Test-Taking Strategy: Eliminate option 1 because of the absolute term "all." Eliminate option 4 because 3 days is a lengthy period to remain isolated, particularly if antibiotics have been initiated. Select option 3 over option 2 knowing that cool, not warm, compresses decrease pain and irritation.

Level of Cognitive Ability: Application
Phase of Nursing Process: Implementation
Client Needs: Physiological Integrity
Content Area: Child Health

Reference

Ashwill, J., & Droske, S. (1997). *Nursing care of children: Principles and practice.* Philadelphia: W. B. Saunders, p. 1337.

---

222. A child is admitted to the hospital with a diagnosis of suspected *Pneumococcus* pneumonia. The nurse should prepare to

1 Have a chest x-ray done to determine how much consolidation there is in the lungs.
2 Allow the child to go to the playroom to play with other children.
3 Monitor the child's respiratory rate and breath sounds.
4 Start antibiotic therapy immediately.

Answer: 3

Rationale: A complication of *Pneumococcus* pneumonia can be a pleural effusion, so the respiratory status of the child needs to be monitored. Option 1 is medical management, not nursing care. Antibiotic therapy should not be started until cultures are obtained. The child should not be allowed in the playroom at this time.

Test-Taking Strategy: Option 3 addresses assessment, the first step of the Nursing Process. This option also addresses the ABCs. It is also the option that is directly related to the child's diagnosis.

Level of Cognitive Ability: Application
Phase of Nursing Process: Planning
Client Needs: Physiological Integrity
Content Area: Child Health

Reference

Wong, D. (1995). *Whaley and Wong's Nursing care of infants and children* (5th ed.). St. Louis: Mosby–Year Book, pp. 1400–1401.

---

223. The nurse admits a client suspected of bulimia nervosa. When performing the admission assessment, the nurse is aware that, characteristic of bulimia, the client

1 Overeats for the enjoyment of food.
2 Binge eats, then purges.
3 Overeats in response to losing control over a weight loss diet.
4 Is accepting of body size.

Answer: 2

Rationale: Options 1, 3, and 4 are true of the obese person who may binge eat. Individuals with bulimia nervosa develop cycles of binge eating followed by purging. They seldom attempt to diet and have no sense of loss of control.

Test-Taking Strategy: Eliminate options 1 and 3 because they are similar. Knowledge of the definition of bulimia can direct you to option 2. If you had difficulty with this question, take time now to review the characteristics associated with this disorder.

Level of Cognitive Ability: Analysis
Phase of Nursing Process: Analysis
Client Needs: Physiological Integrity
Content Area: Mental Health

Reference
Black, J., & Matassarin-Jacobs, E. (1997). *Medical-surgical nursing: Clinical management for continuity of care* (5th ed.). Philadelphia: W. B. Saunders, pp. 1759–1760.

---

224. A client who has experienced a cerebrovascular accident has partial hemiplegia of the left leg. The straight leg cane formerly used by the client is not quite sufficient now. The nurse interprets that the client could benefit from the somewhat greater support and stability provided by a

1 Quad-cane.
2 Wooden crutch.
3 Lofstrand crutch.
4 Wheelchair.

Answer: 1

Rationale: A quad-cane may be used by the client requiring greater support and stability than is provided by a straight leg cane. The quad-cane provides a four-point base of support and is indicated for use by clients with partial or complete hemiplegia. Neither crutches nor a wheelchair is indicated for use with this client. A Lofstrand crutch is useful for clients with bilateral weakness.

Test-Taking Strategy: Giving a wheelchair to a client with partial hemiplegia is excessive and is eliminated first. Wooden crutches are not indicated because there is no restriction in weight bearing. A Lofstrand crutch is useful with bilateral weakness. This leaves the quad cane as the correct option.

Level of Cognitive Ability: Analysis
Phase of Nursing Process: Analysis
Client Needs: Physiological Integrity
Content Area: Adult Health/Neurological

Reference
Potter, P., & Perry, A. (1997). *Fundamentals of nursing: Concepts, process, and practice* (4th ed.). St. Louis: Mosby–Year Book, p. 935.

---

225. The nurse is caring for the client who develops compartment syndrome from a severely fractured arm. The client asks the nurse how this can happen. The nurse's response is based on the understanding that

1 An injured artery causes impaired arterial perfusion through the compartment.
2 The fascia expands with injury, causing pressure on underlying nerves and muscles.
3 A bone fragment has injured the nerve supply in the area.
4 Bleeding and swelling cause increased pressure in an area that cannot expand.

Answer: 4

Rationale: Compartment syndrome is caused by bleeding and swelling within a compartment, which is lined by fascia that does not expand. The bleeding and swelling put pressure on the nerves, muscles, and blood vessels in the compartment, triggering the symptoms.

Test-Taking Strategy: A basic understanding of the concept of a compartment is needed to answer this question. Option 1 should be eliminated first because it is not due to an arterial injury. Knowing that the fascia itself cannot expand eliminates option 2. To discriminate between the last two, it is necessary to know that bleeding and swelling cause the symptoms, not a nerve injury.

Level of Cognitive Ability: Analysis
Phase of Nursing Process: Analysis
Client Needs: Physiological Integrity
Content Area: Adult Health/Musculoskeletal

Reference
Black, J., & Matassarin-Jacobs, E. (1997). *Medical-surgical nursing: Clinical management for continuity of care* (5th ed.). Philadelphia: W. B. Saunders, p. 2139.

226. The client has undergone fasciotomy to treat compartment syndrome of the leg. The nurse would provide which type of wound care to the fasciotomy site?

1 Dry sterile dressings
2 Moist sterile saline dressings
3 Hydrocolloid dressings
4 One half strength povidone-iodine (Betadine) dressings

Answer: 2

Rationale: The fasciotomy site is not sutured but is left open to relieve pressure and edema. The site is covered with moist sterile saline dressings. After 3–5 days, when perfusion is adequate and edema subsides, the wound is débrided and closed.

Test-Taking Strategy: This question can be answered by knowing what a fasciotomy involves and knowing the basics of wound care. With fasciotomy, the skin is not sutured closed but left open for pressure relief. Moist tissue needs to remain moist, which eliminates option 1. A hydrocolloid dressing is not indicated for use with clean, open incisions, which eliminates option 3. The incision is clean, not dirty, so there should be no reason to require povidone-iodine. Knowing that povidone-iodine can be irritating to normal tissues is an additional reason to choose option 2 over option 4.

Level of Cognitive Ability: Application
Phase of Nursing Process: Implementation
Client Needs: Physiological Integrity
Content Area: Adult Health/Musculoskeletal

Reference

Smeltzer, S., & Bare, B. (1996). *Brunner and Suddarth's Textbook of medical-surgical nursing* (8th ed.). Philadelphia: Lippincott-Raven, p. 1917.

227. The nurse is caring for a client who was recently admitted for anorexia nervosa. When the nurse enters the room, the client is engaged in rigorous pushups. Which of the following nursing actions would be best?

1 Allow the client to complete the exercise program
2 Tell the client that he or she is not allowed to exercise rigorously
3 Interrupt the client and offer to take the client for a walk
4 Interrupt the client and weigh immediately

Answer: 3

Rationale: Clients with anorexia nervosa are frequently preoccupied with rigorous exercise and push themselves beyond normal limits to work off caloric intake. The nurse must provide for appropriate exercise as well as place limits on rigorous activities.

Test-Taking Strategy: Knowledge of the seriousness of anorexia nervosa is essential in answering this question. Focus on the need for the nurse to set firm limits with clients who have this disorder yet provide and guide the client to perform appropriate exercise. Review interventions for clients with this disorder if you had difficulty with this question.

Level of Cognitive Ability: Application
Phase of Nursing Process: Implementation
Client Needs: Physiological Integrity
Content Area: Mental Health

Reference

Haber, J. (1997). *Comprehensive psychiatric nursing* (5th ed.). St. Louis: Mosby–Year Book, pp. 561–562.

228. The nurse assesses the peripheral intravenous site dressing and notes that it is damp and that the tape is loose. The first most appropriate nursing action is to

1 Stop the infusion immediately and notify the physician.
2 Check that the tubing is securely attached to the catheter and redress the site.
3 Increase the intravenous flow rate to assess for further leaking.
4 Remove the tape, slow the intravenous rate, and discontinue the intravenous line.

Answer: 2

Rationale: If there is leakage at the intravenous site, the nurse should first locate the source. The nurse should assess the site further to be certain that all connections are secure. One should not increase the flow rate. Although it is true that it may leak more, it may also cause more tissue damage if the intravenous line was infiltrating. Although the infusion most likely will need to be stopped, the physician does not need to be notified. Slowing and discontinuing the intravenous line is also premature. The intravenous line must first be assessed as to the cause of the leaking.

Test-Taking Strategy: The stem of the question contains the key words "first" and "most appropriate." Remember that the priority is to determine the cause of the leaking. Further assessment is needed before intervening. Remember that assessment is the first step of the nursing process.

Level of Cognitive Ability: Application
Phase of Nursing Process: Implementation
Client Needs: Physiological Integrity
Content Area: Fundamental Skills

Reference
Kozier, B., Glenora, E., & Blais, K. (1995). *Fundamentals of nursing: Concepts, process, and practice* (5th ed.). Menlo Park, CA: Addison-Wesley, p. 1104.

---

229. The nurse assists the physician with the removal of a chest tube. During removal of the chest tube, the nurse instructs the client to

1 Breathe out forcefully.
2 Breathe in deeply.
3 Hold his or her breath.
4 Breathe normally.

Answer: 3

Rationale: Instruct the client in the Valsalva maneuver so that the client can hold his or her breath and bear down as the physician removes the tube. This increases intrathoracic pressure, thereby lessening the potential for air to enter the pleural space.

Test-Taking Strategy: Eliminate options 2 and 4 because they are similar in that breathing causes air to enter the pleural space. From the remaining two options, eliminate option 1 because of the word "forcefully." Review the procedure for the removal of chest tubes if you had difficulty with this question.

Level of Cognitive Ability: Application
Phase of Nursing Process: Implementation
Client Needs: Physiological Integrity
Content Area: Adult Health/Respiratory

Reference
Black, J., & Matassarin-Jacobs, E. (1997). *Medical-surgical nursing: Clinical management for continuity of care* (5th ed.). Philadelphia: W. B. Saunders, pp. 1165–1166.

---

230. The nurse assesses the water seal chamber of a closed chest drainage system and notes fluctuations in the chamber. This finding indicates that

1 An air leak is present.
2 The tubing is kinked.
3 The lung has reexpanded.
4 The system is functioning as expected.

Answer: 4

Rationale: Fluctuations (tidaling) in the water seal chamber are normal during inhalation and exhalation until the lung reexpands and the client no longer requires chest drainage. If fluctuations are absent, it could indicate an air leak, kinking, or reexpansion of the lung.

Test-Taking Strategy: Knowledge regarding the functioning of chest tube drainage systems is required to answer this question. Review the normal expectations and the indications of complications if you had difficulty with this question.

Level of Cognitive Ability: Analysis
Phase of Nursing Process: Analysis
Client Needs: Physiological Integrity
Content Area: Adult Health/Respiratory

Reference

Black, J., & Matassarin-Jacobs, E. (1997). *Medical-surgical nursing: Clinical management for continuity of care* (5th ed.). Philadelphia: W. B. Saunders, pp. 1163–1164.

---

231. When a depressed client does not respond to antidepressant medication, what treatment modality may be prescribed?

1 Electroconvulsive therapy
2 Psychosurgery
3 Insulin therapy medication
4 Neuroleptic medication

Answer: 1

Rationale: Electroconvulsive therapy is an effective treatment for severe depression. Psychosurgery is rarely performed and would not treat depression. Insulin coma therapy is outmoded. Neuroleptics or major tranquilizers are not effective in the treatment of depression.

Test-Taking Strategy: Knowledge of treatment measures for depression is required to answer this question. Eliminate option 2 first as being the most invasive. From this point, knowledge that insulin coma therapy and neuroleptics are not used can assist in directing you to the correct option. Review treatment measures for depression if you had difficulty with this question.

Level of Cognitive Ability: Analysis
Phase of Nursing Process: Analysis
Client Needs: Physiological Integrity
Content Area: Mental Health

Reference

Carson, V., & Arnold, E. (1996). *Mental health nursing: The nurse-patient journey.* Philadelphia: W. B. Saunders, p. 785.

---

232. The nurse in the mental health unit is preparing a client for psychotherapy. A form of psychotherapy in which the client enacts situations that are of emotional significance is termed

1 Reality therapy.
2 Short-term psychotherapy.
3 Psychoanalytic therapy.
4 Psychodrama.

Answer: 4

Rationale: Psychodrama is the only option that involves enactment of emotionally charged situations. Reality therapy is used for clients with cognitive impairment. Both short-term dynamic psychotherapy and psychoanalytic psychotherapy depend on techniques drawn from psychoanalysis.

Test-Taking Strategy: The key phrase is "the client enacts situations." This should assist in providing you the definition of psychodrama. If you had difficulty with this question, take time now to review these types of therapy.

Level of Cognitive Ability: Analysis
Phase of Nursing Process: Analysis
Client Needs: Physiological Integrity
Content Area: Mental Health

Reference

Carson, V., & Arnold, E. (1996). *Mental health nursing: The nurse-patient journey.* Philadelphia: W. B. Saunders, pp. 412–413.

233. The client arrives in the emergency room after being in an automobile accident. The client was physically unharmed yet was hyperventilating and complaining of dizziness and nausea. In addition, the client appeared confused and had difficulty focusing on what was going on. The nurse would assess the client's level of anxiety as

1 Mild.
2 Moderate.
3 Severe.
4 Panic.

Answer: 3

Rationale: The person whose anxiety is assessed as severe is unable to solve problems and has a poor grasp of what's happening in the environment. Somatic symptoms are usually present. The individual with mild anxiety is only mildly uncomfortable and may even find performance enhanced. The individual with moderate anxiety grasps less information about a situation and has some difficulty problem solving. The individual in panic demonstrates markedly disturbed behavior and may lose touch with reality.

Test-Taking Strategy: Knowledge regarding the characteristics of the various levels of anxiety can assist in answering this question. Focus on the signs and symptoms presented in the question. You should be able to eliminate options 1 and 4 easily. The fact that the client has difficulty focusing on what was going on should direct you to option 3. Review these characteristics related to the levels of anxiety if you had difficulty with this question.

Level of Cognitive Ability: Analysis
Phase of Nursing Process: Assessment
Client Needs: Physiological Integrity
Content Area: Mental Health

Reference
Carson, V., & Arnold, E. (1996). *Mental health nursing: The nurse-patient journey.* Philadelphia: W. B. Saunders, pp. 695–696.

234. A child is admitted to the hospital with a diagnosis of acute rheumatic fever. Which of the following blood laboratory findings would confirm the likelihood of this disorder?

1 Increased leukocyte count
2 Decreased hemoglobin count
3 Increased antistreptolysin-O (ASO) titer
4 Decreased erythrocyte sedimentation rate

Answer: 3

Rationale: Children suspected of having rheumatic fever are tested for streptococcal antibodies. The most reliable and best standardized test is an elevated or rising antistreptolysin-O (ASO) titer.

Test-Taking Strategy: Knowledge of the clinical manifestations associated with rheumatic fever is required to answer this question. You can easily eliminate options 2 and 4. Remember that an increased leukocyte count indicates the presence of infection but is not specific in confirming a particular diagnosis. This should direct you to option 3.

Level of Cognitive Ability: Analysis
Phase of Nursing Process: Assessment
Client Needs: Physiological Integrity
Content Area: Child Health

Reference
Ashwill, J., & Droske, S. (1997). *Nursing care of children: Principles and practice.* Philadelphia: W. B. Saunders, p. 658.

235. A 5-year-old child is admitted to the hospital for heart surgery to repair tetralogy of Fallot. The nurse notes that the child has clubbed fingers and knows that the clubbing is most likely due to

1 Peripheral hypoxia.
2 Delayed physical growth.
3 Chronic hypertension.
4 Destruction of bone marrow.

Answer: 1

Rationale: Clubbing, a thickening and flattening of the tips of the fingers and toes, is thought to occur because of a chronic tissue hypoxemia and polycythemia.

Test-Taking Strategy: Use the ABCs to answer the question. Hypoxia relates to oxygenation, a concern with this disorder. If you had difficulty with this question, take time now to review the manifestations associated with tetralogy of Fallot.

Level of Cognitive Ability: Analysis
Phase of Nursing Process: Analysis
Client Needs: Physiological Integrity
Content Area: Child Health

Reference

Ashwill, J., & Droske, S. (1997). *Nursing care of children: Principles and practice.* Philadelphia: W. B. Saunders, p. 924.

---

236. A newly admitted elderly client is placed in Buck's traction. The nurse needs to monitor frequently the client's

1. Vital signs.
2. Mental state.
3. Range of motion.
4. Neurovascular status.

Answer: 4

Rationale: The neurovascular status of the extremity of the client in Buck's traction must be assessed every 2 hours for the first 24 hours. Elderly clients are especially at risk for neurovascular compromise because many already have disorders that affect the peripheral vascular system. The client's physiological status determines the frequency of vital signs, not the presence or absence of Buck's traction. Although clients in some types of traction do become depressed after a few days or weeks, Buck's traction is usually used preoperatively, which typically involves a few hours or 1–2 days at the most. Range of motion of the involved leg is contraindicated in hip fractures.

Test-Taking Strategy: Knowledge regarding Buck's traction and its use on clients with hip fractures can assist you in answering this question correctly. You should easily be able to eliminate options 2 and 3. Although vital signs are the most global option, neurovascular status is specific to the use of traction. Review nursing care of the client in traction if you had difficulty with this question.

Level of Cognitive Ability: Application
Phase of Nursing Process: Assessment
Client Needs: Physiological Integrity
Content Area: Adult Health/Musculoskeletal

Reference

Black, J., & Matassarin-Jacobs, E. (1997). *Medical-surgical nursing: Clinical management for continuity of care* (5th ed.). Philadelphia: W. B. Saunders, pp. 2138–2139.

---

237. The client who has a renal mass asks the nurse why an ultrasound has been scheduled, as opposed to other diagnostic tests that may be ordered. The nurse formulates a response on the basis of the understanding that

1. An ultrasound can differentiate a solid mass from a fluid-filled cyst.
2. An ultrasound is much more cost-effective than other diagnostic tests.
3. All other tests are more invasive than an ultrasound.
4. All other tests require more elaborate postprocedure care.

Answer: 1

Rationale: A significant advantage of an ultrasound is that it can differentiate a solid mass from a fluid-filled cyst. It is noninvasive and does not require any special aftercare. There are other diagnostic tests, such as magnetic resonance imaging and computed tomography scanning, which are also noninvasive (unless contrast material is used) and which require no special aftercare. Ultrasound, however, can discriminate between solid and fluid masses most optimally.

Test-Taking Strategy: Eliminate options 3 and 4 first because it is unlikely that any response with the word "all" in it is likely to be true. To differentiate between the remaining two options, knowing that ultrasonography uses sound waves reflected back from tissues of different densities may help you to choose correctly.

Level of Cognitive Ability: Analysis
Phase of Nursing Process: Analysis
Client Needs: Physiological Integrity
Content Area: Adult Health/Renal

Reference

Black, J., & Matassarin-Jacobs, E. (1997). *Medical-surgical nursing: Clinical management for continuity of care* (5th ed.). Philadelphia: W. B. Saunders, p. 1565.

238. The client has been admitted with acute glomerulonephritis. The nurse first assesses the client for a recent history of

1. Bleeding ulcer.
2. Hypertension.
3. Fungal infection.
4. Streptococcal infection.

Answer: 4

Rationale: The predominant cause of acute glomerulonephritis is infection with beta-hemolytic streptococcus 3 weeks before the onset of symptoms. Other infectious agents that could trigger the disorder besides bacteria include viruses or parasites. Hypertension and bleeding ulcer are not precipitating causes.

Test-Taking Strategy: Knowing that infection is a common trigger for glomerulonephritis helps you to eliminate options 1 and 2 first. To discriminate between options 3 and 4, it is necessary to know that streptococcal infections particularly are a common cause of this problem. This is an important concept for this topic. If you chose incorrectly, take a few moments now to review this disorder.

Level of Cognitive Ability: Application
Phase of Nursing Process: Assessment
Client Needs: Physiological Integrity
Content Area: Adult Health/Renal

Reference

Black, J., & Matassarin-Jacobs, E. (1997). *Medical-surgical nursing: Clinical management for continuity of care* (5th ed.). Philadelphia: W. B. Saunders, p. 1630.

---

239. A male client has just been admitted to the emergency room with chest pain. Serum enzyme levels are drawn. Results are reported as follows: creatine phosphokinase (CPK), 295 U/mL; CPK-MB, 10%; LDH, 80 U/liter with LDH_2 exceeding LDH_1. The nurse concludes that these results are compatible with

1. New-onset myocardial infarction.
2. Myocardial infarction of at least 3 days' duration.
3. Unstable angina.
4. Prinzmetal's angina.

Answer: 1

Rationale: CPK and its cardiac isoenzyme CPK-MB is the most sensitive indicator of myocardial damage. Levels begin to rise 3–6 hours after onset of chest pain, peak at approximately 24 hours, and return to normal in about 3 days. Normal values for men are 12–70 U/mL, with CPK-MB 0%–5% of total CPK. LDH begins to rise in 24 hours, peaks at 48–72 hours, and returns to normal in 7–10 days. LDH_1 rises above the level of LDH_2 with myocardial infarction. The levels portrayed in the question are consistent with new-onset myocardial infarction.

Test-Taking Strategy: You need to know which enzymes elevate with myocardial infarction and their associated time frames. There is no permanent myocardial damage with unstable angina or Prinzmetal's angina; the elevated enzymes rule these options out.

Level of Cognitive Ability: Analysis
Phase of Nursing Process: Analysis
Client Needs: Physiological Integrity
Content Area: Adult Health/Cardiovascular

Reference

Ignatavicius, D. D., Workman, M. L., & Mishler, M. A. (1995). *Medical-surgical nursing: A nursing process approach* (2nd ed.). Philadelphia: W. B. Saunders, p. 799.

---

240. The client with heart failure has cardiomegaly on chest x-ray. As part of cardiac assessment, the nurse would position the stethoscope to auscultate the apical rate

1. At the normal point of maximal impulse (PMI).
2. Slightly upward and medial to the normal PMI.
3. Slightly downward and medial to the normal PMI.
4. Lateral to the normal PMI.

Answer: 4

Rationale: The PMI, where the apical rate is auscultated, is normally located in the fifth intercostal space, midclavicular line. With heart failure, the heart enlarges, shifting the PMI laterally.

Test-Taking Strategy: A knowledge of thoracic landmarks is needed to answer this question correctly. Review them, if needed; then, remembering the position of the heart in the thoracic cavity, picture the displacement if the heart is enlarged.

Level of Cognitive Ability: Application
Phase of Nursing Process: Assessment
Client Needs: Physiological Integrity
Content Area: Adult Health/Cardiovascular

Reference

Black, J., & Matassarin-Jacobs, E. (1997). *Medical-surgical nursing: Clinical management for continuity of care* (5th ed.). Philadelphia: W. B. Saunders, p. 1280.

---

241. The nurse is caring for a client receiving bolus feedings via a Levin nasogastric tube. As the nurse is finishing the feeding, the client asks for the bed to be positioned flat to sleep. Which of the following positions is the most appropriate choice for this client at this time?

1 Head of bed flat with client in the supine position for at least 30 minutes
2 Head of bed elevated 35–40 degrees with client in the right lateral position for at least 30 minutes
3 Head of bed elevated 45–60 degrees with client in the supine position for at least 60 minutes
4 Head of bed in semi-Fowler's with client in the left lateral position for at least 60 minutes

Answer: 2

Rationale: Aspiration is a possible complication associated with nasogastric tube feeding. The head of the bed is elevated 35–40 degrees for at least 30 minutes after bolus tube feeding to prevent vomiting and aspiration. The right lateral position uses gravity to facilitate gastric retention to prevent vomiting. The flat supine position is to be avoided for the first 30 minutes after a tube feeding.

Test-Taking Strategy: There are three components to each answer including the level of elevation of the head, the client's position, and the duration. Option 1 can be ruled out immediately because this position could result in aspiration. Option 4 is ruled out because of the supine position and the longer duration. Options 2 and 4 are the same elevation, but the right lateral position is the correct position, and 30 minutes is the correct duration.

Level of Cognitive Ability: Application
Phase of Nursing Process: Implementation
Client Needs: Physiological Integrity
Content Area: Fundamental Skills

Reference

Lewis, S., Collier, I., & Heitkemper, M. (1996). *Medical-surgical nursing: Assessment and management of clinical problems* (4th ed.). St. Louis: Mosby–Year Book, pp. 1115–1118.

---

242. The nurse is caring for a client with acute pancreatitis and a history of alcoholism. Which of the following assessment data would be a sign of paralytic ileus?

1 Firm, nontender mass palpable at the lower right costal margin
2 Severe, constant pain with rapid onset
3 Inability to pass flatus
4 Loss of anal sphincter control

Answer: 3

Rationale: An inflammatory reaction such as acute pancreatitis can cause paralytic ileus, the most common form of nonmechanical obstruction. Inability to pass flatus is a clinical manifestation of paralytic ileus. Option 1 is the description of the physical finding of liver enlargement. The liver is usually enlarged in cases of cirrhosis or hepatitis. Although this client may have an enlarged liver, an enlarged liver is not a sign of paralytic ileus or intestinal obstruction. Pain is associated with paralytic ileus, but the pain usually presents as a more constant generalized discomfort. Pain that is severe, constant, and rapid in onset is more likely caused by strangulation of the bowel. Loss of sphincter control is not a sign of paralytic ileus.

Test-Taking Strategy: Knowledge of the clinical manifestations and abdominal physical assessment findings of paralytic ileus can assist you in answering this question. Remember, in this situation you are looking for symptoms of paralytic ileus and not chronic alcoholism. Knowledge of the definition of paralytic ileus can direct you to the correct option. Review the signs of paralytic ileus if you had difficulty with this question.

Level of Cognitive Ability: Analysis
Phase of Nursing Process: Assessment
Client Needs: Physiological Integrity
Content Area: Adult Health/Gastrointestinal

Reference

Lewis, S., Collier, I., & Heitkemper, M. (1996). *Medical-surgical nursing: Assessment and management of clinical problems* (4th ed.). St. Louis: Mosby–Year Book, pp. 1235–1237.

---

243. After performing an initial abdominal assessment on a client with a diagnosis of cholelithiasis, the nurse reports that the bowel sounds are normal. Which of the following descriptions best describes "normal bowel sounds"?

1 Waves of loud gurgles auscultated in all four quadrants
2 Very high-pitched loud rushes auscultated especially in one or two quadrants
3 Relatively high-pitched clicks or gurgles auscultated in all four quadrants
4 Low-pitched swishing auscultated in one or two quadrants

Answer: 3

Rationale: Although frequency and intensity of bowel sounds vary depending on the phase of digestion, normal bowel sounds are relatively high-pitched clicks or gurgles. Loud gurgles (borborygmi) indicate hyperperistalsis. Bowel sounds are more high pitched and loud (hyperresonance) when the intestines are under tension, such as in intestinal obstruction. A swishing or buzzing sound represents turbulent blood flow associated with a bruit. No aortic bruits should be heard.

Test-Taking Strategy: A knowledge of normal auscultation findings for bowel sounds is helpful in answering this question. Normally, bowel sounds should be audible in all four quadrants; therefore, options 2 and 4 can be eliminated. From the remaining two options, select option 3 because it is more thoroughly descriptive of normal bowel sounds.

Level of Cognitive Ability: Analysis
Phase of Nursing Process: Assessment
Client Needs: Physiological Integrity
Content Area: Adult Health/Gastrointestinal

Reference

Lewis, S., Collier, I., & Heitkemper, M. (1996). *Medical-surgical nursing: Assessment and management of clinical problems* (4th ed.). St. Louis: Mosby–Year Book, pp. 1085, 1089.

---

244. The nurse is assigned to care for a client with nephrotic syndrome. The nurse assesses which of the following most important parameters on a daily basis?

1 Total protein levels
2 Weight
3 BUN
4 Activity tolerance

Answer: 2

Rationale: The client with nephrotic syndrome typically presents with edema, hypoalbuminemia, and proteinuria. The nurse carefully assesses the fluid balance of the client, which includes daily monitoring of weight, intake and output, edema, and girth measurements. Albumin levels are monitored as they are ordered, as are BUN and creatinine levels. The client's activity level is adjusted according to the amount of edema and water retention. As edema increases, the client's activity level should be restricted.

Test-Taking Strategy: Begin to answer this question by eliminating options 1 and 3 first. Nephrotic syndrome is a chronic condition, and daily levels of albumin (not total protein or BUN) may be most helpful during acute episodes. Of the two remaining, knowing that the activity level is adjusted according to the volume of fluid retention helps you to choose option 2 as the correct parameter to monitor on a daily basis.

Level of Cognitive Ability: Application
Phase of Nursing Process: Assessment
Client Needs: Physiological Integrity
Content Area: Adult Health/Renal

Reference

Black, J., & Matassarin-Jacobs, E. (1997). *Medical-surgical nursing: Clinical management for continuity of care* (5th ed.). Philadelphia: W. B. Saunders, p. 1635.

245. The client is being admitted to the nursing unit with urolithiasis and ureteral colic. The nurse assesses the client for pain that is

1 Dull and aching in the costovertebral area.
2 Sharp and radiating posteriorly to the spinal column.
3 Excruciating, wave-like, and radiating toward the genitalia.
4 Aching and cramp-like throughout the abdomen.

Answer: 3

Rationale: The pain of ureteral colic is due to movement of a stone through the ureter and is sharp, excruciating, and wave-like, radiating to the genitalia and thigh. The stone causes reduced flow of urine, and the urine also contains blood because of its abrasive action on urinary tract mucosa. Stones in the renal pelvis cause pain that is a deep ache in the costovertebral area. Renal colic is characterized by pain that is acute, with nausea and vomiting and tenderness over the costovertebral area.

Test-Taking Strategy: Begin to answer this question by eliminating option 4 because this pattern of pain is nonspecific and is the least likely to be the correct answer. Likewise, knowing that no pattern of pain includes radiation to the spinal column helps you to eliminate option 2 next as an unlikely choice. To discriminate between options 1 and 3, recall the anatomical location of the kidneys and the ureters. Because the kidneys are located in the posterior abdomen near the ribcage, pain in the costovertebral area is more likely to be associated with stones in the renal pelvis. Sharp, wave-like pain that radiates toward the genitalia is more consistent with the location of the ureters in the abdomen. With this in mind, choose option 3 over option 1 as the correct answer.

Level of Cognitive Ability: Application
Phase of Nursing Process: Assessment
Client Needs: Physiological Integrity
Content Area: Adult Health/Renal

Reference

Smeltzer, S., & Bare, B. (1996). *Brunner and Suddarth's Textbook of medical-surgical nursing* (8th ed.). Philadelphia: Lippincott-Raven, p. 1207.

246. The nurse is assessing the client with left-sided heart failure. The client states that it is necessary to use three pillows under the head and chest at night to be able to breathe comfortably while sleeping. The nurse documents that the client is experiencing

1 Dyspnea on exertion.
2 Dyspnea at rest.
3 Orthopnea.
4 Paroxysmal nocturnal dyspnea.

Answer: 3

Rationale: Dyspnea is a subjective problem that can range from an awareness of breathing to physical distress and does not necessarily correlate with the degree of heart failure. Dyspnea can be exertional or occur at rest. Orthopnea is a more severe form of dyspnea, requiring the client to assume a three-point position while upright and use pillows to support the head and thorax at night. Paroxysmal nocturnal dyspnea is a severe form of dyspnea occurring suddenly at night because of rapid fluid reentry into the vasculature from the interstitium during sleep.

Test-Taking Strategy: This questions seeks understanding of the different degrees of dyspnea. Eliminate options 1 and 4 because the stem mentions nothing about exertion or a sudden (paroxysmal) event. Select option 3 over option 2 because the client is sleeping "comfortably" with the use of pillows.

Level of Cognitive Ability: Application
Phase of Nursing Process: Assessment
Client Needs: Physiological Integrity
Content Area: Adult Health/Cardiovascular

Reference

Black, J., & Matassarin-Jacobs, E. (1997). *Medical-surgical nursing: Clinical management for continuity of* care (5th ed.). Philadelphia: W. B. Saunders, p. 1281.

247. The nurse witnesses a client going into pulmonary edema. The client exhibits respiratory distress, but the BP is stable at this time. As an immediate action before help arrives, the nurse would plan first to

1 Suction the client vigorously.
2 Place the client in high Fowler's position.
3 Begin assembling medications that are anticipated to be given.
4 Call the respiratory therapy department for a ventilator.

Answer: 2

Rationale: The client in pulmonary edema is placed in high Fowler's position, if the BP is adequate. Vigorous suctioning may deplete the client of vital oxygen at a time when the respiratory system is compromised. Assembling medications is useful but not critical to the immediate well-being of the client. The client may or may not need mechanical ventilation.

Test-Taking Strategy: The words "respiratory distress" and "first" would assist in eliminating options 3 and 4. Option 2 is preferable because it enhances the client's respirations, whereas option 1 may impair oxygenation, as implied by the word "vigorously" in that option.

Level of Cognitive Ability: Application
Phase of Nursing Process: Planning
Client Needs: Physiological Integrity
Content Area: Adult Health/Cardiovascular

Reference
Ignatavicius, D. D., Workman, M. L., & Mishler, M. A. (1995). *Medical-surgical nursing: A nursing process approach* (2nd ed.). Philadelphia: W. B. Saunders, p. 901.

---

248. The client is suspected of developing cardiogenic shock. The nurse would assess for which of the following peripheral vascular manifestations?

1 Flushed, dry skin with bounding pedal pulses
2 Warm, moist skin with irregular pedal pulses
3 Cool, dry skin with alternating weak and strong pedal pulses
4 Cool, clammy skin with weak or thready pedal pulses

Answer: 4

Rationale: Classic signs of cardiogenic shock include increased pulse (weak and thready); decreased BP; falling urinary output; signs of cerebral ischemia (confusion, agitation); and cool, clammy skin.

Test-Taking Strategy: This question tests basic knowledge of signs and symptoms of shock. The word "clammy" in option 4 should provide you with the clue in selecting this option. Review the signs of shock if you had difficulty with this question. You are likely to find questions related to shock on NCLEX-RN.

Level of Cognitive Ability: Analysis
Phase of Nursing Process: Assessment
Client Needs: Physiological Integrity
Content Area: Adult Health/Cardiovascular

Reference
Smeltzer, S., & Bare, B. (1996). *Brunner and Suddarth's Textbook of medical-surgical nursing* (8th ed.). Philadelphia: Lippincott-Raven, p. 672.

---

249. The nurse is caring for a client who returns from cardiac surgery with chest tubes in place. The nurse assesses the drainage on an hourly basis and assesses that the client is stable as long as drainage does not exceed how many milliliters over the first 24 hours?

1 100
2 200
3 500
4 1000

Answer: 3

Rationale: Approximately 500 mL of drainage is expected in the first 24 hours after cardiac surgery. Up to 100 mL may be lost in the first hour postoperatively. The nurse measures and records the drainage on an hourly basis. The drainage is initially dark red and becomes more serous over time.

Test-Taking Strategy: Options 1 and 2 are least plausible because the values are so small and should be discarded first. To discriminate between the remaining options, try converting the drainage to liters (i.e., 1000 mL = 1 liter; 500 mL = 0.5 liter). Knowing that there are only about 6 liters of blood circulating in the body, this technique may help you choose option 3 over option 4.

Level of Cognitive Ability: Analysis
Phase of Nursing Process: Assessment
Client Needs: Physiological Integrity
Content Area: Adult Health/Cardiovascular

Reference

Black, J., & Matassarin-Jacobs, E. (1997). *Medical-surgical nursing: Clinical management for continuity of care* (5th ed.). Philadelphia: W. B. Saunders, p. 1359.

---

250. The client with renal cancer is being treated preoperatively with radiation therapy. The nurse evaluates that the client has an understanding of proper care of the skin over the treatment field if the client states an intention to

1 Avoid skin exposure to direct sunlight and chlorinated water.
2 Use lanolin-based cream on the affected skin on a daily basis.
3 Remove the lines or ink marks using a gentle soap after each treatment.
4 Use the hottest water possible to wash the treatment site twice daily.

Answer: 1

Rationale: The client undergoing radiation therapy should avoid washing the site until instructed to do so. The client should then wash using mild soap and warm or cool water and pat the area dry. No lotions, creams, alcohol, or deodorants should be placed on the skin over the treatment site. Lines or ink marks that are placed on the skin to guide the radiation therapy should be left in place. The affected skin should be protected from temperature extremes, direct sunlight, and chlorinated water (as from swimming pools).

Test-Taking Strategy: Begin to answer this question by eliminating options 2 and 4 because they are contraindicated in the care of this client. Knowing that markings used to guide therapy are to be left in place helps you to choose option 1 over option 3.

Level of Cognitive Ability: Analysis
Phase of Nursing Process: Evaluation
Client Needs: Physiological Integrity
Content Area: Adult Health/Oncology

Reference

Black, J., & Matassarin-Jacobs, E. (1997). *Medical-surgical nursing: Clinical management for continuity of care* (5th ed.). Philadelphia: W. B. Saunders, pp. 571, 1673.

---

251. Which of the following sites is best for checking the pulse during cardiopulmonary resuscitation (CPR) in a 6-month-old infant?

1 Femoral
2 Carotid
3 Radial
4 Brachial

Answer: 4

Rationale: The carotid is the most central and accessible artery in children over 1 year of age. The short and often flat neck of the infant, however, renders the carotid pulse difficult to palpate. Therefore, it is preferable to use the brachial pulse, located on the inner side of the upper arm midway between the elbow and shoulder.

Test-Taking Strategy: Recall the principles related to basic life support (CPR) to answer this question. If you had difficulty remembering this information, take time now to review.

Level of Cognitive Ability: Analysis
Phase of Nursing Process: Assessment
Client Needs: Physiological Integrity
Content Area: Child Health

Reference

Ashwill, J., & Droske, S. (1997). *Nursing care of children: Principles and practice.* Philadelphia: W. B. Saunders, p. 326.

252. The client with renal failure is receiving epoetin alfa (Epogen) to support erythropoiesis. The nurse questions the client about compliance with taking which of the following medications, which supports RBC production?

1 Calcium supplement
2 Iron supplement
3 Magnesium supplement
4 Zinc supplement

Answer: 2

Rationale: Iron is needed for RBC production. The client is not receiving the full benefit of this costly therapy with epoetin alfa if iron is not taken.

Test-Taking Strategy: Basic knowledge of concepts related to RBC production and this specific medication is needed to answer this question accurately. Note the relationship of RBC production in the question and iron in the correct option. If needed, review the concepts related to epoetin alfa and RBC production.

Level of Cognitive Ability: Application
Phase of Nursing Process: Implementation
Client Needs: Physiological Integrity
Content Area: Adult Health/Renal

Reference
Monahan, F., & Neighbors, M. (1998). *Medical-surgical nursing: Foundations for clinical practice* (2nd ed.). Philadelphia: W. B. Saunders, p. 469.

---

253. The community health nurse is performing an initial assessment on a client who has arrived home with a permanent pacemaker after cardiac surgery. The nurse assesses the client's knowledge when the nurse

1 Asks the client to take the pulse in the wrist or neck and checks the accuracy of the client's reading.
2 Determines whether the client knows not to operate a microwave oven.
3 Determines whether the client knows that he or she can resume sexual activity immediately.
4 Asks the client to move the arms and shoulders vigorously to check pacemaker functioning.

Answer: 1

Rationale: Clients with permanent pacemakers must be able to take their pulse in the wrist or neck accurately to report any variation in the pulse rate or rhythm to the physician immediately. Clients can safely operate microwave ovens, VCRs, AM-FM radios, electric blankets, lawn mowers, leaf blowers, and cars. Proper grounding must be ensured if the client is to operate an electric typewriter, copying machine, and personal computer. Sexual activity is not resumed until 6 weeks after surgery. The arms and shoulders should not be moved vigorously for 6 weeks after insertion.

Test-Taking Strategy: Knowing the nursing management for permanent pacemakers is important when answering this question. Eliminate option 3 because of the word "immediately" and option 4 because of the word "vigorously." From the remaining two options, select option 1 because of the knowledge that a pacemaker assists in controlling cardiac rate and rhythm.

Level of Cognitive Ability: Application
Phase of Nursing Process: Assessment
Client Needs: Physiological Integrity
Content Area: Adult Health/Cardiovascular

Reference
Luckmann, J. (1997). *Saunders manual of nursing care*. Philadelphia: W. B. Saunders, pp. 1014–1019.

254. A client in a severe major depressive episode is unable to address activities of daily living. The most appropriate nursing intervention would be to

1 Feed, bathe, and dress the client as needed until the client can perform these activities independently.
2 Structure the client's day so that adequate time can be devoted to the client's assuming responsibility for the activities of daily living.
3 Offer the client choices and describe the consequences to the failure to comply with the expectation of maintaining activities of daily living.
4 Have the client's peers confront the client about how the noncompliance in addressing activities of daily living affects the milieu.

Answer: 1

Rationale: The symptoms of major depression include depressed mood, loss of interest or pleasure, changes in appetite and sleep patterns, psychomotor agitation or retardation, fatigue, feelings of worthlessness or guilt, diminished ability to think or concentrate, and recurrent thoughts of death. Often the clients do not have the energy or interest to complete activities of daily living. Option 2 is incorrect because the client still lacks the energy and motivation to do these independently. Option 3 may lead to increased feelings of worthlessness as the client fails to meet expectations. Option 4 increases the client's feelings of poor self-esteem and unworthiness.

Test-Taking Strategy: The key phrase in the question is "unable to." The only option that meets this client need is option 1. Often, severely depressed clients are unable to perform even the simplest of activities of daily living. The nurse assumes this role and completes these tasks with the client.

Level of Cognitive Ability: Analysis
Phase of Nursing Process: Implementation
Client Needs: Physiological Integrity
Content Area: Mental Health

Reference

Antai-Otong, D. (1995). *Psychiatric nursing: Biological and behavioral concepts.* Philadelphia: W. B. Saunders, pp. 170, 183.

255. A pregnant woman at 32 weeks' gestation is admitted to the obstetrical unit for observation after an automobile accident. She is reporting slight vaginal bleeding and mild cramps. Which of the following will the nurse do next to determine the viability of the fetus?

1 Insert an intravenous line and begin an infusion at 125 mL/hour
2 Administer oxygen to the woman with a face mask at 7–10 liters/minute
3 Position and connect the ultrasound transducer and the tocotransducer to the external fetal monitor
4 Position and connect a spiral electrode to the fetal monitor for internal fetal monitoring

Answer: 3

Rationale: External fetal monitoring allows the nurse to determine any change in the fetal heart rate and rhythm that would indicate the fetus is in jeopardy. Internal monitoring is contraindicated when there is vaginal bleeding of unstated cause, especially in preterm labor. Because fetal distress has not been determined at this time, oxygen administration is premature. The amount of bleeding described is insufficient to require intravenous fluid replacement.

Test-Taking Strategy: The client of the question is the fetus. This fact should assist in eliminating options 1 and 2. In addition, using the first step of the nursing process, assessment, can also assist in eliminating options 1 and 2. Of the remaining options, select option 3 because it is the noninvasive measure.

Level of Cognitive Ability: Application
Phase of Nursing Process: Implementation
Client Needs: Physiological Integrity
Content Area: Maternity

Reference

Lowdermilk, D., Perry, S., & Bobak, I. (1997). *Maternity and women's health care* (6th ed.). St. Louis: Mosby–Year Book, pp. 345–346.

256. The nurse is reviewing the results of a sweat test performed on a child with cystic fibrosis. The expected finding would be

1 A sweat sodium concentration less than 40 mEq/liter.
2 A sweat potassium concentration less than 40 mEq/liter.
3 A sweat potassium concentration greater than 40 mEq/liter.
4 A sweat chloride concentration greater than 60 mEq/liter.

Answer: 4

Rationale: The consistent finding of abnormally high sodium and chloride concentrations in the sweat is a unique characteristic of cystic fibrosis. Normally the sweat chloride concentration is less than 40 mEq/liter. A chloride concentration greater than 60 mEq/liter is diagnostic of cystic fibrosis. Potassium concentration is unrelated to the sweat test.

Test-Taking Strategy: Eliminate options 2 and 3 first because the potassium level is unrelated to the sweat test. For the remaining options, knowledge that sweat chloride concentration is elevated will assist in directing you to option 4. Review this important test if you had difficulty with this question.

Level of Cognitive Ability: Analysis
Phase of Nursing Process: Assessment
Client Needs: Physiological Integrity
Content Area: Child Health

Reference
Ashwill, J., & Droske, S. (1997). *Nursing care of children: Principles and practice.* Philadelphia: W. B. Saunders, p. 890.

257. When assessing the correct placement of a Miller-Abbott tube, which of the following will the nurse expect to note?

1 A pH of aspirate greater than 7.0
2 A pH of aspirate less than 7.0
3 The presence of gastric contents when checking residuals
4 The auscultation of air when inserted into the abdomen

Answer: 1

Rationale: The Miller-Abbott tube is an intestinal tube. Ensure intestinal placement by checking the pH of aspirate. A pH reading greater than 7 indicates intestinal contents; one less than 7 indicates gastric contents.

Test-Taking Strategy: Knowledge that the Miller-Abbott tube is an intestinal tube can assist in eliminating options 3 and 4. For the remaining options, recalling that intestinal fluid is alkaline can assist in directing you to option 1. Review the principles associated with placement of a Miller-Abbott tube.

Level of Cognitive Ability: Analysis
Phase of Nursing Process: Assessment
Client Needs: Physiological Integrity
Content Area: Adult Health/Gastrointestinal

Reference
Black, J., & Matassarin-Jacobs, E. (1997). *Medical-surgical nursing: Clinical management for continuity of care* (5th ed.). Philadelphia: W. B. Saunders, p. 1750.

258. The nurse performs a neurovascular assessment on a client with a newly applied cast. Close observation and further evaluation are required if the nurse notes

1 Capillary refill less than 6 seconds.
2 Palpable pulses distal to the cast.
3 Sensation when the area distal to the cast is pinched.
4 Blanching of the nailbed when depressed.

Answer: 1

Rationale: To assess for adequate circulation, depress the nail bed of each finger or toe until it blanches, then release pressure. Optimally the color changes from white to pink rapidly (<3 seconds). If this does not occur, the toes or fingers require close observation and further evaluation. Palpable pulses and sensations distal to the cast are expected. If pulses could not be palpated or if the client complained of numbness or tingling, the physician should be notified.

Test-Taking Strategy: Note the key phrase "close observation and further evaluation." Eliminate options 2, 3, and 4 because these options identify normal expected findings. Option 1 identifies an abnormal or unexpected finding. Review assessment of capillary refill if you had difficulty with this question.

Level of Cognitive Ability: Analysis
Phase of Nursing Process: Assessment
Client Needs: Physiological Integrity
Content Area: Adult Health/Neurological

Reference

Black, J., & Matassarin-Jacobs, E. (1997). *Medical-surgical nursing: Clinical management for continuity of care* (5th ed.). Philadelphia: W. B. Saunders, p. 2092.

---

259. The client undergoes a cholecystectomy and returns from surgery with a T-tube in place. During the first 24 hours after surgery, the nurse would expect how much bile to drain from the T-tube?

1 50–100 mL
2 100–200 mL
3 300–500 mL
4 700–900 mL

Answer: 3

Rationale: In the initial postoperative period, bloody drainage is expected, which changes to green-brown bile. Bile output is 400 mL per day with a gradual decrease in amount. Bile drainage amounts in excess of 1000 mL per day need to be reported to the physician.

Test-Taking Strategy: Knowledge regarding the expectations after cholecystectomy is required to answer this question. Note the key phrase "during the first 24 hours." This provides the clue that the output would be on the higher side, assisting in eliminating options 1 and 2. Attempt to visualize the amounts identified in the remaining options. Option 4 identifies an excessive amount and should be eliminated. Review postoperative expectations after cholecystectomy if you had difficulty with this question.

Level of Cognitive Ability: Analysis
Phase of Nursing Process: Assessment
Client Needs: Physiological Integrity
Content Area: Adult Health/Gastrointestinal

Reference

Black, J., & Matassarin-Jacobs, E. (1997). *Medical-surgical nursing: Clinical management for continuity of care* (5th ed.). Philadelphia: W. B. Saunders, p. 1919.

---

260. The client with Crohn's disease is admitted to the hospital for creation of a Kock pouch. The client asks the nurse about this type of pouch. Which of the following would not be a part of the nurse's description?

1 "The reservoir gradually increases in size and may attain a capacity of 500 mL."
2 "The adjustment to body image is usually less traumatic than for clients with conventional ileostomies."
3 "The intra-abdominal pouch is created from the looped sigmoid colon."
4 "The stoma is covered with a bandage between intubations to absorb leaks or mucus."

Answer: 3

Rationale: The intra-abdominal pouch (reservoir) is created from the looped ileum. It collects feces, making external collection pouches unnecessary. The stoma is covered with a bandage or gauze pad between intubations to absorb leaks or mucus. The reservoir gradually increases in size and may attain a capacity of 500 mL. The adjustment to the body change is usually less traumatic for these clients than for those with conventional ileostomies.

Test-Taking Strategy: Knowledge regarding the purpose and principles related to a Kock pouch is required to answer this question. Review this procedure if you had difficulty with this question.

Level of Cognitive Ability: Analysis
Phase of Nursing Process: Implementation
Client Needs: Physiological Integrity
Content Area: Adult Health/Gastrointestinal

Reference

Black, J., & Matassarin-Jacobs, E. (1997). *Medical-surgical nursing: Clinical management for continuity of care* (5th ed.). Philadelphia: W. B. Saunders, pp. 1807–1808.

261. On assessment of the newborn's skin, which of the following would the nurse document as abnormal?

1 Several creases noted across the palm
2 A single crease across the palm
3 The absence of creases across the palm
4 Two large creases across the palm

Answer: 2

Rationale: A single crease across the palm (simian crease) is most often associated with chromosomal abnormalities, notably Down's syndrome.

Test-Taking Strategy: Knowledge of normal newborn findings is required to answer this question. Knowledge of the characteristics associated with Down's syndrome is also helpful. You are likely to find questions related to normal newborn findings on NCLEX-RN. Review these normal findings if you had difficulty with this question.

Level of Cognitive Ability: Analysis
Phase of Nursing Process: Assessment
Client Needs: Physiological Integrity
Content Area: Maternity

Reference

Nichols, F., & Zwelling, E. (1997). *Maternal-newborn nursing: Theory and practice.* Philadelphia: W. B. Saunders, pp. 312–313.

262. The nurse is caring for a client after segmental resection of the upper lobe of the left lung. The nurse notes 500 mL of grossly bloody drainage in the chest tube drainage system during the first hour after surgery. The nurse is aware that this finding

1 Is expected after this type of surgery.
2 Represents a malfunction of the chest tube drainage system.
3 Indicates the need for autotransfusion.
4 May represent hemorrhage and requires further assessment.

Answer: 4

Rationale: Within the first 2 hours after surgery, 100–300 mL of drainage is expected. An amount of 500 mL is excessive and indicates that hemorrhage may be occurring and that the client requires further assessment. The physician should be notified.

Test-Taking Strategy: The key phrase "grossly bloody drainage" should provide you with the clue that directs you to option 4. Grossly bloody drainage indicates hemorrhage, particularly with the amount of drainage specified in the question.

Level of Cognitive Ability: Analysis
Phase of Nursing Process: Analysis
Client Needs: Physiological Integrity
Content Area: Adult Health/Respiratory

Reference

Polaski, A., & Tatro, S. (1996). *Luckmann's Core principles and practice of medical-surgical nursing.* Philadelphia: W. B. Saunders, p. 609.

263. The nurse is expecting a client from the operating room after a wedge resection of the right lower lobe. In planning for the client's safety, the nurse

1 Removes obstructions to the transport liter.
2 Notifies the pharmacy of the client's location.
3 Places rubber-shod clamps at the bedside.
4 Ascertains the wall suction unit is operational.

Answer: 3

Rationale: After wedge resection, the client has a chest tube. Clamps should always be available at the bedside of a client on closed drainage system so that they can be applied in the event of an accidental disconnection of the drainage tubing. Also, chest tubes are never clamped without specific orders of the physician except for emergencies. Although an operational wall suction is desirable, it does not directly affect the safety of the client. Option 1 relates to safety but is less directly related to the client. Option 2 is unrelated to the issue of the question.

Test-Taking Strategy: This question requires a basic knowledge of the surgical procedure and the postoperative care. The key word is "safety." Use Maslow's hierarchy of needs to prioritize. Remembering that physiological needs come first should direct you to option 3. Review postoperative expectations after wedge resection if you had difficulty with this question.

Level of Cognitive Ability: Application
Phase of Nursing Process: Planning
Client Needs: Physiological Integrity
Content Area: Adult Health/Respiratory

Reference

Polaski, A., & Tatro, S. (1996). *Luckmann's Core principles and practice of medical-surgical nursing.* Philadelphia: W. B. Saunders, p. 611.

---

264. The client begins to drain small amounts of frank bleeding from the tracheostomy tube 24 hours after a supraglottic laryngectomy. The nurse's best action is to

1 Notify the surgeon immediately.
2 Increase the frequency of suctioning.
3 Add moisture to the oxygen delivery system.
4 Document the character and amount of drainage.

Answer: 1

Rationale: Bleeding may be a sign of impending rupture of a vessel. Immediately after laryngectomy, there is a small amount of bleeding from the tracheostomy, which resolves within the first few hours. The bleeding in this instance represents a potential life threat, and the surgeon is needed to evaluate the client further and suture or repair the bleed. Although the other responses may be appropriate, they do not address the urgency of the problem. Failure to notify the surgeon in a timely fashion places the client at risk.

Test-Taking Strategy: Note the key phrases "frank bleeding" and "24 hours after." These phrases should indicate that a potential complication exists. Be alert to key identifiers such as "bleeding." Bleeding of this nature warrants physician notification. Review the complications after laryngectomy if you had difficulty with this question.

Level of Cognitive Ability: Application
Phase of Nursing Process: Implementation
Client Needs: Physiological Integrity
Content Area: Adult Health/Respiratory

Reference

Polaski, A., & Tatro, S. (1996). *Luckmann's Core principles and practice of medical-surgical nursing.* Philadelphia: W. B. Saunders, p. 552.

---

265. The nurse is caring for a client admitted to the surgical nursing unit after right modified radical mastectomy. The nurse would include which of the following in the nursing care plan for this client?

1 Position the client supine with right arm elevated on a pillow
2 Take BP measurements in the right arm only
3 Draw serum laboratory samples from the right arm only
4 Check the right posterior axilla area when assessing the surgical dressing

Answer: 4

Rationale: If there is drainage or bleeding from the surgical site after mastectomy, gravity causes the drainage to seep down and soak the posterior axillary portion of the dressing first. The nurse checks this area to discover early bleeding. The client should be positioned with the head in semi-Fowler's position and the arm elevated on pillows to decrease edema. Edema is likely to occur because lymph drainage channels have been resected during the surgical procedure. BP measurements, venipunctures, and intravenous sites should not involve use of the operative arm.

Test-Taking Strategy: Remember that options that are similar are not likely to be correct. Therefore eliminate options 2 and 3 first. Use knowledge of the effects of gravity to help you choose option 4 over option 1.

Level of Cognitive Ability: Application
Phase of Nursing Process: Planning
Client Needs: Physiological Integrity
Content Area: Adult Health/Oncology

Reference

Burrell, P., Gerlach, M., & Pless, B. (1997). *Adult nursing: Acute and community care* (2nd ed.). Stamford, CT: Appleton & Lange, p. 1818.

266. The client has a Risk for Infection after radical vulvectomy. The nurse would avoid doing which of the following when giving perineal care to this client?

1 Cleanse using warm tap water and a bulb syringe
2 Intermittently expose wound to air
3 Provide perineal care after each voiding and bowel movement
4 Provide prescribed sitz baths after sutures are removed

Answer: 1

Rationale: A sterile solution such as normal saline should be used for perineal care using an aseptic syringe or a water pick. This should be done regularly twice a day and after each voiding and bowel movement. The wound is intermittently exposed to air to permit drying and prevent maceration. Once sutures are removed, sitz baths may be prescribed to stimulate healing and for the soothing effect.

Test-Taking Strategy: The key words in the stem are "avoid" and "perineal care." Begin to answer this question by eliminating options 3 and 4, which are accepted practices. Choose option 1 over option 2 using principles of asepsis and knowledge of conditions for wound infection.

Level of Cognitive Ability: Application
Phase of Nursing Process: Implementation
Client Needs: Physiological Integrity
Content Area: Adult Health/Oncology

Reference
Monahan, F., & Neighbors, M. (1998). *Medical-surgical nursing: Foundations for clinical practice* (2nd ed.). Philadelphia: W. B. Saunders, p. 1829.

---

267. The nurse is assisting the client with hepatic encephalopathy to fill out the dietary menu. The nurse would advise the client to avoid which of the following entree items, which could aggravate the client's condition?

1 Fresh fruit plate
2 Tomato soup
3 Vegetable lasagna
4 Ground beef patty

Answer: 4

Rationale: Clients with hepatic encephalopathy have impaired ability to convert ammonia to urea and must limit intake of protein and ammonia-containing foods in the diet. The client should avoid foods such as chicken, beef, ham, cheese, buttermilk, Idaho potatoes, onions, peanut butter, and gelatin.

Test-Taking Strategy: Recalling that clients with hepatic encephalopathy need to limit the intake of protein can assist in directing you to the correct option. Note that options 1, 2, and 3 are similar in that they address food items of a fruit and vegetable nature. Option 4 is the option that is different.

Level of Cognitive Ability: Application
Phase of Nursing Process: Implementation
Client Needs: Physiological Integrity
Content Area: Adult Health/Gastrointestinal

Reference
Black, J., & Matassarin-Jacobs, E. (1997). *Medical-surgical nursing: Clinical management for continuity of care* (5th ed.). Philadelphia: W. B. Saunders, p. 1893.

---

268. The client with a colostomy is complaining of gas building up in the colostomy bag. The nurse instructs the client that which of the following food items will not aggravate this problem?

1 Beans
2 Cauliflower
3 Potatoes
4 Corn

Answer: 3

Rationale: Gas-forming foods include corn, cauliflower, onions, beans, and cabbage. These should be avoided by the client with a colostomy until tolerance to them is determined.

Test-Taking Strategy: Specific knowledge related to the effects of these foods is needed to answer this question correctly. If needed, take a few moments to review those food items that are gas forming.

Level of Cognitive Ability: Application
Phase of Nursing Process: Implementation
Client Needs: Physiological Integrity
Content Area: Adult Health/Gastrointestinal

Reference
Monahan, F., & Neighbors, M. (1998). *Medical-surgical nursing: Foundations for clinical practice* (2nd ed.). Philadelphia: W. B. Saunders, p. 961.

269. The client receiving TPN complains of nausea, excessive thirst, and increased frequency of voiding. The nurse next assesses which of the following client data?

1 Serum BUN and creatinine
2 Capillary blood glucose
3 Last serum potassium
4 Rectal temperature

Answer: 2

Rationale: The symptoms exhibited by the client are consistent with hyperglycemia. The nurse would need to assess the client's blood glucose level to verify these data. Clients receiving TPN are at risk for hyperglycemia related to the increased glucose load of the solution. The other options do not give any information that would correlate with the client symptoms.

Test-Taking Strategy: To answer this question correctly, you must interpret that the symptoms portrayed by the client are consistent with hyperglycemia, which is a complication of TPN. This would allow you to eliminate each of the incorrect options without difficulty. Review the complications associated with TPN if you had difficulty with this question.

Level of Cognitive Ability: Analysis
Phase of Nursing Process: Assessment
Client Needs: Physiological Integrity
Content Area: Adult Health/Gastrointestinal

Reference

Monahan, F., & Neighbors, M. (1998). *Medical-surgical nursing: Foundations for clinical practice* (2nd ed.). Philadelphia: W. B. Saunders, p. 987.

270. The client admitted with a diagnosis of cirrhosis has massive ascites and has difficulty breathing. The nurse performs which of the following interventions as a priority measure to assist the client with breathing?

1 Auscultate the lung fields every 4 hours
2 Reposition side-to-side every 2 hours
3 Encourage deep-breathing technique every 2 hours
4 Elevate the head of the bed 60 degrees

Answer: 4

Rationale: The client is having difficulty breathing because of upward pressure on the diaphragm from the ascitic fluid. Elevating the head of bed enlists the aid of gravity in relieving pressure on the diaphragm. The other responses are good general measures to promote lung expansion in the client with ascites, but the priority measure is one that relieves diaphragmatic pressure.

Test-Taking Strategy: Note the key word "priority measure" in the stem of the question. This tells you that more than one or all of the options may be partially or totally correct. In this case, every option is a correct nursing action, but elevating the head takes highest priority in providing immediate relief of symptoms.

Level of Cognitive Ability: Application
Phase of Nursing Process: Implementation
Client Needs: Physiological Integrity
Content Area: Adult Health/Gastrointestinal

Reference

Monahan, F., & Neighbors, M. (1998). *Medical-surgical nursing: Foundations for clinical practice* (2nd ed.). Philadelphia: W. B. Saunders, p. 1190.

271. The client with diverticulitis has just been advanced from a liquid diet to solids. The nurse plans to encourage the client to take in foods that are

1 Low in residue.
2 High in protein.
3 Moderate in fat.
4 High in carbohydrates.

Answer: 1

Rationale: The purpose of a low-residue diet with diverticulitis is to allow the bowel to rest while the inflammation subsides. The client should avoid such foods as nuts, corn, popcorn, and raw celery, which are high in roughage.

Test-Taking Strategy: To answer this question correctly, it is necessary to understand this disease process and the therapeutic dietary considerations needed to promote healing. Recalling that diverticulitis indicates inflammation can assist in directing you to the correct option. If this question was difficult, take a few moments to review the diet prescribed for this disorder.

Level of Cognitive Ability: Application
Phase of Nursing Process: Planning
Client Needs: Physiological Integrity
Content Area: Adult Health/Gastrointestinal

Reference

Monahan, F., & Neighbors, M. (1998). *Medical-surgical nursing: Foundations for clinical practice* (2nd ed.). Philadelphia: W. B. Saunders, pp. 1083–1084.

---

272. The client with Cushing's disease is being admitted to the hospital after a stab wound to the abdomen. The nurse places highest priority on which of the following nursing diagnoses developed for this client?

1. Risk for Fluid Volume Deficit
2. Risk for Infection
3. Body Image Disturbance
4. Altered Health Maintenance

Answer: 2

Rationale: The client with a stab wound has a break in the body's first line of defense against infection. The client with Cushing's disease is at great risk for infection because of excess cortisol secretion, subsequent impaired antibody function, and decreased proliferation of lymphocytes. The client may also have an Altered Health Maintenance and Body Image Disturbance, but these are not the highest priority at this time. The client would be at risk for Fluid Volume Excess, not Fluid Volume Deficit, with Cushing's disease.

Test-Taking Strategy: The key words in the stem are "highest priority." This tells you that more than one or all of the options may be partially or totally correct. Eliminate option 1 first because it is the opposite of what is expected with this disorder. From the remaining three options, note that option 2 addresses the physiological need.

Level of Cognitive Ability: Analysis
Phase of Nursing Process: Analysis
Client Needs: Physiological Integrity
Content Area: Adult Health/Endocrine

Reference

Monahan, F., & Neighbors, M. (1998). *Medical-surgical nursing: Foundations for clinical practice* (2nd ed.). Philadelphia: W. B. Saunders, pp. 1286–1289.

---

273. The client had a radical neck dissection with musculocutaneous flap. Twenty-four hours after the procedure, the nurse notes that the flap has a slightly blue hue. The nurse concludes

1. This is a normal expectation.
2. Heat should be applied to the area.
3. Venous circulation is impaired.
4. The client is exhibiting generalized hypoxia.

Answer: 3

Rationale: The blue color is a sign of venous engorgement resulting from venous stasis, which increases local tissue hypoxia and can lead to necrosis of the area affected. This is not a normal expectation. Heat application causes more damage to the tissue. There is no evidence to support option 4.

Test-Taking Strategy: Eliminate option 1 first knowing that this situation is not normal. Eliminate option 4 next because the question does not provide data to support this option. For the remaining options, basic principles associated with the application of heat should assist in eliminating option 2.

Level of Cognitive Ability: Analysis
Phase of Nursing Process: Analysis
Client Needs: Physiological Integrity
Content Area: Adult Health/Integumentary

Reference

Polaski, A., & Tatro, S. (1996). *Luckmann's Core principles and practice of medical-surgical nursing*. Philadelphia: W. B. Saunders, pp. 554, 1394.

274. A female adolescent client is admitted to the inpatient unit after medical stabilization for an overdose of acetaminophen (Tylenol). Her boyfriend broke up with her 2 weeks ago. She stopped eating at that time and has lost 15 pounds. Which of the following would not be a component of the client's plan of care?

1. Offer frequent nutritious snacks
2. Provide meals on an isolation tray that contains no glass or metal utensils
3. Stand the client in front of a mirror to show her how thin she is
4. Offer bland, easy-to-digest foods

Answer: 3

Rationale: The client has been denying herself food as a means of self-harm. Reinforcing her success at this is not therapeutic. Meeting her nutritional needs is the nursing care priority.

Test-Taking Strategy: In answering this question, look for options that meet the basic needs of adequate nutrition. Note the key word "not" in the stem of the question. Option 3 is the only option that does not address nutrition or a physiological need.

Level of Cognitive Ability: Analysis
Phase of Nursing Process: Planning
Client Needs: Physiological Integrity
Content Area: Mental Health

Reference
Wilson, H., & Kneisl, C. (1996). *Psychiatric nursing* (5th ed.). Menlo Park, CA: Addison-Wesley, pp. 427, 599.

---

275. A manic client is placed in a seclusion room after an outburst of violent behavior, including physical assault on another client. As the client is secluded, the nurse should

1. Remain silent because verbal interaction would be too stimulating.
2. Tell the client that the client will be allowed to rejoin the others when he or she can behave.
3. Ask the client if he or she understands why the seclusion is necessary.
4. Inform the client that he or she is being secluded to help regain self-control.

Answer: 4

Rationale: The client is removed to a nonstimulating environment as a result of behavior. Options 1, 2, and 3 are nontherapeutic. In addition, option 2 implies punishment. It is best to inform the client directly of the purpose of the seclusion.

Test-Taking Strategy: Look for the response that presents reality most clearly to the client. Option 4 is the only option that provides a clear and direct purpose of the seclusion.

Level of Cognitive Ability: Application
Phase of Nursing Process: Implementation
Client Needs: Physiological Integrity
Content Area: Mental Health

Reference
Wilson, H., & Kneisl, C. (1996). *Psychiatric nursing* (5th ed.). Menlo Park, CA: Addison-Wesley, p. 831.

---

276. The nurse evaluates the client after treatment for carbon monoxide poisoning. The nurse would document that the treatment has been successful when the

1. Client is awake and talking.
2. Carboxyhemoglobin levels are less than 5%.
3. Heart monitor shows sinus tachycardia.
4. Client is sleeping soundly.

Answer: 2

Rationale: Normal carboxyhemoglobin levels are less than 5%. Clients can be awake and talking with abnormally high levels. Other symptoms of carbon monoxide poisoning are tachycardia, tachypnea, and central nervous system depression.

Test-Taking Strategy: The question asks about carbon monoxide poisoning. Option 2 is the only option that specifically addresses this issue. Review normal carboxyhemoglobin levels if you had difficulty with this question.

Level of Cognitive Ability: Analysis
Phase of Nursing Process: Evaluation
Client Needs: Physiological Integrity
Content Area: Adult Health/Respiratory

Reference
Ruppert, S., Kernicki, J., & Dolan, J. (1996). *Dolan's critical care nursing: Clinical management through the nursing process* (2nd ed.). Philadelphia: F. A. Davis, p. 947.

277. The nurse caring for the client with hepatic encephalopathy assesses for asterixis. To test for asterixis appropriately, the nurse

1 Asks the client to extend an arm, dorsiflex the wrist, and extend the fingers.
2 Checks stools for clay-colored pigmentation.
3 Asks the client to sign his or her name and notes any deterioration.
4 Reviews laboratory serum levels of bilirubin and alkaline phosphatase for elevation.

Answer: 1

Rationale: Asterixis is an abnormal muscle tremor often associated with hepatic encephalopathy. Asterixis is sometimes called "liver flap." Options 2, 3, and 4 are associated with hepatitis but are not signs of asterixis.

Test-Taking Strategy: Knowledge of signs and symptoms of hepatic encephalopathy is important in answering this question. Specifically, knowledge of how to test for this sign is needed. If you are unfamiliar with assessment for asterixis, it is important to review.

Level of Cognitive Ability: Application
Phase of Nursing Process: Assessment
Client Needs: Physiological Integrity
Content Area: Fundamental Skills

Reference
Luckmann, J. (1997). *Saunders manual of nursing care.* Philadelphia: W. B. Saunders, p. 1318.

278. The nurse instructs a preoperative client in the proper use of an incentive spirometer. Postoperative assessment of this client reveals that the incentive spirometry was effective if the client exhibits

1 Coughing.
2 Shallow breaths.
3 Wheezing in one lung field.
4 Unilateral chest expansion.

Answer: 1

Rationale: Incentive devices provide the stimulus for a spontaneous deep breath. Spontaneous deep breathing, using the sustained maximal inspiration concept, reduces atelectasis, opens airways, stimulates coughing, and actively encourages individual participation in recovery. Shallow breaths, wheezing, and unilateral chest expansion indicate that the incentive spirometry was not effective. Wheezing indicates narrowing or obstruction of the airway, and unilateral chest expansion could indicate atelectasis.

Test-Taking Strategy: To answer this question correctly, knowledge of the purpose and effects of incentive spirometry is essential. Options 2, 3, and 4 indicate abnormal findings. Review the purpose of an incentive spirometer if you had difficulty with this question.

Level of Cognitive Ability: Analysis
Phase of Nursing Process: Assessment
Client Needs: Physiological Integrity
Content Area: Fundamental Skills

Reference
Lammon, C. B., Foote, A. W., Leli, P. G., et al. (1995). *Clinical nursing skills.* Philadelphia: W. B. Saunders, pp. 525–527.

279. The client is to be started on prazosin (Minipress). The client asks the nurse why the first three doses must be taken at bedtime. The nurse's response is based on the understanding that during early use, prazosin

1 Can cause dizziness, lightheadedness, or possible syncope.
2 Results in extreme drowsiness.
3 Should be taken when the stomach is empty.
4 Can cause significant dependent edema.

Answer: 1

Rationale: Prazosin is an alpha-adrenergic blocking agent. "First-dose hypotensive reaction" may occur during early therapy, which is characterized by dizziness, lightheadedness, and possible loss of consciousness. This reaction can also occur during periods when the dosage is increased. This effect usually disappears with continued use or when the dosage is decreased.

Test-Taking Strategy: This question is asking about initial reactions to this medication. Knowing that prazosin is an antihypertensive agent, you should anticipate orthostatic hypotension as the most likely problem. This would help you to eliminate each of the incorrect options. Review this medication now if you had difficulty with this question.

Level of Cognitive Ability: Analysis
Phase of Nursing Process: Analysis
Client Needs: Physiological Integrity
Content Area: Pharmacology

Reference

Deglin, J., & Vallerand, A. (1997). *Davis's drug guide for nurses* (5th ed.). Philadelphia: F. A. Davis, p. 997.

---

280. The nurse has applied the prescribed dressing to the leg of a client with an ischemic arterial leg ulcer. The nurse would use which of the following methods of covering the dressing?

1. Apply an ABD pad, and tape it to the skin
2. Apply a Kerlix roll, and tape it to the skin
3. Apply small Montgomery straps, and tie the edges together
4. Apply a Kling roll, and tape the edge of the roll onto the bandage

Answer: 4

Rationale: With an arterial ulcer, the nurse applies tape only to the bandage itself. Tape is never used directly on the skin because it could cause further tissue damage. For the same reason, Montgomery straps could not be applied to the skin (these are generally intended for use on abdominal wounds anyway). Standard dressing technique includes the use of Kling rolls on circumferential dressings.

Test-Taking Strategy: The wording of the question tells you there is only one correct option. If you know that tape is not applied to the skin, you immediately eliminate options 1 and 2. For the same reason, you next eliminate option 3 because the Montgomery straps would need to be adhered to the skin as well.

Level of Cognitive Ability: Application
Phase of Nursing Process: Implementation
Client Needs: Physiological Integrity
Content Area: Adult Health/Cardiovascular

Reference

Ignatavicius, D. D., Workman, M. L., & Mishler, M. A. (1995). *Medical-surgical nursing: A nursing process approach* (2nd ed.). Philadelphia: W. B. Saunders, p. 945.

---

281. Breathing exercises and postural drainage are ordered for the child with cystic fibrosis. The most appropriate plan to implement these procedures includes which of the following?

1. Perform the postural drainage, then the breathing exercises
2. Perform the breathing exercises, then the postural drainage
3. Plan the breathing exercises and the postural drainage so they are scheduled 4 hours apart
4. Perform postural drainage in the morning and breathing exercises in the evening

Answer: 1

Rationale: Breathing exercises are recommended for the majority of children with cystic fibrosis, even for those with minimal pulmonary involvement. The exercises are usually performed twice daily, and they are preceded with postural drainage. The postural drainage mobilizes secretions, and the breathing exercises then assist with expectoration. Exercises to assist with posture and to mobilize the thorax are included, such as swinging the arms and bending and twisting the trunk. The ultimate aim of these exercises is to establish a good habitual breathing pattern.

Test-Taking Strategy: Knowledge that postural drainage and breathing exercises are most effective when performed together can assist in eliminating options 3 and 4. From the remaining two options, consider the effectiveness that each procedure has on the mobilization of secretions. This can assist in directing you to the correct option.

Level of Cognitive Ability: Application
Phase of Nursing Process: Implementation
Client Needs: Physiological Integrity
Content Area: Child Health

Reference

Black, J., & Matassarin-Jacobs, E. (1997). *Medical-surgical nursing: Clinical management for continuity of care* (5th ed.). Philadelphia: W. B. Saunders, pp. 1148–1149.

282. A child is admitted to the pediatric unit with a diagnosis of celiac disease. On the basis of this diagnosis, the nurse will expect that the child's stools will be

1 Dark in color.
2 Abnormally small in amount.
3 Unusually hard.
4 Particularly offensive in odor.

Answer: 4

Rationale: The stools of a child with celiac disease are characteristically malodorous, pale, large (bulky), and soft (loose). Excessive flatus is common, and bouts of diarrhea may occur.

Test-Taking Strategy: Knowledge of the manifestations that occur in celiac disease is required to answer this question. Review these manifestations if you had difficulty with this question. Knowledge of normal expectations is required to assist in directing nursing interventions appropriately.

Level of Cognitive Ability: Analysis
Phase of Nursing Process: Analysis
Client Needs: Physiological Integrity
Content Area: Child Health

Reference
Ashwill, J., & Droske, S. (1997). *Nursing care of children: Principles and practice.* Philadelphia: W. B. Saunders, pp. 732–735.

---

283. The clinic nurse is caring for a client suspected of a diagnosis of pregnancy-induced hypertension. Significant assessment findings in the client with PIH include

1 Glycosuria, hypertension, and obesity.
2 Edema, ketonuria, and obesity.
3 Edema, tachycardia, and ketonuria.
4 Hypertension, edema, and proteinuria.

Answer: 4

Rationale: PIH is the most common hypertensive disorder in pregnancy. It is characterized by the development of hypertension, proteinuria, and edema. Glycosuria and ketonuria occur in diabetes. Tachycardia and obesity are not specifically related to diagnosing PIH.

Test-Taking Strategy: You can easily eliminate options 2 and 3 because they do not address hypertension. For the remaining options, recalling that glycosuria is an indication of diabetes can assist in directing you to option 4. Review the clinical manifestations associated with PIH if you had difficulty with this question. You are likely to find questions related to PIH on NCLEX-RN.

Level of Cognitive Ability: Analysis
Phase of Nursing Process: Assessment
Client Needs: Physiological Integrity
Content Area: Maternity

Reference
Nichols, F., & Zwelling, E. (1997). *Maternal-newborn nursing: Theory and practice.* Philadelphia: W. B. Saunders, p. 643.

---

284. The client who undergoes a gastric resection is at risk for developing dumping syndrome. Which of the following is a symptom of this syndrome?

1 Extreme thirst
2 Bradycardia
3 Dizziness
4 Constipation

Answer: 3

Rationale: Observation for early manifestations of dumping syndrome should occur 5–30 minutes after eating. Symptoms include vasomotor disturbances, such as vertigo, tachycardia, syncope, sweating, pallor, palpitations, and the desire to lie down.

Test-Taking Strategy: Knowledge of the manifestations that occur with dumping syndrome is required to answer this question. If you know that these symptoms are vasomotor in nature, you can easily select the correct option. Review this disorder and the appropriate treatment measures if you had difficulty with this question.

Level of Cognitive Ability: Analysis
Phase of Nursing Process: Assessment
Client Needs: Physiological Integrity
Content Area: Adult Health/Gastrointestinal

Reference
Black, J., & Matassarin-Jacobs, E. (1997). *Medical-surgical nursing: Clinical management for continuity of care* (5th ed.). Philadelphia: W. B. Saunders, p. 1779.

285. When assessing the client for the major postoperative complication after a craniotomy, the nurse would monitor for

1 Restlessness.
2 Bleeding.
3 Hypotension.
4 Bradycardia.

Answer: 1

Rationale: The major postoperative complication is increased ICP from cerebral edema, hemorrhage, or obstruction of the normal flow of CSF. Symptoms of increased ICP include severe headache, deteriorating level of consciousness, restlessness, irritability, and dilated or pinpoint pupils that are slow to react or nonreactive to light. Without prompt recognition and treatment, herniation syndromes develop, and the client could die.

Test-Taking Strategy: Always monitor the neurological client for increased ICP. Remember that changes in the level of consciousness are the first key indicator of increased ICP. Option 1 is the only option that addresses level of consciousness. Review the signs of increased ICP and postoperative complications after craniotomy if you had difficulty with this question. You are likely to find questions related to ICP on NCLEX-RN.

Level of Cognitive Ability: Analysis
Phase of Nursing Process: Assessment
Client Needs: Physiological Integrity
Content Area: Adult Health/Neurological

Reference

Black, J., & Matassarin-Jacobs, E. (1997). *Medical-surgical nursing: Clinical management for continuity of care* (5th ed.). Philadelphia: W. B. Saunders, p. 853.

286. Buck's traction is applied to an elderly client after a hip fracture. The client asks the nurse about the traction. Which of the following provides the best description of this type of traction?

1 Skin traction involving the use of traction attached to the skin and soft tissues
2 Skeletal traction involving the use of surgically inserted pins
3 Circumferential traction involving the use of a belt around the body
4 Plaster traction involving the use of a cast

Answer: 1

Rationale: Buck's traction is a form of skin traction and involves the use of a belt or halter that is attached to the skin and soft tissues. The purpose of this type of traction is to decrease painful muscle spasms that accompany fractures. The weight that is used as a pulling force is limited (5–10 lb), to prevent injury to the skin.

Test-Taking Strategy: Recalling that Buck's traction is a skin traction can assist in eliminating options 2, 3, and 4. Review the purpose and principles related to this type of traction if you had difficulty with this question.

Level of Cognitive Ability: Analysis
Phase of Nursing Process: Analysis
Client Needs: Physiological Integrity
Content Area: Adult Health/Musculoskeletal

Reference

Black, J., & Matassarin-Jacobs, E. (1997). *Medical-surgical nursing: Clinical management for continuity of care* (5th ed.). Philadelphia: W. B. Saunders, pp. 2138–2139.

287. The client arrives in the emergency room with burns to both legs and perineal areas. Using the rule of nines, the nurse would determine that approximately what percentage of the client's body surface has been burned?

1 19%
2 46%
3 37%
4 65%

Answer: 3

Rationale: The most rapid method used to calculate the size of a burn injury in adult clients whose weights are in normal proportion to their heights is the rule of nines. This method divides the body into areas that are in multiples of 9%. Each leg is 18%, each arm is 9%, and the head is 9%. The trunk is 36%, and the perineal area is 1%. Both legs and perineal area equal 37%.

Test-Taking Strategy: Knowledge of the percentages associated with this method of calculating burn injuries is required to answer this question. Memorize these percentages. You are likely to find questions related to this calculation on NCLEX-RN.

Level of Cognitive Ability: Analysis
Phase of Nursing Process: Assessment
Client Needs: Physiological Integrity
Content Area: Adult Health/Integumentary

Reference

Black, J., & Matassarin-Jacobs, E. (1997). *Medical-surgical nursing: Clinical management for continuity of care* (5th ed.). Philadelphia: W. B. Saunders, pp. 2237–2241.

---

288. Skin closure with heterograft is performed on the burn client. The client asks the nurse about the meaning of a heterograft. The nurse bases the response on the knowledge that a heterograft can best be described as

1. Skin from another species.
2. Skin from a cadaver.
3. Skin from the burned client.
4. Skin from a skin bank.

Answer: 1

Rationale: Biological dressings are usually heterograft or homograft material. Heterograft is skin from another species. The most commonly used type of heterograft is pigskin because of its availability and its relative compatibility with human skin. Homograft is skin from another human, which is usually obtained from a cadaver and is provided through a skin bank. Autograft is skin from the client.

Test-Taking Strategy: Knowledge of the types of skin grafts is helpful in answering the question. Options 2, 3, and 4 all relate to grafts from human skin. Option 1 is the option that is different. Review the various types of skin closure grafts if you had difficulty with this question.

Level of Cognitive Ability: Analysis
Phase of Nursing Process: Analysis
Client Needs: Physiological Integrity
Content Area: Adult Health/Integumentary

Reference

Black, J., & Matassarin-Jacobs, E. (1997). *Medical-surgical nursing: Clinical management for continuity of care* (5th ed.). Philadelphia: W. B. Saunders, p. 2256.

---

289. The nurse admits a client who sustained a head injury to the intensive care unit for observation. The most appropriate position for this client is

1. Head elevated on pillow.
2. Left Sims'.
3. Reverse Trendelenburg.
4. Head of bed elevated 30–45 degrees.

Answer: 4

Rationale: The client is positioned to avoid extreme flexion or extension of the neck and to maintain the head in the midline, neutral position. The client is logrolled when turned to avoid extreme hip flexion. The head of the bed is elevated 30–45 degrees. All of these measures are used to enhance venous drainage, which helps prevent increased ICP.

Test-Taking Strategy: The key issue of this question is the concern regarding increased ICP. Bearing this in mind, and considering the principles of gravity, you should easily be able to eliminate options 1, 2, and 3. Review care of the client after a head injury if you had difficulty with this question.

Level of Cognitive Ability: Application
Phase of Nursing Process: Implementation
Client Needs: Physiological Integrity
Content Area: Adult Health/Neurological

Reference

Black, J., & Matassarin-Jacobs, E. (1997). *Medical-surgical nursing: Clinical management for continuity of care* (5th ed.). Philadelphia: W. B. Saunders, p. 853.

290. The nurse assesses the 12th cranial nerve in the client who sustained a cerebrovascular accident. When assessing the 12th cranial nerve, the nurse should ask the client to

1 Extend the arms.
2 Turn the head toward the nurse's arm.
3 Extend the tongue.
4 Focus the eyes on the object held by the nurse.

Answer: 3

Rationale: To assess the function of the 12th cranial (hypoglossal) nerve, the nurse would assess the client's ability to extend the tongue. Impairment of the 12th cranial nerve can occur with a cerebrovascular accident.

Test-Taking Strategy: Knowledge that the 12th cranial nerve is the hypoglossal nerve can assist in directing you to option 3. Review the cranial nerves and the method of testing these nerves if you had difficulty with this question.

Level of Cognitive Ability: Application
Phase of Nursing Process: Assessment
Client Needs: Physiological Integrity
Content Area: Adult Health/Neurological

Reference

Black, J., & Matassarin-Jacobs, E. (1997). *Medical-surgical nursing: Clinical management for continuity of care* (5th ed.). Philadelphia: W. B. Saunders, p. 721.

---

291. The infant is admitted to the pediatric unit with a diagnosis of tracheoesophageal fistula. A typical finding in the infant with tracheoesophageal fistula is

1 Continuous drooling.
2 Diaphragmatic breathing.
3 Slowed reflexes.
4 Passage of large amounts of frothy stool.

Answer: 1

Rationale: Esophageal atresia prevents the passage of swallowed mucus and saliva into the stomach. After fluid has accumulated in the pouch, it flows from the mouth, and the infant then drools continuously. The lack of swallowed amniotic fluid prevents the accumulation of normal meconium; lack of stools results. Responsiveness of the infant to stimulus depends on the overall condition of the infant and is not considered a classic sign of tracheoesophageal fistula. Diaphragmatic breathing is not associated with tracheoesophageal fistula.

Test-Taking Strategy: Knowledge regarding tracheoesophageal fistula is required to answer this question. Eliminate options 3 and 4 by considering the anatomical location of the disorder. For the remaining options, recalling that diaphragmatic breathing is not associated with tracheoesophageal fistula can assist in directing you to the correct option. Review the manifestations associated with tracheoesophageal fistula if you had difficulty with this question.

Level of Cognitive Ability: Analysis
Phase of Nursing Process: Assessment
Client Needs: Physiological Integrity
Content Area: Child Health

Reference

Nichols, F., & Zwelling, E. (1997). *Maternal-newborn nursing: Theory and practice.* Philadelphia: W. B. Saunders, pp. 1364–1365.

---

292. The nurse is determining the need for suctioning in a client with an endotracheal tube attached to a mechanical ventilator. Which of the following observations, if made by the nurse, is not consistent with the need for suctioning?

1 Low peak inspiratory pressure on the ventilator
2 Gurgling sound with respiration
3 Restlessness
4 Presence of rhonchi

Answer: 1

Rationale: Indications for suctioning include moist, wet respirations; restlessness; rhonchi on auscultation of the lungs; visible mucus bubbling in the endotracheal tube; increased pulse and respiratory rates; and increased peak inspiratory pressures on the ventilator. A low peak inspiratory pressure indicates a leak in the mechanical ventilation system.

Test-Taking Strategy: The question asks for an item that is not consistent with the need to be suctioned. Rhonchi and gurgling sounds are obvious indications for suctioning and are therefore eliminated as possible answers to this question. Recalling that restlessness is a sign of hypoxia (which could result from need for suctioning) helps you to eliminate this option also. Because the client needing suctioning would trigger the high-pressure alarm, not the low-pressure alarm, it is the item not consistent with the need for suctioning and is the answer to this question.

Level of Cognitive Ability: Analysis
Phase of Nursing Process: Assessment
Client Needs: Physiological Integrity
Content Area: Adult Health/Respiratory

Reference

Black, J., & Matassarin-Jacobs, E. (1997). *Medical-surgical nursing: Clinical management for continuity of care* (5th ed.). Philadelphia: W. B. Saunders, p. 1175.

---

293. The client is intubated receiving mechanical ventilation. The physician has added 7 cm H_2O of positive end-expiratory pressure (PEEP) to the ventilator settings of the client. The nurse assesses for which of the following expected but adverse effects of PEEP?

1. Systolic BP decreased from 122 to 98 mmHg
2. Heart rate dropped from 78 to 64 beats/minute
3. Decreased peak pressure on the ventilator
4. Temperature increased from 98°F to 100°F rectal

Answer: 1

Rationale: PEEP leads to increased intrathoracic pressure, which, in turn, leads to decreased cardiac output. This is manifested in the client by decreased BP and increased pulse (compensatory). Peak pressures on the ventilator should not be affected, although the pressure at the end of expiration remains positive at the level set for PEEP. Fever indicates respiratory infection or infection from another source.

Test-Taking Strategy: The question asks for an "expected but adverse" effect. Knowing that PEEP increases intrathoracic pressure leads you to look for an item that reflects a consequence of this event. Fever is irrelevant, and option 4 is eliminated first. Because expected effects would be tachycardia, decreased BP, and increased peak pressure on the ventilator, option 1 is the only possible choice.

Level of Cognitive Ability: Application
Phase of Nursing Process: Assessment
Client Needs: Physiological Integrity
Content Area: Adult Health/Respiratory

Reference

Black, J., & Matassarin-Jacobs, E. (1997). *Medical-surgical nursing: Clinical management for continuity of care* (5th ed.). Philadelphia: W. B. Saunders, p. 1182.

---

294. The nurse is assessing the respiratory status of the client after thoracentesis. The nurse would become most concerned with which of the following assessment findings?

1. Respiratory rate of 22 breaths/minute
2. Equal bilateral chest expansion
3. Few scattered wheezes, unchanged from baseline
4. Diminished breath sounds on the affected side

Answer: 4

Rationale: After thoracentesis, the nurse assesses vital signs and breath sounds. The nurse especially notes increased respiratory rates, dyspnea, retractions, diminished breath sounds, or cyanosis, which could indicate pneumothorax. Any of these signs should be reported to the physician.

Test-Taking Strategy: The question asks for the findings that are of most concern, which implies that more than one answer may be completely or partially abnormal. Eliminate options 1 and 2 first because they are normal findings. Option 3 is an abnormality but is unchanged from the client's baseline. Option 4 is correct because diminished breath sounds on the affected side indicate pneumothorax, which is of much concern.

Level of Cognitive Ability: Analysis
Phase of Nursing Process: Assessment
Client Needs: Physiological Integrity
Content Area: Adult Health/Respiratory

Reference

Black, J., & Matassarin-Jacobs, E. (1997). *Medical-surgical nursing: Clinical management for continuity of care* (5th ed.). Philadelphia: W. B. Saunders, p. 1063.

295. The nurse is preparing to administer a Mantoux skin test to a client. The nurse assesses that which of the following areas is the most appropriate area for injection of the medication?

1. Inner aspect of forearm that is not heavily pigmented
2. Inner aspect of forearm that is close to a burn scar
3. Dorsal aspect of the upper arm near a mole
4. Dorsal aspect of the upper arm that has a small amount of hair

Answer: 1

Rationale: Intradermal injections are most commonly given in the inner surface of the forearm. Other sites include the dorsal area of the upper arm or the upper back beneath the scapulae. The nurse finds an area that is not heavily pigmented and is removed from hairy areas or lesions, which could interfere with reading the results.

Test-Taking Strategy: This question tests a fundamental concept of site selection for intradermal injection. You can easily eliminate options 3 and 4. From the remaining two options, use general principles regarding the administration of medications to direct you to option 1. If this question was difficult for you, take a few moments now to review the basics of intradermal injection techniques.

Level of Cognitive Ability: Application
Phase of Nursing Process: Assessment
Client Needs: Physiological Integrity
Content Area: Adult Health/Respiratory

Reference

Ignatavicius, D. D., Workman, M. L., & Mishler, M. A. (1995). *Medical-surgical nursing: A nursing process approach* (2nd ed.). Philadelphia: W. B. Saunders, p. 720.

---

296. The home care nurse is planning therapeutic measures for the client who experienced a rib fracture 2 days earlier. Which of the following items would not be included by the nurse in the nursing care plan?

1. Rest
2. Local heat
3. Ice
4. Analgesics

Answer: 3

Rationale: Common therapies for fractured ribs include rest, analgesics, and local application of heat. Heat has an analgesic effect and speeds resolution of inflammation.

Test-Taking Strategy: This question can be answered most readily by recalling that ice is used only in the first 24 hours after an injury. This can help you to eliminate each of the other incorrect responses. Review client teaching points related to measures in treating a rib fracture if you had difficulty with this question.

Level of Cognitive Ability: Application
Phase of Nursing Process: Planning
Client Needs: Physiological Integrity
Content Area: Adult Health/Respiratory

Reference

Black, J., & Matassarin-Jacobs, E. (1997). *Medical-surgical nursing: Clinical management for continuity of care* (5th ed.). Philadelphia: W. B. Saunders, p. 2526.

---

297. The hospitalized client is dyspneic, and left pneumothorax has been diagnosed by chest x-ray. Which of the following signs or symptoms observed by the nurse most clearly indicates that the pneumothorax is rapidly worsening?

1. Pain with respiration
2. Hypertension
3. Tracheal deviation to the right
4. Tracheal deviation to the left

Answer: 3

Rationale: A pneumothorax is characterized by distended neck veins, displaced PMI, subcutaneous emphysema, tracheal deviation to the unaffected side, decreased fremitus, and worsening cyanosis. The client could have pain with respiration even with milder pneumothorax. The increased intrathoracic pressure would cause the BP to fall, not to rise.

Test-Taking Strategy: Pain and hypertension are the least specific indicators and are therefore eliminated first. The key point to remember in answering this question is that a large pneumothorax causes the trachea to be pushed in the opposite direction, to the unaffected side. In this case, the deviation would be to the right, making option 3 the correct answer.

Level of Cognitive Ability: Analysis
Phase of Nursing Process: Analysis
Client Needs: Physiological Integrity
Content Area: Adult Health/Respiratory

Reference

Black, J., & Matassarin-Jacobs, E. (1997). *Medical-surgical nursing: Clinical management for continuity of care* (5th ed.). Philadelphia: W. B. Saunders, p. 2524.

---

298. The client is admitted with a diagnosis of right lower lobe pneumonia. The nurse auscultates the right lower lobe for which of the following types of breath sounds?

1 Bronchial
2 Bronchovesicular
3 Vesicular
4 Absent

Answer: 1

Rationale: The client with pneumonia has bronchial breath sounds over area(s) of consolidation because the consolidated tissue carries bronchial sounds to the peripheral lung fields. The client may also have crackles in the affected area because of fluid in the interstitium and alveoli.

Test-Taking Strategy: Knowledge of normal breath sounds and how they change with pneumonia is necessary to answer this question correctly. Knowing that vesicular breath sounds are normal in the lung periphery helps you to eliminate this option as the abnormal finding in pneumonia. To discriminate among the other three, you need to know that the pneumonia transmits bronchial breath sounds, heard over the area of consolidation.

Level of Cognitive Ability: Application
Phase of Nursing Process: Assessment
Client Needs: Physiological Integrity
Content Area: Adult Health/Respiratory

Reference

Black, J., & Matassarin-Jacobs, E. (1997). *Medical-surgical nursing: Clinical management for continuity of care* (5th ed.). Philadelphia: W. B. Saunders, p. 1134.

---

299. The nurse assesses the client with AIDS for early signs of Kaposi's sarcoma. The nurse would observe the client for lesion(s) that are

1 Unilateral, raised, and bluish purple in color.
2 Bilateral, flat, and pink turning to dark violet or black in color.
3 Unilateral, red, raised, and resembling a blister.
4 Bilateral, flat, and brownish and scaly in appearance.

Answer: 2

Rationale: Kaposi's sarcoma generally starts with an area that is flat and pink, which changes to a dark violet or black color. The lesions are usually present bilaterally. They may appear in many areas of the body and are treated with radiation, chemotherapy, and cryotherapy.

Test-Taking Strategy: Knowing that Kaposi's sarcoma occurs in a bilateral pattern helps you to eliminate options 1 and 3. Knowledge of the character of the lesions is necessary to discriminate between options 2 and 4. Review the characteristics of this disorder if you had difficulty with this question.

Level of Cognitive Ability: Application
Phase of Nursing Process: Assessment
Client Needs: Physiological Integrity
Content Area: Adult Health/Integumentary

Reference

Black, J., & Matassarin-Jacobs, E. (1997). *Medical-surgical nursing: Clinical management for continuity of care* (5th ed.). Philadelphia: W. B. Saunders, p. 630.

300. The client is suspected of having pleural effusion. The nurse assesses the client for typical manifestations, including

1. Dyspnea at rest and moist, productive cough.
2. Dyspnea on exertion and moist, productive cough.
3. Dyspnea at rest and dry, nonproductive cough.
4. Dyspnea on exertion and dry, nonproductive cough.

Answer: 4

Rationale: Typical assessment findings in the client with a pleural effusion include dyspnea, which usually occurs with exertion, and a dry, nonproductive cough. The cough is caused by bronchial irritation and possible mediastinal shift.

Test-Taking Strategy: Knowing that a pleural effusion is in the pleural space and not the airways may help you to eliminate the options that address the productive cough. This eliminates options 1 and 2. Knowing that dyspnea occurs on exertion before it occurs at rest helps you to choose option 4 over option 3.

Level of Cognitive Ability: Application
Phase of Nursing Process: Assessment
Client Needs: Physiological Integrity
Content Area: Adult Health/Respiratory

Reference

Black, J., & Matassarin-Jacobs, E. (1997). *Medical-surgical nursing: Clinical management for continuity of care* (5th ed.). Philadelphia: W. B. Saunders, pp. 1166–1167.

---

301. The client with pleural effusion had a thoracentesis, and a sample of fluid was sent to the laboratory. Analysis of the fluid reveals a high RBC count. The nurse interprets that this result is most consistent with

1. Trauma.
2. Infection.
3. Congestive heart failure.
4. Liver failure.

Answer: 1

Rationale: Pleural effusion that has a high RBC count may result from trauma and may be treated with placement of a chest tube for drainage. Other causes of pleural effusion include infection, congestive heart failure, liver or renal failure, malignancy, or inflammatory processes.

Test-Taking Strategy: Knowing that infection would be accompanied by WBCs, not RBCs, helps you to eliminate option 2 first. Knowing that the fluid portion of the serum would accumulate with liver failure and cardiac failure helps you to choose trauma as the answer, through the process of elimination.

Level of Cognitive Ability: Analysis
Phase of Nursing Process: Analysis
Client Needs: Physiological Integrity
Content Area: Adult Health/Respiratory

Reference

Black, J., & Matassarin-Jacobs, E. (1997). *Medical-surgical nursing: Clinical management for continuity of care* (5th ed.). Philadelphia: W. B. Saunders, pp. 1166–1167.

---

302. The morning assessment data of a client admitted with a diagnosis of anxiety is reviewed by the nurse. Which assessment findings should be given priority by the nurse?

1. Tearful, withdrawn, oriented times 4, isolated
2. BP, 140/190 mmHg; pulse, 100 beats/minute; respirations, 18 breaths/minute
3. Temperature, 99.4°F; affect bland
4. Fist clenched, pounding table, fearful

Answer: 4

Rationale: Tearful, withdrawn, and isolated and elevated vital signs are abnormal findings but are not life-threatening. Such findings should be monitored with crisis situations. Anxiety symptoms may take a physical harm form, and if these symptoms occur, they are of priority.

Test-Taking Strategy: Use the process of elimination, remembering that client safety and safety of others is the priority. This concept should direct you to option 4. If you had difficulty with this question, take time now to review interventions for anxiety.

Level of Cognitive Ability: Analysis
Phase of Nursing Process: Analysis
Client Needs: Physiological Integrity
Content Area: Mental Health

Reference

Fortinash, K., & Holoday-Worret, P. (1996). *Psychiatric–mental health nursing.* St. Louis: Mosby–Year Book, p. 229.

---

303. A client is admitted to the emergency room with medication-induced anxiety related to overingestion of a prescribed antipsychotic medication. The most important piece of information the nurse should solicit is

1 Name of nearest relative and his or her phone number.
2 Reason for suicide attempt and if the client will attempt again.
3 Length of time on medication and symptom control information.
4 Name of ingested medication and amount ingested.

Answer: 4

Rationale: The relatives and the reason for the suicide attempt are not the most important initial assessment. The length of time on the medication and symptom control are also not the priority in this situation. In an emergency, life-saving facts are solicited first. The name of and the amount of medication ingested are of utmost importance in treating this potentially life-threatening situation.

Test-Taking Strategy: Use Maslow's hierarchy of needs to answer the question. The key term "overingestion" should assist in determining that a physiological need is the issue. Life-saving treatment cannot begin until the medication and amount are identified.

Level of Cognitive Ability: Application
Phase of Nursing Process: Assessment
Client Needs: Physiological Integrity
Content Area: Mental Health

Reference

Potter, P., & Perry, A. (1997). *Fundamentals of nursing: Concepts, process, and practice* (4th ed.). St. Louis: Mosby–Year Book, pp. 137–138.

---

304. The nurse explains to the mother of a newborn the purpose of giving a vitamin K injection to her newborn. The nurse evaluates understanding by the mother of the purpose of the vitamin K when the mother states

1 "The newborn's blood levels are low."
2 "The newborn's liver can't produce vitamin K."
3 "The newborn lacks vitamins."
4 "The newborn lacks intestinal bacteria."

Answer: 4

Rationale: The absence of normal flora needed to synthesize vitamin K in the normal newborn gut results in low levels of vitamin K and creates a transient blood coagulation deficiency between the second and fifth day of life. From a low point at about 2–3 days after birth, these coagulation factors rise slowly but do not approach normal adult levels until 9 months of age or later. Increasing levels of these vitamin K–dependent factors indicate a response to dietary intake and bacterial colonization of the intestines. An injection of vitamin K (AquaMEPHYTON) is given prophylactically on the day of birth to combat the deficiency.

Test-Taking Strategy: Knowledge regarding the synthesis of vitamin K is required to answer this question. This knowledge should assist in directing you to the correct option. Review the purpose of administering vitamin K in the newborn if you had difficulty with this question.

Level of Cognitive Ability: Analysis
Phase of Nursing Process: Evaluation
Client Needs: Physiological Integrity
Content Area: Maternity

Reference

Nichols, F., & Zwelling, E. (1997). *Maternal-newborn nursing: Theory and practice.* Philadelphia: W. B. Saunders, p. 1152.

305. During the administration of magnesium sulfate to the client with preeclampsia, the nurse should particularly assess which of the following?

1 Deep tendon reflexes
2 Apical heart rate
3 Degree of edema
4 Intake and output

Answer: 1

Rationale: Loss of reflexes is often the first sign of developing toxicity. The nurse should assess knee jerk (patellar tendon reflex) for evidence of diminished or absent reflexes.

Test-Taking Strategy: Knowledge of the effects of magnesium sulfate is required to answer this question. Eliminate options 3 and 4 because they are similar in that they reflect fluid balance in the client. Of the remaining options, option 1 is specific to the administration of this medication. Review this important medication and the nursing responsibilities associated with its administration if you had difficulty with this question.

Level of Cognitive Ability: Application
Phase of Nursing Process: Assessment
Client Needs: Physiological Integrity
Content Area: Maternity

Reference

Clark, J., Queener, S., & Karb, V. (1997). *Pharmacologic basis of nursing practice.* St. Louis: Mosby–Year Book, p. 219.

---

306. The nurse notes that a client's urinalysis report contains a notation of positive RBCs. The nurse interprets that this finding is unrelated to which of the following items that is part of the client's clinical picture?

1 Diabetes mellitus
2 Concurrent anticoagulant therapy
3 History of kidney stones
4 History of recent blow to the right flank

Answer: 1

Rationale: Hematuria can be caused by trauma to the kidney, such as with blunt trauma to the lower posterior trunk or flank. Kidney stones can cause hematuria as they scrape the endothelial lining of the urinary system. Anticoagulant therapy can cause hematuria as a side effect. Diabetes mellitus does not cause hematuria, although it can lead to renal failure from prerenal causes.

Test-Taking Strategy: Begin to answer this question by eliminating options 2 and 4, which are most obviously likely to cause RBCs to be found in the urine. To discriminate between the last two, knowing that the scraping of the stones against mucosa could cause minor trauma and bleeding would help you to eliminate this option as well. Thus diabetes mellitus is the item unrelated to positive RBCs in the urine.

Level of Cognitive Ability: Analysis
Phase of Nursing Process: Analysis
Client Needs: Physiological Integrity
Content Area: Adult Health/Renal

Reference

Black, J., & Matassarin-Jacobs, E. (1997). *Medical-surgical nursing: Clinical management for continuity of care* (5th ed.). Philadelphia: W. B. Saunders, pp. 1548–1550.

307. The nurse has an order to ambulate the client with a nephrostomy tube in the hall four times a day. The nurse reasons that the safest way to accomplish this while maintaining the integrity of the nephrostomy tube is to

1 Tie the drainage bag to the client's waist while ambulating.
2 Use a walker to hang the drainage bag from while ambulating.
3 Tell the client to hold the drainage bag lower than the level of the bladder.
4 Change the drainage bag to a leg collection bag.

Answer: 4

Rationale: The safest approach to protect the integrity and safety of the nephrostomy tube with a mobile client is to attach the tube to a leg collection bag. This allows for greater freedom of movement, while alleviating worry over accidental disconnection or dislodgment.

Test-Taking Strategy: Option 1 is the least reasonable and should be eliminated first. Note that the question states the "safest way," which implies that more than one option may be an acceptable alternative. Options 2 and 3 are somewhat helpful but still contain the risk of tension or pulling on the nephrostomy tube by the client during ambulation. The best option is the fourth one, to change the drainage system to a leg bag.

Level of Cognitive Ability: Analysis
Phase of Nursing Process: Analysis
Client Needs: Physiological Integrity
Content Area: Adult Health/Renal

Reference

Smeltzer, S., & Bare, B. (1996). *Brunner and Suddarth's Textbook of medical-surgical nursing* (8th ed.). Philadelphia: Lippincott-Raven, p. 1169.

---

308. The client with newly diagnosed polycystic kidney disease has just finished speaking with the physician about the disorder. The client asks the nurse to explain again what the most serious complication of the disorder might be. In formulating a response, the nurse incorporates the understanding that the most serious complication would be

1 Diabetes insipidus.
2 Syndrome of inappropriate antidiuretic hormone (ADH) secretion.
3 End-stage renal disease.
4 Chronic urinary tract infection.

Answer: 3

Rationale: The most serious complication of polycystic disease is end-stage renal disease, which is managed with dialysis or transplantation. There is no reliable way to predict who will ultimately progress to end-stage renal disease at this time. Chronic urinary tract infections are the most common complication because of the altered anatomy of the kidney and from development of resistant strains of bacteria. Diabetes insipidus and syndrome of inappropriate ADH secretion are unrelated disorders.

Test-Taking Strategy: Begin to answer this question by eliminating options 1 and 2 because they are unrelated disorders and are amenable to treatment. Chronic urinary tract infections, although troubling, are also not the most serious consequence possible, so this is eliminated next. This leaves the remaining option, end-stage renal disease, as the correct answer. You would know that you have chosen correctly because this disorder is life-threatening and requires dialysis for treatment.

Level of Cognitive Ability: Analysis
Phase of Nursing Process: Analysis
Client Needs: Physiological Integrity
Content Area: Adult Health/Renal

Reference

Black, J., & Matassarin-Jacobs, E. (1997). *Medical-surgical nursing: Clinical management for continuity of care* (5th ed.). Philadelphia: W. B. Saunders, pp. 1678–1679.

---

309. The nurse is assigned to care for a client who has returned to the nursing unit after left nephrectomy. The nurse places highest priority on obtaining which of the following assessments?

1 Tolerance for sips of clear liquids
2 Oxygen saturation levels
3 Hourly urine output
4 Ability to turn side-to-side

Answer: 3

Rationale: After nephrectomy, it is imperative to measure the urine output on an hourly basis. This is done to monitor the effectiveness of the remaining kidney and to detect renal failure early if it should occur. The client may also experience significant pain after this surgery, which could impact on the client's ability to reposition, cough, and deep breathe. Therefore, the next most important measurements are vital signs (including oxygen saturation), pain level, and bed mobility. Clear liquids are not given until the client has bowel sounds, which are not referred to in this question.

Test-Taking Strategy: Note the phrase "highest priority" in the stem, which tells you that more than one or all of the options are partially or totally correct. Options 1 and 4 are helpful but are also obviously not of the highest priority, and therefore they are eliminated first. Oxygen saturation levels are an important indicator of tissue perfusion, but urine output is an even more valuable indicator in the client who has undergone surgery of the kidney. Therefore choose option 3 over option 2 as the answer to the question.

Level of Cognitive Ability: Application
Phase of Nursing Process: Assessment
Client Needs: Physiological Integrity
Content Area: Adult Health/Renal

Reference
Black, J., & Matassarin-Jacobs, E. (1997). *Medical-surgical nursing: Clinical management for continuity of care* (5th ed.). Philadelphia: W. B. Saunders, p. 1673.

---

310. The client is admitted to the hospital after being notified that a cadaver kidney has become available for transplantation. The client asks the nurse how the kidney is being stored to ensure it will function once it is transplanted into the client's body. The nurse responds that the kidney is preserved by using

1 A special form of Ringer's lactate solution that is kept at body temperature.
2 Ice packs that are made from normal saline.
3 A chilled electrolyte solution or hypothermic pulsatile perfusion.
4 Balanced salt solution that is carefully maintained at 72°F.

Answer: 3

Rationale: There are two current methods of kidney preservation. The first involves using chilled electrolyte solution to keep the kidney cool and storing it in a cooler for transport. The second involves using cool pulsatile perfusion to keep the kidney chilled while maintaining the effect of pulsatile flow through the organ.

Test-Taking Strategy: Begin to answer this question by recalling that tissue that is hypothermic has fewer metabolic needs. With this in mind, eliminate options 1 and 4 first. Basic knowledge of fluid and electrolyte balance would help you then to choose option 3 over option 2. A chilled electrolyte solution is more physiological than plain normal saline.

Level of Cognitive Ability: Application
Phase of Nursing Process: Implementation
Client Needs: Physiological Integrity
Content Area: Adult Health/Renal

Reference
Black, J., & Matassarin-Jacobs, E. (1997). *Medical-surgical nursing: Clinical management for continuity of care* (5th ed.). Philadelphia: W. B. Saunders, p. 1661.

---

311. The client with cancer is receiving cisplatin (Platinol). Which of the following assessments indicates that the client is having an adverse reaction to the medication?

1 Excessive urination
2 Tinnitus
3 Increased appetite
4 Yellow halos in front of the eyes

Answer: 2

Rationale: An adverse reaction related to the administration of cisplatin, an antineoplastic medication, is ototoxicity with hearing loss. The nurse should assess for this adverse reaction when administering this medication.

Test-Taking Strategy: Knowledge of the adverse effects related to the administration of cisplatin is required to answer this question. Review the effects of this medication and the nursing responsibilities during its administration if you had difficulty with this question.

Level of Cognitive Ability: Analysis
Phase of Nursing Process: Assessment
Client Needs: Physiological Integrity
Content Area: Pharmacology

Reference
Hodgson, B., & Kizior, R. (1998). *Saunders nursing drug handbook 1998*. Philadelphia: W. B. Saunders, pp. 226–228.

312. The nurse is caring for a client with a diagnosis of psychomotor retarded depression. On the basis of this condition, the nurse would expect to note which of the following behaviors in the client?

1. Standing without moving, as if a statue, for long periods of time
2. Slowed walking and talking
3. Verbalization of increasingly angry feelings
4. Rapid pacing back and forth

Answer: 2

Rationale: Slowed walking and talking is characteristic behavior of a retarded depression. The physical symptoms may be explained by the person's pessimistic view of the future, leading to the "psychomotor inhibition" and vegetative signs typically seen with depressed clients. Options 3 and 4 may occur in any agitated state. Option 1 is behavior more likely seen in schizophrenia.

Test-Taking Strategy: The phrase "psychomotor retarded depression" should assist in eliminating options 3 and 4 fairly easily. From the remaining two options, knowledge that option 1 is most likely seen in the client with schizophrenia can assist in directing you to the correct option. Review the characteristics of this disorder now if you had difficulty with this question.

Level of Cognitive Ability: Analysis
Phase of Nursing Process: Assessment
Client Needs: Physiological Integrity
Content Area: Mental Health

Reference

Carson, V., & Arnold, E. (1996). *Mental health nursing: The nurse-patient journey.* Philadelphia: W. B. Saunders, p. 770.

313. It has been 12 hours since the client's delivery of a newborn. The nurse assesses the process of involution and documents that it is progressing normally when palpation of the client's fundus is noted

1. At the level of the umbilicus.
2. Midway between the umbilicus and the symphysis pubis.
3. One finger-breadth below the umbilicus.
4. Two finger-breadths below the umbilicus.

Answer: 1

Rationale: The term "involution" is used to describe the rapid reduction in size and the return of the uterus to a normal condition similar to its prepregnant state. Immediately after the delivery of the placenta, the uterus contracts to the size of a large grapefruit. The fundus is situated in the midline between the symphysis pubis and the umbilicus. Within 6–12 hours after birth, the fundus of the uterus rises to the level of the umbilicus. The top of the fundus remains at the level of the umbilicus for about a day, then descends into the pelvis approximately one finger-breadth on each succeeding day.

Test-Taking Strategy: Knowledge regarding the normal process of involution is required to answer the question. The key phrase "12 hours since the client's delivery" can assist you in selecting the correct option. Attempt to visualize the process of assessment of involution and the expected finding at this time. Review this process now if you had difficulty with this question.

Level of Cognitive Ability: Analysis
Phase of Nursing Process: Assessment
Client Needs: Physiological Integrity
Content Area: Maternity

Reference

Nichols, F., & Zwelling, E. (1997). *Maternal-newborn nursing: Theory and practice.* Philadelphia: W. B. Saunders, p. 996.

314. The client with a gastric tumor is scheduled for a subtotal gastrectomy (Billroth II procedure). The nurse explains the procedure to the client. The best description of this procedure is

1. "The proximal end of the distal stomach is anastomosed to the duodenum."
2. "The antrum of the stomach is removed with the remaining portion anastomosed to the duodenum."
3. "The entire stomach is removed, and the esophagus is anastomosed to the duodenum."
4. "The lower portion of the stomach is removed, and the remainder is anastomosed to the jejunum."

Answer: 4

Rationale: In the Billroth II procedure, the lower portion of the stomach is removed, and the remainder is anastomosed to the jejunum. This technique is preferred for the treatment of duodenal ulcer because recurrent ulceration develops less frequently. The duodenal stump is preserved to permit bile flow to the jejunum.

Test-Taking Strategy: The word "gastrectomy" indicates removal of the stomach. This should assist in eliminating option 1. The word "subtotal" indicates "lower" and "a part of." This should easily direct you to option 4. If you had difficulty with this question, take time now to review this surgical procedure.

Level of Cognitive Ability: Application
Phase of Nursing Process: Implementation
Client Needs: Physiological Integrity
Content Area: Adult Health/Gastrointestinal

Reference

Black, J., & Matassarin-Jacobs, E. (1997). *Medical-surgical nursing: Clinical management for continuity of care* (5th ed.). Philadelphia: W. B. Saunders, pp. 1777–1778.

315. The diabetic client receives Humulin regular insulin 8 units subcutaneously at 7:30 A.M. The nurse would be most alert to signs of hypoglycemia at what time during the day?

1. 9:30–11:30 A.M.
2. 11:30 A.M.–1:30 P.M.
3. 1:30–3:30 P.M.
4. 3:30–5:30 P.M.

Answer: 1

Rationale: Humulin regular insulin is a short-acting insulin. Its onset of action occurs in ½ hour and peaks in 2–4 hours, and its duration of action is 4–6 hours. A hypoglycemia reaction is most likely to occur at peak time, in this situation, between 9:30 and 11:30 A.M.

Test-Taking Strategy: Knowledge regarding the onset, peak, and duration of action of regular insulin is required to answer this question. Recalling that regular insulin is a short-acting insulin can assist in directing you to option 1. Review both NPH and regular insulin if you had difficulty with this question. You are likely to find questions related to these medications on NCLEX-RN.

Level of Cognitive Ability: Analysis
Phase of Nursing Process: Analysis
Client Needs: Physiological Integrity
Content Area: Pharmacology

Reference

Hodgson, B., & Kizior, R. (1998). *Saunders nursing drug handbook 1998.* Philadelphia: W. B. Saunders, pp. 530–531.

316. The nurse prepares a postoperative plan of care for the client scheduled for hypophysectomy. Which of the following would not be a component of the plan?

1. Mouth care
2. Coughing and deep breathing
3. Monitoring intake and output
4. Daily weights

Answer: 2

Rationale: Toothbrushing, sneezing, coughing, nose blowing, and bending are activities that should be avoided postoperatively in the client who underwent a hypophysectomy. These activities interfere with the healing of the incision and can disrupt the graft.

Test-Taking Strategy: Consider the anatomical location of the surgical procedure when answering this question. Remember that when an option contains two parts, both parts have to be correct. Although coughing and deep breathing are usually a normal component of postoperative care, in this situation, coughing is contraindicated. Review care after a hypophysectomy if you had difficulty with this question.

Level of Cognitive Ability: Analysis
Phase of Nursing Process: Planning
Client Needs: Physiological Integrity
Content Area: Adult Health/Endocrine

Reference

Black, J., & Matassarin-Jacobs, E. (1997). *Medical-surgical nursing: Clinical management for continuity of care* (5th ed.). Philadelphia: W. B. Saunders, p. 2064.

---

317. The client undergoes a thyroidectomy. The nurse monitors for signs of damage to the parathyroid glands postoperatively. Which of the following would indicate damage to the parathyroid glands?

1 Hoarseness
2 Tingling around the mouth
3 Respiratory distress
4 Neck pain

Answer: 2

Rationale: The parathyroid glands can be damaged or their blood supply impaired during thyroid surgery. Hypocalcemia and tetany result when parathyroid hormone levels decrease. Complaints of tingling around the mouth or of the toes or fingers and muscular twitching are signs of calcium deficiency. Additional later signs of hypocalcemia are positive Chvostek's and Trousseau's signs.

Test-Taking Strategy: Knowledge of the clinical manifestations associated with damage to the parathyroid glands is required to answer this question. Recalling that hypocalcemia results when parathyroid hormone levels decrease may assist in directing you to the correct option. Review postoperative care after thyroidectomy and the signs of parathyroid damage if you had difficulty with this question.

Level of Cognitive Ability: Analysis
Phase of Nursing Process: Assessment
Client Needs: Physiological Integrity
Content Area: Adult Health/Endocrine

Reference

Black, J., & Matassarin-Jacobs, E. (1997). *Medical-surgical nursing: Clinical management for continuity of care* (5th ed.). Philadelphia: W. B. Saunders, pp. 2023–2024.

---

318. The nurse is caring for a client who is comatose. The nurse notes in the chart that the client is exhibiting decerebrate posturing. Decerebrate posturing can best be described as

1 The extension of the extremities after a stimulus.
2 The flexion of the extremities after a stimulus.
3 Upper extremity flexion with lower extremity extension.
4 Upper extremity extension with lower extremity flexion.

Answer: 1

Rationale: Decerebrate posturing, which can occur with upper brain stem injury, is the extension of the extremities after a stimulus.

Test-Taking Strategy: Knowledge regarding posturing is required to answer this question. "Decerebrate" may also be known as extension, and recalling this concept can assist in directing you to option 1. Review posturing and its relationship to neurological disorders if you had difficulty with this question.

Level of Cognitive Ability: Analysis
Phase of Nursing Process: Assessment
Client Needs: Physiological Integrity
Content Area: Adult Health/Neurological

Reference

Black, J., & Matassarin-Jacobs, E. (1997). *Medical-surgical nursing: Clinical management for continuity of care* (5th ed.). Philadelphia: W. B. Saunders, p. 723.

319. The nurse teaches the postpartum client about observation of lochia. The nurse evaluates the client's understanding when the client says that on the second postpartum day, the lochia should be

1 Yellow.
2 White.
3 Pink.
4 Red.

Answer: 4

Rationale: The uterus rids itself of the debris remaining after birth through a discharge called lochia, which is classified according to its appearance and contents. Lochia rubra is dark red in color. It occurs for the first 2–3 days and contains epithelial cells; erythrocytes; leukocytes; shreds of decidua; and occasionally fetal meconium, lanugo, and vernix caseosa. Lochia should not contain large clots; if it does, the cause should be investigated without delay.

Test-Taking Strategy: The key phrase is "second day postpartum." This should guide you to option 4. If you had difficulty with this question, take time now to review the normal postpartum assessment findings.

Level of Cognitive Ability: Analysis
Phase of Nursing Process: Evaluation
Client Needs: Physiological Integrity
Content Area: Maternity

Reference
Nichols, F., & Zwelling, E. (1997). *Maternal-newborn nursing: Theory and practice.* Philadelphia: W. B. Saunders, pp. 768–769.

320. The nurse is caring for a depressed client who is being treated with an MAO inhibitor. The nurse monitors the client for hypertensive crisis. Should a hypertensive crisis occur, the medication most likely to be administered would be

1 Metoprolol tartrate (Lopressor).
2 Prazosin hydrochloride (Minipress).
3 Furosemide (Lasix).
4 Phentolamine mesylate (Regitine).

Answer: 4

Rationale: Although all of the medications identified in the options decrease BP, phentolamine mesylate acts quickly and is administered intravenously for a hypertensive crisis.

Test-Taking Strategy: Knowledge of the action and use of these medications is required to answer this question correctly. If you know which medication is rapid-acting, you can select the correct option. Review MAO inhibitors and hypertensive crisis now.

Cognitive Level of Ability: Analysis
Phase of Nursing Process: Analysis
Client Needs: Physiological Integrity
Content Area: Pharmacology

Reference
Clark, J., Queener, S., & Karb, V. (1997). *Pharmacologic basis of nursing practice.* St. Louis: Mosby–Year Book, pp. 662–663.

321. The infant with a dislocated hip is placed in Bryant's traction. Which of the following assessments would be a component of the plan while the infant is in traction?

1 Skin integrity over the scapulae
2 Pin sites at the tibia
3 Security of the pelvic belt
4 Pressure over the hip joint

Answer: 1

Rationale: The infant in Bryant's traction is supine with both legs elevated at a 90-degree angle. The buttocks should just clear the mattress. The scapulae, fibula, shoulders, and Achilles tendons are pressure points because of positioning and skin traction application. There are no pin sites with Bryant's traction. Pelvic traction is the only traction using a pelvic belt. No constructive devices are placed over or near the hip joint with Bryant's traction.

Test-Taking Strategy: Remembering that Bryant's traction is a continuous skin traction can assist in eliminating options 2 and 3. Visualizing the alignment and infant positioning in this traction can direct you to option 1. Review the purpose and positioning used in Bryant's traction if you had difficulty with this question.

Level of Cognitive Ability: Application
Phase of Nursing Process: Assessment
Client Needs: Physiological Integrity
Content Area: Child Health

Reference

Ashwill, J., & Droske, S. (1997). *Nursing care of children: Principles and practice.* Philadelphia: W. B. Saunders, p. 1100.

---

322. The nurse is caring for a client who had a total knee replacement. Postoperatively, which of the following nursing assessments is of highest priority?

1 Bladder distention
2 Homan's sign
3 Extremity shortening
4 Heel breakdown

Answer: 2

Rationale: Deep vein thrombosis is a potentially serious complication of lower extremity surgery. Checking Homan's sign is an assessment for this complication. Although bladder distention may occur postoperatively, option 1 is incorrect because the question does not provide enough information to select this response. Extremity lengthening or shortening may occur as a result of knee replacement but is not the highest priority nursing assessment. In addition, heel breakdown is not the highest priority.

Test-Taking Strategy: Use the ABCs to answer the question. Assessment for deep vein thrombosis involves circulation. Review postoperative assessment after total knee replacement if you had difficulty with this question.

Level of Cognitive Ability: Application
Phase of Nursing Process: Assessment
Client Needs: Physiological Integrity
Content Area: Adult Health/Musculoskeletal

Reference

Black, J., & Matassarin-Jacobs, E. (1997). *Medical-surgical nursing: Clinical management for continuity of care* (5th ed.). Philadelphia: W. B. Saunders, p. 1434.

---

323. The nurse is assessing a client's cigarette smoking habit. The client admits to smoking ¾ pack per day for the past 10 years. The nurse would assess that the client has a smoking history of how many pack-years?

1 0.75 pack-years
2 7.5 pack-years
3 15 pack-years
4 30 pack-years

Answer: 2

Rationale: The standard method for quantifying smoking history is to multiply the number of packs smoked per day by the number of years of smoking. The number is recorded as the number of pack-years. The number of pack-years for the client who has smoked ¾ pack per day for 10 years is calculated as 0.75 (¾) packs × 10 years = 7.5 pack-years.

Test-Taking Strategy: This question tests a fundamental concept of history taking related to smoking. This is an important item to memorize if you have not done so already.

Level of Cognitive Ability: Analysis
Phase of Nursing Process: Assessment
Client Needs: Physiological Integrity
Content Area: Adult Health/Respiratory

Reference

Black, J., & Matassarin-Jacobs, E. (1997). *Medical-surgical nursing: Clinical management for continuity of care* (5th ed.). Philadelphia: W. B. Saunders, p. 1039.

324. The nurse is assessing the client with a nursing diagnosis of Impaired Gas Exchange. Which of the following would be an unexpected assessment finding for this client?

1 Dyspnea when ambulating to the bathroom
2 Oxygen saturation of 88% with pulse oximeter
3 Presence of bibasilar lung crackles
4 Arterial blood gas oxygen level of 88 mmHg

Answer: 4

Rationale: An arterial blood gas oxygen level of 88 mmHg is within the normal range of 80–100 mmHg. Signs and symptoms that correlate with the defining characteristics of this nursing diagnosis include dyspnea and hypoxia. Crackles indicate fluid in the alveoli, which impairs gas exchange at the alveolar level.

Test-Taking Strategy: The wording of this question guides you to look for a normal assessment finding. Eliminate options 1 and 3 first because they obviously are abnormal findings. To discriminate between options 2 and 4, you need to know the normal values for oxygen saturation and the partial pressure of arterial oxygen. Because the normal oxygen saturation level is greater than 95%, and the normal arterial oxygen level is 80–100 mmHg, select option 4 as the correct answer.

Level of Cognitive Ability: Analysis
Phase of Nursing Process: Assessment
Client Needs: Physiological Integrity
Content Area: Adult Health/Respiratory

References

Cox, H., Hinz, M., Lubno, M., et al. (1997). *Clinical applications of nursing diagnosis: Adult, child, women's, psychiatric, gerontic, and home health considerations* (3rd ed.). Philadelphia: F. A. Davis, p. 327.

Smeltzer, S., & Bare, B. (1996). *Brunner and Suddarth's Textbook of medical-surgical nursing* (8th ed.). Philadelphia: Lippincott-Raven, p. 513.

325. The client with a history of respiratory disease is ambulating with the nurse to the doorway of the hospital room. The client becomes pale and dyspneic. The nurse has the client sit and measures vital signs. The respiratory rate is 32 breaths/minute, oxygen saturation is 90%, and the heart rate has increased from 76 to 98 beats/minute. The nurse interprets that this client is experiencing

1 Impaired physical mobility.
2 Activity intolerance.
3 Ineffective breathing pattern.
4 Ineffective airway clearance.

Answer: 2

Rationale: Activity intolerance is characterized by exertional dyspnea, adverse changes in BP or heart rate with activity, and fatigue. Ineffective breathing pattern occurs when the rate, timing, depth, or rhythm of breathing is insufficient to maintain optimal ventilation. Ineffective airway clearance occurs when the client is unable to clear secretions from the airway. Impaired physical mobility occurs when the client is limited in physical movement and has limited muscle strength, range of motion, or coordination.

Test-Taking Strategy: Each of these nursing diagnoses can apply to the client experiencing dyspnea. The question mentions nothing about the pattern of breathing or secretions, so eliminate options 3 and 4 first. Note that the stem tells you that the item triggering the dyspnea is ambulation, which guides you to select Activity Intolerance over Impaired Physical Mobility as your answer.

Level of Cognitive Ability: Analysis
Phase of Nursing Process: Analysis
Client Needs: Physiological Integrity
Content Area: Adult Health/Respiratory

Reference

Cox, H., Hinz, M., Lubno, M., et al. (1997). *Clinical applications of nursing diagnosis: Adult, child, women's, psychiatric, gerontic, and home health considerations* (3rd ed.). Philadelphia: F. A. Davis, pp. 250, 261, 269, 362.

326. The nurse is conducting a health history on a client with hyperparathyroidism. Which of the following questions would elicit the most accurate information about this condition from the client?

1. "Have you had problems with diarrhea lately?"
2. "Do you have tremors in your hands?"
3. "Are you experiencing pain in your joints?"
4. "Do you notice swelling in your legs at night?"

Answer: 3

Rationale: Hyperparathyroidism causes an oversecretion of parathyroid hormone, which causes excessive osteoblast growth and activity within the bones. When bone reabsorption is increased, calcium is released from the bones into the blood causing hypercalcemia. The bones suffer demineralization as a result of calcium loss, leading to bone and joint pain and pathological fractures.

Test-Taking Strategy: Knowledge regarding the pathophysiology associated with hyperparathyroidism is required to answer the question. Eliminate options 1 and 2 first because they provide information about hypoparathyroidism. Knowledge regarding hyperparathyroidism directs you to option 3 because option 4 is unrelated to this condition.

Level of Cognitive Ability: Application
Phase of Nursing Process: Assessment
Client Needs: Physiological Integrity
Content Area: Adult Health/Endocrine

Reference

Polaski, A., & Tatro, A. (1996). *Luckmann's Core principles and practice of medical-surgical nursing.* Philadelphia: W. B. Saunders, p. 1222.

---

327. An 18-year-old client seeks medical attention for intermittent episodes in which the fingers of both hands become cold, pale, and numb, after which they become reddened and swollen with a throbbing, achy pain. The nurse further assesses the client to see if these episodes occur with

1. Exposure to heat.
2. Being in a relaxed environment.
3. Prolonged episodes of inactivity.
4. Ingestion of coffee or chocolate.

Answer: 4

Rationale: Raynaud's disease is a bilateral form of intermittent arteriolar spasm that can be classified as obstructive or vasospastic. Episodes are characterized by pallor, cold, numbness, and possible cyanosis, followed by erythema, tingling, and aching pain. Attacks are triggered by exposure to cold, nicotine, caffeine, trauma to the fingertips, and stress.

Test-Taking Strategy: The symptoms that the client describes occur with vasoconstriction, so you can use your knowledge of events that precipitate vasoconstriction to answer this question. Thus you can rapidly eliminate options 1, 2, and 3 because these events are unlikely to cause vasoconstriction.

Level of Cognitive Ability: Analysis
Phase of Nursing Process: Assessment
Client Needs: Physiological Integrity
Content Area: Adult Health/Cardiovascular

Reference

Black, J., & Matassarin-Jacobs, E. (1997). *Medical-surgical nursing: Clinical management for continuity of care* (5th ed.). Philadelphia: W. B. Saunders, p. 1431.

---

328. The client is admitted with a diagnosis of pericarditis. The nurse assesses the client for which manifestation that differentiates pericarditis from other cardiopulmonary problems?

1. Chest pain that worsens on inspiration
2. Pericardial friction rub
3. Anterior chest pain
4. Weakness and irritability

Answer: 2

Rationale: A pericardial friction rub is heard when there is inflammation of the pericardial sac, during the inflammatory phase of pericarditis. Chest pain that worsens on inspiration is characteristic of both pericarditis and pleurisy. Anterior chest pain may be experienced with angina pectoris and myocardial infarction. Weakness and irritability are nonspecific complaints and could accompany a wide variety of disorders.

Test-Taking Strategy: The key word in the stem of this question is "differentiates." This tells you that the correct answer is one that is unique to this health problem. This key word should assist in eliminating options 3 and 4 easily. Of the remaining options, option 2 is specific to pericarditis. Review the characteristics associated with pericarditis if you had difficulty with this question.

Level of Cognitive Ability: Analysis
Phase of Nursing Process: Assessment
Client Needs: Physiological Integrity
Content Area: Adult Health/Cardiovascular

Reference

Monahan, F., & Neighbors, M. (1998). *Medical-surgical nursing: Foundations for clinical practice* (2nd ed.). Philadelphia: W. B. Saunders, p. 238.

---

329. The ambulatory care nurse is assessing the client with chronic sinusitis. The nurse interprets that which of the following client manifestations is unrelated to this problem?

1 Purulent nasal discharge
2 Chronic cough
3 Headache more pronounced in the evening
4 Anosmia

Answer: 3

Rationale: Chronic sinusitis is characterized by persistent purulent nasal discharge, a chronic cough because of nasal discharge, anosmia (loss of smell), nasal stuffiness, and headache that is worse on arising after sleep.

Test-Taking Strategy: The wording of the question tells you that there is only one correct option. Use knowledge of signs and symptoms of upper respiratory problems to answer this question. Review these signs and symptoms if you had difficulty with this question.

Level of Cognitive Ability: Analysis
Phase of Nursing Process: Assessment
Client Needs: Physiological Integrity
Content Area: Adult Health/Respiratory

Reference

Monahan, F., & Neighbors, M. (1998). *Medical-surgical nursing: Foundations for clinical practice* (2nd ed.). Philadelphia: W. B. Saunders, p. 603.

---

330. The client who just underwent tonsillectomy is becoming slightly restless, with an increasing pulse rate and slight pallor. The nurse notes that the client is swallowing frequently. Which of the following interpretations is most appropriately made by the nurse?

1 The client needs pain medication
2 The client may have postoperative bleeding or hemorrhage
3 This is an expected postoperative finding
4 The client most likely has some mild postoperative edema

Answer: 2

Rationale: Signs of postoperative hemorrhage include pallor, restlessness, frequent swallowing, large amounts of bloody drainage or vomitus, increasing pulse rate, and falling BP. These signs should be reported to the surgeon.

Test-Taking Strategy: Eliminate options 3 and 4 first because they are totally incorrect. Use concepts related to hemorrhage and shock, and focus on the signs presented in the question to discriminate between the final two options. Review postoperative complications after tonsillectomy if you had difficulty with this question.

Level of Cognitive Ability: Analysis
Phase of Nursing Process: Analysis
Client Needs: Physiological Integrity
Content Area: Adult Health/Respiratory

Reference

Monahan, F., & Neighbors, M. (1998). *Medical-surgical nursing: Foundations for clinical practice* (2nd ed.). Philadelphia: W. B. Saunders, p. 607.

331. The client has impaired verbal communication as a result of temporary tracheostomy after a conservation laryngectomy. In planning for communication with this client, the nurse would avoid which of the following methods as least helpful for this particular client?

1 Use of hand or finger signals
2 Nodding and shaking head for "yes" and "no"
3 Use of picture board
4 Use of pencil and paper

Answer: 2

Rationale: After laryngectomy, the client should not be asked to nod or shake the head because these are painful for the client. The use of eye blink, hand, or finger signals is acceptable. Other helpful methods include use of pencil and paper, word or picture board, flash cards, and magic slate.

Test-Taking Strategy: Remember that options that are similar are not likely to be correct. In this question, each of the incorrect options involves use of the hands. The correct option, which is determined using the key words "least helpful," is the one that involves movement of the head during communication. Be alert to the diagnosis stated in the question when selecting an option.

Level of Cognitive Ability: Application
Phase of Nursing Process: Planning
Client Needs: Physiological Integrity
Content Area: Adult Health/Respiratory

Reference

Monahan, F., & Neighbors, M. (1998). *Medical-surgical nursing: Foundations for clinical practice* (2nd ed.). Philadelphia: W. B. Saunders, pp. 621–622.

---

332. The client with pneumonia has anorexia as a result of effort required for eating while dyspneic and decreased taste sensation. Which of the following actions by the nurse would be most helpful in increasing the client's appetite?

1 Push fluids to 3 liters/day
2 Keep water at the bedside
3 Encourage a diet high in protein
4 Provide mouth care before meals

Answer: 4

Rationale: The client with pneumonia may experience decreased taste sensation as a result of sputum expectoration. To minimize this adverse effect, the nurse should provide oral hygiene before meals. The client should also have small, frequent meals because of dyspnea. Increased oral fluids and keeping water at the bedside are good measures to prevent fluid deficit associated with pneumonia, but they do nothing to alleviate anorexia.

Test-Taking Strategy: The key words in the question are "most helpful" and "appetite." Remember that options that are similar are not likely to be correct. This helps you to eliminate options 1 and 2. Use basic nursing knowledge related to hygiene and focus on the issue "increase the appetite" to choose correctly between the two remaining options.

Level of Cognitive Ability: Application
Phase of Nursing Process: Implementation
Client Needs: Physiological Integrity
Content Area: Adult Health/Respiratory

Reference

Monahan, F., & Neighbors, M. (1998). *Medical-surgical nursing: Foundations for clinical practice* (2nd ed.). Philadelphia: W. B. Saunders, p. 646.

---

333. The ambulatory care nurse is seeing large numbers of clients whose chief complaint is the presence of flu-like symptoms. Which of the following recommendations by the nurse is least helpful in working with these clients?

1 "Increase intake of liquids."
2 "Take antipyretics for fever."
3 "Get a flu shot immediately."
4 "Get plenty of rest."

Answer: 3

Rationale: Immunization against influenza is a prophylactic measure and is not used to treat flu symptoms. Treatment for the flu includes getting rest, drinking fluids, and taking in nutritious foods and beverages. Medications such as antipyretics and analgesics may also be used for symptom management.

Test-Taking Strategy: Use knowledge of primary, secondary, and tertiary prevention measures to choose the correct answer to this question. The wording of the question tells you that there is only one correct answer. Recalling that a flu shot is a prophylactic measure can assist in directing you to the correct option.

Level of Cognitive Ability: Application
Phase of Nursing Process: Implementation
Client Needs: Physiological Integrity
Content Area: Adult Health/ Respiratory

Reference

Monahan, F., & Neighbors, M. (1998). *Medical-surgical nursing: Foundations for clinical practice* (2nd ed.). Philadelphia: W. B. Saunders, pp. 649–650.

---

334. The nurse is beginning to ambulate a client with a nursing diagnosis of Activity Intolerance, who was admitted for bacterial endocarditis. The nurse evaluates that the client is best tolerating the exercise if which of the following parameters is noted by the nurse?

1 Pulse rate that increases from 68 to 94 beats/minute
2 BP that increases from 114/82 to 118/86 mmHg
3 Minimal chest pain rated "1" on the pain scale
4 Mild dyspnea after walking 10 feet

Answer: 2

Rationale: General indicators that a client is tolerating exercise include an absence of chest pain or dyspnea, a pulse rate increase of less than 20 beats/minute, and a BP change of less than 10 mmHg.

Test-Taking Strategy: Begin to answer this question by eliminating options 3 and 4 first because they represent abnormal data. Choose option 2 over option 1 using basic physical assessment skills. Remember the key phrase, "best tolerating the exercise," in the question. Option 2 reflects the least physiological change as a result of the exercise.

Level of Cognitive Ability: Analysis
Phase of Nursing Process: Evaluation
Client Needs: Physiological Integrity
Content Area: Adult Health/Cardiovascular

Reference

Monahan, F., & Neighbors, M. (1998). *Medical-surgical nursing: Foundations for clinical practice* (2nd ed.). Philadelphia: W. B. Saunders, p. 235.

---

335. The client at risk for PVCs is placed on a cardiac monitor. The nurse assesses the client's rhythm to detect PVCs by looking for

1 Premature beats followed by a compensatory pause.
2 QRS complexes that are short and narrow.
3 Inverted P waves before the QRS complexes.
4 A P wave preceding every QRS complex.

Answer: 1

Rationale: PVCs are abnormal ectopic beats originating in the ventricles. They are characterized by an absence of P waves, wide and bizarre QRS complexes, and a compensatory pause that follows the ectopy.

Test-Taking Strategy: To answer this question accurately, it is necessary to have a baseline understanding of this fairly common but potentially deadly ventricular dysrhythmia. Note the relationship of "PVCs" in the question and "premature beats" in the correct answer. If this question was difficult, review the characteristics of a PVC.

Level of Cognitive Ability: Analysis
Phase of Nursing Process: Assessment
Client Needs: Physiological Integrity
Content Area: Adult Health/Cardiovascular

Reference

Monahan, F., & Neighbors, M. (1998). *Medical-surgical nursing: Foundations for clinical practice* (2nd ed.). Philadelphia: W. B. Saunders, p. 248.

336. The client with angina pectoris had been given nitroglycerin tablets to take sublingually for chest pain. The client states a dislike for the medication because it causes headache. The nurse makes which of the following interpretations about the client's statement?

1. This is a common but unhealthy response to the medication
2. This is a common response that will diminish as tolerance to nitroglycerin increases
3. This response is due to cerebral hypoxia induced by the medication
4. This is an extremely adverse reaction and should be reported to the physician

Answer: 2

Rationale: Headache is a common side effect of nitroglycerin related to its vasodilator properties. The incidence of headache diminishes over time as the client develops tolerance to the medication. The client should be encouraged to continue its use as needed and to take acetaminophen or aspirin for headache, according to the preference of the prescribing physician.

Test-Taking Strategy: Specific knowledge about the side effects of nitroglycerin is needed to answer this question correctly. Options 3 and 4 can be easily eliminated because of the words "extremely" and "hypoxia." Remember, nitroglycerin dilates vessels and relieves hypoxia to the cardiac tissue. Option 1 is not totally correct; therefore eliminate that option. If you had difficulty with this question, review the key concepts related to nitroglycerin at this time.

Level of Cognitive Ability: Analysis
Phase of Nursing Process: Analysis
Client Needs: Physiological Integrity
Content Area: Adult Health/Cardiovascular

Reference

Monahan, F., & Neighbors, M. (1998). *Medical-surgical nursing: Foundations for clinical practice* (2nd ed.). Philadelphia: W. B. Saunders, p. 266.

---

337. The client is experiencing pulmonary edema as an exacerbation of chronic left-sided heart failure. The nurse assesses this client for which of the following manifestations?

1. Distended neck veins
2. Peripheral pitting edema
3. Weight loss
4. Bilateral crackles

Answer: 4

Rationale: The client with pulmonary edema presents primarily with symptoms that are respiratory in nature because the blood flow is stagnant in the lungs and lies behind the left side of the heart from a circulatory standpoint. The client would experience weight gain from fluid retention, not weight loss. Distended neck veins and peripheral pitting edema are classic signs of right-sided heart failure.

Test-Taking Strategy: Use knowledge of circulatory dynamics to answer this question. Knowing that blood flow is stagnant behind the area of failure allows you to eliminate each of the incorrect options systematically. With heart failure, to remember the signs and symptoms, remember "left, lungs" and "right, systemic."

Level of Cognitive Ability: Application
Phase of Nursing Process: Assessment
Client Needs: Physiological Integrity
Content Area: Adult Health/Cardiovascular

Reference

Monahan, F., & Neighbors, M. (1998). *Medical-surgical nursing: Foundations for clinical practice* (2nd ed.). Philadelphia: W. B. Saunders, p. 270.

---

338. The nurse suspects an air embolism in a client with a multilumen catheter. Which of the following assessment findings will not be noted if air embolism is present?

1. Hypotension.
2. Chest pain.
3. A "churning" sound heard over the right ventricle on auscultation.
4. Rales heard in the lung bases on auscultation.

Answer: 4

Rationale: All clients with intravenous lines are at risk for air embolism. Because an air embolism can be fatal, it is essential that the nurse monitor for the presence of chest pain, coughing, hypotension, cyanosis, and hypoxia. In addition, if the client does have an air embolism, auscultation over the right ventricle may reveal a churning "windmill" sound.

Test-Taking Strategy: Use the process of elimination, noting the key word "not" in the stem of the question. Remember that the issue of the question is "air" embolism. Remembering that fluid produces rales heard in the lung bases can assist in directing you to option 4 as the answer to this question as it is stated. If you are unfamiliar with the clinical indications of an air embolism, review them now.

Level of Cognitive Ability: Analysis
Phase of Nursing Process: Assessment
Client Needs: Physiological Integrity
Content Area: Fundamental Skills

Reference

Luckmann, J. (1997). *Saunders manual of nursing care.* Philadelphia: W. B. Saunders, p. 260.

---

339. The client has suffered an inferior wall myocardial infarction. The nurse evaluates that the client is remaining free of the most common complications of this type of myocardial infarction if the client does not develop signs of

1 Cardiogenic shock.
2 Ventricular tachycardia.
3 PVCs.
4 Heart block.

Answer: 4

Rationale: Conduction disturbances involving the SA node, AV node, and the proximal bundle of His are the most common complications of inferior wall myocardial infarction. Ventricular dysrhythmias and cardiogenic shock are most common with anterior wall myocardial infarction.

Test-Taking Strategy: Remember that options that are similar are not likely to be correct. This guides you to eliminate options 2 and 3 because they are both ventricular in nature. An understanding of the coronary circulation is necessary to discriminate correctly between options 1 and 4. Review the complications associated with inferior wall myocardial infarction if you had difficulty with this question.

Level of Cognitive Ability: Analysis
Phase of Nursing Process: Evaluation
Client Needs: Physiological Integrity
Content Area: Adult Health/Cardiovascular

Reference

Monahan, F., & Neighbors, M. (1998). *Medical-surgical nursing: Foundations for clinical practice* (2nd ed.). Philadelphia: W. B. Saunders, pp. 293–294.

---

340. When ambulating a client, the best position for the nurse in assisting the client is to

1 Stand behind the client.
2 Stand in front of the client.
3 Stand on the unaffected side of the client.
4 Stand on the affected side of the client.

Answer: 4

Rationale: When walking with clients, the nurse should stand on the affected side and grasp the security belt in the midspine area of the small of the back. The nurse should position the free hand at the shoulder area so that the client can be pulled toward the nurse in the event that there is a forward fall. Instruct the client to look up and outward rather than at his or her feet.

Test-Taking Strategy: Recalling that support is needed on the affected side can assist in directing you to the correct option. On the basis of this concept, option 3 can be eliminated. Eliminate options 1 and 2 because neither position places the nurse in a strategic position should the client lose balance and begin to fall frontward or backward. Review this procedure now if you had difficulty with this question.

Level of Cognitive Ability: Analysis
Phase of Nursing Process: Implementation
Client Needs: Physiological Integrity
Content Area: Fundamental Skills

Reference

Lammon, C. B., Foote, A. W., Leli, P. G., et al. (1995). *Clinical nursing skills.* Philadelphia: W. B. Saunders, pp. 236–237.

341. The nurse assesses the height of the cane before ambulating the client. The top of the cane should be parallel to the

1. Greater trochanter of the femur.
2. Midline between the greater trochanter and the waist.
3. Waistline.
4. Uppermost level of the thigh.

Answer: 1

Rationale: The top of the cane should reach the level of the greater trochanter of the client's femur.

Test-Taking Strategy: Visualize each of the positions described in the options. Eliminate option 3 because this position would be too high. Conversely, eliminate option 4 because this position is too low. Again, visualize the remaining options. You can easily realize that the position in option 2 is also too high to provide safety and comfort in ambulating with a cane.

Level of Cognitive Ability: Analysis
Phase of Nursing Process: Assessment
Client Needs: Physiological Integrity
Content Area: Fundamental Skills

Reference

Lammon, C. B., Foote, A. W., Leli, P. G., et al. (1995). *Clinical nursing skills.* Philadelphia: W. B. Saunders, p. 238.

---

342. Which of the following nursing interventions would receive highest priority in caring for the client with wrist restraints?

1. Providing range-of-motion exercises
2. Removing the restraints periodically
3. Applying lotion to the skin under the restraints
4. Assessing color, sensation, and pulses distal to the restraints

Answer: 4

Rationale: Assessing color, sensation, and pulses distal to the restraint identifies the complication of neurovascular compromise that is associated with the use of restraints. Of the options presented, this is the priority. All of the other interventions should also be implemented. Remember that restraints, if used, should be removed at least every 2 hours or as specified by the agency policy and procedure.

Test-Taking Strategy: Use the ABCs to answer the question. Assessing color, sensation, and pulses is the highest priority because it determines circulation.

Level of Cognitive Ability: Application
Phase of Nursing Process: Implementation
Client Needs: Physiological Integrity
Content Area: Fundamental Skills

Reference

Lammon, C. B., Foote, A. W., Leli, P. G., et al. (1995). *Clinical nursing skills.* Philadelphia: W. B. Saunders, p. 292.

---

343. When administering an intramuscular injection in the gluteal muscle, the best position for the client to assume to relax the muscle is

1. On the side with knee of uppermost leg flexed.
2. On the side with knee of lowermost leg flexed.
3. Prone with a toe in position.
4. Sims' with a toe in position.

Answer: 3

Rationale: A prone toe in position promotes internal rotation of the hips, which relaxes the muscle and makes the injection less painful. Options 1, 2, and 4 do not relax the muscle.

Test-Taking Strategy: The key phrase is "relax the muscle." Visualize each position described in the options. You should be able to select the correct option easily. If you are unfamiliar with the position for administering intramuscular medications, review the procedure now.

Level of Cognitive Ability: Application
Phase of Nursing Process: Implementation
Client Needs: Physiological Integrity
Content Area: Fundamental Skills

Reference

Lammon, C. B., Foote, A. W., Leli, P. G., et al. (1995). *Clinical nursing skills.* Philadelphia: W. B. Saunders, p. 621.

344. The nurse plans to give a medication by intravenous bolus through the primary line of an intravenous line. The nurse notes that the medication is incompatible with the primary intravenous solution. The most appropriate nursing action to administer the medication safely is to

1. Call the physician for an order to change the route of the medication.
2. Start a new intravenous line for the medication.
3. Flush the tubing before and after the medication with normal saline.
4. Flush the tubing before and after the medication with sterile water.

Answer: 3

Rationale: When giving a medication by intravenous bolus, if the medication is incompatible with the intravenous solution, flush the tubing before and after the bolus with infusions of normal saline. Option 1 is inappropriate. Option 2 is premature and not necessary. Sterile water is not used for an intravenous flush.

Test-Taking Strategy: Option 1 can be easily eliminated because in this situation, it is not an appropriate action. Option 2 is not necessary and may only cause discomfort for the client. For the remaining options, remember that normal saline is physiologically similar to body fluid and is the best choice.

Level of Cognitive Ability: Application
Phase of Nursing Process: Implementation
Client Needs: Physiological Integrity
Content Area: Fundamental Skills

Reference

Luckmann, J. (1997). *Saunders manual of nursing care.* Philadelphia: W. B. Saunders, pp. 257–258.

345. The most appropriate method to administer eardrops to the infant is to

1. Pull up and back on the auricle, and direct the solution toward the wall of the ear canal.
2. Pull down and back on the auricle, and direct the solution onto the eardrum.
3. Pull down and back on the earlobe, and direct the solution toward the wall of the canal.
4. Pull up and back on the earlobe, and direct the solution toward the wall of the canal.

Answer: 3

Rationale: The infant should be turned on the side with affected ear uppermost. With the nondominant hand, pull down and back on the earlobe. Rest the wrist of the dominant hand on the infant's head. Administer the medication aiming it at the wall of the canal rather than directly onto the eardrum. The infant should be held or positioned with the affected ear uppermost for 10–15 minutes to retain the solution. In the adult, pull up and back on the auricle to straighten the auditory canal.

Test-Taking Strategy: Basic safety principles related to the administration of ear medications should assist in eliminating option 2. Visualizing the procedures identified in the remaining options can assist in directing you toward the correct option. Option 1 is eliminated because it is the adult procedure. It would be difficult to pull up and back on an earlobe; therefore, eliminate option 4. Review the procedure for administering ear medications in an infant and adult if you had difficulty with this question.

Level of Cognitive Ability: Application
Phase of Nursing Process: Planning
Client Needs: Physiological Integrity
Content Area: Pharmacology

Reference

Ashwill, J., & Droske, S. (1997). *Nursing care of children: Principles and practice.* Philadelphia: W. B. Saunders, pp. 498–499.

346. The physician initiates levodopa therapy for the client with Parkinson's disease. A few days after the client starts the medication, the client complains of nausea and vomiting. The nurse's best instruction to the client is that

1 This is an expected side effect of the medication.
2 Eating a high-protein snack before taking the medication helps to prevent the nausea.
3 Taking an antiemetic such as prochlorperazine (Compazine) helps to prevent the nausea.
4 The nausea and vomiting will decrease when the medication dose is stabilized.

Answer: 2

Rationale: The best instruction by the nurse is that high-protein snacks prevent the nausea. Antiemetics from the phenothiazine class should not be used because they block the therapeutic action of dopamine. Options 1 and 4 are inaccurate.

Test-Taking Strategy: The issue of the question is to identify a measure that can assist the client to relieve the nausea. With this in mind, you can easily eliminate options 1 and 4. Nonpharmacological approaches are more appropriate than pharmacological ones; therefore select option 2 as the best instruction to the client.

Level of Cognitive Ability: Application
Phase of Nursing Process: Implementation
Client Needs: Physiological Integrity
Content Area: Pharmacology

Reference
Clark, J., Queener, S., & Karb, V. (1997). *Pharmacologic basis of nursing practice.* St. Louis: Mosby–Year Book, p. 700.

---

347. A client seeks treatment in an ambulatory clinic for a complaint of hoarseness that has lasted for 6 weeks. On the basis of the symptom, the nurse interprets that the client is at risk of having

1 Laryngeal cancer.
2 Acute laryngitis.
3 Bronchogenic cancer.
4 Thyroid cancer.

Answer: 1

Rationale: Hoarseness is a common early sign of laryngeal cancer but not of bronchogenic or thyroid cancer. Hoarseness that lasts for 6 weeks is not associated with an acute problem, such as laryngitis.

Test-Taking Strategy: Begin to answer this question by eliminating option 2 because an acute problem would not generally last for 6 weeks. To discriminate among the other options, knowing that the vocal cords are in the larynx makes option 1 preferable to the others.

Level of Cognitive Ability: Analysis
Phase of Nursing Process: Analysis
Client Needs: Physiological Integrity
Content Area: Adult Health/Respiratory

Reference
Black, J., & Matassarin-Jacobs, E. (1997). *Medical-surgical nursing: Clinical management for continuity of care* (5th ed.). Philadelphia: W. B. Saunders, p. 1082.

---

348. The client is admitted to the nursing unit after lobectomy. The nurse notes that in the first hour after admission the chest tube drainage was 75 mL. During the second hour, the drainage has dropped to 5 mL. The nurse interprets that

1 The lung has fully reexpanded.
2 This is normal.
3 The client needs to cough and deep breathe.
4 The tube may be occluded.

Answer: 4

Rationale: Chest tube drainage in the first 24 hours after thoracic surgery may total 500–1000 mL. The sudden drop in drainage between the first and second hour indicates that the tube is possibly occluded and requires further assessment by the nurse.

Test-Taking Strategy: Option 1 is the least plausible and is eliminated first. Needing to cough and deep breathe is a response that is unrelated to the problem in the stem and is eliminated next. Knowing that the drainage should not drop so radically in 1 hour makes you think that the chest tube has become occluded somehow, making option 4 the correct choice. Review the concepts related to chest tube drainage systems if you had difficulty with this question.

Level of Cognitive Ability: Analysis
Phase of Nursing Process: Analysis
Client Needs: Physiological Integrity
Content Area: Adult Health/Respiratory

Reference
Black, J., & Matassarin-Jacobs, E. (1997). *Medical-surgical nursing: Clinical management for continuity of care* (5th ed.). Philadelphia: W. B. Saunders, p. 1163.

349. The nurse is auscultating the chest of a client with new onset of pleurisy. The client does not have a pleural friction rub, which was auscultated the previous day. The nurse interprets that this is most likely due to

1 Decreased inflammatory reaction at the site.
2 The deep breaths that the client is taking.
3 Accumulation of pleural fluid in the inflamed area.
4 Effectiveness of medication therapy.

Answer: 3

Rationale: Pleural friction rub is auscultated early in the course of pleurisy, before pleural fluid accumulates. Once fluid accumulates in the inflamed area, there is less friction between the visceral and parietal lung surfaces, and the pleural friction rub disappears.

Test-Taking Strategy: Eliminate option 2 first, which would intensify the pain. Options 1 and 4 are similar in tone and since the stem states that the problem is new in onset, these should be eliminated next. This leaves option 3, which is correct. Fluid accumulation in the area provides a buffer between the lung and chest wall surfaces, which eliminates the friction rub.

Level of Cognitive Ability: Analysis
Phase of Nursing Process: Analysis
Client Needs: Physiological Integrity
Content Area: Adult Health/Respiratory

Reference

Smeltzer, S., & Bare, B. (1996). *Brunner and Suddarth's Textbook of medical-surgical nursing* (8th ed.). Philadelphia: Lippincott-Raven, p. 502.

---

350. The client is admitted to the nursing unit with a diagnosis of pleurisy. The nurse assesses the client for which of the following characteristic symptoms of this disorder?

1 Early morning fatigue
2 Dyspnea that is relieved by lying flat
3 Pain that worsens when the breath is held
4 Knife-like pain that worsens on inspiration

Answer: 4

Rationale: A typical symptom with pleurisy is a knife-like pain that worsens on inspiration. This is due to the friction caused by the rubbing together of inflamed pleural surfaces. This pain usually disappears when the breath is held because these surfaces stop moving. The client does not experience early morning fatigue or dyspnea relieved by lying flat.

Test-Taking Strategy: Option 2 is eliminated first because dyspnea is not relieved by lying flat. Option 1 is eliminated next because fatigue, if it were to occur, would not be present in the morning, when clients are most well rested. To discriminate between options 3 and 4, keep in mind that pleurisy results from inflammation of the pleura. Because the visceral and parietal lung pleura glide over one another with respiration, it is expected that chest movement precipitates or intensifies the pain. With this in mind, eliminate option 3 and choose option 4.

Level of Cognitive Ability: Application
Phase of Nursing Process: Assessment
Client Needs: Physiological Integrity
Content Area: Adult Health/Respiratory

Reference

Smeltzer, S., & Bare, B. (1996). *Brunner and Suddarth's Textbook of medical-surgical nursing* (8th ed.). Philadelphia: Lippincott-Raven, p. 502.

REFERENCES

Ashwill, J., & Droske, S. (1997). *Nursing care of children: Principles and practice*. Philadelphia: W. B. Saunders.

Antai-Otong, D. (1995). *Psychiatric nursing: Biological and behavioral concepts*. Philadelphia: W. B. Saunders.

Ball, J., & Bindler, R. (1995). *Pediatric nursing: Caring for children*. Stamford, CT: Appleton & Lange.

Barry, P. (1996). *Psychosocial nursing: Care of physically ill patients and their families* (3rd ed.). Philadelphia: Lippincott-Raven.

Black, J., & Matassarin-Jacobs, E. (1997). *Medical-surgical nursing: Clinical management for continuity of care* (5th ed.). Philadelphia: W. B. Saunders.

Brent, N. (1997). *Nurses and the law*. Philadelphia: W. B. Saunders.

Burrell, L., Gerlach, M., & Pless, B. (1997). *Adult nursing: Acute and community care* (2nd ed.). Stamford, CT: Appleton & Lange.

Carson, V., & Arnold, E. (1996). *Mental health nursing: The nurse-patient journey*. Philadelphia: W. B. Saunders.

Clark, J., Queener, S., & Karb, V. (1997). *Pharmacologic basis of nursing practice*. St. Louis: Mosby–Year Book.

Cox, H., Hinz, M., Lubno, M., et al. (1997). *Clinical applications of nursing diagnosis: Adult, child, women's, psychiatric, gerontic, and home health considerations* (3rd ed.). Philadelphia: F. A. Davis.

Craven, R., & Hirnle, C. (1996). *Fundamentals of nursing: Human health and function* (2nd ed.). Philadelphia: Lippincott-Raven.

Deglin, J., & Vallerand, A. (1997). *Davis's drug guide for nurses* (5th ed.). Philadelphia: F. A. Davis.

Fortinash, K., & Holoday-Worret, P. (1996). *Psychiatric-mental health nursing*. St. Louis: Mosby–Year Book.

Haber, J. (1997). *Comprehensive psychiatric nursing* (5th ed.). St. Louis: Mosby–Year Book.

Hartshorn, J., Sole, M., & Lamborn, M. (1997). *Introduction to critical care nursing* (2nd ed.). Philadelphia: W. B. Saunders.

Hodgson, B., & Kizior, R. (1998). *Saunders nursing drug handbook 1998*. Philadelphia: W. B. Saunders.

Ignatavicius, D. D., Workman, M. L., & Mishler, M. A. (1995). *Medical-surgical nursing: A nursing process approach* (2nd ed.). Philadelphia: W. B. Saunders.

Johnson, B. (1997). *Psychiatric-mental health nursing: Adaptation and growth* (4th ed.). Philadelphia: Lippincott-Raven.

Kee, J., & Hayes, E. (1997). *Pharmacology: A nursing process approach* (2nd ed.). Philadelphia: W. B. Saunders.

Kozier, B., Glenora, E., & Blais, K. (1995). *Fundamentals of nursing: Concepts, process, and practice* (5th ed.). Menlo Park, CA: Addison-Wesley.

Lammon, C. B., Foote, A. W., Leli, P. G., et al. (1995). *Clinical nursing skills*. Philadelphia: W. B. Saunders.

LeMone, P., & Burke, K. (1996). *Medical-surgical nursing: Critical thinking in client care*. Menlo Park, CA: Addison-Wesley.

Lewis, S., Collier, I., & Heitkemper, M. (1996). *Medical-surgical nursing: Assessment and management of clinical problems* (4th ed.). St. Louis: Mosby–Year Book.

Lowdermilk, D., Perry, S., & Bobak, I. (1997). *Maternity and women's health care* (6th ed.). St. Louis: Mosby–Year Book.

Luckmann, J. (1997). *Saunders manual of nursing care*. Philadelphia: W. B. Saunders.

Mauro, J. (1996). *Neurologic instant nursing assessment*. Albany, NY: Delmar.

McKenry, L., & Salerno, E. (1998). *Mosby's pharmacology in nursing* (20th ed.). St. Louis: Mosby-Year Book.

Monahan, F., & Neighbors, M. (1998). *Medical-surgical nursing: Foundations for clinical practice* (2nd ed.). Philadelphia: W. B. Saunders.

National Council of State Boards of Nursing. (1997). *Plan for the National Council Licensure Examination for Registered Nurses*. Chicago: Author.

Nichols, F., & Zwelling, E. (1997). *Maternal-newborn nursing: Theory and practice*. Philadelphia: W. B. Saunders.

Olds, S., London, M., & Ladewig, P. (1996). *Maternal-newborn nursing* (5th ed.). Menlo Park, CA: Addison-Wesley.

O'Toole, M. (Ed.). (1997). *Miller-Keane Encyclopedia and dictionary of medicine, nursing, and allied health* (6th ed.). Philadelphia: W. B. Saunders.

Phillips, L. (1997). *Manual of IV therapeutics* (2nd ed.). Philadelphia: F. A. Davis.

Phipps, W., Cassmeyer, V., Sands, J., et al. (1995). *Medical-surgical nursing: Concepts and clinical practice* (5th ed.). St. Louis: Mosby–Year Book.

Pillitteri, A. (1995). *Maternal and child health nursing: Care of the childbearing and childrearing family* (2nd ed.). Philadelphia: Lippincott-Raven.

Pinnell, N. (1996). *Nursing pharmacology*. Philadelphia: W. B. Saunders.

Polaski, A., & Tatro, S. (1996). *Luckmann's Core principles and practice of medical-surgical nursing*. Philadelphia: W. B. Saunders.

Potter, P., & Perry, A. (1997). *Fundamentals of nursing: Concepts, process, and practice* (4th ed.). St. Louis: Mosby–Year Book.

Reeder, S., Martin, L., & Koniak-Griffin, D. (1997). *Maternity nursing* (18th ed.). Philadelphia: Lippincott-Raven.

Ruppert, S., Kernicki, J., & Dolan, J. (1996). *Dolan's Critical care nursing: Clinical management through the nursing process* (2nd ed.). Philadelphia: F. A. Davis.

Smeltzer, S., & Bare, B. (1996). *Brunner and Suddarth's Textbook of medical-surgical nursing* (8th ed.). Philadelphia: Lippincott-Raven.

Spradley, B., & Allender, J. (1996). *Community health nursing: Concepts and practice*. (4th ed.). Philadelphia: Lippincott-Raven.

Thompson J., McFarland, G., Hirsch, J., & Tucker, S. (1997). *Mosby's clinical nursing* (4th ed.). St. Louis: Mosby–Year Book.

Townsend, M. C. (1996). *Psychiatric–mental health nursing: Concepts of care* (2nd ed.). Philadelphia: F. A. Davis.

Wilson, K., & Kneisl, C. (1996). *Psychiatric nursing* (5th ed.). Menlo Park, CA: Addison-Wesley.

Wong, D. (1995). *Whaley and Wong's Nursing care of infants and children* (5th ed.). St. Louis: Mosby–Year Book.

Wong, D. (1997). *Whaley and Wong's Essentials of pediatric nursing* (5th ed.). St. Louis: Mosby–Year Book.

Wong, D., & Perry, S. (1998). *Maternal-child nursing care*. St. Louis: Mosby–Year Book.

CHAPTER 12

Psychosocial Integrity

Psychosocial Integrity is a major category of Client Needs. The two subcategories of this Client Needs component are (1) Coping and Adaptation and (2) Psychosocial Adaptation.

COPING AND ADAPTATION

Coping is the process of contending with life difficulties in an effort to overcome or work through them. Adaptation is a dynamic, ongoing, life-sustaining process by which human beings adjust to environmental changes. The Coping and Adaptation subcategory encompasses content related to the nurse's role in promoting the client's ability to cope with, adapt to, and/or solve problems in situations related to illnesses or stressful events. The proportion of test questions in the Coping and Adaptation subcategory of NCLEX-RN is 5%–11%.

BOX 12–1. Coping and Adaptation

- Mental Health Concepts
- Religious and Spiritual Influences on Health
- Support Systems
- Counseling Techniques
- Coping Mechanisms
- Stress Management
- Situational Role Changes
- Sensory/Perceptual Alterations
- Grief and Loss
- Unexpected Body Image Changes

PSYCHOSOCIAL ADAPTATION

Psychosocial adaptation is an ongoing process by which humans sustain a balance in their mental and emotional states of being and in their interactions with their social and cultural environments. The Psychosocial Adaptation subcategory includes content related to the nurse's role in managing and providing care with acute or chronic mental illnesses. The proportion of test questions in the Psychosocial Adaptation subcategory of NCLEX-RN is 5%–11%.

BOX 12–2. Psychosocial Adaptation

- Psychopathology
- Behavioral Interventions
- Crisis Intervention
- Therapeutic Milieu
- Chemical Dependency
- Domestic Violence
- Child Abuse/Neglect
- Elder Abuse/Neglect
- Sexual Abuse

PRACTICE TEST

1. The young adult male client with spinal cord injury (SCI) tells the nurse, "It's so depressing that I'll never get to have sex again." The nurse replies in a realistic way by making which of the following statements to the client?

1. "You're young, so you'll adapt to this more easily than if you were older."
2. "It must feel horrible to know you can never have sex again."
3. "It is still possible to have a sexual relationship, but it is different."
4. "Because of body reflexes, sexual functioning will be no different than before."

Answer: 3

Rationale: It is possible to have a form of sexual expression after SCI, but it is different from what the client experienced before the injury. Males may experience reflex erections, although they may not ejaculate. Females can have adductor spasm. Sexual counseling may help the client to adapt to changes in sexuality after SCI.

Test-Taking Strategy: To answer this question accurately, it is necessary to understand the altered physiological processes after SCI. Eliminate options 2 and 4 first because they are false. Choose option 3 over option 1 because option 1 is a statement that is a communication block. It does not promote continued discussion of the client's concerns.

Level of Cognitive Ability: Application
Phase of Nursing Process: Implementation
Client Needs: Psychosocial Integrity
Content Area: Adult Health/Neurological

Reference
Monahan, F., & Neighbors, M. (1998). *Medical-surgical nursing: Foundations for clinical practice* (2nd ed.). Philadelphia: W. B. Saunders, pp. 826–827.

---

2. The family member of a client with a brain tumor is distraught and feeling guilty for not encouraging the client to seek medical evaluation earlier. The nurse would incorporate which of the following items in formulating a response to the client's statement?

1. It is true that brain tumors are easily recognizable
2. The symptoms of brain tumor may be easily attributed to another cause
3. Brain tumors are never detected until very late in their course
4. There are no symptoms of brain tumor

Answer: 2

Rationale: Signs and symptoms of brain tumor vary, depending on location, and may easily be attributed to another cause. Symptoms include headache, vomiting, visual disturbances, and change in intellectual abilities or personality. Seizures occur in some clients. The family requires support to assist them in the normal grieving process.

Test-Taking Strategy: Eliminate options 3 and 4 first because they contain the absolute words "never" and "no," respectively. To discriminate between the two remaining options, it is necessary to know that the symptoms of brain tumor may be easily attributed to another cause and can be vague.

Level of Cognitive Ability: Application
Phase of Nursing Process: Planning
Client Needs: Psychosocial Integrity
Content Area: Adult Health/Neurological

Reference
Monahan, F., & Neighbors, M. (1998). *Medical-surgical nursing: Foundations for clinical practice* (2nd ed.). Philadelphia: W. B. Saunders, pp. 828–829.

3. The male client is in a hip spica cast for a fracture of the hip. On the day after the cast has been applied, the nurse finds the client surrounded by papers from his brief case and planning a phone meeting. The nurse's interaction with the client should be based on the knowledge that

1 Setting limits on a client's behavior is an essential aspect of the nursing role.
2 Not keeping up with his job will increase his stress level.
3 Immediate involvement in his job will keep him from becoming bored while on bed rest.
4 Rest is an essential component in bone healing.

Answer: 4

Rationale: Rest is an essential component of bone healing. Nurses can help clients understand the importance of rest and find ways to balance work demands to promote healing. Nurses cannot demand these changes but need to encourage clients to choose them. Doing work may relieve stress; however, in the immediate postcast period, it may not be physically therapeutic. Stress should be kept at a minimum in order to promote bone healing.

Test-Taking Strategy: The key issue of the question is "rest." Option 4 is the most global response and addresses the issue of the question.

Level of Cognitive Ability: Analysis
Phase of Nursing Process: Planning
Client Needs: Psychosocial Integrity
Content Area: Adult Health/Musculoskeletal

Reference
Black, J., & Matassarin-Jacobs, E. (1997). *Medical-surgical nursing: Clinical management for continuity of care* (5th ed.). Philadelphia: W. B. Saunders, p. 2149.

---

4. When a charge nurse observes an unlicensed assistive person (UAP) talking in an unusually loud voice to a client with delirium, which of these actions should the nurse take?

1 Speak to the UAP immediately while in the client's room to solve the problem
2 Inform the client that everything is all right
3 Ascertain the dementia client's safety, calmly ask the UAP to join you outside the room, and inform the UAP that his or her voice was unusually loud
4 Explain to the UAP that yelling in the client's room is tolerated only if the client is talking loudly

Answer: 3

Rationale: The nurse must ascertain that the client is safe and then discuss the matter with the UAP in an area away from the hearing of the client. If the client heard the conversation, the client may become more confused or agitated.

Test-Taking Strategy: In option 1, the nurse speaks to the UAP in the client room. This strategy could add to the client's confusion and embarrasses the UAP. By informing the client that everything will be all right, the nurse is using a block to therapeutic communication. The statement to the UAP that the only time he or she can talk loudly to the client is when the client is loud can add to the client's confusion.

Level of Cognitive Ability: Application
Phase of Nursing Process: Implementation
Client Needs: Psychosocial Integrity
Content Area: Mental Health

Reference
Varcarolis, E. M. (1998). *Foundations of psychiatric mental health nursing* (3rd ed.). Philadelphia: W. B. Saunders, pp. 317–318.

---

5. A teenager who has celiac disease presents with profuse, watery diarrhea after a pizza party last night. The client states, "I don't want to be different from my friends." The nursing diagnosis most appropriate is

1 Knowledge Deficit.
2 Fluid Volume Deficit.
3 Risk for Altered Self Esteem.
4 Celiac Crisis.

Answer: 3

Rationale: The client expresses concern about being "different." The assessment data provided do not support a diagnosis of knowledge deficit or a fluid volume deficit. Celiac crisis is a medical diagnosis.

Test-Taking Strategy: Remember that this question asks for a nursing diagnosis; thus a medical diagnosis would not be an option, and therefore eliminate option 4. Focus on the client's feelings of being "different." Look for answers that focus on the client as a worthy human being or that are directed toward feelings.

Level of Cognitive Ability: Analysis
Phase of Nursing Process: Analysis
Client Needs: Psychosocial Integrity
Content Area: Child Health

Reference
Wong, D. (1995). *Whaley and Wong's Nursing care of infants and children* (5th ed.). St. Louis: Mosby–Year Book, p. 1479.

6. Which of these nursing measures included in the plan of care for a 1-month-old hospitalized for intussusception would be most effective to provide psychosocial support for the parent-child relationship?

   1 Encourage the parents to go home and get some sleep
   2 Encourage the parents to room in with their infant
   3 Provide educational materials
   4 Initiate home nutritional support as early as possible

Answer: 2

Rationale: Rooming in is effective in reducing separation anxiety and preserving the parent-child relationship. Parents are under stress when a child is ill and hospitalized. Telling a parent to go home and sleep will not relieve this stress. Educational materials, although beneficial, will not provide psychosocial support of the parent-child relationship. Home nutritional support is not usually necessary.

Test-Taking Strategy: Use the process of elimination and focus on the key phrase "provide psychosocial support." This should direct you to the correct option.

Level of Cognitive Ability: Application
Phase of Nursing Process: Planning
Client Needs: Psychosocial Integrity
Content Area: Child Health

Reference

Wong, D., & Perry, S. (1998). *Maternal-child nursing care.* St. Louis: Mosby–Year Book, p. 1430.

7. The parents of an infant son who will have an inguinal hernia repair make the following comments. Which one of these comments would require follow-up by a nurse?

   1 "I understand surgery will repair the hernia."
   2 "The day nurse told me to give him sponge baths for a few days after surgery."
   3 "I'll need to buy extra diapers because we'll need to change them more frequently now."
   4 "I don't know if he will be able to father a child."

Answer: 4

Rationale: The anatomical location of hernias frequently causes more psychological concern to the parents than does the actual condition or treatment. Options 1, 2, and 3 all indicate the parents' accurate understanding.

Test-Taking Strategy: Focus on the key phrase "would require follow-up." Options 1, 2, and 3 do not require follow-up, whereas option 4 reflects parental fear and identifies a need for further assistance.

Level of Cognitive Ability: Analysis
Phase of Nursing Process: Analysis
Client Needs: Psychosocial Integrity
Content Area: Child Health

Reference

Wong, D. (1995). *Whaley and Wong's Nursing care of infants and children* (5th ed.). St. Louis: Mosby–Year Book, pp. 492–494.

8. The nurse is leading a crisis intervention group. The clients are high school students; a classmate recently committed suicide at the school. The clients are experiencing disbelief. Students reviewed details about finding the student dead in a bathroom. With the nurse's perception of such data collection, the nurse would immediately

   1 Inquire how students recovered from death in the past.
   2 Reinforce students' sense of growth through this death.
   3 Reinforce students' ability to work through this death event.
   4 Inquire about the students' perception of their classmate's suicide/problem.

Answer: 4

Rationale: It is essential to determine the students' view. Inquiring about the students' perception of the death will identify specifically the appraisal of the suicide and the meaning of the perception. Options 2 and 3 are similar in terms of attempts to foster clients' self-esteem. Such an approach is premature at this point. Although option 1 is exploratory, it does not address the "here and now" appraisal in terms of their classmate's suicide. Although the nurse is interested in how clients have coped in the past, this inquiry is not the most immediate.

Test-Taking Strategy: Consider the issue of the question and select the response that deals with the "here and now." The nurse must first determine the client's perception or appraisal of the stressful event. Review the phases of crisis and nursing process steps now if you had difficulty with this question!

Level of Cognitive Ability: Application
Phase of Nursing Process: Implementation
Client Needs: Psychosocial Integrity
Content Area: Mental Health

Reference

Johnson, B. (1997). *Psychiatric–mental health nursing: Adaptation and growth* (4th ed.). Philadelphia: Lippincott-Raven, p. 795.

9. The client has been hospitalized and has participated in substance abuse therapy group sessions. Upon discharge, the client has consented to participate in Alcoholics Anonymous community groups. The nurse is monitoring the client's response to the substance abuse sessions. Which of the following statements by the client would best indicate to the nurse that the client has well assimilated session topics and coping response styles and has processed information effectively for self-use?

1 "I know I'm ready to be discharged; I feel like I can say 'no' and leave a group of friends if they are drinking. . . . No problem."
2 "This group has really helped a lot. I know it will be different when I go home. But I'm sure that my family and friends will all help me like the people in this group have. . . . They'll all help me. . . . I know they will. . . . They won't let me go back to old ways."
3 "I'm looking forward to leaving here; I know that I will miss all of you. So, I'm happy and I'm sad. I'm excited and I'm scared. I know it will be different out there. I know I have to make new friends and not hang around the local pubs. I know that I have to work hard to be strong and that everyone isn't going to be as helpful as you people. I know it isn't going to be easy. But, I'm going to try as hard as I can. . . ."
4 "I'll keep all my appointments; go to all my AA groups; I'll do everything I'm supposed to. . . . Nothing will go wrong that way. . . ."

Answer: 3

Rationale: In the defense mechanism of denial, the person denies reality. There can be varying degrees of this denial. In option 3 the client is expressing real concern and ambivalence about discharge from the hospital. The client is realistic in the appraisal about the changes that the client will have to initiate in lifestyle, as well as the fact that the client has to work hard, cultivate new friendships, and find new meeting places.

Test-Taking Strategy: Select the option that identifies the most realistic client verbalization. Knowing that in denial a person is unable to face reality, you can eliminate option 1, which is blatant denial. In option 2, the client is relying heavily on others; the client's locus of control is external. In option 4, the client is concrete and procedure-oriented; again the client denies that "nothing will go wrong that way" if the client follows all the directions. The client denies self and the value of self-input and choice within interactions.

Level of Cognitive Ability: Analysis
Phase of Nursing Process: Evaluation
Client Needs: Psychosocial Integrity
Content Area: Mental Health

Reference

Johnson, B. (1997). *Psychiatric–mental health nursing: Adaptation and growth* (4th ed.). Philadelphia: Lippincott-Raven, p. 8.

10. A client recovering from a head injury becomes agitated at times. Which action will most likely calm this client?

1 Turn on the television to a musical program
2 Offer the client a favorite stuffed animal
3 Assign the client a new task to master
4 Make the client aware that the behavior is undesirable

Answer: 2

Rationale: Decreasing environmental stimuli aids in reducing agitation for the head-injured client. Option 1 increases stimuli. Option 3 does not simplify the environment; a new task may be frustrating. Option 4 identifies a nontherapeutic approach. The correct option helps to distract the client with motor activity: holding the stuffed animal.

Test-Taking Strategy: Use the process of elimination to identify options that may increase stimulation, agitation, and frustration. This should assist in directing you to the correct option!

Level of Cognitive Ability: Application
Phase of Nursing Process: Implementation
Client Needs: Psychosocial Integrity
Content Area: Adult Health/Neurological

Reference

Smeltzer, S., & Bare, B. (1996). *Brunner and Suddarth's Textbook of medical-surgical nursing* (8th ed.). Philadelphia: Lippincott-Raven, p. 1708.

11. A recovering post-stroke client has become irritable and angry about limitations. Which is the best approach by the nurse to help the client regain motivation to succeed?

1 Allow longer and more frequent visitation by spouse
2 Use supportive and kind statements to correct behavior
3 State that with your experience, you know how he or she feels
4 Ignore the behavior, knowing that the client is grieving

Answer: 2

Rationale: Post-stroke clients have many and varied needs. The client may need behavior pointed out so that correction can take place, as well as support and praise for accomplishments. Spouses of post-stroke clients are often grieving; therefore more visitation may not be helpful. Short visits are often encouraged. Stating that you know how someone feels is inappropriate. In option 4 the client may be grieving or may have damage to cerebral inhibitory centers. The behavior should not be ignored.

Test-Taking Strategy: Use therapeutic communication techniques to assist the client to express feelings and to provide the nurse appropriate opportunities to offer the client support. Option 2 is the only option that addresses clients' feelings and supportive care!

Level of Cognitive Ability: Application
Phase of Nursing Process: Implementation
Client Needs: Psychosocial Integrity
Content Area: Adult Health/Neurological

Reference

Black, J., & Matassarin-Jacobs, E. (1997). *Medical-surgical nursing: Clinical management for continuity of care* (5th ed.). Philadelphia: W. B. Saunders, p. 806.

---

12. The client is admitted with a broken hip and is experiencing periods of confusion. The nurse reviews the hospital procedures for developing a plan of care for clients with altered thought processes. The nurse wants to avoid any negligent acts. The psychosocial outcome that has the highest priority in the individualized care plan is

1 Improved sleep patterns.
2 Increased ability to concentrate and make decisions.
3 Independently meeting self-care needs.
4 Reducing family fears and anxiety.

Answer: 2

Rationale: The client needs to be able to concentrate and make decisions. Once the client is able to do that, the nurse can work with the client to achieve the other outcomes. The client is the center of the nurse's concern. Options 1, 3, and 4 are goals secondary to option 2.

Test-Taking Strategy: Look at the option that will have the greatest impact on the client's ability to function. Option 4 can be easily eliminated because it does not address the client of the question. Option 1 is unrelated to the primary issue. Option 3 is unrealistic at this time, considering the word "independently." Option 2 will make the greatest difference in the client's ability to achieve options 1, 3, and 4.

Level of Cognitive Ability: Analysis
Phase of Nursing Process: Planning
Client Needs: Psychosocial Integrity
Content Area: Adult Health/Musculoskeletal

Reference

McFarland, G., & McFarlane, E. (1997). *Nursing diagnosis and intervention*. St. Louis: Mosby–Year Book, pp. 471–478.

---

13. The client is a young woman dying from breast cancer. A defining characteristic of anticipatory grief is present when the client

1 Verbalizes unrealistic goals and plans for the future.
2 Discusses thoughts and feelings related to loss.
3 Has prolonged emotional reactions and outbursts.
4 Ignores untreated medical conditions that require treatment.

Answer: 2

Rationale: The nurse can analyze the client's stage of grief by observing behavior. This is extremely important because the appropriate nursing diagnoses need to be developed so that the plan of care is appropriate. Options 1, 3, and 4 are examples of dysfunctional grieving.

Test-Taking Strategy: Note that options 1, 3, and 4 identify dysfunctional behaviors. Note the words "unrealistic," "prolonged," and "ignores" in these options. Review the stages of grief and anticipatory grief now if you had difficulty with this question!

Level of Cognitive Ability: Analysis
Phase of Nursing Process: Analysis
Client Needs: Psychosocial Integrity
Content Area: Adult Health/Oncology

Reference

McFarland, G., & McFarlane, E. (1997). *Nursing diagnosis and intervention.* St. Louis: Mosby–Year Book, pp. 684–686.

---

14. The nurse determines that a gravida 3, para 3 client is beginning to experience shock and hemorrhage secondary to a partial inversion of the uterus. The nurse pages the obstetrician stat and calls for assistance. The client asks in an apprehensive voice, "What is happening to me? I feel so funny and I know I am bleeding. Am I dying?" The nurse bases the response on the fact that the client is feeling

1 Panic secondary to shock.
2 Fear and anxiety related to unexpected and ambiguous sensations.
3 Anticipatory grieving related to fear of dying.
4 Depression related to postpartum hormonal changes.

Answer: 2

Rationale: Feelings of loss of control resulting from knowledge deficit are common causes of anxiety. The unknown is the most common cause of fear. Apprehension and feelings of impending doom are also associated with shock, but the case situation does not suggest panic at this point. Anticipatory grieving occurs when there is knowledge of the impending loss, but it is not operative in a sudden situational crisis such as this one. It is far too early for the onset of postpartum depression.

Test-Taking Strategy: Use the process of elimination. Note the relationship between "I feel so funny" in the question and "unexpected and ambiguous sensations" in the correct option.

Level of Cognitive Ability: Analysis
Phase of Nursing Process: Analysis
Client Needs: Psychosocial Integrity
Content Area: Maternity

Reference

Lowdermilk, D., Perry, S., & Bobak, I. (1997). *Maternity and women's health care* (6th ed.). St. Louis: Mosby–Year Book, pp. 896, 1109.

---

15. The perinatal home health nurse has just assessed the fetal status of a client with a diagnosis of partial placental abruption at 20 weeks' gestation. The client is experiencing new bleeding and reports less fetal movement. The nurse informs the client that the nonstress test and fetal heart rate are not reassuring and that the nurse will now contact the doctor for an order for immediate transfer to the hospital. The client begins to cry quietly while holding her abdomen with her hands. She murmurs, "No, no, you can't go, my little man." The nurse recognizes the client's behavior as an indication of

1 Pain related to abdominal tetany.
2 Cognitive confusion secondary to shock.
3 Grieving, anticipatory related to perceived potential loss.
4 Situational crisis: death of fetus related to fear and loss.

Answer: 3

Rationale: Anticipatory grieving occurs when a client has knowledge of an impending loss. Fetal distress associated with placental abruption indicates a grade II abruption in which 20%–50% of the placenta may be detached. The larger the percentage of separation of the placenta, the greater the threat to the fetus, resulting in increasing signs of fetal distress. Anticipatory grieving is appropriate when any signs of fetal distress accelerate. The first stages of anticipatory grieving may be characterized by shock, emotional numbness, disbelief, and strong emotions such as tears, screaming, or anger.

Test-Taking Strategy: Options 1 and 2 can be eliminated because there is no indication of pain or confusion. Note that in this situation, there is a situational crisis with feelings of grief, but no loss has occurred at this point; therefore, eliminate option 4.

Level of Cognitive Ability: Application
Phase of Nursing Process: Analysis
Client Needs: Psychosocial Integrity
Content Area: Maternity

Reference

Lowdermilk, D., Perry, S., & Bobak, I. (1997). *Maternity and women's health care* (6th ed.). St. Louis: Mosby–Year Book, pp. 778, 1109.

16. A postoperative client has been vomiting, and ileus has been diagnosed. The physician orders insertion of a nasogastric tube. The nurse explains the purpose and insertion procedure to the client. The client says to the nurse, "I'm not sure I can take any more of this treatment." The most appropriate response by the nurse is

1. "It is your right to refuse any procedure. I'll notify the physician."
2. "You are feeling tired and frustrated with your recovery from surgery?"
3. "If you don't have this tube put down, you will just continue to vomit."
4. "Let's just put the tube down so you can get well."

Answer: 2

Rationale: In option 2, the nurse is sharing a client's frame of reference—an important component in a nurse-client relationship. This approach assists clients in expressing and exploring their feelings, which can lead to problem-solving. The other options are examples of barriers to effective communication in that the nurse does not address the client's concerns.

Test-Taking Strategy: With a communication question, identify options that are examples of therapeutic communication tools or blocks to communication. Option 2 is an open-ended question and is a communication tool. It also focuses on the client's feelings!

Level of Cognitive Ability: Application
Phase of Nursing Process: Implementation
Client Needs: Psychosocial Integrity
Content Area: Adult Health/Gastrointestinal

Reference

Lammon, C. B., Foote, A. W., Leli, P. G., et al. (1995). *Clinical nursing skills.* Philadelphia: W. B. Saunders, p. 418.

---

17. A client is admitted with a bowel obstruction secondary to a recurrent malignancy. The physician inserts a Miller-Abbott tube. After the procedure, the client asks the nurse, "Do you think this is worth all this trouble?" The most appropriate action or response by the nurse is

1. The nurse stays with the client and is silent.
2. "Are you wondering whether you are going to get better?"
3. "Let's give this tube a chance."
4. "I remember a case similar to yours, and the tube relieved the obstruction."

Answer: 2

Rationale: The nurse uses therapeutic communication tools in assisting a client with a chronic terminal illness to express feelings. The nurse listens attentively to the client and uses clarifying and focusing to assist the client in expressing her or his feelings. Responding with inappropriate silence (option 1), changing the subject (option 3), and offering false reassurance (option 4) are examples of barriers to communication.

Test-Taking Strategy: With communication questions, identify the use of therapeutic communication tools, as found in option 2, and blocks to communication, as in options 1, 3, and 4. Option 2 encourages the client to verbalize.

Level of Cognitive Ability: Application
Phase of Nursing Process: Implementation
Client Needs: Psychosocial Integrity
Content Area: Adult Health/Oncology

Reference

Black, J., & Matassarin-Jacobs, E. (1997). *Medical-surgical nursing: Clinical management for continuity of care* (5th ed.). Philadelphia: W. B. Saunders, p. 58.

18. The nurse explains to a client receiving total parenteral nutrition (TPN) that Intralipid 20%, an intravenous fat emulsion, will also be administered three times per week. The client states to the nurse, "I was always overweight until I had this illness. I'm not sure I want to get that fat. The other IVs are probably enough." Which is the best initial response by the nurse?

1 "Fatty acids are essential for life. You'll develop deficiencies without the fats."
2 "I think you need to discuss this decision with the physician."
3 "Tell me how being ill has affected the way you think of yourself."
4 "I understand what you mean. I've dieted most of my life."

Answer: 3

Rationale: Clients receiving long-term parenteral nutrition are at risk for development of essential fatty acid deficiency. However, the client's response requires more than an informational response initially. The nurse uses tools of therapeutic communication to assist the client to express feelings and deal with aspects of illness and treatment. The nurse listens carefully to what the client is saying. The nurse asks for more information and clarifies to assist the client to explore concerns. Blocks to communication, such as giving opinions and giving information too soon, will not assist the client in coping effectively.

Test-Taking Strategy: Be aware of the key phrase "initial response." With communication questions, identify the use of therapeutic tools, as in option 3, clarifying. Eliminate blocks to communication, as found in options 2 and 4. Information about essential fatty acids as in option 1 can be given after the client is encouraged to express feelings.

Level of Cognitive Ability: Analysis
Phase of Nursing Process: Implementation
Client Needs: Psychosocial Integrity
Content Area: Fundamental Skills

Reference
Black, J., & Matassarin-Jacobs, E. (1997). *Medical-surgical nursing: Clinical management for continuity of care* (5th ed.). Philadelphia: W. B. Saunders, p. 58.

---

19. The client has terminal cancer and is using narcotic analgesics for pain relief. The client is concerned about becoming addicted to the pain medication. The home health care nurse allays this anxiety by

1 Explaining to the client that his or her fears are justified but should be of no concern in the final stages of care.
2 Encouraging the client to hold off as long as possible between doses of pain medication.
3 Telling the client to take lower doses of medications even though the pain is not well controlled.
4 Explaining to the client that addiction rarely occurs in people who are taking medication to relieve pain.

Answer: 4

Rationale: Clients who are taking narcotics often have well-founded fears about addiction, even in the presence of pain. The nurse has a responsibility to give correct information about the likelihood of addiction while still maintaining adequate pain control. Addiction is rare in people who are taking medication to relieve pain. Allowing the client to be in pain, as in options 2 and 3, is not acceptable nursing practice. Option 1 is correct only in that it acknowledges the client's fear, but addressing the final stages of care is inappropriate at this time.

Test-Taking Strategy: Eliminate options 2 and 3, as these are not acceptable nursing practices. Eliminate option 1 because it is only partially correct. Review pain management now if you had difficulty with this question!

Level of Cognitive Ability: Application
Phase of Nursing Process: Implementation
Client Needs: Psychosocial Integrity
Content Area: Adult Health/Oncology

Reference
Como, N. (1995). *Home health nursing pocket consultant.* St. Louis: Mosby–Year Book, p. 278.

20. The client is highly anxious about receiving chest physical therapy (CPT) for the first time at home. In planning for the client's care, the home health care nurse proceeds by reassuring the client that

1 There are no risks associated with this procedure.
2 CPT will resolve all of the client's respiratory symptoms.
3 CPT will assist in mobilizing secretions to enhance more effective breathing.
4 CPT will assist the client to cough more effectively.

Answer: 3

Rationale: There are risks associated with this procedure; they include cardiac, gastrointestinal, neurological, and pulmonary complications. Pulmonary risks range from fractured ribs to flail chest, pulmonary embolism, or severe dyspnea and anxiety. CPT is an intervention to assist in clearing secretions and will not resolve all respiratory symptoms. CPT will assist the client to cough, indirectly, if the secretions have been mobilized and the cough stimulus is present.

Test-Taking Strategy: Eliminate options 1 and 2 because they contain the absolute terms "no" and "all." The issue of the question is the purpose of CPT. Focusing on the issue will assist in directing you to select option 3 over option 4. Review the purpose of CPT now if you had difficulty with this question!

Level of Cognitive Ability: Application
Phase of Nursing Process: Planning
Client Needs: Psychosocial Integrity
Content Area: Adult Health/Respiratory

Reference

Como, N. (1995). *Home health nursing pocket consultant.* St. Louis: Mosby–Year Book, pp. 220–227.

21. The client with myocardiopathy stops eating, takes long naps, and turns away from the nurse when the nurse talks to the client. The most appropriate nursing diagnosis for this client would be

1 Activity Intolerance.
2 Intractable Pain.
3 Noncompliance.
4 Depression.

Answer: 4

Rationale: Depression is a common problem of clients who have long-term and debilitating illness. Options 1, 2, and 3 are not described by the symptoms present in the question and therefore are not the appropriate nursing diagnoses.

Test-Taking Strategy: When a question asks for the selection of an appropriate nursing diagnosis, direct yourself to the correct option by identifying the data presented in the question. According to the data presented, the only appropriate diagnosis is depression!

Level of Cognitive Ability: Analysis
Phase of Nursing Process: Analysis
Client Needs: Psychosocial Integrity
Content Area: Adult Health/Cardiovascular

Reference

Black, J., & Matassarin-Jacobs, E. (1997). *Medical-surgical nursing: Clinical management for continuity of care* (5th ed.). Philadelphia: W. B. Saunders, p. 1342.

22. Which short-term psychosocial outcome is important for a pregnant client hospitalized for stabilization of diabetes?

1 Teach the client and family about diabetes and its implications
2 Provide emotional support and education about altered family processes related to the pregnant women's hospitalization
3 Protect from risk of injury secondary to convulsions
4 Be alert to the risks of early labor and birth

Answer: 2

Rationale: The short-term psychosocial well-being of the family is at risk because of the hospitalization of a diabetic mother. Teaching about diabetes is a long-term goal related to diabetes. Options 3 and 4 are unrelated to diabetes and are more related to pregnancy-induced hypertension.

Test-Taking Strategy: Eliminate options 3 and 4 because they are unrelated to diabetes. From the remaining two options, note the phrase "short-term psychosocial outcome." This should direct you to option 2 because option 1 is a long-term outcome.

Level of Cognitive Ability: Analysis
Phase of Nursing Process: Analysis
Client Needs: Psychosocial Integrity
Content Area: Maternity

Reference

Olds, S., London, M., & Ladewig, P. (1996). *Maternal-newborn nursing: A family-centered approach* (5th ed.). Menlo Park, CA: Addison-Wesley, pp. 35–40.

---

23. A new parent is trying to make the decision whether to have her baby boy circumcised. Which of the following is the best response to assist the mother in making a decision?

1 "I had my son circumcised, and I am so glad!"
2 "Circumcision is a difficult decision, but your physician is the best, and you know it's better to get it done now than later!"
3 "Circumcision is a difficult decision. There are various controversies surrounding circumcision. Here, read this pamphlet that discusses the pros and cons, and we will talk after you read, to answer any questions that you have."
4 "You know, they say it prevents cancer and sexually transmitted diseases, so I would definitely have my son circumcised!"

Answer: 3

Rationale: Various controversies have surrounded circumcision. Providing written information to the client will give the mother the information she needs to make an educated and informed decision. Options 1, 2, and 4 identify nontherapeutic communication techniques in that they offer a personal opinion and advice to the client.

Test-Taking Strategy: Options 1 and 4 are similar. In addition, options 1, 2, and 4 are communication blocks because the nurse is providing a personal opinion to the client. The nurse should provide educational material and answer questions pertaining to the education of the mother. The nurse's personal thoughts and feelings should not be part of the educational process. Informed decision making is the key point when selecting the correct option in this question.

Level of Cognitive Ability: Application
Phase of Nursing Process: Implementation
Client Needs: Psychosocial Integrity
Content Area: Maternity

Reference

Lowdermilk, D., Perry, S., & Bobak, I. (1997). *Maternity and women's health care* (6th ed.). St. Louis: Mosby–Year Book, pp. 1163–1164.

---

24. The nurse is planning care for a client who is experiencing anxiety after a myocardial infarction. Which nursing intervention should be included in the plan of care?

1 Provide detailed explanations of all procedures
2 Administer cyclobenzaprine (Flexeril) to promote relaxation
3 Limit family involvement during the acute phase
4 Answer questions with factual information

Answer: 4

Rationale: Accurate information reduces fear, strengthens the nurse-client relationship, and assists the client in dealing realistically with the situation. Option 1, providing detailed information, may increase the client's anxiety. Information should be provided simply and clearly. Option 2, Flexeril, is a skeletal muscle relaxant and is used in the short-term treatment of muscle spasms. Option 3, limiting family involvement, may not be helpful; the client's family may be a source of support for the client.

Test-Taking Strategy: Avoid selecting options with strong adjectives, such as "detailed," as in option 1. Option 1 would be a plausible answer if "detailed" were omitted. Eliminate option 2 because medication should not be the first intervention to alleviate anxiety. In addition, this particular medication is used to relieve muscle spasms. Of the remaining two options, eliminate option 3 because limiting family involvement does not reduce anxiety in all situations.

Level of Cognitive Ability: Application
Phase of Nursing Process: Planning
Client Needs: Psychosocial Integrity
Content Area: Adult Health/Cardiovascular

Reference

Black, J., & Matassarin-Jacobs, E. (1997). *Medical-surgical nursing: Clinical management for continuity of care* (5th ed.). Philadelphia: W. B. Saunders, pp. 1272.

25. A client recovering from an acute myocardial infarction will be discharged the following day. Which client action on the evening before discharge suggests that the client is in the denial phase of grieving and that a nursing diagnosis of Grieving is still applicable for the client?

1 Requests a sedative for sleep at 10:00 P.M.
2 Expresses hesitancy to leave the hospital
3 Walks up and down three flights of stairs unsupervised
4 Consumes 25% of foods and fluids for supper

Answer: 3

Rationale: Ignoring activity limitations and avoidance of lifestyle changes are signs of denial in the stages of grieving. Walking three flights of stairs should be a supervised activity during this phase of the recovery process. Option 1 is an appropriate client action on the evening before discharge. Option 2, expressing hesitancy to leave, may be a manifestation of anxiety or fear, not of denial. Option 4, anorexia, is a manifestation of depression, not denial.

Test-Taking Strategy: The key word in the question is "denial." Use the process of elimination. Option 1 is appropriate. Option 2 identifies anxiety or fear. Option 4 identifies depression. Option 3 is the only option that suggests denial in the client.

Level of Cognitive Ability: Analysis
Phase of Nursing Process: Evaluation
Client Needs: Psychosocial Integrity
Content Area: Adult Health/Cardiovascular

Reference

Doenges, M. E., Moorhouse, M. F., & Geissler, A. C. (1997). *Nursing care plans: Guidelines for planning and documenting patient care* (4th ed.). Philadelphia: F. A. Davis, p. 788.

---

26. Which of the following statements, if made by the client, indicates a positive coping mechanism to be used during treatment for Hodgkin's disease?

1 "I have selected a wig even though I will miss my own hair."
2 "I know that losing my hair won't bother me."
3 "I will not leave the house bald."
4 "I will be one of the few who don't lose their hair."

Answer: 1

Rationale: A combination of radiation and chemotherapy often causes alopecia in clients with Hodgkin's disease. In order to use positive coping mechanisms, the client must identify personal feelings and use problem-solving in positive interventions to deal with side effects.

Test-Taking Strategy: Note that the question seeks for a positive coping mechanism. Options 2, 3, and 4 involve avoidance and denial. Option 1 is the only option that addresses a positive coping mechanism.

Level of Cognitive Ability: Analysis
Phase of Nursing Process: Evaluation
Client Needs: Psychosocial Integrity
Content Area: Adult Health/Oncology

Reference

Black, J., & Matassarin-Jacobs, E. (1997). *Medical-surgical nursing: Clinical management for continuity of care* (5th ed.). Philadelphia: W. B. Saunders, pp. 1502–1503.

27. A client is admitted with diabetic ketoacidosis (DKA). The client's daughter says to the nurse, "My mother died last month, and now this. I've been trying to follow all of the instructions from the doctor. What have I done wrong?" The nurse's best response would be

1. "Maybe we can keep your father in the hospital for a while longer to give you a rest."
2. "An emotional stress, such as your mother's death, can trigger DKA even though you are following the prescribed regimen to the letter."
3. "You should talk to the social worker about getting you someone at home who is more capable in managing a diabetic's care."
4. "Tell me what you think you did wrong."

Answer: 2

Rationale: Environment, infection, or an emotional stressor can initiate the pathophysiological mechanism of DKA. Option 1 is not cost effective. Options 3 and 4 substantiate the daughters' feelings of guilt and incompetence. Option 2 assists in relieving the daughter's guilt and provides an accurate statement regarding DKA.

Test-Taking Strategy: Note that the daughter, not the client, is the subject of the question. This will assist in eliminating option 1 in addition to the fact that this option is not cost effective. Options 3 and 4 devalue the client (the daughter) and block therapeutic communication.

Level of Cognitive Ability: Application
Phase of Nursing Process: Implementation
Client Needs: Psychosocial Integrity
Content Area: Adult Health/Endocrine

Reference

Ignatavicius, D. D., Workman, M. L., & Mishler, M. A. (1995). *Medical-surgical nursing: A nursing process approach* (2nd ed.). Philadelphia: W. B. Saunders, p. 1860.

28. The nurse has been working with a victim of rape in an outpatient setting for the past 4 weeks. When planning the short-term goals for these sessions, which of the following is inappropriate?

1. The client will resolve feelings of fear and anxiety related to the rape trauma
2. The client will experience healing of the physical wounds that were incurred at the time of the rape
3. The client will verbalize feelings about the rape event
4. The client will participate in the treatment plan by keeping appointments and following through with treatment options

Answer: 1

Rationale: Short-term goals will include the beginning stages of dealing with the rape trauma. Clients will be expected initially to keep appointments, participate in care, begin to explore feelings, and begin to heal physical wounds that were inflicted at the time of the rape.

Test-Taking Strategy: Note the key word "inappropriate" and key phrase "the short-term goals." Use the process of elimination, considering each option and the possibility that the option statement can be achieved over the short term. Note the word "resolve" in option 1. This word should provide you with the clue that this option is a long-term goal.

Level of Cognitive Ability: Analysis
Phase of Nursing Process: Planning
Client Needs: Psychosocial Integrity
Content Area: Mental Health

Reference

Carson, V., & Arnold, E. (1996). *Mental health nursing: The nurse-patient journey.* Philadelphia: W. B. Saunders, p. 1095.

29. The client is admitted to a surgical unit with a diagnosis of cancer. The client is scheduled for surgery in the morning. When the nurse enters the room and begins the surgical preparation, the client states, "I'm not having surgery. You must have the wrong person! My test results were negative. I'll be going home tomorrow." The nurse recognizes that the ego defense mechanism that may be operating here is

1. Psychosis.
2. Denial.
3. Delusions.
4. Displacement.

Answer: 2

Rationale: By definition, ego defense mechanisms are operations outside of a person's awareness that the ego calls into play to protect against anxiety. Denial is the defense mechanism that "blocks out" painful or anxiety-inducing events or feelings. In this case, the client cannot deal with the upcoming surgery for cancer and, therefore, denies that he or she is ill.

Test-Taking Strategy: Options 1 and 3 are eliminated immediately because these are not ego defense mechanisms. Displacement is acting out in anger or frustration with people who did not arouse those feelings. Therefore, eliminate option 4. Review ego defense mechanisms now if you had difficulty with this question!

Level of Cognitive Ability: Analysis
Phase of Nursing Process: Analysis
Client Needs: Psychosocial Integrity
Content Area: Adult Health/Oncology

Reference

Carson, V., & Arnold, E. (1996). *Mental health nursing: The nurse-patient journey.* Philadelphia: W. B. Saunders, p. 579.

---

30. A community health nurse working in an industrial setting has received a memorandum indicating that a large number of employees will be laid off in the next 2 weeks. An analysis of previous layoffs suggested that workers experienced role crises, indecision, and depression. Using the analyzed data, the nurse should begin to

1 Help the workers acquire unemployment benefits to avoid a gap in income.
2 Reduce the staff in the occupational health department of the industrial setting.
3 Notify the insurance carriers of the upcoming event to assist with potential health alterations.
4 Identify referral, counseling, and vocational rehabilitative services for the employees being laid off.

Answer: 4

Rationale: Analysis of data should lead to a comprehensive conclusion based directly on the data. In this case, option 4 is the only analytical conclusion. The other distracters may or may not need to occur. The nurse would need to know more about the industry to determine whether option 1, 2 or 3 would be necessary or possible.

Test-Taking Strategy: Options 1, 2, and 3 are more industry-specific, and the nurse would need to know more about the industrial setting than is presented in the question. In addition, option 4 is the global answer.

Level of Cognitive Ability: Analysis
Phase of Nursing Process: Planning
Client Needs: Psychosocial Integrity
Content Area: Mental Health

Reference

Clemen-Stone, S., Eigsti, D., & McGuire, S. (1995). *Comprehensive community health nursing: Family, aggregate, and community practice* (4th ed.). St. Louis: Mosby–Year Book, pp. 680–681.

---

31. A primigravida client comes to the clinic, and a urinary tract infection has been diagnosed. She has repeatedly verbalized concern regarding safety of the fetus. Which of the following nursing diagnoses is most appropriate at this time?

1 Pain
2 Impaired Tissue Integrity
3 Urinary Tract Infection
4 Fear

Answer: 4

Rationale: The primary concern for this client is safety of her fetus, not herself. The priority nursing diagnosis at this time is option 4. Option 3 is a medical diagnosis and outside the scope of nursing practice. Pain and impaired tissue integrity are commonly seen in clients experiencing urinary tract infections, but the stem includes no data to support either of the options.

Test-Taking Strategy: Avoid medical diagnoses as in option 3, because they are outside the scope of nursing practice. In addition, note that options 1, 2, and 3 are similar in that they are all physiological. Option 4 is different, addressing a psychosocial issue. The data in the stem supports only option 4.

Level of Cognitive Ability: Analysis
Phase of Nursing Process: Analysis
Client Needs: Psychosocial Integrity
Content Area: Maternity

Reference

Lowdermilk, D., Perry, S., & Bobak, I. (1997). *Maternity and women's health care* (6th ed.). St. Louis: Mosby–Year Book, p. 749.

32. When planning interventions for counseling the pregnant client with newly diagnosed sickle cell anemia, the most important psychosocial intervention at this time would be which of the following?

1. Provide all information regarding the disease initially
2. Allow the client to be alone if she is crying
3. Provide emotional support
4. Avoid the topic of the disease at all costs

Answer: 3

Rationale: Probably the most important of all nursing functions is providing emotional support to the client and family during the counseling process. Option 1 overwhelms the client with information while the client is trying to cope with the news of the disease. Option 2 is appropriate only if the client requests to be alone. If she did not request to be alone, the nurse is abandoning the client in time of need. Option 4 is similar to option 1 and is nontherapeutic. Supportive therapy allows the client to express feeling, explore alternatives, and make decisions in a safe, caring environment.

Test-Taking Strategy: Eliminate options 1 and 4 because of the words "all" and "avoid." In addition, these actions are nontherapeutic. For the remaining two options, remember that the client's feelings are the priority and that an extremely important role of the nurse is to provide emotional support!

Level of Cognitive Ability: Application
Phase of Nursing Process: Planning
Client Needs: Psychosocial Integrity
Content Area: Maternity

Reference

Lowdermilk, D., Perry, S., & Bobak, I. (1997). *Maternity and women's health care* (6th ed.). St. Louis: Mosby–Year Book, p. 130.

---

33. The neonatal intensive care nurse is caring for a newborn with suspected erythroblastosis fetalis immediately after delivery. The nurse would make which of the following statements to the parents at this time?

1. "You must have many concerns. Please ask me any questions as I explain your newborn's care."
2. "This is a common neonatal problem; you shouldn't be concerned."
3. "There is no need to worry. We have the most updated equipment in this hospital."
4. "Your newborn is very sick. The next 24 hours are most crucial."

Answer: 1

Rationale: Parental anxiety is expected related to the care of the newborn with hyperbilirubinemia from erythroblastosis fetalis or blood incompatibilities. This anxiety results from a lack of knowledge regarding the disease process, treatment, and expected outcomes. Parents need to be encouraged to verbalize concerns and participate in care as appropriate.

Test-Taking Strategy: Eliminate options 2 and 3 because they are similar and say basically the same thing. In addition, they are blocks to communication. Option 4 is worded to frighten the parents. Remember to address clients' feelings and concerns. Option 1 is the only option that encourages communication.

Level of Cognitive Ability: Application
Phase of Nursing Process: Implementation
Client Needs: Psychosocial Integrity
Content Area: Maternity

Reference

Lowdermilk, D., Perry S., & Bobak, I. (1997). *Maternity and women's health care* (6th ed.). St. Louis: Mosby–Year Book, pp. 1046–1047.

34. The school nurse is weighing all the high school students. One of the teenagers, who has type I diabetes, has gained 15 pounds since last year with no gain in height. The nurse also notices the student eating alone in the cafeteria at lunch time. On the basis of this data, the nurse is most concerned that the student may have

1 Bulimia nervosa.
2 Suicidal thoughts.
3 An alcohol abuse problem.
4 An insulin deficiency.

Answer: 2

Rationale: Diabetic teenagers are at risk for depression and suicide, which is frequently manifested by changing insulin and eating patterns. Social isolation is another clue. Remember that weight loss is a symptom of type I diabetes, so an insulin deficiency would have the same effect. Bulimic clients may be of normal weight but control weight gain by purging. Alcohol abuse is more likely to be related to weight loss.

Test-Taking Strategy: Use the data presented in the question in selecting the correct option. Eliminate options 1, 3, and 4 because of weight gain. This leaves option 2.

Level of Cognitive Ability: Analysis
Phase of Nursing Process: Analysis
Client Needs: Psychosocial Integrity
Content Area: Child Health

Reference
Wong, D. (1995). *Whaley and Wong's Nursing care of infants and children* (5th ed.). St. Louis: Mosby–Year Book, pp. 910, 926, 1785.

---

35. A school nurse is teaching a class of high school students about the risk of sexually transmitted diseases (STD). What opening statement will best encourage participation within the group?

1 "At the end of the class, condoms will be distributed to everyone in the class."
2 "The topic today is very personal. For this reason, anything shared with the group will remain confidential."
3 "Please feel free to share your personal experiences with the group."
4 "Our goal today is to describe ways to prevent acquiring a sexually transmitted disease."

Answer: 2

Rationale: The correct answer states the rules for confidentiality, which will help develop a trust in sharing sensitive issues with the group. Option 1 may be an incentive for those attending to stay, but participation is not necessary to get the reward. Option 3 offers the opportunity but no protection of confidentiality. Option 4 is a good introduction to the topic but doesn't foster trust, especially with those who may already have an STD.

Test-Taking Strategy: The issues of the question are confidentiality, trust building, and sharing. Eliminate option 4, which focuses on content, and option 1, which addresses format. Option 2 is more global and directly addresses the issue of confidentiality.

Level of Cognitive Ability: Application
Phase of Nursing Process: Implementation
Client Needs: Psychosocial Integrity
Content Area: Child Health

Reference
Wong, D. (1997). *Whaley and Wong's Essentials of pediatric nursing* (5th ed.). St. Louis: Mosby–Year Book, pp. 498, 500.

36. The nurse is planning care for the client with an intrauterine fetal demise. Which of the following is not an appropriate goal for this client?

1. The woman and her family will express their grief about the loss of their desired infant
2. The woman and her family will discuss plans for going home without the infant
3. The woman and her family will contact their pastor or grief counselor for support after discharge
4. The woman will recognize that thoughts of worthlessness and suicide are normal after a loss

Answer: 4

Rationale: It is important for the nurse to assess whether the couple is undergoing the normal grieving process. Signs that are a cause for concern and not part of the normal grieving process include thoughts of worthlessness and suicide. The woman should be referred to a mental heath provider if she exhibits any of these symptoms.

Test-Taking Strategy: Use the process of elimination seeking a nonappropriate goal. You should easily be directed to option 4 because thoughts of suicide and worthlessness are cause for concern. These feelings are not "normal" but instead are indicative of a serious problem.

Level of Cognitive Ability: Analysis
Phase of Nursing Process: Analysis
Client Needs: Psychosocial Integrity
Content Area: Maternity

Reference

Nichols, F., & Zwelling, E. (1997). *Maternal-newborn nursing: Theory and practice.* Philadelphia: W. B. Saunders, pp. 636, 903.

37. A client with severe pre-eclampsia is admitted to the hospital. She is a student at a local college and insists on continuing her studies while in the hospital, despite being instructed to rest. The nurse notes that the client studies about 19 hours a day between numerous visits from fellow students, families, and friends. Which nursing approach should initially be included in the plan of care?

1. Instructing the client that the health of the baby is more important than her studies at this time
2. Asking her why she is not complying with the order of bed rest
3. Including a significant other in helping the client understand the need for bed rest
4. Developing a routine with the client to balance studies and rest needs

Answer: 4

Rationale: With both options 1 and 2, the nurse is judging the client's opinion and asking probing questions. This will cause a breakdown in communication. Option 3 persuades the client's significant others to disagree with the client's action. This could cause problems with the client's self-esteem and with relationships with significant others. Option 4 involves the client in the decision making.

Test-Taking Strategy: The focus of the question needs to be on the client. The client needs to be involved in the decision making and the planning of care. Eliminate options 1, 2, and 3 because these are blocks to communication and to a therapeutic nurse-client relationship. Option 4 is the most thorough nursing action because it addresses rest and studies and involves the client in the decision-making process.

Level of Cognitive Ability: Application
Phase of Nursing Process: Planning
Client Needs: Psychosocial Integrity
Content Area: Maternity

Reference

Fortinash, K., & Holoday-Worret, P. (1996). *Psychiatric–mental health nursing.* St. Louis: Mosby–Year Book, pp. 159–161.

38. A pregnant client has a new diagnosis of gestational diabetes. She cries during the remainder of the interview and keeps repeating, "What have I done to cause this? If I could only live my life over." Which nursing diagnosis should direct nursing care at this time?

1 Self Concept Disturbance related to a complication of pregnancy
2 Knowledge Deficit related to diabetic self-care during pregnancy
3 Body Image Disturbance related to complications of pregnancy
4 Risk for Injury to the Fetus related to maternal distress

Answer: 1

Rationale: The client is putting the blame for the diabetes upon herself, lowering her self-concept or image. She is expressing fear and grief. Knowledge Deficit is an important nursing diagnosis for this client, but not immediately. The client will not be able to comprehend information at this time. There are no data to support the nursing diagnoses in options 3 and 4.

Test-Taking Strategy: Use the data presented in the question to assist you in selecting the correct option. The phrase "what have I done" should assist in eliminating options 2 and 4. For the remaining two options, this important phrase should direct you to option 1. In addition, a Body Image Disturbance is most often associated with a physical change, which is not the case in this situation.

Level of Cognitive Ability: Analysis
Phase of Nursing Process: Analysis
Client Needs: Psychosocial Integrity
Content Area: Maternity

Reference

Reeder, S., Martin, L., & Koniak-Griffin, D. (1997). *Maternity nursing: Family, newborn, and women's health care* (18th ed.). Philadelphia: Lippincott-Raven, pp. 855–860.

39. The community health nurse visits an obese adult client who has a sprained right ankle. The client is using a cane to ambulate but has not exercised for over 1 week and has missed the last two rehabilitation appointments. The client says, "I'm getting therapy for my ankle and I do my exercises three times a day." Which of the following responses would indicate that the nurse is using the most therapeutic communication technique to instruct?

1 "Sounds good to me. Have you made all of your appointments?"
2 "You say you are following your exercise plan, yet you've missed the last two appointments with the physical therapist?"
3 "Show me how you do your exercises. I want to determine whether you're doing them correctly."
4 "You must keep your appointments. I already know that you've missed two appointments with the therapist."

Answer: 2

Rationale: The nurse employs the therapeutic communication technique of sharing perceptions. Sharing perceptions involves asking the client to verify the nurse's understanding of what the client is feeling, thinking, or doing. In addition, concreteness, which involves the use of specific terminology or information in the therapeutic dialogue, is used. Its purpose is to assist the client in stopping the vagueness and the generalization and to support the client in attending to specific problem areas that are currently being avoided. In this situation, the client is employing avoidance. By sharing perceptions, the nurse is assisting the client to begin problem-solving.

Test-Taking Strategy: Use the process of elimination. In option 1, the nurse is nontherapeutic in giving approval and is mirroring the client's avoidance and passivity by not dealing directly with the problem of missed appointments. In option 3, the nurse is therapeutic in the attempt to engage the client and have the client restart the exercises, but this needs to occur in a helpful, trusting environment. In this intervention, the nurse is ordering the client to perform the exercises, which could lead to resistance and, eventually, a regressive struggle. In option 4, the nurse is demanding a behavior that can also lead to resistance.

Level of Cognitive Ability: Analysis
Phase of Nursing Process: Implementation
Client Needs: Psychosocial Integrity
Content Area: Adult Health/Musculoskeletal

Reference

Antai-Otong, D. (1995). *Psychiatric nursing: Biological and behavioral concepts.* Philadelphia: W. B. Saunders, pp. 270–276.

40. The client says to the nurse, "I'm going to die, and I wish my family would stop hoping for a 'cure'! I get so angry when they carry on like this! After all, I'm the one who's dying." The most therapeutic response by the nurse is

1 "You're feeling angry that your family continues to hope for you to be 'cured'?"
2 "I think we should talk more about your anger with your family."
3 "Well, it sounds like you're being pretty pessimistic."
4 "Have you shared your feelings with your family?"

Answer: 1

Rationale: Reflection is the therapeutic communication technique that redirects the client's feelings back in order to validate what the client is saying. In this case, the client may be able to "see" the dynamics involved in the client-family relationship. Questions that the client will be able to deal with more effectively include exploring the client's unwillingness to maintain hope and the client's anger regarding the family's hopefulness.

Test-Taking Strategy: Use therapeutic communication techniques to answer the question. Option 1 uses the therapeutic technique of reflection. In option 2, the nurse attempts to use focusing, but the attempt to discuss central issues seems premature. In option 3, the nurse makes a judgment and is nontherapeutic in the one-to-one relationship. In option 4, the nurse is attempting to assess the client's ability to openly discuss feelings with family members. Although this is an appropriate communication and assessment for this client, the timing is somewhat premature and closes off facilitation of the client's feelings.

Level of Cognitive Ability: Application
Phase of Nursing Process: Implementation
Client Needs: Psychosocial Integrity
Content Area: Mental Health

Reference

Antai-Otong, D. (1995). *Psychiatric nursing: Biological and behavioral concepts.* Philadelphia: W. B. Saunders, pp. 270–276.

---

41. The nurse calls for the laboratory results performed on the client. The technician says, "The client's anti-insulin antibody test is positive. It shows IgG, IgM, and IgE." Which of the following responses would be the most professional communication technique by the nurse?

1 "Well, that explains why the insulin isn't working well for the client."
2 "The client will have to go without insulin, I guess."
3 "I'll notify the physician. Does this indicate an insulin resistance or allergy?"
4 "Hello! Now what will the doctor order for the client?"

Answer: 3

Rationale: Dialogue between professionals is assertive, nonjudgmental, and caring. In the correct option, the nurse states the intervention to be implemented (calling the physician) and questions the technician about the laboratory results. The anti-insulin antibody test detects the insulin antibodies in the blood of a diabetic who is being treated with insulin. Immunoglobulin G (IgG) is the most common anti-insulin antibody. Immunoglobulin M (IgM) is thought to be part of the process for insulin resistance, and immunoglobulin E (IgE) is thought to be part of the process for insulin allergy.

Test-Taking Strategy: This question tests your knowledge of appropriate professional communications with colleagues and other health care providers. Use the process of elimination. Options 1 and 2 make quick conclusions that are unprofessional. Option 4 is a histrionic interpretation that is also unprofessional.

Level of Cognitive Ability: Analysis
Phase of Nursing Process: Implementation
Client Needs: Psychosocial Integrity
Content Area: Fundamental Skills

Reference

Antai-Otong, D. (1995). *Psychiatric nursing: Biological and behavioral concepts.* Philadelphia: W. B. Saunders, pp. 270–276.

42. The nurse is caring for an adult client who says, "I don't want to talk with you. You're only a nurse, I'll wait for my doctor." Which of the following responses would be the most therapeutic communication technique by the nurse?

1. "I'll leave you now and call your physician."
2. "I'm assigned to work with you. Your doctor placed you in my hands."
3. "So you're saying that you want to talk to your physician?"
4. "I'm angry with the way you've dismissed me. I am your nurse, not your servant."

Answer: 3

Rationale: The nurse uses the therapeutic communication of reflection to redirect the client's feelings back for validation. Notice that the nurse does not reflect a negative response in option 3 but focuses on the client's desire to talk with the physician.

Test-Taking Strategy: This question tests your knowledge of the appropriate therapeutic communication for clients who are using a defensive communication that is aimed to drive others away. You can easily eliminate options 2 and 4 because these are certainly nontherapeutic responses. Option 1 is a social response and intervention that reinforces the client's continuation of this behavior. Remember that this question is a classic one that assesses your commitment to the professional nursing code. The nurse places the client's well-being first and foremost while engaged in nursing care.

Level of Cognitive Ability: Analysis
Phase of Nursing Process: Implementation
Client Needs: Psychosocial Integrity
Content Area: Fundamental Skills

Reference

Antai-Otong, D. (1995). *Psychiatric nursing: Biological and behavioral concepts.* Philadelphia: W. B. Saunders, pp. 270–276.

43. A female client and her newborn infant have undergone human immunodeficiency virus (HIV) testing, and for both clients the test results have turned out positive. The news is devastating, and the mother is crying. According to crisis intervention techniques, the most appropriate action at this time is to

1. Call an HIV counselor and make an appointment for them.
2. Describe the progressive stages and treatments for HIV.
3. Examine with the mother how she got HIV.
4. Listen quietly while the mother talks and cries.

Answer: 4

Rationale: This client has just received devastating news and needs to have someone present with her as she begins to cope with this issue. The nurse needs to sit and actively listen while the mother talks and cries. Calling an HIV counselor may be helpful, but it is not what the client needs at this time. The other options are not appropriate for this stage of coping with the news that both she and the baby are HIV-positive.

Test-Taking Strategy: Use the process of elimination to answer the question. Note the key phrase "at this time." Options 2 and 3 can easily be eliminated. From the remaining two options, remember to address the client's feelings and to support the client. This should assist in directing you to the correct option. The nurse could sit and listen and provide support before even considering the other options, because this would be the most caring response and therefore the best nursing action.

Level of Cognitive Ability: Application
Phase of Nursing Process: Analysis
Client Needs: Psychosocial Integrity
Content Area: Maternity

Reference

Nichols, F., & Zwelling, E. (1997). *Maternal-newborn nursing: Theory and practice.* Philadelphia: W. B. Saunders, pp. 1187–1188.

44. The community health nurse visits a recently widowed, retired military man who is estranged from his only child because he was discharged from the service for being "gay." When the nurse visits, the ordinarily immaculate house is in chaos, and the client is disheveled, with alcohol on his breath. Which of the following responses by the nurse would be the most therapeutic communication technique?

1. "You seem to be having a very troubling time."
2. "I can see this isn't a good time to visit."
3. "What are you doing? How much are you drinking and for how long?"
4. "Do you think your wife would want you to behave like this?"

Answer: 1

Rationale: The most therapeutic communication is the one that helps the client explore his situation and express his feelings. Option 1 identifies the use of reflection and will assist the client to begin to ventilate feelings. As the client begins to do so, the nurse or a therapist can assist the client to discuss the reasons behind alienation from his only child.

Test-Taking Strategy: This question tests your knowledge of the proper timing and use of therapeutic or facilitative communications for clients who are responding to loss with maladaptation (drinking, poor hygiene, etc.) and may be depressed. In option 2, the nurse uses humor to avoid therapeutic intimacy and effective problem solving. In option 3, the nurse uses social communication (probably to minimize the anxiety of the nurse rather than the client). In option 4, the nurse uses admonishment and tries to shame the client, which is not therapeutic or professional. This social communication belittles the client, will cause anger, and may evoke "acting out" by the client.

Level of Cognitive Ability: Application
Phase of Nursing Process: Implementation
Client Needs: Psychosocial Integrity
Content Area: Mental Health

Reference

Antai-Otong, D. (1995). *Psychiatric nursing: Biological and behavioral concepts.* Philadelphia: W. B. Saunders, pp. 270–276.

---

45. The client says to the nurse, "I don't do anything right. I'm such a loser." The most appropriate response is

1. "You do things right all the time."
2. "Everything will get better."
3. "You don't do anything right?"
4. "You are not a loser, you are sick."

Answer: 3

Rationale: Option 3 enables the client to tell you more. With this statement, the nurse can learn more about what the client really means. This option repeats the client's statement.

Test-Taking Strategy: Use the process of elimination and therapeutic communication techniques to select the correct option. Only option 3 allows the communication to stay open. Options 1, 2, and 4 are closed statements and do not encourage the client to explore further.

Level of Cognitive Ability: Application
Phase of Nursing Process: Implementation
Client Needs: Psychosocial Integrity
Content Area: Mental Health

Reference

Johnson, B. (1997). *Psychiatric–mental health nursing: Adaptation and growth.* (4th ed.). Philadelphia: Lippincott-Raven, pp. 556–557.

---

46. The client who is experiencing suicidal thoughts greets the nurse with the following statement: "It just doesn't seem worth it anymore. Why not just end it all?" The nurse may further assess the client by using which of the following responses?

1. "I'm sure your family is worried about you."
2. "I know you have had a stressful night."
3. "Did you sleep at all last night?"
4. "What do you mean by that?"

Answer: 4

Rationale: Option 4 allows the client to tell you more about what the current thoughts are. Option 1 is false reassurance and may close communication. Options 2 and 3 change the subject and may close communication.

Test-Taking Strategy: This communication question is asking for the best response. It is also asking for a response that will further assess. Use the nursing process to select the correct option. Options 1 and 2 can be easily eliminated because they do not reflect assessment. Both options 3 and 4 relate to further assessment, but option 4 is directly related to the issue of the question.

Level of Cognitive Ability: Application
Phase of Nursing Process: Assessment
Client Needs: Psychosocial Integrity
Content Area: Mental Health

Reference

Johnson, B. (1997). *Psychiatric–mental health nursing: Adaptation and growth* (4th ed.). Philadelphia: Lippincott-Raven, pp. 866–871.

---

47. A mother says to the nurse, "I am afraid that my child might have another febrile seizure." Which response by the nurse is most therapeutic?

1 "Why worry about something that you cannot control?"
2 "Most children will never experience a second seizure."
3 "Tell me what frightens you the most about seizures."
4 "Acetaminophen [Tylenol] can prevent another seizure from occurring."

Answer: 3

Rationale: Option 3 is the only response that is an open-ended statement that provides the mother with an opportunity to express feelings. Option 1 is incorrect because it blocks communication by giving a flippant response to an expressed fear. Options 2 and 4 are incorrect because the nurse is giving false assurance that a seizure will not recur or can be prevented in this child.

Test-Taking Strategy: Note the key phrase in the stem "most therapeutic." Use the process of elimination seeking the option that is an example of therapeutic communication. Options 1, 2, and 4 violate principles of therapeutic communication and actually block communication.

Level of Cognitive Ability: Analysis
Phase of Nursing Process: Implementation
Client Needs: Psychosocial Integrity
Content Area: Child Health

Reference

Wong, D. (1995). *Whaley and Wong's Nursing care of infants and children* (5th ed.). St. Louis: Mosby–Year Book, pp. 189, 191.

---

48. A mother has just given birth to a baby who has a cleft lip and palate. When planning to talk to this mother, a nurse should recognize that this client must be allowed to work through which of these emotions before maternal bonding can occur?

1. Anger
2. Grief
3. Guilt
4. Depression

Answer: 2

Rationale: The mother must first be assisted to grieve for the anticipated child that she did not have. Once this is accomplished, the mother can begin to focus on bonding with the infant she gave birth to. Options 1, 3, and 4 are incorrect because each is only one component of the grief process.

Test-Taking Strategy: The key words in the stem are "to work through...before maternal bonding can occur." The reader must know that grief is an emotional process. Options 1, 3, and 4 are incorrect because each is only one component of the grief process. Option 2 is the most global response.

Level of Cognitive Ability: Analysis
Phase of Nursing Process: Planning
Client Needs: Psychosocial Integrity
Content Area: Maternity

Reference

Wong, D. (1995). *Whaley and Wong's Nursing care of infants and children* (2nd ed.). St. Louis: Mosby–Year Book, pp. 436, 995.

49. An infant who has been diagnosed with acute chalasia is admitted to the hospital. During the nursing history the mother tells the nurse, "I am concerned that I am somehow causing the baby to vomit after feeding." In view of this statement, which nursing diagnosis is most appropriate?

1. Anxiety related to hospitalization of infant for chalasia
2. Noncompliance related to denial that chalasia is a physiological defect
3. Knowledge Deficit related to lack of exposure to feeding a child with chalasia
4. Altered Parenting related to unrealistic expectation of self

Answer: 4

Rationale: The infant is vomiting because of a physiological problem that is not caused by the parent. The misconception that the mother is responsible for the problem may result in a decreased perception of her ability to adequately parent the child. The nurse should assist the parent to understand that she is not responsible for the child's gastroesophageal reflux. Option 1 is incorrect because the mother's statement does not reflect symptoms of anxiety regarding the child's hospitalization; the mother states a concern about her behavior. Option 2 is incorrect; there is no evidence that the mother has ever been told that chalasia is a physiological problem or that she is using incorrect feeding methods. Option 3 is incorrect because there are no data in the question to support this nursing diagnosis.

Test-Taking Strategy: The reader must correctly interpret from the mother's statement that she is blaming herself for the child's health problem. As a result, the mother is at risk for altered parenting. Focusing on this issue, you should be able to easily eliminate options 1, 2, and 3.

Level of Cognitive Ability: Analysis
Phase of Nursing Process: Analysis
Client Needs: Psychosocial Integrity
Content Area: Child Health

Reference

Wong, D. (1995). *Whaley and Wong's Nursing care of infants and children* (5th ed.). St. Louis: Mosby–Year Book, pp. 1460, 1462.

---

50. A client scheduled for cardiac stress testing expresses a fear of his or her heart "giving out" during the procedure. Which client behavior indicates ineffective nurse-client communication?

1. Client asks numerous questions about the stress test
2. Client verbally expresses fears regarding own mortality
3. Client is frustrated because the test needs to be performed
4. Client does not talk about procedure

Answer: 4

Rationale: Expressions of fear, anxiety, and frustration are examples of effective client communication. These expressions are identified in options 1, 2, and 3. Refusal to speak is a physical barrier to effective communication.

Test-Taking Strategy: Note the key phrase "ineffective nurse-client communication." Options 1, 2, and 3 contain evidence of effective communication. Not talking certainly indicates ineffective communication.

Level of Cognitive Ability: Analysis
Phase of Nursing Process: Assessment
Client Needs: Psychosocial Integrity
Content Area: Adult Health/Cardiovascular

Reference

Varcarolis, E. M. (1998). *Foundations of psychiatric mental health nursing* (3rd ed.). Philadelphia: W. B. Saunders, p. 184.

51. According to standard coronary care unit (CCU) orders, the client with uncomplicated myocardial infarction (MI) may begin progressive activity after 3 days. The client, who experienced an MI 4 days ago, refuses to let his or her legs dangle at the bedside, saying, "If my doctor tells me to do it, I will. Otherwise I won't." The nurse determines that the client is likely displaying

1 Anger.
2 Denial.
3 Dependency.
4 Depression.

Answer: 3

Rationale: Clients may experience numerous emotional and behavioral responses after MI. Dependency is one response that may be manifested by the client's refusal to perform any tasks or activities unless approved by the physician.

Test-Taking Strategy: Use the data identified in the question to determine the correct option. Begin by eliminating options 2 and 4 first. Although the client's statement may express anger to some degree, it most specifically addresses dependency.

Level of Cognitive Ability: Analysis
Phase of Nursing Process: Analysis
Client Needs: Psychosocial Integrity
Content Area: Adult Health/Cardiovascular

Reference

Lewis, S., Collier, I., & Heitkemper, M. (1996). *Medical-surgical nursing: Assessment and management of clinical problems* (4th ed.). St. Louis: Mosby–Year Book, p. 922.

---

52. The nurse is assessing a 45-year-old client admitted for urinary calculi. The client received 4 mg of morphine sulfate (MS) approximately 2 hours previously. The client states to the nurse, "I'm scared to death that it'll come back. That was the worst pain I ever had. Like a knife going from my right side to my groin." Which of the following nursing diagnoses would be appropriate for the nurse to make regarding this statement?

1 Pain, Acute, related to presence of calculus in right ureter
2 Knowledge Deficit related to lack of information about disease process
3 Anxiety related to anticipation of recurrent severe pain
4 Urinary Retention related to obstruction of urinary tract by calculi

Answer: 3

Rationale: The client has stated, "I'm scared to death that it'll come back." The anticipation of the recurring pain threatens the client's psychological integrity. There is no evidence that the client has a calculus in the right ureter. There is also no evidence that either urinary retention or knowledge deficit exists.

Test-Taking Strategy: Use the data presented in the question to assist in answering the question. Note the key phrase "I'm scared to death that it'll come back." This should assist in directing you to the key word, "anxiety," in the correct option!

Level of Cognitive Ability: Analysis
Phase of Nursing Process: Analysis
Client Needs: Psychosocial Integrity
Content Area: Adult Health/Renal

Reference

Wilson, H., & Kneisl, C. (1996). *Psychiatric nursing* (5th ed.). Menlo Park, CA: Addison-Wesley, p. 72.

---

53. The nurse observes the parents at the bedside of their female infant, who was born at 27 weeks' gestation and is small for gestational age (SGA). The infant's mother states, "She is so tiny and fragile. I'll never be able to hold her with all those tubes." The nurse interprets the mother's statement as being relevant to which of the following nursing diagnoses?

1 Impaired Adjustment
2 Risk for Caregiver Strain
3 Ineffective Family Coping
4 Risk for Altered Parenting

Answer: 4

Rationale: One of the nursing diagnoses for the parents of a high-risk neonate, such as a preterm SGA infant, is Risk for Altered Parenting. The initial foci of intervention for parents of a preterm SGA infant are assessing and assisting parent-infant bonding. Failure of a tiny, ill infant to exhibit normal newborn characteristics can interfere with parent infant bonding. Option 1 involves nonacceptance of a health status change or an inability to solve problems or set a goal. Option 2 addresses the strain of a caregiver, which during the initial hospitalization is too early to apply. Option 3 involves identification of ineffective coping. At this time, there are inadequate data for these diagnoses, although they may become relevant at a later time.

Test-Taking Strategy: Use the data presented in the question to assist in answering the question. Eliminate options 1 and 3 first because these are actual nursing diagnoses that do not exist. In selecting from the remaining two options, note the key phrase "I'll never be able to hold her." This should assist in directing you to the key phrase, "Altered Parenting," in the correct option.

Level of Cognitive Ability: Analysis
Phase of Nursing Process: Analysis
Client Needs: Psychosocial Integrity
Content Area: Maternity

Reference

Olds, S., London, M., & Ladewig, P. (1996). *Maternal-newborn nursing: A family-centered approach* (5th ed.). Menlo Park, CA: Addison-Wesley, p. 928.

---

54. After vaginal delivery of a male infant who is large for gestational age (LGA), the nurse wraps the infant in a warm blanket and hands him to his mother. The mother demonstrates reluctance to touch the baby because of her verbalized concern over his facial bruising. To enhance attachment, the nurse responds

1. "Because the bruising is painful, it is advisable that you not touch the baby's face."
2. "The bruising is caused by polycythemia, which usually leads to jaundice."
3. "It is a normal finding in large babies and nothing to be concerned about."
4. "The bruising is temporary, and it is important to interact with your infant."

Answer: 4

Rationale: The mother of an LGA infant with facial bruising may be reluctant to interact with the infant because of concern about causing additional pain to the infant. The bruising is temporary. Option 1 advises the mother not to touch the baby's face because the bruising is painful; however, touch is an important component of the attachment process. Touching the infant gently with fingertips should be encouraged. Option 2 is incorrect; the LGA infant may have polycythemia, which can contribute to bruising, but the bruising is not caused by the polycythemia. Although option 3 appears to be an appropriate response, it does not address the issue of the question.

Test-Taking Strategy: Use the process of elimination. Eliminate options 2 and 3 first because they do not specifically address the issue of attachment. For the remaining two options, note the phrase "not touch" in option 1 and note the relationship of the word "attachment" in the stem of the question and the word "interact" in the correct option.

Level of Cognitive Ability: Application
Phase of Nursing Process: Implementation
Client Needs: Psychosocial Integrity
Content Area: Maternity

Reference

Pillitteri, A. (1995). *Maternal and child health nursing: Care of the childbearing and childrearing family* (2nd ed.). Philadelphia: Lippincott-Raven, p. 746.

---

55. The client with myasthenia gravis is ready to return home. The client confides that she is concerned that her husband will no longer find her physically attractive. In the plan of care, the nurse would include

1. Ecouraging the client to start a support group.
2. Insisting that the client reach out and face this fear.
3. Telling the client not to dwell on the negative.
4. Encouraging the client to share her feelings with her husband.

Answer: 4

Rationale: Sharing feelings with her husband directly addresses the issue of the question. Encouraging the client to start a support group will not address the client's immediate and individual concerns. Options 2 and 3 are blocks to communication and avoid the client's concern.

Test-Taking Strategy: Focus on the issue of the question and use the process of elimination. Option 4 is the only option that addresses the client's immediate concern. Remember to address the client's feelings and concerns first!

Level of Cognitive Ability: Application
Phase of Nursing Process: Planning
Client Needs: Psychosocial Integrity
Content Area: Adult Health/Neurological

Reference

Carpenito, L. (1997). *Nursing diagnosis: Application to clinical practice* (7th ed.). Philadelphia: Lippincott-Raven, pp. 765, 769.

56. A 9-year-old child is hospitalized for 2 months after a car accident. The best way to promote psychosocial development of this child is to plan for

1. Tutoring to keep the child up with school work.
2. A phone to call family and friends.
3. Computer games, TV, and videos at the bedside.
4. A portable radio and tape player with headphones.

Answer: 1

Rationale: The developmental issue of the school-age child is industry versus inferiority. The child achieves success by mastering skills and knowledge. Maintaining school work provides for accomplishment and prevents feelings of inferiority as a result of lagging behind the class. The other options provide diversion and are of lesser importance for a child of this age.

Test-Taking Strategy: Note the age of the child and determine the developmental task for this child. Options 2, 3, and 4 address social and diversional issues, whereas option 1 specifically addresses psychosocial development. Review growth and development related to the school-age child now if you had difficulty with this question!

Level of Cognitive Ability: Application
Phase of Nursing Process: Planning
Client Needs: Psychosocial Integrity
Content Area: Child Health

Reference

Wong, D. (1997). *Whaley and Wong's Essentials of pediatric nursing* (5th ed.). St. Louis: Mosby–Year Book, pp. 534, 643.

---

57. The client who is in halo traction says to the visiting nurse, "I can't get used to this contraption. I can't see properly on the side, and I keep misjudging where everything is." The most therapeutic response by the nurse would be

1. "Halo traction involves many difficult adjustments. Practice scanning with your eyes after standing up, before you move."
2. "No one ever gets used to that thing! It's horrible. Many of our sports people who are in it complain vigorously."
3. "Why do you feel like this when you could have died from a broken neck? This is the way it is for several months. You need to accept it more, don't you think?"
4. "If I were you, I would have had the surgery rather than suffer like this."

Answer: 1

Rationale: The therapeutic communication technique that the nurse employs is reflection. The nurse then offers a problem-solving strategy that helps increase peripheral vision for clients in halo traction. Options 2, 3, and 4 are inappropriate responses and block communication.

Test-Taking Strategy: Use the process of elimination, seeking the option that represents a therapeutic communication technique. In option 2, the nurse provides a social response that contains emotionally charged language, which would increase the client's anxiety. In option 3, the nurse uses excessive questioning and gives advice, which are nontherapeutic. In option 4, the nurse undermines the client's faith in the medical treatment being employed by giving advice that is insensitive and unprofessional.

Level of Cognitive Ability: Application
Phase of Nursing Process: Implementation
Client Needs: Psychosocial Integrity
Content Area: Adult Health/Neurological

Reference

Stuart, G., & Laraia, M. (1998). *Principles and practice of psychiatric nursing* (6th ed.). St. Louis: Mosby–Year Book, pp. 17–61.

58. An elderly client has been admitted with a hip fracture. The nurse prepares a plan for the client and identifies desired outcomes. Which client response most appropriately supports a positive adjustment to the alterations experienced in mobility?

1 "I wish you nurses would leave me alone! You are always telling me what to do!"
2 "What took you so long? I called for you 30 minutes ago."
3 "Hurry up and go away. I want to be alone."
4 "I've found it difficult to concentrate since the doctor talked with me about the surgery tomorrow."

Answer: 4

Rationale: Option 1 demonstrates acting out by the client. Option 2 is a demanding response. Option 3 demonstrates withdrawal behavior. Demanding, acting-out, and withdrawn clients haven't coped with or adjusted to injury or disease. Option 4 is reflective of a person with moderate anxiety evidenced by difficulty in concentrating. This client statement most appropriately supports a positive adjustment.

Test-Taking Strategy: Focus on the issue: "positive adjustment." You should easily be able to eliminate options 1, 2, and 3. Remember that age and limited mobility, combined with medications, often contribute to anxiety and confusion. This should assist in directing you to option 4.

Level of Cognitive Ability: Analysis
Phase of Nursing Process: Evaluation
Client Needs: Psychosocial Integrity
Content Area: Adult Health/Musculoskeletal

Reference

Burrell, L., Gerlach, M., & Pless, B. (1997). *Adult nursing: Acute and community care* (2nd ed.). Stamford, CT: Appleton & Lange, pp. 1628–1629.

---

59. The nurse is caring for a client facing several weeks of cast therapy. The nurse analyzes social supports on the basis of the client's need for several weeks of limited mobility. The nurse correctly identifies the most appropriate nursing diagnosis as

1 Anxiety.
2 Ineffective Coping (Family).
3 Self Care Deficit.
4 Powerlessness.

Answer: 3

Rationale: Chronic illness presents a unique and often frustrating challenge for clients. Activities may need to be planned around the availability of assistance. There is no evidence in the question that anxiety exists; nor are there data that address ineffective family coping. Although powerlessness may be experienced by a client facing several weeks of limited mobility, there are no data that support this nursing diagnosis.

Test-Taking Strategy: Note the key phrase "need for several weeks of limited mobility." In addition, use the data presented in the question to identify the correct option. Options 1 and 2 can be easily eliminated. From the remaining two options, select option 3 over option 4. Powerlessness does not always occur in clients with limited mobility. It is most likely that a self-care deficit would be present.

Level of Cognitive Ability: Analysis
Phase of Nursing Process: Analysis
Client Needs: Psychosocial Integrity
Content Area: Adult Health/Musculoskeletal

Reference

Carpenito, L. (1995). *Nursing care plans and documentation.* Philadelphia: Lippincott-Raven, pp. 38–39, 651.

60. A client comes to the free clinic after losing all personal belongings in a flood. After identifying one of the client's nursing diagnoses as Ineffective Individual Coping, the nurse and client plan goals. Which of the following is the least realistic goal?

1. The client will identify a realistic perception of stressors
2. The client will develop adaptive coping patterns
3. The client will express and share feelings regarding the present crisis
4. The client will stop blaming himself or herself for the lack of flood insurance

Answer: 4

Rationale: Options 1, 2, and 3 identify a positive movement toward increased self-esteem and problem solving. Option 4 is unrealistic, and there are no data in the question to support this goal.

Test-Taking Strategy: Note the key phrase "least realistic." The words "realistic" and "adaptive" and the phrase "express and share feelings" in options 1, 2, and 3 respectively, identify positive goals. This should assist in directing you to option 4. In addition, there is nothing in the question which indicates that the client lacked flood insurance, as option 4 reflects.

Level of Cognitive Ability: Analysis
Phase of Nursing Process: Planning
Client Needs: Psychosocial Integrity
Content Area: Mental Health

Reference

Antai-Otong, D. (1995). *Psychiatric nursing: Biological and behavioral concepts.* Philadelphia: W. B. Saunders, p. 147.

---

61. A client who has a spinal cord injury and is paralyzed from the neck down frequently makes lewd sexual suggestions and uses profanity. The nurse realizes that the client is inappropriately using the defense mechanism of displacement and identifies the most appropriate nursing diagnosis for this client to be

1. Ineffective Individual Coping.
2. Risk for Disuse Syndrome.
3. Impaired Environmental Interpretation Syndrome.
4. Body Image Disturbance.

Answer: 1

Rationale: The definition of Ineffective Individual Coping is the "state in which an individual demonstrates impaired adaptive behaviors and problem-solving abilities in meeting life's demands and roles." Because the client is displacing feelings onto the environment instead of using them in a constructive manner, this nursing diagnosis clearly applies in this situation. Options 2 and 3 have no bearing on this situation. Option 4 may be a factor, but it has nothing to do with the displacement that the client is currently using.

Test-Taking Strategy: Use the data found in the question to identify the correct option. Focus on the defense mechanism of displacement as identified in the question. Focusing on this issue and the definition of displacement should assist in directing you to the correct option. Review defense mechanisms now if you had difficulty with this question!

Level of Cognitive Ability: Analysis
Phase of Nursing Process: Analysis
Client Needs: Psychosocial Integrity
Content Area: Mental Health

Reference

Iyer, P., Taptich, B., & Bernocchi-Losey, D. (1995). *Nursing process and nursing diagnosis.* Philadelphia: W. B. Saunders, p. 378.

---

62. The best way to help parents of a premature baby develop attachment behaviors is to

1. Encourage parents to touch and speak to their baby.
2. Place family pictures in the infant's view.
3. Report only positive qualities and progress to parents.
4. Provide information on infant development and stimulation.

Answer: 1

Rationale: Parents' involvement through touch and voice establishes and initiates the bonding process in the relationship. Their active participation builds confidence and supports the parenting role. Providing information and emphasizing positives are not incorrect, but they do not relate to the attachment process. Family pictures are ineffective for an infant.

Test-Taking Strategy: Read the situation and stem carefully to identify the clients as the parents and the issue as attachment. The stem asks for the best response, so this will involve the parents in attachment behaviors. The only option that addresses attachment behaviors is option 1.

Level of Cognitive Ability: Application
Phase of Nursing Process: Implementation
Client Needs: Psychosocial Integrity
Content Area: Maternity

Reference

Wong, D. (1997). *Whaley and Wong's Essentials of pediatric nursing* (5th ed.). St. Louis: Mosby–Year Book, p. 247.

---

63. A 16-year-old is admitted with hyperglycemia from failure to follow the diet, insulin, and glucose-monitoring regimens. The client states, "I'm fed up with having my life ruled by doctors' orders and machines!" A priority nursing diagnosis is

1 Altered Nutrition, Greater Than Body Requirements, related to high blood glucose.
2 Altered Family Process related to chronic illness.
3 Altered Thought Process related to personal crisis.
4 Ineffective Management of Therapeutic Regimen related to feelings of loss of control.

Answer: 4

Rationale: Adolescents strive for identity and independence, and the situation describes a common fear of loss of control. The correct diagnosis relates to the issues of the question, which are failure to follow the prescribed regimen and feelings of powerlessness. There is no indication of altered family or thought process in the situation. The nutrition diagnosis is inaccurate and limited.

Test-Taking Strategy: Use the data in the situation to assist in directing you to the correct option. Eliminate option 1 because there are no data indicating greater than body requirements. Eliminate option 2 because there are no data to support an altered family process. Eliminate option 3 because although the client may be experiencing a personal crisis, there is no evidence of altered thought process. This leaves option 4 as the correct option.

Level of Cognitive Ability: Analysis
Phase of Nursing Process: Analysis
Client Needs: Psychosocial Integrity
Content Area: Child Health

Reference

Wong, D. (1997). *Whaley and Wong's Essentials of pediatric nursing* (5th ed.). St. Louis: Mosby–Year Book, pp. 612–613.

---

64. A client angrily tells the nurse that the doctor purposefully provided wrong information. Which of the following responses would hinder therapeutic communication?

1 "I'm certain the doctor would not lie to you."
2 "Can you describe the information that you are referring to?"
3 "I'm not sure what information you are referring to."
4 "Perhaps it would be helpful to talk to your doctor about this."

Answer: 1

Rationale: Option 1 hinders communication by disagreeing with the client. This technique could make the client defensive and block further communication. Options 2 and 3 attempt to clarify what the client is referring to. Option 4 attempts to explore if the client is comfortable talking to the doctor about this issue and encourages direct confrontation.

Test-Taking Strategy: Use the process of elimination noting the key word "hinder." Disagreeing with or challenging a client's response will hinder or block therapeutic communication. Select responses that address client concerns, seek clarification, acknowledge their feelings, or encourage open and direct communication.

Level of Cognitive Ability: Analysis
Phase of Nursing Process: Implementation
Client Needs: Psychosocial Integrity
Content Area: Fundamental Skills

Reference

Varcarolis, E. M. (1998). *Foundations of psychiatric mental health nursing* (3rd ed.). Philadelphia: W. B. Saunders, p. 193.

65. A client with major depression says to the nurse, "I should have died. I've always been a failure." The most therapeutic response by the nurse is

1 "I see a lot of positive things in you."
2 "Feeling like a failure is part of your illness."
3 "You've been feeling like a failure for some time now?"
4 "You still have a great deal to live for."

Answer: 3

Rationale: Responding to the feelings expressed by a client is an effective therapeutic communication technique. The correct option is an example of the use of restating. Options 1, 2, and 4 block communication because they minimize the client's experience and do not facilitate exploration of the client's expressed feelings.

Test-Taking Strategy: Knowledge of the techniques that facilitate therapeutic communication will help you choose the correct option. Select an option that directly addresses clients' feelings and concerns. Option 3 is the only option that is stated in the form of a question, is open-ended, and thus will encourage the verbalization of feelings.

Level of Cognitive Ability: Application
Phase of Nursing Process: Implementation
Client Needs: Psychosocial Integrity
Content Area: Mental Health

Reference

Haber, J. (1997). *Comprehensive psychiatric nursing* (5th ed.). St. Louis: Mosby–Year Book, p. 131.

---

66. Two months after a right mastectomy for breast cancer, the client comes to the office for a follow-up appointment. The client was told, after the diagnosis of cancer in the right breast, that the risk for cancer in the left breast existed. When asked about the breast self-examination practices since the surgery, the client replies, "I don't need to do that any more." This response may indicate

1 Change in body image.
2 Change in family role.
3 Denial.
4 Grief and mourning.

Answer: 3

Rationale: The coping strategy of denying or minimizing a health problem is manifested in anxiety-producing health situations, especially those that may be life-threatening. Denial can lead to avoidance of self-care measures such as performing breast self-examination.

Test-Taking Strategy: Use the data presented in the question to select the correct option. Note the client statement "I don't need to do that any more." Eliminate options 1 and 2 because they are not directly related to the client statement. Of the remaining two options, select option 3 over option 4 on the basis of the client's statement, which reflects denial. Review the indicators of denial now if you had difficulty with this question!

Level of Cognitive Ability: Analysis
Phase of Nursing Process: Analysis
Client Needs: Psychosocial Integrity
Content Area: Adult Health/Oncology

Reference

Smeltzer, S., & Bare, B. (1996). *Brunner and Suddarth's Textbook of medical-surgical nursing* (8th ed.). Philadelphia: Lippincott-Raven, pp. 122–131.

---

67. In planning for care of the client dying of cancer, one of the nurse's goals was to have the client verbalize acceptance of impending death. Which of the following statements indicates to the nurse that this goal has been reached?

1 "I'll be ready to die when my children finish school."
2 "I just want to live until my 100th birthday."
3 "I want to see my daughter. Then I'll be ready to die."
4 "I'd like to have my family here when I die."

Answer: 4

Rationale: Acceptance is often characterized by plans for death. Often the client wants loved ones near. Options 1, 2, and 3 all reflect the bargaining stage of coping wherein the client tries to negotiate with his or her God or with fate.

Test-Taking Strategy: Note the similarity in options 1, 2, and 3. All these options demonstrate negotiating for something else to happen before death occurs. Option 4 is the option that is different and the option that reflects acceptance.

Level of Cognitive Ability: Analysis
Phase of Nursing Process: Evaluation
Client Needs: Psychosocial Integrity
Content Area: Adult Health/Oncology

Reference

Smeltzer, S., & Bare, B. (1996). *Brunner and Suddarth's Textbook of medical-surgical nursing* (8th ed.). Philadelphia: Lippincott-Raven, pp. 130–131.

68. Which of the following nursing interventions would the nurse implement for the oncology client with a nursing diagnosis of Body Image Disturbance related to alopecia?

1 Teach proper dental hygiene with the use of a foam toothbrush
2 Teach the importance of rinsing the mouth after eating
3 Teach the use of wigs, which are often covered by insurance
4 Teach the use of cosmetics to hide medication-induced rashes

Answer: 3

Rationale: The temporary or permanent thinning or loss of hair known as alopecia is common in oncology clients receiving chemotherapy. This often causes body image disturbance that can be easily addressed by the use of wigs, hats, or scarves.

Test-Taking Strategy: Knowledge of the definition of alopecia will quickly direct you to option 3. Eliminate options 1 and 2 because they are addressing a similar issue. Select option 3 over option 4 because cosmetics are not always prescribed for use when a client has a rash.

Level of Cognitive Ability: Application
Phase of Nursing Process: Implementation
Client Needs: Psychosocial Integrity
Content Area: Adult Health/Oncology

Reference
Smeltzer, S., & Bare, B. (1996). *Brunner and Suddarth's Textbook of medical-surgical nursing* (8th ed.). Philadelphia: Lippincott-Raven, p. 292.

---

69. A client with aldosteronism has developed renal failure and says to the nurse, "This means that I will die very soon." The most appropriate response by the nurse is

1 "Why do you feel this way?"
2 "You will do just fine."
3 "You sound discouraged today."
4 "I read that death is a beautiful experience."

Answer: 3

Rationale: Option 3 uses the therapeutic communication technique of reflection, and it clarifies and encourages further expression of the client's feelings. Option 1 may cause defensiveness and block communication. Options 2 and 4 deny the client's concerns and provide false reassurance.

Test-Taking Strategy: Remember to identify the use of communication blocks, such as the use of cliché, false reassurance, and requesting explanation. You can easily eliminate options 2 and 4. Avoid the use of the word "why" when communicating with a client. Option 3 facilitates the client's expression of feelings.

Level of Cognitive Ability: Application
Phase of Nursing Process: Implementation
Client Needs: Psychosocial Integrity
Content Area: Adult Health/Endocrine

Reference
Taylor, C., Lillis, C., & LeMone, P. (1997). *Fundamentals of nursing: The art and science of nursing care* (3rd ed.). Philadelphia: Lippincott-Raven, pp. 371, 374.

---

70. The nurse is admitting a client with a recent bilateral adrenalectomy. Which of the following interventions is essential for the nurse to include in the client's plan of care?

1 Preventing social isolation
2 Discussing changes in body image
3 Considering occupational therapy
4 Avoiding stressful situations

Answer: 4

Rationale: Adrenalectomy could lead to adrenal insufficiency. Adrenal hormones are essential in maintaining homeostasis in response to stressors. Options 1, 2, and 3 do not represent life-threatening situations.

Test-Taking Strategy: A key word in the stem is "essential" and indicates the need to prioritize. Remember that according to Maslow's hierarchy of needs theory, physiological needs come first. The stress reaction involves physiological processes. Review the effects of an adrenalectomy now if you had difficulty with this question!

Level of Cognitive Ability: Analysis
Phase of Nursing Process: Planning
Client Needs: Psychosocial Integrity
Content Area: Adult Health/Endocrine

Reference
LeMone, P., & Burke, K. (1996). *Medical-surgical nursing: Critical thinking in client care.* Menlo Park, CA: Addison-Wesley, pp. 690, 692.

71. Which statement made by a client with anorexia nervosa would indicate to the nurse that treatment has been effective?

1 "I no longer have a weight problem."
2 "I don't want to starve myself anymore."
3 "I'll eat until I don't feel hungry."
4 "My friends and I went out to lunch today."

Answer: 4

Rationale: Anorexia nervosa usually affects adolescent girls who try to establish identity and control by self-imposed starvation. Options 1, 2, and 3 are verbalizations of the client's intentions. Option 4 is a measurable action that can be verified.

Test-Taking Strategy: Note the key phrase "treatment has been effective." Select an option that is measurable and can be verified. Option 4 is the only measurable action.

Level of Cognitive Ability: Analysis
Phase of Nursing Process: Evaluation
Client Needs: Psychosocial Integrity
Content Area: Mental Health

Reference
Potter, P., & Perry, A. (1997). *Fundamentals of nursing: Concepts, process, and practice* (4th ed.). St. Louis: Mosby–Year Book, p. 243.

72. A client with cancer is placed on permanent total parenteral nutrition (TPN). For what reason must the nurse consider psychosocial support when planning care for this client?

1 Death is imminent
2 TPN requires disfiguring surgery for permanent port implantation
3 The client will need to adjust to the idea of living without eating by the usual route
4 Nausea and vomiting occur regularly with this type of treatment and will prevent the client from social activity

Answer: 3

Rationale: Permanent TPN is indicated for clients who can no longer absorb nutrients via the enteral route. These clients will no longer take nutrition orally. Options 1, 2, and 4 are false. There is no indication in the question that death is imminent; permanent port implantation is not disfiguring; and TPN does not cause nausea and vomiting.

Test-Taking Strategy: Note the word "permanent" in the question. Option 3 states "living without eating." These are similar thoughts. You can easily eliminate option 1 because there are no data to support this option. Knowledge regarding TPN and port implantation will assist in eliminating options 2 and 4 as inaccurate statements.

Level of Cognitive Ability: Analysis
Phase of Nursing Process: Planning
Client Needs: Psychosocial Integrity
Content Area: Adult Health/Oncology

Reference
Burrell, L., Gerlach, M., & Pless, B. (1997). *Adult nursing: Acute and community care* (2nd ed.). Stamford, CT: Appleton & Lange, p. 1354.

73. The client who is to be discharged with a temporary colostomy says to the nurse, "I know I've changed this thing once, but I just don't know how I'll do it by myself when I'm home alone. Can't I stay here until the doctor puts it back?" Which of the following is the most therapeutic response by the nurse?

1. "So you're saying that while you've practiced changing your colostomy bag once, you don't feel comfortable on your own yet?"
2. "Well, your insurance will not pay for a longer stay just to practice changing your colostomy, so you'll have to fight it out with them."
3. "Going home to care for yourself still feels pretty overwhelming? I will schedule you for home visits until you're feeling more comfortable."
4. "This is only temporary, but you need to hire a nurse companion until your surgery."

Answer: 3

Rationale: The client is expressing feelings of helplessness and abandonment. Option 3 assists in meeting this need. Option 1 restates but then focuses on the issue of helplessness. Option 2 provides what is probably accurate information, but the phrase "just to practice" can be interpreted by the client as belittling. Option 4 provides information that the client already knows and then problem-solves by using a client-centered action that would probably overwhelm the client.

Test-Taking Strategy: Focus on the issue of the question, fear and dependency. You can easily eliminate options 2 and 4. In selecting from the remaining two options, remember the issue of the question and address the client's feelings and concerns. Option 1 is restating but then focuses on the issue of helplessness. Option 3 addresses both fear and dependency needs.

Level of Cognitive Ability: Analysis
Phase of Nursing Process: Implementation
Client Needs: Psychosocial Integrity
Content Area: Adult Health/Gastrointestinal

Reference

Antai-Otong, D. (1995). *Psychiatric nursing: Biological and behavioral concepts.* Philadelphia: W. B. Saunders, pp. 543–576.

---

74. The parents of a newborn with congenital hypothyroidism and Down's syndrome tell the nurse how sad they are that their child was born with these problems. They had many plans for a normal child and now these will need to be adjusted. On the basis of these statements, the nurse should plan to address the nursing diagnosis

1. Grieving, Anticipatory.
2. Grieving, Dysfunctional.
3. Adjustment, Impaired.
4. Family Coping, Ineffective.

Answer: 1

Rationale: Anticipatory grieving is the intellectual and emotional responses and behaviors with which individuals and families work through the process of modifying self-concept with the perception of potential loss. Defining characteristics include expressions of sorrow and distress at potential loss. Dysfunctional grieving or impaired adjustment are abnormal responses to changes in health status. The nursing diagnosis of ineffective family coping is used when a usually supportive person is providing insufficient, ineffective, or compromised support, comfort, assistance, or encouragement.

Test-Taking Strategy: According to principles of therapeutic communication, the word "sad" should immediately lead you to one of the options related to grieving. There were no pathological expressions of grief stated. Down's syndrome and congenital hypothyroidism are birth defects that lead to impaired intellectual functioning that will require adaptations to different life expectations. Realizing this should assist in directing you to the correct option.

Level of Cognitive Ability: Analysis
Phase of Nursing Process: Analysis
Client Needs: Psychosocial Integrity
Content Area: Maternity

Reference

Cox, H., Hinz, M., Lubno, M., et al. (1997). *Clinical applications of nursing diagnosis: Adult, child, women's, psychiatric, gerontic, and home health considerations* (3rd ed.). Philadelphia: F. A. Davis, pp. 594, 705, 721.

---

75. When a client with a diagnosis of schizophrenia is unable to speak although nothing is wrong with the organs of communication, the condition is referred to as

1 Pressured speech.
2 Verbigeration.
3 Poverty of speech.
4 Mutism.

Answer: 4

Rationale: Mutism is absence of verbal speech. The client does not communicate verbally despite intact physical structural ability to speak. Withdrawn clients may be mute, immobile, or reclusive. Pressured speech refers to rapidity of speech, reflecting the client's racing thoughts. Verbigeration is the purposeless repetition of words or phrases. Poverty of speech means diminished amounts of speech or monotonic replies.

Test-Taking Strategy: Focus on the issue: "unable to speak." This should assist in easily eliminating options 1 and 2. Knowledge that poverty of speech indicates a diminished amount of speech will assist in eliminating option 3. If you had difficulty with this question, take time now to review altered thought and speech patterns!

Level of Cognitive Ability: Analysis
Phase of Nursing Process: Analysis
Client Needs: Psychosocial Integrity
Content Area: Mental Health

Reference

Carson, V., & Arnold, E. (1996). *Mental health nursing: The nurse-patient journey.* Philadelphia: W. B. Saunders, p. 990.

---

76. A client tells the nurse, "I am a spy for the FBI. I am an eye, an eye in the sky." The nurse recognizes that this is an example of

1 Loosened associations.
2 Tangential speech.
3 Clang associations.
4 Echolalia.

Answer: 3

Rationale: Repetition of words or phrases that are similar in sound and in no other way (rhyming) is one of the patterns of altered thought and language seen in schizophrenia. Clang associations often take the form of rhyming.

Test-Taking Strategy: The question asks you to select the response that indicates a specialized form of loosened association. Therefore, eliminate option 1, which is global. Knowledge that rhyming occurs only in clang forms of loosened associations will assist you in eliminating options 2 and 4. Review altered thought and language patterns in schizophrenia now if you had difficulty with this question!

Level of Cognitive Ability: Analysis
Phase of Nursing Process: Assessment
Client Needs: Psychosocial Integrity
Content Area: Mental Health

Reference

Haber, J. (1997). *Comprehensive psychiatric nursing* (5th ed.). St. Louis: Mosby–Year Book, p. 576.

77. The nurse is planning the discharge of a young client with newly diagnosed insulin-dependent diabetes. The client tells the nurse that she or he is concerned about self-administering insulin while in school with other students around. Which statement by the nurse best supports the client's need at this time?

1 "You could contact the school nurse, who could provide a private area for you to take your insulin."
2 "You could leave school early and take your insulin at home."
3 "You shouldn't be embarrassed by your diabetes. Lots of people have this disease."
4 "Oh, don't worry about that! You'll do fine!"

Answer: 1

Rationale: In the therapeutic caring relationship, the nurse offers information that will promote or assist the client to reach a decision that optimizes a sense of well-being. Option 2 requires a change in lifestyle. Options 3 and 4 are inappropriate statements and are similar in that both are blocks to communication. In planning this client's role transition, the nurse serves as a problem-solver in assisting the client to adapt to her or his illness.

Test-Taking Strategy: The issue of the question relates to a concern of self-administering insulin while in school. Eliminate options 3 and 4 because they do not enhance communications. Select option 1 because it promotes the client's ability to continue the current lifestyle, whereas option 2 changes the lifestyle.

Level of Cognitive Ability: Analysis
Phase of Nursing Process: Planning
Client Needs: Psychosocial Integrity
Content Area: Child Health

Reference

Potter, P., & Perry, A. (1997). *Fundamentals of nursing: Concepts, process, and practice* (4th ed.). St. Louis: Mosby–Year Book, p. 243.

---

78. The nurse is preparing a client for a parathyroidectomy. The client states, "I guess I'll have to learn to love wearing a scarf after this surgery!" Which nursing diagnosis would be appropriate to identify in the plan of care that addresses this client's need?

1 Alteration in Comfort related to surgical interruption of body tissue
2 Body Image Disturbance related to perceived negative effect of surgical incision
3 High Risk for Impaired Mobility related to limited movement secondary to neck surgery
4 Denial related to poor coping mechanisms

Answer: 2

Rationale: The client's statement reflects a psychosocial concern regarding appearance after surgery; thus Body Image Disturbance would be an appropriate choice. Options 1 and 3 identify biophysical nursing diagnoses, and option 4 would be inappropriate because the client is addressing the concern rather than avoiding it.

Test-Taking Strategy: Use the process of elimination. The client is expressing a concern. Keeping that in mind, you could eliminate option 4 because denial is a way of avoiding concerns. Options 1 and 3 are physiological nursing diagnoses and unrelated to the issue.

Level of Cognitive Ability: Analysis
Phase of Nursing Process: Analysis
Client Needs: Psychosocial Integrity
Content Area: Fundamental Skills

Reference

Potter, P., & Perry, A. (1997). *Fundamental of nursing: Concepts, process, and practice* (4th ed.). St. Louis: Mosby–Year Book, p. 390.

---

79. The husband of a client with Graves' disease expresses concern regarding his wife's health because during the past 3 months, she has been experiencing nervousness, inability to concentrate even on trivial tasks, and outbursts of temper. On the basis of this information, which of the following nursing diagnoses would be the most appropriate for the client?

1 Ineffective Individual Coping
2 Alteration in Sensory Perception
3 Social Isolation
4 Grieving

Answer: 1

Rationale: Frequently, family and friends may report that the client with Graves' disease has become more irritable or depressed, especially upon discharge from the hospital. The signs and symptoms in the question are supporting data for a nursing diagnosis of Ineffective Individual Coping and are not related to options 2, 3, and 4. The question does not offer data to support options 2, 3, and 4.

Test-Taking Strategy: Identify data in the question that supports the nursing diagnosis. There is no information offered in the question that provides evidence for options 2, 3, and 4. If you do not know the answer, look for a similar word or phrase such as "inability" in the question and "ineffective" in option 1.

Level of Cognitive Ability: Analysis
Phase of Nursing Process: Analysis
Client Needs: Psychosocial Integrity
Content Area: Adult Health/Endocrine

Reference

Ignatavicius, D. D., Workman, M. L., & Mishler, M. A. (1995). *Medical-surgical nursing: A nursing process approach* (2nd ed.). Philadelphia: W. B. Saunders, pp. 1836–1837, 1843.

---

80. The client who was admitted for recurrent thyroid storm is preparing for discharge. The client is anxious about the illness and at times emotionally labile. Which of the following approaches would be most appropriate for the nurse to include in the care plan for this client?

1 Avoid teaching the client anything about the disease until he or she is emotionally stable
2 Assist the client in identifying coping skills, support systems, and potential stressors
3 Reassure the client that everything will be fine once he or she is in the home environment
4 Confront the client and explain that he or she must control the outbursts if he or she wants to go home

Answer: 2

Rationale: It is not abnormal for clients who experience hyperthyroidism/thyroid storm to continue to be anxious and emotionally labile at the time of discharge. Confrontation in option 4 will only heighten anxiety. In addition, options 1 and 3 block communication by either avoiding the issue or providing false reassurance. The best intervention the nurse can do is to help the client cope with these changes in behavior and perhaps anticipate potential stressors so that symptoms will not be as severe.

Test-Taking Strategy: Eliminate options 3 and 4 because they are blocks to communication. Note the key phrase "anxious about the illness." Eliminate option 1 because it is unrelated to addressing the client's anxiety. When confronted with psychosocial issues, always select the option that address the client's feelings and concerns!

Level of Cognitive Ability: Application
Phase of Nursing Process: Planning
Client Needs: Psychosocial Integrity
Content Area: Adult Health/Endocrine

Reference

Ignatavicius, D. D., Workman, M. L., & Mishler, M. A. (1995). *Medical-surgical nursing: A nursing process approach* (2nd ed.). Philadelphia: W. B. Saunders, p. 1843.

---

81. Upon discharge from the hospital, a priority nursing diagnosis for a client hospitalized with severe iatrogenic hypoparathyroidism would be

1 Alteration in Comfort related to cold intolerance secondary to decreased metabolical rate.
2 Constipation related to decreased peristaltic action secondary to decreased metabolical rate.
3 High Risk for Impaired Skin Integrity related to edema.
4 Anxiety related to the need for lifelong dietary interventions to control the disease.

Answer: 4

Rationale: Medical management of hypoparathyroidism is aimed at correcting the hypocalcemia. This is accomplished with prescribed medications as well as with lifelong compliance to dietary guidelines, which include consumption of foods high in calcium but low in phosphorus. Knowing that the interventions are lifelong can create some anxiety for the client, and this problem needs to be addressed before discharge. The other options are unrelated to this condition.

Test-Taking Strategy: The question asks you to select a priority nursing diagnosis related to hypoparathyroidism. Knowledge of hypoparathyroidism will assist in eliminating options 1, 2, and 3 because these options are unrelated to the disorder. Knowledge that dietary changes are necessary and are lifelong will assist in directing you to option 4. Take time now to review the teaching points related to this disorder if you had difficulty with this question!

Level of Cognitive Ability: Analysis
Phase of Nursing Process: Analysis
Client Needs: Psychosocial Integrity
Content Area: Adult Health/Endocrine

Reference

Ignatavicius, D. D., Workman, M. L., & Mishler, M. A. (1995). *Medical-surgical nursing: A nursing process approach* (2nd ed.). Philadelphia: W. B. Saunders, pp. 1853–1854.

82. A 12-year-old client was diagnosed with tuberculosis (TB) 6 months ago and is seen every other week by a home health nurse. Which of the following behaviors would suggest to the nurse that the client is experiencing a disruption in the development of self-concept?

1 The client enjoys a part-time baby sitting job
2 The client enjoys playing chess and mastering new skills with this game
3 The client interacts well with peer group
4 The client has an intimate relationship with a significant other

Answer: 4

Rationale: A sense of industry is appropriate for this age group and may be exhibited by having a part-time job. The increase in self-esteem associated with skill mastery is an important part of development for the school-age child. Positive peer interaction is also appropriate. The formation of intimate relationships would not be expected until early adulthood.

Test-Taking Strategy: Use the process of elimination focusing on normal growth and development. Note the age of the client in the question. This will assist in eliminating options 1, 2, and 3. Review normal growth and development and developmental tasks associated with this age group now if you had difficulty with this question!

Level of Cognitive Ability: Analysis
Phase of Nursing Process: Analysis
Client Needs: Psychosocial Integrity
Content Area: Child Health

Reference

Potter, P., & Perry, A. (1997). *Fundamentals of nursing: Concepts, process, and practice* (4th ed.). St. Louis: Mosby–Year Book, p. 395.

83. A client with newly diagnosed tuberculosis (TB) will be on respiratory isolation in the hospital for at least 2 weeks. Which of the following would be vital in preventing psychosocial distress for the client?

1 Remove the calendar and clock in the room so that the client will not obsess about time
2 Note whether the client has visitors
3 Give the client a roommate with TB who persistently tries to talk
4 Instruct all staff not to touch the client

Answer: 2

Rationale: The nurse should note whether the client has adequate visitation and social contact because the presence of others can offer positive stimulation. The calendar and clock are needed to promote orientation to time. A roommate who insists on talking could create sensory overload. Touch may be important in order to help the client feel socially acceptable.

Test-Taking Strategy: Note the key phrase "preventing psychosocial distress." By the process of elimination and considering the basic principles related to sensory overload and deprivation, you can easily eliminate options 1, 3, and 4.

Level of Cognitive Ability: Application
Phase of Nursing Process: Planning
Client Needs: Psychosocial Integrity
Content Area: Adult Health/Respiratory

Reference

Potter, P., & Perry, A. (1997). *Fundamentals of nursing: Concepts, process, and practice* (4th ed.). St. Louis: Mosby–Year Book, pp. 1000–1001.

84. The nurse is interviewing a client with chronic obstructive pulmonary disease (COPD), who has a respiratory rate of 35 and is experiencing extreme dyspnea. Which of the following nursing diagnoses would be appropriate for this client?

1 Impaired Verbal Communication related to physical barrier
2 Ineffective Individual Coping related to client's inability to handle a situational crisis
3 Impaired Verbal Communication related to neurological deficit
4 Ineffective Individual Coping related to COPD

Answer: 1

Rationale: A client may suffer physical or psychological alterations that impair communication. To speak spontaneously and clearly, a person must have an intact respiratory system. Extreme dyspnea is a physical alteration affecting speech.

Test-Taking Strategy: Option 1 clearly addresses the problem that the client is experiencing. Option 2 is judgmental and inappropriate. There is nothing to indicate that the client has a neurological deficit. Option 4 is a medical diagnosis. Be very careful with questions addressing nursing diagnoses. Avoid nursing diagnoses that address a medical diagnosis. Remember that NCLEX is a nursing examination!

Level of Cognitive Ability: Analysis
Phase of Nursing Process: Analysis
Client Needs: Psychosocial Integrity
Content Area: Adult Health/Respiratory

Reference
Potter, P., & Perry, A. (1997). *Fundamentals of nursing: Concepts, process, and practice* (4th ed.). St. Louis: Mosby–Year Book, p. 252.

85. The client was injured as a result of passing out from drinking alcohol and falling into the coals of a fire. A fourth-degree circumferential burn wound to the left leg resulted from this accident. In report, the nurse is told that the client just signed consent for amputation of the limb and that the procedure is scheduled for tomorrow. During the nursing assessment, the client is sullen and withdrawn. What is the most appropriate nursing action at this time?

1 Let the client have some time alone to grieve over the future loss of the limb
2 Teach the client that the injury was a result of alcohol abuse and refer him or her for counseling
3 Inform the physician of the client's depression and request medication to assist the client in coping with the diagnosis
4 Reflect back to the client that he or she appears upset

Answer: 4

Rationale: Reflection statements tend to elicit deeper awareness of feelings. In addition, option 4 validates the perception that the client is upset. A well-timed reflection can reveal an emotion that has escaped the client's notice. Option 2 is inappropriate and a block to communication. Options 1 and 3 jump to interventions before the situation is assessed.

Test-Taking Strategy: Use the therapeutic communication techniques to answer the question. Select the option that encourages the client to express feelings and talk more. Avoid options that provide unsolicited advice and jump to conclusions and judgmental biases, leaving the client isolated or encouraging him or her to escape from confronting the situation.

Level of Cognitive Ability: Application
Phase of Nursing Process: Implementation
Client Needs: Psychosocial Integrity
Content Area: Mental Health

Reference
Carson, V., & Arnold, E. (1996). *Mental health nursing: The nurse-patient journey.* Philadelphia: W. B. Saunders, p. 196.

86. Which of the following statements, if made by a client with left-sided Bell's palsy, requires further psychosocial exploration by the nurse?

1 "My left eye is tearing a lot."
2 "I have trouble closing my left eyelid."
3 "I can't taste anything on the left side."
4 "I don't know how I'll live with the effects of this stroke for the rest of my life."

Answer: 4

Rationale: Bell's palsy is an inflammatory condition involving the facial nerve (cranial nerve VII). Although it results in facial paralysis, it is not the same as a stroke or a cerebrovascular accident (CVA). Bell's palsy is a temporary condition in about 80% of the clients affected. Symptoms resolve in several weeks to months. It is important to be positive with clients who have Bell's palsy and correct any misconceptions. Many clients fear that they have had a CVA when the symptoms of Bell's palsy appear, and they commonly believe that the paralysis is permanent. It is important for the nurse to assess these fears and formulate a plan for helping these clients deal with them.

Test-Taking Strategy: Use the process of elimination. Note the key phrase "requiring further psychosocial exploration." Options 1, 2, and

3 reflect expected assessment findings in clients with Bell's palsy. Option 4 identifies an inaccurate understanding of the disorder and requires further psychosocial exploration.

Level of Cognitive Ability: Analysis
Phase of Nursing Process: Assessment
Client Needs: Psychosocial Integrity
Content Area: Adult Health/Neurological

Reference

Ignatavicius, D. D., Workman, M. L., & Mishler, M. A. (1995). *Medical-surgical nursing: A nursing process approach* (2nd ed.). Philadelphia: W. B. Saunders, p. 1242.

---

87. A client with newly diagnosed diabetes mellitus has a nursing diagnosis of Altered Health Maintenance related to anxiety regarding the self-administration of insulin. Initially, the nurse should plan to

1 Teach the family member to give the client the insulin.
2 Use an orange for the client to inject into until the client is less anxious.
3 Insert the needle and have the client push in the plunger and remove the needle.
4 Give the injection until the client feels confident enough to do so by himself or herself.

Answer: 3

Rationale: Some clients find it difficult to insert a needle into their own skin. For these clients, the nurse might assist by selecting the site and inserting the needle. Then, as a first step in self-injection, the client can push in the plunger and remove the needle. Options 1 and 4 place the client into a dependent role. Option 2 is not realistic, in view of the issue of the question.

Test-Taking Strategy: The issue of the question is based on the general principle of diabetes management that the client is responsible for his or her own self-care. The correct answer addresses this issue and yet takes into consideration that the client is anxious about the self-administration of insulin. The nurse is put into a helping/guiding situation, which is exactly the role that the nurse should be in during education of the client.

Level of Cognitive Ability: Application
Phase of Nursing Process: Planning
Client Needs: Psychosocial Integrity
Content Area: Adult Health/Endocrine

Reference

Black, J., & Matassarin-Jacobs, E. (1997). *Medical-surgical nursing: Clinical management for continuity of care* (5th ed.). Philadelphia: W. B. Saunders, p. 1980.

---

88. A client in labor has HIV and says to the nurse, "I know I will have a sick-looking baby." Which of the following would be the most appropriate response by the nurse?

1 "There is no reason to worry. Our neonatal unit offers the latest treatments available."
2 "You have concerns about how HIV will affect your baby?"
3 "You are very sick, but your baby may not be."
4 "All babies are beautiful. I am sure your baby will be, too."

Answer: 2

Rationale: Option 2 is the most therapeutic response and the response that will elicit the best information. It addresses the therapeutic communication technique of paraphrasing. Parents need to know that their baby will not look sick from HIV at birth and that there will be a period of uncertainty before it is known whether the baby has acquired the infection.

Test-Taking Strategy: Use therapeutic communication techniques. Eliminate option 1 because you would not tell the client "there is no reason to worry." Options 3 and 4 provide false reassurances. Option 2 is an open-ended question that will provide an opportunity for the client to verbalize concerns.

Level of Cognitive Ability: Analysis
Phase of Nursing Process: Implementation
Client Needs: Psychosocial Integrity
Content Area: Maternity

Reference

Nichols, F., & Zwelling, E. (1997). *Maternal-newborn nursing: Theory and practice.* Philadelphia: W. B. Saunders, p. 1500.

89. The client who is scheduled for an abdominal peritoneoscopy asks the visiting nurse, "The doctor told me to restrict food and liquids at least 8 hours before this procedure and to use a Fleet enema 4 hours before entering the hospital. Do people ever get into trouble after this procedure?" Which of the following is the most therapeutic response by the nurse?

1 "Any invasive procedure brings risk with it. You need to report any shoulder pain immediately."
2 "There are relatively few problems, especially if you are having local anesthesia, but vaginal bleeding should be reported immediately."
3 "Trouble? There is never any trouble with this procedure. That's why the surgeon will use local anesthesia."
4 "You seem to understand the preparation very well. Are you concerned about the risks related to this procedure?"

Answer: 4

Rationale: Abdominal peritoneoscopy is performed to directly visualize the liver, gallbladder, spleen, and stomach after the insufflation of nitrous oxide. During the procedure, a rigid laparoscope is inserted through a small incision in the abdomen. A microscope in the endoscope allows visualization of the organs and provides a way to collect a specimen for biopsy or to remove small tumors. The most therapeutic response is one which facilitates the client's expression of feelings and directly addresses the client's concerns.

Test-Taking Strategy: Use the process of elimination. In option 1, the nurse uses a platitude, which would only serve to increase the client's anxiety. In option 3, the nurse states that there are no problems associated with this procedure. This is an absolute and does not contain correct information. In option 2, the nurse provides an answer that is true. However, option 4 is the most therapeutic response because it supports the data provided in the question and provides an opportunity for the client to verbalize concerns.

Level of Cognitive Ability: Analysis
Phase of Nursing Process: Implementation
Client Needs: Psychosocial Integrity
Content Area: Adult Health/Gastrointestinal

Reference

Antai-Otong, D. (1995). *Psychiatric nursing: Biological and behavioral concepts.* Philadelphia: W. B. Saunders, pp. 270–276.

90. In assessing the client's emotional needs during a precipitate labor, the nurse can anticipate the client having

1 Less pain and anxiety than with a normal labor.
2 A need for support in maintaining a sense of control.
3 Fewer fears regarding the effect on the infant.
4 A sense of satisfaction regarding the quick labor.

Answer: 2

Rationale: The client experiencing a precipitate labor may have more difficulty maintaining control because of abrupt onset and quick progression. This may be very different from previous labor experiences; therefore the client needs support from the nurse in order to understand and adapt to the rapid progression. The contractions often increase in intensity quickly, adding to the pain, anxiety, and lack of control. The client may also have an increased amount of concern about the effect of the labor on the baby. Lack of control over the situation, combined with increased pain and anxiety, can result in a decreased level of satisfaction with the labor and delivery experience.

Test-Taking Strategy: Options 1, 3, and 4 imply a positive effect of the experience of precipitate labor. Note the key phrase "need for support" in option 2. Psychosocial questions often address the client's needs for support.

Level of Cognitive Ability: Analysis
Phase of Nursing Process: Assessment
Client Needs: Psychosocial Integrity
Content Area: Maternity

Reference

Nichols, F., & Zwelling, E. (1997). *Maternal-newborn nursing: Theory and practice.* Philadelphia: W. B. Saunders, p. 890.

91. The nurse is planning care for the client who presents in active labor with a history of a previous classical cesarean delivery. She complains of a "tearing" sensation in the lower abdomen. The client is upset and expresses concern for the safety of her baby. The most appropriate response from the nurse would be

1 "Don't worry, you are in good hands."
2 "I can understand that you are fearful. We are doing everything possible for your baby."
3 "You'll have to talk to your doctor about that."
4 "I don't have time to answer questions now. We'll talk later."

Answer: 2

Rationale: Clients have a concern for the safety of their baby during labor and delivery, especially when a problem arises. A calm attitude with realistic reassurances is an important aspect of client care. Dismissing or ignoring the client's concerns can lead to increased fear and lack of cooperation.

Test-Taking Strategy: Avoid answers that block therapeutic communication. Option 1 uses a cliché and false reassurance. Options 3 and 4 attempt to place the client's feelings "on hold." Choose the option that reflects acceptance of the client's feelings and provides realistic reassurances. Option 2 is the "most appropriate" response!

Level of Cognitive Ability: Analysis
Phase of Nursing Process: Planning
Client Needs: Psychosocial Integrity
Content Area: Maternity

Reference

Nichols, F., & Zwelling, E. (1997). *Maternal-newborn nursing: Theory and practice.* Philadelphia: W. B. Saunders, pp. 706–708.

---

92. During an initial physical assessment of a newborn male, an undescended testicle (cryptorchidism) is discovered and this finding is shared with the parents. If this condition is not corrected, which of the following could have a psychosocial impact?

1 Infertility
2 Malignancy
3 Feminization
4 Atrophy

Answer: 1

Rationale: Infertility could occur in this disorder because sperm production is decreased in the undescended testes. The psychological effects of an "empty scrotum" could affect the client's perception of self and the ability to reproduce.

Test-Taking Strategy: Options 2 and 4 are possible physical consequence of failure to treat cryptorchidism, not psychosocial consequences; therefore, eliminate these options. Since all hormones responsible for secondary sex characteristics continue to be secreted directly into the blood stream, option 3 is not correct. This leaves option 1 as the correct option.

Level of Cognitive Ability: Analysis
Phase of Nursing Process: Assessment
Client Needs: Psychosocial Integrity
Content Area: Maternity

Reference

Ashwill, J., & Droske, S. (1997). *Nursing care of children: Principles and practice.* Philadelphia: W. B. Saunders, p. 797.

---

93. Cranial surgery is performed on an adolescent who sustained a head injury. Which psychosocial complication would be of most concern to the nurse?

1 Short-term memory loss
2 Head area shaved for the surgical procedure
3 Administration of phenobarbital (Luminal) medication
4 Residual headaches

Answer: 2

Rationale: Body image is a main focus for the adolescent age group. Appearance is very important and is linked with peer acceptance. Loss of hair in the area of the head alters the adolescent's appearance. Option 1 could be a problem if memory loss interferes with remembering friends' names, directions, or school performance, but this is not as obvious as hair loss. Phenobarbital administration does not have psychosocial implications unless the adolescent refuses to take the medication. Residual headaches can be controlled by medication and stress reduction techniques.

Test-Taking Strategy: Remember that the adolescents' focus at this stage of growth and development is body image and how peers perceive them. On the basis of this issue, you can easily eliminate options 3 and 4. Of the remaining two options, select option 2 because this is the most physically obvious alteration in body image.

Level of Cognitive Ability: Analysis
Phase of Nursing Process: Analysis
Client Needs: Psychosocial Integrity
Content Area: Child Health

Reference

Ashwill, J., & Droske, S. (1997). *Nursing care of children: Principles and practice.* Philadelphia: W. B. Saunders, p. 157.

---

94. The mother with an infant with hydrocephalus is concerned about the complication of mental retardation. The mother makes this statement to the nurse: "I'm not sure if I can care for my baby at home." The most appropriate response by the nurse would be which of the following?

1 "There is no reason to worry. You have a good pediatrician."
2 "Mothers instinctively know what is best for their babies."
3 "You have concerns about your baby's condition and care?"
4 "All babies have individual needs."

Answer: 3

Rationale: Paraphrasing is restating the mother's message in the nurse's own words. Option 3 addresses the therapeutic technique of paraphrasing. The mother is reaching out for understanding. In the nurse's response in options 1 and 2, the nurse is offering false reassurance, and these types of responses will block communication. In option 4, the nurse is minimizing the social needs involved with the baby's diagnosis, which is harmful for the nurse-parent relationship.

Test-Taking Strategy: Use therapeutic communication techniques and the process of elimination to answer the question. Option 3 is the only therapeutic technique and addresses paraphrasing. This is the only option that will provide the client an opportunity to verbalize concerns.

Level of Cognitive Ability: Analysis
Phase of Nursing Process: Implementation
Client Needs: Psychosocial Integrity
Content Area: Maternity

Reference

Potter, P., & Perry, A. (1997). *Fundamentals of nursing: Concepts, process, and practice* (4th ed.). St. Louis: Mosby–Year Book, pp. 240–254.

---

95. A preschooler is just diagnosed with impetigo. The child's mother tells the nurse, "But my children take baths every day." The most appropriate response by the nurse is which of the following?

1 "You are concerned about how your child got impetigo?"
2 "There is no need to worry, we will not tell daycare why your child is absent."
3 "Not only do you have to do a better job in keeping the children clean, you must also wash your hands more frequently."
4 "You should have seen the doctor before the wound became infected, then you would not have had to worry about the child's having impetigo."

Answer: 1

Rationale: By paraphrasing what the parent tells the nurse, the nurse is addressing the parent's thoughts. Option 1 is the therapeutic technique of paraphrasing. All the other options are blocks to therapeutic communication by making the parent feel guilty for the child's illness.

Test-Taking Strategy: Use therapeutic communication techniques and the process of elimination to answer the question. Option 1 is the only therapeutic technique and addresses paraphrasing. This is the only option that will provide the client an opportunity to verbalize concerns. Options 2, 3, and 4 are blocks to communication.

Level of Cognitive Ability: Analysis
Phase of Nursing Process: Implementation
Client Needs: Psychosocial Integrity
Content Area: Child Health

Reference

Potter, P., & Perry, A. (1997). *Fundamentals of nursing: Concepts, process, and practice* (4th ed.). St. Louis: Mosby–Year Book, pp. 240–254.

96. Which is the best way to address the cultural needs of a child and family when the child is admitted to a health care facility?

1 Ask questions and explain to the family why the questions are being asked
2 Explain to the family that while the child is being treated, they need to discontinue cultural practices because they may be harmful to the child
3 Ignore cultural needs because they are not important to health care professionals
4 Address only the issues that directly affect the nurse's care of that child

Answer: 1

Rationale: When caring for individuals from different cultures, it is important to ask questions about their specific cultural needs and means of treatment. An understanding of a family's beliefs and health practices is essential for successful interventions for that particular family. Options 2, 3, and 4 ignore the cultural beliefs and values of the client.

Test-Taking Strategy: This question addresses gathering of subjective data relative to a family's cultural needs. Options 2, 3, and 4 are judgmental. In addition, these options are all similar in that they ignore the cultural practices and values of the client. Option 1 addresses the psychosocial needs of the family and the child; thus it is the best choice.

Level of Cognitive Ability: Analysis
Phase of Nursing Process: Assessment
Client Needs: Psychosocial Integrity
Content Area: Child Health

Reference

Wong, D. (1995). *Whaley and Wong's Nursing care of infants and children* (5th ed.). St. Louis: Mosby–Year Book, pp. 42–49.

---

97. A client with a T1 spinal cord injury has just learned that the cord was completely severed. The client says, "I'm no good to anyone. I might as well be dead." The most appropriate response by the nurse is

1 "It makes me uncomfortable when you talk this way."
2 "I'll ask the psychologist to see you about this."
3 "You're not a useless person at all."
4 "You are feeling pretty bad about things right now?"

Answer: 4

Rationale: Restating and reflecting keeps the communication open and shows interest that will encourage the client to expand on current feelings of unworthiness and loss that require exploration. The conversation must continue in order to enable the nurse to assess for suicidal thoughts. The nurse can block communication by showing discomfort or disapproval or by postponing discussion of issues. Grief is a common reaction to loss of function. The nurse can facilitate grieving through open communication.

Test-Taking Strategy: Use therapeutic communication techniques and the process of elimination. Review these nursing statements, considering the effect that they may produce on the client. Options 1, 2, and 3 clearly block communication. Option 4 identifies the therapeutic communication technique of restating and reflecting.

Level of Cognitive Ability: Application
Phase of Nursing Process: Implementation
Client Needs: Psychosocial Integrity
Content Area: Adult Health/Neurological

Reference

Smeltzer, S., & Bare, B. (1996). *Brunner and Suddarth's Textbook of medical-surgical nursing* (8th ed.). Philadelphia: Lippincott-Raven, pp. 332–334.

98. The nurse enters the room of a client with myocardial infarction (MI) and finds the client quietly crying. After determining that there is no physiological reason for the client's distress, the nurse replies

1. "Do you want me to call your daughter?"
2. "Can you tell me a little about what has you so upset?"
3. "I understand how you feel. I'd cry, too, if I had a major heart attack."
4. "Try not to be so upset. Psychological stress is bad for your heart."

Answer: 2

Rationale: Clients with MI often have a nursing diagnosis of Anxiety or Fear. The nurse allows the client to express concerns by showing genuine interest and concern and by facilitating communication, using therapeutic communication techniques.

Test-Taking Strategy: Select an option that has an exploratory approach, because the question does not identify why the client is upset. This technique helps you methodically eliminate each of the incorrect options. Options 1, 3, and 4 do not address the client's feelings or promote client verbalization.

Level of Cognitive Ability: Application
Phase of Nursing Process: Implementation
Client Needs: Psychosocial Integrity
Content Area: Adult Health/Cardiovascular

Reference

Potter, P., & Perry, A. (1997). *Fundamentals of nursing: Concepts, process, and practice* (4th ed.). St. Louis: Mosby–Year Book, p. 241.

---

99. A client with a recent complete T4 spinal cord transection tells the nurse that he or she will walk as soon as spinal shock abates. Which of the following will provide the most accurate basis for planning a response?

1. In order to speed acceptance, the client needs reinforcement that he or she will not walk again
2. The client needs to move through the grieving process rapidly in order to benefit from rehabilitation
3. The client is projecting by insisting that walking is the rehabilitation goal
4. Denial can be protective while the client deals with the anxiety created by the new disability

Answer: 4

Rationale: During the adjustment period in the first few weeks after spinal cord injury, clients may use denial as a defense mechanism. Denial may decrease anxiety temporarily and is a normal part of grieving. After spinal shock abates, denial may impair rehabilitation if its use is prolonged or excessive. However, rehabilitation programs include psychological counseling to deal with grief.

Test-Taking Strategy: Knowledge of the physiological effects of a T4 spinal injury will assist in answering the question. Use the process of elimination. The phrases "speed acceptance," "move through the grieving process rapidly," and "walking is the rehabilitation goal" should be indicators that these are incorrect options. Focus on the client's statement, which is an indication of denial.

Level of Cognitive Ability: Analysis
Phase of Nursing Process: Planning
Client Needs: Psychosocial Integrity
Content Area: Adult Health/Neurological

Reference

Smeltzer, S., & Bare, B. (1996). *Brunner and Suddarth's Textbook of medical-surgical nursing* (8th ed.). Philadelphia: Lippincott-Raven, p. 1805.

---

100. Maladaptive coping behavior may occur in response to a loss or change in the body in association with surgery. The nurse should include which of these actions in the nursing care plan?

1. Explain to the client that open grieving is abnormal
2. Discourage sharing feelings with others who have had similar experiences
3. Encourage the client to express feelings about body changes
4. Advise the client to seek psychological treatment immediately

Answer: 3

Rationale: Surgical incisions can alter a client's body image. The onset of problems with coping with these changes may occur in the immediate or extended postoperative stage. Nursing interventions primarily involve providing psychological support. Draw the client and significant others into discussions of anticipated changes about how they believe these postoperative changes will affect their lives. Encourage the expression of feelings.

Test-Taking Strategy: All of these interventions relate to the psychosocial aspects of postoperative care. Remember that answers that block communication, such as giving advice in option 4 and showing disapproval in options 1 and 2, indicate incorrect responses. Always focus on the client's feelings first, as in option 3.

Level of Cognitive Ability: Application
Phase of Nursing Process: Planning
Client Needs: Psychosocial Integrity
Content Area: Fundamental Skills

Reference

Black, J., & Matassarin-Jacobs, E. (1997). *Medical-surgical nursing: Clinical management for continuity of care* (5th ed.). Philadelphia: W. B. Saunders, p. 492.

---

101. The client with pulmonary edema exhibits severe anxiety. The nurse is preparing to carry out the medically prescribed orders. Which approach should the nurse plan to best meet the needs of the client in a holistic manner?

1. Leave the client alone while gathering required equipment and medications
2. Give the client the call bell and encourage its use if the client feels worse
3. Ask a family member to stay with the client
4. Stay with the client and ask another nurse to gather equipment and supplies not already in the room

Answer: 4

Rationale: Pulmonary edema is accompanied by extreme fear and anxiety. Because the client typically experiences a sense of impending doom, the nurse should remain with the client as much as possible.

Test-Taking Strategy: The word "holistic" in the stem guides you to consider both physical and emotional well-being of the client. Options 1 and 2 do not provide for the psychological needs of the client in distress. Family members (option 3) may provide emotional support to the client but are not able to respond to physiological needs and symptoms. In fact, they are typically in psychological distress themselves. Option 4 is the best option.

Level of Cognitive Ability: Application
Phase of Nursing Process: Planning
Client Needs: Psychosocial Integrity
Content Area: Adult Health/Respiratory

Reference

Smeltzer, S., & Bare, B. (1996). *Brunner and Suddarth's Textbook of medical-surgical nursing* (8th ed.). Philadelphia: Lippincott-Raven, p. 662.

---

102. The family of a client with myocardial infarction complicated by cardiogenic shock is visibly anxious and upset about the client's condition. The nurse would plan to do which of the following to give the best support to the family?

1. Insist that they go home to sleep at night, to keep up their own strength
2. Provide flexibility with visiting times according to the client's condition and family's needs
3. Offer them coffee and other beverages on a regular basis
4. Ask the hospital chaplain to sit with them until the client's condition stabilizes

Answer: 2

Rationale: The use of flexible visiting hours meets the needs of both client and family in reducing the anxiety levels of both. Insisting that the family go home is nontherapeutic. Offering the family beverages does not provide support. Although a chaplain may provide support, it is unrealistic for the chaplain to stay until the client stabilizes; in addition, the religious preference of the family may not be compatible with this option.

Test-Taking Strategy: The question asks for the "best" method of support. Options 1 and 4 may or may not be helpful, depending on the client and family situation. Coffee and beverages, although probably helpful to many visitors, do not provide the best support and can also be obtained in the hospital cafeteria. This leaves option 2 as the choice with most universal value.

Level of Cognitive Ability: Application
Phase of Nursing Process: Planning
Client Needs: Psychosocial Integrity
Content Area: Adult Health/Cardiovascular

Reference

Smeltzer, S., & Bare, B. (1996). *Brunner and Suddarth's Textbook of medical-surgical nursing* (8th ed.). Philadelphia: Lippincott-Raven, p. 659.

103. The client with premature ventricular contractions says to the nurse, "I'm so afraid something bad will happen." Which of the following actions by the nurse would probably be of most immediate help to the client?

1 Giving reassurance that nothing will happen to the client
2 Telephoning the client's family
3 Having a staff member stay with the client
4 Using television to distract the client

Answer: 3

Rationale: When a client experiences fear, the nurse can provide a calm, safe environment by offering appropriate reassurance, therapeutic use of touch, and by having someone remain with the client as much as possible.

Test-Taking Strategy: Use the process of elimination. Options 1 and 4 should be eliminated quickly. The phrase "of most immediate help" guides you to select option 3 over option 2.

Level of Cognitive Ability: Analysis
Phase of Nursing Process: Implementation
Client Needs: Psychosocial Integrity
Content Area: Adult Health/Cardiovascular

Reference

Cox, H., Hinz, M., Lubno, M., et al. (1997). *Clinical applications of nursing diagnosis: Adult, child, women's, psychiatric, gerontic, and home health considerations* (3rd ed.). Philadelphia: F. A. Davis, p. 514.

104. The client with Raynaud's disease tells the nurse that he or she has a stressful job and does not handle stressful situations well. The nurse should encourage the client to

1 Change jobs.
2 Consider a stress-management program.
3 Seek help from a psychologist.
4 Use ear plugs to minimize environmental noise.

Answer: 2

Rationale: Stress can trigger the vasospasm that occurs with Raynaud's disease, so referral to stress-management programs or use of biofeedback training may be helpful. Option 1 is unrealistic. Option 3 is not necessarily required at this time. Option 4 does not specifically address the issue.

Test-Taking Strategy: This question tests the concept of managing stress. With many disorders, including Raynaud's, clients benefit from stress-management programs, which teach clients a variety of techniques for reducing or minimizing stress. This question is straightforward, and you should be able to eliminate each of the incorrect options in turn. Note the word "consider" in the correct option. This provides the client with both assistance and the opportunity to make an independent decision.

Level of Cognitive Ability: Application
Phase of Nursing Process: Implementation
Client Needs: Psychosocial Integrity
Content Area: Adult Health/Cardiovascular

Reference

Black, J., & Matassarin-Jacobs, E. (1997). *Medical-surgical nursing: Clinical management for continuity of care* (5th ed.). Philadelphia: W. B. Saunders, p. 1432.

105. The client with a history of pulmonary emboli is scheduled for insertion of an inferior vena cava filter. The nurse checks on the client 1 hour after the physician has explained the procedure and obtained consent from the client. The client is lying in bed, wringing the hands, and says to the nurse, "I'm not sure about this. What if it doesn't work and I'm just as bad off as before?" The nurse formulates which of the following nursing diagnoses for the client?

1 Fear related to potential risks and outcome of surgery
2 Anxiety related to fear of death
3 Ineffective Individual Coping related to treatment regimen
4 Knowledge Deficit related to surgical procedure

Answer: 1

Rationale: This client has indicated that the surgical procedure and its outcome are the objects of fear. Anxiety is used when the client cannot identify the source of the uneasy feelings. Ineffective Individual Coping is appropriate when the client is not making needed adaptations to deal with daily life. Knowledge Deficit is characterized by a lack of appropriate information.

Test-Taking Strategy: The stem gives no evidence to support options 3 or 4, so they can be eliminated first. Knowledge of the meanings of the words "fear" and "anxiety" helps you to easily discriminate between these two choices. Select option 1 over option 2 because the client statement supports fear related to potential risks and outcome of surgery. The fear of death is not addressed.

Level of Cognitive Ability: Analysis
Phase of Nursing Process: Analysis
Client Needs: Psychosocial Integrity
Content Area: Adult Health/Respiratory

Reference

Cox, H., Hinz, M., Lubno, M., et al. (1997). *Clinical applications of nursing diagnosis: Adult, child, women's, psychiatric,herontic, and home health considerations* (3rd ed.). Philadelphia: F. A. Davis, pp. 496–497, 514.

106. The client has an oral endotracheal tube attached to a mechanical ventilator and is about to begin the weaning process. The nurse interprets that which of the following items, which were previously useful in minimizing the client's anxiety, should now be limited?

1 Television
2 Radio
3 Family visitors
4 Antianxiety medications

Answer: 4

Rationale: Antianxiety medications and narcotic analgesics are used cautiously in the client being weaned from a mechanical ventilator. These medications may interfere with the weaning process by suppressing the respiratory drive. The client may exhibit anxiety during the weaning process as well for a variety of reasons, and therefore distractions such as radio, television, and visitors are still very useful.

Test-Taking Strategy: To answer this question accurately, you need to reflect on items that could interfere with the client's strength, endurance, and respiratory drive in maintaining independent ventilation. Using this as the guideline, you would realize that the only possible option is option 4. The side effects of these medications could include sedation, which could interfere with optimal respiratory function.

Level of Cognitive Ability: Analysis
Phase of Nursing Process: Analysis
Client Needs: Psychosocial Integrity
Content Area: Adult Health/Respiratory

Reference

Black, J., & Matassarin-Jacobs, E. (1997). *Medical-surgical nursing: Clinical management for continuity of care* (5th ed.). Philadelphia: W. B. Saunders, p. 1180.

107. The client scheduled for pulmonary angiography is fearful about the procedure and asks the nurse whether the procedure involves significant pain and radiation exposure. The nurse gives a response to the client that provides reassurance, according to the understanding that

1. The procedure is somewhat painful, but there is minimal exposure to radiation.
2. Discomfort may occur with needle insertion, and there is minimal exposure to radiation.
3. There is absolutely no pain, although a moderate amount of radiation must be used to get accurate results.
4. There is very mild pain throughout the procedure, and the exposure to radiation is negligible.

Answer: 2

Rationale: Pulmonary angiography involves minimal exposure to radiation. The procedure is painless, although the client may feel discomfort with insertion of the needle for the catheter that is used for dye injection.

Test-Taking Strategy: Knowing that radiation exposure is minimal helps you to eliminate option 3 first. It is helpful to know that the only discomfort occurs with needle insertion. From the remaining 3 options, option 2 is most accurate in providing the client with a description of what may cause discomfort.

Level of Cognitive Ability: Analysis
Phase of Nursing Process: Implementation
Client Needs: Psychosocial Integrity
Content Area: Adult Health/Respiratory

Reference

Black, J., & Matassarin-Jacobs, E. (1997). *Medical-surgical nursing: Clinical management for continuity of care* (5th ed.). Philadelphia: W. B. Saunders, p. 1062.

---

108. The nurse is caring for the anxious client with an open pneumothorax and a sucking chest wound. An occlusive dressing has been applied to the site. Which of the following interventions planned by the nurse would have the greatest overall immediate benefit?

1. Encouraging the client to cough and breathe deeply
2. Staying with the client
3. Interpreting the arterial blood gas report
4. Distracting the client with television

Answer: 2

Rationale: Staying with the client has a twofold benefit. First, the presence of the nurse relieves the anxiety of the dyspneic client. In addition, the nurse must stay with the client to observe respiratory status after application of the occlusive dressing. It is possible that the dressing could convert the open pneumothorax to a closed (tension) pneumothorax, with sudden decline in respiratory status and mediastinal shift. If this occurs, the nurse is present and able to remove the dressing immediately.

Test-Taking Strategy: Eliminate option 4 first, since the client is in distress. Coughing and deep breathing may be eliminated for the same reason, because they have no immediate benefit for the client who is in distress. Of the two remaining plausible answers, you would select staying with the client because the question states that the client is anxious. The blood gas report can be interpreted in the client's room, anyway.

Level of Cognitive Ability: Application
Phase of Nursing Process: Planning
Client Needs: Psychosocial Integrity
Content Area: Adult Health/Respiratory

Reference

Black, J., & Matassarin-Jacobs, E. (1997). *Medical-surgical nursing: Clinical management for continuity of care* (5th ed.). Philadelphia: W. B. Saunders, p. 2524.

109. The client with acquired immunodeficiency syndrome (AIDS) shares with the nurse feelings of social isolation since the diagnosis was made. The nurse plans to suggest which of the following strategies as the most useful way to decrease the client's stated loneliness?

1. Using Internet on the computer to facilitate communication while maintaining isolation
2. Use of television and newspapers to maintain a feeling of being "in touch" with the world
3. Contacting any of the support groups available in the local region for clients with HIV
4. Reinstituting contact with the client's family, who live in a distant city

Answer: 3

Rationale: The nurse encourages the client to maintain social contact and support and assists the client in reducing barriers to social contact. This can include educating the client's family about the disease and transmission and suggesting use of community resources and support groups.

Test-Taking Strategy: Eliminate options 1 and 2 first because they do not actually decrease the client's physical isolation and loneliness. These options maintain a measure of distance between the client and others. To discriminate between the last two, note that option 3 is the more pragmatic approach. There are no data in the question that indicate loss of contact with the family, and the logistics of distance make this the less likely solution to the client's current feelings of isolation.

Level of Cognitive Ability: Application
Phase of Nursing Process: Planning
Client Needs: Psychosocial Integrity
Content Area: Adult Health/Respiratory

Reference

Ignatavicius, D. D., Workman, M. L., & Mishler, M. A. (1995). *Medical-surgical nursing: A nursing process approach* (2nd ed.). Philadelphia: W. B. Saunders, pp. 508, 524.

110. The client has an initial positive result of an enzyme-linked immunosorbent assay (ELISA) test for human immunodeficiency virus (HIV). The client begins to cry and asks the nurse what this means. The nurse is able to provide support to the client, using knowledge that

1. The client is HIV-positive but the disease has been detected early.
2. The client is HIV-positive but the client's CD4 cell count is high.
3. There is a high rate of false-positive results with this test and more testing is needed before diagnosing the client's status as HIV positive.
4. There are occasional false-positive readings with this test, which can be cleared up by repeating it one more time.

Answer: 3

Rationale: If the ELISA test results are positive, the test is repeated. If it is positive a second time, the Western blot (a more specific test) is done to confirm the finding. The client is not considered HIV-positive unless the Western blot is positive. (Some laboratories also run the Western blot a second time with a new specimen before making a final determination). The ELISA is fast and relatively inexpensive, but it carries a high false-positive rate.

Test-Taking Strategy: To answer this question correctly, it is necessary to know that HIV infection is not diagnosed with a single laboratory test. With this in mind, eliminate options 1 and 2 first. To choose correctly between options 3 and 4, it is necessary to understand that the ELISA would be repeated and a Western blot would then be done to confirm these results.

Level of Cognitive Ability: Analysis
Phase of Nursing Process: Analysis
Client Needs: Psychosocial Integrity
Content Area: Adult Health/Respiratory

Reference

Black, J., & Matassarin-Jacobs, E. (1997). *Medical-surgical nursing: Clinical management for continuity of care* (5th ed.). Philadelphia: W. B. Saunders, p. 611.

111. The home care nurse is making home visits to an elderly client with urinary incontinence who is very disturbed by the incontinent episodes. The nurse explores the client's home situation to determine environmental barriers to normal voiding. Which of the following items, if assessed by the nurse, may be contributing to the client's problem?

1 Presence of hand railings in the bathroom
2 Having one bathroom on each floor of the home
3 Nightlight present in the hall between bedroom and bathroom
4 Bathroom located on the second floor, bedroom on the first floor

Answer: 4

Rationale: Having a bathroom on the second floor and the bedroom on the first floor may pose a problem for the elderly client with incontinence. Both the need to negotiate the stairs and the distance may interfere with reaching the bathroom in a timely manner. It is more helpful to the incontinent client to have a bathroom on the same floor as the bedroom or to have a commode rented for use. The presence of nightlights and hand railings is helpful to the client in reaching the bathroom quickly and safely.

Test-Taking Strategy: Begin to answer this question by eliminating option 1 as obviously helpful. Option 2 is also helpful and cannot be the answer to the question as stated. Because option 3 is more helpful than option 4, at least for nighttime voiding, option 4 must be the correct answer. This option can be causing the disturbing problem for the client.

Level of Cognitive Ability: Analysis
Phase of Nursing Process: Assessment
Client Needs: Psychosocial Integrity
Content Area: Fundamental Skills

Reference

Black, J., & Matassarin-Jacobs, E. (1997). *Medical-surgical nursing: Clinical management for continuity of care* (5th ed.). Philadelphia: W. B. Saunders, pp. 1550–1551.

112. The client with cancer of the bladder has a nursing diagnosis of Fear related to uncertain outcome of upcoming cystectomy and urinary diversion. The nurse assesses that this diagnosis still applies if the client makes which of the following statements?

1 "I'm so afraid I won't live through all this."
2 "What if I have no help at home after going through this awful surgery?"
3 "I'll never feel like myself once I can't go to the bathroom normally."
4 "I wish I'd never gone to the doctor at all."

Answer: 1

Rationale: In order for Fear to be an actual diagnosis, the client must be able to identify the object of fear. In this question, the client is expressing a fear of death related to cancer. The statement in option 2 reflects risk for impaired home maintenance management. Option 3 reflects a body image disturbance. Option 4 is vague and nonspecific; further exploration would be necessary to associate this statement with a nursing diagnosis.

Test-Taking Strategy: The diagnostic statement includes wording about the uncertain outcome of surgery. Because option 4 is a general statement, it should be eliminated first. Options 2 and 3 focus on the self after surgery but do not contain statements about an uncertain outcome. By elimination, option 1 is correct. The client expresses a fear of dying after enduring the ordeal of surgery.

Level of Cognitive Ability: Analysis
Phase of Nursing Process: Assessment
Client Needs: Psychosocial Integrity
Content Area: Adult Health/Renal

Reference

Black, J., & Matassarin-Jacobs, E. (1997). *Medical-surgical nursing: Clinical management for continuity of care* (5th ed.). Philadelphia: W. B. Saunders, p. 1552.

113. The client with nephrotic syndrome asks the nurse, "Why should I even bother trying to control my diet and the edema? It doesn't really matter what I do, if I can never get rid of this kidney problem anyway!" The nurse selects which of the following most appropriate nursing diagnostic labels in formulating a nursing diagnostic statement for this client?

1 Powerlessness
2 Ineffective Individual Coping
3 Anxiety
4 Body Image Disturbance

Answer: 1

Rationale: Powerlessness is used when the client believes that personal actions will not affect an outcome in any significant way. Ineffective Individual Coping is used when the client has impaired adaptive abilities or behaviors in meeting the demands or roles expected from the individual. Anxiety is used when the client has a feeling of unease with a vague or undefined source. Body Image Disturbance occurs when there is an alteration in the way the client perceives body image.

Test-Taking Strategy: Begin to answer this question by eliminating option 3 first as the least likely of all the options. The client makes no statement that refers to body image, so option 4 is eliminated next. It may be difficult to choose between the last two choices. However, note the statement "It doesn't really matter what I do. . . ." This implies the client has a sense of no control of the situation and is the basis for choosing Powerlessness over Ineffective Individual Coping as the most appropriate nursing diagnosis.

Level of Cognitive Ability: Analysis
Phase of Nursing Process: Analysis
Client Needs: Psychosocial Integrity
Content Area: Adult Health/Renal

Reference

Cox, H., Hinz, M., Lubno, M., et al. (1997). *Clinical applications of nursing diagnosis: Adult, child, women's, psychiatric, gerontic, and home health considerations* (3rd ed.). Philadelphia: F. A. Davis, pp. 496, 506, 545, 735.

114. The client with renal cell carcinoma of the left kidney is scheduled for nephrectomy. The right kidney appears normal at this time. The client is anxious about whether dialysis will ultimately be a necessity. The nurse would plan to use which of the following pieces of information in discussions with the client?

1 There is absolutely no chance of needing dialysis because of the nature of the surgery
2 Dialysis could become likely, but it depends on how well the client complies with fluid restriction after surgery
3 One kidney is adequate to meet the needs of the body as long as it has normal function
4 There is a strong likelihood that the client will need dialysis within 5–10 years

Answer: 3

Rationale: Fears about having only one functioning kidney are common in clients who must undergo nephrectomy for renal cancer. These clients need emotional support and reassurance that the remaining kidney should be able to fully meet the body's metabolical needs, as long as it has normal function.

Test-Taking Strategy: Begin to answer this question by eliminating option 1. An option that contains the phrase "absolutely no chance" is not likely to be correct. Knowing that there is no need for fluid restriction with a functioning kidney guides you to eliminate option 2 next. To discriminate between the last two options, remember that an individual can donate a kidney without adverse consequences or the need for dialysis. Applying that knowledge to this question would guide you to choose option 3 over option 4.

Level of Cognitive Ability: Analysis
Phase of Nursing Process: Planning
Client Needs: Psychosocial Integrity
Content Area: Adult Health/Renal

Reference

Black, J., & Matassarin-Jacobs, E. (1997). *Medical-surgical nursing: Clinical management for continuity of care* (5th ed.). Philadelphia: W. B. Saunders, p. 1672.

115. The charge nurse is supervising a new RN providing care to a client with end-stage heart failure. The client is withdrawn, is reluctant to talk, and shows little interest in participating in hygienic care or activities. Which statement, if made by the new RN to the client, indicates that the new RN needs further teaching in the use of therapeutic communication skills?

1 "You are very quiet today."
2 "Why don't you feel like getting up for your bath?"
3 "What are your feelings right now?"
4 "These dreams you mentioned: what are they like?"

Answer: 2

Rationale: When the nurse asks a "why" question of the client, the nurse is requesting an explanation for feelings and behaviors when the client may not know the reason. Requesting an explanation is a nontherapeutic technique of communication. In option 1 the nurse is using the therapeutic communication technique of acknowledging the client's behavior. In option 3 the nurse is encouraging assessment of emotions or feelings, which is a therapeutic communication technique. In option 4 the nurse is using the therapeutic communication technique of exploring. Exploring is asking the client to describe something in more detail or to discuss it more fully.

Test-Taking Strategy: Note the key phrase "needs further teaching in the use of therapeutic communication skills." Use the process of elimination, seeking the option that is a block to communication. The word "why" in option 2 should easily guide you to this option as the correct answer to this question as it is stated.

Level of Cognitive Ability: Analysis
Phase of Nursing Process: Evaluation
Client Needs: Psychosocial Integrity
Content Area: Adult Health/Cardiovascular

Reference
Potter, P., & Perry, A. (1997). *Fundamentals of nursing: Concepts, process, and practice* (4th ed.). St. Louis: Mosby–Year Book, pp. 240–246.

---

116. The plan of care for a client with a diagnosis of acute pulmonary edema should include strategies for

1 Decreasing cardiac output.
2 Increasing fluid volume.
3 Promoting a positive body image.
4 Reducing anxiety.

Answer: 4

Rationale: When cardiac output falls as a result of acute pulmonary edema, the sympathetic nervous system is stimulated. Stimulation of the sympathetic nervous system results in the flight-or-fight reaction, which further impairs cardiac function. The goal of treatment is to increase cardiac output. Fluid volume should be decreased. Altered body image is not a common problem experienced by clients with acute pulmonary edema.

Test-Taking Strategy: Knowledge of the care of clients with acute pulmonary edema is needed to assist you in answering this question. Consider the physiological manifestations of this condition in order to eliminate the incorrect options. Knowledge that severe dyspnea occurs should assist in directing you to the correct option.

Level of Cognitive Ability: Application
Phase of Nursing Process: Planning
Client Needs: Psychosocial Integrity
Content Area: Adult Health/Cardiovascular

Reference
Black, J., & Matassarin-Jacobs, E. (1997). *Medical-surgical nursing: Clinical management for continuity of care* (5th ed.). Philadelphia: W. B. Saunders, pp. 1288–1289.

117. The client with acute renal failure (ARF) is having trouble remembering information and instructions because of the elevated blood urea nitrogen (BUN) level. The nurse would avoid doing which of the following when communicating with this client?

1 Giving simple, clear directions
2 Explaining treatments, using understandable language
3 Including the family in discussions related to care
4 Giving thorough, complete explanations of treatment options

Answer: 4

Rationale: The client with ARF may have difficulty remembering information and instructions because of anxiety and because of an increased BUN level. Communications should be clear, simple, and understandable. The family is included whenever possible. It is the physician's responsibility to explain treatment options.

Test-Taking Strategy: The wording of this question guides you to select a response that is not helpful to the communication process. Knowledge of the basic principles of effective communication would allow you to recognize that options 1, 2, and 3 are helpful in maintaining effective communication. Therefore, these are eliminated as possible choices, and option 4 is the answer to the question as stated.

Level of Cognitive Ability: Application
Phase of Nursing Process: Implementation
Client Needs: Psychosocial Integrity
Content Area: Adult Health/Renal

Reference

Black, J., & Matassarin-Jacobs, E. (1997). *Medical-surgical nursing: Clinical management for continuity of care* (5th ed.). Philadelphia: W. B. Saunders, p. 1641.

---

118. The rehabilitation nurse witnesses the postoperative coronary artery bypass client and spouse arguing after a rehabilitation session. The most appropriate statement by the nurse in identifying the feelings of the client would be

1 "You seem upset. . . ."
2 "You shouldn't get upset. It'll affect your heart."
3 "Oh, don't let this get you down."
4 "It will seem better tomorrow. Smile."

Answer: 1

Rationale: Acknowledging the client's feelings without inserting your own values or judgments is a method of therapeutic communication. Therapeutic communication techniques assist the flow of communication and always focus on the client. Options 2, 3, and 4 do not encourage verbalization by the client.

Test-Taking Strategy: Use communication techniques that do not block or belittle the client's feelings. Open-ended statements allow the client to verbalize, giving the nurse a direction or clarification of the true feelings.

Level of Cognitive Ability: Analysis
Phase of Nursing Process: Assessment
Client Needs: Psychosocial Integrity
Content Area: Adult Health/Cardiovascular

Reference

Potter, P., & Perry, A. (1997). *Fundamentals of nursing: Concepts, process, and practice* (4th ed.). St. Louis: Mosby–Year Book, pp. 240–246.

---

119. An acutely psychotic client displays increased motor activity. Which of the following medications, if prescribed, would the nurse administer?

1 Sertraline hydrochloride (Zoloft)
2 Haloperidol (Haldol)
3 Chloral hydrate
4 Isocarboxazid (Marplan)

Answer: 2

Rationale: Antipsychotics are used to treat acute and chronic psychosis, especially when the client has increased psychomotor activity. A fast-acting, injectable agent would be the medication of choice. Antidepressants (Zoloft and Marplan) and hypnotics (chloral hydrate) are not indicated for the presenting condition.

Test-Taking Strategy: The stem of the question clues the reader to the situation in the presenting case and the classification of medication needed. The distracters can be eliminated if the actions of the four choices are known. Options 1, 3, and 4 can be eliminated because of their action. Review these medications now if you had difficulty with this question!

Level of Cognitive Ability: Application
Phase of Nursing Process: Implementation
Client Needs: Psychosocial Integrity
Content Area: Pharmacology

Reference

Townsend, M. (1996). *Psychiatric–mental health nursing: Concepts of care* (2nd ed.). Philadelphia: F. A. Davis, p. 283.

---

120. A client is admitted with a diagnosis of panic disorder. The nurse would anticipate that the physician's order for a benzodiazepine would include

1 Imipramine (Tofranil).
2 Alprazolam (Xanax).
3 Bupropion (Wellbutrin).
4 Doxepin (Sinequan).

Answer: 2

Rationale: Options 1, 3, and 4 are classified as antidepressants and act by stimulating the central nervous system (CNS) to elevate mood. Xanax, a benzodiazepine antianxiety agent, depresses the CNS and induces relaxation in clients with panic disorders.

Test-Taking Strategy: Knowledge regarding panic disorders and the medications identified in each of the options is necessary to answer this question. Take time now to review these medications if you had difficulty with this question!

Level of Cognitive Ability: Analysis
Phase of Nursing Process: Analysis
Client Needs: Psychosocial Integrity
Content Area: Pharmacology

Reference

Wilson, H., & Kneisl, C. (1996). *Psychiatric nursing* (5th ed.). Menlo Park, CA: Addison-Wesley, p. 929.

---

121. The client with long-standing empyema is to undergo decortication to remove the inflamed tissue, pus, and debris. The nurse offers emotional support to the client on the basis of the understanding that

1 The client is likely to be in excruciating pain after surgery.
2 The client will probably have chronic dyspnea after the surgery.
3 Chest tubes will be in place after surgery for some time, and the healing process is slow.
4 This problem may decrease the client's life expectancy.

Answer: 3

Rationale: The client undergoing decortication to treat empyema needs ongoing support by the nurse. This is especially true because the client will have chest tubes in place after surgery, which must remain until the formerly pus-filled space is completely obliterated. This usually takes a considerable amount of time and may be discouraging to the client. Progress is monitored by chest x-ray.

Test-Taking Strategy: Option 4 is the least likely response and is eliminated first. Option 1 is discarded next because no client should be in "excruciating" pain postoperatively. To choose between the remaining two options, it is necessary to know that the client will need chest tubes and that it may take some time for full healing to occur. Knowing that the client has chest tubes after thoracic surgery may be sufficient to help you discriminate between these last two options as well.

Level of Cognitive Ability: Analysis
Phase of Nursing Process: Implementation
Client Needs: Psychosocial Integrity
Content Area: Adult Health/Respiratory

Reference

Smeltzer, S., & Bare, B. (1996). *Brunner and Suddarth's Textbook of medical-surgical nursing* (8th ed.). Philadelphia: Lippincott-Raven, p. 503.

122. The client who has never been hospitalized before is having trouble initiating the stream of urine. Knowing that there is no pathological reason for this difficulty, the nurse avoids which of the following as the least helpful method of assisting the client?

1 Encouraging fluid intake
2 Providing privacy during voiding
3 Assisting the client to a commode behind a closed curtain
4 Closing the bathroom door during voiding

Answer: 3

Rationale: Lack of privacy is a key issue that may inhibit the ability of the client to void in the absence of known pathological processes. Using a commode behind a curtain may inhibit voiding in some people. Use of a bathroom is preferable, and encouraging fluid intake will aid in urinary elimination.

Test-Taking Strategy: This question is fairly straightforward in wording and tests a basic principle related to lack of privacy during elimination. Option 4 is most helpful and therefore is eliminated first, in view of the wording of the question. Knowing that options 1 and 2 are standard measures, you would then pick option 3 as the least helpful method of assisting the client with elimination.

Level of Cognitive Ability: Application
Phase of Nursing Process: Implementation
Client Needs: Psychosocial Integrity
Content Area: Adult Health/Renal

Reference
Black, J., & Matassarin-Jacobs, E. (1997). *Medical-surgical nursing: Clinical management for continuity of care* (5th ed.). Philadelphia: W. B. Saunders, p. 1551.

---

123. The client tells the nurse, "My doctor says I can have the surgery and go home the same day, but I'm afraid. My husband's dead, and my son is 3000 miles away. I'm alone, and what happens if something goes wrong? I'm not supposed to be up walking unless absolutely necessary." Which of the following responses would be the most therapeutic communication for the nurse to employ?

1 "I know, I know. They say, 'Managed care is no care'! Have you got an alarm system so if you fall, it will alert someone to come? If worse comes to worse, call me and I'll come immediately."
2 "Don't worry. This procedure is done all the time without any problems. You'll be fine!"
3 "Your concern is well voiced. I advise you to call your son and insist he come home immediately! You can't be too careful."
4 "You seem very concerned about going home without help. Have you discussed your concerns with your doctor?

Answer: 4

Rationale: The client in this question has articulated concerns that are appropriate. In option 4, the nurse uses reflection to direct the client's feelings and concerns. In option 1, the nurse is ventilating the nurse's own anger, frustration, and powerlessness. In addition, the nurse is trying to solve problems for the client but is overly controlling and takes the decision making out of the client's hands. In option 2, the nurse provides false reassurance and then minimizes the client's concerns. In option 3, the nurse is projecting the client's own fears, and the problem-solving suggested by the nurse is histrionic and provokes fear and anxiety.

Test-Taking Strategy: Use therapeutic communication techniques to answer the question. By the process of elimination, you should easily be able to eliminate options 1, 2, and 3. Remember that the priority is to address the client's feelings!

Level of Cognitive Ability: Analysis
Phase of Nursing Process: Implementation
Client Needs: Psychosocial Integrity
Content Area: Fundamental Skills

Reference
Antai-Otong, D. (1995). *Psychiatric nursing: Biological and behavioral concepts.* Philadelphia: W. B. Saunders, pp. 543–576.

124. In the nursing assessment, the client says, "My doctor just told me that my cancer has spread and that I have less than 6 months." Which of the following responses would be the most therapeutic communication technique for this client?

1. "I know it seems desperate, but there have been a lot of breakthroughs. Something might come along in a month or so to change your status drastically."
2. "I hope you'll focus on the fact that your doctor says you have a good 6 months to live and that you'll think of how you'd like to live."
3. "I am sorry. There are no easy answers in times like this, are there?"
4. "I am sorry. Would you like to discuss this with me some more?"

Answer: 4

Rationale: The client has just received very difficult news. The nurse can assume that the client is still in the beginning stage of shock and denial. In the correct option, the nurse encourages the client to ventilate. Option 1 provides a social communication and false hope. Option 2 is patronizing and stereotypical. Option 3 expresses the nurse's feelings rather than facilitates the client's feelings.

Test-Taking Strategy: This question tests your knowledge of the most therapeutic communication technique to apply for this client. You can easily eliminate options 1 and 2. Of the remaining two options, note that option 4 is providing the opportunity for the client to express feelings!

Level of Cognitive Ability: Analysis
Phase of Nursing Process: Implementation
Client Needs: Psychosocial Integrity
Content Area: Adult Health/Oncology

Reference

Antai-Otong, D. (1995). *Psychiatric nursing: Biological and behavioral concepts.* Philadelphia: W. B. Saunders, pp. 543–576.

---

125. The client with an endotracheal tube gets easily frustrated when trying to communicate personal needs to the nurse. The nurse interprets that which of the following methods for communication may be the easiest for the client?

1. Have the family interpret needs
2. Use a picture or word board
3. Use a pad and paper
4. Devise a system of hand signals

Answer: 2

Rationale: The client with an endotracheal tube in place cannot speak. The nurse devises an alternative communication system with the client. Use of a picture or word board is the simplest method of communication, as it requires only pointing at the word or object. A pad and pencil is an acceptable alternative, but it requires more client effort and more time. The use of hand signals may not be a reliable method, as it may not meet all needs and is subject to misinterpretation. The family does not need to bear the burden of communicating the client's needs, and they may not understand them either.

Test-Taking Strategy: This question is most easily answered by focusing on the words "easily frustrated" and "easiest." Options 3 and 4 are obviously not the "easiest" and are therefore eliminated first. Because the family may not necessarily know what the client is trying to communicate, this option could add to the client's frustration. By elimination, the picture or word board is the easiest and the least frustrating for the client.

Level of Cognitive Ability: Analysis
Phase of Nursing Process: Analysis
Client Needs: Psychosocial Integrity
Content Area: Adult Health/Respiratory

Reference

Black, J., & Matassarin-Jacobs, E. (1997). *Medical-surgical nursing: Clinical management for continuity of care* (5th ed.). Philadelphia: W. B. Saunders, p. 1175.

126. The community health nurse visits a client who is receiving total parenteral nutrition (TPN) in the home. The client states, "I really miss eating with my family at dinner." Which is the best response by the nurse?

1. "It is normal to miss something as basic as eating."
2. "I think in a few weeks you will probably be allowed to eat a little."
3. "Tell me more about how you feel about dinner time?"
4. "You could sit with your family at mealtime anyway even if you do not eat."

Answer: 3

Rationale: The nurse uses tools of therapeutic communication to assist the client to express feelings and deal with aspects of illness and treatment. The nurse uses clarifying and focusing to encourage the client to explore concerns. Blocks to communication such as giving opinions and changing the subject will stop the client from exploring the reason for the distress.

Test-Taking Strategy: Read the stem carefully. Be aware of the key phrase "best response." With communication questions, identify the use of therapeutic communication tools, as in option 3, and eliminate options that are blocks to communication, as in options 1, 2, and 4. Always focus on clients' feelings first!

Level of Cognitive Ability: Application
Phase of Nursing Process: Implementation
Client Needs: Psychosocial Integrity
Content Area: Fundamental Skills

Reference

Potter, P., & Perry, A. (1997). *Fundamentals of nursing: Concepts, process, and practice* (4th ed.). St. Louis: Mosby–Year Book, pp. 240–246.

---

127. The client has been receiving maprotiline (Ludiomil). The nurse notifies the health care provider if which of the following client responses to the medication is noted?

1. Increased sense of well-being
2. Reported decrease in anxiety
3. Increased drowsiness
4. Increased appetite

Answer: 3

Rationale: Maprotiline is a tricyclic antidepressant used to treat various forms of depression and anxiety. The client is also often in psychotherapy while on this medication. Expected effects of the medication include improved sense of well-being, appetite, and sleep, as well as a reduced sense of anxiety. Common side effects to report to the health care provider include drowsiness, lethargy, and fatigue.

Test-Taking Strategy: To answer this question accurately, it is necessary to know that maprotiline is an antidepressant. With this in mind, note that options 1, 2, and 4 are positive responses. Review this medication now if you had difficulty with this question!

Level of Cognitive Ability: Analysis
Phase of Nursing Process: Implementation
Client Needs: Psychosocial Integrity
Content Area: Pharmacology

Reference

Deglin, J., & Vallerand, A. (1997). *Davis's drug guide for nurses* (5th ed.). Philadelphia: F. A. Davis, p. 728.

128. The client who is to undergo thoracentesis is afraid of not being able to tolerate the procedure. The nurse interprets that the client needs honest support and reassurance, which can best be accomplished by which of the following statements?

1. "The procedure only takes 1–2 minutes, so you might try to get through it by mentally counting up to 120."
2. "The needle is a little uncomfortable going in, but this is controlled by rhythmically breathing in and out. I'll be with you to coach your breathing."
3. "The needle hurts when it goes in, but you must remain still. I'll stay with you throughout the entire procedure and help you hold your position."
4. "I'll be right by your side, but the procedure will be totally painless as long as you don't move."

Answer: 3

Rationale: The needle insertion for thoracentesis is painful for the client. The nurse tells the client how important it is to remain still during the procedure so that the needle won't injure visceral pleura or lung tissue. The nurse reassures the client during the procedure and helps the client maintain the proper position.

Test-Taking Strategy: Knowing that the client must remain still during the procedure helps you eliminate option 2 first. Knowing that the procedure is painful for the client and takes longer than 1–2 minutes helps you eliminate options 1 and 4. Review this procedure now if you had difficulty with this question!

Level of Cognitive Ability: Analysis
Phase of Nursing Process: Analysis
Client Needs: Psychosocial Integrity
Content Area: Adult Health/Respiratory

Reference

Black, J., & Matassarin-Jacobs, E. (1997). *Medical-surgical nursing: Clinical management for continuity of care* (5th ed.). Philadelphia: W. B. Saunders, p. 1063.

---

129. The client with chronic respiratory failure is dyspneic. The client responds to the dyspnea with anxiety, which worsens the feelings of dyspnea on the part of the client. The nurse would teach the client which of the following methods to best interrupt the dyspnea-anxiety-dyspnea cycle?

1. Relaxation and breathing techniques
2. Biofeedback and coughing techniques
3. Guided imagery and limiting fluids
4. Distraction and increased dietary carbohydrates

Answer: 1

Rationale: The anxious client with dyspnea should be taught interventions to decrease anxiety, which include relaxation, biofeedback, guided imagery, and distraction. This will stop the escalation of feelings of dyspnea. The dyspnea can be further controlled by teaching the client respiratory techniques, which include pursed-lip and diaphragmatic breathing. Coughing techniques are useful, but breathing techniques are more effective. Limiting fluids will thicken secretions and is not indicated. Increased dietary carbohydrates will increase production of CO_2 by the body, which is also not indicated.

Test-Taking Strategy: Because the first part of every response is helpful for anxiety reduction, you must focus on the second part of each option to determine the correct choice. Limiting fluids and increasing carbohydrates are contraindicated and are therefore eliminated. Breathing techniques are more effective than coughing techniques, which helps you to choose option 1 over option 2.

Level of Cognitive Ability: Application
Phase of Nursing Process: Implementation
Client Needs: Psychosocial Integrity
Content Area: Adult Health/Respiratory

Reference

Ignatavicius, D. D., Workman, M. L., & Mishler, M. A. (1995). *Medical-surgical nursing: A nursing process approach* (2nd ed.). Philadelphia: W. B. Saunders, p. 689.

130. The client who has had drainage of a pleural effusion is in pain. The nurse would not include which of the following interventions in providing support to this client?

1 Offering verbal support and reassurance
2 Assisting the client to find positions of comfort
3 Leaving the client alone for an extended rest period
4 Providing pain medication for the client

Answer: 3

Rationale: The pain associated with drainage of pleural effusion is minimized by the nurse, who positions the client for comfort and administers analgesics for relief of pain. The nurse also offers verbal support and understanding. All of these measures help the client to cope with the pain and discomfort associated with this problem. It is least helpful to leave the client alone for extended periods, as the client may experience continued pain, which may be augmented by isolation.

Test-Taking Strategy: The wording of the question guides you to look for an option that should be avoided by the nurse. Basic knowledge of pain management techniques allows you to eliminate each of the incorrect options. Basic principles of nursing care will assist in directing you to option 3.

Level of Cognitive Ability: Application
Phase of Nursing Process: Implementation
Client Needs: Psychosocial Integrity
Content Area: Fundamental Skills

Reference

Smeltzer, S., & Bare, B. (1996). *Brunner and Suddarth's Textbook of medical-surgical nursing* (8th ed.). Philadelphia: Lippincott-Raven, p. 503.

131. The nurse is caring for a client who has just experienced a pulmonary embolism. The client is restless and very anxious. The nurse would plan to use which approach in communicating with this client?

1 Explaining each treatment in great detail
2 Having the family reinforce the nurse's directions
3 Giving simple, clear directions and explanations
4 Speaking very little to the client until the crisis is over

Answer: 3

Rationale: The client who has suffered pulmonary embolism is fearful and anxious. The nurse effectively communicates with this client by staying with the client; providing simple, accurate information; and behaving in a calm, efficient manner. Options 1, 2, and 4 will produce more anxiety for the client and family.

Test-Taking Strategy: Options 1 and 4 represent the least effective communication strategies, overall, and may be eliminated first. Of the two remaining, having the family reinforce the directions places stress on the family and provides too much sensory input for the client; thus option 3 is the correct answer. The nurse gives simple, clear information to the client who is in distress.

Level of Cognitive Ability: Application
Phase of Nursing Process: Planning
Client Needs: Psychosocial Integrity
Content Area: Adult Health/Respiratory

Reference

Black, J., & Matassarin-Jacobs, E. (1997). *Medical-surgical nursing: Clinical management for continuity of care* (5th ed.). Philadelphia: W. B. Saunders, p. 1129.

132. The client with bone metastasis after previous lung resection for cancer is considering megavitamin and diet therapy because the original surgery did not provide a cure. The client asks the nurse for an opinion of these therapies. In formulating a response, the nurse incorporates which of the following concepts?

1 The client's right to justice and the nurse's obligation to project parentalism
2 The client's right to privacy and the nurse's obligation to uphold the law
3 The client's right to freedom of speech and the nurse's obligation to support the client
4 The client's right to autonomy and the nurse's obligation to behave ethically

Answer: 4

Rationale: The client has the right to autonomy, or the exercise of personal choice. At the same time, the nurse has the obligation to behave ethically. Unconventional cancer treatments have not been proven effective, may be toxic to the client, and may be extremely expensive. The nurse balances the client's right to self-determination with the obligation to share with the client knowledge about the ineffectiveness of these methods. Privacy is the right of a client to be free from intrusion by someone into their own personal affairs. Justice is the ethical principle of treating people fairly.

Test-Taking Strategy: Begin to answer this question by eliminating options 1 and 2, which are the two options that do not relate to the issue of the question. Of the remaining two, you would pick option 4 by knowing that the nurse must behave ethically and that the client ultimately has freedom of choice (autonomy).

Level of Cognitive Ability: Analysis
Phase of Nursing Process: Planning
Client Needs: Psychosocial Integrity
Content Area: Fundamental Skills

Reference

Smeltzer, S., & Bare, B. (1996). *Brunner and Suddarth's Textbook of medical-surgical nursing* (8th ed.). Philadelphia: Lippincott-Raven, p. 289.

---

133. The emergency room nurse is admitting a client with carbon monoxide poisoning from a suicide attempt. The nurse plans to ensure that which of the following most needed services is put in place for the client?

1 Pulmonary rehabilitation
2 Occupational therapy
3 Psychiatric consultation
4 Neurological consultation

Answer: 3

Rationale: The client with carbon monoxide poisoning as a result of a suicide attempt should have a psychiatric consultation. The necessity of a neurological consultation would depend on the sequelae to the nervous system from the carbon monoxide poisoning. Occupational therapy and pulmonary rehabilitation are not indicated.

Test-Taking Strategy: Note the phrase "most needed" in the stem of the question. Eliminate occupational therapy first because there is no indication of the need for that service. The client will need respiratory therapy but not pulmonary rehabilitation, so that is eliminated next. A neurological consultation could be beneficial, but only if the client suffers long-term central nervous system (CNS) damage from this suicide attempt. The obvious correct answer is the psychiatric consultation. This client is most in need of this service at this time.

Level of Cognitive Ability: Application
Phase of Nursing Process: Planning
Client Needs: Psychosocial Integrity
Content Area: Mental Health

Reference

Smeltzer, S., & Bare, B. (1996). *Brunner and Suddarth's Textbook of medical-surgical nursing* (8th ed.). Philadelphia: Lippincott-Raven, p. 2025.

134. The nurse is caring for a young adult diagnosed with sarcoidosis. The client is angry and tells the nurse there is no point in learning disease management, inasmuch as there is no possibility of ever being cured. The nurse formulates which of the following nursing diagnoses for this client?

1 Impaired Thought Processes
2 Altered Health Maintenance
3 Anxiety
4 Powerlessness

Answer: 4

Rationale: The client with powerlessness expresses feelings of having no control over a situation or outcome. Altered health maintenance involves the inability to seek out help that is needed to maintain health. Anxiety is a vague sense of unease. Impaired thought processes involve disruption in cognitive abilities or thought.

Test-Taking Strategy: In evaluating the stem of the question, it is clear that the client is lashing out because of anger over a situation in which the client has little control. All the incorrect nursing diagnoses should be eliminated fairly easily. If this question was difficult, take a few moments to review the definitions of these various nursing diagnoses.

Level of Cognitive Ability: Analysis
Phase of Nursing Process: Analysis
Client Needs: Psychosocial Integrity
Content Area: Adult Health/Respiratory

Reference

Cox, H., Hinz, M., Lubno, M., et al. (1997). *Clinical applications of nursing diagnosis: Adult, child, women's, psychiatric, gerontic, and home health considerations* (3rd ed.). Philadelphia: F. A. Davis, pp. 29, 476, 545.

---

135. The nurse is caring for the client with silicosis who has massive pulmonary fibrosis. The nurse gives anticipatory guidance to the client about common periodic emotional reactions to chronic respiratory disease. Which of the following reactions would the nurse not include in discussions with the client?

1 Anxiety
2 Ineffective coping
3 Depression
4 Suicidal ideation

Answer: 4

Rationale: Common emotional reactions to advanced silicosis may be the same as for chronic airflow limitation and include anxiety, ineffective coping, and depression. Suicidal ideation is not a normal response with this condition. However, if it does appear, it warrants attention.

Test-Taking Strategy: This question is straightforward in approach and tests a fundamental concept in dealing with chronic illness. If this question was difficult, take a few moments to review the common emotional reactions that occur in chronic diseases!

Level of Cognitive Ability: Application
Phase of Nursing Process: Implementation
Client Needs: Psychosocial Integrity
Content Area: Adult Health/Respiratory

Reference

Ignatavicius, D. D., Workman, M. L., & Mishler, M. A. (1995). *Medical-surgical nursing: A nursing process approach* (2nd ed.). Philadelphia: W. B. Saunders, pp. 710, 726.

---

136. The client immobilized in skeletal leg traction complains of being bored and restless. On the basis of these complaints, the nurse formulates which of the following nursing diagnoses for this client?

1 Diversional Activity Deficit
2 Powerlessness
3 Self Care Deficit
4 Impaired Physical Mobility

Answer: 1

Rationale: A major defining characteristic of diversional activity deficit is expression of boredom by the client. The question does not identify difficulties with coordination, range of motion, or muscle strength, which would indicate impaired physical mobility. The question also does not relate the client's feelings of inability to perform activities of daily living (self-care deficit) or lack of control (powerlessness).

Test-Taking Strategy: The key to answering this question lies in the complaints of boredom and restlessness. Comparing these complaints to each of the listed nursing diagnoses, you should be able to eliminate each of the incorrect options systematically.

Level of Cognitive Ability: Analysis
Phase of Nursing Process: Analysis
Client Needs: Psychosocial Integrity
Content Area: Adult Health/Musculoskeletal

Reference

Cox, H., Hinz, M., Lubno, M., et al. (1997). *Clinical applications of nursing diagnosis: Adult, child, women's, psychiatric, gerontic, and home health considerations* (3rd ed.). Philadelphia: F. A. Davis, p. 301.

---

137. The client being mechanically ventilated after experiencing a fat embolus is visibly anxious. The nurse should

1 Encourage the client to sleep until arterial blood gas results improve.
2 Ask a family member to stay with the client at all times.
3 Ask the physician for an order for succinylcholine.
4 Provide reassurance to the client and give small doses of morphine intravenously (IV) as prescribed.

Answer: 4

Rationale: The nurse always speaks to the client calmly and provides reassurance to the anxious client. Morphine is often prescribed for pain and anxiety for the client receiving mechanical ventilation.

Test-Taking Strategy: In option 1, the nurse does nothing to reassure or help the client, so it is incorrect. Family members are also stressed. It is not beneficial to ask the family to take on the burden of remaining with the client at all times. Succinylcholine (option 3) is a paralyzing agent but has no antianxiety properties. Thus option 4 is the answer to the question. The nurse communicates with the client to relieve anxiety and can provide the client with prescribed morphine, which alleviates anxiety while helping the client tolerate the ventilator.

Level of Cognitive Ability: Application
Phase of Nursing Process: Implementation
Client Needs: Psychosocial Integrity
Content Area: Adult Health/Respiratory

Reference

Smeltzer, S., & Bare, B. (1996). *Brunner and Suddarth's Textbook of medical-surgical nursing* (8th ed.). Philadelphia: Lippincott-Raven, p. 1917.

---

138. The nurse is assessing a confused elderly client admitted with a hip fracture. Which of the following data obtained by the nurse would not place the client at more risk for altered thought processes?

1 Stress induced by the fracture
2 Hearing aid available and in working order
3 Unfamiliar hospital setting
4 Eyeglasses left at home

Answer: 2

Rationale: Confusion in the elderly client with hip fracture could result from the unfamiliar hospital setting, stress caused by the fracture, concurrent systemic diseases, cerebral ischemia, or side effects of medications. Use of eyeglasses and hearing aids enhances the client's interaction with the environment and can reduce disorientation.

Test-Taking Strategy: The wording of the question asks you to look for an option that will keep the client at the highest possible level of functioning from a cognitive perspective. Stress from the fracture (option 1) and an unfamiliar setting (option 3) are not likely to help the client's functional level and are eliminated as possible choices. Both eyeglasses and hearing aids are useful adjuncts in communicating by a client. Because the eyeglasses were left at home, they are of no use at the current time. The working hearing aid is the answer to the question.

Level of Cognitive Ability: Analysis
Phase of Nursing Process: Assessment
Client Needs: Psychosocial Integrity
Content Area: Fundamental Skills

Reference

Smeltzer, S., & Bare, B. (1996). *Brunner and Suddarth's Textbook of medical-surgical nursing* (8th ed.). Philadelphia: Lippincott-Raven, p. 1930.

139. A client is admitted to the nursing unit after a left below-the-knee amputation that followed a crush injury to the foot and lower leg. The client tells the nurse, "I think I'm going crazy. I can feel my left foot itching." The nurse interprets the client's statement to be

1 A normal response and indicates the presence of phantom limb sensation.
2 A normal response and indicates the presence of phantom limb pain.
3 An abnormal response and indicates the client needs more psychological support.
4 An abnormal response and indicates the client is in denial about the limb loss.

Answer: 1

Rationale: Phantom limb sensations are felt in the area of the amputated limb. These can include itching, warmth, and cold. The sensations are caused by intact peripheral nerves in the area amputated. Whenever possible, clients should be prepared for these sensations. The client may also feel painful sensations in the amputated limb, called phantom limb pain. The origin of the pain is less understood, but the client should be prepared for this, too, whenever possible.

Test-Taking Strategy: Knowing that sensation and pain may be felt in the residual limb helps you to eliminate options 3 and 4 first, because the sensations are not abnormal responses. You would select option 1 over option 2 because the client has described an itching sensation but has not complained of pain in the residual limb.

Level of Cognitive Ability: Analysis
Phase of Nursing Process: Analysis
Client Needs: Psychosocial Integrity
Content Area: Adult Health/Neurological

Reference

Black, J., & Matassarin-Jacobs, E. (1997). *Medical-surgical nursing: Clinical management for continuity of care* (5th ed.). Philadelphia: W. B. Saunders, p. 1421.

140. The client who has had spinal fusion and insertion of hardware is extremely concerned with the perceived lengthy rehabilitation period. The client expresses concerns about finances and ability to return to prior employment. The nurse understands that the client's needs could best be addressed by referral to the

1 Surgeon.
2 Clinical nurse specialist.
3 Social worker.
4 Physical therapist.

Answer: 3

Rationale: After spinal surgery, concerns about finances and employment are best handled by referral to a social worker. This individual has the best well-rounded information about resources available to the client. The physical therapist has the best knowledge of techniques for increasing mobility and endurance. An occupational therapist would have knowledge of techniques for activities of daily living and items related to occupation, but this is not one of the options. The clinical nurse specialist and surgeon do not have information related to financial resources.

Test-Taking Strategy: An understanding of the roles of the various members of the health care team helps you to answer this question quickly and without hesitation. In fact, it is the need for information related to finances that is the real key to answering this question and points to the social worker as the optimal resource in this instance.

Level of Cognitive Ability: Analysis
Phase of Nursing Process: Analysis
Client Needs: Psychosocial Integrity
Content Area: Fundamental Skills

Reference

Black, J., & Matassarin-Jacobs, E. (1997). *Medical-surgical nursing: Clinical management for continuity of care* (5th ed.). Philadelphia: W. B. Saunders, p. 923.

141. The client who has experienced nonunion of a fracture is scheduled for bone grafting with cadaver bone. The client appears restless and anxious about the procedure. After determining that the client understands the surgical procedure, the nurse next explores

1 Concern about the level of postoperative pain.
2 Potential worry about hepatitis or HIV infection.
3 Whether the client needs a PRN order for an antianxiety agent.
4 The availability of assistance for the client upon discharge.

Answer: 2

Rationale: Clients who use cadaver bone can develop psychological problems as a result of worry about contracting HIV infection or hepatitis from the cadaver bone. Clients need reassurance and information about the donor screening that is done to ensure that this does not occur.

Test-Taking Strategy: Options 3 and 4 are the least likely options of the four available, so these are eliminated first. Both options 1 and 2 are realistic possibilities. Assessment of the level of pain that will be experienced in the postoperative period should be included as part of the basic preparation of the client for surgery. Knowing that a common concern is contracting disease from cadaver bone leads you to select this option over concern about postoperative pain. In addition, option 2 is specific to the information contained in the question.

Level of Cognitive Ability: Application
Phase of Nursing Process: Assessment
Client Needs: Psychosocial Integrity
Content Area: Adult Health/Musculoskeletal

Reference

Black, J., & Matassarin-Jacobs, E. (1997). *Medical-surgical nursing: Clinical management for continuity of care* (5th ed.). Philadelphia: W. B. Saunders, pp. 2145–2146.

142. The client is fearful about having an arm cast removed. Which of the following actions by the nurse would be the most helpful?

1 Telling the client that the saw makes a frightening noise
2 Reassuring the client that no one has had an arm lacerated yet
3 Stating that the hot cutting blades cause burns only very rarely
4 Showing the client the cast cutter and explaining how it works

Answer: 4

Rationale: Because of misconceptions about the cast cutting blade, clients may be fearful of having a cast removed. The nurse should show the cast cutter to the client before it is used and explain that the client may feel heat, vibration, and pressure. The cast cutter resembles a small electric saw with a circular blade. The nurse should reassure the client that the blade does not cut like a saw but instead cuts the cast by vibrating side to side.

Test-Taking Strategy: Note that the question asks for the "most helpful" action, which tells you that more than one option may be partially or totally correct. Option 2 gives no information, although it may be well-intentioned, and is eliminated first. Options 1 and 3 give accurate information but are not reassuring. Option 4 gives the client the most reassurance because it best prepares the client for what will occur when the cast is removed.

Level of Cognitive Ability: Application
Phase of Nursing Process: Implementation
Client Needs: Psychosocial Integrity
Content Area: Adult Health/Musculoskeletal

Reference

Black, J., & Matassarin-Jacobs, E. (1997). *Medical-surgical nursing: Clinical management for continuity of care* (5th ed.). Philadelphia: W. B. Saunders, p. 2152.

143. The client has several fractures of the lower leg and has been placed in an external fixation device. The client is upset about the appearance of the leg, which is very edematous and misshapen. The nurse formulates which of the following nursing diagnoses for the client?

1 Body Image Disturbance
2 Activity Intolerance
3 Risk for Impaired Physical Mobility
4 Social Isolation

Answer: 1

Rationale: The client is at risk for body image disturbance related to a change in the structure and function of the affected leg. There are no data in the stem to support a diagnosis of Activity Intolerance or Social Isolation. The client does have actual impaired mobility because of the fixation device.

Test-Taking Strategy: The key words in the stem include "external fixation device," "edematous," and "misshapen." In view of these descriptions, the defining characteristics for Body Image Disturbance match most readily. The only other option that is plausible given the information in the stem is Impaired Physical Mobility. However, this is an actual problem for the client, whereas option 3 identifies this as a risk diagnosis, and thus option 3 is incorrect.

Level of Cognitive Ability: Analysis
Phase of Nursing Process: Analysis
Client Needs: Psychosocial Integrity
Content Area: Adult Health/Musculoskeletal

Reference

Ignatavicius, D. D., Workman, M. L., & Mishler, M. A. (1995). *Medical-surgical nursing: A nursing process approach* (2nd ed.). Philadelphia: W. B. Saunders, p. 1464.

---

144. The client with narcolepsy has been prescribed dextroamphetamine (Dexedrine). The client complains to the nurse that the client cannot sleep well anymore at night and does not want to take the medication any longer. Before making any specific comment, the nurse plans to investigate whether the client takes the medication at which of the following proper time schedules?

1 At least 6 hours before bedtime
2 Two hours before bedtime
3 After supper each night
4 Just before going to sleep

Answer: 1

Rationale: Dextroamphetamine is a CNS stimulant that acts by releasing norepinephrine from nerve endings. To prevent disturbances with sleep, the client should take the medication at least 6 hours before going to bed at night.

Test-Taking Strategy: To answer this question successfully, you should remember that this medication causes CNS stimulation. This medication effect interferes with sleep. Knowing this, you would evaluate each of the options in terms of how far removed the scheduled dose is from the client's bedtime. Evaluating the question in this manner helps you eliminate each of the other incorrect options easily.

Level of Cognitive Ability: Application
Phase of Nursing Process: Planning
Client Needs: Psychosocial Integrity
Content Area: Pharmacology

Reference

Deglin, J., & Vallerand, A. (1997). *Davis's drug guide for nurses* (5th ed.). Philadelphia: F. A. Davis, pp. 339, 341.

145. The client was just told by the primary care physician that the client will have an exercise stress test to evaluate status after recent episodes of more severe chest pain. As the nurse enters the examining room, the client states, "Maybe I shouldn't bother going. I wonder if I should just take more medication instead." The nurse's best response would be

1 "Can you tell me more about how you're feeling?"
2 "Don't worry. Emergency equipment is available if it should be needed."
3 "Most people tolerate the procedure well without any complications."
4 "Don't you really want to control your heart disease?"

Answer: 1

Rationale: Anxiety and fear are often present before stress testing. The nurse uses questioning as a communication method to explore the client's feelings and concerns.

Test-Taking Strategy: Options 2 and 3 are statements, not questions, and therefore limit communication, so eliminate them first. The correct answer is open-ended and is the only option that is phrased to engender trust and sharing of concerns by the client.

Level of Cognitive Ability: Application
Phase of Nursing Process: Implementation
Client Needs: Psychosocial Integrity
Content Area: Adult Health/Cardiovascular

Reference

Potter, P., & Perry, A. (1997). *Fundamentals of nursing: Concepts, process, and practice* (4th ed.). St. Louis: Mosby–Year Book, pp. 241–242.

146. The nurse is giving the client with left-sided heart failure home care instructions for use after hospital discharge. The client interrupts, saying, "What's the use? I'll never remember all of this, and I'll probably die anyway!" The nurse interprets that the client's response is most likely a result of

1 The teaching strategies used by the nurse.
2 Anger about the new medical regimen.
3 Insufficient financial resources to pay for the medications.
4 Anxiety about the ability to manage the disease process at home.

Answer: 4

Rationale: Anxiety often develops after heart failure. The fear of death can persist, and there is often a long, difficult period of adjustment. Anxiety and fear further tax the failing heart. The nurse should take time to explore the concerns and fears of the client.

Test-Taking Strategy: The client's statement comes suddenly in the middle of receiving self-care instructions. There is no evidence in the stem to support options 1 or 3. Note the key phrase "I'll never remember all this" in the question. This key phrase should easily direct you to option 4.

Level of Cognitive Ability: Analysis
Phase of Nursing Process: Analysis
Client Needs: Psychosocial Integrity
Content Area: Adult Health/Cardiovascular

Reference

Black, J., & Matassarin-Jacobs, E. (1997). *Medical-surgical nursing: Clinical management for continuity of care* (5th ed.). Philadelphia: W. B. Saunders, p. 1289.

147. Before initiating intravenous (IV) therapy, the nurse notes nonverbal signs of anxiety in the client. In order to help relieve client anxiety, the nurse should explain the procedure of IV initiation. Which of the following would be most appropriate for the nurse to say to the client?

1 "I'll be starting an IV line that will add fluid directly to your blood stream."
2 "I will be starting an IV line, and it should not hurt much."
3 "A No. 18 angiocatheter will be inserted into your arm so fluid can be administered."
4 "Try not to worry. This procedure won't take long and will be over with before you know it."

Answer: 1

Rationale: The first option is correct in that it explains what an IV line is in simple terms. The second option contains incorrect information and gives the client unwarranted reassurance, inasmuch as initiating an IV can be painful. The term "No. 18 gauge angiocatheter" is medical and may not be understood by the client. Suggesting that the client not worry is a cliché and blocks client communication of fears and feelings.

Test-Taking Strategy: Remember that the basics of good communication include avoiding the use of medical jargon and terminology that clients may not understand. Always avoid responses that will block communication. Never use a response that avoids or downplays a client's feelings or concerns, and always be truthful with information given to clients, avoiding unwarranted and false reassurance. Using these communication principles will assist in directing you to the correct option!

Level of Cognitive Ability: Analysis
Phase of Nursing Process: Implementation
Client Needs: Psychosocial Integrity
Content Area: Fundamental Skills

Reference

Potter, P., & Perry, A. (1997). *Fundamentals of nursing: Concepts, process, and practice* (4th ed.). St. Louis: Mosby–Year Book, pp. 240–246.

---

148. A client scheduled for an implanted catheter for intermittent chemotherapy treatments says, "I'm not sure if I can handle having a tube coming out of me all the time. What will my friends think?" Which of the following should the nurse plan to do first?

1 Show the client various central line tubes and catheters
2 Explain that an implanted port is not visible under the skin
3 Notify the physician of the client's concerns
4 Explain that the client's friends probably will not see the tube under the clothing

Answer: 2

Rationale: What the client says in the scenario shows that the client needs to be educated about the implanted port. An implanted port is placed under the skin and is not visible. There is no tubing coming out. Tubing is used only when the port is accessed intermittently and the IV line is connected. Showing the client various other tubes will not be beneficial because the client will not be using them. It is premature to notify the physician. Option 4 does not correct the client's confusion regarding the implanted port.

Test-Taking Strategy: Read the case situation carefully to understand that client education is the issue of the question. Knowledge of implanted catheters is essential in answering this question. Review the concepts related to implanted catheters and the teaching/learning process now if you had difficulty with this question!

Level of Cognitive Ability: Application
Phase of Nursing Process: Planning
Client Needs: Psychosocial Integrity
Content Area: Fundamental Skills

Reference

Phillips, L. (1997). *Manual of IV therapeutics* (2nd ed.). Philadelphia: F. A. Davis, p. 418.

149. A client displays signs of anxiety. When explaining to the client that the intravenous (IV) line will need to be discontinued because of an infiltration, the nurse should say which of the following?

1 "This will be a totally painless experience. It is nothing to worry about."
2 "I'm sure it will be a real relief for you just as soon as I discontinue this IV for good."
3 "Just relax and take a deep breath. This procedure will not take long and will be over soon."
4 "I can see that you're anxious. Removal of the IV shouldn't be painful; however, the IV will need to be restarted in another location."

Answer: 4

Rationale: Although discontinuing an IV line is a painless experience, it is not therapeutic to tell a client not to worry. Option 2 does not acknowledge the client's feelings and does not tell the client that an infiltrated IV line will need to be restarted. Option 3 does not address the client's feelings. The correct option addresses the client's anxiety and honestly informs the client that the IV line will need to be restarted. This option uses the therapeutic technique of giving information, as well as acknowledging the client's feelings.

Test-Taking Strategy: When answering communication questions, remember to use therapeutic techniques. Avoid choices with communication blocks such as placing a client's feelings on hold or devaluing the client's feelings. Also, avoid clichés and giving false reassurance. Always focus on the client's feelings.

Level of Cognitive Ability: Analysis
Phase of Nursing Process: Implementation
Client Needs: Psychosocial Integrity
Content Area: Fundamental Skills

Reference
Potter, P., & Perry, A. (1997). *Fundamentals of nursing: Concepts, process, and practice* (4th ed.). St. Louis: Mosby–Year Book, pp. 240–246.

---

150. A toddler with suspected conjunctivitis is crying and refuses to sit still during the eye examination. Which of the following is the most appropriate nursing statement to the child?

1 "If you will sit still, the exam will be over soon."
2 "Would you like to see my flashlight?"
3 "I know you are upset. We can do this exam later."
4 "Don't be scared, the light won't hurt you."

Answer: 2

Rationale: Fears in this age group can be decreased by getting the child actively involved in the examination. Option 1 gives advice and ignores the client's feelings. Option 3, although acknowledging feelings, puts off the inevitable. Option 4 tells the child how to feel.

Test-Taking Strategy: Use knowledge regarding the stages of growth and development to answer the question. Note that the child is a toddler. Using the child's developmental level and the techniques of communication, you can easily be directed to the correct option. Review growth and development in relation to the toddler now if you had difficulty with this question!

Level of Cognitive Ability: Analysis
Phase of Nursing Process: Implementation
Client Needs: Psychosocial Integrity
Content Area: Child Health

Reference
Ashwill, J., & Droske, S. (1997). *Nursing care of children: Principles and practice.* Philadelphia: W. B. Saunders, p. 206.

---

151. The client with acute pyelonephritis is scheduled for a voiding cystourethrogram. The client is timid by nature. The nurse interprets that this client would most likely benefit from increased support and teaching about the procedure because

1 Radiopaque contrast is injected into the blood stream.
2 Radioactive material is inserted into the bladder.
3 The client must lie on an x-ray table in a cold, barren room.
4 The client must void while the micturition process is filmed.

Answer: 4

Rationale: Having to void in the presence of others can be very embarrassing for clients and may actually interfere with the client's ability to void. The nurse teaches the client about the procedure to try to minimize stress from lack of preparation and gives the client encouragement and emotional support. Screens may be used in the radiology department to try to provide a modicum of privacy during this procedure.

Test-Taking Strategy: Begin to answer this question by eliminating options 1 and 2, because the contrast material is inserted into the bladder by means of a catheter. To discriminate between options 3 and 4, you must know that the client has to void to allow filming of the movement of urine through the lower urinary tract. Review this procedure now if you had difficulty with this question!

Level of Cognitive Ability: Analysis
Phase of Nursing Process: Analysis
Client Needs: Psychosocial Integrity
Content Area: Adult Health/Renal

Reference

Black, J., & Matassarin-Jacobs, E. (1997). *Medical-surgical nursing: Clinical management for continuity of care* (5th ed.). Philadelphia: W. B. Saunders, pp. 1564, 1629.

---

152. The nurse shares with the psychiatrist that he or she thinks that a severely depressed client would benefit greatly from electroconvulsive therapy (ECT). This assessment is valid because

1 ECT provides the most rapid relief of any treatment for severe depression.
2 The client has not been started on any medications.
3 The client is well nourished.
4 The client is not suicidal.

Answer: 1

Rationale: Option 1 is a true statement. Option 2 is incorrect because medications should be attempted before trying ECT. Most severely ill clients who fail to respond to medications respond to ECT. Clients at high risk for malnutrition are good candidates for ECT. Suicidal clients are equally good candidates for ECT.

Test-Taking Strategy: To answer this question correctly, you need to apply characteristics of clients that make them the best candidates for ECT. Option 1 is the only correct option. Note the relationship between depression in the question and in the correct option. Review ECT now if you had difficulty with this question!

Level of Cognitive Ability: Application
Phase of Nursing Process: Assessment
Client Needs: Psychosocial Integrity
Content Area: Mental Health

Reference

Carson, V., & Arnold, E. (1996). *Mental health nursing: The nurse-patient journey.* Philadelphia: W. B. Saunders, p. 785.

---

153. The female client in a manic state emerges from her room. She is topless and is making sexual remarks and gestures toward staff and peers. The best initial nursing response is

1 Quietly approach the client, escort her to her room and assist her in getting dressed.
2 Approach the client in the hallway and insist that she go to her room.
3 Confront the client on the inappropriateness of her behaviors and offer her a time-out.
4 Ask the other clients to ignore her behavior; eventually she will return to her room.

Answer: 1

Rationale: A person who is experiencing mania lacks insight and judgment, has poor impulse control, and is highly excitable. The nurse must take control without creating increased stress or anxiety in the client. A quiet, firm approach while distracting the client (walking her to her room and assisting her to get dressed) achieves the goal of having her dressed appropriately and preserving her psychosocial integrity.

Test-Taking Strategy: The goal of the interaction is to have the client dress appropriately. Option 4 is immediately discarded as a selection. Although options 1, 2, and 3 are all similar, "insisting" that the client go to her room may meet with a great deal of resistance, and confronting the client and offering her a consequence of "time-out" may be meaningless to her.

Level of Cognitive Ability: Application
Level of Nursing Process: Implementation
Client Needs: Psychosocial Integrity
Content Area: Mental Health

Reference

Varcarolis, E. M. (1998). *Foundations of psychiatric mental health nursing* (3rd ed.). Philadelphia: W. B. Saunders, pp. 600–604, 606–607.

154. The client underwent cardiac surgery 48 hours ago. The client is disoriented, believes the nurse is a cousin, and stated there were ants crawling on the wall. The nurse reports to the oncoming shift nurse that this client is experiencing signs and symptoms consistent with

1 Postcardiotomy syndrome.
2 Dressler's syndrome.
3 Cerebrovascular insufficiency.
4 Neurosis.

Answer: 1

Rationale: Postcardiotomy syndrome may result from anxiety, sleep deprivation, sensory overload, and interruption of day-night pattern. Symptoms include perceptual distortions, hallucinations, disorientation, and paranoid delusions. Dressler's syndrome is a form of pericarditis that occurs after myocardial infarction. Cerebrovascular insufficiency would be marked by signs and symptoms similar to transient ischemic attacks (TIAs). A neurosis is a faulty or inefficient way of coping with a stressor.

Test-Taking Strategy: Knowledge regarding the complications associated with cardiac surgery is necessary to answer this question. Note the relationship between "underwent cardiac" and "postcardiotomy." This should assist in directing you to option 1.

Level of Cognitive Ability: Application
Phase of Nursing Process: Assessment
Client Needs: Psychosocial Integrity
Content Area: Adult Health/Cardiovascular

Reference

Black, J., & Matassarin-Jacobs, E. (1997). *Medical-surgical nursing: Clinical management for continuity of care* (5th ed.). Philadelphia: W. B. Saunders, p. 1267.

155. Both the client, who had cardiac surgery, and the family express anxiety about how to cope with the recuperative process once they are home alone after discharge. The nurse would plan to tell the client and family about which available resource?

1 Local library
2 United Way
3 American Heart Association Mended Heart's Club
4 American Cancer Society Reach for Recovery

Answer: 3

Rationale: Most clients and families benefit from knowing that there are available resources to help them cope with the stress of self-care management at home. These can include telephone contact with the surgeon, cardiologist, and nurse; cardiac rehabilitation programs; and community support groups such as the American Heart Association Mended Hearts Club (a nationwide program with local chapters).

Test-Taking Strategy: Of the four options, three list organizations and one is a library. Eliminate the library first because the client and family need resources to cope, which implies the need for interactive processes. Focusing on the type of surgery addressed in the question will easily direct you to option 3.

Level of Cognitive Ability: Application
Phase of Nursing Process: Planning
Client Needs: Psychosocial Integrity
Content Area: Adult Health/Cardiovascular

Reference

Smeltzer, S., & Bare, B. (1996). *Brunner and Suddarth's Textbook of medical-surgical nursing* (8th ed.). Philadelphia: Lippincott-Raven, p. 716.

156. The elderly client who has never been hospitalized before is ordered to have a 12-lead electrocardiogram (ECG). The nurse could best plan to alleviate the client's anxiety by giving which of the following explanations?

1 "The ECG can give the doctor information about what might be wrong with your heart."
2 "It's important to lie still during the procedure."
3 "It should only take about 20 minutes to complete the ECG tracings."
4 "The ECG electrodes are painless and will record the electrical activity of the heart."

Answer: 4

Rationale: The ECG involves the use of painless electrodes, which are applied to the chest and limbs. It takes less than 5 minutes to complete and requires the client to lie still. The ECG measures the heart's electrical activity to determine rate, rhythm, and a variety of abnormalities.

Test-Taking Strategy: Option 3 is an incorrect statement and is eliminated first. Of those remaining, options 1 and 2 are factual statements, but they are not stated to reduce anxiety. Option 4 is the only statement constructed to be reassuring to the client.

Level of Cognitive Ability: Application
Phase of Nursing Process: Planning
Client Needs: Psychosocial Integrity
Content Area: Adult Health/Cardiovascular

Reference

Potter, P., & Perry, A. (1997). *Fundamentals of nursing: Concepts, process, and practice* (4th ed.). St. Louis: Mosby–Year Book, p. 1390.

---

157. The spouse of a client scheduled for insertion of an automatic implantable cardioverter-defibrillator (AICD) expresses anxiety about what would happen if the device discharges during physical contact. The nurse would plan to tell the spouse that

1 Physical contact should be avoided whenever possible.
2 A warning device sounds before countershock so there is time to move away.
3 The spouse would not feel or be harmed by the countershock.
4 The shock would be felt, but it would not cause the spouse any harm.

Answer: 4

Rationale: Clients and families are often fearful about activation of the AICD. Their fears are about the device itself and also the occurrence of life-threatening dysrhythmias that trigger its function. Family members need reassurance that even if the device activates while they are touching the client, the level of the charge is not high enough to harm the family member, although it will be felt. The AICD emits a warning beep when the client is near magnetic fields, which could possibly deactivate it, but does not beep before countershock.

Test-Taking Strategy: This question is difficult to answer without knowledge of the device. However, of the four choices, options 1 and 2 are the least likely, and so these should be eliminated first. Of the two remaining choices, option 4 is the more plausible one, if you reflect on each of those options. Review the concepts related to this device now if you had difficulty with this question!

Level of Cognitive Ability: Application
Phase of Nursing Process: Planning
Client Needs: Psychosocial Integrity
Content Area: Adult Health/Cardiovascular

Reference

Ignatavicius, D. D., Workman, M. L., & Mishler, M. A. (1995). *Medical-surgical nursing: A nursing process approach* (2nd ed.). Philadelphia: W. B. Saunders, p. 884.

158. The client who is scheduled for permanent transvenous pacemaker insertion says to the nurse, "I know I need it, but I'm not sure this surgery is the best idea." Which of the following responses will best help the nurse assess the client's preoperative concerns?

1. "Has anyone taught you about the procedure yet?"
2. "You sound concerned about the procedure. Can you tell me more about what has you concerned?"
3. "You sound unnecessarily worried. Has anyone told you that the technology is quite advanced now?"
4. "How does your family feel about the surgery?"

Answer: 2

Rationale: Anxiety is common in the client with the need for pacemaker insertion. This can be related to fear of life-threatening dysrhythmias or related to the surgical procedure. The nurse must use communication techniques that will help the client identify the source of anxiety and discuss specific concerns.

Test-Taking Strategy: The question is really asking for the communication strategy that will best help identify the client's concerns. Eliminate options 1 and 3 because they are closed-ended and not exploratory. Option 4 is not indicated because it asks about the family and deflects attention from the client's concerns. Option 2 is correct because it is open-ended and uses clarification as a communication technique to explore the client's concerns.

Level of Cognitive Ability: Application
Phase of Nursing Process: Assessment
Client Needs: Psychosocial Integrity
Content Area: Adult Health/Cardiovascular

Reference

Black, J., & Matassarin-Jacobs, E. (1997). *Medical-surgical nursing: Clinical management for continuity of care* (5th ed.). Philadelphia: W. B. Saunders, p. 1322.

---

159. The client with superficial varicose veins says to the nurse, "I hate these things. They're so ugly. I wish I could get them to go away." The nurse's best response would be

1. "You should try sclerotherapy. It's great."
2. "What have you been told about varicose veins and their management?"
3. "There's not much you can do once you get them."
4. "I understand how you feel, but you know, they really don't look too bad."

Answer: 2

Rationale: The client is expressing distress about physical appearance and has a risk for body image disturbance. The nurse assesses self-management of the condition as a means of empowering the client, which ultimately can help in adapting to the body change.

Test-Taking Strategy: With questions that deal with client's feelings, look for options that facilitate sharing of information and concerns by the client. In this question, all of the incorrect choices cut off or limit further comments by the client, as well-intentioned as some of them may be. In addition, option 2 is worded to gather assessment data.

Level of Cognitive Ability: Application
Phase of Nursing Process: Assessment
Client Needs: Psychosocial Integrity
Content Area: Adult Health/Cardiovascular

Reference

Cox, H., Hinz, M., Lubno, M., et al. (1997). *Clinical applications of nursing diagnosis: Adult, child, women's, psychiatric, gerontic, and home health considerations* (3rd ed.). Philadelphia: F. A. Davis, p. 507.

---

160. The client says to the nurse, "My obstetrician has just told me I'm going to deliver several babies. It looks like there are five of them!" The most therapeutic response by the nurse is

1. "Congratulations! You and your husband must be very excited!"
2. "Way to go, girl! You and your husband better get some 'R and R' now!"
3. "Oh, how wonderful! You must be on Cloud Nine!"
4. "Oh, my. How are you, your husband, and families feeling?"

Answer: 4

Rationale: The client has just been informed that she is expecting not one but five babies. You have learned that both positive and negative life events create anxiety. In option 4, the nurse asks an open-ended question that will allow the client to verbalize feelings without fear of being judged.

Test-Taking Strategy: This question tests your knowledge of the appropriate therapeutic communication technique to employ to allow clients to ventilate feelings. In option 1, the nurse gives a response that conforms to social norms but also gives approval, which might prevent the client from vocalizing negative responses. Option 2 is another cliché response that confers approval and again might prevent the client from verbalizing negative responses. In addition, the humor of the remark is fairly indiscriminate. Option 3 is another social response that would not facilitate the client's expression of feelings, concerns, or anxieties.

Level of Cognitive Ability: Application
Phase of Nursing Process: Implementation
Client Needs: Psychosocial Integrity
Content Area: Maternity

Reference

Antai-Otong, D. (1995). *Psychiatric nursing: Biological and behavioral concepts.* Philadelphia: W. B. Saunders, pp. 543–576.

---

161. A client who has been diagnosed with chronic renal failure has been told that hemodialysis will be required. The client becomes angry and withdrawn and states, "I'll never be the same now." The nurse formulates which of the following nursing diagnoses for this client?

1 Altered Thought Processes
2 Body Image Disturbance
3 Anxiety
4 Noncompliance

Answer: 2

Rationale: The client with any renal disorder, such as renal failure, may become angry and depressed as a result of the permanence of the alteration. Because of the physical change and the change in lifestyle that may be necessary to manage a severe renal condition, the client may experience body image disturbance.

Test-Taking Strategy: Options 1 and 4 are eliminated first, because the client is not cognitively impaired (option 1) or refusing to undergo therapy (option 4). To discriminate between the last two, note that the client's statement focuses on self, which is consistent with Body Image Disturbance. You would select this option over Anxiety because the client is able to identify the cause of concern.

Level of Cognitive Ability: Analysis
Phase of Nursing Process: Analysis
Client Needs: Psychosocial Integrity
Content Area: Adult Health/Renal

Reference

Black, J., & Matassarin-Jacobs, E. (1997). *Medical-surgical nursing: Clinical management for continuity of care* (5th ed.). Philadelphia: W. B. Saunders, p. 1552.

---

162. The nurse observes the client, who is recovering from cardiogenic shock secondary to an anterior myocardial infarction, crying silently. What action by the nurse would best explore the client's feelings?

1 Enter the room and stand quietly at the bedside
2 Sit by the client and discuss the news of the day
3 Sit quietly by the client
4 Assure the client that the condition will improve

Answer: 3

Rationale: Sitting quietly by the client conveys caring and acceptance. Therapeutic communication techniques assist with flow of communication and always focus on the client.

Test-Taking Strategy: Option 1 may or may not encourage the client to ventilate feelings. Options 2 and 4 do not address the client's feelings and ignore the client's behavior.

Level of Cognitive Ability: Analysis
Phase of Nursing Process: Assessment
Client Needs: Psychosocial Integrity
Content Area: Adult Health/Cardiovascular

Reference

Smith, S., & Duell, D. (1996). *Clinical nursing skills* (4th ed.). Stamford, CT: Appleton & Lange, p. 66.

163. A client with the diagnosis of hyperparathyroidism says to the nurse, "I can't stay on this diet. It is too difficult for me." When intervening in this situation, the nurse should respond

1. "It is very important that you stay on this diet to avoid forming renal calculi."
2. "It really isn't difficult to stick to this diet. Just avoid milk products."
3. "Why do you think you find this diet plan difficult to adhere to?"
4. "You are having a difficult time staying on this plan. Let's discuss this."

Answer: 4

Rationale: By paraphrasing this client's statement, the nurse can encourage the client to reveal emotions. The nurse also sends feedback to the client that the message was understood. An open-ended statement or question such as this prompts an informative response.

Test-Taking Strategy: For communication questions, communication blocks are incorrect answers. Option 1 is giving advice, which cuts off communication. Option 2 devalues the client's feelings. Option 3 is requesting information that the client may not be able to express.

Level of Cognitive Ability: Application
Phase of Nursing Process: Implementation
Client Needs: Psychosocial Integrity
Content Area: Adult Health/Endocrine

Reference

Potter, P., & Perry, A. (1997). *Fundamentals of nursing: Concepts, process, and practice* (4th ed.). St. Louis: Mosby–Year Book, pp. 242–246.

---

164. A nurse is caring for a client with newly diagnosed type 1 diabetes. In order to develop an effective teaching plan, it would be most important to assess this client for

1. The client's knowledge of the diabetic diet.
2. The expressions of denial of having diabetes.
3. Fear of performing insulin administration.
4. Feeling depressed about lifestyle changes.

Answer: 2

Rationale: When diabetes is first discovered, the client usually goes through the phases of grief: denial, fear, anger, bargaining, depression, and acceptance. Denial is the phase that is the most detrimental to the teaching/learning process. If the client is denying the fact that he or she has diabetes, the client probably will not listen to discussions about the disease or how to manage it. Denial must be identified before the nurse can develop a teaching plan.

Test-Taking Strategy: All of the options may be appropriate to assess; however, note that options 1, 3, and 4 are related to very specific components of the teaching. Option 2 is the most global, and in view of the principles of teaching and learning, this aspect needs to be assessed before the implementation of teaching.

Level of Cognitive Ability: Application
Phase of Nursing Process: Assessment
Client Needs: Psychosocial Integrity
Content Area: Adult Health/Endocrine

Reference

Potter, P., & Perry, A. (1997). *Fundamentals of nursing: Concepts, process, and practice* (4th ed.). St. Louis: Mosby–Year Book, p. 377.

165. When planning an education program for a client taking conjugated estrogen (Premarin), the nurse plans to address psychosocial adaptation by including which of the following pieces of information?

1 The client should notify the physician if migraine headaches occur
2 Premarin may cause mood and affect changes, and the medication may need to be discontinued if depression occurs
3 Estrogen should be used with caution by clients with a family history of breast or reproductive cancer
4 Premarin may cause hyperglycemia, and the client needs to be informed of signs/symptoms to report to the physician

Answer: 2

Rationale: Conjugated estrogen can cause changes in client affect, mood, and behavior. Aggression and/or depression can also occur. Options 1, 3, and 4 are correct but address physiological needs. Option 2 is the only psychological need noted.

Test-Taking Strategy: Identify the key word "psychosocial" in the stem of the question. Then read all four options and eliminate the options that address physiological issues, not psychosocial. Even if you do not know the side effects of Premarin, you can correctly answer this question by using this strategy.

Level of Cognitive Ability: Application
Phase of Nursing Process: Planning
Client Needs: Psychosocial Integrity
Content Area: Pharmacology

Reference
Hodgson, B., & Kizior, R. (1998). *Saunders nursing drug handbook 1998.* Philadelphia: W. B. Saunders, pp. 255–257.

166. The client with newly diagnosed diabetes mellitus type I has been seen for 3 consecutive days in the emergency department with hyperglycemia. While undergoing the physical assessment, the client says to the nurse, "I'm sorry to keep bothering you every day, but I just can't give myself those awful shots." The nurse's best response is

1 "You must learn to give yourself the shots."
2 "I couldn't give myself a shot either."
3 "I'm sorry you are having trouble with your injections. Has someone given you instructions on them?"
4 "Let me see if the doctor can change your medication."

Answer: 3

Rationale: It is important to determine and deal with a client's underlying fear of self-injection. The nurse should determine whether a knowledge deficit exists. Scare tactics should not be used. Positive reinforcement is necessary instead of focusing on negative behaviors. The nurse should not offer a change in regimen that can't be accomplished.

Test-Taking Strategy: Focus on communication tools and the issue of the question. Options 1 and 2 are not therapeutic, and option 4 may give false reassurance of a change in medication. Option 3 focuses on the issue of the question and is the therapeutic response.

Level of Cognitive Ability: Application
Phase of Nursing Process: Implementation
Client Needs: Psychosocial Integrity
Content Area: Adult Health/Endocrine

Reference
Potter, P., & Perry, A. (1997). *Fundamentals of nursing: Concepts, process, and practice* (4th ed.). St. Louis: Mosby–Year Book, pp. 240–254.

167. The nurse requests that the diabetic client ask his or her significant other(s) to attend an educational conference on self-administration of insulin. The client questions why significant others need to be included. The nurse's best response would be

1 "Clients and families often work together to develop strategies for the management of diabetes."
2 "Family members can take you to the doctor."
3 "Family members are at risk for developing diabetes."
4 "Nurses need someone to call and check on a client's progress."

Answer: 1

Rationale: Families and/or significant others may be included in diabetes education to assist with adjustment to the diabetic regimen.

Test-Taking Strategy: Use the process of elimination. Although options 2 and 3 may be accurate, they are not the most appropriate responses in relation to the issue of the question. Option 4 devalues the client, disregards the issue of independence, and promotes powerlessness.

Level of Cognitive Ability: Application
Phase of Nursing Process: Implementation
Client Needs: Psychosocial Integrity
Content Area: Adult Health/Endocrine

Reference
Potter, P., & Perry, A. (1997). *Fundamentals of nursing: Concepts, process, and practice* (4th ed.). St. Louis: Mosby–Year Book, pp. 240–254.

168. A 22-year-old female client has recently received a diagnosis of polycystic kidney disease. The nurse has a series of discussions with the client that are intended to help her adjust to the disorder. The nurse would plan to include which of the following items as part of one of these discussions?

1 Ongoing fluid restriction
2 Depression about massive edema
3 Risk of hypotensive episodes
4 Need for genetic counseling

Answer: 4

Rationale: Adult polycystic disease is a hereditary disorder that is inherited as an autosomal dominant trait. Because of this, the client should have genetic counseling, as should the extended family. Ongoing fluid restriction is unnecessary. Massive edema is not part of the clinical picture for this disorder. The client is likely to have hypertension, not hypotension.

Test-Taking Strategy: Because massive edema and the need for fluid restriction are not part of the clinical picture for the client with polycystic kidney disease, options 1 and 2 are eliminated first as possible answers. To choose correctly between options 3 and 4, you would need to know either that this disorder is hereditary in nature or that the client would exhibit hypertension, not hypotension. Knowing either of these pieces of information would enable you to choose correctly between these two remaining options.

Level of Cognitive Ability: Application
Phase of Nursing Process: Planning
Client Needs: Psychosocial Integrity
Content Area: Adult Health/Renal

Reference

Black, J., & Matassarin-Jacobs, E. (1997). *Medical-surgical nursing: Clinical management for continuity of care* (5th ed.). Philadelphia: W. B. Saunders, pp. 1678–1679.

---

169. The nurse is admitting a client who is to undergo ureterolithotomy for urinary calculi removal. The nurse would not include which of the following assessments in determining the client's readiness for surgery?

1 Understanding of surgical procedure
2 Knowledge of postoperative activities
3 Feelings or anxieties about the surgical procedure
4 Need for a visit from a support group

Answer: 4

Rationale: Ureterolithotomy is removal of a calculus from the ureter through either a flank or abdominal incision. Because no urinary diversion is created during this procedure, the client has no need for a visit from a member of a support group. The client should have an understanding of the same items as for any surgery, which includes knowledge of the procedures, expected outcome, and postoperative routines and discomfort. The client should also be assessed for any concerns or anxieties before surgery.

Test-Taking Strategy: The wording of the question guides you to select an assessment that is either incorrect or unnecessary. Eliminate options 1 and 3 first because both are indicated assessments in the preoperative period. Knowing that this procedure does not involve urinary diversion helps you choose option 4 over option 2 as the correct answer. The client does need to know about postoperative activities but does not need a visit from a support group.

Level of Cognitive Ability: Application
Phase of Nursing Process: Assessment
Client Needs: Psychosocial Integrity
Content Area: Adult Health/Renal

Reference

Black, J., & Matassarin-Jacobs, E. (1997). *Medical-surgical nursing: Clinical management for continuity of care* (5th ed.). Philadelphia: W. B. Saunders, p. 1597.

170. Which of the following therapeutic communication skills would be the most therapeutic if a dying client's husband says to the nurse, "I don't think I can come anymore and watch her die. It's 'chewing me up' too much!"?

1 "I wish you'd focus on your wife's pain rather than yours. I know it's hard, but this isn't about what's happening to you, you know."
2 "I know it's hard for you, but she would know if you're not there, and you'd feel guilty all the rest of your days."
3 "It's hard to watch someone you love die. You've been here with your wife every day. Are you taking any time for yourself?"
4 "I think you're making the right decision. Your wife knows you love her. You don't have to come. I'll take care of her."

Answer: 3

Rationale: The husband is the client of this question. The most therapeutic response is the one that reflects the nurse's understanding of the client's stress and emotional pain. The nurse observes the client's caring and suggests that the client take time for himself, which is simply an act of symbolically "giving permission." This can be helpful to clients who have punishing egos.

Test-Taking Strategy: This question tests your knowledge of the therapeutic communication skills to employ for a caregiver who is experiencing stress. Option 1 is an example of a nontherapeutic, judgmental attitude. Option 2 makes statements that the nurse cannot know are true (the wife may, in fact, not know whether the husband visits) and predicting guilt feelings is not appropriate. Option 4 is inappropriate because it fosters dependency and gives advice, which is nontherapeutic.

Level of Cognitive Ability: Analysis
Phase of Nursing Process: Implementation
Client Needs: Psychosocial Integrity
Content Area: Fundamental Skills

Reference
Antai-Otong, D. (1995). *Psychiatric nursing: Biological and behavioral concepts.* Philadelphia: W. B. Saunders, pp. 543–576.

171. The elderly client at the retirement center spits her food out, throws it on the floor at the Thanksgiving dinner in the community dining room, and yells, "This turkey is dry and cold! I can't stand the food here!" Which of the following would be the most therapeutic communication response by the nurse?

1 "Let me get you another serving that is more to your liking. Would you like to come visit the chef and select your own serving?"
2 "I think you had better return to your apartment, where a new meal will be served to you there."
3 "Now look what you've done! You're ruining this meal for the whole community. Aren't you ashamed of yourself?"
4 "One of the things that the residents of this group agreed was that anyone who did not use appropriate behavior would be asked to leave the dining room. Please leave now."

Answer: 1

Rationale: Selecting the most therapeutic response is difficult here. Although the nurse may feel annoyed that this client is behaving inappropriately, the most professional response is to realize that the behavior stems from some troubled feelings with which the client is struggling. The chief concern of the nurse must be to assist all the clients in the dining room. If the nurse orders the angry client out of the dining room, it might provoke another "temper tantrum," which would increase what must already be uncomfortable feelings on the part of the group in the dining room. Asking the client to accompany the nurse to the kitchen respects the client's need for control, removes the angry client from the dining room, and may offer the nurse an opportunity to assess what is happening to the client.

Test-Taking Strategy: This question tests your knowledge of the therapeutic communication technique for clients who are explosive and behave inappropriately. Option 2 could provoke a regressive struggle between the nurse and client and cause more explosive behavior on the client's part. Option 3 is angry, aggressive, nontherapeutic communication and is humiliating to the client. In option 4, the nurse is authoritative, but trying to expel the client would not be appropriate, and it might set up an aggressive struggle between the nurse and the client.

Level of Cognitive Ability: Analysis
Phase of Nursing Process: Implementation
Client Needs: Psychosocial Integrity
Content Area: Fundamental Skills

Reference
Antai-Otong, D. (1995). *Psychiatric nursing: Biological and behavioral concepts.* Philadelphia: W. B. Saunders, pp. 543–576.

172. The physician orders a follow-up visit for an elderly client with emphysema. When the community health nurse arrives, the client is smoking. Which of the following statements, if made by the nurse, would be most therapeutic?

1. "Well, I can see you never got to the Stop Smoking clinic!"
2. "I notice that you are smoking. Did you explore the Stop Smoking Program at the Senior Citizens Center?"
3. "I wonder if you realize that you are slowly killing yourself? Why prolong the agony? You can just jump off the bridge!"
4. "I'm glad I caught you smoking! Now that your secret is out, let's decide what you are going to do."

Answer: 2

Rationale: Emphysema clients need to avoid smoking and all airborne irritants. The nurse observes the client's maladaptive behavior (but does not make judgmental comments) and explores an adaptive strategy with the client without being overly controlling. This communication technique places the decision making in the client's hands and provides an avenue for the client to share what may be expressions of frustration at an inability to stop what is essentially a physiological addiction.

Test-Taking Strategy: This question tests your knowledge of the therapeutic communication technique for the nurse to employ for clients who are failing to make adaptive decisions regarding health. Option 1 is an intrusive use of sarcastic humor that demeans the client. Option 3 is preachy, judgmental, and an excellent example of a countertransference issue for the nurse. Option 4 sounds like a disciplinary remark and places a barrier between the nurse and client within the therapeutic relationship.

Level of Cognitive Ability: Analysis
Phase of Nursing Process: Implementation
Client Needs: Psychosocial Integrity
Content Area: Adult Health/Respiratory

Reference

Antai-Otong, D. (1995). *Psychiatric nursing: Biological and behavioral concepts.* Philadelphia: W. B. Saunders, pp. 543–576.

---

173. The client is to have arterial blood gases measured. While the nurse is performing the Allen test, the client says to the nurse, "What are you doing? No one else has done that!" On the basis of the understanding of the nursing care plan, the nurse's most therapeutic communication technique would be

1. "This is a routine precautionary step that simply makes certain your circulation is intact before I obtain a blood sample."
2. "Oh? You have questions about this? You should insist that they all do this procedure before drawing up your blood."
3. "I assure you that I am doing the correct procedure. I cannot account for what others do."
4. "This step is crucial to safe blood withdrawal. I would not let anyone take my blood until they did this."

Answer: 1

Rationale: The Allen test is performed to assess collateral circulation in the hand before drawing blood from a percutaneous puncture of an artery or from an indwelling arterial catheter. The nurse's most therapeutic communication technique is giving information for client teaching. Notice that the nurse does not engage in a defensive posture but rather offers the information, as a client advocate should do. In this way, the client is empowered with the knowledge and can know what to expect in treatment.

Test-Taking Strategy: This question tests your knowledge of the Allen test and the most therapeutic communication to employ when the client questions nursing actions. Option 2 is aggressive and controlling as well as nontherapeutic in its disapproving stance. Option 3 is defensive and nontherapeutic in offering false reassurance. Option 4 demonstrates client advocacy that is overly controlling and quite aggressive and undermining of treatment.

Level of Cognitive Ability: Analysis
Phase of Nursing Process: Implementation
Client Needs: Psychosocial Integrity
Content Area: Adult Health/Cardiovascular

References

Antai-Otong, D. (1995). *Psychiatric nursing: Biological and behavioral concepts.* Philadelphia: W. B. Saunders, pp. 543–576.
Luckmann, J. (1997). *Saunders manual of nursing care.* Philadelphia: W. B. Saunders, pp. 917–920.

174. The client is complaining of difficulty concentrating, having outbursts of anger, and feeling "keyed up" all the time and that peer relations are poor. The nurse obtaining the client's history discovers that the symptoms started about 6 months ago. The client reveals that his or her best friend was killed in a drive-by shooting while they were sitting on the porch talking. The nurse suspects the client is experiencing

1 Obsessive-Compulsive Disorder.
2 Panic Disorder.
3 Post Traumatic Stress Disorder.
4 Social Phobia.

Answer: 3

Rationale: Post Traumatic Stress Disorder (PTSD) is a response to an event that would be markedly distressing to almost anyone. Characteristic symptoms include sustained level of anxiety, difficulty sleeping, irritability, difficulty concentrating, or outbursts of anger. Obsessive-Compulsive Disorder refers to some repetitive thoughts or behaviors. Panic Disorder and Social Phobia are characterized by fear of a specific object or situation.

Test-Taking Strategy: Knowledge about the disorders listed will help you answer this question. Both options 2 and 4 have similar symptoms, so they should be eliminated as possible answers. The information described in the question is not characteristic of an obsessive-compulsive disorder.

Level of Cognitive Ability: Analysis
Phase of Nursing Process: Assessment
Client Needs: Psychosocial Integrity
Content Area: Mental Health

Reference

Carson, V., & Arnold, E. (1996). *Mental health nursing: The nurse-patient journey.* Philadelphia: W. B. Saunders, pp. 702–706.

175. A client who is reported by staff to be very demanding says to the nurse, "I can't get any help with my care! I call and call, but the nurses never answer my light. Last night one of them told me she had 'other patients besides me'! I'm very sick, but the nurses don't care!" Which of the following therapeutic communication skills would be the most therapeutic response by the nurse?

1 "I think you are being very impatient. The nurses work very hard and come as quickly as they can."
2 "I can hear your anger. That nurse had no right to speak to you that way. I will report her to the Director. It won't happen again."
3 "It's hard to be in bed and have to ask for help. You ring for a nurse who never seems to help?"
4 "You poor thing! I'm so sorry this happened to you. That nurse should be killed!"

Answer: 3

Rationale: In option 3, the nurse displays empathy as she shares perceptions. Sharing perceptions asks the client to validate the nurse's understanding of what the client is feeling and thinking. It opens the door for the client to share concerns, fears, and anxieties.

Test-Taking Strategy: This question tests your knowledge of therapeutic communications for a client who is reported by the nursing staff to be "demanding." In option 1, the nurse is assertive and certainly defends the nursing staff. In option 2, the nurse expresses the client's frustration by labeling the client's feelings as "angry" and disapproving of the nursing staff. Option 4 is sympathetic and inappropriate regarding the negative comment about another nurse.

Level of Cognitive Ability: Analysis
Phase of Nursing Process: Implementation
Client Needs: Psychosocial Integrity
Content Area: Fundamental Skills

Reference

Stuart, G., & Laraia, M. (1998). *Principles and practice of psychiatric nursing* (6th ed.). St. Louis: Mosby–Year Book, pp. 17–61.

176. The nurse is caring for a client with an alcohol abuse disorder. The client attempted suicide before hospital admission. In reviewing the client's discharge outcomes, the most positive outcome recognized by the nurse is that the client states that he or she will

1 Continue to attend Alcoholics Anonymous (AA) meetings.
2 Take a biofeedback class.
3 Start an exercise program.
4 Learn to play golf.

Answer: 1

Rationale: Suicide rates are higher among clients who abuse alcohol. All of the other outcomes deserve support by the nurse, but option 1 will help the client abstain from alcohol and provide the client with a support group. Option 1 is the most positive outcome.

Test-Taking Strategy: Use the process of elimination to arrive at a choice between options 1 and 2. Both are therapeutic, but AA has a greater potential to provide impulse control.

Level of Cognitive Ability: Analysis
Phase of Nursing Process: Evaluation
Client Needs: Psychosocial Integrity
Content Area: Mental Health

Reference

Wilson, H., & Kneisl, C. (1996). *Psychiatric nursing* (5th ed.). Menlo Park: CA: Addison-Wesley, p. 593.

---

177. An English-speaking Hispanic male with a newly applied long leg cast has a right proximal fractured tibia. During rounds that night, the nurse finds the client restless, withdrawn, and quiet. Which of the following initial nurse statements would be most appropriate?

1 "Are you uncomfortable?"
2 "Tell me what you are feeling."
3 "I'll get you pain medication right away."
4 "You'll feel better in the morning."

Answer: 2

Rationale: Option 2 is open-ended and makes no assumptions about the client's psychological or emotional state. Option 1 is incorrect because males in traditional standard Hispanic cultures practice "machismo" in which stoicism is valued, so this client may deny any pain when asked. Client assessment is necessary before intervention, so option 3 would be incorrect. False reassurance is never therapeutic, and thus option 4 is incorrect.

Test-Taking Strategy: A long leg cast on the right leg will preclude driving and possibly work for approximately 4 weeks, so this client may be concerned about a variety of issues. The word "initial" in the question tells you that assessment and prioritization with the therapeutic communication techniques is needed. Knowledge of fracture healing, casting, and therapeutic communication techniques is helpful in answering this question.

Level of Cognitive Ability: Application
Phase of Nursing Process: Implementation
Client Needs: Psychosocial Integrity
Content Area: Adult Health/Musculoskeletal

Reference

DeLaune, S., & Ladner, P. (1998). *Fundamentals of nursing: Standards and practice.* Albany, NY: Delmar, p. 124.

178. A client was started on oral anticoagulant therapy while hospitalized. The client is now being discharged to home and is intermittently confused. The nurse would evaluate that the client has the best support system for successful anticoagulant therapy monitoring if the client

1 Has a good friend living next door who would take the client to the doctor.
2 Has a home health aide coming to the house for 9 weeks.
3 Lives with the daughter and son-in-law.
4 Was going to have blood work drawn in the home by a local laboratory.

Answer: 3

Rationale: The client taking anticoagulant therapy should be informed about the medication, its purpose, and the necessity of taking the proper dose at the specified times. The client who is intermittently confused may need support systems in place to enhance compliance with therapy.

Test-Taking Strategy: Successful anticoagulant therapy in essence has three components: taking the medication properly, having proper follow-up medical care, and having serial follow-up blood work. As this question is written, option 1 facilitates only medical care, option 2 facilitates only reminding the client to take the medication, and option 4 facilitates only blood work. Option 3 is the best choice, in view of the situation in the question.

Level of Cognitive Ability: Analysis
Phase of Nursing Process: Evaluation
Client Needs: Psychosocial Integrity
Content Area: Adult Health/Cardiovascular

Reference

Smeltzer, S., & Bare, B. (1996). *Brunner and Suddarth's Textbook of medical-surgical nursing* (8th ed.). Philadelphia: Lippincott-Raven, p. 759.

---

179. The client who has undergone successful femoral-popliteal bypass grafting to the leg says to the nurse, "I hope everything goes well after this and I don't lose my leg. I'm so afraid that I'll have gone through this for nothing." The nurse's best response would be

1 "I can understand what you mean. I'd be nervous too, if I were in your shoes."
2 "Stress isn't helpful for you. You should probably just relax and try not to worry unless something actually happens."
3 "Complications are possible, but you have a good deal of control if you make the lifestyle adjustments we talked about."
4 "This surgery is so successful that I wouldn't be concerned at all if I were you."

Answer: 3

Rationale: Clients frequently fear that they will ultimately lose a limb or become debilitated in some other way. The nurse reassures the client that participation in exercise, diet, and medication therapy, along with smoking cessation, can limit further plaque development.

Test-Taking Strategy: Option 1 feeds into the client's anxiety and is not therapeutic. Option 4 gives false reassurance, which is incorrect. Option 2 is meant to be reassuring but offers no suggestions to empower the client. Option 3, the correct option, acknowledges the client's concerns and empowers the client to improve health, which will ultimately reduce concern about the risk of complications.

Level of Cognitive Ability: Application
Phase of Nursing Process: Implementation
Client Needs: Psychosocial Integrity
Content Area: Adult Health/Cardiovascular

Reference

Ignatavicius, D. D., Workman, M. L., & Mishler, M. A. (1995). *Medical-surgical nursing: A nursing process approach* (2nd ed.). Philadelphia: W. B. Saunders, p. 946.

180. A client in the coronary care unit is about to undergo pericardiocentesis for a rapidly accumulating pericardial effusion. The nurse could best plan to alleviate the apprehension of the client by

1 Staying beside the client and giving information and encouragement during the procedure.
2 Talking to the client from the foot of the bed to be available to get added supplies.
3 Telling the client that the nurse will take care of another assigned client at this time, so as to be available once the procedure is complete.
4 Telling the client to watch television during the procedure as a distraction.

Answer: 1

Rationale: Clients who develop sudden complications are in situational crisis and need therapeutic intervention. Staying with the client and giving information and encouragement are part of building and maintaining trust in the nurse-client relationship.

Test-Taking Strategy: Options 3 and 4 distance the nurse from the client in the psychosocial as well as physical sense, and should be eliminated immediately. Option 1 is preferable to option 2. The nurse should ask another caregiver to be available to get extra supplies if needed.

Level of Cognitive Ability: Analysis
Phase of Nursing Process: Planning
Client Needs: Psychosocial Integrity
Content Area: Adult Health/Cardiovascular

Reference

Potter, P., & Perry, A. (1997). *Fundamentals of nursing: Concepts, process, and practice* (4th ed.). St. Louis: Mosby–Year Book, p. 248.

181. The nurse has formulated a nursing diagnosis of Body Image Disturbance for the male client taking spironolactone (Aldactone). The nurse based this diagnosis on assessment of which of the following side effects of the medication?

1 Edema and hirsutism
2 Weight gain and hair loss
3 Alopecia and muscle atrophy
4 Decreased libido and gynecomastia

Answer: 4

Rationale: The nurse should be alert to the fact that the client taking spironolactone may experience body image changes as a result of threatened sexual identity. These are related to decreased libido, gynecomastia in males, and hirsutism in females.

Test-Taking Strategy: Knowledge regarding the side effects associated with the administration of this medication is necessary to answer this question. Review now if you had difficulty with this question!

Level of Cognitive Ability: Application
Phase of Nursing Process: Assessment
Client Needs: Psychosocial Integrity
Content Area: Pharmacology

Reference

Hodgson, B., & Kizior, R. (1998). *Saunders nursing drug handbook 1998.* Philadelphia: W. B. Saunders, pp. 942–944.

182. Which of the following statements would be most appropriate for the nurse in talking with the client who is recovering from the signs and symptoms of autonomic dysreflexia?

1 "I'm sure you now understand the importance of preventing this from occurring."
2 "Now that this problem is taken care of, I'm sure you'll be fine."
3 "How could your home care nurse let this happen?"
4 "I have some time if you would like to talk about what happened to you."

Answer: 4

Rationale: Offering time to the client encourages the client to discuss feelings. The three distracters are blocks to therapeutic communication. Options 1 and 3 show disapproval, and option 2 gives false reassurance.

Test-Taking Strategy: Use the process of elimination and select the option that does not indicate a block to communication. Always address the client's concerns and feelings first!

Level of Cognitive Ability: Analysis
Phase of Nursing Process: Analysis
Client Needs: Psychosocial Integrity
Content Area: Adult Health/Neurological

Reference

Potter, P., & Perry, A. (1997). *Fundamentals of nursing: Concepts, process, and practice* (4th ed.). St. Louis: Mosby–Year Book, pp. 242–245.

183. While assisting a spinal cord–injured client with activities of daily living, the client states, "I can't do this; I wish I were dead." The nurse's best response would be which of the following?

1 "Let's wash your back now."
2 "You wish you were dead?"
3 "I'm sure you are frustrated, but things will work out just fine for you."
4 "Why do you say that?"

Answer: 2

Rationale: Clarifying is a therapeutic technique involving restating what was said in order to get additional information. Option 1 is changing the subject. In option 3, false reassurance is offered. By asking why, in option 4, the nurse puts the client on the defensive. Options 1, 3, and 4 are nontherapeutic and block communication.

Test-Taking Strategy: Identify statements that indicate the blocks to communication and eliminate these options. Option 2 identifies clarifying and restating and is the only option that will encourage the client to verbalize feelings and concerns.

Level of Cognitive Ability: Analysis
Phase of Nursing Process: Implementation
Client Needs: Psychosocial Integrity
Content Area: Adult Health/Neurological

Reference

Potter, P., & Perry, A. (1997). *Fundamentals of nursing: Concepts, process, and practice* (4th ed.). St. Louis: Mosby–Year Book, pp. 242–245.

184. During an assessment of a 30-year-old client, the client says, "I want to die; I think about it sometimes, but I don't know how in the world to do it. My mother gave me this ring; I love it so; I think I'll give it to my grandchildren." Which of the following reflects an accurate suicide assessment?

1 There is no suicide risk noted during the assessment
2 There is minimal suicide risk
3 Suicide has been attempted unsuccessfully
4 The risk for suicide exists, and continued assessment is needed

Answer: 4

Rationale: The phrase "I want to die" indicates a suicide risk. Minimal risk cannot be determined. Any self-harm language must be viewed as serious. This situation gives no date related to self-harm history. The acknowledgment of no formal suicide plan and statement of plans for the future indicate that a suicide risk assessment must be ongoing.

Test-Taking Strategy: Note the key client phrases that indicate the risk for suicide. This should assist in eliminating option 1. There are no data to support option 3. Focusing on the statements made by the client will easily direct you to option 4. Review suicide assessment now if you had difficulty with this question!

Level of Cognitive Ability: Analysis
Phase of Nursing Process: Analysis
Client Needs: Psychosocial Integrity
Content Area: Mental Health

Reference

Fortinash, K., & Holoday-Worret, P. (1996). *Psychiatric–mental health nursing.* St. Louis: Mosby–Year Book, p. 623.

185. Family members awaiting the outcome of a suicide attempt are tearful. Which response by the nurse would be most therapeutic to the family at this time?

1 "Don't worry, you have nothing to feel guilty about."
2 "Everything possible is being done."
3 "Let me check to see how long it will be before you can see your loved one."
4 "I can see you are worried."

Answer: 4

Rationale: Options 1, 2, and 3 are communication blocks. Option 1 labels the family's behavior without their validation. Option 2 uses clichés and false reassurance. Option 3 focuses on an important issue at an inappropriate time. Option 4 presents therapeutic communication and uses the technique of clarifying.

Test-Taking Strategy: Identify the use of therapeutic communication tools. Identify statements that indicate the blocks to communication and eliminate these options. Option 4 identifies clarifying and is the only option that will encourage the family to verbalize feelings and concerns.

Level of Cognitive Ability: Analysis
Phase of Nursing Process: Implementation
Client Needs: Psychosocial Integrity
Content Area: Mental Health

Reference

Fortinash, K., & Holoday-Worret, P. (1996). *Psychiatric–mental health nursing.* St. Louis: Mosby–Year Book, p. 623.

186. Which of the following is important to include in caring for an 11-year-old child who has been abused?

1 Encourage the child to fear the abuser
2 Provide a care environment that allows for the development of trust
3 Teach the child to make wise choices when confronted with an abusive situation
4 Have the child point out the abuser if that person should visit while the child is hospitalized

Answer: 2

Rationale: The abused child usually requires long-term therapeutic support. The environment provided during the child's healing must include one in which trust and caring are provided for the child.

Test-Taking Strategy: Options 3 and 4 ask the child to behave with a maturity beyond that which would be expected for an 11-year-old. Option 1 reinforces fear, which, although a legitimate response to abuse, should not be encouraged. Option 2 is the option that is most appropriate because it provides the child with a nurturing and supportive environment in which to begin the healing process.

Level of Cognitive Ability: Application
Phase of Nursing Process: Implementation
Client Needs: Psychosocial Integrity
Content Area: Child Health

Reference

Carson, V., & Arnold, E. (1996). *Mental health nursing: The nurse-patient journey.* Philadelphia: W. B. Saunders, p. 1068.

187. The nurse assesses an elderly client for signs of potential abuse. Which of the following psychosocial factors place the client at risk for abuse?

1 The client is completely dependent on family members for receiving food and medicine
2 The client shows signs and symptoms of depression
3 The client resides in a low-income neighborhood
4 The client has a chronic illness

Answer: 1

Rationale: Elder abuse is sometimes the result of frustration of adult children who find themselves caring for dependent parents. Increasing demands by parents for care and financial support can cause resentment and be burdensome.

Test-Taking Strategy: Knowledge of the risk factors involved with elder abuse are essential for answering this question. Option 4 could be eliminated because the question asked for a psychosocial factor rather than a physical factor. Option 3 can be immediately eliminated as a possibility because issues of abuse are not bound to socioeconomic status. Note the key word "dependent" in option 1. This should direct you to select this option. If you had difficulty with this question, take time now to review the risk factors associated with elder abuse!

Level of Cognitive Ability: Analysis
Phase of Nursing Process: Assessment
Client Needs: Psychosocial Integrity
Content Area: Mental Health

Reference

Johnson, B. (1997). *Psychiatric–mental health nursing: Adaptation and growth* (4th ed.). Philadelphia: Lippincott-Raven, pp. 829–834.

188. The nurse is caring for a dying client who says, "What would you say if I asked you to be the executor for my will?" Which of the following responses would be the most therapeutic communication technique by the nurse?

1 "Why, I'd be honored to be the executor of your will."
2 "Is there any money in it? I adore money, but I am honest."
3 "Your confidence in me is an honor, but I would like to understand more about your thinking."
4 "I'd say, 'great'! No worries. I'll carry out your will just as you want me to."

Answer: 3

Rationale: The nurse uses the therapeutic communication of seeking clarification. The client's question reflects the fact that the client has been thinking about the will and how best to obtain an executor. What is unknown is why the client is asking the nurse to be executor of the will and other specific and important information. In addition, the nurse would want to investigate the legal ramifications that could arise if such a position were accepted.

Test-Taking Strategy: This question tests your knowledge of the therapeutic communication technique to employ for a client who is requesting that the nurse perform a legal service. In option 1, the nurse responds with a social communication with no assessment of the consequences, which demonstrates a lack of critical thinking and exploration of motivation or client needs. In option 2, the nurse uses histrionic language and crass ideation. In option 4, the nurse provides false reassurance, which is nontherapeutic.

Level of Cognitive Ability: Analysis
Phase of Nursing Process: Analysis
Client Needs: Psychosocial Integrity
Content Area: Fundamental Skills

Reference

Antai-Otong, D. (1995). *Psychiatric nursing: Biological and behavioral concepts.* Philadelphia: W. B. Saunders, pp. 270–276.

---

189. The client who is suffering from urticaria (hives) and pruritus says to the nurse, "What am I going to do? I'm getting married next week and I'll probably be covered in this rash and itching like crazy." Which of the following is the most therapeutic response by the nurse?

1 "You're very troubled that this will extend into your wedding?"
2 "It's probably just due to prewedding jitters."
3 "The antihistamine will help a great deal, just you wait and see."
4 "I hope your husband-to-be has a sense of humor."

Answer: 1

Rationale: The therapeutic communication technique that the nurse uses is reflection. This technique presents themes that have emerged in the interaction and allows the client to view them from another perspective. Urticaria (hives), a skin reaction in the upper dermis appearing as a wheal surrounded by a flare (areas of redness caused by vasodilation) and pruritus (itching) can be caused by medications, food, chemical allergies, viral infections, and malignancies, or they can be hereditary.

Test-Taking Strategy: This question tests your knowledge of the therapeutic communication technique for a client experiencing skin reactions. Antihistamines, mild analgesics, and cold compresses are used to treat these reactions. In option 2, the nurse minimizes the client's anxiety and fears. In option 3, the nurse talks about antihistamines and asks the client to "wait and see." This is nontherapeutic because the nurse is making promises that may not be kept and because the response is closed-ended and shuts off the client's expression of feelings. In option 4, the nurse uses humor inappropriately and with insensitivity.

Level of Cognitive Ability: Analysis
Phase of Nursing Process: Implementation
Client Needs: Psychosocial Integrity
Content Area: Adult Health/Integumentary

Reference

Stuart, G., & Laraia, M. (1998). *Principles and practice of psychiatric nursing* (6th ed.). St. Louis: Mosby–Year Book, pp. 17–61.

---

190. A client with a spinal cord injury makes the following comments. Which comment warrants additional intervention by the nurse?

1 "I'm so angry this happened to me."
2 "I know I will have to make major adjustments in my life."
3 "I would like my family members to be here for my teaching sessions."
4 "I'm really looking forward to going home."

Answer: 1

Rationale: It is important to allow a client with a spinal cord injury to verbalize feelings. If the client indicates a desire to discuss feelings, the nurse should respond therapeutically. Options 2 and 3 indicate that the client understands that changes will be occurring and that family involvement is desirable. Nothing in the question indicates that the client will not be going home; therefore, this statement does not require further intervention.

Test-Taking Strategy: In general, an opportunity to discuss the client's feelings is an appropriate answer. Three options are similar in that the client expresses positive acceptance. When distracters are similar, usually they are not the correct responses. In option 1, the client expresses a feeling warranting a need.

Level of Cognitive Ability: Analysis
Phase of Nursing Process: Analysis
Client Needs: Psychosocial Integrity
Content Area: Adult Health/Neurological

Reference

Hartshorn, J., Sole, M., & Lamborn, M. (1997). *Introduction to critical care nursing.* Philadelphia: W. B. Saunders, p. 289.

191. The nurse is caring for a client with a grade II cerebral aneurysm rupture. The client becomes restless and anxious before visiting hours. The nurse determines that the client's response is likely related to

1. The severity of the aneurysm rupture
2. Ineffective family coping
3. Body image disturbance
4. Spiritual distress

Answer: 3

Rationale: A grade II cerebral aneurysm rupture is a mild hemorrhage in which the client remains alert but has nuchal rigidity with possible neurological deficits, depending on the area of the hemorrhage. Because these clients remain alert, they are acutely aware of the neurological deficits and frequently have some degree of body image disturbance.

Test-Taking Strategy: Knowledge of cerebral aneurysm is helpful in answering this question. Notice the key phrase "before visiting hours." This should assist in directing you to the correct option.

Level of Cognitive Ability: Analysis
Phase of Nursing Process: Analysis
Client Needs: Psychosocial Integrity
Content Area: Adult Health/Neurological

Reference

Thompson, J., McFarland, G., Hirsch, J., & Tucker, S. (1997). *Mosby's clinical nursing*. St. Louis: Mosby–Year Book, pp. 295–299.

---

192. In planning care for the client with thromboangiitis obliterans (Buerger's disease), the nurse would incorporate measures to help the client cope with lifestyle changes needed to control the disease process. The nurse can best accomplish this by recommending a

1. Smoking cessation program.
2. Pain management clinic.
3. Consultation with a dietitian.
4. Referral to a medical social worker.

Answer: 1

Rationale: Smoking is highly detrimental to clients with Buerger's disease, and such clients are urged to stop completely. Because smoking is a form of chemical dependency, referral to a smoking cessation program may be helpful for many clients. For many clients, symptoms are relieved or alleviated once smoking stops.

Test-Taking Strategy: Knowledge of the effects of smoking on clients with this disorder is needed to answer this question correctly. Because treatment goals are the same as for peripheral vascular disease, option 1 may be selected easily even without thorough familiarity with this disorder.

Level of Cognitive Ability: Analysis
Phase of Nursing Process: Planning
Client Needs: Psychosocial Integrity
Content Area: Adult Health/Cardiovascular

Reference

Smeltzer, S., & Bare, B. (1996). *Brunner and Suddarth's Textbook of medical-surgical nursing* (8th ed.). Philadelphia: Lippincott-Raven, p. 738.

193. When examination of a 14-year-old pregnant client reveals bruises and bleeding in the genital area, cigarette burns on the chest, rope burns on the buttocks, and multiple old fractures, the client says, "I'm afraid to go home! My stepfather will be angry with me for telling on him!" The nurse's most therapeutic communication to the client is

1. "I am sorry that this has happened to you, but you will be safe here. Your physician has admitted you until further plans can be made."
2. "You can't go back there with that lecher. How do you think your mother will react?"
3. "You must know that your presence in the house will only tease your stepfather more."
4. "Let's keep this between you, me, and the physician until we can formulate further plans to assist you."

Answer: 1

Rationale: A child who is found to be physically and sexually assaulted should be admitted to the hospital. This will provide time for a more comprehensive evaluation while simultaneously protecting the child from further abuse. The correct option assures the client of protection from abuse.

Test-Taking Strategy: This question requires you to apply your knowledge of childhood physical and sexual abuse within a dysfunctional family. In option 2, the nurse does not respond with a calm and reassuring communication style, nor does the nurse maintain a professional attitude. Option 3, which holds an innuendo, appears to accuse the victim of "teasing" the stepfather and is incorrect. It is also judgmental, controlling, and demeaning. The legal and ethical responsibilities for the nurse in such cases are carefully prescribed, with protection built in for confidentiality for reporting the situation to protective services. The nurse's suggestion in option 4 is not only wrong but is also collusive and passive in its stance.

Level of Cognitive Ability: Application
Phase of Nursing Process: Implementation
Client Needs: Psychosocial Integrity
Content Area: Child Health

Reference

Antai-Otong, D. (1995). *Psychiatric nursing: Biological and behavioral concepts.* Philadelphia: W. B. Saunders, pp. 407–426.

194. The nurse is caring for a 15-year-old female client admitted with diagnosis of physical and sexual abuse by her father. That evening, the father angrily approaches the nurse and says, "I'm taking my daughter home. She's told me what you people are up to, and 'we're out of here'!" Which of the following would be the most therapeutic response by the nurse?

1. "Over my dead body you will! She's here, and here she stays until the doctor says different, so get off my floor or I'll call hospital security and the police!"
2. "Listen to me. If you attempt to take your daughter from this unit, the police will only bring her back."
3. "Your daughter is ill and needs to be here. I know you want to help her to recover and that you will work to help everyone straighten out the circumstances that caused this. Go to the chapel and pray for your daughter and for your soul."
4. "You seem very upset. Let's talk at the nurse's station. I want to help you. I know you're very concerned and want to help your daughter. It will be best if you agree to let your daughter stay here for now."

Answer: 4

Rationale: When a child suspected of being abused is admitted to the hospital for further evaluation and protection, the physician usually attempts to get the parents to agree to the admission. If the parents refuse to agree to the admission, the hospital can request an immediate court order to retain the child for a specific length of time.

Test-Taking Strategy: This question assesses your knowledge of the policies and procedures involved in the care and protection of children at risk and in therapeutic communication techniques. In option 1, the nurse is angry and verbally abusive. It is clear that the nurse has decided that the father is guilty of child abuse, and yet the child is there for further evaluation. In addition, the nurse is so aggressive and challenging that she may antagonize the father and become a victim of violence as well. In option 2, the command to listen is somewhat demanding. Option 3 seems pompous and lecturing.

Level of Cognitive Ability: Analysis
Phase of Nursing Process: Implementation
Client Needs: Psychosocial Integrity
Content Area: Child Health

Reference

Antai-Otong, D. (1995). *Psychiatric nursing: Biological and behavioral concepts.* Philadelphia: W. B. Saunders, pp. 407–426.

195. The client with peripheral arterial disease is being discharged to home. The client is occasionally forgetful about medication, exercise, and diet instructions; needs daily dressing changes to a small open area on the leg; has limited endurance for activities of daily living (ADLs); and lives alone in a one-story house. To best assist the client to adapt to self-care and disease management, the nurse initiates a request to the physician for which follow-up services to be provided in the home?

1 Nursing, home health aide, physical therapy
2 Nursing, home health aide, speech therapy
3 Nursing, home health aide, and occupational therapy
4 Nursing, physical therapy, and occupational therapy

Answer: 1

Rationale: Home health care agencies provide a variety of services to clients, depending on individual need. The multidisciplinary team includes a nurse; home health aides; social workers; and physical, occupational, and speech therapists. Nurses provide skilled nursing services, including assessments. Home health aides can assist clients with ADLs, and physical therapists assist in rehabilitation and increasing musculoskeletal endurance. The occupational therapist would train clients to adapt to physical handicaps through new vocational skills and adaptive techniques for ADLs.

Test-Taking Strategy: The question tells you that the client needs daily dressing changes (with which a nurse can help), is forgetful about exercise program and has limited endurance (with which a physical therapist can help), and needs assistance with ADLs (which can be provided by a home health aide).

Level of Cognitive Ability: Application
Phase of Nursing Process: Implementation
Client Needs: Psychosocial Integrity
Content Area: Fundamental Skills

Reference

Potter, P., & Perry, A. (1997). *Fundamentals of nursing: Concepts, process, and practice* (4th ed.). St. Louis: Mosby–Year Book, pp. 72, 84.

196. The client with chronic arterial leg ulcers over the course of a year complains of pain and tells the nurse, "I'm so discouraged. The pain never seems to go away. I can't do anything, and I feel as though I'll never get better." The nurse would formulate which of the following nursing diagnoses for this client?

1 Acute Pain related to effects of leg ischemia
2 Chronic Pain related to nonhealing arterial ulcerations
3 Fatigue related to lack of sleep and frustration with illness
4 Ineffective Individual Coping related to chronic illness

Answer: 2

Rationale: The major focus of the client's complaint is the experience of pain. Pain that has a duration of longer than 6 months is defined as chronic pain, not acute pain. The North American Nursing Diagnosis Association (NANDA) defines fatigue as "a sense of exhaustion and decreased capacity for physical and mental work." NANDA defines ineffective individual coping as "impairment of adaptive behaviors and abilities of a person in meeting life's demands and roles."

Test-Taking Strategy: The focus of the question is on the client's pain. Expressions of discouragement and frustration on the part of the client do not automatically indicate poor coping skills, so eliminate option 4. The stem makes no mention of fatigue as the primary problem, so eliminate option 3. The stem states that the ulcer has been an ongoing problem for about a year, which is the critical piece of data needed to determine chronic pain, not acute pain, as the answer.

Level of Cognitive Ability: Analysis
Phase of Nursing Process: Analysis
Client Needs: Psychosocial Integrity
Content Area: Adult Health/Cardiovascular

Reference

Cox, H., Hinz, M., Lubno, M., et al. (1997). *Clinical applications of nursing diagnosis: Adult, child, women's, psychiatric, gerontic, and home health considerations* (3rd ed.). Philadelphia: F. A. Davis, pp. 320, 453, 735.

197. The client with valvular heart disease is being considered for mechanical valve replacement. Which of the following items does the nurse know is essential to assess before the surgery is done?

1 The likelihood of the client's experiencing body image problems
2 The ability to participate in a cardiac rehabilitation program
3 The physical demands of the client's lifestyle
4 The ability to comply with anticoagulant therapy for life

Answer: 4

Rationale: Mechanical valves carry the associated risk of thromboemboli, which necessitates long-term anticoagulation with warfarin (Coumadin).

Test-Taking Strategy: The word "essential" in the stem guides you to look for a critical item. Option 1 is important but not critical. Next, not all clients who undergo cardiac surgery need cardiac rehabilitation, so option 2 may be eliminated. Knowing that mechanical valves are thrombogenic, you will then easily pick the option related to anticoagulant therapy as the correct choice of the two remaining options.

Level of Cognitive Ability: Analysis
Phase of Nursing Process: Assessment
Client Needs: Psychosocial Integrity
Content Area: Adult Health/Cardiovascular

Reference

Smeltzer, S., & Bare, B. (1996). *Brunner and Suddarth's Textbook of medical-surgical nursing* (8th ed.). Philadelphia: Lippincott-Raven, p. 685.

---

198. The client who has a history of depression has been prescribed nadolol (Corgard) in the management of angina pectoris. Which of the following items is a priority when the nurse plans to counsel this client about the effects of nadolol?

1 High incidence of hypoglycemia
2 Possible exacerbation of depression
3 Risk of tachycardia
4 Probability of fatigue

Answer: 2

Rationale: Clients with depression or a history of depression have experienced an exacerbation of depression after beginning therapy with beta-adrenergic blocking agents. These clients should be monitored carefully if these agents are prescribed.

Test-Taking Strategy: This question guides your response, in that it tells you the client has a history of depression. Option 3 is incorrect because the medication would cause bradycardia, not tachycardia. Fatigue is a possible side effect, but this is not a priority item. Hypoglycemia is a sign that is masked with beta-blockers, and so option 1 also is incorrect. Review this medication now if you had difficulty with this question!

Level of Cognitive Ability: Application
Phase of Nursing Process: Planning
Client Needs: Psychosocial Integrity
Content Area: Pharmacology

Reference

Hodgson, B., & Kizior, R. (1998). *Saunders nursing drug handbook 1998.* Philadelphia: W. B. Saunders, pp. 712–714.

199. The nurse is caring for a client with terminal cancer of the throat. The family approaches the nurse and tells that nurse that they have spoken to the physician about taking their loved one home. The nurse plans to coordinate discharge planning. Which of the following services would be most supportive to the client and family?

1 American Cancer Society
2 American Lung Association
3 Hospice care
4 Local religious and social organizations

Answer: 3

Rationale: Hospice care provides an environment that emphasizes caring rather than curing. The emphasis is on palliative care. One of the major goals of hospice care is that the client be free of pain and other symptoms that do not allow clients to maintain the quality of their lives. An interdisciplinary approach is used.

Test-Taking Strategy: Knowledge regarding the goals and services provided by hospice care will assist in answering the question. Think about what each support service presented in the options will provide in meeting this client's needs. This will assist in directing you to option 3.

Level of Cognitive Ability: Analysis
Phase of Nursing Process: Planning
Client Needs: Psychosocial Integrity
Content Area: Adult Health/Oncology

Reference
DeLaune, S., & Ladner, P. (1998). *Fundamentals of nursing: Standards and practice.* Albany, NY: Delmar, p. 552.

200. The community health nurse is visiting a shelter for the homeless to provide health services and education. The nurse plans the visit knowing that which of the following health problems are least likely experienced by the homeless population?

1 Diabetes
2 Tuberculosis
3 Parasitic infestations
4 Gastrointestinal disturbances

Answer: 4

Rationale: Diabetes, AIDS, respiratory and cardiovascular diseases, and parasitic infestations are the most common health problems experienced by the homeless population.

Test-Taking Strategy: Try to think about the environmental conditions that the homeless individual is exposed to in answering this question. Options 2 and 3 can easily be eliminated, in view of the crowded living conditions that exist and the close physical contact and sharing that occur with the homeless in shelters. From the remaining two options, select option 1 over option 4 because the homeless individual lacks regularly scheduled nutritious meals, rest, and exercise, all of which contribute to the development of diabetes.

Level of Cognitive Ability: Analysis
Phase of Nursing Process: Planning
Client Needs: Psychosocial Integrity
Content Area: Fundamental Skills

Reference
DeLaune, S., & Ladner, P. (1998). *Fundamentals of nursing: Standards and practice.* Albany, NY: Delmar, p. 131.

REFERENCES

Antai-Otong, D. (1995). *Psychiatric nursing: Biological and behavioral concepts.* Philadelphia: W. B. Saunders.

Ashwill, J., & Droske, S. (1997). *Nursing care of children: Principles and practice.* Philadelphia: W. B. Saunders.

Black, J., & Matassarin-Jacobs, E. (1997). *Medical-surgical nursing: Clinical management for continuity of care* (5th ed.). Philadelphia: W. B. Saunders.

Burrell, L., Gerlach, M., & Pless, B. (1997). *Adult nursing: Acute and community care* (2nd ed.). Stamford, CT: Appleton & Lange.

Carpenito, L. (1995). *Nursing care plans and documentation.* Philadelphia: Lippincott-Raven.

Carpenito, L. (1997). *Nursing diagnosis: Application to clinical practice* (7th ed.). Philadelphia: Lippincott-Raven.

Carson, V., & Arnold, E. (1996). *Mental health nursing: The nurse-patient journey.* Philadelphia: W. B. Saunders.

Clemen-Stone, S., Eigsti, D., & McGuire, S. (1995). *Comprehensive community health nursing: Family, aggregate, and community practice* (4th ed.). St. Louis: Mosby–Year Book.

Como, N. (1995). *Home health nursing pocket consultant.* St. Louis: Mosby–Year Book.

Cox, H., Hinz, M., Lubno, M., et al. (1997). *Clinical applications of nursing diagnosis: Adult, child, women's, psychiatric, gerontic, and home health considerations* (3rd ed.). Philadelphia: F. A. Davis.

Deglin, J., & Vallerand, A. (1997). *Davis's drug guide for nurses* (5th ed.). Philadelphia: F. A. Davis.

DeLaune, S., & Ladner, P. (1998). *Fundamentals of nursing: Standards and practice.* Albany, NY: Delmar.

Doenges, M. E., Moorhouse, M. F., & Geissler, A. C. (1997). *Nursing care plans: Guidelines for planning and documenting patient care* (4th ed.). Philadelphia: F. A. Davis.

Fortinash, K., & Holoday-Worret, P. (1996). *Psychiatric–mental health nursing.* St. Louis: Mosby–Year Book.

Haber, J. (1997). *Comprehensive psychiatric nursing* (5th ed.). St. Louis: Mosby–Year Book.

Hartshorn, J., Sole, M., & Lamborn, M. (1997). *Introduction to critical care nursing.* Philadelphia: W. B. Saunders.

Hodgson, B., & Kizior, R. (1998). *Saunders nursing drug handbook 1998.* Philadelphia: W. B. Saunders.

Ignatavicius, D. D., Workman, M. L., & Mishler, M. A. (1995). *Medical-surgical nursing: A nursing process approach* (2nd ed.). Philadelphia: W. B. Saunders.

Iyer, P., Taptich, B., & Bernocchi-Losey, D. (1995). *Nursing process and nursing diagnosis.* Philadelphia: W. B. Saunders.

Johnson, B. (1997). *Psychiatric mental health: Adaptation and growth* (4th ed.). Philadelphia: Lippincott-Raven.

Lammon, C. B., Foote, A. W., Leli, P. G., et al. (1995). *Clinical nursing skills.* Philadelphia: W. B. Saunders.

LeMone, P., & Burke, K. (1996). *Medical-surgical nursing: Critical thinking in client care.* Menlo Park, CA: Addison-Wesley.

Lewis, S., Collier, I., & Heitkemper, M. (1996). *Medical-surgical nursing: Assessment and management of clinical problems* (4th ed.). St. Louis: Mosby–Year Book.

Lowdermilk, D., Perry, S., & Bobak, I. (1997). *Maternity and women's health care* (6th ed.). St. Louis: Mosby–Year Book.

Luckmann, J. (1997). *Saunders manual of nursing care.* Philadelphia: W. B. Saunders.

McFarland, G., & McFarlane, E. (1997). *Nursing diagnosis and intervention.* St. Louis: Mosby–Year Book.

Monahan, F., & Neighbors, M. (1998). *Medical-surgical nursing: Foundations for clinical practice* (2nd ed.). Philadelphia: W. B. Saunders.

National Council of State Boards of Nursing. (1997). *Plan for the National Council Licensure Examination for Registered Nurses.* Chicago: Author.

Nichols, F., & Zwelling, E. (1997). *Maternal-newborn nursing: Theory and practice.* Philadelphia: W. B. Saunders.

Olds, S. London, M., & Ladewig, P. (1996). *Maternal-newborn nursing: A family-centered approach* (5th ed.). Menlo Park, CA: Addison-Wesley.

Phillips, L. (1997). *Manual of IV therapeutics* (2nd ed.). Philadelphia: F. A. Davis.

Pillitteri, A. (1995). *Maternal and child health nursing: Care of the childbearing and childrearing family* (2nd ed.). Philadelphia: Lippincott-Raven.

Potter, P., & Perry, A. (1997). *Fundamentals of nursing: Concepts, process, and practice* (4th ed.). St. Louis: Mosby–Year Book.

Reeder, S., Martin, L., & Koniak-Griffin, D. (1997). *Maternity nursing: Family, newborn, and women's health care* (18th ed.). Philadelphia: Lippincott-Raven.

Smeltzer, S., & Bare, B. (1996). *Brunner and Suddarth's Textbook of medical-surgical nursing* (8th ed.). Philadelphia: Lippincott-Raven.

Smith, S., & Duell, D. (1996). *Clinical nursing skills* (4th ed.). Stamford, CT: Appleton & Lange.

Stuart, G., & Laraia, M. (1998). *Principles and practice of psychiatric nursing* (6th ed.). St. Louis: Mosby–Year Book.

Taylor, C., Lillis, C., & LeMone, P. (1997). *Fundamentals of nursing: The art and science of nursing care* (3rd ed.). Philadelphia: Lippincott-Raven.

Thompson, E. (1995). *Maternity and pediatric nursing* (2nd ed.). Philadelphia: W. B. Saunders.

Thompson, J., McFarland, G., Hirsch, J., & Tucker, S. (1997). *Mosby's clinical nursing.* St. Louis: Mosby–Year Book.

Townsend, M. (1996). *Psychiatric–mental health nursing: Concepts of care* (2nd ed.). Philadelphia: F. A. Davis.

Varcarolis, E. M. (1998). *Foundations of psychiatric mental health nursing* (3rd ed.). Philadelphia: W. B. Saunders.

Wilson, H., & Kneisl, C. (1996). *Psychiatric nursing* (5th ed.). Menlo Park, CA: Addison-Wesley.

Wong, D. (1995). *Whaley and Wong's Nursing care of infants and children* (5th ed.). St. Louis: Mosby–Year Book.

Wong, D. (1997). *Whaley and Wong's Essentials of pediatric nursing* (5th ed.). St. Louis: Mosby–Year Book.

Wong, D., & Perry, S. (1998). *Maternal-child nursing care.* St. Louis: Mosby–Year Book.

CHAPTER 13

Health Promotion and Maintenance

Health Promotion and Maintenance is a major category of Client Needs. The two subcategories of this Client Needs component are (1) Growth and Development Throughout the Life Span and (2) Prevention and Early Detection of Disease.

GROWTH AND DEVELOPMENT THROUGHOUT THE LIFE SPAN

The Growth and Development Throughout the Life Span subcategory includes content related to the nurse's role in assisting the client and significant others through the normal expected stages of growth and development, from conception through advanced old age. The proportion of test questions in the Growth and Development Throughout the Life Span subcategory of NCLEX-RN is 7%–13%.

BOX 13–1. Growth and Development Throughout the Life Span

Human Sexuality
Family Systems
Family Planning
Ante-/Intra-/Postpartum and Newborn
Developmental Stages and Transitions
Aging Process
Expected Body Image Changes

PREVENTION AND EARLY DETECTION OF DISEASE

The Prevention and Early Detection of Disease subcategory includes content related to the nurse's role in managing and providing care for clients in need of prevention and early detection of health problems. The proportion of test questions in the Prevention and Early Detection of Disease subcategory of NCLEX-RN is 5%–11%.

BOX 13–2. Prevention and Early Detection of Disease

Health and Wellness
Disease Prevention
Techniques of Physical Assessment
Health Screening
Health Promotion Programs
Immunizations
Lifestyle Choices

PRACTICE TEST

---

1. The teaching plan for a client who is receiving phenelzine sulfate (Nardil) should include which of these instructions?

1 Avoid aged cheeses
2 Avoid cherries and blueberries
3 Avoid digitalis preparations
4 Avoid vasodilators

Answer: 1

Rationale: Nardil is in the monoamine oxidase (MAO) inhibitor class of antidepressant medications. Clients taking MAO inhibitors must avoid aged cheeses, alcoholic beverages, avocados, bananas, caffeinated drinks, chocolate, meat tenderizers, pickled herring, raisins, sour cream, yogurt, and soy sauce. The medication classifications they should avoid are amphetamines, antiasthmatic agents, tricyclic antidepressants, and serotonin reuptake inhibitor (SRI) antidepressants. They should also avoid antihistamines, antihypertensive medications, levodopa, and meperidine.

Test-Taking Strategy: Knowledge regarding this medication is necessary to answer this question. All the food and medication groups listed in options 2, 3, and 4 are allowed. If you had difficulty with this question, take time now to review this medication!

Level of Cognitive Ability: Application
Phase of Nursing Process: Planning
Client Needs: Health Promotion and Maintenance
Content Area: Pharmacology

Reference

Hodgson, B., & Kizior, R. (1998). *Saunders nursing drug handbook 1998.* Philadelphia: W. B. Saunders, pp. 813–815.

---

2. The home care nurse visits a child with a diagnosis of celiac disease. Which of these findings, if identified in the client, would best indicate that a gluten-free diet is being maintained and has been effective?

1 The client is free of diarrhea
2 The client is free of bloody stools
3 Dietary tolerance of wheat and rye
4 Balanced fluids and electrolytes

Answer: 1

Rationale: Watery diarrhea is a frequent clinical manifestation of celiac disease. The absence of diarrhea indicates effective treatment. The grains of wheat and rye contain gluten and are not allowed. A balance in fluids and electrolytes does not necessarily demonstrate improved status of celiac disease. Bloody stools are not ordinarily a manifestation of celiac disease.

Test-Taking Strategy: The issue of the question is the lack of signs and symptoms related to celiac disease. The question requires knowledge of clinical manifestations of celiac disease. If you had difficulty with this question, take time now to review the manifestations of this disorder!

Level of Cognitive Ability: Analysis
Phase of Nursing Process: Evaluation
Client Needs: Health Promotion and Maintenance
Content Area: Child Health

Reference

Ashwill, J., & Droske, S. (1997). *Nursing care of children: Principles and practice.* Philadelphia: W. B. Saunders, pp. 733–734.

---

3. Which of the following strategies would be included in teaching the parents how to reduce the chance of infection after surgical repair of an inguinal hernia?

1 Change the diapers as soon as they become damp
2 Report a fever immediately
3 Soak the infant in a tub bath twice a day for the next 5 days
4 Restrict the infant's physical activity

Answer: 1

Rationale: Changing diapers as soon as they become damp helps reduce the chance of irritation or infection of the incision. Parents are instructed to change diapers more frequently than usual during the day and once or twice during the night. A fever could indicate the presence of an infection. Parents are instructed to give the child sponge baths instead of tub baths for 2–5 days. There are no restrictions placed on the infant's or the toddler's activity.

Test-Taking Strategy: The question asks for strategies to prevent infection. Eliminate the options that are obviously incorrect. Considering the word "prevention," you can eliminate options 2 and 3. From the remaining options, consider the anatomical location of a hernia. Option 1 is the best choice!

Level of Cognitive Ability: Application
Phase of Nursing Process: Planning
Client Needs: Health Promotion and Maintenance
Content Area: Child Health

Reference

Wong, D. (1995). *Whaley and Wong's Nursing care of infants and children* (5th ed.). St. Louis: Mosby–Year Book, pp. 492–494.

---

4. The client had thoracic surgery 2 days ago and has a chest tube in place. The client is clinically stable and is eager to increase activity to "get better" more quickly. Which of the following activities could the nurse plan for the client to promote optimal mobility?

1 Bed rest with repositioning every 2 hours
2 Dangling at the bedside three times a day
3 Getting out of bed to the chair twice daily
4 Ambulating in the hall three to four times a day with assistance

Answer: 4

Rationale: Once the client's condition is stabilized, the client may ambulate regularly. Early ambulation improves respiratory status and is also good for the client's circulation and morale.

Test-Taking Strategy: This question tests the concept of permissible activity for the client with a chest tube. The fact that the chest tubes do not necessitate bed rest is the first concept to have in mind. Next, because it is 2 days after the client had surgery, the client should be able to get out of bed. Combining these concepts would lead you to eliminate each of the incorrect options. Review activities allowed with a client with a chest tube now if you had difficulty with this question!

Level of Cognitive Ability: Application
Phase of Nursing Process: Planning
Client Needs: Health Promotion and Maintenance
Content Area: Adult Health/Respiratory

Reference

Black, J., & Matassarin-Jacobs, E. (1997). *Medical-surgical nursing: Clinical management for continuity of care* (5th ed.). Philadelphia: W. B. Saunders, pp. 1161, 1165.

---

5. The client is experiencing difficulty using an incentive spirometer. The nurse teaches the client that which of the following variables may interfere with effective use of the device?

1 Breathing through the nose
2 Forming a tight seal around the mouthpiece with the lips
3 Inhaling slowly
4 Removing the mouthpiece to exhale

Answer: 1

Rationale: Incentive spirometry is not effective if the client breathes through the nose. The client should exhale, form a tight seal around the mouthpiece, inhale slowly, hold for the count of three, and remove the mouthpiece to exhale. The client should repeat the exercise approximately 10 times every hour for best results.

Test-Taking Strategy: This question tests a fundamental concept of incentive spirometry use. Note the phrase "may interfere." This may assist in directing you to the correct option. If this question was difficult, take a few moments to review this procedure!

Level of Cognitive Ability: Application
Phase of Nursing Process: Implementation
Client Needs: Health Promotion and Maintenance
Content Area: Adult Health/Respiratory

Reference

Taylor, C., Lillis, C., & LeMone, P. (1997). *Fundamentals of nursing: The art and science of nursing care* (3rd ed.). Philadelphia: Lippincott-Raven, p. 1330.

6. The client with respiratory failure has a knowledge deficit related to positions used to breathe more easily. The nurse plans to teach the client to

1. Lie on the side with the head of the bed at a 45-degree angle.
2. Sit bolt upright in bed with the arms crossed over the chest.
3. Sit on the edge of the bed with the arms leaning on an overbed table.
4. Sit in a reclining chair tilted slightly back with the feet elevated.

Answer: 3

Rationale: Proper positioning can decrease episodes of dyspnea in a client. Such positions include sitting upright while leaning on an overbed table, sitting upright in a chair with the arms resting on the knees, and leaning against a wall while standing.

Test-Taking Strategy: Option 1 restricts expansion of the lateral wall of a lung and is eliminated first. Option 2 restricts movement of the anterior and posterior walls and is also eliminated. Option 3 is preferred to option 4 because it does not restrict expansion of any lung segment, whereas option 4 restricts posterior lung expansion.

Level of Cognitive Ability: Application
Phase of Nursing Process: Planning
Client Needs: Health Promotion and Maintenance
Content Area: Adult Health/Respiratory

Reference

Ignatavicius, D. D., Workman, M. L., & Mishler, M. A. (1995). *Medical-surgical nursing: A nursing process approach* (2nd ed.). Philadelphia: W. B. Saunders, pp. 689, 697.

7. The client with acquired immunodeficiency syndrome (AIDS) has a nursing diagnosis of Fatigue. The nurse would plan to teach the client which of the following strategies to conserve energy after discharge?

1. Stand in the shower instead of taking a bath
2. Bathe before eating breakfast
3. Sit for as many activities as possible
4. Group all tasks to be performed early in the morning

Answer: 3

Rationale: The client is taught to conserve energy by sitting for as many activities as possible, including dressing, shaving, preparing food, and ironing. The client should also sit in a shower chair instead of standing while bathing. The client needs to prioritize activities (e.g., eating breakfast before bathing) and should follow each major activity with a period of rest. Frequent short rest periods are more effective than few long ones. Finally, aerobic exercise in careful moderation can decrease fatigue and increase endurance.

Test-Taking Strategy: Answer this question by analyzing the amount of exertion required by the client in performing each of the activities in the options. Options 1 and 4 are obviously taxing for the client and are eliminated first. To choose between the remaining alternatives, bathing may take away energy that could be used for eating and is thus not helpful. This leaves option 3 as the best possible response to the question.

Level of Cognitive Ability: Application
Phase of Nursing Process: Planning
Client Needs: Health Promotion and Maintenance
Content Area: Adult Health/Respiratory

Reference

Black, J., & Matassarin-Jacobs, E. (1997). *Medical-surgical nursing: Clinical management for continuity of care* (5th ed.). Philadelphia: W. B. Saunders, p. 633.

8. The nurse has taught the client with pleurisy about strategies to promote comfort during recuperation. The nurse evaluates that the client has understood the instructions if the client verbalizes that he or she will

1. Try to take only small, shallow breaths.
2. Splint the chest wall during coughing and deep breathing.
3. Lie as much as possible on the unaffected side.
4. Take as much pain medication as possible.

Answer: 2

Rationale: The client with pleurisy should splint the chest wall during coughing and deep breathing, which is necessary to prevent atelectasis. The client may also lie on the affected side to minimize movement of the affected chest wall. The client should not take only small, shallow breaths because this promotes atelectasis. The client should take medication prudently to allow coughing and deep breathing and adequate levels of comfort.

Test-Taking Strategy: Option 4 is obviously incorrect and is eliminated first. Taking small, shallow breaths (option 1) would promote atelectasis and is not indicated. Lying on the unaffected side would stretch the chest wall on the affected side, increasing discomfort. Thus the only reasonable choice is option 2: to splint the chest wall during coughing and deep breathing. This promotes lung expansion while minimizing client discomfort.

Level of Cognitive Ability: Analysis
Phase of Nursing Process: Evaluation
Client Needs: Health Promotion and Maintenance
Content Area: Adult Health/Respiratory

Reference

Smeltzer, S., & Bare, B. (1996). *Brunner and Suddarth's Textbook of medical-surgical nursing* (8th ed.). Philadelphia: Lippincott-Raven, p. 502.

---

9. After diagnosis of trigeminal neuralgia, a client is started on a regimen of carbamazepine (Tegretol). The nurse teaches the client about the medication. The nurse knows that the client understands the teaching specific to this medication if the client states,

1 "I will report a fever or sore throat to my doctor"
2 "If I notice a pink color to my urine, I will stop the medication and call my doctor"
3 "I must brush my teeth frequently to avoid damage to my gums"
4 "If I notice ringing in my ears that doesn't stop, I'll seek medical attention"

Answer: 1

Rationale: Aplastic anemia is a serious side effect of carbamazepine. Assessments also include mouth ulcers and easy bruising. Common words used to describe hematuria are "a smoky or red color"; "pink" is not a usual description for blood in the urine. Options 2 and 3 relate to side effects of phenytoin, another medication used to treat trigeminal neuralgia. Option 4 relates a side effect of baclofen, a third medication sometimes used to treat this condition.

Test-Taking Strategy: Knowledge of the side effects of carbamazepine is necessary to answer this question. If you had difficulty with this question, take time now to review the side effects of this medication and the laboratory tests that need monitoring!

Level of Cognitive Ability: Analysis
Phase of Nursing Process: Evaluation
Client Needs: Health Promotion and Maintenance
Content Area: Pharmacology

Reference

Hodgson, B., & Kizior, R. (1998). *Saunders nursing drug handbook 1998.* Philadelphia: W. B. Saunders, pp. 144–146.

---

10. The director of nursing has presented a class on conflict management to staff nurses. Which behaviors by the nurses indicate that they are managing conflict effectively?

1 Lower work performance
2 Lower agency productivity
3 High-quality group decisions
4 High absenteeism and lateness

Answer: 3

Rationale: Conflict is part of any situation in which persons with differing interests, motivations, abilities, and temperaments must work together. The ability of groups to make quality decisions has a major impact on the care that clients receive and on the tone of the workplace.

Test-Taking Strategy: Use the process of elimination, noting that options 1, 2, and 4 are similar in that they identify a negative response. Option 3 is the only option that reflects a positive outcome.

Level of Cognitive Ability: Analysis
Phase of Nursing Process: Evaluation
Client Needs: Health Promotion and Maintenance
Content Area: Fundamental Skills

Reference

Rocchiccioli, J., & Tilbury, M. (1998). *Clinical leadership in nursing.* Philadelphia: W. B. Saunders, pp. 157–163.

11. The nurse has just completed initial client teaching with a woman who has been admitted in active first-stage labor. Which of the following evaluation criteria will the nurse use to determine whether the client has understood the education, aimed at identifying and providing early intervention in the event of a prolapse of the umbilical cord?

1 The client will verbalize the definition of a prolapsed umbilical cord
2 The client will turn on her call light for the nurse and stay in bed in a side-lying position if she feels a large gush of fluid from her vagina
3 A healthy baby will be delivered by cesarean section after the occurrence of a prolapsed umbilical cord
4 The client will watch the fetal heart monitor closely for changes in the fetal heart rate and rhythm

Answer: 2

Rationale: A prolapsed cord is most likely to occur just after the rupture of membranes when gravity washes the cord in front of the presenting part. A side-lying or low semi-Fowler's position will decrease the effect of gravity until the nurse has reassessed the condition of the fetus. Although the nursing assessment will include data from the fetal monitor, interpreting a fetal monitor pattern is a highly skilled process that a client cannot be expected to master. Watching the fetal monitor closely is usually a sign of anxiety in the client.

Test-Taking Strategy: This is a risk-prevention question, so the focus is teaching-learning. Eliminate option 1 because knowing the definition of a prolapsed cord will not prevent it from happening. Eliminate option 4 because the mother cannot be expected to watch a fetal monitor. Of the remaining options, option 3 is unrelated to providing early intervention. If you had difficulty with this question, take time now to review interventions for prolapsed cord!

Level of Cognitive Ability: Analysis
Phase of Nursing Process: Evaluation
Client Needs: Health Promotion and Maintenance
Content Area: Maternity

Reference

Lowdermilk, D., Perry, S., & Bobak, I. (1997). *Maternity and women's health care* (6th ed.). St. Louis: Mosby–Year Book, p. 973.

---

12. The nurse is conducting an educational session on prevention of vena cava syndrome (hypotensive syndrome) for couples during early pregnancy. Which of the following will be a priority expected outcome for this session?

1 The clients will be able to describe the vena cava syndrome
2 The clients will state comfortable lying positions for a pregnant woman
3 The clients will demonstrate nonsupine positions appropriate for rest for a pregnant woman
4 The clients will ask clarification questions about the effect of vena cava syndrome

Answer: 3

Rationale: The pressure of the enlarging uterus displaces and compresses abdominal vessels (iliac vessels, the interior vena cava, and possibly the aorta). Lying in a supine position accentuates the compression, often causing hypotension and bradycardia (vena cava syndrome) because of the decrease in venous return and cardiac output. Vena cava syndrome is prevented by not lying on the back (supine).

Test-Taking Strategy: Demonstration of the desired outcome is a good measurement of the ability to implement self-care. Note the word "demonstrate" in the correct option. If you had difficulty with this question, take time now to review measures that will prevent vena cava syndrome!

Level of Cognitive Ability: Analysis
Phase of Nursing Process: Evaluation
Client Needs: Health Promotion and Maintenance
Content Area: Maternity

Reference

Reeder, S., Martin, L., & Koniak Griffin, D. (1997). *Maternity nursing: Family, newborn, and women's health care* (18th ed.). Philadelphia: Lippincott-Raven, p. 374.

13. The nurse teaches a preoperative client about the nasogastric tube that will be inserted in preparation for surgery. The nurse evaluates that the client understands when the tube will be removed when the client states,

1 "When the gastrointestinal system is healed enough"
2 "When I can tolerate food without vomiting"
3 "When the bowels begin to function again and I begin to pass gas"
4 "When the doctor says so"

Answer: 3

Rationale: Nasogastric tubes are discontinued when the normal function returns to the gastrointestinal (GI) tract. Option 1 is incorrect because the tube will be removed before GI healing. Option 4 does not determine client interest or effective teaching. Option 2 is incorrect because food would not be administered unless bowel function returns!

Test-Taking Strategy: Use the process of elimination. Option 4 can be easily eliminated. Eliminate option 1, considering the time factor associated with healing of the GI tract. Knowing that food would not be administered unless bowel function returns will assist in the selection of option 3 over option 2. If you had difficulty with this question, take time now to review the use and care of the nasogastric tube!

Level of Cognitive Ability: Analysis
Phase of Nursing Process: Evaluation
Client Needs: Health Promotion and Maintenance
Content Area: Adult Health/Gastrointestinal

Reference

Black, J., & Matassarin-Jacobs, E. (1997). *Medical-surgical nursing: Clinical management for continuity of care* (5th ed.). Philadelphia: W. B. Saunders, pp. 1780–1781.

14. A client receives Intralipid 20% intravenously in the home. The client's spouse manages the infusion. The community health nurse discusses potential adverse reactions and side effects of the therapy with the client and the spouse. The nurse expects the spouse to verbalize that in case of a suspected adverse reaction, the priority action is to

1 Take a blood pressure.
2 Stop the infusion.
3 Contact the nurse.
4 Contact the local area emergency response team.

Answer: 2

Rationale: Intravenous fat emulsions can cause hypersensitivity reactions, including chest pain, chills, and shock. It is important to stop the infusion and limit the adverse response before obtaining additional assistance.

Test-Taking Strategy: Note the word "priority" and the key phrase "potential adverse reactions." Remembering that the priority action when an adverse reaction occurs is to stop the intravenous infusion will assist in directing you to the correct option. If you had difficulty with this question, take time now to review the adverse reactions of fat emulsion therapy!

Level of Cognitive Ability: Analysis
Phase of Nursing Process: Evaluation
Client Needs: Health Promotion and Maintenance
Content Area: Fundamental Skills

Reference

Wilson, B., Shannon, M., & Stang, C. (1997). *Nurses' drug guide.* Stamford, CT: Appleton & Lange, pp. 555–557.

15. The client with a cerebral vascular accident (CVA) is prepared for discharge from the hospital. The physician has prescribed range-of-motion for the client's right side. In planning for the client's care, the home health care nurse

1 Considers the use of active, passive, or active-assisted exercises in the home.
2 Implements range-of-motion exercises to the point of pain for the client.
3 Encourages the client to be dependent on the home health care nurse to complete the exercise program.
4 Develops a schedule of range-of-motion exercises every 2 hours while awake even if the client is fatigued.

Answer: 1

Rationale: The home health care nurse must consider all forms of range of motion for the client. Even if the client has right hemiplegia, the client can assist in some of his or her own rehabilitative care. In addition, the goal in home health care nursing is for the client to assume as much self-care and independence as possible. The nurse needs to teach so that the client becomes self-reliant, so option 3 is incorrect. Options 2 and 4 are clearly incorrect from a physiological standpoint.

Test-Taking Strategy: Basic knowledge of exercise and range of motion would assist in eliminating options 2 and 4 because they are incorrect. Option 1 is an all-inclusive answer and focuses on planning strategies, which is what the question asks. Dependency is not in the best interest of a client's sense of health promotion, which eliminates option 3. Review basic knowledge related to range-of-motion exercises now if you had difficulty with this question!

Level of Cognitive Ability: Application
Phase of Nursing Process: Planning
Client Needs: Health Promotion and Maintenance
Content Area: Adult Health/Neurological

Reference
Black, J., & Matassarin-Jacobs, E. (1997). *Medical-surgical nursing: Clinical management for continuity of care* (5th ed.). Philadelphia: W. B. Saunders, pp. 807–808.

16. Caregiver strain is a frequent occurrence in home health care when clients may be significantly dependent on someone for their personal and health care needs. Evaluating caregiver strain encompasses

1 Feedback from the client as to the coping abilities of the caregiver.
2 Subjective and objective assessment of the caregiver and client.
3 Waiting until the caregiver expresses concern about the significant responsibility in caring for the client.
4 Making a referral to the home health care agency social worker to complete the assessment.

Answer: 2

Rationale: Client discussion with the nurse provides some subjective evidence of caregiver strain. Waiting for the caregiver to become exhausted or incapable of caring for the client may be too late in the home setting and lead to compromised care for the client or well-being of the caregiver. The nurse can both objectively and subjectively assess the client first and would include client feedback. Feedback is one important mechanism but just a part of the evaluation process. Waiting until there is a problem is a reactionary answer to the question. The nurse has the responsibility to evaluate the client and caregiver concerns so that the social worker can be referred to if a problem or potential problem surfaces.

Test-Taking Strategy: Use the steps of the Nursing Process. Option 2 addresses obtaining data and, in addition, is all-inclusive, including subjective and objective data and both the client and caregiver.

Level of Cognitive Ability: Analysis
Phase of Nursing Process: Evaluation
Client Needs: Health Promotion and Maintenance
Content Area: Fundamental Skills

Reference
Rice, R. (1996). *Home health nursing practice: Concepts and application* (2nd ed.). St. Louis: Mosby–Year Book, p. 29.

17. The client is to be discharged on warfarin (Coumadin) therapy. Which statement by the client would indicate that further teaching is needed?

1 "This medicine thins my blood and allows me to clot slower"

2 "I need to have a prothrombin time checked in 2 weeks"

3 "If I notice any increased bleeding or bruising, I need to call my doctor"

4 "I need to increase foods high in vitamin K in my diet"

Answer: 4

Rationale: Warfarin sodium (Coumadin) is an oral anticoagulant that is used mainly to prevent thromboembolic events, such as thrombophlebitis, pulmonary embolism, and embolism formation caused by atrial fibrillation. Oral anticoagulants prolong the clotting time and are monitored by the prothrombin time (PT) and, more recently, a new laboratory test called the International Normalized Ratio (INR). Client education should include signs and symptoms of toxic effects and dietary restrictions, such as limiting foods high in vitamin K (leafy green vegetables, liver, cheese, and egg yolk), because these increase clotting times.

Test-Taking Strategy: The question asks for the statement that indicates the need for further teaching; thus the correct statements can be eliminated. A basic understanding of the purpose of Coumadin therapy and the role that vitamin K plays in the clotting mechanism would reveal option 4 as the most likely answer. If you had difficulty with this question, take time now to review client education points related to this medication!

Level of Cognitive Ability: Analysis
Phase of Nursing Process: Evaluation
Client Needs: Health Promotion and Maintenance
Content Area: Pharmacology

Reference

Kee, J., & Hayes, E. (1997). *Pharmacology: A nursing process approach* (2nd ed.). Philadelphia: W. B. Saunders, pp. 172, 521–525.

18. The client is taking prazosin (Minipress). Which of the following statements by the client would support the nursing diagnosis of Noncompliance with Medication Therapy?

1 "I don't understand why I have to keep taking the pills when my blood pressure is normal"

2 "I can't see the numbers on the label to know how much salt is in the food"

3 "If I feel dizzy, I skip my dose for a few days"

4 "If I have a cold, I shouldn't take any OTC [over-the-counter] remedies without consulting my doctor"

Answer: 3

Rationale: Side effects of prazosin are dizziness and impotence. The client needs to be instructed to call the physician if these side effects occur. Withholding medication will cause an abrupt rise of blood pressure. Option 1 indicates a knowledge deficit. Option 2 indicates self-care deficit. Option 4 is accurate information.

Test-Taking Strategy: Be careful reading the question stem. This question is looking for a statement to support a nursing diagnosis of Noncompliance with Medication Therapy. Focus on this nursing diagnosis when selecting the correct option. Eliminate options 1 and 2 first. Eliminate option 4 next because this is an accurate statement.

Level of Cognitive Ability: Analysis
Phase of Nursing Process: Assessment
Client Needs: Health Promotion and Maintenance
Content Area: Pharmacology

Reference

Hodgson, B., & Kizior, R. (1998). *Saunders nursing drug handbook 1998.* Philadelphia: W. B. Saunders, pp. 851–852.

19. A 64-year-old client is being treated for an atrial dysrhythmia with quinidine gluconate (Quinidex). Which statement would indicate to the nurse that discharge instructions have been effective?

1 "If I miss a dose, I take two doses of the medication at the next scheduled time"
2 "If I miss a dose, I should call my doctor"
3 "If I miss a dose, I should take the dose as soon as I remember"
4 "If I miss a dose, I should take the next prescribed dose as usual"

Answer: 4

Rationale: The client should be cautioned not to take an extra dose. Teach the client to take the medication if remembered within 2 hours of the missed dose or to omit the dose and then resume the normal schedule. Quinidine needs to be taken exactly as prescribed, around the clock. Option 4 is the best option.

Test-Taking Strategy: Eliminate option 1 because this action is inaccurate and could cause toxic effects. Be cautious about responses that have the client call the doctor. Although they are sometimes the correct responses, be certain that an independent nursing action is not a more appropriate choice. Option 3 is similar to option 1; therefore eliminate this option. If you had difficulty with this question, take time now to review the basic principles associated with medication administration!

Level of Cognitive Ability: Analysis
Phase of Nursing Process: Evaluation
Client Needs: Health Promotion and Maintenance
Content Area: Pharmacology

Reference

Hodgson, B., & Kizior, R. (1998). *Saunders nursing drug handbook 1998.* Philadelphia: W. B. Saunders, pp. 894–896.

20. A teenager returns to the gynecological (GYN) clinic for a follow-up visit for a sexually transmitted disease (STD). Which of the following statements, if made by the client, indicates the need for further teaching?

1 "I always make sure my boyfriend uses a condom"
2 "I know you won't tell my parents I'm sick"
3 "My boyfriend doesn't have to come in for treatment, does he?"
4 "I finished all the antibiotic, just like you said"

Answer: 3

Rationale: In treating STDs, all the sexual contacts must be found and treated with medication. Clients should always use a condom with any sexual contact. Any treatment at a GYN clinic for teenagers is confidential, and parents won't be contacted, even if the client is under 18 years of age. Any client should always finish the medication ordered by the health care provider.

Test-Taking Strategy: The question asks you to select the response indicating need for further teaching. Knowledge of "safe sex" and the treatment of STDs will assist in answering this question. Review this content now if you had difficulty with this question!

Level of Cognitive Ability: Analysis
Phase of Nursing Process: Evaluation
Client Needs: Health Promotion and Maintenance
Content Area: Child Health

Reference

Wong, D. (1997). *Whaley and Wong's Essentials of pediatric nursing* (5th ed.). St. Louis: Mosby–Year Book, pp. 500, 501.

21. The nurse is preparing to teach the client with newly diagnosed diabetes about blood glucose monitoring. The nurse would plan to teach the client to report glucose levels that exceed

1 150 mg/dL.
2 200 mg/dL.
3 250 mg/dL.
4 350 mg/dL.

Answer: 3

Rationale: It is standard practice to teach the client to report blood glucose levels that exceed 250 mg/dL unless otherwise instructed by the physician. Options 1 and 2 do not warrant reporting, whereas option 4 is dangerously high, and the level should have been reported before it became that high.

Test-Taking Strategy: It is necessary to have a basic understanding of blood glucose monitoring and the ramifications of the results if you are to answer this question correctly. Review this common area of teaching for diabetic clients if you had difficulty with this question!

Level of Cognitive Ability: Application
Phase of Nursing Process: Planning
Client Needs: Health Promotion and Maintenance
Content Area: Adult Health/Endocrine

Reference

Lewis, S., Collier, I., & Heitkemper, M. (1996). *Medical-surgical nursing: Assessment and management of clinical problems* (4th ed.). St. Louis: Mosby–Year Book, p. 1458.

---

22. The client who suffers from gastritis asks the nurse at a screening clinic about analgesics that will not cause epigastric distress. The nurse would plan to tell the client to take which of the following medications?

1 Bufferin
2 Tylenol
3 Excedrin
4 Ascriptin

Answer: 2

Rationale: Aspirin is irritating to the gastrointestinal tract of the client with a history of gastritis. The client should be advised to take analgesics that do not contain aspirin, such as acetaminophen (Tylenol). The other medications listed contain aspirin. Another category of medications that is irritating to the gastrointestinal tract is the nonsteroidal anti-inflammatory drugs (NSAIDs).

Test-Taking Strategy: To answer this question accurately, it is necessary to be familiar with the ingredients of common pain relief products. Options 1, 3, and 4 all are aspirin-containing medications, so eliminate these options. Review these medications now if you had difficulty with this question!

Level of Cognitive Ability: Application
Phase of Nursing Process: Planning
Client Needs: Health Promotion and Maintenance
Content Area: Pharmacology

Reference

Lewis, S., Collier, I., & Heitkemper, M. (1996). *Medical-surgical nursing: Assessment and management of clinical problems* (4th ed.). St. Louis: Mosby–Year Book, p. 796.

---

23. The client receives a diagnosis of thromboangiitis obliterans (Buerger's disease). The nurse places highest priority on teaching the client about modifications of which of the following risk factors?

1 Exposure to cold
2 Exposure to heat
3 Diet low in vitamin C
4 Cigarette smoking

Answer: 4

Rationale: Buerger's disease occurs predominantly in men between 25 and 40 years of age who smoke cigarettes. A familial tendency is noted, but cigarette smoking is consistently a factor. Symptoms of the disease improve with smoking cessation. Another aspect of client teaching with this disorder involves avoiding trauma to the limbs.

Test-Taking Strategy: To answer this question accurately, it is necessary to know that smoking is the major risk factor for Buerger's disease. If needed, take a few moments now to review this disorder!

Level of Cognitive Ability: Application
Phase of Nursing Process: Planning
Client Needs: Health Promotion and Maintenance
Content Area: Adult Health/Cardiovascular

Reference

Lewis, S., Collier, I., & Heitkemper, M. (1996). *Medical-surgical nursing: Assessment and management of clinical problems* (4th ed.). St. Louis: Mosby–Year Book, p. 1053.

24. The client has a new prescription for timolol (Betimol). The nurse would evaluate that the client has not fully understood instructions given about the medication if the client stated that he or she would

1 Take the pulse daily and, if it were less than 60, withhold the dose.
2 Use caution with driving, because drowsiness is a side effect.
3 Taper or discontinue the medication once the client feels well.
4 Have enough medication on hand to last through weekends and vacations.

Answer: 3

Rationale: Common client teaching points about beta-adrenergic blocking agents include taking the pulse daily and withholding the dose if the rate is under 60 (and notify the physician), not discontinuing or changing medication dose, keeping enough medication on hand so as not to run out, changing positions slowly, not taking over-the-counter medications (especially decongestants or cough and cold preparations) without consulting physician, and carrying medical identification stating that a beta-blocker is in use.

Test-Taking Strategy: This question is worded so as to make you look for an incorrect response. Option 1 is a correct action, and option 2 is a known effect of the medication, so these are eliminated first. A client should not run out of any prescribed medications, which eliminates option 4. This leaves option 3 as the correct answer, which is also an important point for many prescribed medications. Antihypertensive medications should never be tapered or discontinued by the client without physician approval.

Level of Cognitive Ability: Analysis
Phase of Nursing Process: Evaluation
Client Needs: Health Promotion and Maintenance
Content Area: Pharmacology

Reference

Hodgson, B., & Kizior, R. (1998). *Saunders nursing drug handbook 1998.* Philadelphia: W. B. Saunders, pp. 994–996.

---

25. The nurse has completed giving medication instructions to the client receiving benazepril (Lotensin). The nurse would evaluate that the client needs further instruction if the client stated that he or she would

1 Change positions slowly.
2 Report signs and symptoms of infection at once.
3 Monitor blood pressure every week.
4 Use salt substitutes and foods high in potassium.

Answer: 4

Rationale: The client taking an angiotensin converting enzyme (ACE) inhibitor is instructed to take the medication exactly as prescribed, monitor blood pressure weekly, and continue with other lifestyle changes to control hypertension. The client should change positions slowly to avoid orthostatic hypotension; report fever, mouth sores, and sore throat (signs of neutropenia) to the physician; and avoid salt substitutes and foods high in potassium (which can cause hyperkalemia).

Test-Taking Strategy: This question is worded to make you seek an incorrect statement. Knowing that options 1 and 3 are standard instructions with antihypertensive therapy, you would eliminate these first. To choose correctly between the two remaining options, you need to know that side effects of this medication include neutropenia and hyperkalemia.

Level of Cognitive Ability: Analysis
Phase of Nursing Process: Evaluation
Client Needs: Health Promotion and Maintenance
Content Area: Pharmacology

Reference

Hodgson, B., & Kizior, R. (1998). *Saunders nursing drug handbook 1998.* Philadelphia: W. B. Saunders, pp. 100–101.

26. The nurse has given the client information about the use of sublingual nitroglycerin tablets. The client has an order for PRN use if chest pain occurs. The nurse would evaluate that the client understands the instructions if the client stated that he or she would

1 Avoid using the medication until chest pain actually begins and intensifies.
2 Take aspirin to treat headache that occurs with early use.
3 Discard unused tablets 6 months after the bottle is opened.
4 Keep in a pocket close to the body.

Answer: 3

Rationale: Nitroglycerin may be self-administered sublingually 5–10 minutes before an activity that triggers chest pain. Tablets should be discarded 6 months after opening the bottle. Nitroglycerin is very unstable and is affected by heat and cold, so it should not be kept close to the body (warmth); rather, it should be kept in a jacket pocket or purse. Headache often occurs with early use and diminishes in time. Acetaminophen (Tylenol) may be used to treat headache.

Test-Taking Strategy: This question is worded in the affirmative, so you are looking for a correct statement. Knowing that nitroglycerin is unstable helps you eliminate option 4. It is good practice to take nitroglycerin before activities or stressors that cause chest pain, because this prevents or reduces myocardial ischemia. Aspirin is not the best analgesic to take for headache because it is irritating to the stomach and could interfere with other medications that a client could be taking.

Level of Cognitive Ability: Analysis
Phase of Nursing Process: Evaluation
Client Needs: Health Promotion and Maintenance
Content Area: Pharmacology

Reference

Hodgson, B., & Kizior, R. (1998). *Saunders nursing drug handbook 1998.* Philadelphia: W. B. Saunders, pp. 750–753.

27. The nurse has conducted medication instruction with a client receiving lovastatin (Mevacor). The nurse would evaluate that the client understands the effects of the medication if the client stated the need to adhere to periodic evaluation of serum

1 Triglyceride levels and bleeding times.
2 Cholesterol levels and liver function studies.
3 Very low density lipoprotein (VLDL) and blood glucose levels.
4 Cholesterol levels and bleeding times.

Answer: 2

Rationale: Lovastatin is one of a group of medications called reductase inhibitors. Their use results in an increase in high-density lipoprotein (HDL) cholesterol and a decrease in triglycerides, low-density lipoprotein (LDL), and VLDL cholesterol. These medications are converted by the liver to active metabolites and therefore are not used in clients with active hepatic disease or elevated transaminase levels. For this reason, clients are urged to have periodic liver function studies. Periodic cholesterol levels are needed in order to monitor the effectiveness of therapy.

Test-Taking Strategy: To answer this question, you need to know that this agent lowers blood cholesterol. Other medications in the same group have the same suffix (statin), which could enable you to recognize them on sight. If you know this and know that cholesterol is synthesized in the liver, it may make it easier to eliminate each of the incorrect options. Review this medication now if you had difficulty with this question!

Level of Cognitive Ability: Analysis
Phase of Nursing Process: Evaluation
Client Needs: Health Promotion and Maintenance
Content Area: Pharmacology

Reference

Hodgson, B., & Kizior, R. (1998). *Saunders nursing drug handbook 1998.* Philadelphia: W. B. Saunders, pp. 612–613.

28. The community health nurse visits a client at home. Clonazepam (Klonopin) has been prescribed for the client. The nurse teaches the client about the medication. Which of the following statements, if made by the client, indicates that further teaching is necessary?

1 "I can take my medicine at bedtime to reduce the effects of drowsiness"
2 "My drowsiness will decrease over time with continued treatment"
3 "I need to take my medicine with food to decrease stomach problems"
4 "If I experience slurred speech, it will disappear in 8 weeks"

Answer: 4

Rationale: Clients who are experiencing signs and symptoms of toxicity with the administration of clonazepam (Klonopin) exhibit slurred speech, sedation, confusion, respiratory depression, hypotension, and eventually coma. Remember that with prolonged high doses, physical or psychological dependence may occur. Options 1, 2, and 3 all represent an accurate understanding of the medication

Test-Taking Strategy: Knowledge of clonazepam (Klonopin) and its side effects is necessary to answer the question. If you had difficulty with this question, take time now to review this medication!

Level of Cognitive Ability: Analysis
Phase of Nursing Process: Evaluation
Client Needs: Health Promotion and Maintenance
Content Area: Pharmacology

Reference

Hodgson, B., & Kizior, R. (1998). *Saunders nursing drug handbook 1998.* Philadelphia: W. B. Saunders, pp. 238–240.

---

29. The community health nurse visits a client at home. Dipyridamole (Persantine), 400 mg PO daily, has been ordered for the client. The nurse teaches the client about the medication. Which of the following statements, if made by the client, indicates that the instruction was successful?

1 "If I take this medicine with my warfarin (Coumadin), it will protect my artificial heart valve"
2 "This medication will help protect me from having a heart attack"
3 "This medication will help protect me from having a stroke"
4 "This medication will help me to keep my blood pressure down"

Answer: 1

Rationale: Dipyridamole (Persantine) combined with warfarin is employed to protect clients' artificial heart valves. This medication is currently being studied for prosthetic heart valves and for its use in preventing thromboembolism in clients with a history of venous and arterial thrombosis and in clients with a history of recent myocardial infarction (MI), cerebral infarction, or embolus. It has not yet been definitely determined to be effective in the prevention of heart attacks or strokes.

Test-Taking Strategy: This question tests your knowledge of the use of Persantine, one of the antiplatelet medications. Options 2, 3, and 4 are incorrect because there is no evidence that it is effective as a prophylaxis in preventing heart attacks or strokes or in keeping blood pressure down. Review the use of this medication now if you had difficulty with this question!

Level of Cognitive Ability: Analysis
Phase of Nursing Process: Evaluation
Client Needs: Health Promotion and Maintenance
Content Area: Pharmacology

Reference

Lehne, R. (1998). *Pharmacology for nursing care* (3rd ed.). Philadelphia: W. B. Saunders, p. 544.

30. A client has received a prescription for a phenothiazine, an antipsychotic, in the psychiatrist's office. Which of the following client comments indicates an understanding of the need for intervention while taking this medication?

1. "If I start to talk funny or feel that my tongue is swollen, I should call my doctor"
2. "If I get very, very thirsty, I should increase what I drink and call the doctor"
3. "If my knees feel weak, I should stop my pills and call my doctor"
4. "If I get nauseated, I have to take my pills with food and let my doctor know"

Answer: 1

Rationale: Phenothiazines are likely to cause neuromuscular (extrapyramidal) side effects, such as dysphagia, protrusion of the tongue, laryngeal spasm, or dystonia involving the inner structures of the throat. A dry mouth, weakness, and nausea may occur, and the client should be taught measures to alleviate these side effects. The physician would not need to be notified.

Test-Taking Strategy: For this question, you need to know that abnormal motor behaviors may be caused as side effects to phenothiazines. Although all the options identify side effects, only option 1 warrants physician notification. If you had difficulty with this question, take time to review this medication!

Level of Cognitive Ability: Analysis
Phase of Nursing Process: Evaluation
Client Needs: Health Promotion and Maintenance
Content Area: Pharmacology

Reference

Haber, J. (1997). *Comprehensive psychiatric nursing* (5th ed.). St. Louis: Mosby–Year Book, pp. 265, 266.

---

31. The nurse is caring for the mother of a preterm infant. Discharge planning for the preterm infant should begin

1. When the discharge date is set.
2. When the parents feel comfortable with and can demonstrate adequate care of their infant.
3. When the mother is in labor.
4. After stabilization of the infant in the early stages of hospitalization.

Answer: 4

Rationale: Discharge planning begins in the early stages of hospitalization. Determination of the services, needs, supplies, and equipment requirements cannot wait until the day of discharge.

Test-Taking Strategy: Discharge planning always begins upon admission. Option 1 and 2 are incorrect because it is much too late to make the plans that need to be made. Option 3 is incorrect because the outcome of the delivery is not known. Note the key phrase "early stages of hospitalization" in the correct option.

Level of Cognitive Ability: Application
Phase of Nursing Process: Planning
Client Needs: Health Promotion and Maintenance
Content Area: Maternity

Reference

Nichols, F., & Zwelling, E. (1997). *Maternal-newborn nursing: Theory and practice.* Philadelphia: W. B. Saunders, p. 1383.

---

32. Before discharge of a client recovering from an acute inferior myocardial infarction (MI) with recurrent angina, the nurse teaches the client to

1. Avoid sexual intercourse for at least 10 weeks.
2. Replace sublingual nitroglycerin tablets yearly.
3. Recognize the side effects of aspirin, which include tinnitus and hearing loss.
4. Participate in an exercise program that includes overhead lifting and reaching.

Answer: 3

Rationale: After an acute MI, many clients are instructed to take one aspirin daily. Side effects include tinnitus, hearing loss, epigastric distress, gastrointestinal bleeding, and nausea. Option 1 is incorrect because sexual intercourse may be resumed 4–8 weeks after MI if the physician agrees. Option 2 is incorrect because clients should be advised to purchase a new supply of nitroglycerin tablets every 6–9 months, and expiration dates should be checked. Option 4 is incorrect because activities which include lifting and reaching over the head should be avoided, inasmuch as they reduce cardiac output.

Test-Taking Strategy: The process of elimination can be used to identify incorrect responses. Note the time limits in options 1 and 2: "10 weeks" and "yearly" are excessive, so eliminate these options. In the remaining two options, "overhead lifting and reaching" in option 4 should indicate that this is an incorrect option. If you had difficulty with this question, take time now to review client teaching points after MI!

Level of Cognitive Ability: Application
Phase of Nursing Process: Implementation
Client Needs: Health Promotion and Maintenance
Content Area: Adult Health/Cardiovascular

Reference

Black, J., & Matassarin-Jacobs, E. (1997). *Medical-surgical nursing: Clinical management for continuity of care* (5th ed.). Philadelphia: W. B. Saunders, pp. 1256, 1265.

---

33. The nurse has explained the reason that the physician has chosen laser surgery to treat the client's cervical cancer. Which statement, if made by the client, indicates a correct understanding?

1. "I have too much cancer to be removed with surgery"
2. "I want to be asleep during my procedure"
3. "The doctor could see all the edges of my cancer clearly and my curettage sample was normal"
4. "I am young and the laser keeps cervical tissue from regrowing"

Answer: 3

Rationale: Laser therapy is performed in an outpatient setting and is used when all boundaries of the lesion are visible and the endocervical curettage findings are normal.

Test-Taking Strategy: Eliminate option 1 first because laser surgery would not be the treatment choice if the cancer was extensive. Laser therapy does not prevent regrowth, so option 4 is incorrect. Laser surgery is painless, so eliminate option 2 because the client would not be under anesthesia. Option 3 is the most global response, which is often the correct answer. If you had difficulty with this question, take time now to review the indications for laser surgery.

Level of Cognitive Ability: Analysis
Phase of Nursing Process: Evaluation
Client Needs: Health Promotion and Maintenance
Content Area: Adult Health/Oncology

Reference

Smeltzer, S., & Bare, B. (1996). *Brunner and Suddarth's Textbook of medical-surgical nursing* (8th ed.). Philadelphia: Lippincott-Raven, pp. 2250–2255.

---

34. The nurse is reviewing teaching needs for an elderly insulin-dependent diabetic client with a history of diabetic ketoacidosis (DKA). Which of the following statements, if made by the client's wife, indicates that further teaching is necessary?

1. "If the grandchildren are sick, they probably shouldn't come to visit"
2. "I should call the doctor if he has nausea and/or abdominal pain lasting for more than 1 or 2 days"
3. "If he is vomiting, I shouldn't give him any insulin"
4. "I should bring him to the office if he develops a fever"

Answer: 3

Rationale: Infection is a precipitating factor for DKA; therefore options 1, 2, and 4 are accurate statements. Stopping insulin administration is another precipitating factor of DKA.

Test-Taking Strategy: Identify that the question is asking for the negative option. Eliminate options 1 and 4 first because both relate to infection and are therefore similar. For the remaining two options, recall the causes of DKA. This should assist in directing you to the correct option. If you had difficulty with this question, take time now to review the precipitating factors associated with DKA!

Level of Cognitive Ability: Analysis
Phase of Nursing Process: Evaluation
Client Needs: Health Promotion and Maintenance
Content Area: Adult Health/Endocrine

Reference

Black, J., & Matassarin-Jacobs, E. (1997). *Medical-surgical nursing: Clinical management for continuity of care* (5th ed.). Philadelphia: W. B. Saunders, pp. 1908–1981.

35. The nurse is evaluating client understanding of postdischarge activity instructions after insertion of an automatic internal cardioverter-defibrillator (AICD). The nurse realizes that further instruction is needed if the client makes which of the following statements?

1. "I should try to avoid doing strenuous things that would make my heart rate go up to or above the rate cutoff on the AICD"
2. "I should keep away from electromagnetic sources such as transformers, large electrical generators, and metal detectors and should avoid leaning over running motors"
3. "I must limit activities such as swimming, driving, or operating heavy equipment to an hour or two at a time"
4. "I must avoid doing anything in which there would be rough contact with the AICD insertion site"

Answer: 3

Rationale: Postdischarge instructions typically include avoiding tight clothing or belts over AICD insertion sites; avoiding rough contact with the AICD insertion site; and avoiding electromagnetic fields such as with electrical transformers, radio/television/radar transmitters, metal detectors, and running motors of cars or boats. Clients must also alert physicians or dentists of the device because certain procedures such as diathermy, electrocautery, and magnetic resonance imaging may cause device malfunction and thus may need to be avoided. Clients should follow the specific advice of a physician about activities that are potentially hazardous to self or others, such as swimming, driving, or operating heavy equipment.

Test-Taking Strategy: This question is worded to prompt you to look for an incorrect statement. Options 2 and 4 can be eliminated first because they are similar to standard post–pacemaker insertion instructions. Of the remaining two, option 1 is very plausible, whereas option 3 is vague. This may help you make the correct selection, if you are unsure of the answer. Review client teaching points for AICD now if you had difficulty with this question.

Level of Cognitive Ability: Analysis
Phase of Nursing Process: Evaluation
Client Needs: Health Promotion and Maintenance
Content Area: Adult Health/Cardiovascular

Reference

Ignatavicius, D. D., Workman, M. L., & Mishler, M. A. (1995). *Medical-surgical nursing: A nursing process approach* (2nd ed.). Philadelphia: W. B. Saunders, p. 886.

---

36. The nurse is caring for a client who has had a permanent pacemaker inserted. The nurse would plan to incorporate which of the following points in hospital discharge instructions?

1. Wear tight clothing over the generator site to help avoid dislodgment
2. Avoid swimming, to prevent microshock
3. Scanners at security gates will not affect the pacemaker
4. Perform a daily pulse check to monitor pacemaker function

Answer: 4

Rationale: Client instruction after pacemaker insertion typically includes daily pulse check, to wear loose-fitting clothing around the generator, to avoid only contact sports (other activities do not need to be curtailed), to avoid exposure to sources of magnetic fields, and to request hand scanning at airport and other security gates.

Test-Taking Strategy: Wearing tight clothing could cause local trauma and will not prevent catheter dislodgment from the right ventricular wall. The pacemaker generator is insulated by the manufacturer to protect against body moisture. Thus options 1 and 2 are eliminated. Option 3 sounds plausible on the surface, but the client should have hand scanning. Option 4 is the correct answer, inasmuch as it is a universal standard.

Level of Cognitive Ability: Application
Phase of Nursing Process: Planning
Client Needs: Health Promotion and Maintenance
Content Area: Adult Health/Cardiovascular

Reference

Smeltzer, S., & Bare, B. (1996). *Brunner and Suddarth's Textbook of medical-surgical nursing* (8th ed.). Philadelphia: Lippincott-Raven, p. 633.

37. The home care nurse is caring for a client with chronic venous insufficiency resulting from deep vein thrombosis. Which of the following instructions would not be included in the teaching plan implemented for this client?

1. Cross the legs at the knees but not at the ankles
2. Elevate the foot of the bed 6 inches during sleep
3. Avoid prolonged standing or sitting
4. Continue to wear elastic hose for at least 6–8 weeks

Answer: 1

Rationale: Clients with chronic venous insufficiency are advised to avoid crossing the legs, avoid sitting in chairs in which the feet don't touch the floor, and avoid wearing garters or sources of pressure above the legs (such as girdles). The client should wear elastic hose for 6–8 weeks and perhaps for life. The client should sleep with the foot of the bed elevated to promote venous return during sleep.

Test-Taking Strategy: Use the concept of gravity when answering many questions that relate to peripheral vascular problems. Venous problems are characterized by insufficient drainage of blood from the legs returning to the heart. Thus interventions need to be aimed at promoting flow of blood out of the legs and back to the heart. Only option 1 does not promote venous drainage, so it is the correct answer because of the way the question is worded.

Level of Cognitive Ability: Application
Phase of Nursing Process: Implementation
Client Needs: Health Promotion and Maintenance
Content Area: Adult Health/Cardiovascular

Reference

Black, J., & Matassarin-Jacobs, E. (1997). *Medical-surgical nursing: Clinical management for continuity of care* (5th ed.). Philadelphia: W. B. Saunders, p. 1436.

---

38. The nurse is giving discharge instructions to the client with varicose vein stripping and ligation done as outpatient surgery. The nurse would give which of the following directions to the client?

1. Maintain bed rest for the first 3 days
2. Ambulate for 5–10 minutes twice a day beginning the day after surgery
3. Elevate the foot of the bed while in bed
4. Remove elastic hose after 24 hours

Answer: 3

Rationale: Standard postoperative care after vein ligation and stripping consists of bed rest for 24 hours, with ambulation for 5–10 minutes every 2 hours thereafter. Continuous elastic compression of the leg is maintained for 1 week after the procedure, followed by long-term use of elastic hose. The foot of the bed should be elevated to promote venous drainage.

Test-Taking Strategy: Use your knowledge of concepts related to blood flow and immobility to answer this question. Options 1 and 4 will promote venous stasis, so they are eliminated first. Option 2 may look plausible on the surface if you are unfamiliar with this postoperative protocol, but option 3 is so clearly correct that you would choose this as your answer. Review postoperative teaching points after varicose vein stripping and ligation if you had difficulty with this question!

Level of Cognitive Ability: Application
Phase of Nursing Process: Implementation
Client Needs: Health Promotion and Maintenance
Content Area: Adult Health/Cardiovascular

Reference

Smeltzer, S., & Bare, B. (1996). *Brunner and Suddarth's Textbook of medical-surgical nursing* (8th ed.). Philadelphia: Lippincott-Raven, p. 764.

---

39. The nurse is developing a teaching plan for the client with Raynaud's disease. The nurse includes in the plan the information that the symptoms may improve with

1 A high-protein diet to minimize tissue malnutrition.
2 Vitamin K administration to prevent tendencies toward bleeding.
3 Keeping the hands and feet warm and dry to prevent vasoconstriction.
4 Daily cool baths to give an analgesic effect.

Answer: 3

Rationale: Use of measures to prevent vasoconstriction are helpful in managing this disorder. The hands and feet should be kept dry; gloves and warm fabrics (e.g., Thinsulate) should be used in cold weather; and the client should avoid exposure to nicotine and caffeine. Avoidance of situations that trigger stress is also helpful.

Test-Taking Strategy: This question is worded in a straightforward manner. Knowledge of the disorder and the need to promote vasodilation helps you eliminate each of the incorrect options. Review teaching points related to Raynaud's disease now if you had difficulty with this question!

Level of Cognitive Ability: Application
Phase of Nursing Process: Planning
Client Needs: Health Promotion and Maintenance
Content Area: Adult Health/Cardiovascular

Reference

Lewis, S., Collier, I., & Heitkemper, M. (1996). *Medical-surgical nursing: Assessment and management of clinical problems* (4th ed.). St. Louis: Mosby–Year Book, pp. 1053–1054.

---

40. The client with peripheral arterial disease has received instructions from the nurse about how to limit progression of the disease. The nurse would evaluate that the client needs further instruction if which of the following statements was made by the client?

1 "I should walk daily to increase the circulation to my legs"
2 "A warm heating pad on my leg will help soothe the leg pain"
3 "I need to take special care of my feet to prevent injury"
4 "It's too bad I have to cut out butter; I used to love it on all my vegetables"

Answer: 2

Rationale: Long-term management of peripheral arterial disease consists of measures that increase peripheral circulation (exercise), promote vasodilatation (body warmth), relieve pain, and maintain tissue integrity (foot care and nutrition). Application of heat directly to the extremity is contraindicated because the limb may have decreased sensitivity and be more at risk for burns.

Test-Taking Strategy: Knowledge of the concepts used in managing this disorder is needed to answer this question. Using the process of elimination should assist in directing you to option 2 as the answer to this question as it is stated. This is an important area for testing, and many of the concepts have applicability to other content areas as well. If you need to review teaching points related to peripheral arterial disease, do so now!

Level of Cognitive Ability: Analysis
Phase of Nursing Process: Evaluation
Client Needs: Health Promotion and Maintenance
Content Area: Adult Health/Cardiovascular

Reference

Ignatavicius, D. D., Workman, M. L., & Mishler, M. A. (1995). *Medical-surgical nursing: A nursing process approach* (2nd ed.). Philadelphia: W. B. Saunders, p. 941.

---

41. The nurse is planning to teach the hypertensive client about nonfood items that contain sodium and develops a written list for the client. Which of the following would not be included on the list of items whose labels should be carefully evaluated by the client?

1 Demineralized water
2 Antacids
3 Laxatives
4 Toothpaste

Answer: 1

Rationale: Sodium intake can be increased by use of several types of products, including toothpaste and mouthwashes; over-the-counter (OTC) medications such as analgesics, antacids, cough remedies, laxatives, and sedatives; and softened water, as well as some mineral waters. Water that is bottled, distilled, deionized, or demineralized may be used for drinking and cooking. Clients are strongly advised to read labels for sodium content.

Test-Taking Strategy: The wording of the question directs you to seek for an item that is low in sodium. Several OTC medications and products contain significant levels of sodium, and these are good items to remember in answering a question of this nature. Last, look at the word "demineralized," which approximately means having the minerals removed. An option such as this would be a good choice in selecting an item low in sodium.

Level of Cognitive Ability: Application
Phase of Nursing Process: Planning
Client Needs: Health Promotion and Maintenance
Content Area: Adult Health/Cardiovascular

Reference

Lutz, C., & Przytulski, K. (1997). *Nutrition and diet therapy* (2nd ed.). Philadelphia: F. A. Davis, pp. 375–376.

---

42. A client is to be discharged to home after a second operation to repair a recurrent abdominal hernia. The nurse tells the client, "The care for your incision is the same as last time," and leaves the room. A week later, the client is hospitalized for treatment of a serious wound infection. The client may be able to take legal action against the nurse if it is proved that

1 The nurse failed to evaluate the client's ability to appropriately care for the incision.
2 The client did not sign a copy of the postoperative care discharge instructions.
3 The physician instructed the nurse to have the client make an appointment for the following day.
4 The hospital did not allow the client to stay an additional day when requested to do so.

Answer: 1

Rationale: Teaching is a primary role of the nurse in assisting the client to promote and maintain health. The nurse has a moral and legal obligation to evaluate the client's ability to provide appropriate care upon discharge to home or other setting. The question specifically asks about the nurse and not about actions by the hospital or about physician responsibilities, so options 3 and 4 are incorrect. Option 2 in a real situation may have some bearing on the case, but in view of the information here, it is not relevant to the question.

Test-Taking Strategy: Read the stem carefully, and note that the question specifically refers to the nurse's action or inaction. This allows you to immediately eliminate the possible answers that refer to actions by the physician (option 3) and the hospital (option 4). The fact that the client did not sign any discharge instructions (option 2) may be relevant to the situation on further examination, but the stem is asking you to isolate the issue regarding the nurse's practice. Because the client has a legal right to be protected from malpractice and because malpractice can include both acts of omission and acts of commission, option 1 is the only logical response to the question. If you had difficulty with this question, take time now to review the legal responsibilities of the nurse!

Level of Cognitive Ability: Analysis
Phase of Nursing Process: Evaluation
Client Needs: Health Promotion and Maintenance
Content Area: Fundamental Skills

Reference

Wywialowski, E. (1997). *Managing client care* (2nd ed.). St. Louis: Mosby–Year Book, p. 303.

---

43. The nurse is working with a multidisciplinary group of health care providers in the care of an elderly man with recently diagnosed diabetes. Which of the following statements by the client indicates to the nurse that additional assistance from the team members is needed?

1 "I take 50 units of regular insulin every morning and evening"
2 "I can substitute peanut butter for meat tonight"
3 "The Home Health Aide gave me a shower today"
4 "The Social Worker helped me get this emergency call button"

Answer: 1

Rationale: The nurse is responsible for the collaborative efforts of the multidisciplinary care team. There is nothing in option 2, 3, or 4 to indicate that there is anything out of the ordinary. Option 1, however, indicates that the client believes that he is to take an excessively high dose of regular insulin each day. The nurse, pharmacist, physician, and client need to be involved in planning care.

Test-Taking Strategy: An understanding of the role of the nurse as coordinator and manager of care is essential in answering this question correctly. The nurse must evaluate the client's responses to care provided by all members of the multidisciplinary team and recognize statements by the client that may indicate the need for follow-up. In addition, knowledge of usual dosages of insulin and the differences in onset and duration of action is essential. Options 2, 3, and 4 show no evidence that there is a problem. If you had difficulty with this question, take time now to review normal daily insulin prescriptions!

Level of Cognitive Ability: Analysis
Phase of Nursing Process: Evaluation
Client Needs: Health Promotion and Maintenance
Content Area: Adult Health/Endocrine

Reference

Black, J., & Matassarin-Jacobs, E. (1997). *Medical-surgical nursing: Clinical management for continuity of care* (5th ed.). Philadelphia: W. B. Saunders, p. 1974.

---

44. A community health nurse is analyzing evaluation comments after several sessions with a group of high school students on the hazards of tobacco use. Which of the following comments would suggest the need for further teaching?

1 "Both inhalation of tobacco smoke from active smoking and passive smoke inhaled from other people's smoking are public health issues"
2 "Chewing tobacco is a safer method of tobacco use than is smoking the tobacco"
3 "The health of children is at risk when their parents smoke"
4 "Smoking during pregnancy increases the risk of stillbirth and miscarriages"

Answer: 2

Rationale: All forms of tobacco use are health hazards. Options 1, 3, and 4 indicate a good understanding of the health hazards of tobacco use.

Test-Taking Strategy: Use the process of elimination seeking the option that suggests the need for further teaching. This should direct you to option 2. If you had difficulty with this question, take time now to review the hazards of tobacco use!

Level of Cognitive Ability: Analysis
Phase of Nursing Process: Evaluation
Client Needs: Health Promotion and Maintenance
Content Area: Fundamental Skills

Reference

Clemen-Stone, S., Eigsti, D., & McGuire, S. (1995). *Comprehensive community health nursing: Family, aggregate, and community practice* (4th ed.). St. Louis: Mosby–Year Book, pp. 630–634.

---

45. The perinatal client has been instructed on the prevention of genital tract infections. Which of the following statements made by the client would indicate effective teaching by the nurse?

1 "I should avoid the use of condoms"
2 "I can douche anytime I want"
3 "I can wear my tight-fitting jeans"
4 "I should choose underwear with a cotton panel liner"

Answer: 4

Rationale: Condoms should be used to minimize the spread of sexually transmitted infectious diseases. Wearing tight clothes irritates the genital area and does not allow for air circulation. Douching is to be avoided. Wearing items with a cotton panel liner allows for air movement in and around the genital area.

Test-Taking Strategy: This question focuses on how the nurse should monitor or make a judgment concerning a client's response to teaching. Use the process of elimination. Options 1, 2, and 3 are all incorrect statements regarding client self-care. If you had difficulty with this question, take time now to review prevention measures associated with genital tract infections!

Level of Cognitive Ability: Analysis
Phase of Nursing Process: Evaluation
Client Needs: Health Promotion and Maintenance
Content Area: Maternity

Reference

Lowdermilk, D., Perry, S., & Bobak, I. (1997). *Maternity and women's health care* (6th ed.). St. Louis: Mosby–Year Book, p. 749.

46. The nurse is developing goals for the postpartum client with a nursing diagnosis of Risk for Infection. Which of the following goals would be most appropriate for this nursing diagnosis?

1. The client will verbalize a reduction of pain
2. The client will no longer have a positive Homans' sign
3. The client will report symptoms of the infection
4. The client will be able to identify measures to prevent infection

Answer: 4

Rationale: The uterus is theoretically sterile during pregnancy and until the membranes rupture. It is capable of being invaded by pathogens after that rupture. Pain and a positive Homans' sign are not directly related to infection. Symptoms indicate that an infection exists.

Test-Taking Strategy: The question asks for a goal appropriate for the nursing diagnosis identified in the stem. Option 3 implies that an infection has been diagnosed, not that the client is merely at risk for infection. Options 1 and 2 are not appropriate for the identified diagnosis but refer to pain and impaired tissue perfusion, respectively.

Level of Cognitive Ability: Application
Phase of Nursing Process: Planning
Client Needs: Health Promotion and Maintenance
Content Area: Maternity

Reference

Lowdermilk, D., Perry, S., & Bobak, I. (1997). *Maternity and women's health care* (6th ed.). St. Louis: Mosby–Year Book, p. 750.

---

47. The neonatal intensive care unit (NICU) nurse teaches handwashing techniques to parents before their handling of an infant who is receiving antibiotic treatment for a neonatal infection. The nurse evaluates that the parents understand the purpose of handwashing if they state that this is primarily done to

1. Reduce their own fears.
2. Minimize spread of infection to other siblings.
3. Reduce the possibility of environmental infection for their newborn.
4. Allow them an opportunity to communicate with each other and staff.

Answer: 3

Rationale: Appropriate handwashing by staff and parents has been effective in the prevention of nosocomial infections in nursery units. This action also promotes parents' taking an active part in the care of their newborns, thus enhancing attachment behaviors with their compromised infant and reducing risk of additional infection.

Test-Taking Strategy: This question tests your knowledge of the transmission of nosocomial infections within the nursery setting. The nursing action of evaluating parental handwashing is a priority to reduce spread of infection to all neonates within this unit and represents a globally accepted nursing action.

Level of Cognitive Ability: Analysis
Phase of Nursing Process: Evaluation
Clients Needs: Health Promotion and Maintenance
Content Area: Maternity

Reference

Lowdermilk, D., Perry, S., & Bobak, I. (1997). *Maternity and women's health care* (6th ed.). St. Louis: Mosby–Year Book, p. 1085.

---

48. The client is receiving rehabilitative services during pregnancy for alcohol abuse. The nurse would provide supportive care by

1. Encouraging the client to participate in care and to identify supportive nursing strategies that are helpful.
2. Avoiding discussion of the alcohol problem and recovery with the client.
3. Minimizing communication with supportive family members.
4. Encouraging the client to stop counseling once the infant is born.

Answer: 1

Rationale: Supportive nurse-client interactions are established when all members of the health care team work collaboratively to identify appropriate client goals. Women may drink in isolation. Once their problem is personally identified, they frequently benefit from counseling programs and a supportive network during and after pregnancy.

Test-Taking Strategy: Use the process of elimination, seeking the positive option. Option 1 provides the client with an active role in identifying a treatment plan to foster positive outcomes during pregnancy. The other choices create barriers for long-term success and behavioral outcomes.

Level of Cognitive Ability: Application
Phase of Nursing Process: Implementation
Clients Needs: Health Promotion and Maintenance
Content Area: Maternity

Reference

Reeder, S., Martin, L., & Koniak-Griffin, D. (1997). *Maternity nursing: Family, newborn, and women's health* (18th ed.). Philadelphia: Lippincott-Raven, p. 916.

---

49. A teenager with active pulmonary tuberculosis has been receiving multimedication chemotherapy for the past month. The client is being prepared for discharge to home. The nurse determines that respiratory isolation is no longer required and that therapeutic effects have been achieved when

1 Nausea and vomiting have stopped.
2 The Mantoux test (purified protein derivative [PPD]) result is negative.
3 Sputum cultures are negative.
4 Stools are clay-colored.

Answer: 3

Rationale: The primary diagnostic tool for pulmonary tuberculosis is a sputum culture. Reverse results can measure effectiveness. Nausea and vomiting and clay-colored stools are side effects of the medications. Their presence or absence doesn't measure the therapeutic effectiveness of the medication. The Mantoux test is a screening tool, not a diagnostic test for tuberculosis. Because it indicates exposure to the organism but not active disease, the test results will continue to be positive.

Test-Taking Strategy: Remember that the absence of infectious organisms is a desired outcome in communicable diseases. The sputum is the only diagnostic test that will determine absence of infectious organisms. Options 1 and 4 identify side effects. The Mantoux test result will continue to be positive. If you had difficulty with this question, take time now to review the Mantoux test!

Level of Cognitive Ability: Analysis
Phase of Nursing Process: Evaluation
Client Needs: Health Promotion and Maintenance
Content Area: Child Health

Reference

Wong, D. (1997). *Whaley and Wong's Essentials of pediatric nursing* (5th ed.). St. Louis: Mosby–Year Book, pp. 770–771.

---

50. A 9-year-old child has newly diagnosed type I diabetes. The nurse is planning for home care with the child and family. An age-appropriate activity for this child for health maintenance is

1 Independently self-administering insulin.
2 Making independent decisions regarding sliding scale coverage of insulin.
3 Assisting an adult in self-administration of insulin and in glucose monitoring.
4 Administering insulin drawn up by an adult.

Answer: 1

Rationale: School-age children have the cognitive and motor skills to independently administer insulin. Developmentally, they don't have the maturity to make situational decisions (as in option 2) without adult validation. In options 3 and 4, the maximum level of independence appropriate to the level of the child is suppressed.

Test-Taking Strategy: The key word is "independent," which is always encouraged. With children, the activity must be age-appropriate. Eliminate options 3 and 4 first. The remaining two options use the word "independent"; decision making is a cognitive skill, which develops later than motor skills. Therefore, option 1 is the better choice. If you had difficulty with this question, take time now to review growth and development of the 9-year-old!

Level of Cognitive Ability: Application
Phase of Nursing Process: Planning
Client Needs: Health Promotion and Maintenance
Content Area: Child Health

Reference

Wong, D. (1997). *Whaley and Wong's Essentials of pediatric nursing* (5th ed.). St. Louis: Mosby–Year Book, pp. 1055–1056.

51. The nurse has been encouraging intake of oral fluids in the laboring woman to improve hydration. Which of the following represents a successful outcome of this action?

1 A urine specific gravity of 1.020
2 Continued leaking of amniotic fluid during labor
3 Blood pressure of 150/90
4 Ketones in the urine

Answer: 1

Rationale: Urine specific gravity measures the concentration of the urine. During the first stage of labor, the renal system has a tendency to concentrate urine. Labor and birth require hydration and caloric intake to replenish energy expenditure and promote efficient uterine function, as well as general well-being. Adequate nutrition and hydration may be accomplished by oral intake of food and fluids.

Test-Taking Strategy: This question focuses on evaluating the effectiveness of a nursing intervention for health maintenance. An elevated blood pressure and ketones in the urine are not expected outcomes of labor and hydration. Once membranes are ruptured, it is expected that amniotic fluid may continue to leak. If you had difficulty with this question, take time now to review interventions during labor!

Level of Cognitive Ability: Analysis
Phase of Nursing Process: Evaluation
Client Needs: Health Promotion and Maintenance
Content Area: Maternity

Reference
Nichols, F., & Zwelling, E. (1997). *Maternal-newborn nursing: Theory and practice.* Philadelphia: W. B. Saunders, p. 771.

---

52. The nurse has completed a class for diabetic pregnant clients on signs and symptoms of potential complications. The nurse would consider the teaching as effective if a client made which of the following statements?

1 "I'm glad I don't have to worry about developing hypoglycemia while I am pregnant"
2 "I need to watch my weight for any sudden gains because I am prone to pregnancy-induced hypertension"
3 "My insulin dosage should decrease in the last 2 months because I will be using some of the baby's insulin supply"
4 "I should not have ultrasounds done, because I am diabetic"

Answer: 2

Rationale: Hypoglycemia is a problem during pregnancy and needs to be assessed. The incidence of pregnancy-induced hypertension is higher among diabetic pregnant clients than among nondiabetic pregnant clients. Insulin needs will increase during the last trimester because of increased placenta degradation. Ultrasound examinations are done frequently during a diabetic pregnancy to check for congenital anomalies and determine appropriate growth patterns.

Test-Taking Strategy: Options 1 and 4 can be easily eliminated. Remembering that insulin needs will increase during the last trimester will assist in eliminating option 3. Note that the question addresses diabetic pregnant clients. This will assist in directing you to the correct option. If you had difficulty with this question, take time now to review the complications associated with diabetes and pregnancy!

Level of Cognitive Ability: Analysis
Phase of Nursing Process: Evaluation
Client Needs: Health Promotion and Maintenance
Content Area: Maternity

Reference
Reeder, S., Martin, L., & Koniak-Griffin, D. (1997). *Maternity nursing: Family, newborn, and women's health care* (18th ed.). Philadelphia: Lippincott-Raven, pp. 859–861.

---

53. A postpartum client recovering from disseminated intravascular coagulopathy is to be discharged on low dosages of an anticoagulant medication. Discharge teaching should include which of the following priority safety instructions regarding this medication?

1 Avoid any activities that may cause bruising injuries
2 Avoid walking long distances and climbing stairs
3 Avoid taking aspirin
4 Avoid brushing teeth

Answer: 3

Rationale: All of the activities in options 1, 2, and 4 may cause bleeding; however, some may be impossible to avoid. The client needs to be taught to be cautious and report any signs of bleeding. Aspirin can interact with the anticoagulant medication and increase clotting time beyond therapeutic ranges. Avoiding aspirin is the priority.

Test-Taking Strategy: All of the options may cause bleeding. Options 1, 2, and 4 involve activities, whereas option 3 refers to a medication. Note the word "priority" in the question. This should assist in directing you to the correct option. If you had difficulty with this question, take time now to review teaching points related to anticoagulants!

Level of Cognitive Ability: Application
Phase of Nursing Process: Planning
Client Needs: Health Promotion and Maintenance
Content Area: Pharmacology

Reference

Hodgson, B., & Kizior, R. (1998). *Saunders nursing drug handbook 1998.* Philadelphia: W. B. Saunders, pp. 1062–1064.

---

54. Hypoglycemia is a common problem for newborns in the first few hours of life. Which of the following observations by the nurse would indicate the need for further evaluation of hypoglycemia in a full-term infant 24 hours old who had a confirmed episode of hypoglycemia at 1 hour of age?

1 Blood glucose level of 40 mg/dL before the last feeding
2 High-pitched cry and eating 15–20 mL of formula per feeding
3 Weight loss of 4 ounces and dry, peeling skin
4 Breast-feeding 20 minutes or longer and strong sucking

Answer: 2

Rationale: At 24 hours of age, a full-term infant should be able to consume at least 30 mL of formula per feeding. A high-pitched cry is indicative of neurological involvement. Blood glucose levels of 40 mg/dL are acceptable in the first few days of life. Weight loss over the first few days of life and dry, peeling skin are normal findings for full-term infants. Breast-feeding for 20 minutes with strong sucking is an excellent finding. Hypoglycemia causes central nervous system (CNS) symptoms (high-pitched cry) and also is exhibited by lack of strength for eating enough for growth.

Test-Taking Strategy: The question seeks an answer that indicates the need for follow-up care. Knowledge of normal findings in newborns, of hypoglycemia, and of acceptable blood glucose levels is needed to understand the question. Eliminate options 1, 3, and 4 because these are normal findings. The phrase "high-pitched cry" in option 2 should direct you to this choice. If you had difficulty with this question, take time now to review normal findings in newborns!

Level of Cognitive Ability: Analysis
Phase of Nursing Process: Evaluation
Client Needs: Health Promotion and Maintenance
Content Area: Maternity

References

Ashwill, J., & Droske, S. (1997). *Nursing care of children: Principles and practice.* Philadelphia: W. B. Saunders, pp. 562–564.
Nichols, F., & Zwelling, E. (1997). *Maternal-newborn nursing: Theory and practice.* Philadelphia: W. B. Saunders, pp. 1187–1188.

---

55. A newborn infant is suspected to be infected with human immunodeficiency virus (HIV). Most infants have no evidence of an HIV infection at birth. The nurse is preparing to help the parents understand about the disease and how it will affect their infant. Which of the following would be inappropriate for the nurse to include in the teaching?

1 Opportunistic infections occur as early as 4 weeks of age
2 The latency period for infants is equal to the adult latency period
3 Nutrition is a main concern for HIV-positive infants
4 Most newborn HIV infection is attributable to perinatal transmission

Answer: 2

Rationale: The latency period for infants is much shorter than that for adults. This may be a result of their immature immune systems. This also makes them more prone to opportunistic infections that may show up as early as 4 weeks of age. These infants often exhibit failure to thrive and diarrhea, making nutrition a difficult issue for these clients. The most common route of infection for infants is perinatal transmission.

Test-Taking Strategy: This question asks you to determine a plan for client education about the disease process. Knowledge about HIV infection in the newborn is needed to determine the correct answer. If you needed to guess, remember that infants and elderly are most often affected by viral diseases and would therefore have a shorter latency period. If you had difficulty with this question, take time now to review HIV infection in the neonate!

Level of Cognitive Ability: Application
Phase of Nursing Process: Planning
Client Needs: Health Promotion and Maintenance
Content Area: Maternity

Reference

Nichols, F., & Zwelling, E. (1997). *Maternal-newborn nursing: Theory and practice.* Philadelphia: W. B. Saunders, pp. 1187–1188.

56. The depressed client admits that one reason for the depression is that too many demands drain the energy. The client also admits that one reason why the situation is so bad is that the word "no" is not part of the vocabulary when it comes to the requests and needs of others. After 7 days of the client's hospitalization, another client asks for assistance in cleaning the dayroom. Immediately the client says, "No, I can't help you now. I am enjoying the movie." The nurse evaluates this response as

1 A shirking of responsibility.
2 Withdrawal from peers.
3 Increased control over decisions.
4 Decreased cooperation with others.

Answer: 3

Rationale: The client has been unable to refuse requests in the past. Saying "no" now indicates that the client is trying to meet his or her own needs. "No" is being said now without guilt or apology. The client has learned to be more assertive about own needs during the treatment process, and this can help to maintain health upon discharge.

Test-Taking Strategy: Option 3 is the most related to the stem and the information that the client has been unable to say "no" before hospitalization. In that sense, all other options can be eliminated.

Level of Cognitive Ability: Analysis
Phase of Nursing Process: Evaluation
Client Needs: Health Promotion and Maintenance
Content Area: Mental Health

Reference

Johnson, B. (1997). *Psychiatric-mental health nursing: Adaptation and growth* (4th ed.). Philadelphia: Lippincott-Raven, pp. 556–558.

---

57. The suicidal client who was admitted to the unit approximately 7 days ago is preparing for discharge. In evaluating the coping strategies learned during hospitalization, the nurse would recognize which of the following statements, if made by the client, indicates that further teaching needs to occur?

1 "I think this has been a very positive experience in my life"
2 "I know I must continue to take my medications just as prescribed"
3 "I now know that I can't be all things to all people"
4 "I know that I probably won't have depression in the future"

Answer: 4

Rationale: Depression may be a recurring illness for some people. The client needs to understand the symptoms and recognize when or whether treatment needs to begin again. The other comments show that the client has learned some coping skills, such as setting limits, taking medications, and reframing an unpleasant experience into a more positive one.

Test-Taking Strategy: Option 4 is the correct option for this question as stated. Options 1, 2, and 3 are very positive and realistic. A statement such as option 4 is the only unrealistic statement and thus indicates that further teaching is needed.

Level of Cognitive Ability: Analysis
Phase of Nursing Process: Evaluation
Client Needs: Health Promotion and Maintenance
Content Area: Mental Health

Reference

Johnson, B. (1997). *Psychiatric-mental health nursing: Adaptation and growth* (4th ed.). Philadelphia: Lippincott-Raven, pp. 558–561.

---

58. A nurse demonstrates to a mother how to correctly take an axillary temperature to determine whether a child has a fever. Which action by the mother would indicate a need for further teaching?

1 She selects a mercury thermometer with a slender tip
2 She holds the thermometer in the axilla for 1 minute
3 She records the actual temperature reading and route
4 She places the thermometer in the center of the axilla

Answer: 2

Rationale: An axillary temperature should be taken for at least 5 minutes to be most accurate. Options 1, 3, and 4 are correct steps for taking an axillary temperature.

Test-Taking Strategy: The phrase "needs further instruction" is a clue that one option is an incorrect action. The reader must have knowledge of how to correctly obtain an axillary measurement of body temperature. If you had difficulty with this question, take time now to review the procedure for obtaining an axillary temperature!

Level of Cognitive Ability: Analysis
Phase of Nursing Process: Evaluation
Client Needs: Health Promotion and Maintenance
Content Area: Child Health

Reference

Ashwill, J., & Droske, S. (1997). *Nursing care of children: Principles and practice.* Philadelphia: W. B. Saunders, pp. 437-438.

59. A school nurse is teaching an athletic coach how to prevent dehydration in athletes during football practice. Which observation during football practice would indicate that the teaching was ineffective?

1 Scheduled fluid breaks every 30 minutes throughout practice
2 Weighed athletes before, during, and after football practice
3 Asked the athletes to take a salt tablet before football practice
4 Told athletes to drink 16 ounces of fluid per pound lost during practice

Answer: 3

Rationale: Salt tablets should not be taken because they can contribute to dehydration. Option 1 is correct; frequent fluid breaks should be taken to prevent dehydration. Option 2 is correct; early detection of decreased body weight alerts an individual to drink fluids before becoming dehydrated. A 3% or greater fluid loss mandates rehydration before further exercise is done. Option 4 is correct; 16 ounces of fluid should be consumed for every pound lost to prevent dehydration.

Test-Taking Strategy: The key word in the stem is "ineffective." This gives a clue to the reader that one choice is false. The reader must also know principles of fluid and electrolyte balance and causes of dehydration. Options 1, 2, and 4 are measures that prevent the occurrence of dehydration in athletes. If you had difficulty with this question, take time now to review these measures!

Level of Cognitive Ability: Analysis
Phase of Nursing Process: Evaluation
Client Needs: Health Promotion and Maintenance
Content Area: Fundamental Skills

Reference

Wong, D. (1995). *Whaley and Wong's Nursing care of infants and children* (5th ed.). St. Louis: Mosby–Year Book, p. 1840.

---

60. The nurse instructs the client in a low-fat diet. The client would indicate understanding of this diet by choosing

1 Liver, potato salad, and sherbet.
2 Shrimp and bacon salad.
3 Turkey breast, boiled rice, and angel food cake.
4 Lean hamburger steak and macaroni and cheese.

Answer: 3

Rationale: Major sources of fats include organ meats and red meats, salad dressings, eggs, butter, and cheese. All options except the correct one contain high-fat foods.

Test-Taking Strategy: Eliminate options 2 and 4 first because both a hamburger steak and bacon are high in fat. From the remaining two options, look at the foods closely. Option 3 does not contain any high-fat foods. Potato salad will contain mayonnaise, which is high in fat. If you had difficulty with this question, take time now to review those foods that contain fat!

Level of Cognitive Ability: Analysis
Phase of Nursing Process: Evaluation
Client Needs: Health Promotion and Maintenance
Content Area: Fundamental Skills

Reference

Black, J., & Matassarin-Jacobs, E. (1997). *Medical-surgical nursing: Clinical management for continuity of care* (5th ed.). Philadelphia: W. B. Saunders, pp. 1402–1403.

61. Discharge instructions have been given to the client with angina by the nurse. Which statement by the client reveals an understanding of home use of nitroglycerin therapy?

1. "When I have chest pain, I should put a tablet under my tongue. If I have a burning sensation, I should call my doctor immediately"
2. "When I experience chest pain, I can continue what I'm doing. If it doesn't go away in 10 minutes, I should use a nitroglycerin tablet"
3. "When I have pain, I should lie down and place a tablet under my tongue. If unrelieved in 5 minutes, I should take another tablet"
4. "If I use nitroglycerin and the pain does not subside in 15 minutes, I should go to the hospital"

Answer: 3

Rationale: The client taking sublingual nitroglycerin should lie down after taking the medication because lightheadedness and dizziness may occur as a result of postural hypotension, a side effect. The client should use up to three tablets at 5-minute intervals before seeking medical attention.

Test-Taking Strategy: Eliminate option 1 because burning sensation is a common side effect of nitroglycerin. Nitroglycerin should be used with the onset of anginal pain; thus option 2 is incorrect. Option 4 is erroneous in that the client should repeat nitroglycerin if relief is not obtained with the first or second dose. If you had difficulty with this question, take time now to review client teaching related to nitroglycerin!

Level of Cognitive Ability: Analysis
Phase of Nursing Process: Evaluation
Client Needs: Health Promotion and Maintenance
Content Area: Adult Health/Cardiovascular

Reference

Hodgson, B., & Kizior, R. (1998). *Saunders nursing drug handbook 1998.* Philadelphia: W. B. Saunders, pp. 750–753.

---

62. A client has calculi composed of uric acid. The nurse is teaching the client measures to prevent further development of lithiasis. Which of the following statements would indicate that the client understands what foods to avoid?

1. "I would avoid milk and dairy products"
2. "I would avoid foods such as spinach, chocolate, and tea"
3. "I would avoid foods such as fish with fine bones and organ meats"
4. "I need to drink cranberry juice"

Answer: 3

Rationale: With a uric acid stone, the client should limit intake of foods high in purines. Organ meats, sardines, herring, and other high-purine foods are eliminated from the diet. Foods with moderate levels of purines, such as red and white meats and some seafood, are also limited. Options 1 and 2 are recommended dietary changes for calculi composed of calcium phosphate or calcium oxalate. Cranberry juice is commonly recommended to help lower the pH of urine, rendering it more acid, to prevent the development of urinary tract infections. However, uric acid stones form most readily in acid urine, and cranberry juice would therefore be contraindicated in this client with uric acid stone formation.

Test-Taking Strategy: The key phrase is "uric acid." Remembering simply that organ meats contain purines will assist in directing you to the correct option. If you had difficulty with this question, take time now to review foods to avoid with uric acid calculi!

Level of Cognitive Ability: Application
Phase of Nursing Process: Evaluation
Client Needs: Health Promotion and Maintenance
Content Area: Adult Health/Renal

Reference

Black, J., & Matassarin-Jacobs, E. (1997). *Medical-surgical nursing: Clinical management for continuity of care* (5th ed.). Philadelphia: W. B. Saunders, pp. 1597, 1667.

63. The nurse is teaching the insulin-dependent diabetic (IDM) mother of a male infant who is large for gestational age (LGA). The nurse tells the mother that IDM babies who are LGA appear to be more mature because of their large size but that in reality these infants frequently need to be aroused to facilitate nutritional intake and attachment. Which statement, if made by the mother, indicates that further teaching is necessary?

1 "I will talk to my baby when he is in the quiet, alert state"
2 "I will watch my baby closely because I know he may develop hypoglycemia"
3 "I will breast-feed my baby every 2½–3 hours and will implement arousing techniques"
4 "I will allow my baby to sleep throughout the night because he needs his rest"

Answer: 4

Rationale: IDM infants who are LGA tend to be more difficult to arouse and therefore need to be aroused to facilitate nutritional intake and attachment opportunities. Such infants also have problems maintaining a quiet, alert state. It is beneficial for the mother to interact with the infant during those times to enhance and lengthen the quiet, alert state. The LGA infant should be monitored for hypoglycemia. LGA infants need to be aroused for feedings, usually every 2½–3 hours for breast-feeding.

Test-Taking Strategy: Note the key phrase "frequently need to be aroused" in the question. On the basis of this phrase, by the process of elimination, you should easily be directed toward option 4. Options 1, 2, and 3 address observation and arousal, whereas option 4 does not!

Level of Cognitive Ability: Analysis
Phase of Nursing Process: Evaluation
Client Needs: Health Promotion and Maintenance
Content Area: Maternity

Reference

Olds, S., London, M., & Ladewig, P. (1996). *Maternal-newborn nursing: A family-centered approach* (5th ed.). Menlo Park, CA: Addison-Wesley, pp. 925–930.

64. The client has been experiencing muscle weakness over a period of several months. The physician suspects polymyositis. Which statement, if made by the client, correctly identifies a confirmation of test results and this diagnosis?

1 "The physician said if the muscle fibers were thickened, I would have polymyositis"
2 "To have polymyositis, there will be a decrease in elastic tissue"
3 "I will know I have polymyositis if the muscle fibers are inflamed"
4 "The physician said there would be more fibers and tissue with polymyositis"

Answer: 3

Rationale: Option 2 is referring to the decreased elastic tissue in the aorta, seen in Marfan's syndrome. Options 1 and 4 refer to increased fibrous tissue, seen in ankylosis. Option 3 is correct; necrosis and inflammation are seen in muscle fibers and myocardial fibers.

Test-Taking Strategy: Note the issue of the question: polymyositis. The suffix "-itis" indicates inflammation. The only option that addresses inflammation is option 3. If you had difficulty with this question, take time now to review the description of polymyositis!

Level of Cognitive Ability: Analysis
Phase of Nursing Process: Evaluation
Client Needs: Health Promotion and Maintenance
Content Area: Adult Health/Musculoskeletal

Reference

Burrell, L., Gerlach, M., & Pless, B. (1997). *Adult nursing: Acute and community care* (2nd ed.) Stamford, CT: Appleton & Lange, p. 1655.

65. The client has two chest tubes inserted in the right pleural space after thoracic surgery, which are attached to Pleur-Evac drainage systems. The nurse plans to promote optimal respiratory functioning of the client by

1 Milking and stripping the chest tubes once a shift.
2 Maintaining the client on bed rest until chest tube removal.
3 Positioning the client only on the back and on the right side.
4 Encouraging the client to cough and breathe deeply every hour.

Answer: 4

Rationale: The client with chest tubes should be encouraged to cough and breathe deeply every 1–2 hours after surgery. This helps to facilitate drainage of fluid from the pleural space, as well as facilitating the clearance of secretions from the respiratory tract. Milking and stripping of the chest tube is done only when there is occlusion, such as with a small clot; even then, it is done only with a physician's order or when allowed by agency policy. The client is maintained in semi-Fowler's position and may lie on the back or on the nonoperative side. The client may be allowed to lie on the operative side according to surgeon preference, but care must be taken not to compress the chest tube or attached drainage tubing. Ambulation is generally allowed within a day or two and also facilitates optimal respiratory function.

Test-Taking Strategy: The key phrase of the question is "to promote optimal respiratory functioning." Option 1 is somewhat controversial and is eliminated first. Bed rest (option 2) does not promote respiratory function and is eliminated next. Of the two remaining choices, knowing that positioning is done by surgeon preference helps you choose coughing and deep breathing as the correct answer.

Level of Cognitive Ability: Application
Phase of Nursing Process: Planning
Client Needs: Health Promotion and Maintenance
Content Area: Adult Health/Respiratory

Reference

Black, J., & Matassarin-Jacobs, E. (1997). *Medical-surgical nursing: Clinical management for continuity of care* (5th ed.). Philadelphia: W. B. Saunders, pp. 1160–1161, 1165.

---

66. The nurse in an ambulatory clinic administers a Mantoux skin test to a client on a Monday. The nurse plans to have the client return to the clinic to have the results read on

1 Tuesday or Wednesday.
2 Wednesday or Thursday.
3 Thursday or Friday.
4 The following Monday.

Answer: 2

Rationale: The Mantoux skin test for tuberculosis is read in 48–72 hours. The client should return to the clinic on Wednesday or Thursday.

Test-Taking Strategy: This question tests the concept that Mantoux skin test results must be read within 48–72 hours. Memorize this now if the question was difficult for you.

Level of Cognitive Ability: Application
Phase of Nursing Process: Planning
Client Needs: Health Promotion and Maintenance
Content Area: Adult Health/Respiratory

Reference

Ignatavicius, D. D., Workman, M. L., & Mishler, M. A. (1995). *Medical-surgical nursing: A nursing process approach* (2nd ed.). Philadelphia: W. B. Saunders, p. 720.

---

67. The nurse teaches the client with rib fracture to cough and breathe deeply. The client resists directions by the nurse because of the pain. The nurse interprets that the most appropriate nursing action would be to

1 Continue to give the client gentle encouragement to do so.
2 Ask the physician about administering a nerve block to deaden the pain.
3 Explain in detail the potential complications from lack of coughing and deep breathing.
4 Premedicate the client and assist the client to splint the area during these exercises.

Answer: 4

Rationale: Shallow respirations and splinting that occur with rib fracture predispose the client to developing atelectasis and pneumonia. It is essential that the client perform coughing and deep breathing to prevent these complications. The nurse accomplishes this most effectively by premedicating the client with pain medication and assisting the client with splinting during the exercises.

Test-Taking Strategy: Options 2 and 3 are likely to be the most extreme or unrealistic options, respectively, and should be eliminated first. Of the remaining two, premedication and assistance are more likely to be effective than continued gentle encouragement.

Level of Cognitive Ability: Analysis
Phase of Nursing Process: Implementation
Client Needs: Health Promotion and Maintenance
Content Area: Adult Health/Respiratory

Reference

Black, J., & Matassarin-Jacobs, E. (1997). *Medical-surgical nursing: Clinical management for continuity of care* (5th ed.). Philadelphia: W. B. Saunders, p. 2526.

68. The client with chronic airflow limitation (CAL) is admitted to the hospital with exacerbation and has a nursing diagnosis of Ineffective Airway Clearance. The nurse assesses the client to determine the extent of which of the following prehospitalization factors that could have contributed most to this condition?

1 Anxiety level
2 Amount of sleep
3 Fat intake
4 Fluid intake

Answer: 4

Rationale: The client with Ineffective Airway Clearance has ineffective coughing and excess sputum in the airways. The nurse assesses for contributing factors, such as dehydration and lack of knowledge of proper coughing techniques. Reduction of these factors helps limit exacerbations of the disease.

Test-Taking Strategy: Begin to answer this question by noting that the nursing diagnosis is Ineffective Airway Clearance. This should call to mind the concept of sputum production and clearance. You would then evaluate each of the options in terms of their potential ability to inhibit sputum production or clearance. You would eliminate option 3 first as least plausible, followed by options 1 and 2. The fluid intake is the only factor that could affect the viscosity of secretions, thus affecting airway clearance.

Level of Cognitive Ability: Application
Phase of Nursing Process: Assessment
Client Needs: Health Promotion and Maintenance
Content Area: Adult Health/Respiratory

Reference

Black, J., & Matassarin-Jacobs, E. (1997). *Medical-surgical nursing: Clinical management for continuity of care* (5th ed.). Philadelphia: W. B. Saunders, p. 1120.

---

69. The client with acquired immunodeficiency syndrome (AIDS) gets recurrent *Candida* infections of the mouth. The nurse has given instructions to the client to minimize the occurrence of thrush and evaluates that the client understands the material by which of the following client statements?

1 "I should brush my teeth and rinse the mouth once a day"
2 "I should use a strong mouthwash at least once a week"
3 "Increasing red meat in my diet will keep this from recurring"
4 "Adding 8 ounces of yogurt with live cultures to my diet helps to control this"

Answer: 4

Rationale: *Candida* infections can be controlled by adding 8 ounces of yogurt that has live cultures (*Lactobacillus acidophilus*) to the diet. Meticulous routine skin and mouth care is also helpful in preventing recurrence.

Test-Taking Strategy: Eliminate options 1 and 2 first as the least likely choices because the time frames for oral hygiene are too infrequent. In addition, these options are similar. To discriminate between options 3 and 4, it is necessary to know that yogurt contains cultures that will help minimize recurrences. Review teaching points related to the prevention of *Candida* infections now if you had difficulty with this question!

Level of Cognitive Ability: Analysis
Phase of Nursing Process: Evaluation
Client Needs: Health Promotion and Maintenance
Content Area: Adult Health/Respiratory

Reference

Black, J., & Matassarin-Jacobs, E. (1997). *Medical-surgical nursing: Clinical management for continuity of care* (5th ed.). Philadelphia: W. B. Saunders, p. 628.

---

70. The nurse is teaching the client with acquired immunodeficiency syndrome (AIDS) how to avoid foodborne illnesses. The nurse would instruct the client to avoid which of the following items, to prevent infection?

1 Raw oysters
2 Bottled water
3 Products with sorbitol
4 Bananas

Answer: 1

Rationale: The client is taught to avoid raw or undercooked seafood, meat, poultry, and eggs. The client should also avoid unpasteurized milk and dairy products. Fruits that the client peels are safe, as are bottled beverages. The client may be taught to avoid sorbitol, but this is to diminish diarrhea and has nothing to do with foodborne infections.

Test-Taking Strategy: Sorbitol produces diarrhea but is unrelated to foodborne illness, so option 3 is eliminated first. Bottled water is safe, which eliminates option 2. Eliminate option 4 because the client is taught that fruits that are peeled are safe.

Level of Cognitive Ability: Application
Phase of Nursing Process: Implementation
Client Needs: Health Promotion and Maintenance
Content Area: Fundamental Skills

References

Black, J., & Matassarin-Jacobs, E. (1997). *Medical-surgical nursing: Clinical management for continuity of care* (5th ed.). Philadelphia: W. B. Saunders, p. 635.

Lutz, C., & Przytulski, K. (1997). *Nutrition and diet therapy* (2nd ed.). Philadelphia: F. A. Davis, p. 480.

---

71. The client has had a laryngectomy for throat cancer and has started oral intake. The nurse evaluates that the client has tolerated the first stage of dietary advancement if the client takes which of the following types of diet without aspiration or choking?

1 Bland
2 Clear liquids
3 Full liquids
4 Semisolid foods

Answer: 4

Rationale: Oral intake after laryngectomy is started with semisolid foods. Once the client can manage this type of food, liquids may be introduced. Liquids are not given until the risk of aspiration is negligible. A bland diet is not appropriate. The client may not be able to tolerate the texture of some of the solid foods that would be included in a bland diet.

Test-Taking Strategy: Begin to answer this question by eliminating options 2 and 3. For a client with swallowing difficulty for any reason, liquids are the hardest substance to manage. To discriminate between the remaining two options, you need to know that a bland diet provides no control over the consistency or texture of the food. Because the client is just beginning oral intake, the nonpourable pureed diet is preferable because it is most easily moved past the upper airway.

Level of Cognitive Ability: Analysis
Phase of Nursing Process: Evaluation
Client Needs: Health Promotion and Maintenance
Content Area: Adult Health/Oncology

Reference

Black, J., & Matassarin-Jacobs, E. (1997). *Medical-surgical nursing: Clinical management for continuity of care* (5th ed.). Philadelphia: W. B. Saunders, p. 1091.

---

72. The client with histoplasmosis has an order for ketoconazole (Nizoral). The nurse teaches the client to do which of the following while taking this medication?

1 Take the medication on an empty stomach
2 Take the medication with an antacid
3 Avoid exposure to sunlight
4 Limit alcohol to 2 ounces per day

Answer: 3

Rationale: The client should be taught that ketoconazole is an antifungal medication. It should be taken with food or milk, and antacids should be avoided for 2 hours after it is taken, because gastric acid is needed to activate the medication. The client should avoid concurrent use of alcohol, because the medication is hepatotoxic. The client should also avoid exposure to sunlight, because the medication increases photosensitivity.

Test-Taking Strategy: Begin to answer this question by eliminating options 2 and 4. Many medications are not well absorbed if an antacid is given concurrently. There are also many medications with which alcohol use is contraindicated for the duration of the therapy. To discriminate between options 1 and 3, you would need to know that the medication causes photosensitivity reaction and should be taken with food or milk.

Level of Cognitive Ability: Application
Phase of Nursing Process: Implementation
Client Needs: Health Promotion and Maintenance
Content Area: Pharmacology

Reference

Ignatavicius, D. D., Workman, M. L., & Mishler, M. A. (1995). *Medical-surgical nursing: A nursing process approach* (2nd ed.). Philadelphia: W. B. Saunders, pp. 511–512.

73. The nurse is developing a plan of care for a client with a hip spica cast. In the planning, the nurse plans to limit complications of prolonged immobility. The essential part of the client's plan of care is to

1 Provide a daily fluid intake of 1000 mL/24 hours.
2 Monitor for signs of low serum calcium.
3 Maintain the client in a supine position.
4 Limit milk and milk products to meals only.

Answer: 4

Rationale: Daily fluid intake should be 2000 mL or more per day. The nurse should monitor for signs and symptoms of hypercalcemia (i.e., nausea, vomiting, polydipsia, polyuria, lethargy). A supine position increases urinary stasis; therefore, it should be limited or avoided. Limiting milk and milk products to only meals is the best answer.

Test-Taking Strategy: The question tests the nurse's knowledge of the complication and prevention of prolonged immobility. These concepts must be clearly understood in order to plan care for the client. Option 3 should be eliminated immediately in reference to maintaining an immobile client in any one position. If you know the amount of fluid needed daily and the movement of calcium into the blood from the bones, you will determine that option 4 is the best answer. If you had difficulty with this question, take time now to review the complications of immobility!

Level of Cognitive Ability: Application
Phase of Nursing Process: Planning
Client Needs: Health Promotion and Maintenance
Content Area: Adult Health/Musculoskeletal

Reference

Black, J., & Matassarin-Jacobs, E. (1997). *Medical-surgical nursing: Clinical management for continuity of care* (5th ed.). Philadelphia: W. B. Saunders, pp. 2148–2149.

74. The nurse determines that it is safe for a client to come out of seclusion when the nurse hears the client say which of the following?

1 "I am no longer a threat to myself or others"
2 "I need to use the rest room right away"
3 "I'd like to go back to my room and be alone for a while"
4 "I can't breathe in here. The walls are closing in on me"

Answer: 1

Rationale: Option 1 is clearly the best choice of the four options. The client in seclusion must be assessed at regular intervals (usually every 15–30 minutes) for physical needs, safety, and comfort. Option 2 indicates a physical need that could be met with a urinal or bedpan. It does not indicate that the client has calmed down enough to leave the seclusion room. Option 3 could be an attempt to manipulate the nurse. It gives no indication that the client will control himself or herself when alone in the room. Option 4 could be handled by supportive communication or a PRN medication, if indicated. It does not necessitate discontinuing seclusion.

Test-Taking Strategy: The issue of the question is the specific subject content that the question is asking about. In this particular question, the issue involves knowledge of the appropriate seclusion procedure. Review seclusion procedure now if you had difficulty with this question!

Level of Cognitive Ability: Analysis
Phase of Nursing Process: Evaluation
Client Needs: Health Promotion and Maintenance
Content Area: Mental Health

Reference

Carson, V., & Arnold, E. (1996). *Mental health nursing: The nurse-patient journey.* Philadelphia: W. B. Saunders, pp. 348–349.

75. A male client being discharged who initially denied that he drank "2 six packs of beer a day" before admission is now willing to admit that he has a drinking problem. The client states that he will "get some help" so that he will live a healthier lifestyle. The nurse plans for a meeting with a representative of which of the following groups to meet with the client before discharge?

1 Al Anon
2 Alcoholics Anonymous
3 Families Anonymous
4 Fresh Start

Answer: 2

Rationale: Alcoholics Anonymous is a major self-help organization for the treatment of alcoholism. Option 1 is a group for families of alcoholics. Option 3 is for parents of children who abuse substances. Option 4 is for nicotine addicts.

Test-Taking Strategy: If you are unfamiliar with these support groups, note the relationship between "drinking" in the question and "Alcoholics" in the correct option. Familiarize yourself with the purpose of specific support groups now if you had difficulty with this question!

Level of Cognitive Ability: Application
Phase of Nursing Process: Planning
Client Needs: Health Promotion and Maintenance
Content Area: Mental Health

Reference
Townsend, M. (1996). *Psychiatric–mental health nursing: Concepts of care.* Philadelphia: F. A. Davis, p. 395.

---

76. The nurse is planning to teach a teenage client about sexuality. The nurse would begin the instruction by

1 Exploring the client's area of interest and prior knowledge.
2 Providing written information about sexually transmitted diseases.
3 Informing the client of the dangers of pregnancy.
4 Advising the teenager to maintain sexual abstinence until marriage.

Answer: 1

Rationale: The first step in effective communication is establishing trust. By exploring the client's interest and prior knowledge, rapport is established and learning needs are assessed. The other options may be later steps, depending on the data obtained.

Test-Taking Strategy: Use the nursing process and select an option that gathers data. This will direct you to option 1. When teaching, determine motivation, interest, and level of knowledge before providing information. If you had difficulty with this question, take time now to review the principles of teaching and learning!

Level of Cognitive Ability: Application
Phase of Nursing Process: Planning
Client Needs: Health Promotion and Maintenance
Content Area: Child Health

Reference
Ball, J., & Bindler, R. (1995). *Pediatric nursing: Caring for children.* Stamford, CT: Appleton & Lange, pp. 70–71.

---

77. The nurse instructs a parent regarding the appropriate actions to take when the toddler has a temper tantrum. Which statement by the parent shows a successful outcome of the education?

1 "I will send my child to a room alone for 10 minutes after every tantrum"
2 "I will reward my child with candy at the end of each day without a tantrum"
3 "I will give frequent reminders that only bad children have tantrums"
4 "I will ignore tantrums as long as there is no physical danger"

Answer: 4

Rationale: Ignoring a negative attention-seeking behavior is considered the best way to extinguish it, provided that the child is safe from injury. Option 1 gives attention to the tantrum and also exceeds the recommended time of 1 minute per year of age for time-out. Providing candy as rewards is unhealthy and unlikely to be effective at the end of a day. Option 3 is untrue and negative.

Test-Taking Strategy: Knowledge of recommended childrearing practices is necessary to select the correct answer. Use the process of elimination. If you had difficulty with this question, take time now to review interventions for the child who has temper tantrums!

Level of Cognitive Ability: Analysis
Phase of Nursing Process: Evaluation
Client Needs: Health Promotion and Maintenance
Content Area: Child Health

Reference
Wong, D. (1997). *Whaley and Wong's Essentials of pediatric nursing* (5th ed.). St. Louis: Mosby–Year Book, p. 371.

78. The nurse is caring for a male client who has been prescribed disulfiram (Antabuse). Which of the following statements, if made by the client, would indicate the need for further health teaching?

1 "As long as I don't drink alcohol, I'll be fine"
2 "I must be careful taking cold medicines"
3 "I'll have to check my aftershave lotion"
4 "I'll have to be more careful with the ingredients I use for cooking"

Answer: 1

Rationale: Clients who are taking Antabuse must be taught that substances containing alcohol can trigger an adverse reaction. Sources of hidden alcohol include foods (soups, sauces, vinegars), medicine (cold medicine, mouthwashes), and skin preparations (alcohol rubs, aftershave lotions).

Test-Taking Strategy: Knowledge of this medication is necessary to assist you in answering this question. Remember that Antabuse is used with clients who have alcoholism and that any form of alcohol needs to be avoided with this medication. If you are unfamiliar with this medication and the health teaching that is indicated when this medication is prescribed, it would be important for you to review this now!

Level of Cognitive Ability: Analysis
Phase of Nursing Process: Evaluation
Client Needs: Health Promotion and Maintenance
Content Area: Pharmacology

Reference

Hodgson, B., & Kizior, R. (1998). *Saunders nursing drug handbook 1998.* Philadelphia: W. B. Saunders, pp. 339–340.

---

79. Which of the following indicates that the client needs further teaching regarding testicular self-examination (TSE)?

1 "I feel the spermatic cord in back and going up"
2 "I know to report any small lumps"
3 "I examine myself after I take a warm shower"
4 "I examine myself every 2 months"

Answer: 4

Rationale: TSE should be performed every month. Small lumps or abnormalities should be reported. The spermatic cord finding is normal. After a warm bath or shower, the scrotum is relaxed, making it easier to perform TSE.

Test-Taking Strategy: Use the process of elimination. Remembering that breast self-examination needs to be performed monthly may assist in recalling that TSE is also performed monthly. If you had difficulty with this question, take time now to review the procedure for TSE!

Level of Cognitive Ability: Analysis
Phase of Nursing Process: Evaluation
Client Needs: Health Promotion and Maintenance
Content Area: Adult Health/Oncology

Reference

Smeltzer, S., & Bare, B. (1996). *Brunner and Suddarth's Textbook of medical-surgical nursing* (8th ed.). Philadelphia: Lippincott-Raven, p. 1355.

---

80. A nurse should recognize that a client with Cushing's syndrome understands the hospital discharge instructions if the client makes which of these statements?

1 "I need to favor foods low in potassium"
2 "I need to favor aspirin over acetaminophen (Tylenol)"
3 "I need to check the color of my stools"
4 "I need to check the temperature of my legs"

Answer: 3

Rationale: Cortisol stimulates the secretion of gastric acid, and this can result in the development of peptic ulcers and gastrointestinal bleeding. Option 1 is incorrect because potassium-rich foods should be encouraged to correct hypokalemia. Option 2 is incorrect because aspirin can increase the risk for gastric bleeding and skin bruising. Option 4 is incorrect because Cushing's syndrome does not affect temperature changes in lower extremities.

Test-Taking Strategy: A key word in the stem is "understands," which indicates that there is one correct answer. Use the process of elimination; however, if you had difficulty with this question, take time now to review Cushing's syndrome!

Level of Cognitive Ability: Analysis
Phase of Nursing Process: Evaluation
Client Needs: Health Promotion and Maintenance
Content Area: Adult Health/Endocrine

Reference

Black, J., & Matassarin-Jacobs, E. (1997). *Medical-surgical nursing: Clinical management for continuity of care* (5th ed.). Philadelphia: W. B. Saunders, pp. 2052–2053.

---

81. Which nursing intervention is intended to prevent infection in a client receiving total parenteral nutrition (TPN)?

1 Using strict aseptic technique for intravenous site dressing changes
2 Monitoring serum blood urea nitrogen (BUN) daily
3 Weighing the client daily
4 Encouraging increased fluid intake

Answer: 1

Rationale: Strict aseptic technique is vital during dressing changes because the catheter can serve as a direct entry for microorganisms.

Test-Taking Strategy: Note the similar words "infection" in the question and "aseptic" in the option. In addition, the only option that will prevent infection is option 1. If you had difficulty with this question, take time now to review care of a client receiving TPN!

Level of Cognitive Ability: Application
Phase of Nursing Process: Planning
Client Needs: Health Promotion and Maintenance
Content Area: Fundamental Skills

Reference

Black, J., & Matassarin-Jacobs, E. (1997). *Medical-surgical nursing: Clinical management for continuity of care* (5th ed.). Philadelphia: W. B. Saunders, p. 1756.

---

82. A client is on a diet designed to avoid concentrated sugars. The nurse knows that the client understands the diet plan if which of these diets is selected?

1 Strawberry yogurt, lettuce salad, coffee
2 Chicken salad, tomato, Jell-O, tea, and honey
3 Peanut butter and jelly sandwich, sherbet, cola
4 Tuna sandwich, lettuce salad, watermelon, herbal tea

Answer: 4

Rationale: Concentrated sugars are found in fruit yogurt, gelatin desserts, prepared drink mixes, jelly, and sherbet.

Test-Taking Strategy: Some knowledge of sugar content of food is needed. Read each food item in each option, noting that options 1, 2, and 3 contain foods high in concentrated sugars. Review foods containing concentrated sugars now if you had difficulty with this question!

Level of Cognitive Ability: Analysis
Phase of Nursing Process: Evaluation
Client Needs: Health Promotion and Maintenance
Content Area: Fundamental Skills

Reference

Mahan, K., & Escott-Stump, S. (1996). *Krause's Food, nutrition, & diet therapy* (9th ed.). Philadelphia: W. B. Saunders, p. 36.

83. A client with Cushing's syndrome is undergoing a dexamethasone suppression test. Which of the following statements indicates that the client understands this test?

1 "One milligram of dexamethasone is taken orally at night, and serum cortisol levels are measured the next morning and evening"
2 "After an injection of dexamethasone, a 24-hour urine specimen is collected to measure serum cortisol levels"
3 "Blood samples are drawn before and after exercise to evaluate the effect of exercise on serum cortisol levels"
4 "An injection of ACTH [adrenocorticotropic hormone] is given 30 minutes before blood is drawn to measure serum cortisol levels"

Answer: 1

Rationale: The dexamethasone suppression test is performed to evaluate the function of the adrenal cortex. The procedure for this test is to instruct the client to take 1 mg of dexamethasone at 11 P.M. to suppress ACTH formation in time for an 8 A.M. and an 8 P.M. phlebotomy to measure serum cortisol levels.

Test-Taking Strategy: The question asks you to select the response that indicates correct procedure for a dexamethasone suppression test. Cushing's syndrome is a disorder caused by excessive amounts of cortisol. Because the test is a dexamethasone suppression test, you would expect that something is given to suppress cortisol production. With this in mind, option 3 can be eliminated. You then need to make a choice between options 1, 2, and 4. Knowledge of the procedure is then needed to answer the question correctly. If you had difficulty with this question, take time now to review this test!

Level of Cognitive Ability: Analysis
Phase of Nursing Process: Evaluation
Client Needs: Health Promotion and Maintenance
Content Area: Adult Health/Endocrine

Reference

Black, J., & Matassarin-Jacobs, E. (1997). *Medical-surgical nursing: Clinical management for continuity of care* (5th ed.). Philadelphia: W. B. Saunders, p. 2045.

---

84. A client with congestive heart failure and secondary hyperaldosteronism is started on spironolactone (Aldactone) to manage this disorder. The nurse will anticipate the need to instruct the client regarding dosage adjustment of which of the following medications, if it is also being taken by the client?

1 Warfarin sodium (Coumadin)
2 Alprazolam (Xanax)
3 Verapamil (Calan)
4 Potassium chloride (K-Dur)

Answer: 4

Rationale: Spironolactone (Aldactone) is a potassium-sparing diuretic. If the client is taking potassium chloride or another potassium supplement, the risk for hyperkalemia exists. Potassium doses would need to be adjusted while the client is on this medication.

Test-Taking Strategy: The focus of this question is identifying a medication that interacts with spironolactone. Knowledge that spironolactone is a potassium-sparing diuretic would immediately direct you to the correct option. If you had difficulty with this question, take time now to review potassium-sparing diuretics!

Level of Cognitive Ability: Analysis
Phase of Nursing Process: Planning
Client Needs: Health Promotion and Maintenance
Content Area: Adult Health/Cardiovascular

References

Black, J., & Matassarin-Jacobs, E. (1997). *Medical-surgical nursing: Clinical management for continuity of care* (5th ed.). Philadelphia: W. B. Saunders, p. 2056.
Luckmann, J. (1997). *Saunders manual of nursing care*. Philadelphia: W. B. Saunders, p. 1407.

---

85. The nurse is planning health education classes for a group of expectant parents. Included in the teaching plan is prevention of mental retardation caused by congenital hypothyroidism. The most effective means of preventing this disorder is by

1 Adequate protein intake.
2 Limiting alcohol consumption.
3 Genetic testing.
4 Neonatal screening.

Answer: 4

Rationale: Congenital hypothyroidism is the most common preventable cause of mental retardation. Neonatal screening is the only means of early diagnosis. All 50 states require newborns to be screened for congenital hypothyroidism before discharge from the nursery and before 7 days of life.

Test-Taking Strategy: This question is asking you to identify the most effective means of preventing mental retardation caused by congenital hypothyroidism. Options 1 and 2 are appropriate measures for preventing all birth defects. Genetic testing is one means of preventing congenital hypothyroidism; however, there are other causes for this disorder, and so neonatal screening is the more global answer. If you had difficulty with this question, take time now to review congenital hypothyroidism!

Level of Cognitive Ability: Application
Phase of Nursing Process: Planning
Client Needs: Health Promotion and Maintenance
Content Area: Maternity

Reference

Black, J., & Matassarin-Jacobs, E. (1997). *Medical-surgical nursing: Clinical management for continuity of care* (5th ed.). Philadelphia: W B. Saunders, pp. 2005–2006.

---

86. A client being discharged has a history of command hallucinations to harm self or others. The nurse teaches the client about interventions for hallucinations and anxiety. The nurse knows the client understands this teaching when the client says,

1. "It's important for me to take my medication so I won't be anxious"
2. "I will call my clinical specialist when I'm hallucinating so that I can talk about my feelings and plans and not hurt anyone"
3. "I can go to group and talk so that I don't hurt anyone"
4. "If I get enough sleep and eat well, I won't get anxious and hear things"

Answer: 2

Rationale: There may be an increased risk for impulsive and/or aggressive behavior if a client is receiving command hallucinations to harm self or others. Such clients should be asked if they have intentions to hurt themselves or others. Research has shown that as interpersonal and self-care skills improve, hallucinations decrease. Talking about auditory hallucinations can interfere with subvocal muscular activity associated with a hallucination.

Test-Taking Strategy: Use the process of elimination. Options 1, 3, and 4 are all interventions that a client can do to aid wellness. Option 2 is a specific agreement to seek help and evidences self-responsible commitment and control over own behavior.

Level of Cognitive Ability: Analysis
Phase of Nursing Process: Evaluation
Client Needs: Health Promotion and Maintenance
Content Area: Mental Health

Reference

Haber, J. (1997). *Comprehensive psychiatric nursing* (5th ed.). St. Louis: Mosby–Year Book, pp. 580, 592–593.

---

87. A female client who is experiencing disordered thinking about food being poisoned is admitted to the unit. Which communication technique would the nurse plan to use to encourage her to eat dinner?

1. Using open-ended questions and silence
2. Offering opinions about the need to eat
3. Verbalizing reasons that the client may not choose to eat
4. Focusing on self-disclosure of own food preference

Answer: 1

Rationale: Open-ended questions and silence are strategies used to encourage clients to discuss their problems in a descriptive manner. Options 2 and 3 are not helpful to the client because they do not encourage the client to express feelings. Option 4 is not a client-centered intervention.

Test-Taking Strategy: Use the process of elimination. Eliminate options 2 and 3 first because they do not support client expression of feelings. Eliminate option 4 next because it is not a client-centered response. This leaves option 1 as the correct choice.

Level of Cognitive Ability: Application
Phase of Nursing Process: Planning
Client Needs: Health Promotion and Maintenance
Content Area: Mental Health

Reference

Haber, J. (1997). *Comprehensive psychiatric nursing* (5th ed.). St. Louis: Mosby–Year Book, pp. 129, 592–593.

88. The nurse in an outpatient diabetes clinic is monitoring an insulin-dependent client. Today's blood work reveals a glycosylated hemoglobin (HbA_{1c}) concentration of 10%. In evaluating this client's plan of care, how would the nurse interpret this blood work?

1. Normal value, indicating that the client is managing blood glucose control well
2. Low value, indicating that the client is not managing blood glucose control very well
3. High value, indicating that the client is not managing blood glucose control very well
4. The value does not offer information regarding client management of the disease

Answer: 3

Rationale: Glycosylated hemoglobin is a measure of glucose control during the past 6–8 weeks before the test. It is a reliable measure to determine the degree of glucose control in diabetic clients over a period of time and is not influenced by glucose/dietary management a day or two before the test is done. The normal range for HbA_{1c} is 4%–7%; elevated levels indicate poor glucose control.

Test-Taking Strategy: You need to know what information this test provides as well as the normal values or range. This is a relatively new test that is useful for monitoring compliance with diet and insulin. If you had difficulty with this question, take time now to review this important test!

Level of Cognitive Ability: Analysis
Phase of Nursing Process: Evaluation
Client Needs: Health Promotion and Maintenance
Content Area: Adult Health/Endocrine

Reference

Black, J., & Matassarin-Jacobs, E. (1997). *Medical-surgical nursing: Clinical management for continuity of care* (5th ed.). Philadelphia: W B. Saunders, pp. 1960–1961.

---

89. The nurse is instructing an insulin-dependent client about management of hypoglycemic reactions. The nurse instructs the client that hypoglycemia most likely occurs during what time interval after insulin administration?

1. Onset
2. Peak
3. Duration
4. Any time

Answer: 2

Rationale: Insulin reactions are most likely to occur during the peaking of the insulin, when the medication is at its maximum action. Peak action depends upon type of insulin, amount, injection site, and other factors.

Test-Taking Strategy: Remember that insulin is a hypoglycemic agent. The word "peak" means the "highest point." Remembering this should assist in directing you to the correct option. If you had difficulty with this question, take time now to review the occurrence of hypoglycemia when a client is taking insulin!

Level of Cognitive Ability: Application
Phase of Nursing Process: Implementation
Client Needs: Health Promotion and Maintenance
Content Area: Adult Health/Endocrine

Reference

Black, J., & Matassarin-Jacobs, E. (1997). *Medical-surgical nursing: Clinical management for continuity of care* (5th ed.). Philadelphia: W B. Saunders, p. 1989.

90. A client with Graves' disease has in the care plan the nursing diagnosis Altered Nutrition: Less than Body Requirements related to the effects of the hypercatabolical state. Which of the following would indicate a successful outcome for this diagnosis?

1 The client will maintain normal weight or gradually gain weight if it is below normal
2 The client demonstrates knowledge regarding the need to consume a diet high in fat and low in protein
3 The client verbalizes the need to avoid snacking between meals
4 The client discusses the relationship between meal time and blood glucose

Answer: 1

Rationale: As a result of the body's attempt to respond to the demands of hypermetabolism from the elevated levels of thyroid hormones, protein, carbohydrate, and lipid metabolism will be greatly affected. This ultimately causes a state of chronic nutritional and caloric deficiency as a result of the metabolical effects of excessive triiodothyronine (T_3) and thyroxine (T_4). Clinical manifestations associated with this state are weight loss and increased appetite. It is therefore a nutritional goal that the client will not lose any more weight and will gradually return to the ideal body weight if necessary. To accomplish this, the client must be weighed regularly and encouraged to eat frequent high-calorie, high-protein, and high-carbohydrate meals and snacks.

Test-Taking Strategy: Eliminate options that do not relate to the nursing diagnosis. Options 2 and 3 would not be beneficial for a client in a hypercatabolical state. Option 4 can be eliminated because discussing the fluctuation in blood glucose will not assist the client with a hypermetabolical state. If you had difficulty with this question, take time now to review altered nutrition and Graves' disease!

Level of Cognitive Ability: Analysis
Phase of Nursing Process: Planning
Client Needs: Health Promotion and Maintenance
Content Area: Adult Health/Endocrine

Reference
Ignatavicius, D. D., Workman, M. L., & Mishler, M. A. (1995). *Medical-surgical nursing: A nursing process approach* (2nd ed.). Philadelphia: W. B. Saunders, pp. 1834, 1842–1843.

---

91. The nurse is caring for a client who is scheduled to undergo thyroidectomy. Which of the following responses by the client would indicate an understanding of the nurse's instructions?

1 "I will definitely have to continue taking antithyroid medications after this surgery"
2 "I need to place my hands behind my neck when I have to cough or change positions"
3 "I need to turn my head and neck front, back, and laterally every hour for the first 12 hours after surgery"
4 "I expect to experience some tingling of my toes, fingers, and lips after surgery"

Answer: 2

Rationale: The client must be aware that tension needs to be reduced on the suture line; otherwise, hemorrhage may develop. One way of reducing incisional tension is to teach the client how to support the neck when coughing or being repositioned. Likewise, during the postoperative period, clients should avoid any unnecessary movement of the neck. That is why sandbags and pillows are frequently used to support the head and neck. Removal of the thyroid does not necessarily mean that the client will be taking antithyroid medications postoperatively. Finally, tingling in the fingers, toes, and lips is probably caused by injury to the parathyroid gland during surgery resulting in hypocalcemia. These signs and symptoms need to be reported immediately to the nurse to prevent tetany from becoming too severe.

Test-Taking Strategy: Use the process of elimination and knowledge regarding this surgery. Options 1, 3, and 4 can be eliminated first because they are inaccurate. Your only option is to then select 2. If you had difficulty with this question, take time now to review postoperative care after thyroidectomy!

Level of Cognitive Ability: Analysis
Phase of Nursing Process: Evaluation
Client Needs: Health Promotion and Maintenance
Content Area: Adult Health/Endocrine

Reference
Ignatavicius, D. D., Workman, M. L., & Mishler, M. A. (1995). *Medical-surgical nursing: A nursing process approach* (2nd ed.). Philadelphia: W. B. Saunders, p. 1840.

92. The nurse has been preparing a client with chronic obstructive pulmonary disease (COPD) for discharge to home. Which statement, if made by the client, would indicate a need for further teaching in relation to nutrition?

1. "I will certainly try to drink 3 liters of fluid every day"
2. "It's best to eat three large meals a day so I will get all my nutrients"
3. "I will not eat as much cabbage as I once did"
4. "I will rest a few minutes before I eat"

Answer: 2

Rationale: Adequate fluid intake helps to liquefy pulmonary secretions. Large meals distend the abdomen and elevate the diaphragm, which may interfere with breathing. Gas-forming foods may cause bloating, which interferes with normal diaphragmatic breathing. Resting before eating may decrease the fatigue that is often associated with COPD.

Test-Taking Strategy: This question is asking you to select a false response. Fundamental nutrition knowledge suggests that an overdistended abdomen will have deleterious effects on a client's respiratory system. Also, option 2 suggests that the only way to get all of the daily nutrients is by eating three large meals a day; this of course is false. If you had difficulty with this question, take time now to review nutrition and the client with a chronic respiratory disorder!

Level of Cognitive Ability: Analysis
Phase of Nursing Process: Evaluation
Client Needs: Health Promotion and Maintenance
Content Area: Adult Health/Respiratory

Reference

Burrell, L., Gerlach, M., & Pless, B. (1997). *Adult nursing: Acute and community care* (2nd ed.). Stamford, CT: Appleton & Lange, pp. 775–777.

---

93. The nurse is preparing a client with pneumonia for discharge to home. Which statement, if made by the client, would alert the nurse to the fact that the client is in need of further discharge teaching?

1. "I will take all of my antibiotics even if I do feel 100% better"
2. "I understand that it may be weeks before my usual sense of well-being returns"
3. "It is a good idea for me to take a nap every afternoon for the next couple of weeks"
4. "You can toss out that incentive spirometry as soon as I leave for home"

Answer: 4

Rationale: Deep breathing and coughing exercises should be practiced for 6–8 weeks after the client is discharged from the hospital in order to keep the alveoli expanded and promote the removal of lung secretions. If the entire regimen of antibiotics is not taken, the client may suffer a relapse. Adequate rest is needed to maintain progress toward recovery. The period of convalescence with pneumonia is often lengthy, and it may be weeks before the client feels a sense of wholeness.

Test-Taking Strategy: This question asks for the client's statement that indicates inaccurate information regarding the issue in the question. The issue of the question is "pneumonia." Options 1, 2, and 3 are accurate, whereas option 4 is inaccurate. In addition, the use of an incentive spirometer has a direct relationship to the pneumonia, the issue of the question. If you had difficulty with this question, take time now to review teaching points for the client with pneumonia!

Level of Cognitive Ability: Analysis
Phase of Nursing Process: Evaluation
Client Needs: Health Promotion and Maintenance
Content Area: Adult Health/Respiratory

Reference

Lewis, S., Collier, I., & Heitkemper, M. (1996). *Medical-surgical nursing: Assessment and management of clinical problems* (4th ed.). St. Louis: Mosby–Year Book, pp. 631–633.

94. The nurse is planning to teach a client who has newly diagnosed tuberculosis (TB) how to prevent the spread of TB. Which of the following strategies would be least effective in preventing the spread of TB?

1. Teach the client to cover the mouth when coughing
2. Teach the client to sterilize dishes at home
3. Teach the client to properly dispose of tissues
4. Teach the client that close contacts should be tested for TB

Answer: 2

Rationale: Options 1, 3, and 4 would assist in breaking the chain of infection. Not only would option 2 be impractical, but also there is no evidence to suggest that sterilizing dishes would break the chain of infection with pulmonary TB.

Test-Taking Strategy: The issue of the question is to prevent the spread of TB. Use the process of elimination, noting that the stem addresses the phrase "least effective." Review home care principles related to TB, if you had difficulty with this question. You will likely see questions similar to this one on NCLEX-RN!

Level of Cognitive Ability: Application
Phase of Nursing Process: Planning
Client Needs: Health Promotion and Maintenance
Content Area: Adult Health/Respiratory

Reference

Smeltzer, S., & Bare, B. (1996). *Brunner and Suddarth's Textbook of medical-surgical nursing* (8th ed.). Philadelphia: Lippincott-Raven, pp. 496–497.

---

95. The client asks the nurse for a recommendation about how to prevent fires and burn injury. The nurse tells the client that the one single intervention that has been shown to decrease the risk of dying in a residential fire by 50% is

1. The installation of a sprinkler system.
2. Fire extinguishers placed in key areas such as the kitchen, near the furnace, and near the hot water heater.
3. The use of properly functioning smoke detectors.
4. Installation of fire-resistant dry-wall panels throughout the house.

Answer: 3

Rationale: Early detection of smoke and, subsequently, immediate evacuation from the house have been shown to significantly decrease mortality. The installation of a sprinkler system is very expensive and not usually used in residential situations. Fire extinguishers are useful to have in the kitchen for small fires, but it is unrealistic and dangerous to use them to attempt to extinguish large fires. Although fire-resistant products may help slow down a blaze, fire-resistant products can eventually catch fire.

Test-Taking Strategy: Look for the health prevention measure that is simple to implement and will alert people of the need to evacuate a residence. If you had difficulty with this question, take time now to review fire safety!

Level of Cognitive Ability: Application
Phase of Nursing Process: Implementation
Client Needs: Health Promotion and Maintenance
Content Area: Fundamental Skills

Reference

Black, J., & Matassarin-Jacobs, E. (1997). *Medical-surgical nursing: Clinical management for continuity of care* (5th ed.). Philadelphia: W. B. Saunders, p. 2234.

---

96. The nurse makes a home health visit to a client with Bell's palsy. Which of the following statements by this client requires clarification by the nurse?

1. "I have been wearing a facial sling during the daytime"
2. "I wear dark glasses when I go out"
3. "I have started to actively exercise my face a few times a day"
4. "I am staying on a liquid diet"

Answer: 4

Rationale: It is not necessary for a client with Bell's palsy to stay on a liquid diet. This client should be encouraged to chew on the unaffected side. The rest of the options reflect accurate recommendations for managing Bell's palsy.

Test-Taking Strategy: Knowledge regarding Bell's palsy is necessary to answer this question. Knowing that Bell's palsy relates to the face may assist in eliminating options 1 and 3. If you had difficulty with this question, take time now to review interventions associated with this disorder!

Level of Cognitive Ability: Analysis
Phase of Nursing Process: Evaluation
Client Needs: Health Promotion and Maintenance
Content Area: Adult Health/Neurological

Reference

Lewis, S., Collier, I., & Heitkemper, M. (1996). *Medical-surgical nursing: Assessment and management of clinical problems* (4th ed.). St. Louis: Mosby–Year Book, p. 179.

---

97. The home care nurse is reviewing a client's understanding of management of trigeminal neuralgia. Which client statement requires further teaching by the nurse?

1 "Wearing a facial sling will help relieve my symptoms"
2 "I should chew on my good side"
3 "I should use warm mouth wash for oral hygiene"
4 "Taking my Tegretol will help control my pain"

Answer: 1

Rationale: Facial slings help the paralysis of Bell's palsy and are not useful with trigeminal neuralgia. The other statements are true. It is recommended that clients chew on the unaffected side and use warm mouth wash or a water jet for oral hygiene. Antiseizure medications such as carbamazepine (Tegretol) and phenytoin (Dilantin) help control the pain of trigeminal neuralgia.

Test-Taking Strategy: Knowledge regarding trigeminal neuralgia is necessary to answer this question. This will assist in eliminating options 2, 3, and 4. If you had difficulty with this question, take time now to review this disorder!

Level of Cognitive Ability: Analysis
Phase of Nursing Process: Evaluation
Client Needs: Health Promotion and Maintenance
Content Area: Adult Health/Neurological

Reference

Black, J., & Matassarin-Jacobs, E. (1997). *Medical-surgical nursing: Clinical management for continuity of care* (5th ed.). Philadelphia: W. B. Saunders, p. 930.

---

98. Because a type 1 diabetic is at risk for hypoglycemia, the nurse should plan to teach the client and family to

1 Omit the afternoon dose of NPH insulin if the client is exercising.
2 Monitor the urine for acetone.
3 Assess for signs of drowsiness and coma.
4 Keep subcutaneous glucagon on hand.

Answer: 4

Rationale: Glucagon is administered subcutaneously or intramuscularly to release glycogen stores and raise blood glucose levels in hypoglycemia. This medication is useful if the client loses consciousness and is unable to take glucose orally. Family members can be taught to administer this medication and possibly prevent an emergency room visit. The nurse would not instruct a client to omit insulin. Acetone in the urine may indicate hyperglycemia. Although signs of hypoglycemia need to be taught to the client, drowsiness and coma are not the initial and key signs of this disorder.

Test-Taking Strategy: Use the process of elimination. Option 1 can be eliminated first because the nurse would not instruct a client to omit doses. Options 2 and 3 can be eliminated next because they are not related to the issue of hypoglycemia. If you had difficulty with this question, take time now to review signs of hypoglycemia and the appropriate interventions!

Level of Cognitive Ability: Application
Phase of Nursing Process: Planning
Client Needs: Health Promotion and Maintenance
Content Area: Adult Health/Endocrine

Reference

Hodgson, B., & Kizior, R. (1998). *Saunders nursing drug handbook 1998.* Philadelphia: W. B. Saunders, pp. 469–470.

99. The nurse teaches a client about precipitate labor. Which of the following comments by the client would indicate an understanding?

1. "My last labor was only 2 hours long"
2. "I pushed for 2 hours with my last labor"
3. "My contractions always start far apart and gradually get closer"
4. "My doctor wants to induce me to make my labor shorter"

Answer: 1

Rationale: Precipitate labor is defined as labor that lasts 3 hours or less for the entire labor and delivery. It usually has an abrupt, not gradual, onset. Induction, particularly with an oxytocic agent, is contraindicated because of the enhanced stimulatory effects on the uterine muscle and an increased risk for fetal hypoxia.

Test-Taking Strategy: The word "precipitate" should assist in defining this condition. This should assist in eliminating options 2 and 4. Option 3 includes the absolute term "always"; therefore eliminate this option. Review information related to precipitate labor now if you had difficulty answering this question!

Level of Cognitive Ability: Analysis
Phase of Nursing Process: Evaluation
Client Needs: Health Promotion and Maintenance
Content Area: Maternity

Reference

Nichols, F., & Zwelling, E. (1997). *Maternal-newborn nursing: Theory and practice.* Philadelphia: W. B. Saunders, p. 891.

100. The nurse is instructing the client on preventing recurrent episodes of preterm labor. Which statement by the client indicates a need for further teaching?

1. "I will report any feeling of pelvic pressure"
2. "I will adhere to the limitations in activity and stay off my feet"
3. "I will abstain from sexual intercourse"
4. "I will limit my fluid intake to three 8-ounce glasses a day"

Answer: 4

Rationale: Risks for preterm labor include dehydration. A client should not restrict fluids (except for those containing alcohol and caffeine, whose "safe" amounts during pregnancy are not known). A sign of preterm labor may be pelvic pressure without the perception of a contraction. Bed rest and a decrease in activity are often ordered in an attempt to decrease pressure on the cervix and increase uterine blood flow. Mechanical stimulation of the cervix during intercourse can stimulate contractions.

Test-Taking Strategy: Note the phrase "indicates a need for further teaching" in the stem of the question. You should easily be able to identify option 4 as the correct option. It is generally not good practice for the client to limit fluid intake to three 8-ounce glasses a day. Review this content now if you had difficulty answering the question!

Level of Cognitive Ability: Analysis
Phase of Nursing Process: Evaluation
Client Needs: Health Promotion and Maintenance
Content Area: Maternity

Reference

Nichols, F., & Zwelling, E. (1997). *Maternal-newborn nursing: Theory and practice.* Philadelphia: W. B. Saunders, pp. 660–666.

101. The nurse has completed discharge teaching with the parents of a child with glomerulonephritis. Which of the following statements, if made by the parents, indicates that further teaching is necessary?

1. "We'll check the blood pressure every day"
2. "We'll be eating a lot of vegetables and not add extra salt"
3. "It'll be so good to have our child back in karate next week"
4. "We'll test the urine for albumin every week"

Answer: 3

Rationale: After discharge, parents should allow the child to return to his or her normal routine and activities with adequate periods allowed for rest. Karate 1 week after discharge, however, would be too rapid an increase in activities and unrealistic. Options 1, 2, and 4 are correct measures.

Test-Taking Strategy: Use the process of elimination. If you are unfamiliar with this disorder, read the options carefully. It would make sense to select option 3 because karate is an aggressive exercise. If you had difficulty with this question, take time now to review client teaching points for glomerulonephritis!

Level of Cognitive Ability: Analysis
Phase of Nursing Process: Evaluation
Client Needs: Health Promotion and Maintenance
Content Area: Child Health

Reference

Ball, J., & Bindler, R. (1995), *Pediatric nursing: Caring for children*. Stamford, CT: Appleton & Lange, p. 649.

---

102. The nurse is planning discharge teaching for parents of a child who had sustained a head injury and is now on tapering doses of dexamethasone sodium phosphate (Decadron). The nurse would include which of the following statements in the parent teaching?

1 "This medication decreases chances of infections"
2 "This medication is tapered to minimize side effects"
3 "If your child's face becomes puffy, the medication dose needs to be increased"
4 "This medication is tapered to decrease chances of rebounding of the cerebral edema"

Answer: 4

Rationale: Rebounding of cerebral edema is a side effect of abrupt Decadron withdrawal. Option 2 is incorrect because tapering, although required, is not done for the purpose of decreasing side effects. Option 1 is incorrect; Decadron decreases inflammation, not chances of infection. Option 3 is incorrect; facial "mooning" is a common side effect that disappears when Decadron is discontinued.

Test-Taking Strategy: It is also important to understand the principles and impact of tapering. Remembering that tapering is necessary to prevent rebound will assist in directing you to the correct answer. Option 4 is the only correct answer. If you had difficulty with this question, take time now to review this important medication!

Level of Cognitive Ability: Application
Phase of Nursing Process: Planning
Client Needs: Health Promotion and Maintenance
Content Area: Pharmacology

Reference

Hodgson, B., & Kizior, R. (1998). *Saunders nursing drug handbook 1998*. Philadelphia: W. B. Saunders, pp. 296–299.

---

103. A woman comes into the emergency room in a state of severe anxiety after a car accident. The most important nursing intervention would be to

1 Remain with the client.
2 Put the client in a quiet room.
3 Teach the client deep breathing.
4 Encourage the client to talk about feelings and concerns.

Answer: 1

Rationale: If the client is left alone with severe anxiety, she may feel abandoned and become overwhelmed. Placing the client in a quiet room is also indicated, but the nurse must stay with the client. It is not possible to teach the client deep breathing or relaxation until the anxiety decreases. Encouraging the client to discuss concerns and feelings would not take place until the anxiety has decreased.

Test-Taking Strategy: Note the key phrase "severe state of anxiety." Because the anxiety state is "severe," eliminate options 3 and 4. For the remaining two options, the phrase "most important" in the stem of the question should direct you toward option 1.

Level of Cognitive Ability: Application
Phase of Nursing Process: Implementation
Client Needs: Health Promotion and Maintenance
Content Area: Mental Health

Reference

Varcarolis, E. (1998). *Foundations of psychiatric mental health nursing* (3rd ed.). Philadelphia: W. B. Saunders, p. 349.

104. An 18-year-old woman is admitted to an inpatient unit with the diagnosis of anorexia nervosa. Health promotion should focus on

1. Helping the client identify and examine dysfunctional thoughts and beliefs.
2. Emphasizing social interaction with clients who withdraw.
3. Providing a supportive environment.
4. Examining intrapsychic conflicts and past issues.

Answer: 1

Rationale: Health promotion focuses on helping clients identify and examine dysfunctional thoughts, as well as identify and examine values and beliefs that maintain these thoughts. Providing a supportive environment is important but is not as primary as option 1. Emphasizing social interaction is not appropriate at this time. Examining intrapsychic conflicts and past issues is not directly related to the client's problem.

Test-Taking Strategy: Use the process of elimination. Option 1 is the only option that is specifically client centered. This option also focuses on identifying client issues related to the diagnosis.

Level of Cognitive Ability: Application
Phase of Nursing Process: Planning
Client Needs: Health Promotion and Maintenance
Content Area: Mental Health

Reference

Varcarolis, E. (1998). *Foundations of psychiatric mental health nursing* (3rd ed.). Philadelphia: W. B. Saunders, p. 812.

---

105. A nurse is conducting group therapy for sexual addicts. At these meetings, sexual behaviors that would offend many people in the general public are discussed. The nurse knows that a guiding principle for effectively conducting this group is

1. Accepting that sexual aberrations are always the result of inappropriate childhood experiences.
2. Knowledge that being nonjudgmental does not mean that the nurse accepts the values and beliefs of others.
3. Convictions that sexual perverts must be identified publicly and forced to take hormone suppression medications.
4. Knowledge that sexual arousal disorders always result from inadequate psychosocial response during sexual arousal.

Answer: 2

Rationale: A primary characteristic of an effective nurse is a nonjudgmental approach to clients. Nonjudgmental nurses allow clients to talk about feelings, and they respect clients as responsible people capable of making their own decisions. This approach allows clients to communicate openly and does not imply that the nurse accepts or condones the behavior of the client.

Test-Taking Strategy: Options 1 and 4 contain the word "always," which is a clue that it might not be the correct option. Option 3 is blatantly judgmental, so it is obviously not the correct answer. Option 2 is a basic tenet of psychiatric nursing and global in that it can be applied in all specialties.

Level of Cognitive Ability: Analysis
Phase of Nursing Process: Analysis
Client Needs: Health Promotion and Maintenance
Content Area: Mental Health

Reference

Fortinash, K., & Holoday-Worret, P. (1996). *Psychiatric–mental health nursing.* St. Louis: Mosby–Year Book, pp. 149–150.

---

106. Which of the following client outcomes would indicate effective interventions for a client with a C5 spinal cord injury?

1. Regains bladder and bowel control
2. Performs activities of daily living (ADLs) independently
3. Maintains intact skin
4. Independently transfers to and from wheelchair

Answer: 3

Rationale: C5 spinal cord injury results in quadriplegia with no sensation below the clavicle, including most of the arms and hands. The client maintains partial movement of the shoulders and elbows. Maintaining intact skin is a key outcome for clients with spinal cord injuries. The remaining options are inappropriate for this type of client.

Test-Taking Strategy: Eliminate options 2 and 4 first because they are similar. Knowledge of a C5 spinal cord injury will assist in eliminating option 1 because it is unrealistic. If you are unfamiliar with this type of injury, it would be important to review it now!

Level of Cognitive Ability: Analysis
Phase of Nursing Process: Evaluation
Client Needs: Health Promotion and Maintenance
Content Area: Adult Health/Neurological

Reference

Burrell, L., Gerlach, M., & Pless, B. (1997). *Adult nursing: Acute and community care* (2nd ed.). Stamford, CT: Appleton & Lange, p. 953.

---

107. A community health nurse visits the home of a child who is being treated with penicillin for scarlet fever. The mother tells the nurse that the child has voided only a small amount of tea-colored urine since the previous day. The child's appetite has decreased, and the child's face was swollen in the morning. The nurse knows that these new symptoms are

1 Signs of the normal progression of scarlet fever.
2 Nothing to be concerned about.
3 The symptoms of acute glomerulonephritis.
4 Symptoms of an allergic reaction to penicillin.

Answer: 3

Rationale: The symptoms identified in the question indicate glomerulonephritis. Although the child is on penicillin, these are not symptoms of an allergic reaction. These symptoms are not normal and should not be ignored.

Test-Taking Strategy: Knowledge of the complications and the symptoms of scarlet fever and of medication reactions is necessary to answer this question. You can easily eliminate options 2 and 4. From this point, eliminate option 1 because of the word "normal." If you had difficulty with this question, take time now to review the complications of scarlet fever and the symptoms of glomerulonephritis.

Level of Cognitive Ability: Analysis
Phase of Nursing Process: Assessment
Client Needs: Health Promotion and Maintenance
Content Area: Child Health

Reference

Wong, D. (1997). *Whaley and Wong's Essentials of pediatric nursing* (5th ed.). St. Louis: Mosby–Year Book, pp. 410, 411, 967.

---

108. A client who sustained a thoracic cord injury a year ago returns to the clinic with a small reddened area on the coccyx. The client has no sensation in the area. After counseling the client to relieve pressure on the area according to a turning schedule, which action by the nurse is most appropriate?

1 Ask a family member to assess the skin daily
2 Schedule the client to return to the clinic daily for a skin check
3 Teach the client to feel for broken areas
4 Teach the client to use a mirror for skin assessment

Answer: 4

Rationale: The client should be allowed to be as independent as possible. The most effective method of skin self-assessment is to use a special mirror.

Test-Taking Strategy: Independence is the key in rehabilitation of clients. Options 1 and 2 involve others in performing a task that the client can perform independently. Option 3 is an inaccurate assessment technique. Option 4 is the only option that addresses client self-assessment of the issue of the question: redness!

Level of Cognitive Ability: Application
Phase of Nursing Process: Implementation
Client Needs: Health Promotion and Maintenance
Content Area: Adult Health/Neurological

Reference

Smeltzer, S., & Bare, B. (1996). *Brunner and Suddarth's Textbook of medical-surgical nursing* (8th ed.). Philadelphia: Lippincott-Raven, pp. 1806–1808.

109. A client is admitted with a leaking cerebral aneurysm. Which plan should the nurse use during the preoperative period?

1. Encourage the client to be up at least twice per day
2. Allow the client to ambulate to the bathroom
3. Obtain a bedside commode for the client's use
4. Place the client on strict bed rest

Answer: 4

Rationale: The client's activity is kept at a minimum to prevent a Valsalva maneuver. Clients often hold their breath and strain while pulling up to get out of bed. This exertion may cause a rise in blood pressure, which increases bleeding.

Test-Taking Strategy: When time frameworks are given, pay attention. The time period in the question is the preoperative period, during which bleeding can still occur. Clients who have bleeding aneurysms in any vessel will have activity curtailed. Options 1, 2, and 3 are similar in that they all involve out-of-bed (OOB) activity. If you had difficulty with this question, take time now to review aneurysm precautions!

Level of Cognitive Ability: Application
Phase of Nursing Process: Planning
Client Needs: Health Promotion and Maintenance
Content Area: Adult Health/Neurological

Reference

Smeltzer, S., & Bare, B. (1996). *Brunner and Suddarth's Textbook of medical-surgical nursing* (8th ed.). Philadelphia: Lippincott-Raven, p. 1766.

---

110. Many intraoperative nursing activities are focused on protecting the client from electrical, chemical, and physical hazards. Which of the following nursing actions would be inappropriate in minimizing or preventing hazards when electrical equipment is in use?

1. Use only electrical equipment designed for operating room use
2. Assume that the correct attachments for the equipment are being used
3. Ground the client correctly
4. Prevent the pooling of fluids under the client

Answer: 2

Rationale: The use of electricity in surgery introduces hazards of electric shock, power failure, and fire to clients. When electrical equipment is in use, the nurse can minimize or prevent hazards to the client by using only electrical equipment designed for the operating room, grounding the client correctly, testing the equipment before use, verifying (not assuming) that the correct attachments for a piece of equipment are being used, reporting faulty equipment immediately, maintaining humidity levels at 50% or higher to minimize static electricity, and preventing the pooling of fluids under the client.

Test-Taking Strategy: Through the process of elimination, determine that option 2 is the only inappropriate nursing action. The nurse should never "assume" anything. Options 1, 3, and 4 contain nursing actions that are appropriate to prevent electrical hazards and promote the health of the client in the intraoperative area.

Level of Cognitive Ability: Analysis
Phase of Nursing Process: Implementation
Client Needs: Health Promotion and Maintenance
Content Area: Fundamental Skills

Reference

Potter, P., & Perry, A. (1997). *Fundamentals of nursing: Concepts, process, and practice* (4th ed.). St. Louis: Mosby–Year Book, p. 885.

---

111. The client has been prescribed allopurinol (Zyloprim) in the treatment of gouty arthritis. The nurse teaches the client to anticipate which of the following prescriptions during an acute attack?

1. Add colchicine or a nonsteroidal anti-inflammatory drug (NSAID)
2. Double the dose of the allopurinol
3. Stop the allopurinol and take an NSAID
4. Stop the allopurinol and take aspirin

Answer: 1

Rationale: Allopurinol helps prevent attacks of gouty arthritis, but it does not relieve them. Therefore, another medication such as colchicine or an NSAID must be added during this time. Because acute attacks may occur more frequently early in the course of therapy with allopurinol, some physicians recommend taking the two products concurrently during the first 3–6 months anyway.

Test-Taking Strategy: Eliminate options 3 and 4 first because it is unlikely that medication will be stopped. Knowledge that an acute attack of gouty arthritis is painful will assist in selecting option 1 because of the anti-inflammatory action of the NSAID. If you had difficulty with this question, take time now to review interventions for an acute attack of gouty arthritis!

Level of Cognitive Ability: Application
Phase of Nursing Process: Implementation
Client Needs: Health Promotion and Maintenance
Content Area: Pharmacology

Reference

Deglin, J., & Vallerand, A. (1997). *Davis's drug guide for nurses* (5th ed.). Philadelphia: F. A. Davis, p. 28.

---

112. The client is taking propranolol (Inderal) as treatment for hypertension. The nurse teaches the client that concurrent use of which of the following items may aggravate the hypertension?

1 Alcohol
2 Insulin
3 Ephedrine
4 Digoxin (Lanoxin)

Answer: 3

Rationale: Ephedrine is an ingredient in some commonly used nasal decongestant products. Clients taking beta-adrenergic blocking agents such as propranolol should avoid concurrent use of ephedrine because it could cause rebound hypertension and bradycardia. Alcohol has an additive hypotensive effect. Digoxin has an additive bradycardic effect. The insulin effect may be altered by propranolol, which necessitates dosage adjustments of the insulin.

Test-Taking Strategy: To answer this question correctly, it is necessary to understand the effects of the listed items on the cardiovascular system. Focus on the issue of the effect on the hypertension. This would enable you to eliminate each of the incorrect options. If you are unfamiliar with the effects of these items on the blood pressure, review them now!

Level of Cognitive Ability: Application
Phase of Nursing Process: Implementation
Client Needs: Health Promotion and Maintenance
Content Area: Pharmacology

Reference

Deglin, J., & Vallerand, A. (1997). *Davis's drug guide for nurses* (5th ed.). Philadelphia: F. A. Davis, p. 140.

---

113. The client has received a prescription for lisinopril (Prinivil). The nurse teaches the client that which of the following frequent side effects may occur?

1 Hypertension
2 Polyuria
3 Hypothermia
4 Cough

Answer: 4

Rationale: Cough is a frequent side effect of therapy with any of the angiotensin converting enzyme (ACE) inhibitors. Hypertension, not a side effect, is the reason to administer the medication. Fever is an occasional side effect. Proteinuria is another common side effect, but not polyuria.

Test-Taking Strategy: To answer this question accurately, it is necessary to be familiar with this medication and its side effects. If this question was difficult, take a few moments to review the side effects of this medication now.

Level of Cognitive Ability: Application
Phase of Nursing Process: Implementation
Client Needs: Health Promotion and Maintenance
Content Area: Pharmacology

Reference

Deglin, J., & Vallerand, A. (1997). *Davis's drug guide for nurses* (5th ed.). Philadelphia: F. A. Davis, p. 90.

114. Which of the following statements indicate that the client understands the prescribed lithium carbonate (Eskalith) regimen?

1. "My last blood test showed that my salt level is normal"
2. "I keep my medication next to the milk in the refrigerator so that I can remember to take it every day"
3. "It is not difficult to restrict my water intake"
4. "I eat foods with adequate amounts of potassium"

Answer: 1

Rationale: Lithium replaces sodium ions in the cells and induces excretion of sodium and potassium from the body. Client teaching includes maintenance of sodium in the daily diet and increased fluid intake (at least 1–1½ liters/day) during maintenance. Lithium is stored at room temperature and protected from light and moisture. Option 4 is not directly related to this medication.

Test-Taking Strategy: Knowledge regarding this medication is necessary to answer the question. Remembering that lithium is a salt may assist in directing you to the correct option. If you had difficulty with this question, take time now to review this medication. You are likely to find questions related to this medication on NCLEX-RN!

Level of Cognitive Ability: Analysis
Phase of Nursing Process: Evaluation
Client Need: Health Promotion and Maintenance
Content Area: Pharmacology

Reference

Hodgson, B., & Kizior, R. (1998). *Saunders nursing drug handbook 1998.* Philadelphia: W. B. Saunders, pp. 598–600.

---

115. An aged client is given a prescription for haloperidol (Haldol). The nurse instructs the client and family to report any signs of pseudoparkinsonism. Which of the following symptoms would the nurse instruct the family to monitor for?

1. Stooped posture, shuffling gait
2. Muscle weakness, decreased salivation
3. Tremors, hyperreflexia
4. Motor restlessness, aphasia

Answer: 1

Rationale: Pseudoparkinsonism is a common extrapyramidal side effect (EPS) of antipsychotic medications. This condition is characterized by stooped posture, shuffling gait, mask-like facial appearance, drooling, tremors, and pill-rolling motions of fingers. Hyperreflexia and aphasia are not characteristic of pseudoparkinsonism.

Test-Taking Strategy: Knowledge regarding the characteristics of pseudoparkinsonism is necessary to answer the question. Review these characteristics and the effects of antipsychotic medications now if you had difficulty with this question. You are likely to find questions related to these medications on NCLEX-RN!

Level of Cognitive Ability: Application
Phase of Nursing Process: Implementation
Client Needs: Health Promotion and Maintenance
Content Area: Pharmacology

Reference

Wilson, H., & Kneisl, C. (1996). *Psychiatric nursing* (5th ed.). Menlo Park, CA: Addison-Wesley, p. 786.

---

116. A client taking tranylcypromine (Parnate) requests information on foods that are contraindicated with this medication. Which of the following foods can be safely included in the diet?

1. Raisins
2. Smoked fish
3. Yogurt
4. Oranges

Answer: 4

Rationale: Parnate is classified as a monoamine oxidase (MAO) inhibitor, and tyramine-containing food should therefore be avoided. Types of food to be avoided include, but are not limited to, options 1, 2, and 3. In addition, beer, wine, caffeine beverages, pickled meats, yeast preparations, avocados, bananas, and plums are to be avoided. Oranges are permissible.

Test-Taking Strategy: Some knowledge of tyramine-containing food may be necessary to answer this question. Use similar distracters to group possible incorrect choices. Options 1, 2, and 3 are foods that are processed or contain some type of additive. The only natural food is option 4. Bear in mind, however, if option 4 were bananas, avocados, or plums, it would be an incorrect answer. If you had difficulty with this question, take time now to review foods high in tyramine!

Level of Cognitive Ability: Analysis
Phase of Nursing Process: Implementation
Client Needs: Health Promotion and Maintenance
Content Area: Pharmacology

Reference

Hodgson, B., & Kizior, R. (1998). *Saunders nursing drug handbook 1998.* Philadelphia: W. B. Saunders, pp. 1012–1014.

---

117. The client is being discharged to home with a Heimlich (flutter) valve. The nurse teaches the client that if the valve needs to be changed, it is done

1 On inspiration.
2 On expiration.
3 During a Valsalva maneuver.
4 Between inspiration and expiration.

Answer: 3

Rationale: A Heimlich valve is a one-way valve that is used instead of underwater chest drainage in some clients. The client is taught to change the valve during a Valsalva maneuver while the stopcock is turned off. The client is also instructed how to do change dressings, to keep dressing and tubing airtight, and to recognize signs of infection.

Test-Taking Strategy: To answer this question accurately, it is necessary to know the purpose of the Heimlich valve. This enables you to apply the same principles that relate to the care of the client with a chest tube. Review this procedure now if you had difficulty with this question!

Level of Cognitive Ability: Application
Phase of Nursing Process: Implementation
Client Needs: Health Promotion and Maintenance
Content Area: Adult Health/Respiratory

Reference

Monahan, F., & Neighbors, M. (1998). *Medical-surgical nursing: Foundations for clinical practice* (2nd ed.). Philadelphia: W. B. Saunders, pp. 579–580.

---

118. The nurse is giving instructions about foot care to the client with chronic arterial insufficiency. The nurse tells the client to

1 Wear shoes that are snugly fitting.
2 Clean the feet daily, drying them well.
3 Apply moisturizer and powder to feet, especially between toes.
4 Cut the toenails very short to prevent scratching.

Answer: 2

Rationale: Foot care for the client with vascular disease is the same as for clients who are diabetic. This includes daily cleansing of the feet; drying well, especially between toes; applying lotion only to dry areas; wearing shoes that fit well without pressure areas; and keeping the toenails trimmed by cutting straight across the nail. Powder should be avoided, to prevent dryness and resultant cracking of the skin.

Test-Taking Strategy: Recall that both diabetes and vascular disease result in impairment of the tissues of the feet. Using the principles involved in diabetic foot care, you may eliminate each of the incorrect options systematically. Review foot care for the client with vascular disease now if you had difficulty with this question!

Level of Cognitive Ability: Application
Phase of Nursing Process: Implementation
Client Needs: Health Promotion and Maintenance
Content Area: Adult Health/Cardiovascular

Reference

Monahan, F., & Neighbors, M. (1998). *Medical-surgical nursing: Foundations for clinical practice* (2nd ed.). Philadelphia: W. B. Saunders, p. 355.

119. The nurse is giving instructions to the client with peptic ulcer disease about symptom management. The nurse tells the client to

1 Eat slowly and chew food thoroughly.
2 Eat large meals to absorb gastric acid.
3 Limit intake of water.
4 Use aspirin to relieve gastric pain.

Answer: 1

Rationale: The client with a peptic ulcer is taught to eat small, frequent meals to help keep the gastric secretions neutralized. The client should eat slowly and chew thoroughly to prevent excess gastric acid secretion. The client should push fluids to 6 to 8 glasses of water per day to dilute gastric acid. The use of aspirin is avoided because it is irritating to gastric mucosa.

Test-Taking Strategy: To answer this question correctly, you should apply knowledge of concepts related to digestion and knowledge of substances that are known gastric irritants. Review teaching points related to the client with peptic ulcer disease now if you had difficulty with this question!

Level of Cognitive Ability: Application
Phase of Nursing Process: Implementation
Client Needs: Health Promotion and Maintenance
Content Area: Adult Health/Gastrointestinal

Reference

Monahan, F., & Neighbors, M. (1998). *Medical-surgical nursing: Foundations for clinical practice* (2nd ed.). Philadelphia: W. B. Saunders, p. 1032.

---

120. The client with a hiatal hernia asks the nurse for something to drink. The nurse offers the client which of the following items stocked in the nursing unit kitchen?

1 Tomato juice
2 Orange juice
3 Grapefruit juice
4 Apple juice

Answer: 4

Rationale: Substances that are irritating to the client with hiatal hernia include tomato products and citrus fruits, which should be avoided. Because caffeine stimulates gastric acid secretion, beverages that contain caffeine, such as coffee, tea, cola, and cocoa, are also eliminated from the diet.

Test-Taking Strategy: Remember that options that are similar are not likely to be correct. Use this principle of test taking to eliminate options 1, 2, and 3. Apple juice is the least irritating substance.

Level of Cognitive Ability: Application
Phase of Nursing Process: Implementation
Client Needs: Health Promotion and Maintenance
Content Area: Adult Health/Gastrointestinal

Reference

Monahan, F., & Neighbors, M. (1998). *Medical-surgical nursing: Foundations for clinical practice* (2nd ed.). Philadelphia: W. B. Saunders, p. 1044.

---

121. The nurse's discharge plan for the client with seizures includes information about the safe use of phenytoin (Dilantin). The nurse instructs the client to

1 Take the anticonvulsant for life.
2 Not skip a dose without expecting the occurrence of a serious effect.
3 Realize that seizures cannot be completely controlled.
4 Discontinue driving a car.

Answer: 2

Rationale: In 50% of well-controlled cases, the medication may eventually be discontinued. Because 50% of cases can be completely controlled, a client can, in some states, drive a car if the client has had no seizures for a year. Option 2 alerts the client to the seriousness of the condition in that skipping a dose places the client at risk for status epilepticus.

Test-Taking Strategy: Knowledge regarding seizures is necessary to answer the question. You can easily eliminate options 3 and 4. Of the remaining two options, option 2 provides the most complete and accurate statement regarding seizures!

Level of Cognitive Ability: Application
Phase of Nursing Process: Implementation
Client Needs: Health Promotion and Maintenance
Content Area: Pharmacology

Reference

Hodgson, B., & Kizior, R. (1998). *Saunders nursing drug handbook 1998.* Philadelphia: W. B. Saunders, pp. 823–825.

---

122. The client with spinal cord injury (SCI) experiences bladder spasms and reflex incontinence. In preparing for discharge, the nurse instructs the client to

1. Limit fluid intake to 1000 mL in 24 hours.
2. Take own temperature every day.
3. Catheterize self every 2 hours PRN to prevent spasm.
4. Avoid caffeine in the diet.

Answer: 4

Rationale: Caffeine can contribute to bladder spasms and reflex incontinence. Therefore, it should be eliminated from the diet of the client with an SCI. Limiting fluid intake does not prevent spasm and could place the client at further risk of urinary tract infection. Self-monitoring of temperature would be useful in detecting infection, but it does nothing to alleviate bladder spasm. Self-catheterization every 2 hours is too frequent and serves no useful purpose.

Test-Taking Strategy: To answer this question accurately, it is necessary to understand the etiology and preventive measures for bladder spasm and reflex incontinence. Eliminate options 1 and 3 first because they place the client at increased risk of urinary tract infection and are therefore not appropriate. Choose option 4 over option 2 because option 2 would detect infection and does not deal with spasm and incontinence.

Level of Cognitive Ability: Application
Phase of Nursing Process: Implementation
Client Needs: Health Promotion and Maintenance
Content Area: Adult Health/Neurological

Reference

Monahan, F., & Neighbors, M. (1998). *Medical-surgical nursing: Foundations for clinical practice* (2nd ed.). Philadelphia: W. B. Saunders, p. 826.

---

123. The client seeks treatment in an ambulatory care center for symptoms of Raynaud's disease. The nurse instructs the client to

1. Wear protective items, such as gloves and warm socks PRN.
2. Alternate exposures to heat and cold.
3. Decrease cigarette smoking by one half.
4. Continue activity during vasospasm for quicker relief of symptoms.

Answer: 1

Rationale: Treatment for Raynaud's disease includes avoidance of precipitating factors such as cold or damp weather, stress, and cigarettes. The client should get sufficient rest and sleep, protect the extremities by wearing protective clothing, and stop activity during vasospasm.

Test-Taking Strategy: Recall that the symptoms of Raynaud's disease are caused by vasospasm. Eliminate those options that will cause vasospasm. This includes options 2, 3, and 4. Review client teaching points related to Raynaud's disease now if you had difficulty with this question!

Level of Cognitive Ability: Application
Phase of Nursing Process: Implementation
Client Needs: Health Promotion and Maintenance
Content Area: Adult Health/Cardiovascular

Reference

Monahan, F., & Neighbors, M. (1998). *Medical-surgical nursing: Foundations for clinical practice* (2nd ed.). Philadelphia: W. B. Saunders, p. 356.

124. The client with atherosclerosis asks the nurse about dietary modifications to lower risk of heart disease. The nurse encourages the client to eat which of the following foods that the client enjoys?

1. Baked chicken with skin
2. Fresh cantaloupe
3. Broiled cheeseburger
4. Mashed potato with gravy

Answer: 2

Rationale: To lower the risk of heart disease, the diet should be low in saturated fat with the appropriate number of total calories. The diet should include fewer red meats and more white meat, with skin removed. Dairy products used should be low in fat, and foods with high amounts of empty calories should be avoided.

Test-Taking Strategy: Use fat content of the foods in the options as a guide to answering this question. Eliminate options 1 and 3 first, because of the fat content of the described meats. Choose option 2 over option 4 because fresh fruits and vegetables are naturally low in fat.

Level of Cognitive Ability: Application
Phase of Nursing Process: Implementation
Client Needs: Health Promotion and Maintenance
Content Area: Adult Health/Cardiovascular

Reference

Monahan, F., & Neighbors, M. (1998). *Medical-surgical nursing: Foundations for clinical practice* (2nd ed.). Philadelphia: W. B. Saunders, p. 363.

---

125. The client is being discharged to home after angioplasty in which the right femoral area was used as the catheter insertion site. The nurse instructs the client that which of the following signs and symptoms may be expected after the procedure?

1. Coolness or discoloration of the right foot
2. Temperature as high as 101°F
3. Large area of bruising at the right side of the groin
4. Mild discomfort in the right side of the groin

Answer: 4

Rationale: The client may feel some mild discomfort at the catheter insertion site after angioplasty. This is usually well relieved by analgesics such as acetaminophen (Tylenol). The client is taught to report to the physician any neurovascular changes to the affected leg, bleeding or bruising at the insertion site, and signs of local infection such as drainage at the site or increased temperature.

Test-Taking Strategy: The wording of the question guides you to choose an option that is a correct statement. Knowing that bleeding and infection are complications of the procedure guides you to eliminate options 2 and 3. You would choose option 4 over option 1 by knowing either that neurovascular status should not be impaired by the procedure or that the area may be mildly uncomfortable.

Level of Cognitive Ability: Application
Phase of Nursing Process: Implementation
Client Needs: Health Promotion and Maintenance
Content Area: Adult Health/Cardiovascular

Reference

Monahan, F., & Neighbors, M. (1998). *Medical-surgical nursing: Foundations for clinical practice* (2nd ed.). Philadelphia: W. B. Saunders, p. 344.

---

126. The nurse is teaching dietary modifications to the hypertensive client. The nurse encourages which of the following snack foods according to the client's taste?

1. Cheese and crackers
2. Honeydew melon slices
3. Frozen pizza
4. Canned tomato soup

Answer: 2

Rationale: Sodium should be avoided by the client with hypertension. Fresh fruits and vegetables are naturally low in sodium. Hypertensive clients are also advised to keep fat intake to less than 30% of total calories as part of prudent heart living. Each of the incorrect options contain increased amounts of sodium.

Test-Taking Strategy: To answer this question correctly, it is necessary to know the dietary modifications needed with hypertension and to select foods accordingly. The correct answer is not only a fruit but also the only unprocessed food of the choices given. Use this principle as a guide in selecting the correct option.

Level of Cognitive Ability: Application
Phase of Nursing Process: Implementation
Client Needs: Health Promotion and Maintenance
Content Area: Adult Health/Cardiovascular

Reference

Monahan, F., & Neighbors, M. (1998). *Medical-surgical nursing: Foundations for clinical practice* (2nd ed.). Philadelphia: W. B. Saunders, p. 382.

---

127. The nurse is teaching the hypertensive client to recognize signs and symptoms that may occur during periods of elevated blood pressure. Which of the following would not be included by the nurse during the discussion?

1 Early morning headaches
2 Epistaxis
3 Feeling of fullness in the head
4 Blurred vision

Answer: 3

Rationale: Cerebrovascular symptoms of hypertension include early morning headaches, occipital headaches, blurred vision, lightheadedness and vertigo, dizziness, and epistaxis. The client should be aware of these symptoms and report them if they occur. The client should also be taught self-monitoring of blood pressure.

Test-Taking Strategy: Specific knowledge of signs and symptoms related to hypertension is needed to answer this question. Use the process of elimination in selecting the correct option. Option 3 is the most vague option, whereas options 1, 2, and 4 are specific and related to hypertension. If this question was difficult, take a few moments now to review the signs and symptoms of hypertension!

Level of Cognitive Ability: Application
Phase of Nursing Process: Implementation
Client Needs: Health Promotion and Maintenance
Content Area: Adult Health/Cardiovascular

Reference

Monahan, F., & Neighbors, M. (1998). *Medical-surgical nursing: Foundations for clinical practice* (2nd ed.). Philadelphia: W. B. Saunders, p. 375.

---

128. The client is taking iron supplements to correct iron-deficiency anemia. The nurse teaches the client which of the following special considerations while on iron therapy?

1 Avoid taking iron with milk or antacids
2 Limit intake of meat, fish, and poultry
3 Take in a low-fiber diet
4 Limit intake of fluids

Answer: 1

Rationale: The client should avoid taking iron with milk or antacids, which decrease absorption of iron. The client should also avoid taking iron with food if possible. The client should increase natural sources of iron, such as meats, fish, and poultry. Finally, the client should consume sufficient fiber and fluids to prevent constipation as a side effect of therapy.

Test-Taking Strategy: Begin to answer this question by eliminating options 3 and 4, knowing that constipation is a common side effect of iron therapy. An understanding of nutritional contents of meat products would guide you to eliminate option 2 next. This leaves option 1 as the correct answer. Remember that absorption of certain medications is impaired by milk products or antacids.

Level of Cognitive Ability: Application
Phase of Nursing Process: Implementation
Client Needs: Health Promotion and Maintenance
Content Area: Pharmacology

Reference

Monahan, F., & Neighbors, M. (1998). *Medical-surgical nursing: Foundations for clinical practice* (2nd ed.). Philadelphia: W. B. Saunders, p. 470.

129. The client with a colostomy complains to the nurse of appliance odor. The nurse recommends that the client consume which of the following deodorizing foods?

1 Yogurt
2 Mushrooms
3 Cucumbers
4 Eggs

Answer: 1

Rationale: Foods that help to eliminate odor with colostomy include yogurt, buttermilk, spinach, beet greens, and parsley. Foods that cause odor are many and include alcohol, beans, turnips, radishes, asparagus, onions, cucumbers, mushrooms, cabbage, eggs, and fish.

Test-Taking Strategy: Foods that cause gas in the client with normal gastrointestinal function also form gas in the gastrointestinal tract of the client with a colostomy. Use basic nutritional knowledge and principles to answer this question.

Level of Cognitive Ability: Application
Phase of Nursing Process: Implementation
Client Needs: Health Promotion and Maintenance
Content Area: Adult Health/Gastrointestinal

Reference

Monahan, F., & Neighbors, M. (1998). *Medical-surgical nursing: Foundations for clinical practice* (2nd ed.). Philadelphia: W. B. Saunders, p. 1009.

---

130. The nurse is demonstrating colostomy care to a client with a newly created colostomy. The nurse demonstrates correct cutting of the appliance by making the circle how much larger than the client's stoma?

1 1/16 inch
2 1/8 inch
3 1/4 inch
4 1/2 inch

Answer: 2

Rationale: The size of the opening for the appliance is generally cut 1/8 inch larger than the size of the client's stoma. This minimizes the amount of exposed skin but does not cause pressure on the stoma itself.

Test-Taking Strategy: Begin to answer this question by eliminating options 3 and 4 because they leave too much skin area exposed for possible irritation by gastrointestinal contents. You would then choose option 2 over option 1 because 1/16 inch is extremely small and not realistic.

Level of Cognitive Ability: Application
Phase of Nursing Process: Implementation
Client Needs: Health Promotion and Maintenance
Content Area: Adult Health/Gastrointestinal

Reference

Monahan, F., & Neighbors, M. (1998). *Medical-surgical nursing: Foundations for clinical practice* (2nd ed.). Philadelphia: W. B. Saunders, p. 1009.

131. A 10-year-old child has received a diagnosis of type I diabetes. The nurse prepares to educate the family. The child is very active and is often away from the parents. What would be the best nursing intervention to maintain physiological homeostasis for this child ?

1 Teach the child's teacher to monitor insulin requirements and administer the child's insulin
2 Teach the child to monitor insulin requirements and administer own insulin
3 Teach the parents to always be available to monitor the child's insulin requirements
4 Teach all the friends and family involved with the child's activities to monitor the child's insulin requirements

Answer: 2

Rationale: Most children 9 years old or older can understand the principles of monitoring their own insulin requirements according to developmental stage. They are usually responsible enough to determine the appropriate intervention needed to maintain their health.

Test-Taking Strategy: Note that the age of the child indicates that the child is able to take control and responsibility of the health care situation. Eliminate option 4 first because of the absolute word "all" and because this option is unrealistic. Eliminate option 1 next because the teacher will not take responsibility for health care interventions. Eliminate option 3 next because the parents cannot always be available. If you had difficulty with this question, take time now to review growth and development of a 10-year-old!

Level of Cognitive Ability: Application
Phase of Nursing Process: Implementation
Client Needs: Health Promotion and Maintenance
Content Area: Child Health

Reference
Wong, D. (1997). *Whaley and Wong's Essentials of pediatric nursing* (5th ed.). St. Louis: Mosby–Year Book, pp. 1055–1056, 1058.

---

132. When evaluating the effectiveness of client teaching for a client with spinal cord injury, which of the following statements, if made by the client, would indicate the need for additional teaching regarding autonomic dysreflexia?

1 "I need to pay close attention to how frequently my bowels move"
2 "It is best if I avoid tight clothing and lumpy bedclothes"
3 "I should watch for headache, congestion, and flushed skin"
4 "Symptoms I should watch for include fever and chest pain"

Answer: 4

Rationale: Symptoms of autonomic dysreflexia include headache, congestion, flushed skin above the injury and cold skin below it, diaphoresis, nausea, and anxiety. Fever and chest pain are not associated with this condition. Options 1, 2, and 3, if stated by a client, would indicate understanding of the condition.

Test-Taking Strategy: Knowledge of autonomic dysreflexia is necessary to correctly answer this question. Use your nursing knowledge to answer this question. If you are unfamiliar with this syndrome, take time now to review!

Level of Cognitive Ability: Analysis
Phase of Nursing Process: Evaluation
Client Needs: Health Promotion and Maintenance
Content Area: Adult Health/Neurological

Reference
Black, J., & Matassarin-Jacobs, E. (1997). *Medical-surgical nursing: Clinical management for continuity of care* (5th ed.). Philadelphia: W. B. Saunders, pp. 899–900.

133. The nurse is discharging a female client who has a diagnosis of T11 fracture with cord transection. Which of the following would indicate the need for further discharge teaching?

1. The client states that she will have to be careful not to eat as many dairy products
2. The client states that she will wash her hands, perineum, and catheter with soap and water before performing self-catheterization
3. The client jokes about no longer needing to worry about birth control
4. The client verbalizes the need to eat her meals close to the same time every day

Answer: 3

Rationale: Female clients with spinal cord trauma in their reproductive years remain fertile. Contraception is necessary for such clients who are sexually active. However, oral contraceptives may increase the risk for thrombophlebitis. Clients with paralysis should avoid dairy products, to control the formation of urinary calculi. Clients who lack bladder control are taught to self-catheterize, using clean technique. Meals should be at the same time every day and include fiber, warm solid foods, and liquid foods to promote evacuation of the bowel.

Test-Taking Strategy: Key aspects of dealing with a client with spinal cord injury are nutrition and elimination. Options 1, 2, and 4 address these key areas. If you had difficulty with this question, take time now to review teaching points for a client with transection of the cord!

Level of Cognitive Ability: Analysis
Phase of Nursing Process: Evaluation
Client Needs: Health Promotion and Maintenance
Content Area: Adult Health/Neurological

Reference

Burrell, L., Gerlach, M., & Pless, B. (1997). *Adult nursing: Acute and community care* (2nd ed.). Stamford, CT: Appleton & Lange, pp. 961–962.

---

134. Nursing discharge plans for the client who has attempted suicide should focus on which of the following?

1. Weekly follow-up appointments
2. Contracts and immediately available crisis resources
3. Encouraging family and friends to always be present
4. Providing phone numbers for hospital and physician

Answer: 2

Rationale: Crisis times may occur between appointments. No self-control measures have been given to this client. Contracts facilitate clients' feelings of responsibility for keeping a promise. This gives the client control. Option 3 is unrealistic. Providing phone numbers will not ensure available and immediate crisis intervention.

Test-Taking Strategy: The issue of the question relates to the availability of immediate resources for the client if needed. Eliminate option 3 first because this is unrealistic. Options 1 and 4 will not necessarily provide these immediate resources. Note the word "immediately" in the correct option.

Level of Cognitive Ability: Application
Phase of Nursing Process: Planning
Client Needs: Health Promotion and Maintenance
Content Area: Mental Health

Reference

Fortinash, K., & Holoday-Worret, P. (1996). *Psychiatric–mental health nursing*. St. Louis: Mosby–Year Book, pp. 630, 634.

---

135. The nurse is teaching a community group about violence in the family. Which of the following statements by group members would indicate a need for further instruction?

1. Abusers usually have poor self-esteem
2. Abusers use fear and intimidation
3. Abusers are often jealous or self-centered
4. Abuse occurs more in low-income families

Answer: 4

Rationale: Personal characteristics of abusers include low self-esteem, immaturity, dependence, insecurity, and jealousy. Abusers often use fear and intimidation to the point where their victims will do anything just to avoid further abuse. The notion that abuse occurs more in lower socioeconomic groups is a myth.

Test-Taking Strategy: This question calls for the statement that would indicate a need for further education. Therefore you are looking for the incorrect statement. Options 1, 2, and 3 all are true statements. Only answer 4 is incorrect. If you had difficulty with this question, take time now to review the characteristics of an abuser and family violence!

Level of Cognitive Ability: Analysis
Phase of Nursing Process: Evaluation
Client Needs: Health Promotion and Maintenance
Content Area: Mental Health

Reference

Carson, V., & Arnold, E. (1996). *Mental health nursing: The nurse-patient journey.* Philadelphia: W. B. Saunders, pp. 1044–1046.

---

136. A 2-year-old child is a suspected victim of child abuse. You are evaluating the child's parent for educational needs related to growth and development. Which statement made by the parent indicates a need for education on the growth and development stage of the child?

1 "Once my child is potty trained, I can still expect him or her to have some 'accidents' "
2 "When I tell my child to do something once, I don't expect to have to tell him or her again"
3 "My child is expected to try to do things on his or her own, such as dress and feed"
4 "A 2-year-old's vocabulary is usually limited to about 200 words"

Answer: 2

Rationale: One characteristic of abusive parents is that their expectations are too high. As a result, the child cannot live up to the expectations of the parent. Unrealistic expectations result in the disappointment and frustration of the parent. The parent may even believe that the action of the child is intentional or done out of spite. The parent may react in an excessive manner, causing severe injury to the child.

Test-Taking Strategy: Only option 2 contains a statement of concern, thereby indicating a need for the education of the parent. Options 1, 3, and 4 are true statements in that they are appropriate for the 2-year-old. Knowing normal growth and development activities for a 2-year-old is essential to correctly answering the question. If you had difficulty with this question, take time now to review growth and development!

Level of Cognitive Ability: Analysis
Phase of Nursing Process: Evaluation
Client Needs: Health Promotion and Maintenance
Content Area: Child Health

Reference

Ashwill, J., & Droske, S. (1997). *Nursing care of children: Principles and practice.* Philadelphia: W. B. Saunders, pp. 1292–1293

---

137. An elderly client, who is a victim of elder abuse, and the family have been seen in the counseling center weekly for the past month. Which of the following statements, if made by the abusive family members, would indicate that they have learned more positive coping skills?

1 "I will be more careful to make sure that my father's needs are 100% met"
2 "I am so sorry and embarrassed that the abusive event occurred. It won't happen again"
3 "I feel better equipped to care for my father now that I know where to turn if I need assistance"
4 "Now that my father is moving into my home, I will have to stop drinking alcohol"

Answer: 3

Rationale: Elder abuse sometimes results when family members are expected to care for their aging parents. This care can cause the family to become socially overextended, frustrated, or financially depleted. Knowing where to turn in the community for assistance in caring for aging family members can bring the much needed relief. Using these resources is a positive alternative coping strategy of many families.

Test-Taking Strategy: The stem of the question calls for a coping strategy. Only option 3 is a means of coping with the issues. The other responses are statements of good faith or promises, which may or may not be kept in the future. Only option 3 outlines a definitive plan for how to handle the pressure associated with father's care.

Level of Cognitive Ability: Analysis
Phase of Nursing Process: Evaluation
Client Needs: Health Promotion and Maintenance
Content Area: Mental Health

Reference

Carson, V., & Arnold, E. (1996). *Mental health nursing: The nurse-patient journey.* Philadelphia: W. B. Saunders, pp. 1070–1073.

138. Which of the following should the nurse include when teaching a client who has recently been started on a monoamine oxidase (MAO) inhibitor?

1. The client should be told that the medication will begin to alleviate symptoms of depression almost immediately
2. The medication is associated with a high rate of abuse
3. This medication can cause severe drowsiness
4. The client must avoid foods containing tyramine

Answer: 4

Rationale: Although MAO inhibitors usually produce hypotension as a side effect, potentially lethal hypertension can occur if the client eats foods that contain tyramine. Some such foods include aged cheeses, hot dogs, and beer.

Test-Taking Strategy: Knowledge of MAO inhibitors will assist in answering the question. This classification is most commonly associated with the need for education about food-medication interactions. If you had difficulty with this question, take time now to review these interactions!

Level of Cognitive Ability: Application
Phase of Nursing Process: Planning
Client Needs: Health Promotion and Maintenance
Content Area: Pharmacology

Reference
Carson, V., & Arnold, E. (1996). *Mental health nursing: The nurse-patient journey.* Philadelphia: W. B. Saunders, p. 542.

---

139. Which of the following is a reasonable outcome for the elderly client with dementia who has a nursing diagnosis of Self-Care Deficit?

1. The client will be admitted to a nursing home to have activities of daily living (ADLs) needs met
2. The client will function at the highest level of independence possible
3. The client will complete all ADLs independently within a 1- to 1½-hour time frame
4. The nursing staff will attend to all the client's ADL needs during the hospital stay

Answer: 2

Rationale: All clients, regardless of age, need to be encouraged to perform at the highest level of independence possible. This contributes to the client's sense of control and sense of well-being.

Test-Taking Strategy: Options 3 and 4 are eliminated because the word "all" appears in the selections. Option 1 is eliminated because it is not known what the "self-care deficit" entails. To assume on the basis of such little data that the client requires a nursing home level of care would be erroneous!

Level of Cognitive Ability: Analysis
Phase of Nursing Process: Planning
Client Needs: Health Promotion and Maintenance
Content Area: Mental Health

Reference
Luckmann, J. (1997). *Saunders manual of nursing care.* Philadelphia: W. B. Saunders, p. 584.

---

140. The client who takes haloperidol (Haldol), 5 mg at bedtime, also receives benztropine (Cogentin), 1 mg, at the same time. The nurse instructs the client that the Cogentin is given to

1. Combat extrapyramidal side effects (EPS).
2. Enhance sleep.
3. Enhance the effects of Haldol.
4. Enhance the anticholinergic effects of the medications.

Answer: 1

Rationale: Haldol is a neuroleptic medication that may cause the client to experience EPS. Antiparkinsonian medications such as Cogentin are given to decrease the symptoms of EPS.

Test-Taking Strategy: Knowledge regarding the purpose of administering medications in combination is necessary to answer the question. If you had difficulty with this question, take time now to review the purposes of these medications!

Level of Cognitive Ability: Application
Phase of Nursing Process: Implementation
Client Needs: Health Promotion and Maintenance
Content Area: Pharmacology

Reference
Hodgson, B., & Kizior, R. (1998). *Saunders nursing drug handbook 1998.* Philadelphia: W. B. Saunders, pp. 102–104, 486–488.

141. The client has newly diagnosed chronic obstructive pulmonary disease (COPD). The client returns home after a short hospitalization. The home health nurse visits the client and the most important plan is to teach strategies that are designed to

1 Encourage the client's self-concept as an active person.
2 Improve oxygenation and minimize carbon dioxide retention.
3 Identify irritants in the home that interfere with breathing.
4 Promote membership in support groups.

Answer: 2

Rationale: Improving oxygenation and minimizing carbon dioxide retention are the primary objectives of nursing interventions for the client with COPD. The other options are interventions that will help achieve this primary goal.

Test-Taking Strategy: Answering this question requires a fundamental knowledge of COPD. All of the options are important for the client with COPD; however, the question asks for the most important strategy. Eliminate options 1 and 4 first because they are similar. Of the remaining two options, note that option 2 addresses airway.

Level of Cognitive Ability: Application
Phase of Nursing Process: Planning
Client Needs: Health Promotion and Maintenance
Content Area: Adult Health/Respiratory

Reference

Polaski, A., & Tatro, S. (1996). *Luckmann's Core principles and practice of medical-surgical nursing.* Philadelphia: W. B. Saunders, p. 579.

---

142. A client is being discharged after a bronchoscopy that was performed yesterday. In performing the discharge planning, the client makes all the following statements to the nurse. Which statement should the nurse identify as indicating a need for further teaching?

1 "I can expect to cough up bright red blood"
2 "I will stop smoking my cigarettes"
3 "I will get help immediately if I start having trouble breathing"
4 "I will use the throat lozenges as directed by the physician until my sore throat goes away"

Answer: 1

Rationale: After the procedure, the client should be observed for signs of respiratory distress, including dyspnea, changes in respiratory rate, use of accessory muscles, and changes in or absence of lung sounds. Expectorated secretions are inspected for hemoptysis. The client needs to avoid smoking. A sore throat is common, and lozenges would be helpful as directed.

Test-Taking Strategy: Use the process of elimination. Options 2 and 3 can be easily eliminated first. For the remaining two options, remember that bright red bleeding indicates active bleeding. Thus bright red blood and any signs of distress would need to be reported to the physician.

Level of Cognitive Ability: Analysis
Phase of Nursing Process: Evaluation
Client Needs: Health Promotion and Maintenance
Content Area: Adult Health/Respiratory

Reference

Black, J., & Matassarin-Jacobs, E. (1997). *Medical-surgical nursing: Clinical management for continuity of care* (5th ed.). Philadelphia: W. B. Saunders, pp. 1061–1062.

---

143. A client who is on chlorpromazine (Thorazine) is preparing for discharge. In developing a plan of care for the client, the nurse instructs the client

1 To adhere to a strict tyramine-restricted diet.
2 On the signs and symptoms of relapse of depression.
3 To avoid prolonged exposure to the sun.
4 To have the therapeutic blood levels measured, because there is a narrow range between the therapeutic and toxic levels of the medication.

Answer: 3

Rationale: Chlorpromazine is an antipsychotic medication often used in treatment of psychosis. Photosensitivity is sometimes a side effect of the phenothiazine class of antipsychotic medications, to which chlorpromazine (Thorazine) belongs. Options 1, 2, and 4 are unrelated to the administration of this medication.

Test-Taking Strategy: Because chlorpromazine is an antipsychotic, not an antidepressive medication, option 2 can be eliminated. Eliminate option 1 because this option relates to medications that are MAO inhibitors. There is not a narrow range between therapeutic and toxic levels such as with lithium; therefore, eliminate option 4. If you had difficulty with this question, take time now to review this medication!

Level of Cognitive Ability: Application
Phase of Nursing Process: Implementation
Client Needs: Health Promotion and Maintenance
Content Area: Pharmacology

Reference

Hodgson, B., & Kizior, R. (1998). *Saunders nursing drug handbook 1998.* Philadelphia: W. B. Saunders, pp. 210–213.

---

144. A client is being discharged with a heparin lock (intermittent intravenous [IV] catheter) to receive a week of antibiotic IV therapy at home after abdominal surgery. When evaluating the discharge teaching session, which of the following statements by the client indicates the need for further instruction?

1 "I'll examine the IV site frequently"
2 "If the IV site becomes wet or moist, it can air dry"
3 "Pain, redness, and swelling need to be reported to the physician"
4 "If the lock or catheter accidentally comes out, I'll apply pressure at the site"

Answer: 2

Rationale: Clients receiving IV therapy at home need to be instructed on site assessment as well as complications to report to the physician. Clients should also know how to treat critical complications such as bleeding at the IV site. Clients often are expected to change dressings and need to be aware that if the dressing is wet or soiled, it needs to be changed immediately in order to prevent infection.

Test-Taking Strategy: Knowing principles of aseptic care of peripheral IV sites is a top priority for health maintenance in the home. Options 1 and 3 are similar in relating to assessment of the site. You should be able to easily eliminate option 4 on the basis of knowledge related to IV therapy. Review these principles now if you had difficulty with this question!

Level of Cognitive Ability: Analysis
Phase of Nursing Process: Evaluation
Client Needs: Health Promotion and Maintenance
Content Area: Fundamental Skills

Reference

Phillips, L. (1997). *Manual of IV therapeutics* (2nd ed.). Philadelphia: F. A. Davis, pp. 259, 381.

---

145. The home health nurse provides instructions to the client with jaundice who is experiencing pruritus. Which of the following would the nurse not include in the instructions to this client?

1 Wear loose cotton clothing
2 Use tepid water for bathing
3 Maintain a warm environment temperature
4 Avoid alkaline soaps

Answer: 3

Rationale: Pruritus is caused by the accumulation of bile salts in the skin and results from obstructed biliary excretion. Antihistamines may relieve the itching, as will tepid water or emollient baths. The client should avoid alkaline soap and wear loose, soft cotton clothing. The client is instructed to keep the environment cool.

Test-Taking Strategy: Recalling that heat causes vasodilation will assist in answering this question. This principle should direct you to option 3 as the measure to avoid in the treatment of pruritus. If you had difficulty with this question, take time now to review the measures that assist in alleviating pruritus!

Level of Cognitive Ability: Application
Phase of Nursing Process: Implementation
Client Needs: Health Promotion and Maintenance
Content Area: Adult Health/Gastrointestinal

Reference

Black, J., & Matassarin-Jacobs, E. (1997). *Medical-surgical nursing: Clinical management for continuity of care* (5th ed.). Philadelphia: W. B. Saunders, p. 1860.

146. The nurse is instructing the client with hepatitis about measures to control fatigue. Which of the following would not be a component of this teaching plan?

1. Plan rest periods after meals
2. Do not engage in activity to the point of becoming overly tired
3. Perform personal hygiene if not fatigued
4. Complete all daily activities in the morning when the client is most rested

Answer: 4

Rationale: A client with hepatitis has tremendous metabolical demands that lead to fatigue and interfere with ADLs. The nurse encourages ADLs unless they cause excessive fatigue. The client is advised to plan rest periods after activities such as meals. Activities should be spaced throughout the day with frequent planned rest periods. Clients who engage in excessive activity too early in the recovery stage may experience a relapse.

Test-Taking Strategy: Use the basic principles associated with a balance of rest and activities to answer the question. By the process of elimination, the only option that does not provide this balance is option 4. Review measures to alleviate fatigue in the client with hepatitis, if you had difficulty with this question!

Level of Cognitive Ability: Application
Phase of Nursing Process: Implementation
Client Needs: Health Promotion and Maintenance
Content Area: Adult Health/Gastrointestinal

Reference

Black, J., & Matassarin-Jacobs, E. (1997). *Medical-surgical nursing: Clinical management for continuity of care* (5th ed.). Philadelphia: W. B. Saunders, p. 1870.

---

147. The nurse provides home care instruction to the client with multiple sclerosis (MS). Which of the following would the nurse include in the teaching plan?

1. To avoid pregnancy
2. To restrict fluid intake to 1000 mL daily
3. To maintain a low-fiber diet
4. To avoid taking hot baths or showers

Answer: 4

Rationale: Because fatigue can be precipitated by warm temperatures, the client is instructed to take cool baths and maintain a cool environmental temperature. A high-fiber diet and an adequate fluid intake of 2000 mL daily are encouraged in order to prevent alterations in elimination and bowel patterns. The client should not be told to avoid pregnancy, but the nurse should assist the client to make informed decisions regarding pregnancy.

Test-Taking Strategy: Use knowledge regarding the effects of MS in answering the question. Eliminate option 1 first because it is inappropriate to insist that a client avoid pregnancy. Eliminate options 2 and 3 next because these measures are unhealthy for this client and would promote alterations in elimination patterns. Review teaching points related to the client with MS if you had difficulty with this question.

Level of Cognitive Ability: Application
Phase of Nursing Process: Implementation
Client Needs: Health Promotion and Maintenance
Content Area: Adult Health/Musculoskeletal

Reference

Black, J., & Matassarin-Jacobs, E. (1997). *Medical-surgical nursing: Clinical management for continuity of care* (5th ed.). Philadelphia: W. B. Saunders, p. 873.

148. The home care nurse provides instructions to the client with a halo vest. Which of the following instructions would the nurse include in the plan of care?

1. Have the spouse use the metal frame to assist the client to sit up
2. Perform pin care three times a week, using peroxide or alcohol
3. Loosen the bolts once a day for bathing
4. Carry the correct size of wrench to loosen the bolts in an emergency

Answer: 4

Rationale: The metal frame is never used or pulled on for turning or lifting. Pin care should be performed at least once a day either with soap and water on cotton-tipped swabs or with alcohol swabs. The bolts should never be loosened except in an emergency. In fact, the physician should be notified if the bolts loosen. The client is instructed to carry the correct-size wrench in case of an emergency necessitating cardiopulmonary resuscitation (CPR). In such a situation, the anterior portion of the vest, including the anterior bolts, will need to be loosened, and the posterior portion should remain in place to provide stability for the spine during CPR.

Test-Taking Strategy: Try to visualize the appearance of a halo vest. Use knowledge regarding the purpose of this vest in stabilizing a cervical spinal fracture to answer the question. Eliminate option 2 first because pin care should be done at least once a day. Eliminate option 1 because pulling on the frame will disrupt the stabilization of the fracture and possibly lead to serious complications. Bolts should never be loosened except in an emergency situation.

Level of Cognitive Ability: Application
Phase of Nursing Process: Implementation
Client Needs: Health Promotion and Maintenance
Content Area: Adult Health/Neurological

Reference

Black, J., & Matassarin-Jacobs, E. (1997). *Medical-surgical nursing: Clinical management for continuity of care* (5th ed.). Philadelphia: W. B. Saunders, p. 906.

---

149. Haloperidol (Haldol) has been prescribed for a client with Tourette's syndrome. The nurse instructs the client about the medication. Which of the following statements, if made by the client, indicates the need for further education?

1. "It may take 6 weeks before the medication works"
2. "The drowsiness will probably go away as I continue the medication"
3. "I should stop the medication if my vision becomes blurred"
4. "I need to avoid alcohol while taking this medication"

Answer: 3

Rationale: The client needs to be instructed not to abruptly discontinue medication therapy. Inform the client that if visual disturbances occur, the physician should be notified. Options 1, 2, and 4 are accurate statements regarding the medication.

Test-Taking Strategy: Eliminate option 4 first because this is a general principle with most medications. Knowledge that this medication is an antipsychotic will assist in eliminating options 1 and 2. In addition, knowing that the medication should not be abruptly stopped will assist in directing you to option 3.

Level of Cognitive Ability: Analysis
Phase of Nursing Process: Evaluation
Client Needs: Health Promotion and Maintenance
Content Area: Pharmacology

Reference

Hodgson, B., & Kizior, R. (1998). *Saunders nursing drug handbook 1998.* Philadelphia: W. B. Saunders, p. 488.

150. A client with diabetes mellitus has received instructions about foot care. Which of the following statements would indicate that the client needs further instruction about foot care?

1. "The best time to cut my nails is after bathing"
2. "Cotton stockings should be worn to absorb excess moisture"
3. "The cuticles of my nails must be cut to prevent overgrowth"
4. "My feet should be inspected daily with a mirror"

Answer: 3

Rationale: Trimming or cutting the cuticles of the nails can lead to injury to the foot by scratching the skin. Even small injuries can be dangerous to the diabetic client who has decreased peripheral vascular circulation. A manicure stick can be used to gently clean the cuticle. Nails can be cut straight across, and after a bath is the best time because that is when the nails are softest. White cotton stockings are the best stockings, and the client needs to inspect the feet daily.

Test-Taking Strategy: Use the process of elimination, seeking the action that could result in altered skin integrity. Using this principle, eliminate options 1, 2, and 4. Review diabetic foot care now if you had difficulty with this question!

Level of Cognitive Ability: Analysis
Phase of Nursing Process: Evaluation
Client Needs: Health Promotion and Maintenance
Content Area: Adult Health/Endocrine

Reference

Black, J., & Matassarin-Jacobs, E. (1997). *Medical-surgical nursing: Clinical management for continuity of care* (5th ed.). Philadelphia: W. B. Saunders, p. 1999.

---

151. In evaluating a client's understanding about the signs and symptoms of hyperglycemia, which statement by the client best reflects accurate understanding?

1. "I may become diaphoretic and faint"
2. "I need to take an extra Orinase tablet if my blood sugar is greater than 300 mg"
3. "I may notice signs of fatigue, dry skin, increased thirst, and urination"
4. "I should restrict my fluid intake if my blood sugar is greater than 250 mg"

Answer: 3

Rationale: Fatigue, dry skin, polyuria, and polydipsia are classic symptoms of hyperglycemia. Fatigue occurs because of lack of energy from inability of the body to use glucose. Dry skin occurs secondary to dehydration related to polyuria. Polydipsia occurs secondary to fluid loss. Diaphoresis is associated with hypoglycemia. Clients should not take extra oral hypoglycemic agents to reduce an elevated blood glucose level. A client with hyperglycemia becomes dehydrated secondary to the osmotic effect of elevated glucose levels. Therefore, the client must increase fluid intake.

Test-Taking Strategy: In identification of the components of the question, note that the nurse is evaluating understanding of signs and symptoms of hyperglycemia. Of all four options, only two directly address signs and symptoms. Therefore, eliminate the others (options 2 and 4). For the remaining two options, discriminating between signs of hypoglycemia and hyperglycemia will direct you to option 3. Review these signs now if you had difficulty with this question!

Level of Cognitive Ability: Analysis
Phase of Nursing Process: Evaluation
Client Needs: Health Promotion and Maintenance
Content Area: Adult Health/Endocrine

Reference

Lewis, S., Collier, I., & Heitkemper, M. (1996). *Medical-surgical nursing: Assessment and management of clinical problems* (4th ed.). St. Louis: Mosby–Year Book, pp. 1440, 1453, 1465.

152. A client taking famotidine (Pepcid) asks the home health nurse about what would be the best medication to take for a headache. Which of the following would be the best response by the nurse?

1 Aspirin (acetylsalicylic acid, ASA)
2 Ibuprofen (Motrin)
3 Acetaminophen (Tylenol)
4 Naproxen (Naprosyn)

Answer: 3

Rationale: The client is taking famotidine, a histamine receptor antagonist. This implies that the client has a disorder characterized by gastrointestinal (GI) irritation. Of the medications listed, the only one that is not irritating to the GI tract is acetaminophen. The others could aggravate an already existing GI problem.

Test-Taking Strategy: To answer this question accurately, it is important to know the reason behind histamine receptor antagonist use. This would allow you to analyze each of the medications listed according to its effects on the GI tract. Review these medications now if you had difficulty with this question!

Level of Cognitive Ability: Application
Phase of Nursing Process: Implementation
Client Needs: Health Promotion and Maintenance
Content Area: Pharmacology

Reference

Deglin, J., & Vallerand, A. (1997). *Davis's drug guide for nurses* (5th ed.). Philadelphia: F. A. Davis, pp. 593, 598.

153. The nurse is teaching the client taking cyclosporine (Sandimmune) after renal transplantation about key medication information. The nurse tells the client to be especially alert for

1 Signs of infection.
2 Hypotension.
3 GI disturbances.
4 Hair loss.

Answer: 1

Rationale: Cyclosporine is an immunosuppressant medication used to prevent transplant rejection. The client should be especially alert for signs and symptoms of infection while taking this medication and should report them to the physician if experienced. The client is also taught about other side effects of the medication, including hypertension, increased facial hair, tremors, gingival hyperplasia, and GI complaints.

Test-Taking Strategy: To answer this question accurately, it is necessary to know that this medication is an immunosuppressant and that the client is at risk for infection while taking the medication. Review this information if necessary, because this is a key concept in transplant medication therapy!

Level of Cognitive Ability: Application
Phase of Nursing Process: Implementation
Client Needs: Health Promotion and Maintenance
Content Area: Pharmacology

Reference

Deglin, J., & Vallerand, A. (1997). *Davis's drug guide for nurses* (5th ed.). Philadelphia: F. A. Davis, p. 311.

154. The client has undergone surgery for glaucoma. The nurse gives the client which of the following discharge instructions?

1 Wound healing usually takes 12 weeks
2 Expect that vision will be permanently impaired to a small degree
3 A shield or eye patch should be worn to protect the eye
4 The sutures are removed after 1 week

Answer: 3

Rationale: After ocular surgery, the client should wear an eye patch or eyeglasses for protection of the eye. Healing takes place in about 6 weeks. Once the postoperative inflammation subsides, the client's vision should return to preoperative level of acuity. Sutures may be either absorbable or nonabsorbable, but in either case, they are not removed.

Test-Taking Strategy: Eliminate options 1 and 4 first as the least plausible of all the options. To discriminate between options 2 and 3, it is necessary to understand that the eye requires protection after surgery. According to Maslow's hierarchy of needs theory, safety is the most important issue. If you had difficulty with this question, take time now to review postoperative teaching points!

Level of Cognitive Ability: Application
Phase of Nursing Process: Implementation
Client Needs: Health Promotion and Maintenance
Content Area: Adult Health/Eye

Reference

Luckmann, J. (1997). *Saunders manual of nursing care.* Philadelphia: W. B. Saunders, p. 776.

---

155. The client has undergone surgery for cataracts. The nurse instructs the client to call the physician for which of the following complaints?

1 A sudden decrease in vision
2 Eye pain relieved by acetaminophen (Tylenol)
3 Small amounts of dried matter on lashes after sleep
4 Gradual resolution of eye redness

Answer: 1

Rationale: The client should report a noticeable or sudden decrease in vision to the physician. The client is taught to take acetaminophen, which is usually effective in relieving discomfort. The eye may be slightly reddened postoperatively, but this should gradually resolve. Small amounts of dried material may be present on the lashes after sleep. This is expected and should be removed with a warm face cloth.

Test-Taking Strategy: Familiarity with principles of care related to cataract surgery is needed to answer this question accurately. Note the key phrase "sudden decrease" in the correct option. This is the clue that option 1 is correct. If this question was difficult, take a few moments to review this content area now!

Level of Cognitive Ability: Application
Phase of Nursing Process: Implementation
Client Needs: Health Promotion and Maintenance
Content Area: Adult Health/Eye

Reference

Luckmann, J. (1997). *Saunders manual of nursing care.* Philadelphia: W. B. Saunders, p. 770.

---

156. The home health nurse visits a client with a diagnosis of cirrhosis and ascites. Which of the following dietary measures will the nurse review?

1 Decrease in fat intake
2 Decrease in carbohydrates
3 Calorie restriction of 1500 daily
4 Sodium restriction

Answer: 4

Rationale: If the client has ascites, sodium and possibly fluids should be restricted in the diet. Fat restriction is not necessary. Total daily calories should range between 2000 and 3000. The diet should supply sufficient carbohydrates to maintain weight and spare protein. The diet should provide ample protein to rebuild tissue but not enough protein to precipitate hepatic encephalopathy.

Test-Taking Strategy: The key word in the question is "ascites." This should assist in directing you to option 4. If you had difficulty with this question, take time now to review dietary measures for the client with cirrhosis and ascites!

Level of Cognitive Ability: Application
Phase of Nursing Process: Implementation
Client Needs: Health Promotion and Maintenance
Content Area: Adult Health/Gastrointestinal

Reference

Black, J., & Matassarin-Jacobs, E. (1997). *Medical-surgical nursing: Clinical management for continuity of care* (5th ed.). Philadelphia: W. B. Saunders, p. 1882.

157. The nurse is preparing to discharge the client with a diagnosis of multiple myeloma. Which of the following would be included in the discharge teaching plan?

1 To restrict fluid intake to 1500 mL daily
2 To maintain bed rest
3 To maintain a high-calorie, low-fiber diet
4 To notify the physician if anorexia and nausea persist

Answer: 4

Rationale: Clients with multiple myeloma need to be taught to monitor for signs of hypercalcemia and to report them immediately to the physician. Anorexia, nausea, vomiting, polyuria, weakness and fatigue, constipation, and signs of dehydration are signs of moderate hypercalcemia. A fluid intake of 3000 mL daily is necessary to dilute the calcium overload and prevent protein from precipitating in the renal tubules. Activity is encouraged. Although a high-calorie diet is encouraged, a diet low in fiber will lead to constipation.

Test-Taking Strategy: Knowledge that hypercalcemia is a concern in multiple myeloma will assist in directing you to the correct option. Eliminate option 2 first. Next, eliminate option 1 because this amount of fluid is rather low. Finally, eliminate option 3 because of the low-fiber diet stated in the option. Review the signs of hypercalcemia now if you had difficulty in selecting the correct option!

Level of Cognitive Ability: Application
Phase of Nursing Process: Implementation
Client Needs: Health Promotion and Maintenance
Content Area: Adult Health/Oncology

Reference

Black, J., & Matassarin-Jacobs, E. (1997). *Medical-surgical nursing: Clinical management for continuity of care* (5th ed.). Philadelphia: W. B. Saunders, pp. 320, 1500.

158. The nurse provides home care instructions to the client hospitalized for a transurethral resection of the prostate (TURP). Which of the following would the nurse not include in the discharge plan?

1 Avoid strenuous activity for 4–6 weeks
2 Maintain a daily intake of 6–8 glasses of water
3 Avoid lifting items heavier than 25 pounds
4 Include prune juice in the diet

Answer: 3

Rationale: The client needs to be advised to avoid strenuous activity for 4–6 weeks and to avoid lifting items weighing more than 20 pounds. The client needs to consume a high daily intake of at least 6–8 glasses of nonalcoholic fluids to minimize clot formation. Straining during defecation for at least 6 weeks after surgery is avoided in order to prevent bleeding; prune juice is a satisfactory bowel stimulant.

Test-Taking Strategy: Use the process of elimination. Option 1 and 2 can be easily eliminated. Considering the anatomical location of the surgical procedure, it would be reasonable to think that constipation needs to be avoided; therefore, eliminate option 4. Items weighing 25 pounds seem to be rather excessive. Keeping this principle in mind will assist in directing you to option 3. Review TURP discharge teaching points now if you had difficulty with this question!

Level of Cognitive Ability: Application
Phase of Nursing Process: Implementation
Client Needs: Health Promotion and Maintenance
Content Area: Adult Health/Renal

Reference

Black, J., & Matassarin-Jacobs, E. (1997). *Medical-surgical nursing: Clinical management for continuity of care* (5th ed.). Philadelphia: W. B. Saunders, p. 2363.

159. The nurse provides discharge instructions to the client with mastectomy and axillary lymph node dissection. Which of the following would the nurse include in the teaching plan?

1 Avoid the use of insect repellent
2 Cut cuticles on nails carefully, using a clean cuticle scissors
3 Wear protective gloves when doing the dishes
4 Avoid the use of lanolin hand cream on the affected arm

Answer: 3

Rationale: After axillary node dissection, the affected arm may swell and is less able to fight infection. The client should use insect repellent to avoid bites and stings. Picking at or cutting cuticles should never be done. Lanolin hand cream should be applied a few times daily. Protective gloves should be worn while doing dishes and cleaning.

Test-Taking Strategy: The issue of the question relates to preventing altered skin integrity and thus infection. Keeping this concept in mind will assist in the process of eliminating options 1, 2, and 4, which could potentially lead to a skin alteration. Review the client education teaching points related to mastectomy and lymph node dissection if you had difficulty with this question!

Level of Cognitive Ability: Application
Phase of Nursing Process: Implementation
Client Needs: Health Promotion and Maintenance
Content Area: Adult Health/Oncology

Reference

Black, J., & Matassarin-Jacobs, E. (1997). *Medical-surgical nursing: Clinical management for continuity of care* (5th ed.). Philadelphia: W. B. Saunders, p. 2445.

---

160. The camp nurse provides instructions regarding skin protection from the sun to the parents who are preparing their children for a camping adventure. Which of the following would not be included in the instructions?

1 Sunscreens with a skin protection factor (SPF) of 15 or more are recommended
2 Sunscreen will not be required on cloudy days
3 Pack a hat, long-sleeved shirt, and long pants for each child
4 Select tightly woven materials for greater protection from the sun's rays

Answer: 2

Rationale: The sun's rays are as damaging to the skin on cloudy, hazy days as they are on sunny days. Sunscreens with an SPF of 15 or more are recommended and should be applied before exposure to the sun and reapplied frequently and liberally at least every 2 hours. A child should wear a hat, long-sleeved shirt, and long pants when out in the sun. Tightly woven materials provide greater protection from the sun's rays.

Test-Taking Strategy: Recalling that the ultraviolet rays can be damaging regardless of cloudiness or haziness will assist in directing you to option 2. Eliminate options 1, 3, and 4 because these measures provide the greatest protection from the sun. Review guidelines that protect the skin from the damaging rays of the sun now if you had difficulty with this question!

Level of Cognitive Ability: Application
Phase of Nursing Process: Implementation
Client Needs: Health Promotion and Maintenance
Content Area: Fundamental Skills

Reference

Black, J., & Matassarin-Jacobs, E. (1997). *Medical-surgical nursing: Clinical management for continuity of care* (5th ed.). Philadelphia: W. B. Saunders, p. 2224.

161. The client is receiving, on an outpatient basis, a course of chemotherapy for the diagnosis of lung cancer. Which of the following home care instructions would the nurse provide to the client?

1. A bathroom can be shared with other members of the family
2. Urinary and bowel excreta are not considered contaminated
3. Disposable plates and plastic utensils must be used during the entire course of chemotherapy
4. Contaminated linens should be washed separately and then washed a second time with the rest of the laundry

Answer: 4

Rationale: The client may excrete the chemotherapeutic agent for 48 hours or more after administration, depending on the medication administered. Blood, emesis, and excreta may be considered contaminated during this time. The client should not share a bathroom with children or pregnant women during this time. Any contaminated linens or clothing should be washed separately and then washed a second time with the rest of the laundry. All contaminated disposable items should be sealed in plastic bags and disposed of as hazardous waste.

Test-Taking Strategy: Eliminate options 1 and 2 first because the concepts in each are very similar. Eliminate option 3 next because it would seem unreasonable to have to use disposable utensils for the entire course of therapy. Review client teaching points related to chemotherapy if you had difficulty with this question!

Level of Cognitive Ability: Application
Phase of Nursing Process: Implementation
Client Needs: Health Promotion and Maintenance
Content Area: Adult Health/Oncology

Reference

Black, J., & Matassarin-Jacobs, E. (1997). *Medical-surgical nursing: Clinical management for continuity of care* (5th ed.). Philadelphia: W. B. Saunders, p. 580.

162. The home care nurse visits a client with bowel cancer who recently underwent a course of chemotherapy. The client has developed stomatitis. Which of the following instructions would not be a component of the teaching plan for this condition?

1. To drink foods and liquids that are cold
2. To avoid foods with spices
3. To maintain a diet of soft foods
4. To avoid citrus fruits and juices

Answer: 1

Rationale: "Stomatitis" is a term used to describe inflammation and ulceration of the mucosal lining of the mouth. Dietary modifications for this condition include avoiding extremely hot or cold foods, spices, and citrus fruits and juices. The client should be instructed to eat soft foods and take nutritional supplements as prescribed.

Test-Taking Strategy: Note the word "not" in the stem of the question. Knowledge that stomatitis is an inflammation of the mucosal lining of the mouth will assist in eliminating options that include measures that will alleviate further irritation: options 2, 3, and 4. Review client teaching points for stomatitis now if you had difficulty with this question!

Level of Cognitive Ability: Application
Phase of Nursing Process: Implementation
Client Needs: Health Promotion and Maintenance
Content Area: Adult Health/Oncology

Reference

Black, J., & Matassarin-Jacobs, E. (1997). *Medical-surgical nursing: Clinical management for continuity of care* (5th ed.). Philadelphia: W. B. Saunders, p. 583.

163. The home health nurse provides instructions to the postpartum client who has developed breast engorgement. Which of the following instructions would the nurse provide to the client?

1 Feed the infant less frequently, every 4–6 hours, using bottle feeding in between
2 Apply cool packs to both breasts 20 minutes before a feeding
3 Avoid the use of a brassiere during engorgement
4 During feeding, gently massage the breast from the outer areas to the nipple

Answer: 4

Rationale: The client with breast engorgement should be advised to feed frequently, at least every 2½ hours for 15–20 minutes per side. Moist heat should be applied to both breasts for about 20 minutes before a feeding. Between feedings, the mother should wear a supportive brassiere. During a feeding, it is helpful to gently massage the breast from the outer areas to the nipple to stimulate the letdown and flow of milk.

Test-Taking Strategy: Consider the manifestations that occur with engorgement, and eliminate the options that will not assist in alleviating the flow of milk: options 1 and 2. From the remaining 2 options, you would select option 4 over option 3 because massage would assist in the flow of milk. In addition, it would seem likely that a supportive brassiere would be necessary to alleviate the discomfort that occurs with this condition. If you had difficulty with this question, take time now to review the measures used for breast engorgement!

Level of Cognitive Ability: Application
Phase of Nursing Process: Implementation
Client Needs: Health Promotion and Maintenance
Content Area: Maternity

Reference
Nichols, F., & Zwelling, E. (1997). *Maternal-newborn nursing: Theory and practice.* Philadelphia: W. B. Saunders, pp. 1007–1008.

164. A client in the third trimester of pregnancy arrives at the clinic and tells the nurse that she frequently has a backache. Which of the following instructions would the nurse provide to the client to alleviate the backache?

1 Sleep in a supine position and on a firm mattress
2 Wear a maternity girdle
3 Eat small meals frequently
4 Elevate the legs when sitting

Answer: 2

Rationale: To provide relief from backache, the nurse would advise the client to use good posture and body mechanics, to perform pelvic rocking exercises, and to wear flat, supportive shoes. The client would also be instructed to wear a maternity girdle, to avoid overexertion, and to sleep in the lateral position on a firm mattress. Back massage is also helpful. Eating small meals would more specifically assist in the relief of dyspnea. Leg elevation assists the client with varicosities.

Test-Taking Strategy: Use the process of elimination, keeping in mind that the issue of the question is backache. This should assist in eliminating options 3 and 4 because they are unrelated to the relief of backache. For the remaining two options, knowledge that the lateral position is most appropriate for sleeping will assist in directing you to option 2. Review relief measures for backache now if you had difficulty with this question!

Level of Cognitive Ability: Application
Phase of Nursing Process: Implementation
Client Needs: Health Promotion and Maintenance
Content Area: Maternity

Reference
Nichols, F., & Zwelling, E. (1997). *Maternal-newborn nursing: Theory and practice.* Philadelphia: W. B. Saunders, p. 500.

165. The nurse provides dietary instructions for the client receiving spironolactone (Aldactone). Which of the following foods would the nurse instruct the client to avoid while taking this medication?

1 Crackers
2 Shrimp
3 Apricots
4 Popcorn

Answer: 3

Rationale: Aldactone is a potassium-sparing diuretic, and the client needs to avoid foods high in potassium, such as whole-grain cereals, legumes, meat, bananas, apricots, orange juice, potatoes, and raisins. Option 3 is the source of highest levels of potassium and should be avoided.

Test-Taking Strategy: Knowledge regarding the classification of this medication and foods high in potassium is necessary to answer this question. Begin by eliminating options 1 and 4 because they are food items that are similar. Remembering that fruits, vegetables, and fresh meats are high in potassium will assist in directing you to option 3 as the food to avoid.

Level of Cognitive Ability: Application
Phase of Nursing Process: Implementation
Client Needs: Health Promotion and Maintenance
Content Area: Pharmacology

Reference

Hodgson, B., & Kizior, R. (1998). *Saunders nursing drug handbook 1998.* Philadelphia: W. B. Saunders, p. 944.

166. Oral lactulose (Chronulac) is prescribed for the client with a hepatic disorder. The home health nurse provides instructions to the client regarding this medication. Which of the following instructions would not be a component of the teaching plan?

1 Take the medication with milk
2 Increase fluid intake while taking the medication
3 Increase fiber in the diet
4 Notify the physician if nausea occurs

Answer: 4

Rationale: Lactulose retains ammonia in the colon and promotes increased peristalsis and bowel evacuation, expelling ammonia from the colon. It should be taken with water, juice, or milk to aid in softening the stool. An increased fluid intake and a high-fiber diet will promote defecation. The client should be instructed to drink cola or to eat unsalted crackers or dry toast if nausea occurs.

Test-Taking Strategy: Knowledge regarding the action of this medication will assist in directing you to the correct option. Eliminate options 2 and 3 first because they are similar in that both promote defecation. Of the remaining two options, eliminate option 1 because it is a correct action. There are measures that the client can take to relieve nausea before notifying the physician.

Level of Cognitive Ability: Application
Phase of Nursing Process: Implementation
Client Needs: Health Promotion and Maintenance
Content Area: Pharmacology

Reference

Hodgson, B., & Kizior, R. (1998). *Saunders nursing drug handbook 1998.* Philadelphia: W. B. Saunders, p. 944.

167. The client with leukemia receives a course of chemotherapy. The home care nurse scheduled to visit the client receives a telephone call from the client's physician. The physician informs the nurse that the neutrophil count is 600/mm^3. Which of the following instructions will the nurse provide to the client during the home care visit?

1. Avoid eating any raw fruits or vegetables
2. Avoid aspirin or medications containing aspirin
3. Avoid straining at bowel movements
4. Avoid the use of a straight razor for shaving

Answer: 1

Rationale: Neutrophil counts should range between 3000 and 5800/mm^3. A low neutrophil count places the client at risk for infection. When the client is at risk for infection, he or she should avoid exposure to persons with colds or infections. All live plants, flowers, and objects that harbor bacteria, such as stuffed animals, should be removed from the client's environment. The client should be on a low-bacteria diet that excludes raw fruits and vegetables. Options 2, 3, and 4 are measures that would be implemented if the client was at risk for bleeding.

Test-Taking Strategy: Knowledge that a low neutrophil count places the client at risk for infection will assist in directing you to the correct option. Bearing in mind that the issue of the question relates to infection will assist in eliminating options 2, 3, and 4, as these options identify measures that reduce the risk of bleeding.

Level of Cognitive Ability: Application
Phase of Nursing Process: Implementation
Client Needs: Health Promotion and Maintenance
Content Area: Adult Health/Oncology

Reference

Black, J., & Matassarin-Jacobs, E. (1997). *Medical-surgical nursing: Clinical management for continuity of care* (5th ed.). Philadelphia: W. B. Saunders, pp. 1492–1493

168. The child admitted to the hospital for sickle cell crisis is preparing for discharge. The nurse instructs the child and parents on measures to prevent a crisis. Which of the following would not be a component of this teaching plan?

1. Avoid high altitudes and air travel
2. Increase oral fluid intake
3. Notify the physician if vomiting or diarrhea occur
4. Increase the dose of the analgesic as soon as the pain begins

Answer: 4

Rationale: The client should be provided with information on how to prevent crises, such as avoiding high altitudes and flying in nonpressurized planes, because oxygen tension is lowered under these conditions. The client should also take caution against becoming dehydrated and should call a physician if vomiting, diarrhea, high fever, or any other cause of water loss develops. The client should not be instructed to increase analgesics.

Test-Taking Strategy: Knowledge regarding the causes of crises will assist in answering this question. However, using basic principles related to client instructions regarding medications will assist in directing you to option 4. Clients should not be instructed to increase medication unless this is specifically prescribed. If you had difficulty with this question, take time now to review the causes of sickle cell crisis.

Level of Cognitive Ability: Application
Phase of Nursing Process: Implementation
Client Needs: Health Promotion and Maintenance
Content Area: Child Health

Reference

Black, J., & Matassarin-Jacobs, E. (1997). *Medical-surgical nursing: Clinical management for continuity of care* (5th ed.). Philadelphia: W. B. Saunders, p. 1515.

169. The nurse provides instructions to the client who received cryosurgery for a local stage 0 cervical tumor. Which of the following would the nurse include in the discharge plan?

1. Call the physician if a watery discharge occurs
2. Call the physician if the discharge remains odorous after 1 week
3. Avoid tub baths
4. Pain indicates a complication of the procedure

Answer: 3

Rationale: Mild pain may occur and continue for several days after this procedure. A clear watery discharge is expected. This is followed by discharge containing debris that may be malodorous. If the discharge continues longer than 8 weeks, an infection is suspected. Healing takes about 10 weeks. Showers or sponge baths should be taken during this time, and tub baths and sitz baths need to be avoided.

Test-Taking Strategy: Knowledge regarding cryosurgery is necessary to answer this question. If you are unfamiliar with this procedure, consider the anatomical area of the body in terms of where this procedure is performed. It would seem likely that the client would be instructed to avoid tub baths after this procedure. Review teaching points related to this procedure if you had difficulty with this question. You are likely to find a question similar to this one on NCLEX-RN!

Level of Cognitive Ability: Application
Phase of Nursing Process: Implementation
Client Needs: Health Promotion and Maintenance
Content Area: Adult Health/Oncology

Reference

Black, J., & Matassarin-Jacobs, E. (1997). *Medical-surgical nursing: Clinical management for continuity of care* (5th ed.). Philadelphia: W. B. Saunders, p. 2409.

---

170. The home care nurse provides instructions to the client taking digoxin (Lanoxin), 0.25 mg daily. Which of the following client statements would indicate a need for further education?

1. "I will take my prescribed antacid if I become nauseated"
2. "It is important to have my blood drawn when prescribed"
3. "I will check my pulse before I take my medication"
4. "I will carry a medication ID card with me"

Answer: 1

Rationale: Digoxin is an antidysrhythmic. The most common early manifestations of toxicity are GI disturbances such as anorexia, nausea, and vomiting. Digoxin blood levels need to be obtained as prescribed to monitor for therapeutic plasma levels (0.5–2.0 ng/mL). The client is instructed to take the pulse, withhold the medication if the pulse is below 60 beats/minute, and notify the physician. The client is instructed to wear or carry an ID bracelet or card.

Test-Taking Strategy: Use the process of elimination and knowledge regarding digoxin to answer the question. Remembering that GI disturbances are the earliest signs of digoxin toxicity will assist in directing you to option 1. Take time now to review this very important medication if you had difficulty with this question!

Level of Cognitive Ability: Analysis
Phase of Nursing Process: Evaluation
Client Needs: Health Promotion and Maintenance
Content Area: Pharmacology

Reference

Hodgson, B., & Kizior, R. (1998). *Saunders nursing drug handbook 1998.* Philadelphia: W. B. Saunders, pp. 324–326

171. The nurse is caring for a client with possible cholelithiasis who is being prepared for a cholangiogram. The nurse teaches the client about the procedure. Which of the following client statements indicates that the client understands the purpose of a cholangiogram?

1 "They are going to 'look at' my gallbladder and ducts"
2 "This procedure will drain my gallbladder"
3 "My gallbladder will be irrigated"
4 "They will put medication in my gallbladder"

Answer: 1

Rationale: An IV cholangiogram is for diagnostic purposes. It outlines both the gallbladder and the ducts, so gallstones that have moved into the ductal system can be detected. X-rays are used to visualize the biliary duct system after IV injection of radiopaque dye.

Test-Taking Strategy: Knowledge of the pathophysiological processes of cholelithiasis and the purpose of the cholangiogram will assist in answering this question. Note that options 2, 3, and 4 are similar in that they involve some form of treatment. Option 1 involves assessment of the gallbladder. If you had difficulty with this question, take time now to review the purpose of this procedure!

Level of Cognitive Ability: Analysis
Phase of Nursing Process: Evaluation
Client Needs: Health Promotion and Maintenance
Content Area: Adult Health/Gastrointestinal

Reference

Lewis, S., Collier, I., & Heitkemper, M. (1996). *Medical-surgical nursing: Assessment and management of clinical problems* (4th ed.). St. Louis: Mosby–Year Book, pp. 1091, 1298.

---

172. The nurse is providing immediate post-procedure care to a client who underwent thoracentesis to relieve a tension pneumothorax that resulted from rib fractures. The goal is that the client will exhibit normal respiratory functioning. The nurse provides instructions to assist the client toward this goal. Which of the following statements by the client would indicate to the nurse that further instructions are needed?

1 "I will let you know at once if I have trouble breathing"
2 "I will lie on the affected side for an hour"
3 "I can expect a chest x-ray to be done shortly"
4 "I will notify you if I feel a crackling sensation in my chest"

Answer: 2

Rationale: After the procedure, the client is usually turned onto the unaffected side for 1 hour to facilitate lung expansion. Tachypnea, dyspnea, cyanosis, retractions, or diminished breath sounds, which may indicate pneumothorax, should be reported to the physician. A chest x-ray study may be performed to evaluate the degree of lung reexpansion or pneumothorax. Subcutaneous emphysema may follow this procedure because air in the pleural cavity leaks into subcutaneous tissues. The tissues feel like lumpy paper and crackle when palpated (crepitus). Subcutaneous emphysema usually causes no problems unless it is increasing and constricting vital structures such as the trachea.

Test-Taking Strategy: It would be appropriate to teach the client to notify the nurse if there were any signs of distress and that an x-ray is routinely performed. Note the phrase "the affected side for an hour" in option 2. Think about the rationales for nursing prescriptions. The client should be placed on the unaffected side for 1 hour to facilitate lung expansion. Review postprocedure care for a thoracentesis now if you had difficulty with this question!

Level of Cognitive Ability: Analysis
Phase of Nursing Process: Evaluation
Client Needs: Health Promotion and Maintenance
Content Area: Adult Health/Respiratory

Reference

Black, J., & Matassarin-Jacobs, E. (1997). *Medical-surgical nursing: Clinical management for continuity of care* (5th ed.). Philadelphia: W. B. Saunders, pp. 1063–1064.

173. The nurse is trying to determine the client's adjustment to a new diagnosis of coronary heart disease before discharge. Of the following questions, which one should the nurse ask to elicit the most useful response by the client?

1 "Do you have anyone at home to help with housework and shopping?"
2 "How do you feel about the lifestyle changes you are planning to make?"
3 "Do you understand the use of your new medications?"
4 "Are you going to book your follow-up physician visit?"

Answer: 2

Rationale: All questions relate to aspects of posthospital care, but only option 2 explores the client's feelings about the disease. Exploring feelings as the initial assessment will assist in determining the individualized plan of care for the client.

Test-Taking Strategy: Open-ended questions are needed to explore client's reactions or feelings to an identified situation. Close-ended questions generally elicit a "yes" or "no" response exclusively. All of the incorrect options are closed-ended responses. Remember teaching/learning theory. The client's feelings, motivation, and goals are the priority!

Level of Cognitive Ability: Application
Phase of Nursing Process: Implementation
Client Needs: Health Promotion and Maintenance
Content Area: Fundamental Skills

Reference

Potter, P., & Perry, A. (1997). *Fundamentals of nursing: Concepts, process, and practice* (4th ed.). St. Louis: Mosby–Year Book, pp. 241–242.

---

174. The elderly client with coronary artery disease is scheduled for hospital discharge and lives alone. The client states, "I don't know how I'll be able to remember all these instructions and take care of myself once I get home." The nurse should plan which of the following actions to assist the client?

1 Ask an out-of-town relative to stay with the client for a day or so
2 Ask the physician to delay the discharge until the client is better able to manage self-care
3 Ask the social worker to follow up with a telephone call after discharge to ensure the client is progressing
4 Ask the physician for a referral to a home health agency for nursing and home health aide support

Answer: 4

Rationale: With earlier hospital discharge, clients are returning home with greater acuity of problems and may require support from a home health agency until they are independent in functioning.

Test-Taking Strategy: Option 3 does nothing to actively assist the client, and option 2 is not realistic in the current health care environment, so these two are eliminated first. Option 1 may be unrealistic and does not ensure the client continued care until he or she is able to be independent in managing own care. Option 4 is the method of ensuring the client necessary assistance as required.

Level of Cognitive Ability: Analysis
Phase of Nursing Process: Planning
Client Needs: Health Promotion and Maintenance
Content Area: Fundamental Skills

Reference

Black, J., & Matassarin-Jacobs, E. (1997). *Medical-surgical nursing: Clinical management for continuity of care* (5th ed.). Philadelphia: W. B. Saunders, p. 146.

---

175. A client with newly diagnosed angina pectoris asks the nurse how to prevent future angina attacks. The nurse would plan to incorporate which of the following instructions in a teaching session?

1 Eat fewer, larger meals for more efficient digestion
2 Plan all activities for early in the morning, when the client is most rested
3 Adjust medication doses freely until symptoms do not recur
4 Dress appropriately in very cold or very hot weather

Answer: 4

Rationale: Anginal episodes are triggered by events such as eating heavy meals, straining during bowel movements, smoking, overexertion, and experiencing emotional upset or temperature extremes. Medication therapy is monitored and regulated by the physician.

Test-Taking Strategy: The wording of the question indicates that three of the options are incorrect. Basic knowledge of the causes of chest pain and core concepts of medication therapy helps systematically eliminate the incorrect options. If you had difficulty with this question, review teaching points for the client with angina!

Level of Cognitive Ability: Application
Phase of Nursing Process: Planning
Client Needs: Health Promotion and Maintenance
Content Area: Adult Health/Cardiovascular

Reference

Luckmann, J. (1997). *Saunders manual of nursing care*. Philadelphia: W. B. Saunders, p. 1040.

176. The nurse is caring for a client who has just returned to the nursing unit after intravenous pyelography (IVP). The nurse would make which of the following a priority in the postprocedure care of this client?

1. Encouraging increased intake of oral fluids
2. Ambulating the client in the hallway
3. Encouraging the client to try to void frequently
4. Maintaining the client on bed rest

Answer: 1

Rationale: After IVP, the client should consume increased fluids to aid in clearance of the dye used for the procedure. It is unnecessary to void frequently after the procedure. The client is usually allowed activity as tolerated, without any specific activity guidelines.

Test-Taking Strategy: The stem of the question asks for a "priority" of care. Option 3 has no useful purpose and may be eliminated first. To discriminate among the remaining three alternatives, you would choose correctly by knowing that there are no activity guidelines after this procedure. Alternatively, you could choose correctly if you know that fluids are necessary to promote clearance of the dye from the client's system.

Level of Cognitive Ability: Application
Phase of Nursing Process: Planning
Client Needs: Health Promotion and Maintenance
Content Area: Adult Health/Renal

Reference

Black, J., & Matassarin-Jacobs, E. (1997). *Medical-surgical nursing: Clinical management for continuity of care* (5th ed.). Philadelphia: W. B. Saunders, p. 1563.

---

177. The nurse has done a nutritional assessment of the client with cystitis. The nurse interprets that which of the following beverages preferred by the client should be encouraged to minimize recurrence of cystitis?

1. Coffee
2. Tea
3. Water
4. White wine

Answer: 3

Rationale: Caffeine and alcohol can irritate the bladder. Therefore, alcohol- and caffeine-containing beverages as coffee, tea, and cocoa are avoided to minimize risk. Water helps flush bacteria out of the bladder, and an intake of 6–8 glasses per day is encouraged.

Test-Taking Strategy: Option 4 should be eliminated first because alcohol intake is not encouraged in the general sense for any disorder. Options 1 and 2 are similar to each other in that both contain caffeine. Thus it is unlikely that either of these is the answer, and they may be eliminated.

Level of Cognitive Ability: Analysis
Phase of Nursing Process: Analysis
Client Needs: Health Promotion and Maintenance
Content Area: Fundamental Skills

Reference

Black, J., & Matassarin-Jacobs, E. (1997). *Medical-surgical nursing: Clinical management for continuity of care* (5th ed.). Philadelphia: W. B. Saunders, p. 1578.

---

178. The home care nurse has given instructions to the female client with cystitis about measures to prevent recurrence. The nurse evaluates that the client needs further instruction if the client verbalizes that she will

1. Take bubble baths for more effective hygiene.
2. Wear underwear made of cotton or with cotton panels.
3. Drink a glass of water and void after intercourse.
4. Avoid wearing pantyhose while wearing slacks.

Answer: 1

Rationale: Measures to prevent cystitis include increasing fluid intake to 3 liters/day; using an acid-ash diet; wiping front to back after urination; using showers instead of tub baths; drinking water and voiding after intercourse; avoiding bubble baths, feminine hygiene sprays, and perfumed toilet tissue and sanitary pads; and wearing clothes that "breathe" (cotton pants, no tight jeans, no pantyhose under slacks). Other measures include teaching pregnant women to void every 2 hours and teaching menopausal women to use estrogen vaginal creams to restore vaginal pH.

Test-Taking Strategy: Use the process of elimination in selecting the correct option. Eliminate option 3 first, knowing that drinking water is a basic measure to prevent cystitis. Next, eliminate options 2 and 4 because they are similar. Review teaching measures to prevent cystitis now if you had difficulty with this question!

Level of Cognitive Ability: Analysis
Phase of Nursing Process: Evaluation
Client Needs: Health Promotion and Maintenance
Content Area: Fundamental Skills

Reference

Black, J., & Matassarin-Jacobs, E. (1997). *Medical-surgical nursing: Clinical management for continuity of care* (5th ed.). Philadelphia: W. B. Saunders, p. 1573.

---

179. The client with pyelonephritis is being discharged from the hospital. The nurse gives the client discharge instructions to prevent recurrence. The nurse evaluates that the client understands the information that was given if the client states an intention to

1. Report signs and symptoms of urinary tract infection (UTI) if they persist for more than 1 week.
2. Take the prescribed antibiotics until all symptoms subside.
3. Return to the physician's office for scheduled follow-up urine cultures.
4. Modify fluid intake for the day on the basis of the previous day's output.

Answer: 3

Rationale: The client with pyelonephritis should take the full course of antibiotic therapy that has been prescribed and return to the physician's office for follow-up urine cultures if so instructed. The client should learn the signs and symptoms of UTI and report them immediately if they occur. The client should perform all measures that are used to prevent cystitis, which includes forcing fluids to 3 liters/day.

Test-Taking Strategy: Begin to answer this question by eliminating option 1 because UTI symptoms should never go unreported for a week. Option 2 is eliminated next because antibiotics should be taken for the full course of treatment for adequate elimination of the infection. Knowing that the client needs follow-up urine cultures helps you choose option 3 over option 4, which is not an appropriate option.

Level of Cognitive Ability: Analysis
Phase of Nursing Process: Evaluation
Client Needs: Health Promotion and Maintenance
Content Area: Adult Health/Renal

Reference

Black, J., & Matassarin-Jacobs, E. (1997). *Medical-surgical nursing: Clinical management for continuity of care* (5th ed.). Philadelphia: W. B. Saunders, p. 1630.

---

180. The client with nephrotic syndrome needs dietary teaching about how diet can help counteract the effects of altered renal function. The nurse would plan to include which of the following statements in instructions to the client?

1. "Plan to drink at least 8 glasses of water a day"
2. "Add salt during cooking to replace sodium lost in the urine"
3. "Increase your intake of fish"
4. "Increase your intake of fatty foods to prevent protein loss"

Answer: 3

Rationale: The diet in nephrotic syndrome is limited in sodium. This is done to help control edema, which is a predominant part of the clinical picture. Fluids are not limited unless hyponatremia is present. On the other hand, the client is not encouraged to force fluids. Unless the glomerular filtration rate is impaired, protein intake is increased. This helps to replace protein lost in the urine and ultimately helps in controlling edema also. A part of the clinical picture in nephrotic syndrome is hyperlipidemia, which results from the liver's synthesis of lipoproteins in response to hypoalbuminemia. Increasing fatty food intake would not be helpful in this circumstance.

Test-Taking Strategy: Begin to answer this question by recalling that nephrotic syndrome is characterized by fluid retention and hypoalbuminemia. This would help you eliminate options 1 and 2 first as possible choices. Knowing that hyperlipidemia accompanies this clinical picture would help you to choose option 3 over option 4. You could also choose correctly if you knew that hypoalbuminemia is part of the picture and that the food in option 3 is a good source of protein.

Level of Cognitive Ability: Application
Phase of Nursing Process: Planning
Client Needs: Health Promotion and Maintenance
Content Area: Adult Health/Renal

Reference

Black, J., & Matassarin-Jacobs, E. (1997). *Medical-surgical nursing: Clinical management for continuity of care* (5th ed.). Philadelphia: W. B. Saunders, p. 1635.

181. The nurse is giving the client with polycystic kidney disease instructions in replacing elements lost in the urine as a result of impaired kidney function. The nurse instructs the client to increase intake of which of the following in the diet?

1 Sodium and potassium
2 Sodium and water
3 Water and phosphorus
4 Calcium and phosphorus

Answer: 2

Rationale: Clients with polycystic kidney disease waste sodium rather than retain it and therefore need an increase in sodium and water in the diet. Potassium, calcium, and phosphorus levels need no special attention.

Test-Taking Strategy: In reviewing the possible answers to this question, notice that either sodium or phosphorus appears in each of the options. Remember also that when an answer has two parts to it, both of the parts must be correct for the option to be correct. Knowing this, begin to answer this question by eliminating options 3 and 4 first because the disorder causes sodium, not phosphorus, to be wasted. To discriminate between options 1 and 2, you should recall that when the kidney excretes sodium, water is carried with it. This would allow you to choose option 2 over option 1 as the correct answer.

Level of Cognitive Ability: Application
Phase of Nursing Process: Implementation
Client Needs: Health Promotion and Maintenance
Content Area: Adult Health/Renal

Reference

Black, J., & Matassarin-Jacobs, E. (1997). *Medical-surgical nursing: Clinical management for continuity of care* (5th ed.). Philadelphia: W. B. Saunders, p. 1679.

182. The client with AIDS is being treated for tuberculosis with isoniazid (INH). Which of the following nursing actions does the nurse plan in relation to administration of the medication?

1 Administer with antacids to prevent GI distress
2 Administer at least 1 hour before administering an aluminum antacid, to prevent a medication interaction
3 Administer with food to prevent rapid absorption of INH
4 Administer with a corticosteroid to potentiate the effects of INH

Answer: 2

Rationale: Aluminum hydroxide, a common ingredient in antacids, significantly decreases INH absorption. INH should be administered at least 1 hour before aluminum antacids are administered. Food affects the rate of absorption of rifampin (Rifadin), not INH. INH administration with a corticosteroid decreases INH's effects and increases the corticosteroid's effects.

Test-Taking Strategy: In order to effectively answer this question, you would need to know that INH should be given 1 hour before an aluminum antacid is administered. In general, you would not usually administer a medication with an antacid because it would decrease absorption of the medication. In general, most medications are not given together specifically to potentiate one or the other's effects.

Level of Cognitive Ability: Application
Phase of Nursing Process: Planning
Clients Needs: Health Promotion and Maintenance
Content Area: Adult Health/Respiratory

Reference

Hodgson, B., & Kizior, R. (1998). *Saunders nursing drug handbook 1998.* Philadelphia: W. B. Saunders, p 551.

183. The client is treated in the physician's office after a fall, which sprained the ankle. X-ray has ruled out fracture. Before sending the client home, the nurse would plan to teach the client that which of the following items is to be avoided in the next 24 hours?

1 Application of a heating pad
2 Application of an Ace wrap
3 Resting the foot
4 Elevating the ankle on a pillow while sitting or lying down

Answer: 1

Rationale: Soft tissue injuries such as sprains are treated by rest, ice, compression, and elevation (RICE) for the first 24 hours after the injury. Ice is applied intermittently for 20–30 minutes at a time. Heat is not used in the first 24 hours because it could increase venous congestion, which would increase edema and pain.

Test-Taking Strategy: Sprained limbs should be rested and elevated, so options 3 and 4 are ruled out as the items to be avoided after a sprain. Use of an Ace wrap is also helpful in reducing the pain and swelling, so option 2 cannot be the answer either. By the process of elimination, heat must be the item to avoid in the first 24 hours.

Level of Cognitive Ability: Application
Phase of Nursing Process: Planning
Client Needs: Health Promotion and Maintenance
Content Area: Adult Health/Musculoskeletal

Reference

Smeltzer, S., & Bare, B. (1996). *Brunner and Suddarth's Textbook of medical-surgical nursing* (8th ed.). Philadelphia: Lippincott-Raven, p. 1909.

---

184. The nurse has given dietary instructions to a client to minimize the risk of osteoporosis. The nurse would evaluate that the client understands the recommended changes if the client verbalized an intent to increase intake of which of these preferred foods?

1 Rice
2 Yogurt
3 Sardines
4 Chicken

Answer: 2

Rationale: The major dietary source of calcium is dairy foods, including milk, yogurt, and a variety of cheeses and ice cream. Calcium may also be added to certain products, such as orange juice, which are then advertised as being "fortified" with calcium. Calcium supplements are available and recommended for clients with typically low calcium intake.

Test-Taking Strategy: This question is reasonably straightforward. To answer this question, you need to know that dairy products are rich in calcium and that yogurt is a dairy product. None of the other options belongs to that food group.

Level of Cognitive Ability: Analysis
Phase of Nursing Process: Evaluation
Client Needs: Health Promotion and Maintenance
Content Area: Adult Health/Musculoskeletal

Reference

Black, J., & Matassarin-Jacobs, E. (1997). *Medical-surgical nursing: Clinical management for continuity of care* (5th ed.). Philadelphia: W. B. Saunders, pp. 2101–2102.

---

185. The nurse is conducting health screening for osteoporosis. The nurse would focus health promotion measures on the basis of the knowledge that which of the following clients is at greatest risk of developing this disorder?

1 A 36-year-old male who has asthma
2 A 25-year-old female who jogs
3 A sedentary 65-year-old female who smokes cigarettes
4 A 70-year-old male who consumes excessive alcohol

Answer: 3

Rationale: Risk factors for osteoporosis include being female, being postmenopausal, being of advanced age, consuming a low-calcium diet, excessive alcohol intake, being sedentary, and smoking cigarettes. Long-term use of corticosteroids, anticonvulsants, and furosemide also increase risk.

Test-Taking Strategy: Option 2 is eliminated first; the 25-year-old female who jogs (exercise with the long bones) has negligible risk. Option 1 is eliminated next because the only risk factor for the 36-year-old male with asthma might be long-term corticosteroid use. Of the two remaining options, the 65-year-old female has more risk factors (age, gender, postmenopausal status, sedentary lifestyle, smoking) than does the 70-year-old male (age, alcohol consumption).

Level of Cognitive Ability: Analysis
Phase of Nursing Process: Analysis
Client Needs: Health Promotion and Maintenance
Content Area: Adult Health/Musculoskeletal

Reference

Black, J., & Matassarin-Jacobs, E. (1997). *Medical-surgical nursing: Clinical management for continuity of care* (5th ed.). Philadelphia: W. B. Saunders, p. 2102.

186. The client with right-sided weakness needs to learn how to use a cane. The nurse plans to teach the client to position the cane by holding it with the

1. Left hand and placing the cane in front of the left foot.
2. Right hand and placing the cane in front of the right foot.
3. Left hand and 6 inches lateral to the left foot.
4. Right hand and 6 inches lateral to the right foot.

Answer: 3

Rationale: The client is taught to hold the cane on the side opposite the weak side. This is because with normal walking, the opposite arm and leg move together (called reciprocal motion). The cane is placed 6 inches lateral to the fifth toe.

Test-Taking Strategy: Knowing that the cane is held at the client's side, not in front, helps you eliminate options 1 and 2 first. Knowing that the preferred method is to have the cane positioned on the stronger side helps you choose option 3 over option 4. Remember these important points!

Level of Cognitive Ability: Application
Phase of Nursing Process: Planning
Client Needs: Health Promotion and Maintenance
Content Area: Adult Health/Musculoskeletal

Reference

Potter, P., & Perry, A. (1997). *Fundamentals of nursing: Concepts, process, and practice* (4th ed.). St. Louis: Mosby–Year Book, p. 935.

---

187. The nurse has taught the client with a below-the-knee amputation about prosthesis and stump care. The nurse would evaluate that the client has understood the instructions if the client stated that he or she would

1. Wear a clean nylon stump sock daily.
2. Toughen the skin of the stump by rubbing it with alcohol.
3. Prevent cracking of the skin of the stump by applying lotion daily.
4. Use a mirror to inspect all areas of the stump each day.

Answer: 4

Rationale: The client should wear a clean woolen stump sock each day. The stump is cleansed daily with a gentle soap and water and is dried carefully. Alcohol is avoided because it could cause drying or cracking of the skin. Oils and creams are also avoided because they are too softening to the skin for safe prosthesis use. The client should inspect all surfaces of the stump daily for irritation, blisters, or breakdown.

Test-Taking Strategy: Nylon is a synthetic material that does not allow the best air circulation and holds in moisture. For this reason, a stump sock is not made of nylon, and option 1 is incorrect. Either alcohol or lotion can interfere with the natural condition of the skin, increasing the likelihood of breakdown either from drying or from excess moisture. For these reasons, options 2 and 3 are also incorrect. By elimination, the answer is option 4. It is very important that the client assess skin integrity of the stump at least daily.

Level of Cognitive Ability: Analysis
Phase of Nursing Process: Evaluation
Client Needs: Health Promotion and Maintenance
Content Area: Adult Health/Musculoskeletal

Reference

Black, J., & Matassarin-Jacobs, E. (1997). *Medical-surgical nursing: Clinical management for continuity of care* (5th ed.). Philadelphia: W. B. Saunders, p. 1423.

188. The nurse is ambulating a client with a right leg fracture who has an order for partial weight-bearing status. The nurse evaluates that the client demonstrates compliance with this restriction if the client

1 Does not bear weight on the right leg.
2 Allows the right leg to touch the floor.
3 Puts 30%–50% of the weight on the right leg.
4 Puts 60%–80% of the weight on the right leg.

Answer: 3

Rationale: The client who has partial weight-bearing status places 30%–50% of the body weight on the affected limb. Full weight-bearing status is placing full weight on the limb. Non–weight-bearing status does not allow the client to let the limb touch the floor. Touch-down weight-bearing allows the client to let the limb touch the floor but not bear weight. There is no classification for 60%–80% weight-bearing status.

Test-Taking Strategy: To answer this question with ease, you need to be familiar with the different categories of weight-bearing. Begin by eliminating options 1 and 2 first, using general knowledge. The word "partial" to describe weight-bearing does not seem to fit either of these. Option 3 is also a better descriptor than option 4 for partial weight-bearing, which may help you to select this one as the correct answer.

Level of Cognitive Ability: Analysis
Phase of Nursing Process: Evaluation
Client Needs: Health Promotion and Maintenance
Content Area: Adult Health/Musculoskeletal

Reference

Black, J., & Matassarin-Jacobs, E. (1997). *Medical-surgical nursing: Clinical management for continuity of care* (5th ed.). Philadelphia: W. B. Saunders, p. 2156.

189. The nurse is planning measures to increase bed mobility for the client in skeletal leg traction. Which of the following items would the nurse consider to be most helpful for this client?

1 Television
2 Reading materials
3 Overhead trapeze
4 Fracture bedpan

Answer: 3

Rationale: The use of an overhead trapeze is extremely helpful in helping a client to move about in bed and to get on and off the bedpan. The trapeze has the greatest value in increasing overall bed mobility. A fracture bedpan is useful in reducing discomfort with elimination. Television and reading materials are helpful in reducing boredom and providing distraction.

Test-Taking Strategy: Note the phrase "most helpful" in the stem, which is seeking to identify options that will increase bed mobility. Although all options are useful to the client in skeletal traction, the only one that helps with overall bed mobility is the trapeze.

Level of Cognitive Ability: Application
Phase of Nursing Process: Planning
Client Needs: Health Promotion and Maintenance
Content Area: Adult Health/Musculoskeletal

Reference

Smeltzer, S., & Bare, B. (1996). *Brunner and Suddarth's Textbook of medical-surgical nursing* (8th ed.). Philadelphia: Lippincott-Raven, p. 1862.

190. The nurse has given medication instructions to the client beginning anticonvulsant therapy with carbamazepine (Tegretol). The nurse would evaluate that the client understands the use of the medication if the client stated that he or she would

1 Drive as long as it was not at night.
2 Use sunscreen when out of doors.
3 Keep tissues handy because of excess salivation.
4 Discontinue the medication if fever or sore throat occurred.

Answer: 2

Rationale: Carbamazepine acts by depressing synaptic transmission in the central nervous system (CNS). Because of this, the client should avoid driving or performing other activities that require mental alertness until the effect on the client is known. The client should use protective clothing and sunscreen to avoid photosensitivity reactions. The medication may cause dry mouth, and the client should be instructed to provide good oral hygiene and use sugarless candy or gum as needed. The medication should not be abruptly discontinued, because this could cause return of seizures or status epilepticus. Fever and sore throat (signs of leukopenia) should be reported to the physician.

Test-Taking Strategy: Begin to answer this question by recalling that carbamazepine is an anticonvulsant medication with CNS depressant properties. This would lead you to discard option 1 first, because driving in general could be hazardous, but it has nothing to do with night vision. Option 4 is eliminated next because an anticonvulsant is not discontinued just because side effects or infection occurs; rather, the physician should be called. To choose between the remaining alternatives, remembering that carbamazepine causes dry mouth may help you eliminate option 3 and choose option 2 as the answer. Photosensitivity can occur with this medication.

Level of Cognitive Ability: Analysis
Phase of Nursing Process: Evaluation
Client Needs: Health Promotion and Maintenance
Content Area: Pharmacology

Reference
Deglin, J., & Vallerand, A. (1997). *Davis's drug guide for nurses* (5th ed.). Philadelphia: F. A. Davis, p. 216.

---

191. The client with myasthenia gravis has difficulty chewing and has received a prescription for pyridostigmine (Mestinon). The nurse plans to check to see that the client takes the medication

1 Just after meals.
2 Between meals.
3 With meals.
4 30 minutes before meals.

Answer: 4

Rationale: Pyridostigmine is a cholinergic medication used to increase muscle strength for the client with myasthenia gravis. For the client who has difficulty chewing, the medication may be administered 30 minutes before meals to enhance the client's ability to eat.

Test-Taking Strategy: The key to answering this question is the client's difficulty with chewing. Knowing that the medication increases muscle strength may lead you to choose to give the medication 30 minutes before meals, so that the client has the ability to chew the food.

Level of Cognitive Ability: Application
Phase of Nursing Process: Planning
Client Needs: Health Promotion and Maintenance
Content Area: Pharmacology

Reference
Deglin, J., & Vallerand, A. (1997). *Davis's drug guide for nurses* (5th ed.). Philadelphia: F. A. Davis, p. 1041.

---

192. The nurse prepares discharge instructions for a client with rheumatoid arthritis (RA). The instructions focus on measures to lessen discomfort and provide joint protection. Which of the following would be included in the plan of care?

1 Change positions every hour
2 Lift items rather than sliding them
3 Perform prescribed exercises even if the joints are inflamed
4 Avoid stooping, bending, and overreaching

Answer: 4

Rationale: The client with RA should avoid remaining in one position and should change position or stretch every 20 minutes. To reduce efforts by joints, the client should slide objects rather than lift them. The client should avoid exercises and activities other than gentle range-of-motion exercises when the joints are inflamed. The client is instructed to avoid stooping, bending, and overreaching.

Test-Taking Strategy: Basic principles of body mechanics will assist in eliminating option 2 and assist in directing you to the correct option, option 4. Eliminate option 1 because with RA, remaining in one position for 1 hour is stressful to the joints. Eliminate option 3 because of the basic principle that joints should be rested if inflamed. Review principles for joint protection in RA if you had difficulty with this question!

Level of Cognitive Ability: Application
Phase of Nursing Process: Planning
Client Needs: Health Promotion and Maintenance
Content Area: Adult Health/Musculoskeletal

Reference
Black, J., & Matassarin-Jacobs, E. (1997). *Medical-surgical nursing: Clinical management for continuity of care* (5th ed.). Philadelphia: W. B. Saunders, p. 663.

193. The home health nurse visits an elderly client with arthritis. The client complains of difficulty instilling the glaucoma eyedrops because of shaking hands caused by the arthritis. Which of the following instructions would the nurse provide to the client to alleviate this problem?

1 Keep the drops in the refrigerator so that they will thicken and be easier to instill
2 Lie down on a bed or sofa to instill the eyedrops
3 Tilt the head back to instill the eyedrops
4 Inform the client that a family member will have to instill the eyedrops

Answer: 2

Rationale: Elderly clients with arthritis or shaking hands have difficulty instilling their own eyedrops. The elderly client should be instructed to lie down on a bed or sofa. Tilting the head back can lead to loss of balance. Placing eyedrops in a refrigerator should not be done unless specifically prescribed. Eyedrop regimen for glaucoma requires accurate timing, and it is unreasonable to expect a family member to instill the drops. In addition, this discourages client independence.

Test-Taking Strategy: Eliminate option 1 first because eye medication should not be refrigerated unless specifically prescribed. Considering the issue of promoting client independence and the fact that the question does not provide data regarding family, eliminate option 4. Of the remaining two options, select option 2 over option 3 because it provides greater safety for the elderly client.

Level of Cognitive Ability: Application
Phase of Nursing Process: Implementation
Client Needs: Health Promotion and Maintenance
Content Area: Adult Health/Eye

Reference

Black, J., & Matassarin-Jacobs, E. (1997). *Medical-surgical nursing: Clinical management for continuity of care* (5th ed.). Philadelphia: W. B. Saunders, p. 956.

---

194. A scleral buckling procedure is performed on the client with retinal detachment. Which of the following would not be a component of the discharge teaching plan for the client?

1 Clean the eye daily with sterile water and a clean white washcloth
2 Wear an eye shield during naps and at night
3 Avoid vigorous activity and heavy lifting
4 Avoid air travel

Answer: 1

Rationale: In a scleral buckling procedure, the sclera is compressed from the outside by Silastic sponges or silicone bands that are sutured in place permanently. In addition, an intraocular injection of air or gas bubble, or both, may be used to apply pressure on the retina from the inside of the eye to hold the retina in place. If an air or gas bubble has been injected, it may take several weeks to absorb. Vigorous activities, heavy lifting, and air travel are avoided. An eye shield or glasses should be worn during the day, and a shield should be worn during naps and at night. The client is instructed to clean the eye with warm tap water, using a clean washcloth.

Test-Taking Strategy: Reading each option carefully will assist in directing you to the correct option. It is not necessary to use sterile water to clean the eye. In fact, it does not make sense to use a sterile solution with a clean washcloth. Review client teaching points after scleral buckling if you had difficulty with this question!

Level of Cognitive Ability: Application
Phase of Nursing Process: Planning
Client Needs: Health Promotion and Maintenance
Content Area: Adult Health/Eye

Reference

Black, J., & Matassarin-Jacobs, E. (1997). *Medical-surgical nursing: Clinical management for continuity of care* (5th ed.). Philadelphia: W. B. Saunders, pp. 962–964.

195. The newborn receives the first dose of hepatitis B vaccine within 12 hours of birth. The nurse instructs the mother with regard to the immunization schedule for this vaccine. Which of the following instructions would the nurse provide to the mother?

1. The second vaccine is administered at 1–2 months of age and then 4 months after the initial dose
2. The second vaccine is administered at 6 months of age and then 8 months after the initial dose
3. The second vaccine is administered at 8 months of age and then 1 year after the initial dose
4. The second vaccine is administered at 3 years of age and then during the adolescent years

Answer: 1

Rationale: The vaccination schedule for an infant whose mother's hepatitis B status is negative consists of a series of three immunizations given at 0 months (birth), 1–2 months of age, and then 4 months after the initial dose. An infant whose mother's hepatitis B status is positive receives human B immunoglobulin along with the first dose of the hepatitis B vaccine within 12 hours of birth.

Test-Taking Strategy: Knowledge regarding the immunization schedule for hepatitis B vaccine is necessary to answer this question. Take time now to review this schedule if you are unfamiliar with it. You are likely to find questions related to this vaccine on NCLEX-RN!

Level of Cognitive Ability: Application
Phase of Nursing Process: Implementation
Client Needs: Health Promotion and Maintenance
Content Area: Child Health

Reference

Ashwill, J., & Droske, S. (1997). *Nursing care of children: Principles and practice.* Philadelphia: W. B. Saunders, p. 594.

---

196. The school nurse performs health screening for scoliosis on children aged 9–15 years. Which of the following is the appropriate technique for this screening procedure?

1. Have the child stand with the arms extended over the head
2. Have the child stand with weight-bearing on the right leg followed by the left leg
3. Have the child unclothed or wear underpants only so the chest, back, and hips can be clearly seen
4. Take shoulder-to-foot measurements on the right and left sides and compare measurements

Answer: 3

Rationale: The child should be unclothed or wearing underpants only so that the chest, back, and hips can be clearly seen. The child should stand with weight equally on both feet, legs straight, and arms hanging loosely at both sides. Shoulder heights are observed for unequal alignment. Observation for equal leg lengths is also done.

Test-Taking Strategy: With knowledge regarding the anatomical location of this disorder, attempt to visualize the screening procedure identified in each option. This should assist you in eliminating options 1, 2, and 4. If you had difficulty with this question, take time now to review this important screening procedure!

Level of Cognitive Ability: Analysis
Phase of Nursing Process: Assessment
Client Needs: Health Promotion and Maintenance
Content Area: Child Health

Reference

Ashwill, J., & Droske, S. (1997). *Nursing care of children: Principles and practice.* Philadelphia: W. B. Saunders, p. 1141.

---

197. The nurse provides dietary instruction to the parents of a child with a diagnosis of cystic fibrosis. Which of the following would be a component of dietary management and teaching?

1. Low protein
2. Low fat
3. High calorie
4. Low sodium

Answer: 3

Rationale: Children with cystic fibrosis are managed with a high-calorie, high-protein diet; pancreatic enzyme replacement therapy; fat-soluble vitamin supplements; and, if nutritional problems are severe, nighttime gastrostomy feedings or TPN. Fats are not restricted unless steatorrhea cannot be controlled by increased pancreatic enzymes. Sodium intake is unrelated to this disorder.

Test-Taking Strategy: Knowledge regarding the digestive problems and the dietary management in children with cystic fibrosis is necessary to answer this question. If you are unfamiliar with this content, you might select option 3 because children do require calories for growth and development. Review this content now if you had difficulty with this question!

Level of Cognitive Ability: Application
Phase of Nursing Process: Implementation
Client Needs: Health Promotion and Maintenance
Content Area: Child Health

Reference

Ashwill, J., & Droske, S. (1997). *Nursing care of children: Principles and practice.* Philadelphia: W. B. Saunders, p. 891.

---

198. The clinic nurse instructs an adolescent with iron-deficiency anemia about the administration of oral iron preparations. The nurse would instruct the adolescent to take the iron with

1 Water.
2 Milk.
3 Tomato juice.
4 Apple juice.

Answer: 3

Rationale: Iron should be administered with fluids rich in ascorbic acid (vitamin C). Tomato juice contains a high content of ascorbic acid. Vitamin C enhances the absorption of the iron preparation.

Test-Taking Strategy: Knowledge that vitamin C increases the absorption of iron will assist in answering this question. With this concept in mind, you can easily eliminate options 1 and 2. Of the remaining two options, you would select option 3 because this fluid has the highest content of ascorbic acid.

Level of Cognitive Ability: Application
Phase of Nursing Process: Implementation
Client Needs: Health Promotion and Maintenance
Content Area: Child Health

Reference

Ashwill, J., & Droske, S. (1997). *Nursing care of children: Principles and practice.* Philadelphia: W. B. Saunders, p. 968.

---

199. The nurse is conducting a home visit for the client who started taking a sustained-release preparation of procainamide (Pronestyl-SR). The nurse would plan on teaching the client which of the following items about this medication?

1 The client should not crush, chew, or break the sustained-release tablets
2 Presence of tablet wax matrix in stool indicates poor medication absorption
3 The client may take a double dose if the first one is missed
4 Monitoring of pulse rate and rhythm is unnecessary once this medication is begun

Answer: 1

Rationale: Procainamide (Pronestyl) is a group 1A antidysrhythmic that is available in sustained-release form. The sustained-release preparation should not be broken, chewed, or crushed. The SR form has a wax matrix that may be found in the stool and is not significant. If a dose is forgotten, a sustained-release tablet may be taken if remembered within 4 hours (2 hours for regular-acting form); otherwise, the dose should be omitted. The client or family member should be taught to monitor the client's pulse and to report any change in rate or rhythm.

Test-Taking Strategy: The wording of the question lets you know that only one of the options is a correct statement. Knowing that procainamide is an antidysrhythmic, you may eliminate options 3 and 4 first as unlikely. Basic knowledge of administration of sustained-release medications will help you to choose option 1 over option 2.

Level of Cognitive Ability: Application
Phase of Nursing Process: Planning
Client Needs: Health Promotion and Maintenance
Content Area: Pharmacology

Reference

Deglin, J., & Vallerand, A. (1997). *Davis's drug guide for nurses* (5th ed.). Philadelphia: F. A. Davis, pp. 1006–1007.

200. The nurse has given the client with a nephrostomy tube instructions to follow after hospital discharge. The nurse evaluates that the client understands the instructions if the client verbalizes that he or she will drink at least how many glasses of water per day?

1 2–4
2 6–8
3 10–12
4 14–16

Answer: 2

Rationale: The client with a nephrostomy tube needs to have adequate fluid intake to dilute urinary particles that could cause calculus and to provide good mechanical flushing of the kidney and tube. The nurse encourages the client to take in at least 2000 mL fluid per day, which is approximately equivalent to 6–8 glasses of water.

Test-Taking Strategy: This question can be answered most easily by knowing the client needs at least 2 liters of fluid per day and by knowing how to convert ounces to milliliters. You would avoid options in the much higher range because these are unnecessary and could possibly cause undue distention of the renal pelvis.

Level of Cognitive Ability: Analysis
Phase of Nursing Process: Evaluation
Client Needs: Health Promotion and Maintenance
Content Area: Adult Health/Renal

Reference

Smeltzer, S., & Bare, B. (1996). *Brunner and Suddarth's Textbook of medical-surgical nursing* (8th ed.). Philadelphia: Lippincott-Raven, pp. 1169, 1173.

---

201. The client has been given a prescription for cisapride (Propulsid), 20 mg once daily, in the management of gastroesophageal reflux disease (GERD). The nurse instructs the client to take the medication at which of the following times?

1 Before breakfast
2 After breakfast
3 At lunch time
4 At bedtime

Answer: 4

Rationale: Cisapride may be given on a variety of schedules, from QD to QID. When given once a day, it is taken at bedtime. When given QID, it is taken 15 minutes before meals and at bedtime. The medication is a kinetic agent for the gastrointestinal tract and is commonly used in the management of heartburn associated with GERD.

Test-Taking Strategy: To answer this question correctly, it is necessary to know the purpose of the medication. With this in mind, you may easily deduce that the appropriate timing for this once-daily medication is at bedtime. Review this medication now if you had difficulty with this question!

Level of Cognitive Ability: Application
Phase of Nursing Process: Implementation
Client Needs: Health Promotion and Maintenance
Content Area: Pharmacology

Reference

Deglin, J., & Vallerand, A. (1997). *Davis's drug guide for nurses* (5th ed.). Philadelphia: F. A. Davis, pp. 265–266.

---

202. The clinic nurse is providing home care instructions to a female client in whom recurrent trichomoniasis has been diagnosed. Which of the following would the nurse not include in the instructions?

1 Good perineal hygiene
2 Refraining from sexual intercourse
3 Discontinuing treatment if the menstrual cycle begins
4 Take metronidazole (Flagyl) for 7 days

Answer: 3

Rationale: Treatment for a recurrent infection should be continued throughout the menstrual period because the vagina is more alkaline during this time and a flare-up is likely to occur. Options 1, 2, and 4 are correct. The client should refrain from sexual intercourse while the infection remains active. If this is not possible, a condom is recommended.

Test-Taking Strategy: Option 1 and option 2 can be easily eliminated. Of the remaining two options, select option 3 over option 4 because it is unlikely that treatment would be discontinued. If you had difficulty with this question, take time now to review treatment for this protozoal infection.

Level of Cognitive Ability: Application
Phase of Nursing Process: Implementation
Client Needs: Health Promotion and Maintenance
Content Area: Fundamental Skills

Reference

Black, J., & Matassarin-Jacobs, E. (1997). *Medical-surgical nursing: Clinical management for continuity of care* (5th ed.). Philadelphia: W. B. Saunders, pp. 2473–2474.

---

203. The nurse is providing home care instructions to a client recovering from a radical vulvectomy. Which of the following would the nurse not include in the discharge plan?

1 Take showers rather than tub baths
2 Wipe from front to back after a bowel movement
3 Monitor for foul-smelling perineal discharge
4 Notify physician if swelling of the groin or genital area persists for longer than 3 days

Answer: 4

Rationale: The physician needs to be notified if any swelling of the groin or genital area occurs. The client should not wait for 3 days. Options 1, 2, and 3 are accurate instructions. In addition, the client should monitor for pain, redness, or tenderness in the calves and for any signs of infection.

Test-Taking Strategy: Basic hygiene principles will assist in eliminating options 1 and 2. Of the remaining two options, select option 4 over option 3 as the correct answer to this question, as it is stated, because of the time frame noted in this option. Review client teaching points related to a radical vulvectomy if you had difficulty with this question!

Level of Cognitive Ability: Application
Phase of Nursing Process: Implementation
Client Needs: Health Promotion and Maintenance
Content Area: Adult Health/Oncology

Reference

Black, J., & Matassarin-Jacobs, E. (1997). *Medical-surgical nursing: Clinical management for continuity of care* (5th ed.). Philadelphia: W. B. Saunders, p. 2421.

---

204. A client with major depression is considering cognitive therapy. The client says to the nurse, "How does this treatment work?" The nurse's response would be

1 "This type of treatment helps you examine how your thoughts and feelings contribute to your difficulties."
2 "This type of treatment helps you examine how your life experiences have contributed to your problems."
3 "This type of treatment helps you confront your fears by gradually exposing you to them."
4 "This type of treatment will help you relax and develop new coping skills."

Answer: 1

Rationale: Cognitive therapy is frequently used with clients who have depression. This type of therapy is based on exploring the client's subjective experience. It includes examining the client's thoughts and feelings about situations, as well as how these thoughts and feelings contribute and perpetuate the client's difficulties and mood.

Test-Taking Strategy: Focusing on the word "cognitive" will assist you in choosing the correct option. Look for a similar word or phrase used in the stem and repeated in one of the options. Option 1 uses the word "thoughts" in describing the treatment.

Level of Cognitive Ability: Application
Phase of Nursing Process: Implementation
Client Needs: Health Promotion and Maintenance
Content Area: Mental Health

Reference

Carson, V., & Arnold, E. (1996). *Mental health nursing: The nurse-patient journey.* Philadelphia: W. B. Saunders, pp. 376–377.

205. The client with AIDS has a nursing diagnosis of Altered Nutrition: Less Than Body Requirements. The nurse has instructed the client about methods of maintaining and increasing weight. The nurse evaluates that the client would benefit from further instruction if the client stated that he or she would

1 Use low-calorie snacks between meals.
2 Eat small, frequent meals throughout the day.
3 Consume nutrient-dense foods and beverages.
4 Keep easy-to-prepare foods available in the home.

Answer: 1

Rationale: The client should eat small, frequent meals throughout the day. The client also should take in nutrient-dense and high-calorie meals and snacks. The client is encouraged to eat favorite foods to keep intake up and to plan meals that are easy to prepare. The client can also avoid taking fluids with meals, in order to increase food intake before satiety sets in.

Test-Taking Strategy: The wording of the question guides you to look for an answer that is incorrect. Because options 2, 3, and 4 are all plausible responses, option 1 is the answer to the question as stated. The client should choose snacks that are high, not low, in calories.

Level of Cognitive Ability: Analysis
Phase of Nursing Process: Evaluation
Client Needs: Health Promotion and Maintenance
Content Area: Fundamental Skills

Reference

Black, J., & Matassarin-Jacobs, E. (1997). *Medical-surgical nursing: Clinical management for continuity of care* (5th ed.). Philadelphia: W. B. Saunders, pp. 634–635.

---

206. The nurse is caring for the client who had chest tube placement for drainage of empyema. The nurse has given the client instructions about breathing exercises that will best promote respiratory function. The nurse evaluates that the client understands the material if the client properly demonstrates which of the following techniques?

1 Diaphragmatic and pursed-lip breathing
2 Incentive spirometry and quad coughing
3 Deep breathing only
4 Incentive spirometry only

Answer: 1

Rationale: Respiratory exercises that promote normal respiratory function for the client with empyema include diaphragmatic and pursed-lip breathing. These exercises strengthen respiratory muscles and promote gas exchange.

Test-Taking Strategy: Options 3 and 4 are unnecessarily limiting, using the word "only," and are thus eliminated first. Option 2 is eliminated next because the client has no need to learn quad coughing technique. This leaves option 1 as the only remaining alternative.

Level of Cognitive Ability: Analysis
Phase of Nursing Process: Evaluation
Client Needs: Health Promotion and Maintenance
Content Area: Adult Health/Respiratory

Reference

Smeltzer, S., & Bare, B. (1996). *Brunner and Suddarth's Textbook of medical-surgical nursing* (8th ed.). Philadelphia: Lippincott-Raven, pp. 503–504.

---

207. The nurse has given the postoperative thoracotomy client instructions about how to perform arm and shoulder exercises after discharge. The nurse evaluates that the client has not learned the proper techniques if the client is observed performing which of the following movements on the affected side?

1 Moving the arm up over the head and back down
2 Holding the hands crossed in front and raising them over the head
3 Holding the upper arm straight out while moving the forearm up and down
4 Making circles with the wrist

Answer: 4

Rationale: A variety of exercises that involve moving the shoulder and elbow joints are indicated after thoracotomy. These include shrugging the shoulders and moving them back and forth; moving the arms up and down, forward, and backward; holding the hands crossed in front of the waist and then raising them over the head; and holding the upper arm straight out while moving the lower arm up and down. Exercises that move only the wrist joint are of no use after this surgery.

Test-Taking Strategy: The wording of this question guides you to look for either an exercise that is not helpful or one that is done incorrectly. A brief review of the exercises shows that none of them are described incorrectly. In examining each of the options again, note that options 1 and 2 move the shoulder joint. Option 3 moves the shoulder and elbow joint. Option 4 moves only the wrist joint. By the process of elimination, you would choose option 4 as the incorrect response. Because the post-thoractomy client needs to exercise the shoulder joint, there is no other possible answer.

Level of Cognitive Ability: Analysis
Phase of Nursing Process: Evaluation
Client Needs: Health Promotion and Maintenance
Content Area: Adult Health/Respiratory

Reference

Black, J., & Matassarin-Jacobs, E. (1997). *Medical-surgical nursing: Clinical management for continuity of care* (5th ed.). Philadelphia: W. B. Saunders, p. 1158.

---

208. The nurse is teaching the client with histoplasmosis infection about prevention of future exposure to infectious sources. The nurse evaluates that the client needs further instruction if the client states that potential sources include

1 Grape arbors.
2 Mushroom cellars.
3 Floors of chicken houses.
4 Bird droppings.

Answer: 1

Rationale: The client with histoplasmosis is taught to avoid exposure to potential sources of the fungus *Histoplasma capsulatum,* which includes soil of composition conducive to fungal growth, bird droppings (especially those of starlings and blackbirds), floors of chicken houses and bat caves, and mushroom cellars.

Test-Taking Strategy: Eliminate options 3 and 4 first because they are similar. By the process of elimination, the least likely choice is the grape arbor, which is above ground and is not in a dark and damp area. For these reasons, it is the least likely choice for causing infection and is the answer to the question as stated.

Level of Cognitive Ability: Analysis
Phase of Nursing Process: Evaluation
Client Needs: Health Promotion and Maintenance
Content Area: Adult Health/Respiratory

Reference

Black, J., & Matassarin-Jacobs, E. (1997). *Medical-surgical nursing: Clinical management for continuity of care* (5th ed.). Philadelphia: W. B. Saunders, p. 1146.

---

209. The nurse is teaching the client with pulmonary sarcoidosis about long-term ongoing management. The nurse plans to explain which of the following in the instructions?

1 Need for daily corticosteroids
2 Usefulness of home oxygen
3 Need for follow-up chest films every 6 months
4 Importance of using the incentive spirometer daily

Answer: 3

Rationale: The client with pulmonary sarcoidosis needs to have follow-up chest films every 6 months to monitor disease progression. If an exacerbation occurs, treatment is given with systemic corticosteroids. These tend to produce rapid improvement in symptoms. Home oxygen and ongoing use of incentive spirometer are not indicated.

Test-Taking Strategy: Eliminate option 2 first because there is no specific information in the stem to indicate a need for its use. Knowing that corticosteroids are used for exacerbation helps you eliminate this option as well. To discriminate between the last two options, it is necessary to know that serial monitoring with x-ray is needed to track progression of the disease.

Level of Cognitive Ability: Application
Phase of Nursing Process: Planning
Client Needs: Health Promotion and Maintenance
Content Area: Adult Health/Respiratory

Reference

Black, J., & Matassarin-Jacobs, E. (1997). *Medical-surgical nursing: Clinical management for continuity of care* (5th ed.). Philadelphia: W. B. Saunders, p. 1150.

210. The nurse has taught the client with silicosis about situations to avoid in order to prevent exposure to silica dust. The nurse evaluates that the client understands the instructions if the client verbalizes that he or she will give up or wear a mask for which of the following hobbies?

1 Pottery making
2 Woodworking
3 Painting
4 Gardening

Answer: 1

Rationale: Exposure to silica dust occurs with activities such as pottery making and building stone masonry. Exposure to the finely ground silica, such as is used with soaps, polishes, and filters, is also dangerous.

Test-Taking Strategy: To answer this question, it is necessary to have an understanding of the materials that could give off silica dust. Eliminate gardening first because silica exposure does not occur with this activity. Knowing that it is not inhaled in fumes, you may then eliminate woodworking or painting. By elimination, then, you may choose the pottery making as the correct answer. This makes sense because pottery is made from clay.

Level of Cognitive Ability: Analysis
Phase of Nursing Process: Evaluation
Client Needs: Health Promotion and Maintenance
Content Area: Adult Health/Respiratory

Reference
Ignatavicius, D. D., Workman, M. L., & Mishler, M. A. (1995). *Medical-surgical nursing: A nursing process approach* (2nd ed.). Philadelphia: W. B. Saunders, p. 725.

---

211. The nurse is conducting dietary teaching with the client who is hypocalcemic. The nurse encourages the client to increase intake of which of the following foods that the client enjoys?

1 Apples
2 Chicken breast
3 Yogurt
4 Cooked pasta

Answer: 3

Rationale: Products that are naturally high in calcium are dairy products, including milk, cheese, ice cream, and yogurt. High-calcium foods generally have more than 100 mg of calcium per serving. The other options are foods that are low in calcium, which means that they have less than 25 mg of calcium per serving.

Test-Taking Strategy: Knowledge of the calcium content of specific foods is needed to answer this question accurately. If this question was difficult, take a few moments to review this area. As a general rule, recall that dairy products are naturally high in calcium.

Level of Cognitive Ability: Application
Phase of Nursing Process: Implementation
Client Needs: Health Promotion and Maintenance
Content Area: Fundamental Skills

Reference
Black, J., & Matassarin-Jacobs, E. (1997). *Medical-surgical nursing: Clinical management for continuity of care* (5th ed.). Philadelphia: W. B. Saunders, p. 318.

---

212. The client is diagnosed with hyperphosphatemia. The nurse encourages the client to limit intake of which of the following items that is aggravating the condition?

1 Bananas
2 Grapes
3 Coffee
4 Carbonated beverages

Answer: 4

Rationale: Foods that are naturally high in phosphates should be avoided by the client with hyperphosphatemia. These include fish, eggs, milk products, vegetables, whole grains, and carbonated beverages.

Test-Taking Strategy: Specific knowledge related to the phosphate content of foods is needed to answer this question correctly. If needed, take a few moments to review these foods and fluids!

Level of Cognitive Ability: Application
Phase of Nursing Process: Implementation
Client Needs: Health Promotion and Maintenance
Content Area: Fundamental Skills

Reference
Black, J., & Matassarin-Jacobs, E. (1997). *Medical-surgical nursing: Clinical management for continuity of care* (5th ed.). Philadelphia: W. B. Saunders, p. 318.

213. The nurse is caring for the client who has sustained thoracic burns and smoke inhalation and is at risk for impaired gas exchange. The nurse avoids which of the following actions as the least helpful in caring for this client?

1. Repositioning the client from side to side every 2 hours
2. Positioning the client only on the back with head of bed at 45-degree angle
3. Suctioning the airway on a PRN basis
4. Providing humidified oxygen and incentive spirometry

Answer: 2

Rationale: Aggressive pulmonary measures are used to prevent respiratory complications in the client who has impaired gas exchange as a result of burn injury. These include turning and repositioning, positioning for comfort, using humidified oxygen, providing incentive spirometry, and suctioning the airway on an as-needed basis. The least helpful measure is to keep the client in one single position. This will ultimately lead to atelectasis and possible pneumonia.

Test-Taking Strategy: Note the key word in the question is "least." This tells you that the answer to the question is an incorrect nursing action. Use basic nursing knowledge of respiratory support measures to eliminate each of the incorrect options. Note the word "only" in the correct option in this question.

Level of Cognitive Ability: Application
Phase of Nursing Process: Implementation
Client Needs: Health Promotion and Maintenance
Content Area: Adult Health/Integumentary

Reference
Smeltzer, S., & Bare, B. (1996). *Brunner and Suddarth's Textbook of medical-surgical nursing* (8th ed.). Philadelphia: Lippincott-Raven, p. 1556.

---

214. The community health nurse provides an educational session on the risk factors for cervical cancer to the women in a local community. Which of the following would the nurse not include as a risk factor of this type of cancer?

1. Occurs most frequently in white women
2. Early age of first intercourse
3. Multiparity
4. Low socioeconomic class

Answer: 1

Rationale: Risk factors for cervical cancer include being black or Native American, prostitution, early first pregnancy, untreated chronic cervicitis, sexually transmitted diseases, postpartum lacerations, partner with a history of penile or prostate cancer, and infection with human papillomavirus. In addition, options 2, 3, and 4 identify risk factors.

Test-Taking Strategy: Knowledge regarding the risk factors for cervical cancer is necessary to answer this question. Take time now to review these risk factors if you had difficulty with this question!

Level of Cognitive Ability: Application
Phase of Nursing Process: Implementation
Client Needs: Health Promotion and Maintenance
Content Area: Adult Health/Oncology

Reference
Black, J., & Matassarin-Jacobs, E. (1997). *Medical-surgical nursing: Clinical management for continuity of care* (5th ed.). Philadelphia: W. B. Saunders, p. 2406.

---

215. The high school nurse teaches the female students how to prevent pelvic inflammatory disease (PID). Which of the following would be a component of the instructions?

1. Single sexual partners should be avoided
2. To consult with gynecologist regarding placement of an intrauterine device (IUD)
3. To douche monthly
4. To avoid unprotected intercourse

Answer: 4

Rationale: Primary prevention for PID includes avoiding unprotected intercourse, avoiding multiple sexual partners, avoiding the use of an IUD, and avoiding douching.

Test-Taking Strategy: Use the principle of exposure of the pelvic area as a cause of leading to infection. With this concept in mind, you should be able to eliminate options 1, 2, and 3. Review preventive measures for PID now if you had difficulty with this question!

Level of Cognitive Ability: Application
Phase of Nursing Process: Implementation
Client Needs: Health Promotion and Maintenance
Content Area: Fundamental Skills

Reference
Black, J., & Matassarin-Jacobs, E. (1997). *Medical-surgical nursing: Clinical management for continuity of care* (5th ed.). Philadelphia: W. B. Saunders, p. 2406.

216. The nurse provides discharge teaching to a client after a vasectomy. Which of the following statements, if made by the client, would indicate a need for further education?

1 "If I have pain or swelling, I can use an ice bag and take Tylenol"
2 "I can use a scrotal support if I need to"
3 "I can resume sexual intercourse whenever I want"
4 "I don't need to practice birth control any longer"

Answer: 4

Rationale: After vasectomy, the client must continue to use means of birth control until the follow-up semen analysis shows azoospermia, because live sperm are left in the ampulla of vas deferens. Options 1, 2, and 3 are appropriate.

Test-Taking Strategy: Considering the purpose of a vasectomy should assist in directing you to option 4. Options 1 and 2 can be easily eliminated because these measures assist in alleviating discomfort or swelling after the procedure. Option 3 can be eliminated because there would be no reason to avoid sexual intercourse unless the client was experiencing discomfort.

Level of Cognitive Ability: Analysis
Phase of Nursing Process: Evaluation
Client Needs: Health Promotion and Maintenance
Content Area: Fundamental Skills

Reference
Black, J., & Matassarin-Jacobs, E. (1997). *Medical-surgical nursing: Clinical management for continuity of care* (5th ed.). Philadelphia: W. B. Saunders, p. 2378

217. The physician in a community clinic diagnoses prostatitis in the client. The nurse provides home care instructions to the client. Which of the following statements, if made by the client, would indicate a need for further education?

1 "I need to take the anti-inflammatory medications as prescribed"
2 "The hot sitz baths will help my condition"
3 "I need to avoid sexual activity for 1 week"
4 "There are no restrictions in my diet"

Answer: 3

Rationale: Interventions include anti-inflammatory agents or short-term antimicrobial medication. Hot sitz baths are recommended, and normal sexual activity is not discouraged. Dietary restrictions are not recommended unless the client finds them to be associated with manifestations.

Test-Taking Strategy: Eliminate option 1 first, using the general principles associated with medication prescriptions. Option 4 can be eliminated next because there is no specific relationship of diet to this disorder. Of the remaining two options, eliminate option 2 because it seems reasonable that sitz baths would provide comfort.

Level of Cognitive Ability: Analysis
Phase of Nursing Process: Evaluation
Client Needs: Health Promotion and Maintenance
Content Area: Adult Health/Renal

Reference
Black, J., & Matassarin-Jacobs, E. (1997). *Medical-surgical nursing: Clinical management for continuity of care* (5th ed.). Philadelphia: W. B. Saunders, p. 2373.

218. The nursing instructor asks the student to identify the risk factors and methods of prevention of prostate cancer. Which of the following, if stated by the nursing student, would indicate a need to review this information?

1 Men older than 50 should be monitored with a yearly digital rectal examination
2 Men older than 50 should be monitored with a prostate-specific antigen (PSA assay)
3 A high-fat diet will assist in preventing this type of cancer
4 Employment in fertilizer, textile, and rubber industries increases the risk of prostate cancer

Answer: 3

Rationale: A high intake of dietary fat is a risk factor for prostate cancer. Options 1, 2, and 4 are accurate statements regarding the risks and prevention measures related to this type of cancer.

Test-Taking Strategy: Use the process of elimination and general risk factors related to cancer prevention to answer the question. By the wording of this question, you are looking for the option that is an incorrect statement. This should assist in directing you to option 3 as the correct answer for this question as it is stated.

Level of Cognitive Ability: Analysis
Phase of Nursing Process: Evaluation
Client Needs: Health Promotion and Maintenance
Content Area: Adult Health/Renal

Reference
Black, J., & Matassarin-Jacobs, E. (1997). *Medical-surgical nursing: Clinical management for continuity of care* (5th ed.). Philadelphia: W. B. Saunders, p. 2366.

219. The clinic nurse provides information to a married couple regarding measures to prevent infertility. Which of the following measures would not be a component of the discussion?

1 Avoid excessive intake of alcohol
2 Decrease exposure to environmental hazards
3 Eat a nutritious diet
4 Maintain warmth to the scrotum

Answer: 4

Rationale: Keeping the testes cool by avoiding hot baths and tight clothing appears to improve the sperm count. Avoiding factors that depress spermatogenesis, such as the use of drugs (e.g., alcohol and marijuana), exposure to occupational and environmental hazards, and maintaining good nutrition, is a key component in preventing infertility.

Test-Taking Strategy: Eliminate option 3 first because maintenance of a nutritious diet is important in all situations. Eliminate options 1 and 2 next because these factors affect spermatogenesis. Remembering that heat decreases numbers of viable sperm will assist in directing you to the correct option. Review the measures that prevent infertility now if you have difficulty with this question!

Level of Cognitive Ability: Application
Phase of Nursing Process: Implementation
Client Needs: Health Promotion and Maintenance
Content Area: Maternity

Reference

Black, J., & Matassarin-Jacobs, E. (1997). *Medical-surgical nursing: Clinical management for continuity of care* (5th ed.). Philadelphia: W. B. Saunders, p. 2347.

220. The nurse educates a client preparing for discharge after a total hip replacement. Which of the following statements, if made by the client, would indicate a need for further education?

1 "I need to place a pillow between my knees when I lie down"
2 "I need to wear a support stocking on my unaffected leg"
3 "I should not sit in one position for longer than 2 hours"
4 "I cannot drive a car for 6 weeks"

Answer: 3

Rationale: The client needs to be instructed not to sit continuously for longer than 1 hour. The client should be instructed to stand, stretch, and take a few steps periodically. The client cannot drive a car for 6 weeks after surgery unless authorized by a physician. A support stocking should be worn on the unaffected leg and an Ace bandage on the affected leg until there is no swelling in the legs or feet and full activities are resumed. The legs are abducted by placing a pillow between them when the client lies down.

Test-Taking Strategy: Recalling standard measures related to the postoperative period will assist in eliminating option 4. Knowing that leg abduction is maintained postoperatively during hospitalization may assist in eliminating option 1. For the remaining two options, note the time frame of 2 hours in option 3. This is a rather lengthy time period for this client to remain in one position. Review teaching points after total hip replacement now if you had difficulty with this question!

Level of Cognitive Ability: Analysis
Phase of Nursing Process: Evaluation
Client Needs: Health Promotion and Maintenance
Content Area: Adult Health/Musculoskeletal

Reference

Black, J., & Matassarin-Jacobs, E. (1997). *Medical-surgical nursing: Clinical management for continuity of care* (5th ed.). Philadelphia: W. B. Saunders, p. 2116.

221. The nurse is preparing to administer intravenous ampicillin sodium (Omnipen) to a pregnant woman who has had ruptured membranes for more than 20 hours. The client asks the nurse why the medication is being given. The best response by the nurse is to tell the client that it will prevent

1 Early-onset neonatal group B streptococcus (GBS) disease.
2 Transmission of a sexually transmitted disease to her partner.
3 The development of chorioamnionitis.
4 Maternal rheumatic fever.

Answer: 1

Rationale: One of the Centers for Disease Control and Prevention (CDC) treatment guidelines for early-onset neonatal GBS disease and maternal illness includes providing intrapartum antibiotics to women who develop risk conditions at the time of labor or rupture of membranes. A major risk factor is prolonged rupture of membranes (longer than 12–18 hours). Other risk factors include prolonged labor, high number of vaginal examinations during labor, low-birth-weight infants, colonized women, premature onset of labor, and premature rupture of membranes.

Test-Taking Strategy: The treatment of GBS in the intrapartum period is focused on avoiding maternal and neonatal infections. The key phrase that should direct you to the correct option is "early onset." If you had difficulty with this question, take time now to review GBS disease!

Level of Cognitive Ability: Application
Phase of Nursing Process: Implementation
Client Needs: Health Promotion and Maintenance
Content Area: Maternity

Reference

Nichols, F., & Zwelling, E. (1997). *Maternal-newborn nursing: Theory and practice.* Philadelphia: W. B. Saunders, pp. 1478–1479.

222. A female client has received a diagnosis of hypothyroidism and is to begin taking thyroid supplements. The nurse instructs the client about the medication. Which of the following statements, if made by the client, would indicate the need for further education?

1 "I need to take my daily dose every night at bedtime"
2 "I need to call my physician if I develop any chest pain"
3 "I need to speak to my physician when I begin to plan for parenthood"
4 "My appetite may increase because of the medication"

Answer: 1

Rationale: The client is instructed to take the medication in the morning to prevent insomnia. Chest pain may indicate overdose, and the physician needs to be notified. The dose needs to be adjusted if the client is pregnant or plans to become pregnant. GI side effects of thyroid supplements include increased appetite, nausea, and diarrhea.

Test-Taking Strategy: You can easily eliminate options 2 and 3 on the basis of basic principles related to medication therapy. Chest pain warrants follow-up, and pregnancy would necessitate a review of the medication dosage. Considering the disorder hypothyroidism, you would expect thyroid hormone to increase body metabolism. This should assist you in selecting option 1 over option 4.

Level of Cognitive Ability: Analysis
Phase of Nursing Process: Evaluation
Client Needs: Health Promotion and Maintenance
Content Area: Adult Health/Endocrine

Reference

Black, J., & Matassarin-Jacobs, E. (1997). *Medical-surgical nursing: Clinical management for continuity of care* (5th ed.). Philadelphia: W. B. Saunders, p. 2016.

223. The clinic nurse instructs the client with diabetes about how to prevent diabetic ketoacidosis (DKA) on days when the client is feeling ill. Which statement, if made by the client, indicates a need for further education?

1 "I need to stop my insulin if I am vomiting"
2 "I need to call my physician if I am ill for more than 24 hours"
3 "I need to eat 10–15 g of carbohydrates every 1–2 hours"
4 "I need to drink small quantities of fluid every 15–30 minutes"

Answer: 1

Rationale: The client needs to be instructed to take insulin even if he or she is vomiting and unable to eat. It is important to self-monitor the blood glucose level more frequently (every 2–4 hours) during illness. If the premeal blood glucose level is higher than 250 mg/dL, the client should test for urine ketones and contact the physician. Options 2, 3, and 4 are accurate interventions.

Test-Taking Strategy: You should easily be able to eliminate options 2, 3, and 4. In addition, recalling that insulin needs to be taken every day will assist in directing you to option 1.

Level of Cognitive Ability: Analysis
Phase of Nursing Process: Evaluation
Client Needs: Health Promotion and Maintenance
Content Area: Adult Health/Endocrine

Reference

Black, J., & Matassarin-Jacobs, E. (1997). *Medical-surgical nursing: Clinical management for continuity of care* (5th ed.). Philadelphia: W. B. Saunders, p. 2002.

---

224. The nurse is instructing the diabetic client about hypoglycemia. Which of the following statements, if made by the client, would indicate a need for further education?

1 "Hypoglycemia can occur at any time of the day or night"
2 "If hypoglycemia occurs, I need to take my regular insulin as prescribed"
3 "If I feel sweaty or shaky, I might be experiencing hypoglycemia"
4 "I can drink 8 ounces of 2% milk if hypoglycemia occurs"

Answer: 2

Rationale: If a hypoglycemia reaction occurs, the client will need to consume 10–15 g of carbohydrate. Six to eight ounces of 2% milk contains this amount of carbohydrate. Tremors and diaphoresis are signs of mild hypoglycemia. Insulin is not taken as a treatment for hypoglycemia because the insulin will lower the blood glucose. Hypoglycemic reactions can occur at any time of the day or night.

Test-Taking Strategy: Think about the concept that in hypoglycemia the blood glucose level is lowered. Insulin also lowers blood glucose; therefore, it seems reasonable that insulin is not a treatment for this condition. Take time now to review the signs of hypoglycemia and the appropriate interventions if you had difficulty with this question. You are likely to find a question related to this concept on NCLEX-RN!

Level of Cognitive Ability: Analysis
Phase of Nursing Process: Evaluation
Client Needs: Health Promotion and Maintenance
Content Area: Adult Health/Endocrine

Reference

Black, J., & Matassarin-Jacobs, E. (1997). *Medical-surgical nursing: Clinical management for continuity of care* (5th ed.). Philadelphia: W. B. Saunders, p. 1989.

---

225. The client with nephrolithiasis arrives at the clinic for a follow-up visit. The laboratory analysis of the stone that the client passed 1 week ago indicates that the stone is composed of calcium oxalate. Which of the following foods would the nurse instruct the client to avoid?

1 Lentils
2 Spinach
3 Lettuce
4 Pasta

Answer: 2

Rationale: About 80% of stones are composed of calcium oxalate. Foods that raise urinary oxalate excretion include spinach, rhubarb, strawberries, chocolate, wheat bran, nuts, beets, and tea.

Test-Taking Strategy: Knowledge regarding the foods that raise urinary oxalate excretion is necessary to answer this question. If you had difficulty identifying this food, take time now to review this content!

Level of Cognitive Ability: Application
Phase of Nursing Process: Implementation
Client Needs: Health Promotion and Maintenance
Content Area: Adult Health/Renal

Reference

Mahan, K., & Escott-Stump, S. (1996). *Krause's Food, nutrition, & diet therapy* (9th ed.). Philadelphia: W. B. Saunders, p. 778.

226. The nurse provides teaching to a new mother who is about to breast-feed her newborn. Which of the following instructions would not be a component of the teaching?

1 Turn the baby on the side, facing the mother
2 When the baby opens the mouth, draw the baby's head close to the breast so that the nipple goes into the baby's mouth
3 Tilt up the nipple or squeeze the areola, pushing it into the baby's mouth
4 Place a clean finger in the side of the baby's mouth to break the suction before removing the baby from the breast

Answer: 3

Rationale: The mother is instructed to avoid tilting up the nipple or squeezing the areola before pushing it into the baby's mouth. Options 1, 2, and 4 are correct procedures for breast-feeding.

Test-Taking Strategy: Attempt to visualize the descriptions in each of the options. This will help you eliminate options 1, 2, and 4. Careful reading of option 3, noting the word "pushing," suggests force or resistance and should assist in directing you in selecting this option.

Level of Cognitive Ability: Application
Phase of Nursing Process: Implementation
Client Needs: Health Promotion and Maintenance
Content Area: Maternity

Reference
Nichols, F., & Zwelling, E. (1997). *Maternal-newborn nursing: Theory and practice.* Philadelphia: W. B. Saunders, p. 1217.

227. The clinic nurse provides instructions to a mother regarding the care of her child, in whom croup is diagnosed. Which of the following statements, if made by the mother, indicates a need for further education?

1 "I will place a cool-mist humidifier next to my child's bed"
2 "Sips of warm fluids during a croup attack will help"
3 "I will give acetaminophen [Tylenol] for the fever"
4 "I will give cough syrup every night at bed time"

Answer: 4

Rationale: The mother needs to be instructed that cough syrup and cold medicines are not to be administered because they may dry and thicken secretions. Sips of warm fluid will relax the vocal cords and thin mucus. A cool-mist humidifier rather than a steam vaporizer is recommended because of the danger of the child pulling the steam vaporizer over and causing a burn. Tylenol will reduce the fever.

Test-Taking Strategy: Knowledge regarding interventions for croup is helpful in answering this question. Option 3 can be easily eliminated. Remembering that warm fluids will thin secretions will assist in eliminating option 2. For the remaining two options, recalling that cough syrup will dry secretions will assist in directing you to selecting option 4. Review home care instructions for the child with croup if you had difficulty with this question.

Level of Cognitive Ability: Application
Phase of Nursing Process: Implementation
Client Needs: Health Promotion and Maintenance
Content Area: Child Health

Reference
Ashwill, J., & Droske, S. (1997). *Nursing care of children: Principles and practice.* Philadelphia: W. B. Saunders, p. 838.

228. The client with anxiety disorder is taking buspirone (BuSpar), 10 mg three times daily. The client tells the nurse that it is difficult to swallow the tablets. Which of the following would be the best instruction to provide to the client?

1 To purchase the liquid preparation with the next refill
2 To crush the tablets before taking them
3 To call the physician for a change in medication
4 To mix the tablet uncrushed in applesauce

Answer: 2

Rationale: BuSpar may be administered without regard to meals, and the tablets may be crushed. This medication is not available in liquid form. It is premature to advise the client to call the physician for a change in medication without first trying alternative interventions. Mixing the tablet uncrushed in applesauce will not likely facilitate swallowing.

Test-Taking Strategy: You can easily eliminate option 3 first because in most situations there is a nursing intervention that can be instituted first. Next, eliminate option 4 because this instruction will not likely facilitate swallowing. For the remaining two options, it is necessary to know that this medication is not available in liquid form. In addition, tablets can be crushed.

Level of Cognitive Ability: Application
Phase of Nursing Process: Implementation
Client Needs: Health Promotion and Maintenance
Content Area: Pharmacology

Reference

Hodgson, B., & Kizior, R. (1998). *Saunders nursing drug handbook 1998.* Philadelphia: W. B. Saunders, p. 131.

---

229. The nurse caring for a child with congestive heart failure provides instructions to the parents about the administration of digoxin (Lanoxin). Which of the following statements, if made by the mother, indicates the need for further education?

1 "If the child vomits after I give the medication, I will not repeat the dose"
2 "I will check my child's pulse before giving the medication"
3 "I will check the dose of the medication with my husband before I give the medication"
4 "I will mix the medication with food"

Answer: 4

Rationale: The medication should not be mixed with food or formula because this method would not ensure that the child receives the entire dose of medication. Options 1, 2, and 3 are correct. In addition, if a dosage is missed and is not remembered until 4 or more hours later, do not administer that dose. If two or more consecutive doses are skipped, the physician needs to be notified.

Test-Taking Strategy: General principles regarding medication administration to children should assist in directing you to the correct option. Mixing medications with formula or food may alter the effectiveness of the medication and, more important, if the child does not consume the entire formula or food, the total dosage would not be administered.

Level of Cognitive Ability: Analysis
Phase of Nursing Process: Evaluation
Client Needs: Health Promotion and Maintenance
Content Area: Pharmacology

Reference

Ashwill, J., & Droske, S. (1997). *Nursing care of children: Principles and practice.* Philadelphia: W. B. Saunders, p. 955.

---

230. The nurse provides discharge instructions to the mother of a child who was hospitalized for heart surgery. Which of the following would be included in the teaching plan?

1 The child may return to school 1 week after hospital discharge
2 After bathing, rub lotion and sprinkle powder on the incision
3 Allow the child to play outside for short periods of time
4 Notify the physician if the child develops a fever higher than 100.5°F

Answer: 4

Rationale: After heart surgery, the child should not return to school until 3 weeks after hospital discharge, at which time he or she should go to school for half days for the first few days. No creams, lotions, or powders should be placed on the incision until it is completely healed and without scabs. The mother is instructed to keep the child from playing outside for several weeks. The physician needs to be notified if the child develops a fever higher than 100.5°F.

Test-Taking Strategy: Use the process of elimination, bearing in mind the potential for infection. Eliminate option 1 because of the time frame of 1 week. Eliminate option 3 because outside play can expose the child to infection and the risk of injury. Basic principles related to incision care should assist in eliminating option 2.

Level of Cognitive Ability: Application
Phase of Nursing Process: Implementation
Client Needs: Health Promotion and Maintenance
Content Area: Child Health

Reference

Ashwill, J., & Droske, S. (1997). *Nursing care of children: Principles and practice.* Philadelphia: W. B. Saunders, p. 922

231. The clinic nurse provides instructions to the client who will begin taking oral contraceptives. Which of the following statements, if made by the client, would indicate the need for further education?

1 "I will take one pill daily at the same time every day"
2 "I will not need to use an additional birth control method once I start these pills"
3 "If I miss a pill, I need to take it as soon as I remember"
4 "If I miss two pills, I will take them both as soon as I remember and I will take two pills the next day also"

Answer: 2

Rationale: The client needs to be instructed to use a second birth control method during the first pill cycle. Options 1, 3, and 4 are correct. In addition, the client needs to be instructed that if she misses three pills, she will need to discontinue use for that cycle and use another birth control method.

Test-Taking Strategy: Knowledge regarding guidelines for oral contraceptive use is necessary to answer this question. It seems reasonable, however, that during the first pill cycle, a second birth control method would need to be used to prevent conception. Review these guidelines now if you had difficulty with this question!

Level of Cognitive Ability: Analysis
Phase of Nursing Process: Evaluation
Client Needs: Health Promotion and Maintenance
Content Area: Pharmacology

Reference

Nichols, F., & Zwelling, E. (1997). *Maternal-newborn nursing: Theory and practice.* Philadelphia: W. B. Saunders, p. 258

---

232. The nurse is providing dietary instructions to the client hospitalized for acute pancreatitis. Which of the following foods would the nurse instruct the client to avoid?

1 Lentil soup
2 Bagel
3 Chili
4 Watermelon

Answer: 3

Rationale: The client needs to avoid alcohol, coffee and tea, spicy foods, and heavy meals, all of which stimulate pancreatic secretions and produces attacks of pancreatitis. Instruct the client in the benefit of eating small, frequent meals that are high in protein, low in fat, and moderate to high in carbohydrates.

Test-Taking Strategy: Use the process of elimination, noting that options 1, 2, and 4 are foods that are moderately bland. Option 3, chili, is a spicy food.

Level of Cognitive Ability: Application
Phase of Nursing Process: Implementation
Client Needs: Health Promotion and Maintenance
Content Area: Adult Health/Gastrointestinal

Reference

Black, J., & Matassarin-Jacobs, E. (1997). *Medical-surgical nursing: Clinical management for continuity of care* (5th ed.). Philadelphia: W. B. Saunders, p. 1926.

---

233. The home health care nurse visits a client who recently received a diagnosis of cirrhosis. The nurse provides home care management instructions to the client. Which of the following statements, if made by the client, indicates a need for further education?

1 "I will take acetaminophen [Tylenol] if I get a headache"
2 "I will obtain adequate rest"
3 "I do not need to restrict fat in my diet"
4 "I should monitor my weight on a regular basis"

Answer: 1

Rationale: Tylenol is avoided because it can cause fatal liver damage in the client with cirrhosis. Adequate rest and nutrition are important. Fat restriction is not necessary, and the diet should supply sufficient carbohydrates with a total daily calorie intake of 2000–3000. The client's weight should be monitored on a regular basis.

Test-Taking Strategy: Options 2 and 4 can be easily eliminated. Recalling that Tylenol is a hepatotoxic agent will assist in directing you to the correct option. Review medications that are restricted or are avoided in clients with cirrhosis now if you had difficulty with this question!

Level of Cognitive Ability: Analysis
Phase of Nursing Process: Evaluation
Client Needs: Health Promotion and Maintenance
Content Area: Adult Health/Gastrointestinal

Reference

Black, J., & Matassarin-Jacobs, E. (1997). *Medical-surgical nursing: Clinical management for continuity of care* (5th ed.). Philadelphia: W. B. Saunders, p. 1882.

234. The client who has a history of gout is also diagnosed with urolithiasis. The stones are determined to be of uric acid type. The nurse gives the client instructions in foods to limit, which include

1 Liver.
2 Apples.
3 Carrots.
4 Milk.

Answer: 1

Rationale: Foods containing high amounts of purines should be avoided in the client with uric acid stones. This includes limiting or avoiding organ meats, such as liver, brain, heart, kidney, and sweetbreads. Other foods to avoid include herring, sardines, anchovies, meat extracts, consommés, and gravies. Foods that are low in purines include all fruits, many vegetables, milk, cheese, eggs, refined cereals, sugars and sweets, coffee, tea, chocolate, and carbonated beverages.

Test-Taking Strategy: To answer this question, begin by examining the options and classifying the types of food sources they represent. Options 2 and 3 represent foods that are grown, whereas options 1 and 4 represent foods that derive from animal sources. Because purines are end products of protein metabolism, you would eliminate options 2 and 3 first. To discriminate between options 1 and 4, you would need to know that organ meats such as liver provide a greater quantity of purines than does milk. With this in mind, you would choose option 1 over option 4.

Level of Cognitive Ability: Application
Phase of Nursing Process: Implementation
Client Needs: Health Promotion and Maintenance
Content Area: Adult Health/Renal

Reference

Lutz, C., & Przytulski, K. (1997). *Nutrition and diet therapy* (2nd ed.). Philadelphia: F. A. Davis, p. 400.

---

235. The home health nurse is making follow-up home visits to the client after nephrectomy. Which of the following best indicates that the client understands concepts related to self-care?

1 States that he or she will change the dressing if it gets wet in the shower
2 Indicates that the surgeon should be called if the temperature exceeds 102°F
3 Wipes the portable suction drain port with alcohol sponges before emptying and reclosing the port
4 Stays in bed as much as possible after discharge

Answer: 3

Rationale: The self-care needs of the client after nephrectomy resemble those of clients after any other surgical procedure. The client should report signs and symptoms of infection, increase activity gradually, and keep the surgical dressing dry and intact. If the client is discharged with a portable suction drain, the port should be cleansed before it is emptied and again before the port is closed after the bulb is recharged.

Test-Taking Strategy: Eliminate option 4 first as the most incorrect self-care action. Option 1 is eliminated next because the dressing should not be allowed to get wet. To discriminate between options 2 and 3, knowing that a fever should be reported even before it climbs to 102°F guides you to choose option 3 as the correct answer. Alternatively, if you know proper procedure for emptying a portable suction apparatus, you would also choose correctly.

Level of Cognitive Ability: Analysis
Phase of Nursing Process: Evaluation
Client Needs: Health Promotion and Maintenance
Content Area: Adult Health/Renal

Reference

Black, J., & Matassarin-Jacobs, E. (1997). *Medical-surgical nursing: Clinical management for continuity of care* (5th ed.). Philadelphia: W. B. Saunders, pp. 492, 1672.

236. The client tells the nurse that the client gets dizzy and lightheaded with each use of the incentive spirometer. The nurse asks the client to demonstrate the use of the device, expecting that the client is

1 Not forming a tight seal around the mouthpiece.
2 Inhaling too slowly.
3 Not resting adequately between breaths.
4 Rebreathing exhaled air.

Answer: 3

Rationale: If the client does not breathe normally between incentive spirometer breaths, then hyperventilation and fatigue can result. Hyperventilation is the most common cause of respiratory alkalosis, which is characterized by lightheadedness and dizziness.

Test-Taking Strategy: To answer this question easily, evaluate each of the possible responses to see whether they would be expected to cause dizziness or lightheadedness. In doing so, you will see that only option 3, not resting adequately between breaths, could result in hyperventilation, decreased carbon dioxide levels, and subsequent dizziness or lightheadedness. Options 1 and 2 would result in ineffective use, and option 4 would result in mental cloudiness.

Level of Cognitive Ability: Analysis
Phase of Nursing Process: Analysis
Client Needs: Health Promotion and Maintenance
Content Area: Adult Health/Respiratory

Reference

Black, J., & Matassarin-Jacobs, E. (1997). *Medical-surgical nursing: Clinical management for continuity of care* (5th ed.). Philadelphia: W. B. Saunders, p. 333.

237. The nurse is participating in a health screening clinic. The nurse interprets that which of the following clients participating in the screening has the greatest need for instruction to lower the risk of developing respiratory disease?

1 A 50-year-old smoker with cracked asbestos lining on basement pipes in the home
2 A 40-year-old smoker who works in a hospital
3 A 36-year-old who works with pesticides
4 A 25-year-old who does woodworking as a hobby

Answer: 1

Rationale: Smoking greatly enhances the client's risk of developing some form of respiratory disease. Other risk factors include exposure to harmful chemicals, airborne toxins, and dust or fumes. The client at greatest risk has two identified risk factors, one of which is smoking.

Test-Taking Strategy: Begin to answer this question by eliminating options 3 and 4, since the most harmful risk factor for the respiratory system is smoking. You would select option 1 over option 2 because asbestos is a substance that is toxic to the lungs, if particles are inhaled. In this particular question also, two risk factors are identified, which put this client at greater risk than the others, each of whom has one factor identified.

Level of Cognitive Ability: Analysis
Phase of Nursing Process: Analysis
Client Needs: Health Promotion and Maintenance
Content Area: Adult Health/Respiratory

Reference

Black, J., & Matassarin-Jacobs, E. (1997). *Medical-surgical nursing: Clinical management for continuity of care* (5th ed.). Philadelphia: W. B. Saunders, p. 1039.

238. The nurse has conducted teaching with the client who has experienced pulmonary embolism about methods to prevent recurrence after discharge. The nurse evaluates that the instructions have been effective if the client states an intention to

1 Continue to wear supportive hose.
2 Limit intake of fluids.
3 Cross the legs only at the ankle but not the knee.
4 Sit down whenever possible.

Answer: 1

Rationale: Recurrence of pulmonary embolism can be minimized by wearing elastic or supportive hose, which enhances venous return. The client also enhances venous return by avoiding crossing the legs at the knee or ankle, interspersing periods of sitting with walking, and doing active foot and ankle exercises. The client should also take in sufficient fluids to prevent hemoconcentration and hypercoagulability.

Test-Taking Strategy: This question tests a fundamental concept of measures to promote good venous circulation. Option 4 can be easily eliminated first. Noting the words "limit" in option 2 and "cross" in option 3 will assist in eliminating these options. If this question was difficult, take a few moments to review these very important concepts!

Level of Cognitive Ability: Analysis
Phase of Nursing Process: Evaluation
Client Needs: Health Promotion and Maintenance
Content Area: Adult Health/Respiratory

Reference

Smeltzer, S., & Bare, B. (1996). *Brunner and Suddarth's Textbook of medical-surgical nursing* (8th ed.). Philadelphia: Lippincott-Raven, p. 529.

---

239. The female client is being discharged to home with an indwelling urinary catheter after surgical repair of the bladder after trauma. The nurse evaluates that the client understands the principles of catheter management if the client states that she will

1 Cleanse the perineal area with soap and water once a day.
2 Keep the drainage bag lower than the level of the bladder.
3 Limit fluid intake so that the bag won't become full so quickly.
4 Coil the tubing and place under the thigh when sitting, to avoid tugging on the bladder.

Answer: 2

Rationale: The perineal area should be cleansed twice daily and after each bowel movement with soap and water. The drainage bag should be lower than the level of the bladder, and the tubing should be free of kinks and compression. Adequate fluid intake is necessary to prevent infection and to provide natural irrigation of the catheter from increased urine flow.

Test-Taking Strategy: Option 4 is eliminated first as incorrect because sitting on coiled tubing could cause compression and obstruct drainage. Option 3 may be eliminated next because increased fluids are helpful. To discriminate between options 1 and 2, knowing that option 1 is insufficient in frequency would guide you to choose option 2 as correct. You could also choose option 2 as correct by knowing that option 2 is consistent with principles of catheter management.

Level of Cognitive Ability: Analysis
Phase of Nursing Process: Evaluation
Client Needs: Health Promotion and Maintenance
Content Area: Adult Health/Renal

Reference

Black, J., & Matassarin-Jacobs, E. (1997). *Medical-surgical nursing: Clinical management for continuity of care* (5th ed.). Philadelphia: W. B. Saunders, p. 1619.

---

240. The home health nurse is planning to make a home visit to a client who has had a creation of an ileal conduit. The nurse plans to include which of the following items about ostomy care in discussions with the client?

1 Cut an opening in the faceplate of the appliance that is slightly smaller than the stoma
2 Plan to do appliance changes in the late evening hours
3 Appliance odor from urine breakdown to ammonia can be minimized by limiting fluids
4 To cleanse the skin around the stoma, use gentle soap and water; rinse and dry well

Answer: 4

Rationale: The skin around the stoma is cleansed at each appliance change with a gentle, nonresidue soap and water. The skin is rinsed and then dried thoroughly. The appliance should be changed early in the morning because that is when urine production is slowest, as a result of no fluid intake during sleep. The appliance is cut so that the opening is not more than 3 mm larger than the stoma. An opening smaller than the stoma will prevent application of the appliance. Fluids are encouraged to dilute the urine, decreasing the incidence of odor.

Test-Taking Strategy: Begin to answer this question by eliminating option 3. Fluid limitation will not limit ammonia odor; in fact; decreased fluids will increase the concentration of the urine, making it stronger. Option 1 is eliminated next, because an appliance cut in this way will be too small to fit over the stoma. It may be difficult to choose between options 2 and 4. To choose correctly, you would need to realize that option 4 is completely correct, or you would need to recall that urine flow is slowest in the early morning as a result of decreased intake during the night. Either of these thought processes would lead you to choose the correct answer to this question.

Level of Cognitive Ability: Application
Phase of Nursing Process: Planning
Client Needs: Health Promotion and Maintenance
Content Area: Adult Health/Renal

Reference

Black, J., & Matassarin-Jacobs, E. (1997). *Medical-surgical nursing: Clinical management for continuity of care* (5th ed.). Philadelphia: W. B. Saunders, p. 1592.

241. A 24-year-old female with a familial history of heart disease comes to the physician's office, asking to begin oral contraceptive therapy for birth control. The nurse would next inquire whether the client

1 Has taken oral contraceptives before.
2 Exercises regularly.
3 Eats a low-cholesterol diet.
4 Is currently a smoker.

Answer: 4

Rationale: Oral contraceptive use is a risk factor for heart disease, particularly when it is combined with cigarette smoking. Regular exercise and keeping total cholesterol levels under 200 mg/dL are general measures to decrease cardiovascular risk.

Test-Taking Strategy: All options are partially correct because they relate either to cardiovascular disease risk factors or medication history. The question asks you to prioritize which option is most important by including the word "next" in the stem. Smoking is the item that is linked with oral contraceptive as a risk factor for cardiovascular disease.

Level of Cognitive Ability: Analysis
Phase of Nursing Process: Assessment
Client Needs: Health Promotion and Maintenance
Content Area: Adult Health/Cardiovascular

Reference

Black, J., & Matassarin-Jacobs, E. (1997). *Medical-surgical nursing: Clinical management for continuity of care* (5th ed.). Philadelphia: W. B. Saunders, p. 1239.

---

242. The nurse is implementing measures to maintain adequate peripheral tissue perfusion in the client after cardiac surgery. Which of the following actions would not be included by the nurse in giving care to this client?

1 Range-of-motion (ROM) exercises for the feet
2 Application of compression stockings
3 Leg elevation while sitting in chair
4 Use of knee gatch

Answer: 4

Rationale: After surgery, measures are taken to prevent venous stasis. They include applying elastic stockings or leg wraps, use of pneumatic compression boots, discouraging leg crossing, avoiding knee gatch, performing passive and active ROM, and omitting pillows in the popliteal space. Leg elevation while sitting will promote venous drainage and help postoperative edema.

Test-Taking Strategy: The use of the word "not" in the stem guides you to look for an incorrect choice. The use of knee gatch is contraindicated because it puts pressure on blood vessels in the popliteal area, impeding venous return. Knowledge of standard nursing care procedures helps you answer this question correctly.

Level of Cognitive Ability: Application
Phase of Nursing Process: Implementation
Client Needs: Health Promotion and Maintenance
Content Area: Adult Health/Cardiovascular

Reference

Smeltzer, S., & Bare, B. (1996). *Brunner and Suddarth's Textbook of medical-surgical nursing* (8th ed.). Philadelphia: Lippincott-Raven, p. 708.

243. The nurse is planning to teach a client with atrial fibrillation about the need to begin long-term anticoagulant therapy. Which of the following explanations would the nurse use to best describe the reasoning for this therapy?

1. "Because of this dysrhythmia, blood backs up in the legs and puts you at risk for blood clots, also called deep vein thrombosis"
2. "The antidysrhythmic medications you are taking cause blood clots as a side effect, so you need this medication to prevent them"
3. "Because the atria are 'quivering,' blood flows sluggishly through them, and clots can form along the heart wall, which could then loosen and travel to the lungs or brain"
4. "This dysrhythmia decreases the amount of blood flow coming from the heart, which can lead to formation of blood clots in the brain"

Answer: 3

Rationale: A severe complication of atrial fibrillation is the development of mural thrombi. The blood stagnates in the "quivering" atria, as a result of the loss of organized atrial muscle contraction and "atrial kick," which can account for up to 30% of the cardiac output. The blood that pools in the atria can then clot, which increases the risk of pulmonary and cerebral emboli.

Test-Taking Strategy: Option 2 is the least plausible and should be discarded first. Note the key word "fibrillation" in the question and the word "quivering" in the correct option. Review this content now if you had difficulty with this question!

Level of Cognitive Ability: Application
Phase of Nursing Process: Planning
Client Needs: Health Promotion and Maintenance
Content Area: Adult Health/Cardiovascular

Reference

Black, J., & Matassarin-Jacobs, E. (1997). *Medical-surgical nursing: Clinical management for continuity of care* (5th ed.). Philadelphia: W. B. Saunders, p. 1302.

244. The clinic nurse is providing instructions to a client in the third trimester of pregnancy about relief measures related to heartburn. Which of the following instructions would the nurse provide to the client?

1. Eat fatty foods only once a day in the morning
2. Avoid milk and hot tea
3. Chew gum
4. Use antacids that contain sodium

Answer: 3

Rationale: Measures to provide relief of heartburn include small frequent meals, avoiding fatty fried foods, avoiding coffee, and avoiding cigarettes. Mild antacids can be used if they do not contain aspirin or sodium. Frequent sips of milk, hot tea, or water are helpful. Gum is also helpful in the relief of heartburn.

Test-Taking Strategy: Eliminate option 4 first, because sodium will lead to edema and should be avoided. Eliminate option 1 next on the basis of basic nutritional principles that fatty and fried foods should be avoided. Knowledge that milk and hot tea can be soothing to the GI tract will assist in eliminating option 2 and direct you to option 3 as the answer to this question.

Level of Cognitive Ability: Application
Phase of Nursing Process: Implementation
Client Needs: Health Promotion and Maintenance
Content Area: Maternity

Reference

Nichols, F., & Zwelling, E. (1997). *Maternal-newborn nursing: Theory and practice.* Philadelphia: W. B. Saunders, p. 501.

245. The nurse provides instructions regarding home care to the parents of a 3-year-old child hospitalized with hemophilia. Which of the following would not be a component of the teaching plan?

1. Do not leave the child unattended
2. Pad table corners in the home
3. Remove household items that can tip over
4. Avoid immunizations and dental hygiene

Answer: 4

Rationale: The nurse needs to stress the importance of immunizations, dental hygiene, and routine well-child care. Options 1, 2, and 3 are appropriate. The parents are also instructed in the event of blunt trauma, especially trauma involving the joints, and to apply prolonged pressure to superficial wounds until the bleeding has stopped.

Test-Taking Strategy: Knowledge that bleeding is a concern in this disorder will assist in eliminating options 1, 2, and 3, which include measures of protection and safety for the child. If you had difficulty with this question, take time now to review care to the child with hemophilia!

Level of Cognitive Ability: Application
Phase of Nursing Process: Implementation
Client Needs: Health Promotion and Maintenance
Content Area: Child Health

Reference

Ashwill, J., & Droske, S. (1997). *Nursing care of children: Principles and practice.* Philadelphia: W. B. Saunders, p. 981.

---

246. The nurse provides instructions to the client taking clorazepate (Tranxene) for management of an anxiety disorder. Which of the following instructions would the nurse provide to the client?

1 Drowsiness is a side effect that usually disappears with continued therapy
2 If dizziness occurs, call the physician
3 Smoking increases the effectiveness of the medication
4 If GI disturbances occur, discontinue the medication

Answer: 1

Rationale: The client should be instructed that if dizziness occurs, the client should change positions slowly, from lying to sitting before standing. Smoking reduces medication effectiveness. GI disturbance is an occasional side effect, and the medication can be given with food if this occurs.

Test-Taking Strategy: Eliminate options 3 and 4 first. The client should never be instructed to smoke or instructed to discontinue medication. Eliminate option 2 next because episodes of dizziness commonly occur with antianxiety medications and interventions to alleviate the dizziness should be told to the client. Select option 1 because drowsiness is commonly associated with antianxiety medications and normally disappears with continued therapy.

Level of Cognitive Ability: Application
Phase of Nursing Process: Implementation
Client Needs: Health Promotion and Maintenance
Content Area: Pharmacology

Reference

Hodgson, B., & Kizior, R. (1998). *Saunders nursing drug handbook 1998.* Philadelphia: W. B. Saunders, p. 243.

---

247. The client with chlamydial infection has received instructions on self-care and prevention of further infection. The nurse evaluates that the client needs further reinforcement if the client states that he or she will

1 Reduce the chance of reinfection by limiting the number of sexual partners.
2 Use latex condoms to prevent disease transmission.
3 Return to the clinic as requested for follow-up culture in 1 week.
4 Use doxycycline prophylactically to prevent symptoms of chlamydia.

Answer: 4

Rationale: Antibiotics are not taken prophylactically to prevent chlamydia. The risk of reinfection can be reduced by limiting the number of sexual partners and by the use of condoms. In some instances, follow-up culture is requested in 4–7 days to confirm a cure.

Test-Taking Strategy: The wording of the question guides you to look for an incorrect response. Options 1 and 2 are the most obviously correct and are therefore eliminated as possible answers to the question. Knowing the basic principles of antibiotic therapy directs you to option 4, inasmuch as antibiotics are not used intermittently at will for prophylaxis of this infection.

Level of Cognitive Ability: Analysis
Phase of Nursing Process: Evaluation
Client Needs: Health Promotion and Maintenance
Content Area: Fundamental Skills

Reference

Black, J., & Matassarin-Jacobs, E. (1997). *Medical-surgical nursing: Clinical management for continuity of care* (5th ed.). Philadelphia: W. B. Saunders, p. 2470.

248. The client with prostatitis asks the nurse, "Why do I need to take a stool softener? The problem is with my urine, not my bowels!" Which of the following is the best response by the nurse?

1 "Being constipated puts you at more risk for developing complications of prostatitis"
2 "This is a standard medication order for anyone with an abdominal problem"
3 "This will keep the bowel free of feces, which will help decrease the swelling inside"
4 "This will help you avoid constipation, because straining is painful with prostatitis"

Answer: 4

Rationale: Stool softeners are ordered for the client with prostatitis to prevent constipation, which is painful. Constipation does not cause complications of prostatitis or decrease swelling. Stool softeners are not a standard medication order.

Test-Taking Strategy: The response in option 2 is nonspecific and nonhelpful and may be eliminated first. Because the bowel is never "free of feces," option 3 may be eliminated next. In comparing the remaining two options, option 4 sounds reasonable, whereas there is no logic to the response in option 1. Therefore, you would select option 4 as correct.

Level of Cognitive Ability: Application
Phase of Nursing Process: Implementation
Client Needs: Health Promotion and Maintenance
Content Area: Adult Health/Renal

Reference

Black, J., & Matassarin-Jacobs, E. (1997). *Medical-surgical nursing: Clinical management for continuity of care* (5th ed.). Philadelphia: W. B. Saunders, p. 2372.

249. The client with Parkinson's disease has begun therapy with levodopa (L-dopa). The nurse evaluates that the client understands the action of the medication if the client verbalizes that results may not be apparent for

1 24 hours.
2 2–3 days.
3 1 week.
4 2–3 weeks.

Answer: 4

Rationale: Signs and symptoms of Parkinson's disease usually begin to resolve within 2–3 weeks of starting therapy, although in some clients marked improvement may not be seen for up to 6 months. Clients need to understand this concept to aid in compliance with medication therapy.

Test-Taking Strategy: To answer this question accurately, you need to know when the medication begins to produce the expected effects. If this question was difficult, you should probably take a few moments to briefly review this medication!

Level of Cognitive Ability: Analysis
Phase of Nursing Process: Evaluation
Client Needs: Health Promotion and Maintenance
Content Area: Pharmacology

Reference

Deglin, J., & Vallerand, A. (1997). *Davis's drug guide for nurses* (5th ed.). Philadelphia: F. A. Davis, p. 694.

250. The nurse in the physician's office is reviewing the results of a client's phenytoin (Dilantin) level in a sample drawn that morning. The nurse would evaluate that the client had a therapeutic medication level if the client's result was

1 3 μg/mL.
2 8 μg/mL.
3 15 μg/mL.
4 24 μg/mL.

Answer: 3

Rationale: The therapeutic range for serum phenytoin levels is 10–20 μg/mL in clients with normal serum albumin levels and renal function. A level below this range indicates that the client is not receiving sufficient medication and is at risk for seizure activity. The medication dose should be adjusted upward. A level above this range indicates that the client is entering the toxic range and is at risk for toxic side effects of the medication. In this case, the dose should be adjusted downward.

Test-Taking Strategy: To answer this question accurately, you need to know the therapeutic medication level. This would be a helpful value range to memorize now because you are likely to find questions related to this content on NCLEX-RN!

Level of Cognitive Ability: Analysis
Phase of Nursing Process: Evaluation
Client Needs: Health Promotion and Maintenance
Content Area: Pharmacology

Reference

Deglin, J., & Vallerand, A. (1997). *Davis's drug guide for nurses* (5th ed.). Philadelphia: F. A. Davis, p. 965.

---

251. The nurse is planning to teach the client with a fractured leg in a long leg cast about appropriate dietary measures. Which of the following suggestions would be least helpful to the client?

1 Consume a high-protein diet
2 Consume a well-balanced diet
3 Make sure to increase dietary fiber
4 Drink extra amounts of fluids

Answer: 1

Rationale: In clients who wear casts, mobility is decreased to some degree, and they should optimize nutrition to aid in healing. This can be accomplished by increasing intake of dietary fiber, drinking extra fluids, and consuming a well-balanced diet.

Test-Taking Strategy: The concepts that are useful in answering this question relate to wound healing and decreased mobility. The wording of the question is such that you are looking for an incorrect item. Knowing that wound healing requires balanced nutrition helps you eliminate option 2. With decreased mobility there is a risk of constipation; increased fluid and dietary fiber are necessary to prevent this. Therefore, the option that does not fit with these requirements is the high-protein diet, which is the answer to the question as stated. Remember that the question asks for the item that will be least helpful!

Level of Cognitive Ability: Application
Phase of Nursing Process: Planning
Client Needs: Health Promotion and Maintenance
Content Area: Adult Health/Musculoskeletal

Reference

Black, J., & Matassarin-Jacobs, E. (1997). *Medical-surgical nursing: Clinical management for continuity of care* (5th ed.). Philadelphia: W. B. Saunders, p. 2151.

---

252. The nurse is participating in a prostate screening clinic. The nurse interprets that a client understands the educational information that was shared if the nurse overhears the client tell another participant that

1 Increased intake of green, leafy vegetables is helpful.
2 A daily supplement of vitamin E will prevent benign prostatic hypertrophy (BPH).
3 An annual prostate examination after age 40 is best for early detection.
4 Cigarette smoking triples the chance of developing BPH.

Answer: 3

Rationale: Increasing age is the major risk factor for developing BPH. The etiology is currently thought to be alteration in androgen levels, although the exact cause is still unknown. Increased intake of yellow vegetables and some elements of the Japanese diet may be helpful in reducing risk. Vitamin E and cigarette smoking have no known relationship with BPH. Early detection is the only method of prevention (and is actually secondary prevention). This is accomplished by annual prostate examination after the age of 40.

Test-Taking Strategy: This question tests knowledge of risk factors for development of BPH. Knowing that advancing age is the prime risk factor, you may systematically eliminate options 1, 2, and 4. Because the setting of the question is a prostate screening clinic, your attention is automatically drawn to detection, which would also guide you to choose option 3 as correct.

Level of Cognitive Ability: Analysis
Phase of Nursing Process: Evaluation
Client Needs: Health Promotion and Maintenance
Content Area: Adult Health/Renal

Reference

Black, J., & Matassarin-Jacobs, E. (1997). *Medical-surgical nursing: Clinical management for continuity of care* (5th ed.). Philadelphia: W. B. Saunders, p. 2350.

253. The client is being discharged to home after prostatectomy. The nurse plans to teach the client which of the following points as part of discharge teaching?

1 Drink 10–15 glasses of water a day to minimize clot formation
2 Mowing the lawn is allowed after 1 week
3 Notify the physician if fever, increased pain, or inability to void occurs
4 Avoid lifting more than 50 pounds for 4–6 weeks after surgery

Answer: 3

Rationale: The client should notify the physician if there are any signs of infection, bleeding, or urinary obstruction. Lifting more than 20 pounds is prohibited for 4–6 weeks after surgery. Other strenuous activities that could increase intra-abdominal tension are also restricted, such as mowing the lawn. The client should drink 6–8 glasses of water or nonalcoholic beverages per day to minimize the risk of clot formation.

Test-Taking Strategy: Begin to answer this question by eliminating option 1 as excessive fluid intake. Knowing that the activities outlined in options 2 and 4 are excessive guides you to eliminate them next. This leaves option 3 as correct. The client should notify the physician if signs of infection or obstruction occur.

Level of Cognitive Ability: Application
Phase of Nursing Process: Planning
Client Needs: Health Promotion and Maintenance
Content Area: Adult Health/Renal

Reference
Black, J., & Matassarin-Jacobs, E. (1997). *Medical-surgical nursing: Clinical management for continuity of care* (5th ed.). Philadelphia: W. B. Saunders, p. 2363.

254. The nurse is teaching the client with acute renal failure (ARF) to include proteins in the diet that are considered high quality. Which of the following foods that the client enjoys would the nurse discourage, because it is a low-quality protein source?

1 Eggs
2 Broccoli
3 Chicken
4 Fish

Answer: 2

Rationale: High-quality proteins come from animal sources and include such foods as eggs, chicken, meat, and fish. Low-quality proteins derive from plant sources and include vegetables and foods made from grains. Because the renal diet is limited in protein, it is important that the proteins ingested are of high quality.

Test-Taking Strategy: In comparing the possible options, note that option 2 (broccoli) is the only choice that does not derive from an animal source. Chicken, eggs, and fish are similar in that they are or derive from animal sources, whereas broccoli is a plant. This makes option 2 the correct choice.

Level of Cognitive Ability: Application
Phase of Nursing Process: Implementation
Client Needs: Health Promotion and Maintenance
Content Area: Adult Health/Renal

Reference
Black, J., & Matassarin-Jacobs, E. (1997). *Medical-surgical nursing: Clinical management for continuity of care* (5th ed.). Philadelphia: W. B. Saunders, p. 1640.

255. The home care nurse visits a client with a cardiovascular accident (CVA) with unilateral neglect recently discharged from the hospital. The nurse provides instructions to the family regarding care. Which of the following would be included in the nurse's instructions?

1 Place personal items directly in front of the client
2 Assist the client from the affected side
3 Assist the client to groom the unaffected side first
4 Discourage the client from scanning the environment

Answer: 2

Rationale: Unilateral neglect is a pattern of lack of awareness of body parts such as paralyzed arms or legs. Initially, adapt the environment to the deficit by focusing on the client's unaffected side. Keep personal items on the unaffected side. Gradually begin to focus the client's attention to the affected side. Assist the client from the affected side and have the client groom the affected side first. Cue the client to scan the entire environment.

Test-Taking Strategy: Understanding the physiological alteration that occurs in unilateral neglect will assist in directing you to option 2. Take time now to review interventions associated with unilateral neglect, if you had difficulty with this question!

Level of Cognitive Ability: Application
Phase of Nursing Process: Implementation
Client Needs: Health Promotion and Maintenance
Content Area: Adult Health/Neurological

Reference

Black, J., & Matassarin-Jacobs, E. (1997). *Medical-surgical nursing: Clinical management for continuity of care* (5th ed.). Philadelphia: W. B. Saunders, p. 806.

---

256. The nurse has completed discharge teaching for the client who has had surgery for lung cancer. The nurse evaluates that the client has not understood all of the essential elements of home management if the client verbalizes that he or she will

1 Sit up and lean forward to breathe more easily.
2 Deal with any increases in pain independently.
3 Avoid exposure to crowds.
4 Call the physician if there is increased temperature or shortness of breath.

Answer: 2

Rationale: Health teaching includes using positions that facilitate respiration, such as sitting up and leaning forward; avoiding exposure to crowds or persons with respiratory infections; and reporting signs and symptoms of respiratory infection or increases in pain.

Test-Taking Strategy: This question is worded to elicit a statement that is incorrect. Options 1 and 3 are obviously correct and are therefore eliminated as possible answers. For the two remaining options, knowing that the client should report signs of infection, difficulty breathing, and increased pain would help you to choose option 2 over 4, according to the wording of this question.

Level of Cognitive Ability: Analysis
Phase of Nursing Process: Evaluation
Client Needs: Health Promotion and Maintenance
Content Area: Adult Health/Oncology

Reference

Ignatavicius, D. D., Workman, M. L., & Mishler, M. A. (1995). *Medical-surgical nursing: A nursing process approach* (2nd ed.). Philadelphia: W. B. Saunders, p. 750.

---

257. The nurse is evaluating the nutritional status of the client after radical neck dissection. The nurse evaluates that the client has maintained adequate nutritional status if the client maintains what percentage of body weight?

1 100
2 95
3 90
4 80

Answer: 3

Rationale: The nurse evaluates that the client has maintained adequate nutritional status if the client does not lose more than 10% of body weight. Mathematically, this is the same as maintaining 90% of body weight.

Test-Taking Strategy: This is an example of a type of question for which either you know the standard or you do not. In this case, the standard maximal weight loss is 10%. This is a useful item to memorize.

Level of Cognitive Ability: Analysis
Phase of Nursing Process: Evaluation
Client Needs: Health Promotion and Maintenance
Content Area: Fundamental Skills

Reference

Smeltzer, S., & Bare, B. (1996). *Brunner and Suddarth's Textbook of medical-surgical nursing* (8th ed.). Philadelphia: Lippincott-Raven, p. 848.

---

258. The nurse has given the client with a nonplaster (fiberglass) leg cast instructions on cast care at home. The nurse would evaluate that the client needs further instruction if the client makes which of the following statements?

1 "I should avoid walking on wet, slippery floors"
2 "It's OK to wipe dirt off the top of the cast with a damp cloth"
3 "I'm not supposed to scratch the skin underneath the cast"
4 "If the cast gets wet, I can dry it with a hair dryer turned to the warmest setting"

Answer: 4

Rationale: Client instructions should include to avoid walking on wet, slippery floors to prevent falls. Surface soil on a cast may be removed with a damp cloth. If the cast gets wet, it can be dried with a hair dryer set to a cool setting to prevent skin breakdown. If the skin under the cast itches, cool air from a hair dryer may be used to relieve it. The client should never scratch under a cast, because of risk of skin breakdown and ulcer formation.

Test-Taking Strategy: Options 1 and 3 are certainly true and are therefore eliminated as potential answers, in view of the wording of this question. Knowledge of nonplaster cast material is needed to discriminate between the last two. A fiberglass cast may be wiped with a damp cloth because it is water resistant. It may be helpful to remember never to use a hair dryer on a cast, or on the skin under any cast, with the dryer set at the warmest setting. Only cool settings are used, in order to prevent burns.

Level of Cognitive Ability: Analysis
Phase of Nursing Process: Evaluation
Client Needs: Health Promotion and Maintenance
Content Area: Adult Health/Musculoskeletal

Reference

Smeltzer, S., & Bare, B. (1996). *Brunner and Suddarth's Textbook of medical-surgical nursing* (8th ed.). Philadelphia: Lippincott-Raven, p. 1853.

---

259. A child is seen in the health care clinic, and initial testing for HIV is performed because of the child's exposure to HIV infection. Which of the following home care instructions would the nurse provide to the parents of the child?

1 Avoid all immunizations until the diagnosis is established
2 Avoid sharing toothbrushes
3 Wipe up any blood spills with soap and water and allow to air dry
4 Wash hands with half-strength bleach if they come in contact with the child's blood

Answer: 2

Rationale: Immunizations must be kept up to date, and the child should receive inactivated polio vaccine. Blood spills are wiped up with a paper towel; the area is then washed with soap and water, rinsed with bleach and water, and allowed to air dry. Hands are washed with soap and water if they come in contact with blood. Parents are instructed that toothbrushes are not to be shared.

Test-Taking Strategy: Eliminate option 1 first because of the word "all." Eliminate option 3 next on the basis of the knowledge that blood spills need to be cleaned with a bleach solution. Eliminate option 4 because bleach would be very irritating and caustic to the skin. If you had difficulty with this question, take time now to review home care instructions for the child exposed to HIV infection!

Level of Cognitive Ability: Application
Phase of Nursing Process: Implementation
Client Needs: Health Promotion and Maintenance
Content Area: Child Health

Reference

Ashwill, J., & Droske, S. (1997). *Nursing care of children: Principles and practice.* Philadelphia: W. B. Saunders, p. 647.

260. A client is ready to be discharged to home health care for continued intravenous (IV) therapy in the home. The best way to evaluate the client's ability to care for the IV site is to

1 Ask the client to verbalize IV site care.
2 Have the client change the IV dressing.
3 Review the entire discharge plan with the client again.
4 Demonstrate the dressing change again for the client one last time before discharge.

Answer: 2

Rationale: Acquisition of psychomotor skills is best evaluated by observing how a client can carry out a procedure. The client may be able to verbalize how to do the procedure but may not be able to actually perform the psychomotor function. Reviewing the entire plan again and demonstrating it again will not evaluate the client's ability.

Test-Taking Strategy: Read the stem carefully to be certain that you know what the question is asking. The stem contains the key words "evaluate" and "client's ability." The correct answer needs to show some type of client-active evaluation. This narrows the options down to 1 and 2. Active demonstration by the client is always the best method of evaluating a psychomotor skill. Remember this concept about the teaching/learning process!

Level of Cognitive Ability: Analysis
Phase of Nursing Process: Evaluation
Client Needs: Health Promotion and Maintenance
Content Area: Fundamental Skills

Reference
Leahy, J., & Kizilay, P. E. (1998). *Foundations of nursing practice: A nursing process approach.* Philadelphia: W. B. Saunders, p. 253.

---

261. Which of the following remarks from a client with an implanted vascular access port indicates a need for further discharge instruction?

1 "If the site becomes red, I will notify my physician"
2 "I should keep the site clean and dry"
3 "I should pump the port daily to maintain patency"
4 "The port will need to be flushed with saline to maintain patency"

Answer: 3

Rationale: An implanted port does not need to be pumped in order to maintain patency. The site does need to be kept clean and dry, and the physician would need to be notified of signs and symptoms of infection. Saline needs to be flushed into the site to maintain patency.

Test-Taking Strategy: It is essential to know the basics necessary to care for an implanted port in order to answer this question. Take the time now to review these concepts if you need to!

Level of Cognitive Ability: Analysis
Phase of Nursing Process: Evaluation
Client Needs: Health Promotion and Maintenance
Content Area: Fundamental Skills

Reference
Phillips, L. (1997). *Manual of IV therapeutics* (2nd ed.). Philadelphia: F. A. Davis, pp. 421, 427.

---

262. The client is being discharged to home after application of a plaster leg cast. The nurse would evaluate that the client understands proper care of the cast if the client states that he or she will

1 Avoid getting the cast wet.
2 Use the fingertips to lift and move the leg.
3 Cover the casted leg with warm blankets.
4 Use a padded coat hanger end to scratch under the cast.

Answer: 1

Rationale: A plaster cast must remain dry to keep its strength. The cast should be handled with the palms of the hands, not the fingertips, until fully dry. Air should circulate freely around the cast to help it dry. The cast also gives off heat as it dries. The client should never scratch under the cast; a hair dryer with a cool setting may be used to eliminate an itch.

Test-Taking Strategy: Knowledge of cast care is needed to answer this question. Knowing that a wet cast can be dented with the fingertips, causing pressure underneath, helps you discard option 2 first. Knowing that the cast needs to dry helps you eliminate option 3 next. Option 4 is dangerous to skin integrity and is immediately eliminated. This leaves option 1 as correct. Plaster casts, once they have dried after application, should not become wet.

Level of Cognitive Ability: Analysis
Phase of Nursing Process: Evaluation
Client Needs: Health Promotion and Maintenance
Content Area: Adult Health/Musculoskeletal

Reference

Smeltzer, S., & Bare, B. (1996). *Brunner and Suddarth's Textbook of medical-surgical nursing* (8th ed.). Philadelphia: Lippincott-Raven, pp. 1849–1850, 1853.

---

263. The nurse is planning to teach the client with below-the-knee amputation about skin care to prevent breakdown. Which of the following points would the nurse include while developing the teaching plan?

1 A stump sock must be worn at all times and changed twice a week
2 The residual limb is washed gently and dried every other day
3 The socket of the prosthesis is washed with a bactericidal agent daily
4 The socket of the prosthesis must be dried carefully before it is used

Answer: 4

Rationale: A stump sock must be worn at all times to absorb perspiration and is changed daily. The residual limb is washed, dried, and inspected for breakdown twice each day. The socket of the prosthesis is cleansed with a mild detergent, rinsed, and dried carefully each day. A bactericidal agent would not be used.

Test-Taking Strategy: To answer this question accurately, you need the baseline knowledge that the prosthesis is cared for daily and that the stump is cared for twice a day. With this in mind, you can eliminate option 1 easily. Wearing a stump sock for 3–4 days is excessive and not conducive to maintaining intact, clean skin. Option 2 is eliminated for the same reason: the frequency of care is insufficient, inasmuch as it should be done twice daily. To discriminate between options 3 and 4, you should know that a mild cleanser is used. Even without this knowledge, you may be able to pick the correct option by knowing that the prosthesis should be fully dry before use.

Level of Cognitive Ability: Application
Phase of Nursing Process: Planning
Client Needs: Health Promotion and Maintenance
Content Area: Adult Health/Musculoskeletal

Reference

Smeltzer, S., & Bare, B. (1996). *Brunner and Suddarth's Textbook of medical-surgical nursing* (8th ed.). Philadelphia: Lippincott-Raven, p. 1943.

---

264. The nurse has completed instructions on diet and fluid restriction for the client with chronic renal failure. The nurse would evaluate that the client best understands the information presented if the client selected which of the following desserts from the dietary menu?

1 Angel food cake
2 Ice cream
3 Sherbet
4 Jell-O

Answer: 1

Rationale: Dietary fluid includes anything that is liquid at room temperature. This includes items such as ice cream, sherbet, and Jell-O. With clients on a fluid-restricted diet, it is helpful to avoid such "hidden" fluids to whatever extent is possible. This allows the client more fluid for drinking, which can help alleviate thirst.

Test-Taking Strategy: Options that are similar are not likely to be correct. Evaluation of each of the options shows that there is a greater amount of fluid in each of the incorrect options. In addition, these items are fluid at room temperature and therefore must be counted as fluid in the daily allotment. This knowledge helps you eliminate all of the incorrect choices immediately.

Level of Cognitive Ability: Analysis
Phase of Nursing Process: Evaluation
Client Needs: Health Promotion and Maintenance
Content Area: Adult Health/Renal

Reference

Black, J., & Matassarin-Jacobs, E. (1997). *Medical-surgical nursing: Clinical management for continuity of care* (5th ed.). Philadelphia: W. B. Saunders, p. 1656.

265. What is the most important concept to teach a client in order to prevent peripheral intravenous (IV) infections when receiving home IV therapy?

1 Assess the IV site carefully every day for redness and edema
2 Re-dress the IV site daily, cleansing it with alcohol
3 Carefully wash hands with antibacterial soap before working with the IV site or equipment
4 Change IV tubing and fluid containers daily

Answer: 3

Rationale: Although assessment of the IV site is important, it will not actively prevent an infection. IV sites do not need to be re-dressed daily unless the dressing becomes soiled or loose. Although IV containers should be changed daily, tubing needs to be changed only every 48–72 hours, according to the Centers for Disease Control and Prevention guidelines. It is extremely important for the client to realize the absolute necessity of handwashing before working with IV fluids.

Test-Taking Strategy: The stem of this question contains the key phrase "most important." Read the stem carefully to discover that infection prevention is the concept to be taught to the client. Eliminate option 1, which assesses for but does not prevent infection. Also remember the concepts related to client safety and the importance of aseptic technique in the home setting. The top priority in infection prevention always includes proper handwashing technique.

Level of Cognitive Ability: Application
Phase of Nursing Process: Planning
Client Needs: Health Promotion and Maintenance
Content Area: Fundamental Skills

Reference
Phillips, L. (1997). *Manual of IV therapeutics* (2nd ed.). Philadelphia: F. A. Davis, p. 172.

266. The nurse has given instructions to the client with chronic renal failure about reducing pruritus from uremia. The nurse evaluates that the client needs further information if the client states that he or she will use which of the following items for skin care?

1 Mild soap
2 Oil in the bath water
3 Astringent facial cleansing pads
4 Lanolin-based lotion

Answer: 3

Rationale: The client with chronic renal failure often has dry skin, accompanied by itching (pruritus) from uremia. The client should use mild soaps, lotions, and bath water oils to reduce dryness without increasing skin irritation. Products that contain perfumes or alcohol increase dryness and pruritus and should be avoided.

Test-Taking Strategy: The wording of the question guides you to look for an incorrect response on the part of the client. Options 2 and 4 are similar in nature and should therefore be eliminated. You would choose option 3 over option 1 as the correct answer to the question knowing that the client should avoid products irritating to the skin.

Level of Cognitive Ability: Analysis
Phase of Nursing Process: Evaluation
Client Needs: Health Promotion and Maintenance
Content Area: Adult Health/Renal

Reference
Black, J., & Matassarin-Jacobs, E. (1997). *Medical-surgical nursing: Clinical management for continuity of care* (5th ed.). Philadelphia: W. B. Saunders, p. 1656.

267. The client who is scheduled for implantation of an automatic internal defibrillator-cardioverter (AICD) asks the nurse why there is a need to keep a diary and what to put in it. In formulating a reply, the nurse understands that the ultimate purpose of the diary is to

1 Provide a count of the number of shocks delivered.
2 Document events that precipitate a countershock.
3 Record a variety of data useful for the physician in medical management.
4 Analyze which activities to avoid.

Answer: 3

Rationale: The client with an AICD maintains a log or diary, recording date, time, activity before the shock and any symptoms experienced, number of shocks delivered, and how the client felt after the shock. The information is used by the physician to adjust the medical regimen, especially medication therapy, which must be maintained after AICD insertion.

Test-Taking Strategy: The question asks you about the "ultimate" purpose of the log or diary, which implies that the correct response is comprehensive in nature. Each of the incorrect options lists one of the items that should be logged in the diary, but the correct response is the only one that could be considered an "all-purpose" response. Option 3 is the global response!

Level of Cognitive Ability: Analysis
Phase of Nursing Process: Analysis
Client Needs: Health Promotion and Maintenance
Content Area: Adult Health/Cardiovascular

Reference

Ignatavicius, D. D., Workman, M. L., & Mishler, M. A. (1995). *Medical-surgical nursing: A nursing process approach* (2nd ed.). Philadelphia: W. B. Saunders, p. 886.

268. The nurse is evaluating a hypertensive client's understanding of dietary modifications to control the disease process. The nurse would evaluate the client's understanding as satisfactory if the client made which of the following meal selections?

1 Scallops, French fries, salad with blue cheese dressing
2 Corned beef, fresh carrots, boiled potato
3 Hot dog in a bun, sauerkraut, baked beans
4 Turkey, baked potato, salad with oil and vinegar

Answer: 4

Rationale: Foods from the meat group that are higher in sodium include bacon, luncheon meat, chipped or corned beef, kosher meat, smoked or salted meat and fish, and a variety of shellfish.

Test-Taking Strategy: Eliminate the hot dog and corned beef first (options 2 and 3) as highly processed meats, which would be higher in sodium (the sauerkraut in option 3 is high in sodium also). The shellfish and the commercial dressing help you eliminate option 1 next. Review foods high in sodium now if you had difficulty with this question!

Level of Cognitive Ability: Analysis
Phase of Nursing Process: Evaluation
Client Needs: Health Promotion and Maintenance
Content Area: Adult Health/Cardiovascular

Reference

Lutz, C., & Przytulski, K. (1997). *Nutrition and diet therapy* (2nd ed.). Philadelphia: F. A. Davis, p. 378.

269. The nurse is developing a teaching plan for the client who will be taking warfarin (Coumadin) indefinitely. Which of the following suggestions should not be included in the plan by the nurse?

1 Use a soft toothbrush
2 Avoid drinking alcohol while on Coumadin
3 Carry identification about the medication being taken
4 Use only a straight razor

Answer: 4

Rationale: Client instructions for oral anticoagulant therapy include taking the medication only as prescribed and at the same time each day; not taking other medications (including over-the-counter [OTC] medications) without physician approval; avoiding alcohol; notifying all caregivers about the medication; carrying a MedicAlert bracelet or card; reporting any signs of bleeding (and preventing them whenever possible); and adhering to schedule for follow-up blood work.

Test-Taking Strategy: Measures to teach clients taking anticoagulant therapy generally deal with prevention of bleeding and interference with medication effects. Because only option 4 represents a danger in one of these areas, it is the option to select.

Level of Cognitive Ability: Application
Phase of Nursing Process: Planning
Client Needs: Health Promotion and Maintenance
Content Area: Pharmacology

Reference

Lehne, R. (1998). *Pharmacology for nursing care* (3rd ed.). Philadelphia: W. B. Saunders, p. 550.

---

270. The home care nurse has given instructions to the client recently discharged from the hospital with an arterial ischemic leg ulcer. The nurse would evaluate that further instruction is needed if the client made which of the following statements?

1 "I should wear shoes and socks at all times"
2 "I should cut my toenails straight across"
3 "I should raise my legs above the level of my heart periodically"
4 "I should apply lanolin to my feet"

Answer: 3

Rationale: Foot care instructions for the client with peripheral arterial ischemia are the same instructions given to the diabetic client. The client with arterial disease, however, should avoid raising the legs above heart level unless instructed to do so as part of an exercise program (such as Buerger-Allen exercises) or unless venous stasis is also present.

Test-Taking Strategy: Use principles related to care of clients with peripheral arterial disease to answer this question. The word "ischemia" in the stem indicates that gravity is needed to enhance blood flow. With these two items in mind, you can eliminate all of the incorrect options systematically.

Level of Cognitive Ability: Analysis
Phase of Nursing Process: Evaluation
Client Needs: Health Promotion and Maintenance
Content Area: Adult Health/Cardiovascular

Reference

Ignatavicius, D. D., Workman, M. L., & Mishler, M. A. (1995). *Medical-surgical nursing: A nursing process approach* (2nd ed.). Philadelphia: W. B. Saunders, p. 946.

---

271. The hemodialysis client has received instructions on fluid restriction to prevent excessive weight gain from fluid retention between hemodialysis treatments. The nurse evaluates that the client understands the fluid restriction if the client states that he or she will limit fluid intake to the amount of the daily urine output (if any) plus

1 200 mL.
2 400 mL.
3 1000 mL.
4 2000 mL.

Answer: 3

Rationale: The usual allowable daily fluid intake of the client undergoing hemodialysis is the total of the daily urine output plus 1000 mL. In the client with renal failure who has not yet begun dialysis, the allotment may be reduced to the 24-hour output plus 500 mL.

Test-Taking Strategy: Recall that a significant problem with renal failure is fluid retention. This is why hemodialysis is generally done three times per week. With this in mind, you may eliminate option 4 as excessive. At the same time, remember that an allotment of 200 or 400 mL per day in the client undergoing scheduled hemodialysis would be insufficient to meet the body's needs. This leaves option 3, which prevents both fluid overload and fluid volume deficit.

Level of Cognitive Ability: Analysis
Phase of Nursing Process: Evaluation
Client Needs: Health Promotion and Maintenance
Content Area: Adult Health/Renal

Reference

Black, J., & Matassarin-Jacobs, E. (1997). *Medical-surgical nursing: Clinical management for continuity of care* (5th ed.). Philadelphia: W. B. Saunders, p. 1656.

272. The client with chronic renal failure is about to begin hemodialysis therapy. The client asks the nurse about the frequency and scheduling of hemodialysis treatments. The nurse's response is based on an understanding that the typical schedule is

1 5 hours of treatment 2 days per week.
2 3–4 hours of treatment 3 days per week.
3 2–3 hours of treatment 5 days per week.
4 2 hours of treatment 6 days per week.

Answer: 2

Rationale: The typical schedule for hemodialysis is 3–4 hours of treatment 3 days per week. Individual adjustments may be made according to variables such as the size of the client, type of dialyzer, rate of blood flow, and personal client preferences.

Test-Taking Strategy: The question asks about a "typical" dialysis schedule. This is important fundamental knowledge for the nurse to have. If needed, memorize this information now.

Level of Cognitive Ability: Analysis
Phase of Nursing Process: Analysis
Client Needs: Health Promotion and Maintenance
Content Area: Adult Health/Renal

Reference
Black, J., & Matassarin-Jacobs, E. (1997). *Medical-surgical nursing: Clinical management for continuity of care* (5th ed.). Philadelphia: W. B. Saunders, p. 1653.

---

273. A client is being discharged with a peripheral intravenous (IV) site for continued home IV therapy. In planning for the discharge, the nurse should teach the client which of the following to help prevent phlebitis and infiltration?

1 Gently massage the area around the site daily
2 Cleanse the site daily with alcohol
3 Keep the cannula stabilized or anchored properly with tape
4 Immobilize the extremity until the IV therapy is discontinued

Answer: 3

Rationale: The principles of maintaining IV therapy at home are the same as in the acute care area. It is extremely important to ensure that the IV site is anchored properly in order to reduce the risk of phlebitis and infiltration. Massaging the site may actually contribute to catheter movement and tissue damage. Dressings surrounding peripheral IV sites are changed and cleansed at various times (usually every 2–5 days), depending on facility protocols. Most dressings are to remain intact unless the dressing becomes wet, soiled, or loose. Immobilizing the extremity is not routinely necessary for peripheral IV sites. Armboards are used only if a site is near a joint and the IV line is positional.

Test-Taking Strategy: Read all of the options carefully. The question deals with prevention and how to prevent complications without harming the client. Remember client safety when reading options. Review interventions related to phlebitis and infiltration now if you had difficulty with this question!

Level of Cognitive Ability: Application
Phase of Nursing Process: Planning
Client Needs: Health Promotion and Maintenance
Content Area: Fundamental Skills

Reference
Ignatavicius, D. D., Workman, M. L., & Mishler, M. A. (1995). *Medical-surgical nursing: A nursing process approach* (2nd ed.). Philadelphia: W. B. Saunders, p. 283.

---

274. The nurse is planning to teach the client with a leg cast how to stand on crutches. The nurse plans to incorporate into written instructions to tell the client to place the crutches

1 8 inches to the front and side of the client's toes.
2 3 inches to the front and side of the client's toes.
3 20 inches to the front and side of the client's toes.
4 15 inches to the front and side of the client's toes.

Answer: 1

Rationale: The classic tripod position is taught to the client before instructions on gait are given. The crutches are placed anywhere from 6 to 10 inches in front and to the side of the client, depending on the client's body size. This provides a wide enough base of support to the client and improves balance.

Test-Taking Strategy: Three inches (option 2) and 20 inches (option 3) are too short and too long, respectively. These two options should be eliminated first. Of the two remaining, 8 inches is more in keeping with the normal length of a stride than is 15 inches for someone wearing a cast, and it is the answer to the question. Review this procedure now if you had difficulty with this question. You are likely to find a question related to this procedure on NCLEX-RN!

Level of Cognitive Ability: Application
Phase of Nursing Process: Planning
Client Needs: Health Promotion and Maintenance
Content Area: Adult Health/Musculoskeletal

Reference

Potter, P., & Perry, A. (1997). *Fundamentals of nursing: Concepts, process, and practice* (4th ed.). St. Louis: Mosby–Year Book, p. 936.

---

275. The nurse is giving instructions to the client who is beginning therapy with digoxin (Lanoxin). The nurse would teach the client to

1 Monitor blood pressure once a week.
2 Measure weight each morning before breakfast.
3 Take the pulse daily.
4 Have electrolyte levels measured weekly.

Answer: 3

Rationale: Clients taking digoxin should take the pulse each day and notify the physician if the heart rate drops below 60 beats/minute or exceeds 100 beats/minute.

Test-Taking Strategy: Digoxin is not an antihypertensive, so eliminate option 1 first. The client may need to take a daily weight (option 2) for the condition underlying digoxin therapy, but it is not absolutely necessary for safe use of the medication. Weekly electrolyte measurement (option 4) is excessive, which leaves you with the correct answer, which is a "golden rule" of digoxin therapy.

Level of Cognitive Ability: Application
Phase of Nursing Process: Implementation
Client Needs: Health Promotion and Maintenance
Content Area: Pharmacology

Reference

Deglin, J., & Vallerand, A. (1997). *Davis's drug guide for nurses* (5th ed.). Philadelphia: F. A. Davis, p. 371.

---

276. The nurse has completed client teaching with the hemodialysis client about self-monitoring between hemodialysis treatments. The nurse evaluates that the client best understands the information given if the client states that he or she will record on a daily basis

1 Pulse and respiratory rate.
2 Intake and output and weight.
3 Blood urea nitrogen (BUN) and creatinine levels.
4 An activity log.

Answer: 2

Rationale: The client on hemodialysis should monitor fluid status between hemodialysis treatments. This can be accomplished by recording intake and output and measuring weight on a daily basis. Ideally, the hemodialysis client should not gain more than 0.5 kg (1 kg = 2.2 pounds) of weight per day.

Test-Taking Strategy: To answer this question accurately, it is necessary to understand the pathophysiological processes of renal failure and the impact on the client's bodily functions. With this in mind, you would choose the option that relates to monitoring of fluid retention, which is option 2. Option 4 is not indicated. The client does not have the need and may not have the ability to screen laboratory results (option 3). Although it is helpful for the client to monitor own vital signs, it is not the best indicator of fluid status, which is the focus of the question.

Level of Cognitive Ability: Analysis
Phase of Nursing Process: Evaluation
Client Needs: Health Promotion and Maintenance
Content Area: Adult Health/Renal

Reference

Ignatavicius, D. D., Workman, M. L., & Mishler, M. A. (1995). *Medical-surgical nursing: A nursing process approach* (2nd ed.). Philadelphia: W. B. Saunders, p. 2126.

277. Diltiazem (Cardizem) is prescribed for the client with Prinzmetal's angina. The clinic nurse develops a teaching plan for the client with regard to this medication. Which of the following would not be a component of the plan?

1. Call the physician if shortness of breath occurs
2. Rise slowly when getting out of bed in the morning
3. Take the medication after meals
4. Avoid activities that require alertness until your body gets use to the medication

Answer: 3

Rationale: Cardizem is a calcium channel blocker. It is administered before meals and at bed time as prescribed. Hypotension can occur, and the client is instructed to rise slowly. The client should avoid tasks that require alertness until a response to the medication is established. The client should call the physician if an irregular heartbeat, shortness of breath, pronounced dizziness, nausea, or constipation occurs.

Test-Taking Strategy: Knowledge regarding this medication is necessary to answer the question. Knowing that it is used for angina may assist in eliminating options 1, 2, and 4 because many of the cardiac medications lower blood pressure. Review this medication now if you had difficulty with this question!

Level of Cognitive Ability: Analysis
Phase of Nursing Process: Planning
Client Needs: Health Promotion and Maintenance
Content Area: Pharmacology

Reference

Hodgson, B., & Kizior, R. (1998). *Saunders nursing drug handbook 1998.* Philadelphia: W. B. Saunders, pp. 327–328.

---

278. The clinic nurse explains the risk factors associated with breast cancer to a client. Which of the following would not be a part of the explanation?

1. Late age at menarche
2. Nulliparity
3. A prior history of breast cancer
4. A family history of breast cancer

Answer: 1

Rationale: Factors that increase the risk of breast cancer include early age at menarche, especially younger than 12; late age at menopause or more than 40 years of menses; and first full-term pregnancy after the age of 30–35. Options 2, 3, and 4 are also risk factors.

Test-Taking Strategy: You should easily be able to eliminate options 3 and 4 as risk factors for breast cancer. Remembering that a greater number of years of menses increases the risk will assist in directing you to option 1 as the correct answer to this question as it is stated. Review these risk factors now if you had difficulty with this question!

Level of Cognitive Ability: Application
Phase of Nursing Process: Implementation
Client Needs: Health Promotion and Maintenance
Content Area: Adult Health/Oncology

Reference

Luckmann, J. (1997). *Saunders manual of nursing care.* Philadelphia: W. B. Saunders, pp. 1522–1523.

279. A male infant had a pyloromyotomy 18 hours ago. Clear liquid feedings are being tolerated. The physician orders progression to breast milk, limiting the initial feeding to 10 minutes total. Which of the following responses by a nursing mother indicates the need for further instruction?

1 "I nursed him for 10 minutes as you suggested, even though he still acts hungry"
2 "Since he hasn't had any milk for over a day, I let him nurse for 10 minutes on each side"
3 "Could you make an arrangement for me to use a breast pump? I would like to save milk for when he is back to his regular feedings"
4 "I nursed him for a total of 10 minutes and recorded the time and his weight on the clipboard in the bathroom"

Answer: 2

Rationale: The infant who has had a pyloromyotomy performed will resume feedings within 24 hours postoperatively. Clear liquids containing glucose and electrolytes are offered in small quantities at frequent intervals, progressing to breast milk or infant formula, as ordered by the physician. An order of 2 ounces of formula may be ordered for a bottle-fed baby. The intake of a breast-fed baby is controlled by limiting the nursing time. Both bottle-fed and breast-fed babies can be expected to act hungry after these limited feedings. Increased amounts will be ordered as the infant demonstrates the ability to tolerate the milk feedings. The nursing mother who allows her infant to nurse twice as long as instructed demonstrates a need for additional information.

Test-Taking Strategy: The question asks for the mother's statement that indicates a need for more information regarding the infant's feedings. The key phrase "limiting the initial feeding to 10 minutes total" should assist in directing you to the correct option!

Level of Cognitive Ability: Analysis
Phase of Nursing Process: Evaluation
Client Needs: Health Promotion and Maintenance
Content Area: Child Health

Reference

Wong, D. (1995). *Whaley and Wong's Nursing care of infants and children* (5th ed.). St. Louis: Mosby–Year Book, p. 1476.

---

280. The client with a history of rheumatic heart disease asks the nurse why the client must tell the dentist about this condition before dental cleaning or other work. The nurse's response is based on the knowledge that

1 The client is susceptible to reinfection unless prophylactic antibiotic therapy is given before treatment.
2 The client is at risk for episodes of heart failure triggered by stressful events.
3 The dentist should use a lidocaine solution that does not contain epinephrine.
4 The dentist should be aware that the vibration of the drill could cause dysrhythmias.

Answer: 1

Rationale: The client with a history of rheumatic fever is at risk for developing infective endocarditis. The client notifies all physicians and dentists about the history so that prophylactic antibiotic therapy can be given before any invasive procedure or when there is risk of bleeding.

Test-Taking Strategy: Prophylactic antibiotic treatment before any type of invasive procedure is indicated to prevent an episode of endocarditis. Knowledge of this concept should help you methodically eliminate the other options. Review this content now if you had difficulty with this question!

Level of Cognitive Ability: Analysis
Phase of Nursing Process: Analysis
Client Needs: Health Promotion and Maintenance
Content Area: Adult Health/Cardiovascular

Reference

Luckmann, J. (1997). *Saunders manual of nursing care.* Philadelphia: W. B. Saunders, p. 1062.

---

281. The nurse interprets a Mantoux tuberculin skin test result as significant. In order to most accurately diagnose tuberculosis, the nurse should plan to consult with the physician to follow up the skin test with a

1 Chest x-ray.
2 Computed tomographic (CT) scan of the chest.
3 Sputum culture.
4 Complete blood cell (CBC) count.

Answer: 3

Rationale: Although the findings on chest x-ray examination are important, it is not possible to make a diagnosis of tuberculosis solely on the basis of this examination. This is because other diseases can mimic the appearance of tuberculosis. The bacteriological demonstration of tubercle bacilli is essential for establishing a diagnosis. Microscopic examination of stained sputum smears for acid-fast bacilli is usually the first bacteriological study for the presence of tubercle bacilli.

Test-Taking Strategy: An important phrase in this question is "in order to most accurately diagnose tuberculosis." Analyze each option as to its probability of being the most accurate method of diagnosing tuberculosis as a follow-up to the Mantoux skin test. Review the tests used in diagnosing tuberculosis now if you had difficulty with this question!

Level of Cognitive Ability: Application
Phase of Nursing Process: Planning
Client Needs: Health Promotion and Maintenance
Content Area: Adult Health/Respiratory

Reference

Lewis, S., Collier, I., & Heitkemper, M. (1996). *Medical-surgical nursing: Assessment and management of clinical problems* (4th ed.). St. Louis: Mosby–Year Book, pp. 638–639.

---

282. An otherwise healthy client with mitral valve prolapse asks the nurse which type of therapy would be given if the client developed symptoms, such as dizziness, palpitations, or chest pain. The nurse would include which of the following treatments as part of the response?

1 Beta-adrenergic blocking agents and nitrates
2 Calcium channel–blocking agents and cardiac glycosides
3 Beta-adrenergic blocking agents and possible valve replacement
4 Nitrates and possible valve replacement

Answer: 3

Rationale: Treatment of mitral valve prolapse is guided by symptoms. Beta-adrenergic blocking agents may relieve chest pain, syncope, and palpitations. Mitral valve replacement may ultimately become necessary.

Test-Taking Strategy: Knowing that any cardiac valvular problem could ultimately lead to surgical intervention, you would eliminate options 1 and 2 first. Mitral valve prolapse has been linked with autonomic disturbance, with large amounts of catecholamines being produced. The use of beta-adrenergic medications would control this, so option 3 is the correct choice.

Level of Cognitive Ability: Analysis
Phase of Nursing Process: Analysis
Client Needs: Health Promotion and Maintenance
Content Area: Adult Health/Cardiovascular

Reference

Black, J., & Matassarin-Jacobs, E. (1997). *Medical-surgical nursing: Clinical management for continuity of care* (5th ed.). Philadelphia: W. B. Saunders, p. 1347.

---

283. The nurse has given instructions to the client being discharged to home after abdominal aortic aneurysm (AAA) resection. The nurse would evaluate that the client understands the instructions if the client stated that an appropriate activity would be to

1 Lift objects up to 30 pounds.
2 Walk as tolerated, including stairs and out of doors.
3 Mow the lawn.
4 Play a game of 18-hole golf.

Answer: 2

Rationale: The client can walk as tolerated after repair or resection of AAA, including climbing stairs and walking outdoors. The client should not lift objects that weigh more than 15–20 pounds for 6–12 weeks or engage in any activities that involve pushing, pulling, or straining. Driving is also prohibited for several weeks.

Test-Taking Strategy: To answer this question, evaluate each option in terms of the strain it could put on the sutured graft. This will help you eliminate each of the incorrect options successfully. Review discharge instructions after AAA now if you had difficulty with this question!

Level of Cognitive Ability: Analysis
Phase of Nursing Process: Evaluation
Client Needs: Health Promotion and Maintenance
Content Area: Adult Health/Cardiovascular

Reference

Black, J., & Matassarin-Jacobs, E. (1997). *Medical-surgical nursing: Clinical management for continuity of care* (5th ed.). Philadelphia: W. B. Saunders, p. 1428.

---

284. The nurse is planning dietary counseling for the client taking triamterene (Dyrenium). The nurse would plan to include which of the following in a list of foods that are acceptable?

1 Baked potato
2 Bananas
3 Oranges
4 Pears canned in water

Answer: 4

Rationale: Triamterene is a potassium-sparing diuretic, and clients taking this medication should be cautioned against eating foods that are high in potassium, unless they are taking a potassium-losing diuretic with it. Foods high in potassium include many sources, especially unprocessed foods, many vegetables, fruits, and fresh meats. Because potassium is very water-soluble, foods that are prepared in water are often lower in potassium than the same foods cooked another way (e.g., boiled rather than baked potato).

Test-Taking Strategy: To answer this question correctly, you need to know that triamterene is a potassium-sparing diuretic and also which foods are high in potassium (and should therefore be avoided). Review information of high-potassium foods and regarding this medication if you have the need. This type of information will likely be needed in other content areas also, such as renal disorders.

Level of Cognitive Ability: Application
Phase of Nursing Process: Planning
Client Needs: Health Promotion and Maintenance
Content Area: Pharmacology

Reference

Lutz, C., & Przytulski, K. (1997). *Nutrition and diet therapy* (2nd ed.). Philadelphia: F. A. Davis, pp. 390–391.

---

285. Cyclophosphamide (Cytoxan) is prescribed for the client with breast cancer. The nurse provides instructions to the client regarding the medication. Which of the following statements, if made by the client, would indicate a need for further education?

1 "I need to avoid contact with anyone who recently had a live virus vaccine"
2 "If I lose my hair, it will grow back"
3 "If I develop a sore throat, I should notify the physician"
4 "I need to limit my fluid intake while taking this medication"

Answer: 4

Rationale: Hemorrhagic cystitis is an adverse reaction associated with this medication. The client needs to be instructed to consume copious amounts of fluid during therapy. It is important to avoid contact with persons who recently had a live virus vaccine because this medication, an antineoplastic, produces immunosuppression, placing the client at risk for infection. Hair will grow back, although it may have a different color and texture. A sore throat may be an indication of an infection and needs to be reported to the physician.

Test-Taking Strategy: You should easily be able to eliminate option 2. Eliminate options 1 and 3 next because they are similar, in that both relate to the risk of infection. Knowledge that fluids are important may assist in directing you to the correct option. Review the adverse effects of this medication now if you had difficulty with this question!

Level of Cognitive Ability: Analysis
Phase of Nursing Process: Evaluation
Client Needs: Health Promotion and Maintenance
Content Area: Pharmacology

Reference

Hodgson, B., & Kizior, R. (1998). *Saunders nursing drug handbook 1998.* Philadelphia: W. B. Saunders, pp. 273–274.

286. The nurse has reviewed information on the local population. The nurse knows there are groups in the population that are at high risk for infection by *Mycobacterium tuberculosis* (which is the pathogen for tuberculosis). The nurse targets which of the following groups for screening?

1 White Anglo-Saxon Americans
2 Adolescents aged 13–17
3 French Canadians in rural America
4 Elderly clients in long-term care facilities

Answer: 4

Rationale: The elderly are at high risk for infection. Almost half of all new cases of tuberculosis occur in this age group. Other people at risk include children aged 5 years and less, the malnourished, the immunosuppressed, the economically disadvantaged, foreign-born persons, and persons of minority race who lived in a place where tuberculosis is common (e.g., Asia, Pacific Islands).

Test-Taking Strategy: Look for similar distracters. Options 1 and 3 are very similar in nature, which makes them less likely to be correct choices. When considering persons in different age groups, remember that the very young and the very old often belong to a high-risk category.

Level of Cognitive Ability: Analysis
Phase of Nursing Process: Analysis
Client Needs: Health Promotion and Maintenance
Content Area: Adult Health/Respiratory

Reference

Polaski, A., & Tatro, S. (1996). *Luckmann's Core principles and practice of medical-surgical nursing.* Philadelphia: W. B. Saunders, p. 591.

---

287. The community health nurse visits an aged client with osteoarthritis. Indomethacin (Indocin) has been prescribed for the client. The nurse teaches the client about this medication. Which of the following statements, if made by the client, indicates that further teaching is necessary?

1 "I can take a pill whenever I need to for pain"
2 "I need to call the doctor if I notice a rash"
3 "I'll balance rest periods and moderate activity"
4 "I'll watch for any swollen feet or fingers or any gastric distress"

Answer: 1

Rationale: In osteoarthritis, a noninflammatory disorder of the movable joints, pain is aggravated by joint motion, weight-bearing, and/or weather changes. The disease course is described as slow and progressive with no periods of remission or exacerbation. Rest and exercise should be balanced. When pain occurs, the client usually limits movement. A rash should be reported because it could indicate hypersensitivity to the medication. The client should be instructed to monitor for swelling and gastric distress, which this medication can cause.

Test-Taking Strategy: Use the process of elimination to answer the question. You should easily be directed to option 1 because clients should not be instructed to take medication for pain whenever needed. Guidelines regarding time frames for medication should be provided. Review this medication now if you had difficulty with this question!

Level of Cognitive Ability: Analysis
Phase of Nursing Process: Evaluation
Client Needs: Health Promotion and Maintenance
Content Area: Pharmacology

Reference

Black, J., & Matassarin-Jacobs, E. (1997). *Medical-surgical nursing: Clinical management for continuity of care* (5th ed.). Philadelphia: W. B. Saunders, pp. 601–604.

288. The community health nurse plans to visit an elderly client with osteoporosis. The nurse prepares a nursing care plan, and in the planning, the nurse understands that osteoporosis is a condition that

1 Proportionally affects black women more than white women.
2 Does not affect strict vegetarians as much as individuals who eat meat.
3 Does not affect women who were never pregnant as much as women who were.
4 Affects individuals who have blonde hair and fair skin more than others.

Answer: 4

Rationale: This question assesses your understanding of the risk factors for osteoporosis. There are several causative risk factors. Option 4 is the only option that identifies a correct risk factor. Black women are less affected than white and Asian women because they have a higher bone density. Strict vegetarians are at higher risk than individuals who eat meat. Women who were never pregnant are at higher risk than those who were. Additional hereditary factors include having blonde hair and fair skin.

Test-Taking Strategy: This question tests your knowledge of risk factors for osteoporosis that are genetic and those that are related to lifestyle. Take time now to review these important risk factors, if you had difficulty with this question!

Level of Cognitive Ability: Analysis
Phase of Nursing Process: Planning
Client Needs: Health Promotion and Maintenance
Content Area: Adult Health/Musculoskeletal

Reference

Black, J., & Matassarin-Jacobs, E. (1997). *Medical-surgical nursing: Clinical management for continuity of care* (5th ed.). Philadelphia: W. B. Saunders, pp. 2098–2099.

289. The nurse has given instructions on site care to the hemodialysis client who had implantation of a right arm arteriovenous (AV) graft. The nurse evaluates that the client needs further information if the client states that he or she will

1 Avoid carrying heavy objects on the right arm.
2 Sleep on the right side.
3 Report increased temperature, redness, or drainage at the site.
4 Perform range-of-motion exercises routinely with the right arm.

Answer: 2

Rationale: Routine instructions to the client with an AV fistula, graft, or shunt include reporting signs and symptoms of infection, performing routine range-of-motion exercises with the affected extremity, avoiding sleeping with the body weight on the limb with the access site, and avoiding carrying heavy objects or compressing the extremity that has the access site.

Test-Taking Strategy: Note that the wording of the question guides you to look for an incorrect statement on the part of the client. Knowing that options 3 and 4 are part of routine care allows you to eliminate them first as possible answers. To choose correctly between options 1 and 2, it is necessary to understand the adverse effects of pressure on the patency of the access site.

Level of Cognitive Ability: Analysis
Phase of Nursing Process: Evaluation
Client Needs: Health Promotion and Maintenance
Content Area: Adult Health/Renal

Reference

Ignatavicius, D. D., Workman, M. L., & Mishler, M. A. (1995). *Medical-surgical nursing: A nursing process approach* (2nd ed.). Philadelphia: W. B. Saunders, p. 2136.

290. After instructions about administering nitroglycerin ointment (Nitrobid), the nurse evaluates that a client is using correct technique when the client

1. Applies additional ointment if chest pain occurs.
2. Applies the ointment directly to the skin, then gently rubs ointment into skin.
3. Applies the ointment to any non-hairy area of the body.
4. Washes ointment off when bathing and reapplies after bath.

Answer: 3

Rationale: Options 1, 2, and 4 identify incorrect procedure regarding the application of this medication. The medication is used on a regular basis and not specifically for the occurrence of chest pain. The ointment is not rubbed into the skin. It is reapplied only as directed.

Test-Taking Strategy: Knowledge regarding the purpose and administration of this medication is necessary to answer this question. Take time now to review these client teaching points if you had difficulty with this question!

Level of Cognitive Ability: Analysis
Phase of Nursing Process: Evaluation
Client Needs: Health Promotion and Maintenance
Content Area: Pharmacology

Reference

Hodgson, B., & Kizior, R. (1998). *Saunders nursing drug handbook 1998.* Philadelphia: W. B. Saunders, pp. 750–753.

---

291. The nurse is giving medication instructions to the client receiving furosemide (Lasix). The nurse would not include which of the following points in discussion with the client?

1. Avoid the use of salt substitutes
2. Change positions slowly
3. Consume alcohol only after discussion with the physician
4. Be careful not to get overheated in warm weather

Answer: 1

Rationale: Furosemide is a potassium-losing diuretic, so there is no need to avoid high-potassium products, such as salt substitutes. Orthostatic hypotension is a real risk, however, so clients must use caution with changing positions, exposure to warm weather, alcohol ingestion, and prolonged standing.

Test-Taking Strategy: This question is worded to make you look for an incorrect statement. To answer this question correctly, you need to know that furosemide is a potassium-losing diuretic and that diuretic therapy can induce orthostatic hypotension. Knowing these, you can immediately eliminate each of the incorrect options. Review this medication now if you had difficulty with this question!

Level of Cognitive Ability: Application
Phase of Nursing Process: Implementation
Client Needs: Health Promotion and Maintenance
Content Area: Pharmacology

Reference

Hodgson, B., & Kizior, R. (1998). *Saunders nursing drug handbook 1998.* Philadelphia: W. B. Saunders, pp. 452–454.

---

292. The client has been prescribed a clonidine patch (Catapres-TTS). The nurse has instructed the client on the use of the patch. The nurse would note that the client exhibited a need for further instruction if the client

1. Verbalized that he or she would leave the patch in place during bathing or showering.
2. Verbalized that he or she would change the patch every 7 days.
3. Trimmed the patch because one edge was loose.
4. Selected a hairless site on the torso for application.

Answer: 3

Rationale: The clonidine patch should be applied to a hairless site on the torso or upper arm. It is changed every 7 days and is left in place during bathing or showering. The patch should not be trimmed, because this will alter the medication dose. If it becomes slightly loose, it should be covered with an adhesive overlay from the medication package. If it becomes very loose or falls off, it should be replaced. The patch is discarded by folding it in half with the adhesive sides together.

Test-Taking Strategy: The general instructions for use of this type of transdermal system are no different than for several others. Thus you can eliminate options 1 and 4. Option 3 is not standard procedure for transdermal systems. Review this medication now if you had difficulty with this question!

Level of Cognitive Ability: Analysis
Phase of Nursing Process: Evaluation
Client Needs: Health Promotion and Maintenance
Content Area: Pharmacology

Reference

Hodgson, B., & Kizior, R. (1998). *Saunders nursing drug handbook 1998.* Philadelphia: W. B. Saunders, pp. 240–242.

---

293. The nurse has given medication instructions to the hypertensive client receiving nicardipine (Cardene) who also has angina pectoris. The nurse would evaluate that the client needs reinforcement of teaching if the client stated that he or she would

1 Keep track of angina episodes and nitrate use and report if they increased.
2 Ignore edema and weight gain as tolerable side effects of therapy.
3 Report pulse rate of less than 50.
4 Take a missed dose as soon as remembered unless it is almost time for the next dose.

Answer: 2

Rationale: Clients taking calcium channel–blocking agents who also take nitrates should keep track of their use and any angina episodes and should report increases in frequency, severity, and duration of attacks. Clients may take a missed medication dose as soon as it is remembered unless it is almost time for the next dose; otherwise that dose should be omitted. Clients should check their pulse before taking the medication and report to the physician if it is under 50 (unless otherwise ordered by the physician). Weight gain and edema are reported to the physician as signs of right-sided heart failure. Other side effects to report include headaches, rashes, nausea, and vomiting.

Test-Taking Strategy: To answer this question, you must know that nicardipine is a calcium channel–blocking agent and will decrease the force and rate of myocardial contraction. This effect places clients at risk for heart failure, which is the basis for this question. The wording of this question makes you look for an incorrect response. Each of the options is correct except the one concerning signs of right-sided heart failure. Review this medication now if you had difficulty with this question!

Level of Cognitive Ability: Analysis
Phase of Nursing Process: Evaluation
Client Needs: Health Promotion and Maintenance
Content Area: Pharmacology

Reference

Hodgson, B., & Kizior, R. (1998). *Saunders nursing drug handbook 1998.* Philadelphia: W. B. Saunders, pp. 740–741.

---

294. The client is being discharged to home and will be taking cholestyramine (Questran). The nurse knows that further teaching is needed if the client makes which of the following statements?

1 "I need to mix the Questran with juice or applesauce"
2 "I should call my doctor if I develop diarrhea"
3 "I should increase my fluid intake while taking this medication"
4 "I should take this medication with meals"

Answer: 2

Rationale: This medication should not be taken dry and can be mixed in water, juice, carbonated beverages, applesauce, or soup. Common side effects include constipation, nausea, indigestion, and flatulence. Increasing fluids will minimize constipating effects of the medication. Questran must be administered with food to be effective. Diarrhea is not a concern, but severe constipation is.

Test-Taking Strategy: Knowledge regarding this medication is necessary to answer this question. By the process of elimination, select option 2 as the most likely answer because there are normally measures that can be taken for diarrhea other than calling the physician. Review this medication now if you are unfamiliar with it!

Level of Cognitive Ability: Analysis
Phase of Nursing Process: Evaluation
Client Needs: Health Promotion and Maintenance
Content Area: Pharmacology

Reference

Hodgson, B., & Kizior, R. (1998). *Saunders nursing drug handbook 1998.* Philadelphia: W. B. Saunders, pp. 215–217.

295. The nurse is preparing written medication instructions for the client receiving colestipol hydrochloride (Colestid). The nurse would plan to include the need for the client to take which of the following to counteract unintended medication effects?

1. Vitamin D
2. Fat-soluble vitamins
3. B-complex vitamins
4. Vitamin C

Answer: 2

Rationale: Colestipol, a bile-sequestering agent, is used to lower blood cholesterol levels. However, the bile salts (rich in cholesterol) also promote absorption of the fat-soluble vitamins A, D, E, and K, as well as folic acid. With ongoing therapy, the client is at risk of deficiency of these vitamins and is counseled to take appropriate supplements.

Test-Taking Strategy: Note that the options are divided into two sets of answers: the fat-soluble vitamin(s) and the water-soluble vitamins. Because bile-sequestering agents interfere with the absorption of fat-soluble vitamins, it is reasonable to limit your choices to options 1 and 2. Because option 2 is more comprehensive than option 1, you would choose that one as the correct answer.

Level of Cognitive Ability: Application
Phase of Nursing Process: Planning
Client Needs: Health Promotion and Maintenance
Content Area: Pharmacology

Reference
Hodgson, B., & Kizior, R. (1998). *Saunders nursing drug handbook 1998.* Philadelphia: W. B. Saunders, p. 253.

296. The nurse is screening a 39-year-old Caucasian female client. The client has a blood pressure of 152/92 at rest, a total cholesterol level of 190 mg/dL, and a fasting blood glucose level of 114. The nurse would focus attention on which risk factor for coronary artery disease (CAD)?

1. Age
2. Hyperlipidemia
3. Hypertension
4. Glucose intolerance

Answer: 3

Rationale: Hypertension, cigarette smoking, and hyperlipidemia are major risk factors that have been shown through research to be objective predictors of CAD. Glucose intolerance, obesity, and response to stress are contributing factors. Age greater than 40 is a nonmodifiable risk factor. The nurse places priority on major risk factors that can be modified.

Test-Taking Strategy: Risk for CAD is higher with age greater than 40 years, total cholesterol levels greater 200 mg/dL, and diabetes mellitus (random blood glucose level exceeding 120). The client's values in these areas are just within the normal range. Therefore, hypertension (systolic blood pressure >140 mmHg, diastolic blood pressure > 90 mmHg) is the option of choice.

Level of Cognitive Ability: Analysis
Phase of Nursing Process: Assessment
Client Needs: Health Promotion and Maintenance
Content Area: Adult Health/Cardiovascular

Reference
Black, J., & Matassarin-Jacobs, E. (1997). *Medical-surgical nursing: Clinical management for continuity of care* (5th ed.). Philadelphia: W. B. Saunders, pp. 1239, 1962.

297. The client is being discharged to home on warfarin (Coumadin). The nurse knows that further teaching is needed if the client makes which of the following statements?

1. "I can take two acetaminophen [Tylenol] if I get a headache"
2. "If I miss a dose, I should take it as soon as remembered that day"
3. "I should avoid all foods high in vitamin K"
4. "I should use a soft toothbrush"

Answer: 3

Rationale: Clients on Coumadin need to avoid aspirin and ibuprofen because of increased risk for bleeding. If a dose is missed, it should be taken as soon as remembered that day. Missed doses should be reported at the time of laboratory test. The client can have limited and consistent intake of foods high in vitamin K. Because vitamin K is the antidote for Coumadin, alternating amounts of these foods will cause prothrombin levels to fluctuate. Clients should be instructed to use an electric razor and soft toothbrush to minimize risk of bleeding.

Test-Taking Strategy: Note the absolute term "all" in option 3. In addition, recalling the relationship between Coumadin and vitamin K should assist in directing you to this option. Review client teaching points for this very important medication now if you had difficulty with this question!

Level of Cognitive Ability: Analysis
Phase of Nursing Process: Evaluation
Client Needs: Health Promotion and Maintenance
Content Area: Pharmacology

Reference

Hodgson, B., & Kizior, R. (1998). *Saunders nursing drug handbook 1998.* Philadelphia: W. B. Saunders, pp. 1062–1064.

---

298. The client with tuberculosis is preparing for discharge. Which of the following statements indicates to the nurse that further education is necessary?

1 "If I miss a dose of medication because of nausea, I just skip that dose and resume my regular schedule"
2 "I need to eat foods that are high in iron, protein, and vitamin C"
3 "I need to place tissues in a plastic bag when I am home"
4 "I will not need respiratory isolation when I am home"

Answer: 1

Rationale: With current resistant strains of tuberculosis, the nurse must emphasize that noncompliance regarding medication could lead to an infection that is difficult to treat or has total medication resistance. Clients may prevent nausea related to the medications by taking the daily dose at bedtime. Antinausea medications may also prevent this symptom. Options 2, 3, and 4 are correct statements.

Test-Taking Strategy: General principles related to medication administration should assist you in selecting the correct option. These principles should direct you to the option related to skipped medication doses. Review medication therapy and its importance in tuberculosis now if you had difficulty with this question!

Level of Cognitive Ability: Analysis
Phase of Nursing Process: Evaluation
Client Needs: Health Promotion and Maintenance
Content Area: Pharmacology

Reference

Ignatavicius, D. D., Workman, M. L., & Mishler, M. A. (1995). *Medical-surgical nursing: A nursing process approach* (2nd ed.). Philadelphia: W. B. Saunders, pp. 720, 722.

---

299. The nurse has given instructions to the client returning home after arthroscopy of the knee. The nurse would evaluate that the client understands the instructions if the client stated that he or she would

1 Stay off the leg entirely for the rest of the day.
2 Resume regular exercise the following day.
3 Refrain from eating food for the remainder of the day.
4 Report fever or site inflammation to the physician.

Answer: 4

Rationale: After arthroscopy, the client can usually walk carefully on the leg once sensation has returned. The client is instructed to avoid strenuous exercise for at least a few days. The client may resume the usual diet. Signs and symptoms of infection should be reported to the physician.

Test-Taking Strategy: Options 2 and 3 are the least plausible, and may be eliminated first. To differentiate between the remaining two options, you would need to know that the client can walk on the affected leg once sensation has returned. This would help you to eliminate option 1. The client is always taught signs and symptoms of infection to report to the physician.

Level of Cognitive Ability: Analysis
Phase of Nursing Process: Evaluation
Client Needs: Health Promotion and Maintenance
Content Area: Adult Health/Musculoskeletal

Reference

Black, J., & Matassarin-Jacobs, E. (1997). *Medical-surgical nursing: Clinical management for continuity of care* (5th ed.). Philadelphia: W. B. Saunders, p. 256.

300. The community nurse provides an educational session to members of the local community regarding breast self-examination (BSE). Which of the following statements, if made by a client, indicates a need for further education?

1. "I should perform the BSE when I have my period"
2. "It is easiest to perform when I am in the shower when my hands are soapy"
3. "I need to perform this BSE every month"
4. "I'll use the finger pads of my three middle fingers to feel for lumps and thickening"

Answer: 1

Rationale: The best time to perform BSE is after the monthly period when the breasts are not tender and swollen. Options 2, 3, and 4 identify accurate information regarding this very important examination.

Test-Taking Strategy: Knowledge regarding the procedure for BSE is necessary to answer this question. If you had difficulty with this question, take time now to review this procedure. You are likely to find a question related to this procedure on NCLEX-RN!

Level of Cognitive Ability: Analysis
Phase of Nursing Process: Evaluation
Client Needs: Health Promotion and Maintenance
Content Area: Adult Health/Oncology

Reference

Luckmann, J. (1997). *Saunders manual of nursing care*. Philadelphia: W. B. Saunders, p. 1539.

REFERENCES

Ashwill, J., & Droske, S. (1997). *Nursing care of children: Principles and practice*. Philadelphia: W. B. Saunders.

Baer, C., & Williams, B. (1996). *Clinical pharmacology and nursing* (3rd ed.). Springhouse, PA: Springhouse.

Ball, J., & Bindler, R. (1995). *Pediatric nursing: Caring for children*. Stamford, CT: Appleton & Lange.

Black, J., & Matassarin-Jacobs, E. (1997). *Medical-surgical nursing: Clinical management for continuity of care* (5th ed.). Philadelphia: W. B. Saunders.

Burrell, L., Gerlach, M., & Pless, B. (1997). *Adult nursing: Acute and community care* (2nd ed.). Stamford, CT: Appleton & Lange.

Carson, V., & Arnold, E. (1996). *Mental health nursing: The nurse-patient journey*. Philadelphia: W. B. Saunders.

Clemen-Stone, S., Eigsti, D., & McGuire, S. (1995). *Comprehensive community health nursing: Family, aggregate, and community practice* (4th ed.). St. Louis: Mosby–Year Book.

Deglin, J., & Vallerand, A. (1997). *Davis's drug guide for nurses* (5th ed.). Philadelphia: F. A. Davis.

Fortinash, K., & Holoday-Worret, P. (1996). *Psychiatric-mental health nursing*. St. Louis: Mosby–Year Book.

Haber, J. (1997). *Comprehensive psychiatric nursing* (5th ed.). St. Louis: Mosby–Year Book.

Hodgson, B., & Kizior, R. (1998). *Saunders nursing drug handbook 1998*. Philadelphia: W. B. Saunders.

Ignatavicius, D. D., Workman, M. L., & Mishler, M. A. (1995). *Medical-surgical nursing: A nursing process approach* (2nd ed.). Philadelphia: W. B. Saunders.

Johnson, B. (1997). *Psychiatric-mental health nursing: Adaptation and growth* (4th ed.). Philadelphia: Lippincott-Raven.

Kee, J., & Hayes, E. (1997). *Pharmacology: A nursing process approach* (2nd ed.). Philadelphia: W. B. Saunders.

Leahy, J., & Kizilay, P. E. (1998). *Foundations of nursing practice: A nursing process approach*. Philadelphia: W. B. Saunders.

Lehne, R. A. (1998). *Pharmacology for nursing care* (3rd ed.). Philadelphia: W. B. Saunders.

Lewis, S., Collier, I., & Heitkemper, M. (1996). *Medical-surgical nursing: Assessment and management of clinical problems* (4th ed.). St. Louis: Mosby–Year Book.

Lowdermilk, D., Perry, S., & Bobak, I. (1997). *Maternity and women's health care* (6th ed.). St. Louis: Mosby–Year Book.

Luckmann, J. (1997). *Saunders manual of nursing care*. Philadelphia: W. B. Saunders.

Lutz, C., & Przytulski, K. (1997). *Nutrition and diet therapy* (2nd ed.). Philadelphia: F. A. Davis.

Mahan, K., & Escott-Stump, S. (1996). *Krause's Food, nutrition, & diet therapy* (9th ed.). Philadelphia: W. B. Saunders.

Monahan, F., & Neighbors, M. (1998). *Medical-surgical nursing: Foundations for clinical practice* (2nd ed.). Philadelphia: W. B. Saunders.

National Council of State Boards of Nursing. (1997). *Plan for the National Council licensure examination for registered nurses*. Chicago: Author.

Nichols, F., & Zwelling, E. (1997). *Maternal-newborn nursing: Theory and practice*. Philadelphia: W. B. Saunders.

Olds, S., London, M., & Ladewig, P. (1996). *Maternal-newborn nursing: A family-centered approach* (5th ed.). Menlo Park, CA: Addison-Wesley.

Phillips, L. (1997). *Manual of IV therapeutics* (2nd ed.). Philadelphia: F. A. Davis.

Polaski, A., & Tatro, S. (1996). *Luckmann's Core principles and practice of medical-surgical nursing*. Philadelphia: W. B. Saunders.

Potter, P., & Perry, A. (1997). *Fundamentals of nursing: Concepts, process, and practice* (4th ed.). St. Louis: Mosby–Year Book.

Reeder, S., Martin, L., & Koniak-Griffin, D. (1997). *Maternity nursing: Family, newborn, and women's health care* (18th ed.). Philadelphia: Lippincott-Raven.

Rice, R. (1996). *Home health nursing practice: Concepts and application* (2nd ed.). St. Louis: Mosby–Year Book.

Rocchiccioli, J., & Tilbury, M. (1998). *Clinical leadership in nursing*. Philadelphia: W. B. Saunders.

Smeltzer, S., & Bare, B. (1996). *Brunner and Suddarth's Textbook of medical-surgical nursing* (8th ed.). Philadelphia: Lippincott-Raven.

Taylor, C., Lillis, C., & LeMone, P. (1997). *Fundamentals of nursing: The art and science of nursing care* (3rd ed.). Philadelphia: Lippincott-Raven.

Townsend, M. (1996). *Psychiatric–mental health nursing: Concepts of care*. Philadelphia: F. A. Davis.

Varcarolis, E. (1998). *Foundations of psychiatric mental health nursing* (3rd ed.). Philadelphia: W. B. Saunders.

Wilson, H., & Kneisl, C. (1996). *Psychiatric nursing* (5th ed.). Menlo Park, CA: Addison-Wesley.

Wilson, B., Shannon, M., & Stang, C. (1997). *Nurse's drug guide*. Stamford, CT: Appleton & Lange.

Wong, D. (1995). *Whaley and Wong's Nursing care of infants and children* (5th ed.). St. Louis: Mosby–Year Book.

Wong, D. (1997). *Whaley and Wong's Essentials of pediatric nursing* (5th ed.). St. Louis: Mosby–Year Book.

Wywialowski, E. (1997). *Managing client care* (2nd ed.). St. Louis: Mosby–Year Book.